ICD-O—*International Classification of Diseases, Oncology*

ICD-O-2—International Classification of Disease for Oncology, Second Edition

IEC—International Electrotechnical Commission

IEEE—Institute of Electrical and Electronic Engineers

IMS—Indicator Measurement System

IOM—Institute of Medicine

IR—Incidence rate

IRB—Institutional review board

ISO—International Standards Organization

IS/SI—Intensity of Service/Severity of Illness

JAD—Joint Application Development

JCAHO—Joint Commission on Accreditation of Health-care Organizations

LAN—Local area network

LISP—List processing

LTCDS—Long term care data set

MBO—Management by objectives

MDS—Minimum data set

MIB—Medical Information Bureau

MICR—Magnetic ink character reader

MPI—Master patient index

MS/DOS—(Microsoft) Disk Operating System

MSO—Medical staff organization

MSSP—Medical staff services professional

MUMPS—Massachusetts General Hospital Utility Multi-programming System

NAHDO—National Association of Health Data Organizations

NCDB—National Cancer Data Bank

NCHS—National Center for Health Statistics

NCI—National Cancer Institute

NCRA—National Cancer Registrars Association, Inc.

NCVHS—National Committee on Vital and Health Statistics

NHDS—National Hospital Discharge Survey

NI—Nosocomial infections

NIOSH—National Institute for Occupational Safety and Health

NLN—National League for Nursing

NLRA—National Labor Relations Act

NLRB—National Labor Relations Board

NPDB—National Practitioner Data Bank

OBRA—Omnibus Reconciliation Act

OCR—Optical character recognition

OFCCP—Office of Federal Contract Compliance Program

OSHA—Occupational Safety and Health Administration

PACS—Picture archiving and communication system

PC—Personal computer

PC/DOS—(IBM) Disk Operating System

PCE—Potentially compensable events

PCP—Patient care plan

PDCA—Plan, do, check, act

PHS—Public Health Service

PL/1—Programming language one

POMR—Problem-oriented medical record

PPO—Preferred provider organization

PPR—Paper-based patient record

PPS—Prospective payment system

PRO—Peer review organization

PSRO—professional standards review organizations

QA—Quality assurance

QAI—Quality assessment and improvement

QI—Quality improvement

r—Correlation coefficient

R-ADT—Registration–Admission, discharge, transfer

RAI—Resident assessment instrument

RBRVS—Resource-based relative value scale

RFI—Request for information

RFP—Request for proposal

RMRS—Regenstrief Medical Records System

ROI—Return on investment

RR—Relative risk

RSI—Repetitive stress/strain injury

SCSI—Small computer system interface

SEER—Surveillance, epidemiology, and end results

SMR—Standardized mortality ratio

SNDO—Standard Nomenclature of Diseases and Operations

SNOMED—Systematized Nomenclature of Human and Veterinary Medicine

SNOP—Systematized Nomenclature of Pathology

SSA—Social Security Administration

SWOT—Strengths, weaknesses, opportunities, threats

TEFRA—Tax Equity and Fiscal Responsibility Act

TMR—The Medical Record

TN—True negatives

TP—True positives

UACDS—Uniform ambulatory care data set

UB-92—Uniform Bill, 1992

UCDS—Uniform clinical data set

UHDDS—Uniform hospital discharge data set

UM—Utilization management

UNOS—United Network for Organ Sharing

UPIN—Universal personal identification number

UPS—Uninterruptable power supply

UR—Utilization review

VDT—Video display terminal

WAN—Wide area network

WORM—Write once read many

HEALTH INFORMATION:
MANAGEMENT OF A
STRATEGIC
RESOURCE

Managing Editor
MERVAT ABDELHAK, PhD, RRA

Chairman, Health Information Management
  Department and Associate Professor
School of Health and Rehabilitation Sciences
University of Pittsburgh
Pittsburgh, PA

Editors
SARA GROSTICK, MA, RRA

Director, Health Information Management
  Program and Associate Professor
School of Health Related Professions
University of Alabama at Birmingham
Birmingham, AL

MARY ALICE HANKEN, PhD, RRA

Director, Health Information Administration
  Program
School of Public Health and Community Medicine
University of Washington
Seattle, WA

ELLEN JACOBS, MEd, RRA

Director, Health Information Management
  Program and Associate Professor
College of St. Mary
Omaha, NE

HEALTH INFORMATION:
MANAGEMENT OF A
STRATEGIC
RESOURCE

W.B. SAUNDERS COMPANY
A Division of Harcourt Brace & Company
PHILADELPHIA • LONDON • TORONTO • MONTREAL • SYDNEY • TOKYO

W.B. SAUNDERS COMPANY
A Division of Harcourt Brace & Company

The Curtis Center
Independence Square West
Philadelphia, Pennsylvania 19106

Library of Congress Cataloging-in-Publication Data

Health information: management of a strategic resource / [edited by]
Mervat Abdelhak . . . [et al.].

    p.   cm.

  ISBN 0–7216–5132–1

  1. Medical informatics.   2. Information resources management.
I. Abdelhak, Mervat.
  [DNLM: 1. Medical Informatics—organization & administration.
2. Information Services—organization & administration. 3. Delivery
of Health Care—United States. W 26.5 H4337 1996]

R858.H35 1996

610′.285—dc20

DNLM/DLC   95-41998

HEALTH INFORMATION: MANAGEMENT OF A STRATEGIC RESOURCE   ISBN 0–7216–5132–1

Printed in the United States of America.

Last digit is the print number: 9   8   7   6   5   4   3   2

I dedicate this work to my parents, who, even though they are miles and miles away, continue to be my inspiration; to my fiancé Gary Patterson and my sons, Jonathan and Matthew, who are my life; to a very dear friend who passed on in April 1995, Chuck Deaktor, who encouraged and guided me in numerous ways; to my administrative assistant, Patti Grofic, who made it all happen and happen on time; to my colleagues at the University of Pittsburgh, who have stimulated me; and to my co-editors—it has been a joyous experience that I will treasure forever. Thank you all.

Mervat Abdelhak

I dedicate this book to my husband Alan, my son Charles, and my daughter Laura, who are my major sources of encouragement; to my mentor Ms. Gertrude McCalip, who introduced me to the health information management profession at Baptist Hospital in Memphis, TN, many years ago; and to Donna Solvensky, Midge Ray, Gayla Schultz, and Serena Gardner, who supported me while I worked on this project.

Sara Grostick

Encouragement comes in many forms and deserves to be recognized. Thanks to my husband for his support of and participation in one more major undertaking. Thanks to my mother, who died during the project—her unconditional belief in me makes more possible. Thanks to my co-editors—Mervat, Ellen, and Sara—and to Beverli Reding and to the W.B. Saunders staff; you made the work more enjoyable.

Mary Alice Hanken

My participation in this work is due to many individuals and organizations who have supported my advancement in the health information management profession. Thus I dedicate this work to them: first and foremost my parents, who were my first teachers and cheerleaders; my children Danny and Becky, who have continued that support and are just great kids; Rita Finnegan and Margret Amatayakul, who assisted me in achieving professional recognition; faculty and staff at the College of Saint Mary, who have allowed me the freedom and creativity to pursue this endeavor; and to my co-editors, who are inspiring as well as supportive in accomplishing the many tasks that make up this work, and in maintaining our collective and consistent vision of the future of the health information management profession.

Ellen Jacobs

ACKNOWLEDGMENTS

Health Information: Management of a Strategic Resource text and ancillaries, like all other projects, reflect the efforts of many people. For its inception, Lisa Biello, Vice President and Editor-in-Chief, Health Related Professions, of W.B. Saunders Company and Lou Ann Schraffenberger, MA, RRA, then with American Health Information Management Association, were instrumental in getting the editors together. For its creation, a project of this magnitude and scope would not have been possible without the many fine contributors who helped make *Health Information: Management of a Strategic Resource* a reality. A special thank you goes to Beverli Reding for assuming the responsibility of the *Review Manual* and *EXAMaster,* and for her many insights, questions, and suggestions which have strengthened the text and its ancillaries. For its development, a special thanks to Shirley Kuhn, Senior Developmental Editor; Lorraine Kilmer, former Manager and Designer, EDP Team; Risa Clow and Deborah Lyman, Illustrators; Karen Tarasiewicz, Marketing Manager, Health Related Professions; Edna Dick, Project Editor, and Frank Polizzano, Production Manager, EDP Team; and many more people behind the scenes at Saunders who kept us on track and shepherded the manuscript through the publication process. The contributions of these outstanding individuals and the support of many unsung heroes made this project become a reality.

MERVAT ABDELHAK
Managing Editor
SARA GROSTICK
MARY ALICE HANKEN
ELLEN JACOBS

FOREWORD

As a health informatician committed to the concept of the computer-based patient record (CPR), I applaud the four editors of this textbook. For the CPR to succeed, health information professionals must be visionaries and strategists. They must understand the full scope of health information and the role it can and must play in delivering quality health care. Students and practitioners alike can benefit enormously from the content and the philosophy that *Health Information: Management of a Strategic Resource* delivers.

This book comes at an opportune time. Marketplace and governmental efforts are changing the shape of our health care system. Increasingly, the delivery of health care is the responsibility of clinicians from a number of disciplines and professions, located in a number of settings. Rapidly, managed care and care teams are becoming the standard. In this evolving and highly charged environment, health information is a strategic resource, and managing information is essential to the success of the enterprise and to the health of the individual patient.

As we enter the twenty-first century, health information management professionals must play new roles and take on new functions. Technology is changing their profession, and they must change with it, actively seeking new and better ways of conceptualizing and completing their work. As we succeed in implementing the CPR and building networks to help support community-based wellness care, health information —and health information management professionals—will be the very nerve center of the health care enterprise. The editors and contributors to *Health Information: Management of a Strategic Resource* understand this evolving reality and share their vision with their readers.

Designed as a textbook, this important volume includes 19 chapters by more than 30 contributors. In addition to an introduction to health information management and the profession, the book focuses on four key areas—health care data, information management and use, management, and health information systems. Among the topics covered are data collection, registries, and epidemiologic research. Other chapters address areas that are frequently the responsibility of health information managers, such as risk management, legal issues, and financial management.

Throughout this text, the concept of quality recurs, beginning with data quality and on through quality assessment and methods for improving systems. A separate chapter highlights the CPR as a unifying principle, and contributors known for their work with the CPR and health information management offer their viewpoints in a final chapter. Added features include an *Assignment Workbook,* a *Review Manual,* an *EXAMaster* in electronic form, and an instructor's manual—in short, a wide array of teaching materials.

Our move into the future is accelerating. What were future visions just a few years ago are now becoming palpable realities. Networks are linking providers, patients, and payers in the health care enterprise. Individuals are availing themselves of new tools, among them the electronic housecall, faxback services, and personal workstations. Yet all these technologies remain merely the instruments by which data and information are managed.

In this new environment, health information managers play an absolutely crucial role. As professionals, they can help to meet the needs of care providers, managed care organizations, system software developers, and others. For students and practitioners of health information management alike, this new book, *Health Information: Management of a Strategic Resource,* will prove to be an invaluable guide to the topics and tools of their profession. All of us, practitioners and consumers alike, will benefit from the clarity and direction that this publication provides.

To its editors and contributors, our profound thanks.

MARION J. BALL, EdD
Associate Vice President, Information Services,
University of Maryland at Baltimore,
Baltimore, Maryland

PREFACE

Health Information: Management of a Strategic Resource and a set of integrated tools, the *Ancillaries,* are written for health information management students and practitioners who are interested in today's reliable systems and tomorrow's future direction in order to guide and influence practice, education, and research. The purpose of the book is to develop and support health information professionals who believe that their profession is crucial to the success and efficacy of the health care system. *Health Information: Management of a Strategic Resource* helps practitioners and students alike to realize the broader perspective of the scope and domains of health information management practice, understanding the expanded boundaries and roles that exist today, and the opportunities that lie within our reach to influence professional advancement and tomorrow's practice. It is also hoped that this book will aid health information professionals in viewing their profession with confidence, pride, and excitement. Finally, the book may realize its greatest value in expanding the expectations and understanding of other health professionals—administrators, information systems professionals, researchers, policy developers, and others—about the role(s) of health information management professionals and the contributions they make to health care.

In today's fast-changing health care system, health information management professionals must adapt faster; expand their scope and domains of practice; use data, information, and technology in a new way; and assess their performance. Health information management professionals must update their knowledge constantly and approach their expanded roles and functions with a new mindset. This book presents a fresh insight, a new approach in addressing the fundamentals and important issues within the field of health information management. Today's most reliable and workable systems are presented by an impressive list of contributors. Viewpoints toward tomorrow's challenges should stimulate discussion and future action.

The editors designed the book based on a conceptual framework with an agreed-upon set of assumptions rather than presenting a series of chapters with isolated information on tasks, tools, and functions. The following are the underlying assumptions upon which chapter outlines were developed and contributors were selected.

1. Health care will continue to be an information-dependent, market-driven industry.
2. Health information is indeed a strategic resource crucial to the health of individual patients and the population, as well as to the success of the institution or enterprise.
3. Health information professionals are leaders in the design, management, and use of health care data and health information systems.
4. Health care data are to be viewed as a continuum beginning with patient-specific data (clinical data) moving to aggregate data (such as performance data, utilization review and risk management data) to knowledge-based data (used in planning and decision support) to comparative, community-wide data (used in policy development) external to the enterprise or institution.

5. The quality of data and the data-to-information transformation are paramount to the efficacy of any information system; thus, the emphasis is on the use of information that has value in decision making, evaluation, planning, marketing, and policy development.

6. The integration and assimilation of technology in the health information manager's daily functions, if not a reality today, will be real in the next generation of practice.

7. The transition to a computer-based patient record (CPR) is an excellent opportunity, cognate to the scope and domain of practice of health information management professionals.

Health Information: Management of a Strategic Resource is organized into six major sections composed of a total of 19 chapters by 34 contributors. Each chapter begins with a chapter outline, key words, abbreviations defined, and objectives to guide the reader. The glossary provides a comprehensive listing of all the keywords with definitions.

Section I: Foundations of Health Information Management begins with an overview of health care systems, Chapter 1—Health Care Systems, and is followed by Chapter 2—The Health Information Management Profession, which is a review of the HIM profession—its development, structure, goals, and roles from the mid-1800s to today.

Section II: Health Care Data begins with Chapter 3—Patient and Health Care Data, in which the variety of data elements required and/or collected and maintained in the health care industry are presented. Chapter 4—Data Collection addresses the various data collection methods, the users of data systems, and the role of HIM professionals in data collection. Chapter 5—Data Quality addresses the importance of data quality and the role of HIM professionals in developing an institution-wide plan for assessing and improving the quality of health care data. Chapter 6—Data Access and Retention compares and contrasts systems for numbering, storage, and retrieval while applying today's newest technologies to access and storage problems. Chapter 7—Coding and Classification Systems discusses major coding and classification systems currently in use in a variety of health care settings, the use of technology in accomplishing this function, and the relationship between coding and reimbursement.

Section III: Data Management and Use emphasizes the data-to-information transformation and focuses on the use of quality information to improve the decision-making abilities of the enterprise. Chapter 8—Registries presents the necessary components of approved cancer programs using the cancer registry as a model to aid the reader in the development of other disease, medical device, and equipment registries. Chapter 9—Research Statistics and Epidemiology helps the reader in designing research studies and organizing and displaying results, including applications specific to health information management. Chapter 10—Quality Assessment and Improvement describes the various methods for assessing and improving the quality of care and services rendered in today's health care systems, while emphasizing the crucial role of health information management professionals in that area. Chapter 11—Health Law Concepts and Practices addresses the legal issues pertinent to the practice of health information management.

Section IV: Management begins with Chapter 12—Principles of Management which provides the reader with the underpinnings of the practice of management, followed by Chapter 13—Human Relations which focuses on the human factors entailed in creating a productive work environment, including communication, conflict resolution, group dynamics, and the importance of empowerment and the acceptance of human diversity in management. Chapter 14—Human Resources Management explores the societal, legislative, organizational, functional, and personal objectives and activities of human resources management. Performance evaluation, employment law, ergonomics, and career planning are some of the topics addressed. Chapter 15—Financial Management addresses reimbursement methodologies, financial accounting methods, phases in developing strategic and business plans, while emphasizing the role of the health information management professional in such activities. Chapter 16—Methods for Analyzing and Improving Systems addresses standards and methods of improvement, utilizing systems analysis and design processes. Re-engineering and project management methods and activities are also addressed.

Section V: Information Systems begins with Chapter 17—Computer-Based Patient Records—A Unifying Principle, which provides an overview of computer applications in the health care system, while focusing on the CPR and providing a strategic plan to assist health information management professionals in the transition to the CPR system. An opportunity is presented to health information management professionals to assume the leadership role in this transition. Chapter 18—Information Systems Life Cycle addresses the analysis, design, implementation, and evaluation of health information systems, with discussion of the tools and aids used in these phases.

Section VI: Perspectives on Health Care and Health Information Management, Chapter 19—Viewpoints invites leaders in health care and health information management to present their viewpoints on their area of expertise while focusing on the future.

The *Ancillaries,* integrated tools available to students, educators, and practitioners, include an *Assignment Workbook* with 100+ case studies, group exercises, field experience activities, and thought questions; a *Review Manual* with approximately 1,000+ questions and answers, including pretests and chapter reviews, based on Chapters 1 through 18 of the book, as well as providing the reader with helpful test-taking principles, helpful studying techniques, and how to prepare for certification; an *EXAMaster,* an evolving testbank, with 1,000+ questions and answers in electronic form to assist in test construction, scoring, and the generation of grades and test statistics; as well as an *Instructor's Manual* with transparencies, answers to assignments, educational hints, and a list of resources for educators.

We would like to thank the contributors for their willingness to take part in this endeavor and share their expertise. Their insights, suggestions, and questions have greatly strengthened the book and ancillaries, bringing our vision to life.

We shall be grateful to readers who have suggestions for additions or revisions or who are interested in sharing their experiences in using the book and its ancillaries with us. We hope that this book and its ancillaries will be a valuable resource as we move into the twenty-first century and address the challenges that touch all of us.

MERVAT ABDELHAK
Managing Editor
SARA GROSTICK
MARY ALICE HANKEN
ELLEN JACOBS

CONTRIBUTORS

CAROL J. BARR, MA, RRA
Director, Health Information Management Program, University of Central Florida, Orlando, Florida
Human Resources Management

ELIZABETH D. BOWMAN, MPA, RRA
Associate Professor, Department of Health Information Management, The University of Tennessee, Memphis, Memphis, Tennessee
Coding and Classification Systems

MELANIE S. BRODNIK, PhD, RRA
Director and Assistant Professor, Health Information Management and Systems Division, The School of Allied Medical Professions, Ohio State University, Columbus, Ohio
Viewpoints

VIRGINIA K. COBURN, MBA
Adjunct Faculty Lecturer on Health Management and Health Information, Northeastern University; Independent Consultant on Health Management and Policy, Boston, Massachusetts
Health Care Systems

JENNIFER COFER, MA, RRA
Publisher, Opus Communications, Marblehead, Massachusetts
Health Care Systems

JILL CALLAHAN DENNIS, JD, RRA
Principal, Health Risk Advantage, Winfield, Illinois
Health Law Concepts and Practices

W. JACK DUNCAN, MBA, PhD
Professor and University Scholar, Graduate School of Management, Professor of Health Care Organization, School of Public Health, University of Alabama at Birmingham, Birmingham, Alabama
Principles of Management

ROSE T. DUNN, CPA, FACHE, BS, MBA, RRA
Vice President, First Class Solutions, Inc., St. Louis, Missouri
Financial Management

SHIRLEY EICHENWALD, MBA, RRA

Director, Recruiting and Professional Development, Pyramid Health Solutions, Seal Beach, California

Viewpoints

J. MICHAEL FITZMAURICE, PhD

Adjunct Associate Professor, University College; University of Maryland, College Park; Director, Center for Information Technology, Agency for Health Care Policy and Research, Rockville, Maryland

Viewpoints

PETER M. GINTER, MBA, PhD

Professor, Graduate School of Management, Professor, Health Care Organization and Policy, School of Public Health, University of Alabama at Birmingham, Birmingham, Alabama

Principles of Management

MARY ALICE HANKEN, PhD, RRA

Director, Health Information Administration Program, School of Public Health and Community Medicine, University of Washington, Seattle, Washington

The Health Information Management Profession; Viewpoints

SUSAN HELBIG, MA, RRA

Clinical Faculty, Health Information Administration School of Public Health, University of Washington; Director, Patient Data Services, Harborview Medical Center, Seattle, Washington

Viewpoints

MERIDA L. JOHNS, PhD, RRA

Associate Professor and Director, Master of Science in Health Information Management, University of Alabama at Birmingham, Birmingham, Alabama

Information Systems Life Cycle

LYNN KUEHN, MS, RRA

Operations Administrator, Family Health Systems, Milwaukee, Wisconsin

Data Access and Retention

JEANETTE C. LINCK, MA, MPA, RRA

Central Office Coordinator, Michigan Health Information Management Association, Ravenna, Michigan

Patient and Health Care Data

MARTIN MENDELSON, MD, PhD

Clinical Associate Professor of Health Information Administration, School of Public Health and Community Medicine, University of Washington; Occupational Health Physician, DFEOH, US Public Health Service, Seattle, Washington

Viewpoints

GRETCHEN F. MURPHY, MEd, RRA

Senior Project Manager, Group Health Cooperative; Lecturer, Health Information Administration, Department of Health Sciences School of Public Health and Community Medicine, University of Washington, Seattle, Washington

Computer-Based Patient Records—A Unifying Principle

MIDGE NOEL RAY, RN, MSN

Associate Professor, Health Information Management Program, Department of Health Services Administration, School of Health Related Professions, University of Alabama at Birmingham, Birmingham, Alabama

Health Care Systems

WESLEY M. ROHRER III, MBA, PhD

Assistant Professor, Department of Health Information Management, and Associate Dean, School of Health and Rehabilitation Sciences, University of Pittsburgh, Pittsburgh, Pennsylvania

Human Relations

JON L. RUCKLE, MD

Medical Director, Northwest Kinetics, Assistant Clinical Professor of Family Medicine, University of Washington School of Medicine, Tacoma, Washington

Viewpoints

WILLIAM J. RUDMAN, PhD

Associate Professor, School of Health Related Professions (Medical Center), University of Mississippi, Jackson, Mississippi

Human Relations

RITA A. SCICHILONE, MHSA, RRA, CCS

Adjunct Faculty, College of St. Mary; Health Information Program; Consultant, Reimbursement Specialist; Professional Management Midwest, Omaha, Nebraska

Human Resources Management

DONNA J. SLOVENSKY, MA, RRA

Associate Professor, Department of Health Services Administration, School of Health Related Professions, University of Alabama at Birmingham, Birmingham, Alabama

Quality Assessment and Improvement

MARY SPIVEY, MLIS, RRA

Program Coordinator, Health Information Management, Broward Community College, Fort Lauderdale, Florida

Data Collection

MARGARET STEWART, RRA

Manager, Medical Educational Seminars, Medical Association of Georgia, Atlanta, Georgia

Data Access and Retention

MILDRED P. ST. LEGER, BA

Assistant Professor and Director, Health Information Management, College of Health Sciences, Roanoke, Virginia

The Health Information Management Profession

SUE WATKINS, AS, ART, CTR

Director, Tri-Counties Regional Cancer Registry and Health Information Services, Santa Barbara County Health Care Services, Santa Barbara, California
Registries

VALERIE J.M. WATZLAF, PhD, RRA

Assistant Professor, Department of Health Information Management, School of Health and Rehabilitation Sciences, University of Pittsburgh, Pittsburgh, Pennsylvania
Research, Statistics, and Epidemiology

PAMELA K. WEAR, MBA, RRA

Vice President, Health Information Management and Marketing, Innovative Health Systems, Inc., Sacramento, California
Viewpoints

LAWRENCE WEED, MD

PKC Corporation, South Burlington, Vermont
Viewpoints

LINCOLN WEED, JD

Attorney, Groom and Nordberg, Washington, D.C.
Viewpoints

DONNA J. WILDE, MPA, RRA

Professor, Health Care Information Programs, Shoreline Community College, Seattle, Washington
Data Quality

KAREN YOUMANS, MPA, RRA, CCS

Instructor, Health Information Management Program, University of Central Florida, Orlando, Florida
Methods for Analyzing and Improving Systems

CONTENTS

SECTION II HEALTH CARE DATA

5

DATA QUALITY 132
Donna J. Wilde

6

DATA ACCESS AND RETENTION 178
Lynn Kuehn and Margaret Stewart

7

CODING AND CLASSIFICATION SYSTEMS 214

Elizabeth D. Bowman

SECTION III   DATA MANAGEMENT AND USE

8

11

HEALTH LAW CONCEPTS AND PRACTICES

Jill Callahan Dennis

SECTION IV   MANAGEMENT

12
PRINCIPLES OF MANAGEMENT 396
W. Jack Duncan and Peter M. Ginter

13
HUMAN RELATIONS 432
William J. Rudman and Wesley M. Rohrer III

14

Rita A. Scichilone and Carol J. Barr

16

   Karen Youmans

SECTION V   INFORMATION SYSTEMS

SECTION VI   PERSPECTIVES ON HEALTH CARE AND HEALTH INFORMATION MANAGEMENT

SECTION
I

FOUNDATIONS OF HEALTH INFORMATION MANAGEMENT

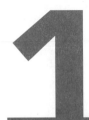

MIDGE NOEL RAY, JENNIFER COFER, and VIRGINIA R. COBURN

KEY WORDS

Accreditation	Certification
Acute care	Claim
Advance directive	Clinical privileges
Ambulatory care	Coinsurance
Ancillary services	Computer-based patient
Assisted living	record
Bed size (bed count)	Continuum of care
Beneficiary	Copayment
Benefit period	Deductible
Capitation	Deemed status
Care	Direct pay, self-pay,
Catchment area	out-of-pocket

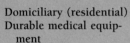

HEALTH CARE SYSTEMS 1

Domiciliary (residential)
Durable medical equipment
Emergency department
Encounter
Episode of care
Fee-for-service
Fiscal intermediary
Gatekeeper
Health
Health care services
Healthy People 2000
Home health care
Hospice
Hospital
Hospital ambulatory care
Hospital inpatient
Hospital patient
Independent living facility
Indigent
Inpatient
Insurance
Licensure
Life care centers
Long-term care
Managed care
Medicaid
Medically indigent
Medicare
Morbidity
Mortality

Multihospital system
Nursing facility
Observation patient
Occasion of service
Osteopath
Out-of-pocket
Outpatient
Palliative care
Patient
Patient assessment
Point of service
Pre-existing condition
Preferred provider organization
Primary care
Prospective payment system
Provider
Rehabilitation
Reimbursement formula
Retrospective payment system
Satellite clinic
Secondary care
Self-pay
Sliding scale fee
Solo practice
Tertiary care
Trauma center
Triage
Usual, customary, and reasonable charges

ABBREVIATIONS

ACF—Administration for Children and Families
ACS—American College of Surgeons
AHA—American Hospital Association
AHIMA—American Health Information Management Association
AMA—American Medical Association
ANA—American Nurses Association
AOA—American Osteopathic Association
CAHEA—Committee on Allied Health Education and Accreditation
CARF—Commission on Accreditation of Rehabilitation Facilities
CDC—Centers for Disease Control and Prevention
CEO—Chief Executive Officer
CFO—Chief Financial Officer
CIO—Chief Information Officer

CHAP—Community Health Accreditation Program
COBRA—Consolidated Omnibus Reconciliation Act
COO—Chief Operating Officer
CPR—Computed-based Patient Record
DHHS—Department of Health and Human Services
DRG—Diagnosis related group
HCFA—Health Care Financing Administration
HMO—Health maintenance organization
JCAHO—Joint Commission on Accreditation of Healthcare Organizations
NLN—National League for Nursing
OSHA—Occupational Safety and Health Administration
PHS—Public Health Service
PPO—Preferred provider organization
SSA—Social Security Administration
TEFRA—Tax Equity and Fiscal Responsibility Act

OBJECTIVES

- Define key words.
- Describe the evolution of the United States health care system beginning with the ancient papyri through *Healthy People 2000*.
- Identify and describe the regulators of health care, including government and nongovernment entities.
- Outline the role of the federal, state, and local governments in the provision of health care.
- Identify legislation that impacts and/or regulates the health care delivery systems in the United States.
- Distinguish between the various health care organizations responsible for providing health care.
- Describe the classification of acute health care facilities, including bed size, ownership and control, population served, and services offered.
- Describe the organizational structures of the hospital as discussed within this chapter.
- Describe the role and responsibilities of the governing body and administrative heads employed in the health care organizations.
- Outline the organizational structure of the professional staff, including the membership, clinical privileges, services, committees, and bylaws.
- Identify and define the scope of the ancillary and support services and departments in health care facilities.
- Describe categories of the health workforce, and address education, licensing and certification requirements, and areas of expertise.
- State current mechanisms of financing health care.
- Describe specific patient care and information technologies and how they impact the health care systems.

Health information management (HIM) is a vital component of the health care delivery system. Therefore, it is crucial for the health information manager to understand the structure of that system. This chapter introduces the reader to the health care delivery system; it covers what the system is like and how it functions and identifies its components. Topics include the history, influencing factors, payers, regulatory agencies, structure, operation, and workforce of health care systems in the United States.

EVOLUTION OF HEALTH CARE SYSTEMS IN THE UNITED STATES

From its inception hundreds of years ago to the present, the health care delivery system has been continually evolving. In the United States, virtually every person is in some way a patient or a consumer of health care at some point in time.[1] Most people are born either in a hospital or outside the hospital with the assistance of a health care professional. Other people come in contact with the health care system in a variety of ways, including physical examination, immunizations, employee physicals, school vision and hearing screens, emergency care, and public health service announcements.

Before proceeding, a few key words need to be defined:

Health—Health is best defined by the World Health Organization as a state of complete physical, mental, and social well-being and not merely the absence of disease or infirmity [1946].

Care—Care is the management of, responsibility for, or the attention to the safety and well-being of another or other persons.

Health care services—Health care services are the processes that contribute to the health and well-being of the person.[2] Services may be provided in a variety of health care settings, such as the hospital, ambulatory care, or home setting, and include nursing, medical, surgical, or other health-related services.

Patient—A patient is an individual, including one who is deceased, who is receiving and/or using or has received health care services.

Inpatient—Inpatient refers to a patient who is receiving health care services and is provided room, board, and continuous nursing service in a unit or area of the hospital.

Outpatient—Outpatient is a patient who is receiving health care services at a hospital without being hospitalized, institutionalized, and/or admitted as an inpatient.

HISTORICAL DEVELOPMENT

Early Forms of Health Care—2700 B.C. to the Eighteenth Century

Health care can be traced back more than 7000 years ago, when primitive tribes would seek out medicine men, who had a reputation for their supernatural powers to rid tribal members of whatever ailed them. Once a medicine man arrived, family and friends would gather around the "patient" for a 4-day ceremony. The ceremony involved prayers, dancing, magic formulas, drumming, and touching. Much like physicians today, medicine men would attempt to remove foreign bodies (stones, splinters), but unlike modern physicians, they would suck out the object. Interestingly, medicine men were often successful with their primitive treatment.[3]

The earliest written records of health care date back to 2700 B.C., to a time when Egyptian physicians and dentists were described in the literature; the physicians were noted to be the best. Still the physicians used supernatural powers for healing; they were trained in temple schools and usually remained priest-physicians. Disease was viewed as being caused by spirits and demons and cured by special gods. In the latter part of Egyptian civilization, there is evidence that one god, Imhotep, was recognized as the new healing god. Imhotep is credited with numerous achievements, including his success as a physician, and, therefore, is called the god of medicine. Information regarding health care during the Egyptian period is documented on papyri, which is material that is made from the papyrus plant. These papyri document medicine from more than 5000 years ago. One of the more famous of these documents is the Edwin Smith Papyrus, which documents a case approach that includes a provisory and final diagnosis, examination techniques, signs of disease, and treatment, which includes magic formulas, prayers, and manipulation[3] (Figure 1–1).

About 2500 years ago, ancient Greek medicine became the forerunner of modern medicine. Much of the medical terminology in use today is derived from the Greek language. Health care in this era was no longer based on supernatural powers and magic potions but had a rational scientific basis. Hippocrates, the father of medicine (460 to 379 B.C.), is regarded as the greatest of the ancient physicians.[3] He is credited with writing more than 50 books that contain notes, surgical procedures, case studies, and conflicting opinions. His approach to disease was naturalistic; he treated the whole person, not just the diseased part.

The concept of hospital as we know it today has its roots in medieval Christendom, when religious orders undertook the task of caring for the sick.[4] The term

Instructions concerning a dislocation of a vertebra of his neck: If you examine a man having a dislocation of a vertebra of his neck, should you find him unconscious of his arms and legs on account of it, while his phallus is erected on account of it and sperm drops from his member without his knowing; his flesh has received wind; his eyes are bloodshot—then you should say concerning him: He has a dislocation of a vertebra of his neck, since he is unconscious of his legs and arms, and his sperm dribbles. An ailment which cannot be treated.

From Ackerknecht, E.H.: Medicine of ancient civilization. *In A Short History of Medicine,* 4th edition, pp 21–26. Baltimore: Johns Hopkins Press, 1982.

FIGURE 1–1. Edwin Smith Papyrus. (From Ackerknecht EH: Medicine of ancient civilization. *In* Ackerknecht EH (ed): A short history of medicine, 4th ed. Baltimore: Johns Hopkins Press, 1982, p 23. Used by permission.)

hospital originated in the fifth century from the Latin word *hospitium*, meaning a place of reception. During the Middle Ages, the hospitium evolved from a Christian tradition of offering weary travelers and guests a place, called hospice, to rest. Hospices were established along the road to the Holy Land for the purpose of providing rest and shelter for those making the pilgrimage to the Holy Land. The hospices were funded by the churches and the wealthy, who viewed the support as doing God's work. Pilgrims traveling to and from the Holy Land caused an epidemic of leprosy to spread into England. As a result, about 200 Lazar houses (hospitals) were built to isolate lepers from the public.[1]

Years after the discovery of North America, Cortez founded the first permanent hospital in 1554 in Mexico, the Jesus of Nazareth Hospital, which is still in operation. The first American hospitals were established in the early 1800s for the purpose of isolating patients who had contagious diseases. These early American hospitals were located in seaports. In the 18th century, hospitals called almshouses were built for the poor and homeless, with the oldest being Pennsylvania Hospital (established in 1752) in Philadelphia. To help pay for health care, the poor or homeless patient performed menial tasks such as scrubbing floors and serving food to other patients. Wealthy Americans received health care in private homes. Because of the serious epidemics, such as typhus, scurvy, smallpox, tuberculosis, and typhoid fever, early American hospitals had an extremely high death rate; admission was considered to be a last resort. It was not until the latter part of the 19th century that hospitals emerged as places to get well.

Health Care in the Nineteenth Century

The first school in America dedicated to training physicians was founded in 1765 in Philadelphia. Before this time, the only training an American physician received was by way of apprenticeship with an older physician. As the population in the United States grew and moved westward, the demand for more hospitals and physicians increased. To meet the growing need for more physicians, a large number of new medical schools were opened, most of which were proprietary. By the 19th century, there were no fewer than 400 medical schools in the United States, most of questionable quality.[3] As a result, a group of highly qualified physicians formed the American Medical Association (AMA) in 1847 for the primary purpose of "cleaning house."[3] The AMA was initially established to examine the poor quality of medical education and questionable ethics of practicing physicians. Today, membership in the AMA is open to any physician in good standing and consists of local, city, and state medical societies. The AMA is dedicated to promoting the science and art of medicine, improving public health, making health care policy, and servicing the professional needs of its members.

The American Hospital Association (AHA) was founded in 1848 for the purpose of promoting public welfare by providing better health care in the hospitals. The AHA membership is composed of both nonprofit and for-profit hospitals. The AHA funds and conducts research and educational programs, maintains data on hospital profiles, and represents the hospital interests in legal and legislative matters, all of which are directed at improving the nation's health care system.

In the late 19th century, states became involved in health care when mental health reformers pushed for insanity to be managed as a medical or mental disorder. State governments established mental institutions for the confinement of the mentally ill rather than housing them in the poorhouses and prisons. However, because of inadequate funding, the mental institutions soon became overcrowded and living conditions were deplorable.

Twentieth-Century Reforms

In the early 1900s, hospitals were funded by private beneficiaries, endowments, and donations. The private sector, however, showed little interest in serving the population as a whole; the assumption was that local government would pay for the poor.[4] Most hospitals were viewed as boardinghouses for the poor and sick; physicians did not take histories and perform physical examinations on admission, and seldom did they document assessments or diagnoses.[5]

Between the 1870s and 1920s, the number of United States hospitals increased from less than 200 to more than 6000. Private benevolence was responsible for establishing hundreds of new hospitals that were not interested in serving the poor. By 1910, there were as many hospitals per 1000 population as there are today, and much like today, part of the population was not being served. Hospitals operated on the principle that the more expensive the care, the more valuable the service, which caused costs to escalate.[4]

In 1910, Abraham Flexner conducted a study funded by the Carnegie Foundation on the quality of medical education in the United States. The famous Flexner Report, published in 1910, identified serious problems and inconsistencies that existed in medical education. As a result, many of the proprietary schools were closed and those that remained open underwent curriculum revision. In addition, the AMA initiated an accreditation process that ranked schools according to their performance. The Flexner Report established a model for medical education that is still used in many medical schools today.[6]

In 1913, the American College of Surgeons (ACS) was founded. One of its purposes was to develop some system of hospital standardization that would improve patient care and recognize those that had the highest ideals.[5] To establish the standards and, thereby, improve quality, the ACS began collecting data on the training of surgeons in schools and hospitals. The data collected came from the health record, and at this point in time, the ACS realized that the documentation was inadequate. In 1917, the ACS established the Hospital Standardization Program, which laid the groundwork for establishing standards of care. In 1919, the ACS reported the findings of the first field test for approving hospitals: "692 hospitals of 100 beds or more had been surveyed and . . . only 89 had met the standards." Furthermore, "some of the most prestigious hospitals in the country failed to meet the most basic standards." After issuing this report, the ACS adopted the *Minimum Standards*, which identified the standards that were essential for the "proper care and treatment of patients in any hospital."[5] They included specifications that established an organized medical staff and required that certain diagnostic and therapeutic facilities be available and that a health record be written for every patient. The standards specified, among other things, that the record be complete, accurate, and accessible.[5] In fact, the standards for health care in use today continue to encompass the documentation requirements identified in 1919 (see Medical Record Specifications Identified in the *Minimum Standards* by the American College of Surgeons, 1919).

Although hospital admissions increased dramatically

Medical Record Specifications Identified in the *Minimum Standards* by the American College of Surgeons, 1919

A complete case record should be developed including the following:

- Patient identification data
- Complaint
- Personal and family history
- History of current illness
- Physical examination
- Special examinations (consultations, radiography, clinical laboratory)
- Provisional or working diagnosis
- Medical and surgical treatments
- Progress notes
- Gross and microscopic findings
- Final diagnosis
- Condition on discharge
- Follow-up
- Autopsy findings in the event of death

Adapted from Minimum Standards, 1919. Bulletin of American College of Surgeons 8:4, 1924.

---

from 1935 to the end of World War II in 1945, the unemployed, disabled, elderly, and others who could not pay were excluded. The economy was growing, and technological advancements continued in the medical field. The need for more hospitals and to make high-quality health care accessible to all Americans increased. In 1946, Senators Lister Hill and Harold H. Burton sponsored the Hospital Survey and Construction Act. This legislation, known as the Hill-Burton Act, provided funding for the construction of hospitals and other health care facilities based on state need. A federal-state planning process was required that included the states' assessment of need for new facilities and the application for Hill-Burton funding.[7] For the next 25 years, as a result of this program, hospital construction and expansion flourished.

In the early 1950s, there was "increasing sophistication in medical care, growing numbers and complexity of hospitals, and rapid emergence of nonsurgical specialties," which burdened the Hospital Standardization Program.[5] As a result, the Joint Commission on Accreditation of Hospitals (JCAH) was founded in 1952 and adopted the Hospital Standardization Program from the ACS.

In the 1950s, Americans began to want more technology that would be accessible to all people at an affordable cost.[4] As advances were made in the medical field, the demand for health care services and the cost to provide those services grew. The attitude became "more is better." In addition, medical advances extended life expectancy, resulting in an increase in the elderly population. With the growing elderly population came a growth in incidence of chronic disease. As hospital care became more expensive, those who were uninsured or underinsured—primarily the poor and the elderly—could not access the health care system. Up to this point, the federal and state governments did little to control hospital costs. However, in 1965, Congress amended the Social Security Act of 1935, Public Law 89-97, establishing both Title XVIII, *Health Insurance for the Aged* (now called Medicare), and Title XIX, which extended the Kerr-Mills Medical Assistance Program (now called Medicaid). **Medicare** is a federally funded program that provides health insurance for elderly people and certain other groups, and Medicaid supports the states in paying for health care for the indigent.[8] An **indigent** is one who is without the means for subsistence—poor or impoverished. At this time, the federal government became a significant player in the health care delivery system because it not only funded and operated the Medicare program but also assisted the states with the Medicaid program. These programs are discussed further under the section on financing health care later in this chapter. In response to the federal government's establishing and regulating the Medicare and Medicaid programs, states began writing more and, in some cases, their first regulatory codes.

In the 1960s, there was a proliferation of various health care facilities, including long-term care, psychiatric and substance abuse facilities, and programs for the developmentally disabled. The JCAH not only redefined the standards to be optimal achievable, as opposed to minimum standards, but also began developing standards for the various types of health care facilities.[5] It was during the late 1980s that the JCAH reflected its broader scope by changing its name to the Joint Commission on Accreditation of Healthcare Organizations (JCAHO; see Historical Landmarks Impacting Health Care Systems).

Complexity of Health Care Today

The health care delivery system in the United States has evolved into a complex system composed of multiple types of facilities, providers, payers, and regulators as well as consumers who are demanding more and better health care. There is a proliferation of sophisticated technology for both medical practice and information management. The technology available in financial, administrative, and clinical information systems impacts on the quality, cost, and efficiency of health care systems. The technological advances in medicine support prevention, early diagnosis, shorter hospital stays, and increased outpatient services and home health care.

In 1992, the cost of health care in the United States reached $838.5 billion, and yet between 37 and 40 million people are uninsured and/or cannot access the system. Those without insurance either cannot afford it or cannot find an insurance company that is willing to sell them a policy at any price. Insurance companies often cancel contracts with patients who have expensive (catastrophic costs) health care needs, as is the case with chronic conditions such as cancers, kidney disease, and heart disease. Those who cannot access the health care system may live in areas where there is little or no health care available or that do not have transportation.

Advances in technology and scientific developments have supported a healthier lifestyle and longer life expectancy. For women, life expectancy has increased from 49.1 years in 1900 to 78.6 years in 1990 and for men, from 49.1 years to 71.8 years. And with the longer life expectancy has come growth in the need for home health and long-term care.

Health care in the 1990s is costly and not accessible to all citizens, and yet consumers are demanding more and better care. As a result, there is tremendous pressure to reform the manner in which health care is delivered to contain the cost and still provide high-quality care to all. The sources of the pressure are numerous. They include the federal government, which is concerned with the cost of health care and its accessibility; the consumers, who have become more educated and are demanding more; the providers, who want to maintain their market share, cut their costs, and realize a profit; and the taxpayers, who are either underinsured or uninsured or who feel overburdened with taxation that finances the health care. The changes that are occurring are evidenced by the shift from inpatient care to outpatient care and by the increase in more alternative health care facilities.

With such problems as the escalating cost of health care, the rising number of uninsured, and the existence of underserved rural areas where medical care is not available, there is great impetus to reform the manner in which health care is delivered in the United States. Various plans for health care reform have been developed by different professional organizations, members of the Congress, state governments, and the federal government. Most of the plans for health care reform address such issues as universal coverage, meaning health care for every citizen; health care costs; and the quality of health care provided.

Healthy People 2000

The United States Department of Health and Human Services (DHHS) has established goals for the year 2000 that promote health and prevention of disease. The report that includes goals based on identified data systems

Historical Landmarks Impacting Health Care Systems

1554	First permanent hospital, Jesus of Nazareth Hospital in Mexico, was founded.
1765	First school in America dedicated to educating and training physicians was established in Philadelphia.
1847	American Medical Association (AMA) was founded for the purpose of improving the quality of medical education and the ethics of practicing medicine.
1848	American Hospital Association was founded for purpose of promoting public welfare by providing improved health care in hospitals.
1910	Flexner Report, published by Abraham Flexner, revealed serious problems that existed in medical education. The report served as an impetus to establishing the accreditation of medical schools by the AMA.
1913	American College of Surgeons (ACS) was founded for the purposes of establishing standards of care and recognizing those hospitals that have high ideals.
1917	ACS established the Hospital Standardization Program, which began testing basic standards of care.
1919	ACS adopted the *Minimum Standards*, which identified factors that are essential to proper care and treatment of hospital patients.
1935	Social Security Act was passed, which provided grants for old age assistance and benefits, unemployment compensation, and aid to dependent children, maternal and child welfare, and other groups. It also established social security.
1946	Hospital Survey and Construction Act (Hill-Burton Act) was passed, which provided funding for the construction of health care facilities and equipment based on state need.
1952	Joint Commission on Accreditation of Hospitals (JCAH) was founded, which adopted the Hospital Standardization Program from the ACS; in the late 1980s, JCAH changed the name to the Joint Commission on Accreditation of Healthcare Organizations.
1953	Department of Health, Education, and Welfare (HEW) was formed for the purpose of addressing issues related to the health, education, and welfare of the people of the United States.
1961	Community Health Services and Facilities Act provided grants for the establishment of voluntary health planning agencies at the local level; it resulted in community health centers to serve low-income areas.
1965	Title III of the Older Americans Act established funding for transportation and for chore, homemaker, and home health aides for the elderly.

is known as **Healthy People 2000**, which is "a statement of national opportunities." Some of the national data systems used to formulate the goals that would lead to a better quality of life include data on adult use of tobacco, continuing survey of individual food intake, national crime survey, and birth and infant death data. To accomplish the goals of *Healthy People 2000,* the states will need to set their own objectives and coordinate those objectives with community involvement and implementation. *Healthy Communities 2000: Model Standards, Guidelines for Community Attainment of Year 2000 Objectives* was developed to provide assistance to state and local governments in reaching their goals.[9]

REGULATORY AGENCIES AND ORGANIZATIONS

External forces that regulate the health care industry include but are not limited to the DHHS, JCAHO, American Osteopathic Association (AOA), Community Health Accreditation Program (CHAP) of the National League for Nursing (NLN), Commission on Accreditation of Rehabilitation Facilities (CARF), Commission on Accreditation of Allied Health Education Programs (CAAHEP), and the state departments of public health. The regulatory activities of health care facilities are primarily directed at quality, utilization, and cost of care,

	Historical Landmarks Impacting Health Care Systems *Continued*
1965	Congress amended the Social Security Act of 1935 (PL 89-97), which established Title XVIII, Health Insurance for the Aged (Medicare), and Title XVIX, Medical Assistance Program (Medicaid).
1970	Occupational Safety and Health Act was passed, which mandated employers to provide a safe and healthy work environment and therefore resulted in the development of standards.
1977	Committee on Allied Health Education and Accreditation (CAHEA) was founded by the AMA for the purpose of accrediting allied health programs; it disbanded in 1994.
1980	HEW was reorganized into the Department of Health and Human Services (DHHS), a federal, cabinet-level department responsible for health issues, including health care and costs, welfare of various populations, occupational safety, and income security plans.
1982	Tax Equity and Fiscal Responsibility Act (TEFRA), PL97-248, established a mechanism for controlling the cost of the Medicare program; TEFRA set a limit on reimbursement and required the development of the prospective payment system.
1985	Consolidated Omnibus Budget Reconciliation Act (COBRA), known as the antidumping statute, established criteria for the transfer and discharge of Medicare and Medicaid patients.
1987	Nursing Home Reform Act, effective in 1990, required nursing facilities (long-term care facilities) to employ sufficient nursing personnel, 24 hours per day, to provide care to each resident according to the care plan.
1989	Omnibus Budget Reconciliation Act brought attention and support to the production and dissemination of scientific and policy-relevant information that improves quality, reduces cost, and enhances effectiveness of health care.
1990	Patient Self-Determination Act resulted from the *Cruzan v. Missouri* (1990) case in which the court upheld patient wishes. The Act increased the public's awareness of state laws governing patient options and rights and advanced directives.
1991	DHHS commissioned the Workgroup on Electronic Data Interchange to identify ways of increasing the number of claims processed electronically, which would reduce administrative costs.
1992	Computer-Based Patient Record Institute was created for the purpose of developing strategy that supports the development and adoption of the computer-based patient record.
1994	Commission on Accreditation of Allied Health Education Programs (CAAHEP) was founded for the purpose of assuming responsibility for the accreditation of allied health programs. CAAHEP is a successor agency of CAHEA, which disbanded in 1994.

whereas the regulatory activities that impact educational programs and the health care workforce are directed at quality and supply.

Federal Government as Regulator

The federal government has been involved in the regulation of the health care systems since the early part of the century, primarily in the consumer's interest. In 1906, the Pure Food and Drug Act was passed because of the unsanitary conditions that prevailed in the food production industry and in 1938, the Food, Drug, and Cosmetic Act was passed to regulate the food, drug, and cosmetic industry. This act mandated manufacturers to prove safety, specify composition and method of manufacture, and provide labeling and package inserts. Interestingly, it was not until 1962 that manufacturers were required to prove efficacy (i.e., how effective a product is).

Current Mechanisms of Regulation

Today the federal government regulates health care in numerous ways, such as the following:

- Its ownership and control of health care facilities

- Its control as a financer of health care programs
- Through legislation that affects health care

All federally owned and operated health care facilities are regulated by the federal government, such as Veterans Affairs medical centers. However, according to Brecher, the "federal government has restricted its role as direct provider at the same time it has expanded its commitments as a financer."[10] There was a time when the federal government owned and operated Public Health Service (PHS) hospitals for the Merchant Marines, but today, these PHS hospitals have been closed and the government contracts for their health care.[10] Therefore, most of the government's regulatory power originates from its funding of health care programs and from legislation that impacts the health care systems.

Department of Health and Human Services

The branch of the federal government that is primarily responsible for the numerous regulatory programs that affect the health industry is the Department of Health and Human Services (DHHS), formerly the Department of Health, Education and Welfare (HEW). HEW, created in 1953, underwent numerous reorganizations that led to the creation of the DHHS in 1980. The organization of the DHHS is quite complex and includes numerous administrations, divisions, offices, centers, and agencies; the highest-ranking official is the secretary of the DHHS, who advises the President of the United States on issues regarding health, welfare, income security plans, and programs and projects of the DHHS. The DHHS has 10 regional offices that work with the states and communities in carrying out various programs.[11]

ORGANIZATION OF DHHS. The organizational structure of the DHHS encompasses four agencies—the Public Health Service (PHS), the Health Care Financing Administration (HCFA), the Social Security Administration (SSA), and the Administration for Children and Families (ACF)—and five offices, some of which are described in Figure 1–2.

OFFICE OF INSPECTOR GENERAL. The responsibility of conducting and monitoring audits, inspections, and investigations regarding programs or projects sponsored by the DHHS is delegated to the inspector general. For example, this office investigates cases of alleged fraud and abuse that occur in Medicare and Medicaid programs and recommends corrective action in such cases.[11]

COMPONENTS OF DHHS

Public Health Service. The PHS manages the following offices.

- Agency for Health Care Policy and Research was established by the Omnibus Budget Reconciliation Act of 1989, which placed greater emphasis on health services research. The primary focus is to produce and disseminate scientific and policy-relevant information that improves the quality, reduces the cost, and enhances the effectiveness of health care.

- Agency for Toxic Substances and Disease Registry is committed to protecting both workers and the public from exposure to and/or the adverse effects of hazardous substances. The agency, among other things, collects, analyzes, and disseminates information regarding mortality, disease, and hazardous substances; establishes registries for long-term follow-up; and develops programs for public response to health emergencies.

- Centers for Disease Control and Prevention (CDC) is concerned with communicable diseases, environmental health, and foreign quarantine activities. CDC also works with state and local agencies regarding these matters and provides consultation, education, and training. For example, the CDC has established recommendations (standards) called "Universal Precautions" that specify how to minimize the risk of contracting acquired immunodeficiency syndrome (AIDS).

- Food and Drug Administration (FDA) is responsible for the safety of foods, drugs, medical devices, cosmetics, and radiation-emitting equipment. Responsibilities include proper labeling, product information, safety, and efficacy.

- Substance Abuse and Mental Health Services Administration is concerned with the effective prevention and treatment of addictive and mental disorders. The administration emphasizes state-of-the-art practice that is based on science, high quality, and access to health care for these disorders.

- Health Resources and Services Administration is primarily involved in the distribution of major grant funding to state governments and the private sector.

- National Institutes of Health is a major research center composed of numerous departments and divisions (e.g., National Institute on Aging, National Center for Nursing Research, National Cancer Institute). It is a major source of funding for health-related research (e.g., aging, cancer, women's health issues, obesity, nutrition).

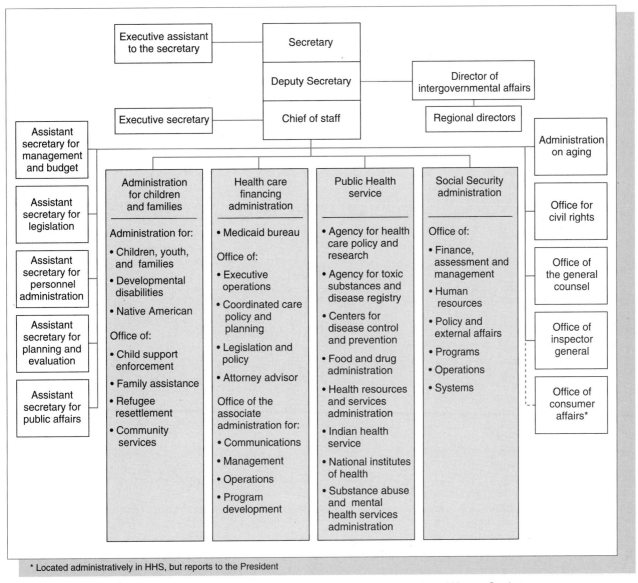

FIGURE 1–2. Organizational structure of the Department of Health and Human Services.

* Located administratively in HHS, but reports to the President

- Indian Health Service is responsible for providing health care through a network of hospitals, health centers, health stations, and school health centers and through contracts with private providers to eligible Native Americans.[11]

Social Security Administration. The SSA manages the social security program for elderly, disabled, and blind people and for survivors (dependents). The social security program is financed by contributions from employees, employers, and self-employed people, which are placed in a fund. When earnings stop or are reduced because of retirement, death, or disability, the fund pays monthly cash amounts to supplement the loss of income.[11]

Administration for Children and Families. The ACF is committed to the "sound development of children, youth, and families" and to supporting activities that improve and enrich these groups. ACF administers and funds state grants regarding such issues as adoption, runaway and homeless youth, prevention and treatment of child abuse, and child welfare services.

Health Care Financing Administration (HCFA). The HCFA is responsible for the Medicare program and the federal government's role in the Medicaid programs, with special emphasis on quality and utilization control.

Through its programs, HCFA is involved in the health care of 67 million people who are elderly, disabled, and/or poor at a projected cost of $230 billion for 1993.[11]

The HCFA has established rules and regulations that govern the Medicare program. To be eligible for Medicare and Medicaid reimbursement, providers must demonstrate compliance with the *Conditions of Participation,* which is the process of certification. **Certification** is the process by which government and nongovernment organizations evaluate educational programs, health care facilities, and individuals as having met predetermined standards. The certification of health care facilities is the responsibility of the states. However, Title XVIII, the Medicare Act, specifies that those facilities accredited by the JCAHO and AOA be deemed in compliance with the Medicare Conditions of Participation for Hospitals[5,12]; those accredited are said to have **deemed status.**

The certification requirements for the various health care facilities were originally published in the Regulation Number 5, Federal Health Insurance for the Aged, *Conditions of Participation.* Revisions to the *Conditions* are published in the *Federal Register.* Compliance with the *Conditions of Participation* is regulated by the states.

Occupational Safety and Health Administration

In 1970, Congress passed the Occupational Safety and Health Act, which mandated employers to provide a safe and healthy work environment. The Occupational Safety and Health Administration (OSHA) is responsible for developing standards and regulations and conducting inspections and investigations to determine compliance and proposes corrective actions for noncompliance in matters related to occupational safety and health.[11] Other agencies involved in establishing standards on occupational safety and health include government agencies, such as the CDC, and professional organizations, such as the ACS. The guidelines, recommendations, and/or standards are directed at protecting employees from occupational health hazards, such as minimizing the risk of contracting tuberculosis or AIDS and limiting injuries that result from poor lighting or wet floors.

Role of States

State governments have regulatory involvement in the health care systems through state-owned and -operated facilities, the funding of medical education and teaching hospitals, the certification of health care facilities according to the "Conditions of Participation," maintenance of public health departments, and licensing of health care facilities and health occupations. Hospital ownership, medical education, certification, and licensing of health occupations are discussed in other sections; therefore, only the states' role in public health departments and in licensing health care facilities are addressed in this section.

State Health Departments

The organization of state health departments varies from state to state but is a joint venture between the state and the local communities. The health care provided is usually directed toward maternal and child health care, communicable diseases, and chronic diseases.[10] The maternal and child care services usually provide obstetric care, family planning, well-baby checkups, vaccinations, and other services. Health care for communicable diseases involves teaching the patient and community about transmission and prevention of certain diseases, diagnosing and treating communicable diseases such as measles and gonorrhea, and tracking the source of the communicable disease. Some of the chronic diseases that the public health department might manage are mental illness, substance abuse, hypertension, and diabetes. HIM professionals need to be knowledgeable about the organization of the state health department in the state where they reside or practice; information is usually available through the county health department.

Licensure of Health Care Facilities

Licensure gives legal approval for a facility to operate or for a person to practice within his or her profession. Virtually every state requires that hospitals, sanatoria, nursing homes, and pharmacies be licensed to operate, although the requirements and standards for licensure may differ from state to state. State licensure is mandatory. Federal facilities such as those of the Department of Veterans Affairs do not require licensure.

Although licensure requirements vary, the health care facilities must meet certain basic criteria that are determined by state regulatory agencies. The standards address such concerns as adequacy of staffing, personnel employed to provide services, physical aspects of the facility (equipment, buildings), and services provided, including health records. Licensure typically is performed annually, and the standards are usually considered to be minimally acceptable for operation.

Legislation

The Consolidated Omnibus Budget Reconciliation Act (COBRA) of 1985 was written out of a concern for the management of indigent patients. The Act, known as the "antidumping" statute, established criteria for facilities and physicians responsible for the transfer and discharge of patients. The act applies to all physicians certified for Medicare or Medicaid (referred to as participating physicians) or physicians responsible for patients in a certified health care facility. The criteria requires that every patient who arrives with an emergency medical condition be evaluated to determine if patient condition warrants therapy or if patient transfer to another health care facility is best for the patient.[13]

In 1989, the Omnibus Budget Reconciliation Act was passed, which emphasizes the production and dissemination of scientific and policy-relevant information that improves the quality, reduces the cost, and enhances the effectiveness of health care. This act promoted the development of outcome measures (criteria) for health care quality.

The Patient Self-Determination Act of 1990 was a result of the Supreme Court's ruling in *Cruzan v. Missouri* (1990) that upheld patient wishes even though the decision meant inevitable death for the patient. The act is intended to increase the public's awareness of the respective state laws governing patient options for health care, patient rights, and advance directives. An **advance directive** is a legal, written document that specifies patient preferences regarding future health care or specifies another person to make medical decisions in the event the patient develops an incurable or irreversible condition and is unable to communicate his or her wishes; the patient must be competent at the time the document is prepared and signed. The advance directive guides the health care team in making decisions about life-sustaining treatment and organ donation and usually designates a person to assume authority for the patient. The statute requires providers to develop written policies and procedures on self-determination and to document in each health record whether or not an advance directive has been signed.[13] The HIM and/or risk management department is responsible for assuring that the proper documentation is in each health record.

Accreditation

The process by which an organization or agency performs an external review and grants recognition to the program of study or institution that meets certain predetermined standards is called **accreditation**. The review process and the standards are devised and regulated by professional organizations such as the JCAHO and the AOA. Although the process is voluntary, there are financial and legal incentives for health care organizations to attain accreditation. Advantages of accreditation are numerous and include the following:

- It is required for reimbursement for certain patient groups.

- It validates the quality of care.

- It provides a competitive edge over nonaccredited facilities.

The HIM department plays a critical role in accreditation because the review of health information data is a major part of the accreditation process. The HIM professional should have access to and be familiar with the standards contained in the most current accreditation manual for the type of health care organization in which she or he is employed.

Joint Commission on Accreditation of Healthcare Organizations

The JCAHO is a private, nonprofit organization that establishes guidelines and standards for the operation and management of health care facilities with emphasis on the health care functions critical to patient care. The standards are "based on the premise that health care organizations exist to maximize the health of the people they serve while using resources efficiently."[14] Once an organization is found to be in substantial compliance with the JCAHO standards, accreditation may be awarded for up to 3 years. Hospitals must undergo a full survey at least every 3 years.

The JCAHO publishes accreditation manuals with standards for hospitals, non–hospital-based psychiatric and substance abuse organizations, long-term care organizations, home care organizations, ambulatory care organizations, and organization-based pathology and clinical laboratory services.[14]

American Osteopathic Association Hospital Accreditation Program

Much like the JCAHO, the AOA accreditation is a voluntary program that accredits osteopathic hospitals. Those hospitals that are accredited are recognized by the DHHS as having "deemed status," and therefore, they are eligible to receive Medicare funds.[16]

Commission on Accreditation of Rehabilitation Facilities

Founded in 1966, CARF is an independent accrediting agency for rehabilitation facilities. **Rehabilitation** is the processes of treatment and education that lead the disabled person in achievement of maximum independence and function and a personal sense of well-being. The mission of CARF is to "serve as the preeminent standards-setting and accrediting body promoting the delivery of quality services to people with disabilities." As a result of this mission, CARF sets and maintains standards directed at improving quality of care, shares aggregate data, identifies competent organizations that provide rehabilitative services, and provides an organized forum in which people served, providers, and others can participate in quality improvement.[15]

Community Health Accreditation Program

The organization that accredits home health agencies is CHAP, a subsidiary of the NLN. Unlike other accrediting bodies, CHAP standards are consumer-oriented, with more emphasis on the patient perspective than on the clinical aspect of care.

Regulatory Mechanisms of Health Occupations

There are numerous agencies, organizations, and legislation that regulate the education and practice of the various health occupations. The regulatory activities include state licensure of practitioners, accreditation of programs, certification of practitioners, and legislation that governs practice. Only a few of these activities are discussed here.

Commission on Accreditation of Allied Health Education Programs

In 1994, CAAHEP was established as the successor agency to the Committee on Allied Health Education and Accreditation (CAHEA). CAHEA, founded in 1977, was disbanded in 1994. The CAAHEP is responsible for accrediting allied health programs, some of which include health information management, physical therapy, speech pathology, and audiology. The different allied health programs develop standards specific to the respective areas. The standards for HIM are printed in the 1994 *Essentials for an Accredited Program for the Health Information Technician and Health Information Manager.* Educational programs utilize these essentials in curriculum development and revision. Those programs in full compliance with the *Essentials* qualify for accreditation.

American Medical Association

The AMA is involved in the accreditation of medical schools, residency programs, and certain allied health programs. It collaborates with the CAAHEP in the accreditation of allied health programs.

AOA Bureau of Professional Education

This bureau is the only accrediting agency for osteopathic medical education in the United States. Accredi-

tation by the AOA is based on standards of educational quality. Programs that are accredited meet or exceed the standards for educational quality that have been established by the AOA. The AOA has certifying boards that offer certification for numerous specialties and procedures that the osteopathic physician may pursue (e.g., nuclear medicine, gynecology, proctology, blood-banking and transfusion medicine, sports medicine, angiography).[16] The AOA also regulates its membership by requiring a minimum number of continuing education credits to retain membership.

National League for Nursing

The accrediting body for schools of nursing that offer diplomas or associate, bachelor, master, and doctoral degrees in nursing is the NLN. The NLN establishes standards for the nursing curriculum, including programs for registered nurses and licensed practical nurses. Although membership in the NLN is open to anyone or any agency interested in nursing, most of the members are licensed practical and registered nurses.

State Licensure of Practitioners

In the licensing of practitioners, states have the right to control the entry into certain professions through licensure and the right to revoke the license. The license itself is a permit issued by the state that authorizes one to practice in a specified area, and without this permission, such practice is illegal.

Each state establishes its own licensing requirements and restricts certain activities to those who are licensed by that state. Licensure requirements involve completion of a program of study and examination by the state. Restrictions are specific for the license. For example, the prescribing and dispensing of medications was at one time restricted to licensed physicians. Today, however, many states have given prescriptive authority to nurse practitioners and others. The health occupations that require licensure to practice include medicine, osteopathy, nursing, nursing home administrators, dentistry, podiatry, and numerous others, depending on the state.[17]

HEALTH CARE DELIVERY SYSTEMS

Issues and Trends

Historically, the biggest provider of care has been the hospital. Today, however, there are enormous pressures to move the focus of care from inpatient to outpatient and to use reduced-stay procedures.[18] The following are some of the issues and trends that have stimulated growth in ambulatory care.

- The cost of health care in the United States has been escalating. The involvement of the federal government in the financing of health care has provided the impetus to better justify hospitalization and to use effective, efficient therapy on an outpatient basis. Almost all diagnostic procedures are now performed in an outpatient setting, whereas in the past, the patient might be admitted to an acute care facility for extensive testing that could require costly days of hospitalization.

- Advances in technology have allowed safer, more effective testing and treatment to be performed on an outpatient basis.[18,19] For example, historically, many abdominal operative procedures were performed solely through a large abdominal incision (laparotomy), which increases the risk, cost, and length of stay. Today, the newer laparoscopic procedure is often an acceptable alternative to the laparotomy. In laparoscopy, a flexible fiberoptic tube is inserted into the abdominal cavity by way of a small puncture wound through which surgical procedures can be accomplished, including exploration, tubal ligations, and prostate cancer staging. This form of endosurgery contributes to more outpatient surgery because it replaces abdominal surgery that involves the 4- to 6-inch incision of a laparotomy.[18]

- Consumers of health care are more educated and demanding higher-quality care and a more comprehensive approach to health care delivery. They are interested in such issues as cost of care, patient rights, living wills, sophisticated diagnostic and therapeutic procedures, and preventive care.

Because of the changes that are occurring in health care systems, both traditional systems and some of the more innovative approaches to health care are discussed. The numerous settings in which health care is provided include physician offices, patient homes, outpatient departments, clinics, acute care hospitals, specialty hospitals, long-term care facilities, and schools. Before discussing the facilities, the reader needs to understand the continuum of care.

Continuum of Care

The **continuum of care** is the full range of health care services provided, moving from the least acute and least intensive to the most acute and most intensive or vice versa.[20] Note that the JCAHO defines the continuum of care as "matching patients' needs with the appropriate level and type of medical, health or social service."[14] The delivery of care falls into one of the following three major levels:

- Primary
- Secondary
- Tertiary

Primary care is most often considered the care provided at the point of first contact (**encounter**) with the health care provider in an ambulatory care setting; the care is continuous and comprehensive and may involve **episodes of care** for a specific condition during a period of relative continuous care. The provider, usually a physician, coordinates and manages all aspects of the patient's health care, including the utilization of consultants and community resources as appropriate.[21] Primary care encompasses preventive care (comprehensive care) and acute care. Health care services directed at preventing disease or injury, minimizing the consequences of existing conditions, and promoting health are the major objectives of preventive care. Annual physical examinations, immunizations, family planning, vision and hearing screens, health education, and early detection of disease are examples of preventive medicine.[21] Acute care, on the other hand, implies the treatment of common illnesses and injuries, such as nausea, vomiting, and abrasions. Providers of primary care are family practitioners, internists, pediatricians, obstetricians, gynecologists, and nurse practitioners; the care is commonly provided in one of many ambulatory care settings. **Secondary care** is a term that is not as widely used as primary or tertiary care but implies care by a specialist, usually through referral from the primary care physician. **Tertiary care** is a term used for the care provided at facilities with advanced technologies and specialized intensive care units, such as teaching institutions and university medical centers. Those institutions that are recognized as providers of tertiary care are often involved in biomedical research. The providers are specialists who are widely recognized for their expertise in specific areas of medicine and include specialists such as endocrinologists, hematologists, oncologists, thoracic surgeons, and neurosurgeons.

Ambulatory Care

Ambulatory care is a comprehensive term for all types of health care provided in an outpatient setting; the patient travels to and from the facility on the same day and is not hospitalized, institutionalized, or admitted as an inpatient.[2] For example, a resident of a nursing home may be transported to the outpatient department at the hospital for a mammogram (radiograph of the breast) and then returned to the nursing home later the same day. This person is a resident (inpatient) of the nursing home but an outpatient of the hospital.

There are two major types of ambulatory (or outpatient) care. They are as follows:

• Care provided in freestanding medical centers that includes physicians' solo, partnership, or group practices; public health department; neighborhood and community health centers (NHCs or CHCs); and urgent care centers

• Care provided in organized settings that function independently of the physicians providing the care. This type of ambulatory care includes hospital-owned clinics, outpatient departments, ambulatory treatment units, emergency rooms, ancillary services, staff health maintenance organizations (HMOs), and urgent care centers.

Note that urgent care centers and others may be in either type of setting, depending on ownership of the facility. The physician may be an employee of the urgent care facility or he or she may be the owner and provider. Figure 1–3 shows the organization of ambulatory care and its components.

Physician Practices

Physician practices have historically been private practice; however, with health care reform, physicians are collaborating, networking, and integrating to form alliances with other providers, including managed care programs, hospitals, and HMOs, all of which are described under the section on financing of health care.

PRIVATE PRACTICE. The term private practice usually refers to physicians or other health care providers who

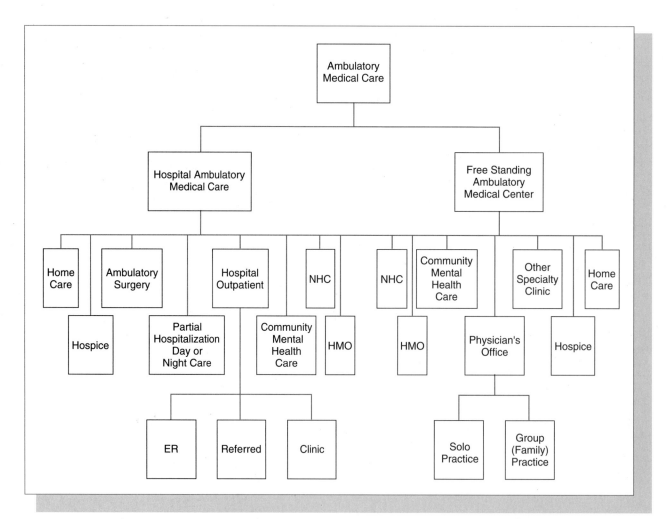

FIGURE 1–3. Organization of ambulatory care.

are established in an independent practice that is for profit. Although providers of health care include numerous professionals (dentists, nurse midwives and practitioners, podiatrists, chiropractors) who can by law practice independently, this discussion focuses on the physician as the provider.

The primary mode by which physicians provide health care is within their private medical office (practice), although this is changing. In the 1990s, there is large-scale purchasing of private physician practices. In 1994, the *American Medical News* published the findings of a survey of 402 hospitals that revealed that 36 per cent of those hospitals have purchased physician practices.[22]

Some physicians are self-employed and legally the sole owners of the practice; this is a **solo practice** and is on the decline. Most physicians in solo practices have an informal arrangement with other physicians to "take call" when they are not available. "Take call" refers to the practice of one physician managing care for another physician's patients, which allows the physician to take time away from work.

A partnership is a legal agreement between two or more physicians to share certain expenses and profits. The term partnership may apply to group practice (three or more physicians) if the group has entered a legal agreement to share certain assets and liabilities as determined by the agreement. The agreement specifies that the physicians are employees of the practice, with all moneys generated and expenses from the practice to be pooled and redistributed to the physicians according to the agreement. The size, composition, organizational structure, and financial arrangements of the groups are highly varied.[21] A more innovative approach to group practices are the "group practices without walls (GPWW)," which are physicians from multiple sites who "share central services and are a unit for contracting purposes, yet have autonomy by keeping their own offices."[23] This concept allows the physician to remain independent and become competitive in the marketplace.

The group practice may be composed of many physicians of the same specialty or it may be a multispecialty group. An example of a same-specialty practice is a group of obstetricians and gynecologists or a group of ophthalmologists. The group shares office space, equipment, nursing and support staff, and patient call (providing care 24 hours a day). The multispecialty group offers services in at least two specialty areas. A women's center is a good example of a multispecialty group practice; the providers at a women's center may include pediatricians, obstetricians, gynecologists, infertility specialists, and gerontologists. Many of the larger groups have their own ancillary services, such as a clinical laboratory and radiology units.

Community Health Centers (Neighborhood Health Centers)

In 1961, the Community Health Services and Facilities Act provided grants for the establishment of voluntary health planning agencies at the local level. These demonstration projects were developed to serve low-income areas. Community health centers were designed to provide comprehensive care in a catchment area that has limited or nonexistent health services for certain populations or special health needs. A **catchment area** is a defined geographic area that is served by a health care program, project, or facility such as a hospital or mental health center.[21] Services provided are usually directed at population groups and range from immunizations, diagnostic testing, and screening to nutrition counseling and family planning.[24]

Funding for community health centers comes from a variety of sources, including moneys from private, state, and federal grants; federal funds from the PHS and Bureau of Community Health Services of DHHS; and funds from local or state health departments. Care at the centers may be provided at no charge or the cost is based on the patient's ability to pay, which is referred to as a **sliding scale fee.**

Community-Based Care

The term community-based care refers to the delivery of services that go beyond an institutional setting and reach out into the community. These services may include adult day care centers, clinics at public schools, visits by medical staff to homeless shelters, house calls to the homebound and elderly, and mobile vans to provide free testing and screening. Community-based programs are financed by a combination of funding that includes Medicare, Medicaid, other federal and state moneys, private donations, and other sources. In 1965, Title III of the Older Americans Act established funding for transportation and for chore, homemaker, and home health aides for the elderly, all of which are forms of community-based care.[25]

Surgicenters and Urgent Care Centers

Freestanding surgical facilities in which minor surgical procedures can be safely performed on the same admission day or on an outpatient basis are called surgicenters. Urgent care, medical walk-in, and convenience care centers are for patients who need routine patient care or have minor but urgent health problems. The facilities usually are open at least 12 hours a day, 7 days a week and do not require appointments. The patient population is composed of those who do not have an established relationship with a physician in the area, those who are not established with any physician, and those whose physician is not accessible at the time of need.

These facilities, surgicenters, urgent care centers, and others are usually for profit and physician- or investor-owned. Facilities that are for profit often operate on a **fee-for-service** basis, which is a payment method in which the cost is based on the provider's estimate of the cost for services rendered; this method of payment usually requires payment in full at the time health care is provided.

Hospital Ambulatory Care

Hospital ambulatory care is "hospital-directed" health care that is provided to patients who are not admitted as inpatients and for which the hospital is responsible, regardless of the location of the health care.[2] Hospital ambulatory care services include satellite clinics, observation units, outpatient departments, ancillary services, and other specialty clinics.

SATELLITE CLINICS. Hospitals may own and operate one or more ambulatory care facilities called **satellite clinics** that are located at distant sites. Satellite clinics are established in areas that are convenient to the patients, such as places of employment, or in areas that are closer to a specific patient population.

OBSERVATION UNIT. The observation unit of the hospital is a unit, department, or beds for the **observation patient** who needs assessment, evaluation, and/or monitoring because of a significant degree of unsteadiness or disability that does not require admission to the hospital as an inpatient. For Medicare patients, HCFA suggests that the physician use 24 hours as a benchmark; that is, if the patient is expected to require hospital care for 24 or more hours, then the physician should admit the patient as an inpatient as opposed to an observation patient. The observation period should not exceed 36 to 48 hours. The patient undergoes an initial assessment, and if the patient meets the inpatient criteria for hospital admission, then the physician should admit the patient as an inpatient and not as an observation patient.[2]

OUTPATIENT DEPARTMENTS. In outpatient departments or clinics of a hospital, primary care or specialized medical care is provided to patients who are not admitted. In addition to primary care, outpatient departments diagnose and treat conditions that are not emergency in nature and yet require intervention within a short period of time, such as earaches, nausea, vomiting, diarrhea, muscle sprains, dizziness, headaches, and pinkeye. The specialty clinics that many hospitals operate include preadmission testing, pediatrics, obstetrics,

gynecology, psychiatry, and surgery; the larger tertiary hospitals may offer clinics for such specialties as low birth weight neonatal care, high-risk pregnancy, sports medicine, and cancer.

Outpatient surgery departments include units within the hospital as well as satellite surgery centers that perform surgery for which admission is not required.

ANCILLARY SERVICES (PROFESSIONAL SERVICE DEPARTMENTS). These services are hospital diagnostic and therapeutic services that are provided to both outpatients and inpatients, excluding room and board. Ancillary services differ from other areas of the hospital because the hospital is able to charge patients or third parties directly and, therefore, generate revenue for the hospital.[1] They are under the direction of physicians and do maintain an abbreviated form of health record.

Ancillary departments provide diagnostic and therapeutic services at the request of a physician (**occasion of service**); the departments include radiology (medical imaging), clinical laboratory, physical therapy, occupational therapy, respiratory therapy, cardiographics, pharmacy, and so on. A patient who needs a fetal ultrasound that her physician is not equipped or trained to perform would be referred to the appropriate ancillary service area, probably diagnostic imaging or radiology, for the procedure. The department that performs the ultrasound bills the patient or the third party payer and sends a report of the procedure to the referring physician.

Emergency Care Area

The **emergency care area** (commonly and hereafter called "ER") is equipped to provide patient care for conditions that are urgent, life-threatening, or potentially disabling. The patient often has suffered the acute onset of a serious condition, such as a myocardial infarction or closed head injury, or has developed a complication of a chronic condition, such as ketoacidosis, which may occur with diabetes mellitus. When the patient arrives, the ER staff triages the patient, which is a rapid assessment to determine the urgency and type of care needed. The term triage is a French word originating from battlefields, where quick decisions had to be made regarding who could wait for care, who needed immediate care, and who was beyond benefiting from care. In the ER, **triage** is the process of sorting out for the purpose of early assessment to determine the urgency and priority for care and to determine the appropriate source of care.[26]

In the United States, emergency patients are a diverse group because the need for care may be anywhere from relatively minor to serious, urgent, or life-threatening. People who do not have access to health care often use the ER for nonemergency problems. The inability to access health care may be due to numerous factors, such as an inability to pay, being either underinsured or uninsured, or not having a health care provider available in the area or at the time of need. In some areas, urgent care centers are not available, and patients use the ER for minor health problems. Triage promotes efficiency and effectiveness in the management of the diverse patient group arriving in the ER.

In the United States, trauma is the leading cause of death in the 34-or-under age-group, and many of those deaths occur in ERs that are not recognized as trauma centers. To minimize the morbidity and mortality rate related to trauma, trauma centers were developed. **Morbidity** is the extent of illness, injury, or disability in a given population, and **mortality** means the death rate in a given population. A **trauma center** is an emergency care center that is specially staffed and equipped to handle trauma patients; most trauma centers are equipped with an air transport system.[1] ERs are accredited according to the level of emergency care, I through IV, that they are capable of providing. The designated level of care is critical to the decision making of emergency personnel (paramedics, emergency medical technicians) in determining which facility is best suited to handle the health care needs of the transported patient. The assigned level of care is based on the center's hours of operation; availability of physicians, nurses, and other trained staff; and access to laboratory, radiology, surgery, anesthesia, equipment, and drugs. Emergency centers ranked as level I offer the most comprehensive emergency care 24 hours a day, with at least one emergency care physician on duty and access to various specialists. Level II and level III emergency services are also staffed 24 hours a day but have more lenient requirements for the availability of specialty physicians and nurses. Level IV centers are not required to operate all hours of the day but must be prepared to render lifesaving care and make referrals to appropriate centers for additional medical services. ERs that are accredited to provide level I or II care are recognized as trauma centers.[1]

Hospitals

There is no single definition of the word hospital, and the hospital of the 90s is undergoing tremendous change because of pressures to contain cost and support continuum of care that is of high quality and accessible to all. The hospital described in this section is a traditional, stand-alone hospital that provides a good foundation regarding the structure of the American hospital.

The American Health Information Management Association has adopted the American Hospital Association's (AHA's) definition of a **hospital**: "health care institution with an organized medical and professional staff and with inpatient beds available round-the-clock, whose primary function is to provide inpatient medical, nursing, and other health-related services to patients for both surgical and nonsurgical conditions, and that usually provides some outpatient services, particularly emergency care."[2] The AHA is primarily a national organization of hospitals and related institutions that is concerned with promotion of public welfare and the provision of high-quality health care. Recognition by the AHA requires that certain criteria listed in the *American Hospital Association Guide* to the health care field be evident in order for a hospital to be an AHA-registered hospital.

The AHA recognizes that accreditation by the JCAHO or certification by DHHS for Medicare exceeds these minimum requirements and therefore waives the registration requirements for those facilities.[27]

Hospitals may be classified in numerous ways (Figure 1-4). Factors include the following:

- Ownership
- Population served
- Number of beds
- Length of stay
- Type
- Patients
- Organization

Ownership

Hospitals are either government-owned (federal, state, or local) or non–government-owned. Government-owned hospitals are not-for-profit, whereas non–government-owned hospitals may be for profit or not-for-profit. Federally owned hospitals receive funding as well as administrative direction from the branch of the government that owns them. The federal government finances health care services and/or facilities for active and retired military personnel, their dependents, veterans, Merchant Marines, native Americans, native Alaskans, and other groups. For some of these groups—for example, the merchant marines—the health care provided is contracted out, whereas other groups, such as the native Americans, have their own government-funded and -operated health care facilities.[10]

The Department of Veterans Affairs medical centers are federally owned health care facilities that provide health benefits to people who have served in the United States military. Eligibility for hospital care requires that the person have a service-related condition or disability and/or be unable to pay for health care. The Department of Defense provides health care for active and retired military personnel and their dependents. The facilities owned and operated by the department include the Army, Navy, Air Force, and Marine Corps, all of

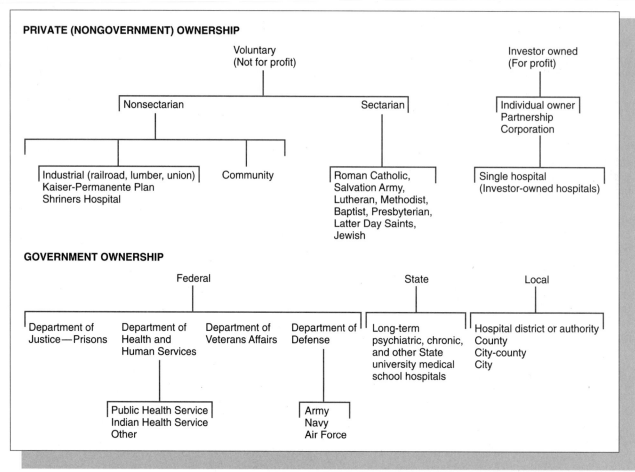

FIGURE 1-4. Classification of hospitals. (From Rakich JS, Longest B Jr, Darr K: Managing health services organizations, 3rd ed. Baltimore: Health Professions Press, 1992. Used by permission.)

which offer comprehensive health care either on military bases or in regional centers. Health care for retired military personnel and the dependents of active members of the armed forces is covered by the Civilian Health and Medical Program of the Uniformed Services. Those in the merchant marine service are covered by Merchant Seamen Health Care.

Although only a few groups have been discussed, the federal government does provide and/or support health care for a number of different populations. For example, native Americans receive health care services through the Indian Health Service of the DHHS.

Much like federally owned hospitals, state, county, and city hospitals are guided by the respective government, depending on the needs of the population served. State hospitals include facilities for mental illness, mental retardation, chronic disease, and medical education. County, district, and city hospitals are usually estab-

lished to meet the health care needs of their community. These facilities are governed by elected officials.

NON–GOVERNMENT-OWNED HOSPITALS. There are two types of non–government-owned hospitals:

- For profit
- Not-for-profit

The for-profit hospitals, also called proprietary, private, or investor-owned, are governed by the individual, partnership, or corporation that owns them. The larger corporations may own numerous hospitals or hospital chains and offer stock that is publicly traded.

The not-for-profit (voluntary) hospitals include those that are owned by churches and religious orders (Catholic and Protestant) and those that are owned by industries, unions, and fraternal organizations. Many hospitals operated by churches and religious orders in the United

States follow church-initiated requirements and may incorporate aspects of the religion into their philosophy about care and leadership of the hospital. For example, Catholic hospitals may prohibit sterilization procedures performed for the purpose of birth control.

Population Served

Many hospitals provide health care for a specific group of people, such as those for children (pediatric hospitals) or women (women's hospitals). In addition, specialty hospitals provide care for specific conditions or diseases, such as mental illness (psychiatric hospitals) or cancer (cancer hospitals).

Bed Size (Bed Count)

The total number of inpatient beds for which the facility is equipped and staffed for patient admissions is its **bed size**. A facility is licensed by the state for a specific number of beds.

Length of Stay

The average length of stay for a hospital determines whether the hospital is classified as a short-term (acute) care facility or long-term care facility. If the average length of stay is less than 30 days, the hospital is classified as a short-term (or acute) care facility; if the average length of stay is 30 or more days, the hospital is classified as a long-term care facility.

Types

According to the AHA, there are four major types of hospitals.

- General
- Specialty
- Rehabilitation and chronic disease
- Psychiatric

Note that some references and literature classify rehabilitation and chronic disease hospitals and psychiatric hospitals as specialty hospitals.

GENERAL HOSPITAL. The general hospital provides "patient services, diagnostic and therapeutic, for a variety of medical conditions."[27] These services include the following:

- Radiographic services for diagnostic purposes
- Clinical laboratory services, including anatomic pathology
- Operating room services

SPECIALTY HOSPITAL. The specialty hospital provides diagnostic and therapeutic services for patients with a specific medical condition. Examples of specialty hospitals are diabetes hospitals, burn centers, cancer institutes, women's centers, sports medicine facilities, and eye foundations.

REHABILITATION AND CHRONIC DISEASE HOSPITAL. The rehabilitation and chronic disease facility must provide diagnostic and therapeutic services to patients who are disabled or handicapped and require restorative and adjustive services. Of critical importance in these facilities are the physical therapy, occupational therapy, and psychological and social work services that are provided.[27]

PSYCHIATRIC HOSPITAL. The primary purpose of the psychiatric hospital is to provide diagnostic and therapeutic services for patients with a mental illness or a psychiatric-related illness. The primary focus of the health care is to provide psychiatric, psychological, and social work services to the patient.

Hospital Patients

People who are receiving and/or utilizing health care services for which the hospital is liable or held accountable are considered to be **hospital patients**. Hospital patients include inpatients, observation patients, ambulatory care patients, emergency patients, and newborn inpatients. To be considered a **hospital inpatient**, the patient must stay overnight (24 or more hours) and be provided room, board, and nursing service in a unit or area of the hospital.[2] All other types of hospital patients are discussed under the appropriate service areas.

Organization

The following discussion is typical of the traditional hospital setting for a general **acute care** facility. However, with health care reform, hospitals are undergoing quantum changes, including the formation of joint ventures and alliances and partnering with managed care organizations, physicians, and other health care organizations. There are numerous organizational schemes by which hospitals operate; only a few are described in this section.

Historically, most hospitals have been organized in a hierarchical form in which the individuals at the top have authority that passes downward through a chain of command (Figure 1–5). This vertical operation gives the governing body the ultimate authority followed by the chief executive officer (CEO). The organization includes a governing body, administration, medical staff, department heads or directors, supervisors, and numerous

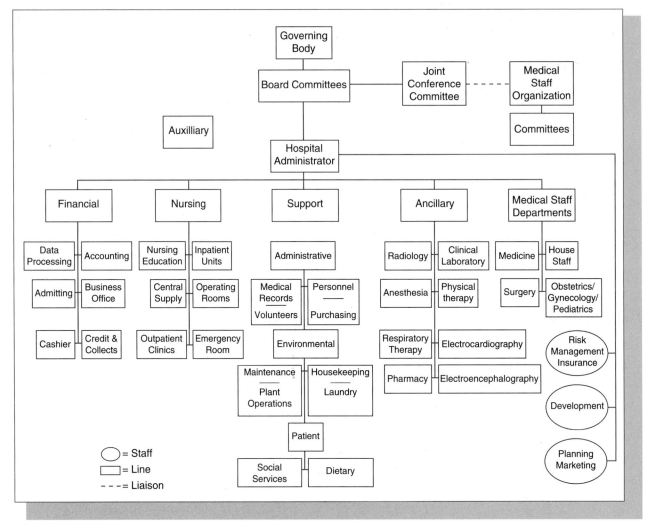

FIGURE 1–5. Hospital organization chart. (From Snook DI: Hospitals: What they are and how they work, 2nd ed. Gaithersburg, MD: Aspen Publishers, 1992. Used by permission.)

subordinates down to the staff and line workers. Communication is fairly restricted to vertical, and according to Kovner, physicians do not fall within the chain of command.[6b]

The matrix organizational scheme is increasing in popularity because it is flexible and supports multidimensional organization. The matrix organization supports general managers who focus on managing people and processes as opposed to strategy and structure. As "the competitive climate grows less stable and less predictable, it is harder for one person alone to succeed in that great visionary role," as is seen in the hierarchical organization.[28] According to Bartlett and Ghoshal, the "CEO as strategic guru is a thing of the past. CEOs must now focus on finding and motivating talent."[28]

The matrix organization gives way to horizontal, informal communications that "capture individual capabil-

ities and motivate the entire organization to respond cooperatively to a complicated and dynamic environment."[28] Employees have dual responsibilities and may have two or more bosses, but they have a shared vision that supports the organization as a whole.

Another type of organizational scheme is product line management. With this model, the hospital may be organized around product line categories, such as obstetric, rehabilitation, and cardiology units, as opposed to departments, such as nursing, pharmacy, and respiratory therapy.

Composition and Structure

Although most hospitals today are forming alliances with other health care providers or are part of multihospital systems, the discussion on the organization is specific to the freestanding hospital. The organizational chart of a typical traditional hospital is shown in Figure 1–5.

The governing body or board, sometimes called the board of trustees, board of governors, or board of directors, has the ultimate legal authority and responsibility for the operation of the hospital, including the quality and cost of care. The governing body of a voluntary (not-for-profit) hospital usually is composed of about 8 (for smaller hospitals) to 25 (for larger hospitals) board members who are not paid. Board membership is made up of private citizens who have a vested interest in their community and perhaps a skill that would be of value to the board.[1] For example, a business executive can provide support for the business aspect, and an attorney would have a better understanding of the legal issues. To help with planning community programs, some community hospital boards are appointing members from the community from the underinsured population.[29] The CEO, medical staff, and other insiders may be members of the governing board but may or may not have voting privileges; the nonvoting members are often referred to as ex officio members.

According to the JCAHO standards, the hospital is required to do the following:[14]

- Have an organized body responsible for governing the organization
- Maintain quality of care
- Provide necessary resources
- Provide for management and planning for the institution

The governing board functions according to bylaws established by the board, has regular meetings with documented minutes of the meetings, and has subcommittees that assist in the responsibilities of the governing board. The bylaws "outline the purposes of the organization, the composition and duties of the governing board, requirements for meetings and notice of meetings," duties and responsibilities of officers and committees, selection of board members and officers, and the revisions and amendments of the bylaws.[6a]

The governing board, especially in larger hospitals, has standing committees and special committees. Standing committees include the executive committee (conducts interim business), finance committee, medical staff, nominating committee, personnel, physician recruitment, and long-range planning. Special committees are created for specific projects or tasks and are disbanded upon completion.[6a]

Having the ultimate responsibility for the quality of patient care, the governing board depends on the HIM department to provide documentation to assist in and support decision making and long-range planning for the hospital. The JCAHO has identified numerous infor-

ation processes for which the governing body and organizational leaders are responsible which include obtaining, managing, and using information to improve patient care, governance, management, and support processes.[14] The governing body and administration depend on the HIM department not only to perform these processes in a timely, accurate manner but also to assure the accessibility, security, confidentiality, and integrity of the data in compliance with internal and external regulations.

Administration

The makeup of the administration or the organizational leaders differs from hospital to hospital, depending on the hospital's size and organizational scheme. Administration may be composed of a wide variety of organizational leaders or only a few, some of whom are briefly described here.

CHIEF EXECUTIVE OFFICER. The CEO, also called hospital administrator or president, is recruited and selected by the governing board. This person is the principal administrative official of the hospital or other health care facility. At one time, the CEO was responsible for the day-to-day operation of the hospital. Today, however, the CEO is not only concerned with the daily operations but must work closely with department heads, project managers, committees, and others to support the mission and achieve the goals of the health care facility.

The CEO serves as a liaison between the governing board and the medical staff. The JCAHO standards stipulates that effective leadership of the hospital:[14]

- develops a strategic plan that supports the organization's mission, vision, and values;
- communicates the mission, vision, and plan throughout the organization; and
- provides the framework to accomplish the goals that fulfill the vision.

Documentation that is necessary to support the strategic plan includes the following:

- Mission statement
- Organizational charts
- Meeting minutes
- Governing body bylaws
- Rules and regulations
- Planning documents
- Reports regarding quality of care, risk management, and utilization review

At least annually, the plan for providing patient care should be reviewed to determine if it meets identified patient needs and is consistent with the hospital mission; the plan should be revised as appropriate.[14] The HIM department is involved in the preparation of much of the documentation, especially the following:

- Clinical information
- Accreditation standards
- Risk management
- Utilization review
- Quality of patient care

CHIEF OPERATING OFFICER. Large hospitals often have several chief operating officers (COOs), also called executive vice president, vice president, or associate administrator, who report directly to the CEO. The COO provides leadership, direction, and administration of operations that is in compliance with the mission and strategic plan of the organization. He or she promotes health care services that are economical, of high quality, and in compliance with regulatory bodies. The coordination of hospital activities, such as ancillary or support services and other functional areas, is often the responsibility of the COO.[1]

CHIEF INFORMATION OFFICER. The chief information officer (CIO) holds an executive position with primary responsibility for information resources management in the organization. He or she is involved in strategic planning, management, design, integration, and implementation of health information systems. Health information systems embrace the financial, administrative, and clinical information needs of the health care facility or organization. In hospitals, the usual departments that report to the CIO are information systems, telecommunications, and management engineering. Other departments that sometimes report to the CIO include HIM, quality assurance, and utilization review.[30]

CHIEF FINANCIAL OFFICER. The financial operations of a health care institution are under the direction of the chief financial officer (CFO), who is sometimes called director of finance or fiscal affairs director. Although the title may vary, this person is often a director or hospital vice president who reports directly to the CEO or some other level in the administration. The CEO and the CFO also report to a finance committee within the governing body of the hospital. The finance committee is an advisory group within the board that is responsible for reviewing the hospital's financial position and making fiscally related decisions. According to the JCAHO, the board and the CEO are responsible for the control and use of all financial resources. The daily financial operation, however, is usually delegated to the CFO.

The financial department of a health care institution, under the direction of the CFO, is responsible for functions such as the accounting, inventory control, payroll, accounts payable and receivable, cash management, billing, credit and collections, budgeting, cost accounting, fund accounting, and internal control.[1] The functions within the finance arena involve the recording and reporting of financial information, the management of cash and other hospital assets, and planning and control. The CFO has overall responsibility for these areas and acts as an adviser to the CEO and the governing board on both daily operational issues and plans for the future.

Medical Staff (Professional Staff Organization)

The medical staff is a formally organized staff of licensed physicians and other licensed providers as permitted by law (e.g., dentists, podiatrists, nurse midwives) with the "delegated authority and responsibility to maintain proper standards of medical care and to plan for continued betterment of that care."[2] The medical staff is governed by its own bylaws, rules, and regulations, which must be approved by the hospital's governing board. The JCAHO standards state that the primary responsibility of the medical staff is the quality of the professional services provided by the members with clinical privileges and the responsibility of being accountable to the governing body. **Clinical privileges** is the permission granted by the governing board to practitioners to provide well-defined patient care services in the granting institution, based on licensure, education, training, experience, competence, health status, and judgment.[14]

The medical staff responsibilities include recommending staff appointments and reappointments, delineating clinical privileges, continuing medical education, and maintaining a high quality of patient care.

The organizational scheme of the medical staff includes officers, committees, and clinical services. The JCAHO requires that there be an executive committee empowered to conduct medical staff business between staff meetings and that is responsible to the governing body. In smaller hospitals, the medical staff as a whole serves as the executive committee. The executive committee is composed of members of the medical staff and an exofficio member from administration, usually the CEO or the CEO's designee. Other committees of the medical staff that may be in place include the following:[17]

- Joint conference committee, which acts as a liaison between the governing body and the medical staff and deliberates on any subject that is of concern to either the medical staff or the governing body
- Credentials committee, which is responsible for reviewing medical staff applications and gather-

ing and verifying data on the applicant, such as education, licensure, experience, competence, and peer review

- Medical Records, which is responsible for the timely completion and quality of information in the health record
- Utilization Review, which is concerned with the resources used in providing patient care (e.g., length of stay, ancillary services)

The members of the medical staff are organized into areas of clinical services and departments that are usually representative of the medical specialties. Each service or department has an appointed director, department head, or chairperson. Each member of the medical staff has "delineated clinical privileges that define the scope of the patient care services they may provide independently in the hospital."[14] The services that are common to most hospitals are internal medicine, surgery, anesthesiology, pediatrics, obstetrics and gynecology, psychiatry, neurology, radiology and diagnostic imaging, and pathology. Each of these are briefly defined in Table 1–1.

The JCAHO standards specify that the medical staff regularly review certain functions that are usually managed by committees. These functions include review of surgical and other invasive procedures, drug usage evaluation, health record review, blood usage review, pharmacy and therapeutics function, risk management activities, infection control, utilization review, safety, and disaster planning.

Essential Services

The JCAHO identifies hospital services that must be provided on a regular basis and that are necessary for patient assessment and care. **Patient assessment** is the "systematic collection and review of patient-specific data."[14] The following services are essential to this function.

NURSING CARE. The nursing service is usually organized under the direction of a nurse executive (director, vice president), with nursing supervisors, department heads, charge nurses, and staff nurses. The nurse executive has the responsibility and authority to establish nursing standards, policies, and procedures that are in compliance with state law and professional standards.

Nursing care standards have been developed by professional organizations, such as the American Nurses' Association; the standards address policies, procedures, and written mechanisms. Although nursing care is integrated and provided throughout various settings, nursing practice itself is regulated by the individual states as stipulated by the Nurse Practice Act of each state.

There are different levels of nursing, including staff nurse, nurse manager, clinical nurse specialist, and private-duty nurse. The staff nurse provides direct patient care in a specific unit with assigned patients. For example, a registered nurse (RN) or a licensed practical nurse (LPN) may be the staff nurse assigned to five patients in the well-baby nursery during the evening shift. The nurse manager may be a head nurse, nursing supervisor, or department head who is responsible for certain units and/or staff. This person makes patient assignments and staffing decisions and is responsible for the quality of care provided by the nursing staff. The clinical nurse specialist is considered an expert in a specialized area, such as neonatology or pain management. This person is an RN with advanced education and/or experience in the area of expertise. The clinical nurse specialist also works in research, education, administration, and consultation.[31] The private-duty nurse is an RN or LPN who is employed by an external agency or individual to provide direct patient care to one patient for 8 to 12 hours over a period of time.

Nursing care is based on a process that involves assessment, diagnosis, outcomes and planning, implementation, and evaluation of patient care,[32] and the documentation in the health record must reflect this process. The HIM department often collaborates with the nursing service in collecting, analyzing, and disseminating data; in developing reports; and in addressing issues related to the health record. Issues of critical importance are the authenticity, completeness, timeliness, integrity, and security of both the paper and the paperless health record.

DIAGNOSTIC RADIOLOGY SERVICES. The diagnostic radiology department (medical imaging department) functions in the diagnosing of diseases and conditions by using ionizing radiation (e.g., radiography, computed tomography, radioactive isotopes), ultrasound, and magnetic resonance imaging. The JCAHO requires health care facilities to provide diagnostic testing, including imaging, that is relevant both to determining the patient's health care needs and to the treatment of the patient.[14] An example of a diagnostic radiology procedure is mammography (breast radiography), which is performed for the purpose of diagnosing breast cancers; an example of a therapeutic procedure is radiation therapy, which is performed for the purpose of treating malignant neoplasms (cancers).

The radiology department is headed by a radiologist who may be called the chief or director of radiology. Under the direction of the radiologist is the technical staff, which includes physicians (radiation therapists, radiation physicists), radiology technologists, radiation therapy technologists, and nuclear medicine technicians.

NUCLEAR MEDICINE. Nuclear medicine may be considered part of the radiology department. It is distin-

TABLE 1-1 EXAMPLES OF MEDICAL AND SURGICAL SERVICES

MEDICAL SERVICES

Service	Description/Examples of Diagnoses and Procedures
Cardiology	Study of the cardiovascular system and treatment of its diseases: rheumatic heart disease, coronary artery disease, myocardial infarction, congestive heart failure
Dermatology	Study and treatment of the skin and diseases/conditions of the skin: basal cell carcinoma, exfoliative dermatitis, pityriasis rosea, biopsies/excisions of lesions, cellulitis, acne vulgaris
Endocrinology	Study and treatment of the endocrine glands: diabetes mellitus (types I and II), thyroiditis, Addison's disease, adrenal virilism
Gastroenterology	Study of the digestive system and treatment of its disorders, including the esophagus, stomach, intestines, liver, pancreas, gallbladder and ulcers, gastroenteritis, pylorospasm, gastritis, Crohn's disease
Hematology	Study and treatment of the blood, blood-forming tissues, and blood disorders: anemias, leukemia, hemophilia, thrombocytopenic purpura, bone marrow biopsy
Infectious disease	Study and treatment of diseases caused by pathogenic microorganisms, including contagious and noncontagious infections: acquired immunodeficiency syndrome, syphilis, tuberculosis, hepatitis, wound infections
Internal medicine	Study and treatment of disease of internal organs, using nonsurgical therapy: hypertension, rheumatoid arthritis, meningitis
Nephrology	Study and treatment of the kidney and its diseases: acute and chronic kidney failure, polycystic kidney disease, nephrolithiasis, pyelonephritis, glomerulonephritis
Neurology	Study and treatment of the nervous system and its diseases: cerebral palsy, brain abscess, cerebrovascular attack, Alzheimer's disease, Parkinson's disease
Oncology	Study and treatment of cancer, including benign and malignant: malignant melanoma, squamous cell carcinoma, multiple myeloma, Hodgkin's disease, leukemia
Pediatrics	Study and care of children, including normal growth and development: chicken pox, cystic fibrosis, pneumonia, immunizations, diarrhea, gastritis, mumps
Psychiatry	Study, diagnosis, and treatment of mental illness: anorexia nervosa, clinical depression, alcohol withdrawal syndrome, senile dementia
Pulmonary medicine	Study, diagnosis, and treatment of lung disorders: pneumonia, chronic obstructive pulmonary disease, asthma, cystic fibrosis, bronchiectasis, respiratory failure
Radiology	Use of radiant energy in the study, diagnosis, and treatment of disease: computed tomography, radiography, echocardiography, magnetic resonance imaging, radiation therapy

guished from radiology, however, because the procedure involves the use of radioisotopes (radionuclides) for diagnosing and treating the patient. Unlike in radiography, the image created in nuclear medicine gives information not only about the structure but also about the function of the organ or tissue under study. Examples of diagnostic procedures performed in nuclear medicine are nuclear scans of the thyroid, heart, and liver and radioimmunoassays, which are used to detect hormones and drugs in blood samples.

The staff in nuclear medicine is under the direction of a physician who specializes in nuclear medicine and includes nuclear medicine technicians and/or staff from the radiology department.

DIETETIC SERVICES. The dietetic service considers all nutritional aspects of the patient and patient care and provides high-quality nutrition to every patient. According to JCAHO, nutritional care must be provided in a timely and effective manner. Such care consists of nutritional assessment, nutritional therapy, diet preparation, distribution and/or administration, nutritional education, and monitoring of the nutritional care of patients.[14]

Nutritional care is interdisciplinary and, therefore, involves not only dietetic services but other members of the health care team as well, such as physicians and nurses. Dietetic services employs clinical dietitians, who are responsible for the therapeutic care of patients. Additional dietary staff are employed to assist with the preparation, serving, and delivery of food and the maintenance of cafeteria services for the staff and visitors.

PATHOLOGY AND CLINICAL LABORATORY SERVICES. This ancillary area assists in the prevention, diagnosis,

TABLE 1-1   EXAMPLES OF MEDICAL AND SURGICAL SERVICES *Continued*

SURGICAL SERVICES

Service	Description/Examples of Diagnoses and Procedures
Anesthesiology	Study and art of anesthesia administration, with and without loss of consciousness: epidural anesthesia, spinal anesthesia, inhalation of ether, analgesia maintenance
Cardiovascular surgery	Surgical specialty of the heart and blood vessels: coronary artery bypass graft, coronary arthrectomy, cardiac catheterization, coronary angioplasty
Gynecology	Surgical specialty concerned with the study of female reproductive and urinary systems and treatment of the disorders: endometriosis, cystitis, herpes genitalia, mastitis, uterine prolapse, infertility
Neurosurgery	Surgical specialty involving the study of the nervous system and treatment of disorders: hydrocephalus, meningomyelocele, brain abscess, carpal tunnel syndrome
Obstetrics	Surgical specialty concerned with the management of pregnancy, including the prenatal, perinatal, and postnatal stages: normal pregnancy, placenta previa, eclampsia, ectopic pregnancy, gestational diabetes
Ophthalmology	Surgical specialty concerned with the study of the eye and treatment of visual problems: cataracts, corneal transplant, diabetic retinopathy, visual acuity, optic nerve damage
Orthopedics	Surgical specialty dealing with the musculoskeletal system, including prevention of disorders and restoration of function: arthritis, fractures, scoliosis, joint replacements, osteomyelitis
Otorhinolaryngology	Surgical specialty dealing with the study and treatment of disorders of the ears, nose, and throat: acute tracheitis, tonsillectomy and adenoidectomy, sinusitis, otitis media, deviated nasal septum
Plastic and reconstructive surgery	Surgical specialty concerned with repair, restoration, and reconstruction of body structures: blepharoplasty, scar revision, liposuction, breast reduction and reconstruction, dermabrasion
Thoracic surgery	Surgical specialty dealing with the study and treatment of the thorax and its disorders: pneumonectomy, diaphragmatic hernia, lung abscess, thoracotomy, bronchial lavage
Urology	Surgical specialty concerned with the study and treatment of the male genitourinary system and female urinary system: vasectomy, nephrolithiasis, benign prostatic hyperplasia, transurethral resection of the prostate

and treatment of disease by examination and study of tissue specimens, blood and body secretions, and wound scrapings and drainage. The pathology and clinical laboratory department functions in serology, histology, cytology, bacteriology, hematology, blood bank, organ bank, biochemistry, and tissue preparation. These departments commonly are subunits of the pathology department.

Pathology and clinical laboratory services employ a variety of health professionals—medical laboratory technologist, medical laboratory technician, histotechnologist, and cytotechnologist—all of whom work under the direction of a pathologist.

EMERGENCY SERVICES. Most emergency care areas have several functional areas, including a trauma area, a casting room, examination rooms, and observation beds. A patient in the ER can be managed in one of the following ways: treated and discharged to home, treated and admitted for observation, treated and admitted to an inpatient unit, assessed and sent to surgery, or stabilized and transferred to another facility.[1]

In the event of death, transferral to the morgue is done.

Emergency services are primarily provided by physicians and RNs who specialize in emergency medicine. The ER is discussed more fully under the section on ambulatory care.

PHARMACEUTICAL SERVICE. The pharmaceutical service is responsible for maintaining an adequate supply of medications, providing nursing units with floor stock, and preparing and dispensing medications with appropriate documentation. Floor stock is an inventory of drugs that is maintained on each nursing unit; the stock varies in each unit, depending on the type of unit (e.g., cardiac intensive care versus a pediatric unit).

The pharmaceutical service is under the direction of a state-licensed pharmacist, who is assisted by pharmaceutical technicians.

PHYSICAL REHABILITATION SERVICES. The diagnosis and treatment of certain musculoskeletal and neuromuscular diseases and conditions are responsibilities of physical medicine and rehabilitation. This area covers physical therapy, occupational therapy, and speech therapy. Physical therapists are state-licensed and trained to use light, heat, cold, water, ultrasound, electricity, and manual manipulation to improve or correct a musculo-skeletal or neuromuscular problem. They often teach the patient exercises that will help to strengthen specific muscle groups or assist the patient to ambulate (walk) with an artificial limb. Occupational therapists work with the patient to minimize the patient's disability and teach the patient how to compensate for the disability. For example, a patient who is permanently confined to a wheelchair and needs to resume housekeeping responsibilities may be taught how to shop for groceries or how to prepare a meal. Speech pathologists are concerned with human communication; they teach the patient how to compensate for the inability to speak. For example, a patient who stutters is taught speech exercises to help control or minimize the stuttering.

RESPIRATORY CARE SERVICES. Respiratory care services encompass diagnostic and therapeutic procedures for a wide variety of patients. Respiratory therapists may administer oxygen, conduct pulmonary function studies, administer bronchodilators, perform chest physiotherapy, analyze arterial blood gases, set up and maintain a mechanical ventilator, and assist in cardiopulmonary resuscitation. These therapists work under the direct order of a physician and provide respiratory care in all patient care areas of the hospital, as necessary.[1]

SOCIAL SERVICES. The department of social services is staffed by medical and psychiatric social workers who work with the patient and family members to help them understand the social, economic, and emotional factors in regard to therapy and recovery; identify and coordinate necessary community and medical care resources; and collaborate with and educate the hospital staff regarding social service concerns. Social workers are often responsible for discharge planning, thereby supporting the continuum of care.

OTHER SERVICES. Information on additional hospital services, such as pastoral care, patient representatives, patient escort, plant technology and safety management, and central supply, may be obtained by surveying area health care facilities. Hospital services vary according to the type and size of the health care organization.

Health Information Management

Although this book is devoted to HIM, a brief discussion is necessary at this point. The HIM department, or medical records department, is primarily responsible for the management of all paper and paperless patient information. It must develop and maintain an information system that is consistent with the mission of the health care facility and in compliance with regulatory and accrediting agencies. The department is responsible for the organization, maintenance, production, and dissemination of information, including data security, integrity, and access.

Home Care (Home Health Care)

Home health care is the provision of medical and nonmedical care in the home or place of residence to promote, maintain, or restore health or to minimize the effect of disease or disability.[2] With the exception of hospice, the location of the health care services distinguishes home health from other types of care facilities and programs. Home care serves multiple purposes, including the integration of institutional and noninstitutional care, the transition for functionally ill patients, and the bridge to other health and non–health-related community services.[33] Home health services are a medical adjunct to acute care, which extends the continuum of care from inpatient to home.

The patient population for home health is dominated by elderly people, even though non-elderly adults as well as children use the service. Home health care for the elderly population is viewed as a cost savings compared with longer hospital stays or long-term care. It is also life-enriching because it enables patients to remain in the comfort of their homes.

Home health has grown rapidly since 1965, which is when the Medicare program was established and allowed reimbursement for home care. The Medicare definition of home health stipulates that the needed nursing care, physical therapy, or speech therapy must be skilled intermittent care provided under a physician's written direction and plan of care in the residence of the homebound client.[8] Simply put, Medicare requires that the home care provided be physician-directed and that it involve regularly scheduled home visits. For example, a home care patient who is receiving oxygen therapy may be initially visited four times a week for 1 week by an RN. One of the goals of therapy is to have the patient or family assume responsibility for care, with visits by the RN being reduced to once or twice a week. On the other hand, if this patient is living alone and needs assistance with self-care, then a nurse's aide, in addition to the RN, may visit every other day to assist with personal care.

Long-Term Care Facilities

Long-term care is health care that is provided over a long period of time (30 or more days) in a non–acute care setting in which the patient resides. The type of care a patient can receive is highly variable and ranges from personal care and social, recreational, and dietary services to skilled nursing care. The patients admitted to long-term care facilities are usually called residents. The term nursing home is a layman's term for any and all long-term care facilities.

Historically, there have been two types of long-term care facilities that provide different levels of nursing care: the skilled-nursing facility (SNF) and the intermediate-care facility (ICF). Although both types provide skilled nursing care and other health care services, the SNF provides a higher level of care to sicker patients than does the ICF.[25] Before 1987, federal requirements were different for the ICF and the SNF in regard to the number, type, and scheduled hours of RNs and LPNs employed.

In 1987, the Nursing Home Reform Act, fully effective in 1990, reduced the differences between the two types of facilities by mandating that intermediate-care facilities provide the same level of care and staffing as skilled-nursing facilities. All long-term care facilities are identified as nursing facilities and required to employ sufficient nursing personnel on a 24-hour basis to provide care to each resident according to the care plan.[34] Among other things, nursing facilities are required to provide skilled nursing care and related services for patients who require medical, nursing, or rehabilitative care; health care services, room, and board are provided around the clock.[25] (In the literature, references to intermediate-care and skilled-nursing facilities remain.)

To be certified as a Medicare or Medicaid provider, a nursing facility must comply with the *Conditions of Participation*. A long-term care facility is licensed by the state to provide a designated level of care, which may simply be personal care, room, and board or may require skilled nursing. A facility may be licensed to provide different levels of care; if so, the number of beds for each level of care is designated.

The patient population in long-term care facilities is primarily elderly people who are unable to live independently but also includes people of all ages who are convalescing or rehabilitating or who have a chronic condition that requires long-term health care services (e.g., Alzheimer's disease, senile dementia).

There are several types of long-term care facilities.

- **Nursing facility.** This is a comprehensive term for a long-term care facility that provides nursing care and related services for residents who require medical, nursing, or rehabilitative care. A sufficient number of nursing personnel must be employed on a 24-hour basis to provide care to residents according to the care plan.

- **Independent living facility.** This type of facility is composed of apartments and condominiums that allow residents to live independently, but assistance (e.g., dietary, health care, social services) is available as needed by residents.

- **Domiciliary (residential).** Supervision, room, and board are provided for people who are unable to live independently. Most residents need assistance with activities of daily living (i.e., bathing, eating, dressing).

- **Life care centers.** Also called retirement communities, these centers provide living accommodations and meals for a monthly fee. They offer a variety of services, including housekeeping, recreation, health care, laundry, and exercise programs.

- **Assisted living.** This type of facility typically offers housing and board with a broad range of personal and supportive care services.

Hospice Care

The concept of hospice, meaning "given to hospitality," dates back to the medieval period when weary travelers were provided a hospice for shelter and rest. Today, a **hospice** is a multidisciplinary health care program that is responsible for the palliative and supportive care of terminally ill patients and their families, with consideration for their physical, spiritual, social, and economic needs. **Palliative care** consists of those health care services that relieve or alleviate patient symptoms and discomforts, such as pain and nausea; it is not curative. The primary goal of a hospice is to allow patients to die with dignity in their homes or a homelike environment. Most hospice patients have cancer, but many hospices accept other terminally ill patients, such as those with acquired immunodeficiency syndrome (AIDS) or end-stage kidney, heart, or lung disease.

The type of program that is suitable often depends on the patient's condition and the support available in the patient's home (Table 1–2). For the patient who remains in the home, most hospices require that a primary caregiver be identified who will assist with care[2]; the primary caregiver may be a spouse, family member, friend, or live-in companion. Other hospice programs, such as skilled-nursing facilities, may have units or beds for hospice patients who are unable to remain in their homes. Hospice patients may require hospitalization for acute symptom management (pain, vomiting, infection) or when the primary care person needs a rest or break (respite).

Hospice programs are physician-directed and multidisciplinary, in that numerous caregivers are involved in providing care. Caregivers for hospice include nurses, social workers, nurse's aides, priests, dietitians, and trained volunteers, who run errands, mow grass, do housekeeping chores, cook, and perform other necessary jobs that allow the patient to remain in the home.

Reimbursement for hospice care comes from Medicare, Medicaid, private pay, third party payers, community funds, and other sources.

TABLE 1-2 MODELS OF HOSPICE CARE

TYPE	DESCRIPTION
Home health agency–based	Owned and operated by private, freestanding home health agencies; care provided in home
Hospital-based	Owned and operated by a hospital: rooms/departments allotted for hospice care; care provided in facility and/or home
Independent community–based	Usually nonprofit; governed by community board, independent; care provided in home
Nursing facility–based	Owned and operated by a nursing facility; rooms/units allotted for hospice care; care provided in facility
Other models	Owned by religious orders, health maintenance organizations, combinations of the above models

Contract Services

The use of contract services by health care organizations is rising. According to the Hospital and Health Networks 1994 survey, 63 per cent of 962 respondents indicated that at least one department was run by contract service compared with 55 per cent in 1993.[35] Contract services include food, laundry, housekeeping, maintenance, medical waste disposal, copy services, transcription, collections, and clinical services such as physical therapy, emergency care, and speech pathology. With the increase in utilization of contract services, providers are expecting improved quality with cost containment.

Multihospital Systems

A health care system composed of two or more hospitals that are owned, managed, or leased by a single organization is called a **multihospital system**.[1] Although multihospital systems vary as to the types of facilities and arrangements that are available, many attempt to provide a continuum of care. The system may include an acute care facility, a long-term care facility, a pediatric hospital, a rehabilitation facility, and a psychiatric hospital.

Health Care Reform of the 1990s

"United States health care expenditures totaled approximately $738 billion in 1991, an increase of more than 10% from 1990"[36]; the result is local, state, and national health care reform initiatives that pressure health care systems to provide more cost-effective care and maintain quality. As a result, hospitals can no longer afford to stand alone and are, therefore, forming alliances, networks, systems, and joint ventures that make them more competitive in the marketplace. These arrangements are directed at providing continuous care of high quality while meeting the needs of the community and controlling cost.

Accountable health plans, coordinated care networks, community care networks, and integrated health systems are comprehensive care models that offer a full range of health care services. The networks include hospitals, primary care physicians, specialty care physicians, and other providers that complement comprehensive health care. An important aspect of the accountable health plans and others is the integration of financing with the delivery of health care and with continuous monitoring of the quality of care.[20]

HEALTH CARE PROFESSIONALS

The health care systems in the United States are labor-intensive, using large numbers of highly skilled health care professionals and practitioners. The rapid increase of new technologies and health care services has resulted in a dramatic increase in new health care occupations.[6] There are more than 200 different health occupations in the United States. The places of employment are just as varied, including hospitals, medical offices, insurance companies, nursing facilities, pharmacies, HMOs, schools, prisons, and pharmaceutical and medical supply companies.

The following attributes help to define the health care professional:[37]

- Certification or licensure is required for membership in the profession.

- A national or regional professional association exists.

- A defined body of scientific knowledge and certain technical skills are required for practice.

- A code of ethics exists.

- Members of the profession practice with a degree of authority and have expertise for decision making in their area of competency.

Health Care Team

Almost all health care is provided by a team of professionals and practitioners. Being a member of the health care team requires that each person be responsible for his or her area of expertise with consideration for the contributions of other team members. The ultimate goal is more comprehensive care for the patient as a whole.[38] The health care team is composed of individuals who work either directly or indirectly to accomplish the goals of patient care. As a member of the health care team, the HIM professional must develop an understanding of the roles, responsibilities, and interface of all members of the health care team.

Terms such as technologist, technician, therapist, paraprofessional, assistant, and aide often are used to describe certain health care providers. Technologist and therapist imply education at or above the bachelor degree level; technician and assistant indicate education or training at or above the associate degree level; and assistant and aide refer to on-the-job training. **Provider** is an all-inclusive generic term for people or institutions that provide health care.

Most health care occupations can be classified into one of the following categories:

* Independent practitioner
* Dependent practitioner
* Supporting staff

The independent practitioner category includes those who by law may provide a range of services without the consent or approval of a third party. The dependent practitioner category includes those who by law may deliver a delimited range of services (often specified by law) under the supervision or authorization of the independent practitioner. Some health occupations may move from one category to another, depending on state law; for example, the physical therapist, nurse practitioner, and nurse midwife may be in either the dependent or the independent category, based on responsibilities and place of employment. The third category is the supporting staff, who function under the supervision or authorization of independent or dependent practitioners.[6] A fourth category that must be identified is the non–care-giving group, which includes all people who have no direct patient contact and yet make significant contributions to the health care systems. Examples of the various groups are shown in Table 1–3.

Physicians

The primary leader of the traditional health care team is most often the physician; some exceptions to this are the independent practices of nurse practitioners, podia-

trists, chiropractors, optometrists, and nurse midwives. A physician is qualified by formal education and legal authority through licensure to practice medicine.[21]

TYPES. There are two types of physicians: Doctor of Medicine (MD) and Doctor of Osteopathic Medicine (DO). Both types of physicians are licensed by each state as medical practitioners who may diagnose, provide treatment, perform surgery, and prescribe medication. They both complete 4 years of medical education, a residency program, and state licensing examinations.[6] DOs emphasize the musculoskeletal system's role in health because it comprises 60 per cent of body mass, and the interdependence of all body systems is emphasized. According to the AOA, the philosophy of osteopathy focuses on the whole body with emphasis on prevention and health and the interrelation of structure and function.[16] The DO practices comprehensive medicine that utilizes manipulative therapy along with more traditional forms of therapy.

MEDICAL EDUCATION AND TRAINING. The framework for medical education as we know it today dates back to 1910, when Abraham Flexner published a report that identified numerous serious deficiencies and inconsistencies in medical education. As a result of the infamous Flexner Report, most medical schools follow the Flexner model.[6]

Today, admission to medical school requires 3 to 4 years of undergraduate work in the sciences and a competitive score on the Medical College Admission Test. Medical school (undergraduate medical education) consists of medical science courses and clinical experience. The medical degree is awarded on completion of medical school. However, a person must still obtain a state license to practice medicine, which requires examination.

LICENSURE. The Federation Licensing Examination (FLEX) is a standardized licensure test developed by the Federation of State Medical Boards of the United States in 1968.[6] The scores for successful completion vary from state to state.

An alternative to the FLEX is an examination developed by the National Board of Medical Examiners (NBME). The NBME is dedicated to preparing and administering high-quality examinations for state licensure, collaborating with the state licensing boards in achieving goals of quality, supporting quality in medical education, and developing and evaluating testing methodologies, medical knowledge, and competence.[21] The three-part NBME examination allows the student to be tested at intervals during training. After passing the NBME or the FLEX examination and completing 1 year of resi-

TABLE 1-3 EXAMPLES OF HEALTH PROFESSIONALS

PROFESSIONAL	CREDENTIAL	BRIEF DESCRIPTION
Cytotechnologist	Certification	Assists pathologists in the microscopic examination of cellular samples from the body to diagnose infectious disease, cancers, and other conditions and identify microorganisms; are employed in pathology departments of hospitals, private or hospital-based laboratories, research laboratories
Emergency medical technician—paramedic	Registration and in some states, licensure	Works under direction of a physician, providing basic and advanced life support to patients including emergency drug administration, IV fluid therapy, ECG interpretation, and assisted ventilation; employed in fire and police departments, ambulance services, hospitals, emergency clinics
Medical assistant	Certification	Multiskilled individual who assists in administrative and clinical areas of ambulatory care; works under the direct supervision of the physician
Medical laboratory technician	Certification	Performs laboratory procedures on blood and other specimens to assist physicians in diagnosis and treatment of disease; works in hospital laboratories, physician offices, and reference/independent laboratories
Medical record administrator (health information manager)	Registration	Designs and maintains health information systems to collect, assess, and disseminate health care data; is employed in administrative/management positions in health care organizations
Medical record technician (health information technician)	Accreditation	Performs medical record functions, including record analysis, data analysis, coding and indexing of diseases and procedures, record storage and retrieval, transcription; is employed in hospitals, ambulatory care settings, insurance companies, health departments, and other health care organizations
Medical technologist	Certification and/or registration	Responsible for analyzing body fluids, tissues, and cells and other specimens to assist physicians in detection, diagnosis, and management of disease; places of employment: hospital laboratories, physician offices, and reference/independent laboratories; can assume positions/roles as researcher, educator, and clinician
Nuclear medicine technologist	Certification and/or registration	Performs imaging procedures involving use of radionuclides for diagnostic, therapeutic, and investigative purposes; works in hospitals, public health, research laboratories, manufacturing companies
Occupational therapy assistant	Certification and in some states, licensure	Works under the direction of an occupational therapist; participates in the assessment and treatment of patients with physical, developmental, and/or psychological deficits; employment opportunities include hospitals, rehabilitation facilities, clinics, nursing homes

TABLE 1-3 EXAMPLES OF HEALTH PROFESSIONALS *Continued*		
PROFESSIONAL	**CREDENTIAL**	**BRIEF DESCRIPTION**
Occupational therapist	Certification and in some states, licensure	Provides assessment and intervention to minimize physical, developmental, and/or psychological deficits that restrict activities of daily living and employment, including promotion of wellness and prevention of illness/injury; employed in hospitals, rehabilitation facilities, clinics, nursing homes
Physical therapist (PT)	Licensure	Uses heat, cold, exercises, electricity, manipulation, and ultraviolet radiation in restoration of function, prevention, of disability, and management of musculoskeletal pain following injury or disease; works in hospitals, private offices, nursing homes and community health centers
Radiographer	Certification	Produces and processes x-rays, including specialized procedures such as angiography, mammography, CT, used in prevention, detection, diagnosis and management of disease, injury, or anomaly; employed in hospitals, outpatient settings, independent/reference laboratories

dency, a medical physician may apply for state licensure, which authorizes him or her to practice medicine.

After graduation from medical school, the physician must complete a residency that consists of several years of training in a teaching hospital; during residency, the physician works under the supervision of licensed physicians. The residency program is considered to be graduate medical education. Depending on the chosen specialty, the residency may vary from 3 to 7 years. Because of the large numbers of physicians who require a residency program, a National Residency Matching Program was established to match applicants with hospital preferences, much like a clearinghouse for the residency program. The hospital's residency programs are accredited by the Accreditation Council on Graduate Medical Education, which is composed of representatives from the public, residents, federal government, and professional organizations, including the AMA, AHA, and American Board of Medical Specialties.[1]

Although there is an increasing demand for more generalists (i.e., family practitioners, general practitioners), many physicians seek certification in a specialty area. There are many specialties and subspecialties in the practice of medicine, such as neurology, hematology, oncology, cardiology, and pediatrics. Examples of surgical specialties and subspecialties are orthopedics, obstetrics, gynecology, and neurosurgery. To become board-certified, the physician must meet certain requirements established by the Board of Certification, which is under the jurisdiction of the specialty. For example, to become board-certified, surgeons must demonstrate additional training time and proven competence and complete rigorous examination. In addition, physicians who are accepted for a fellowship at a specialty college are considered highly respected by the medical profession in their area of expertise.[1]

Nursing

In the United States, nursing is the single largest health care profession, and as of 1992, there were about 2.2 million RNs. They are employed in a wide variety of facilities, including hospitals, physician offices, patient homes, schools, camps, occupational and industrial settings, public health facilities, and private practice.[32] Therefore, it is important to the HIM professional to have a good understanding of the roles and responsibilities of the nurse in regard to health care systems.

Professional nursing is defined by the American Nurses Association (ANA) as "diagnosis and treatment of human responses to actual or potential health problems."[39] Nursing practice includes but is not limited to clinical practice, administration, education, research, consultation, and management.

TYPES AND EDUCATION. The major types of nursing are registered nursing and licensed practical nursing (sometimes called licensed vocational nursing). Table 1–4

TABLE 1-4 EDUCATION FOR PROFESSIONAL NURSES		
DEGREE/LEVEL ATTAINED	**YEARS OF COLLEGE**	**EXAMPLES OF ROLES AND RESPONSIBILITIES**
Doctor of Science in Nursing (DNS) or Doctor of Philosophy (PhD)	3–5 years graduate work (post-baccalaureate) with clinicals	Researcher, educator, administrator, clinician, director of nursing
Master of Science in Nursing (MSN)	5–6 academic years with clinicals	Nurse practitioner, clinical nurse specialist, administrator, director of nursing, supervisor, nurse manager
Baccalaureate degree (BSN)	4 full years with clinicals	Nursing supervisor, head nurse, charge nurse, nurse manager
Associate degree	2 years with clinicals	Charge nurse, nurse manager, staff nurse
Diploma	27–36 months with clinicals	Charge nurse, nurse manager, staff nurse
Licensed practical nurse (LPN)/licensed vocational nurse (LVN)	1 year with clinicals	Staff nurse, nurse manager

outlines the education and training of nurses and their various roles and responsibilities. To practice as an RN, one must graduate from a state-approved school of nursing and pass a state licensing examination.

Nursing education offers a variety of programs and experiences from which potential students can choose. Academic programs for RNs require a bachelor's degree, an associate degree, or a diploma from an approved school of nursing. RNs with advanced degrees (master's, doctoral) usually work more independently as clinical nurse specialists, nurse clinicians, nurse practitioners, and nurse midwives than do those without advanced degrees.

Practical or vocational nurses may choose as little as 1 year of academics integrated with clinical experience and become eligible for licensure as a licensed practical nurse (LPN) or a licensed vocational nurse (LVN). The LPN usually works under the supervision of an RN, a physician, or some other professional authorized by state law.

SPECIALTIES. In addition to the various educational levels of nursing there are many specialties and subspecialties. Some of the specialties include the following:

- Certified nurse midwife—an RN who has completed advanced training in a program accredited by the American College of Nurse-Midwives and who is certified as a nurse midwife. The primary focus of health care is on well-woman gynecologic and low-risk obstetric care, including prenatal, labor and delivery, and postpartum care.[31]

- Certified nurse anesthetist—an RN with specialized training in the administration and control of anesthesia[32] and in the evaluation and management of a patient's physiology during the preoperative, operative, and postoperative periods. Requirements for practice include formal education in a nurse anesthetist program accredited by the American Association of Nurse Anesthetists.

- Nurse practitioner—an RN who is prepared to provide primary and preventive health care services. Nurse practitioners practice in all types of health care settings, such as clinics, hospitals, schools, and private practice. They usually specialize in a specific area, such as family practice, pediatrics, public health, geriatrics, or maternal-infant care. Certification for nurse practitioners is offered by professional organizations such as the National Board of Pediatric Nurse Practitioners.

Allied Health Professionals

The federal government has defined an allied health professional (PL 102-408, the Health Professions Education Amendment of 1991) as a health professional other than an RN or a physician's assistant who (1) has received a certificate; an associate, bachelor's, master's, or doctoral degree; or postdoctoral training in a science relating to health care and (2) shares in the responsibility for the delivery of health care services or related services, including the following:

- Identification, evaluation, and prevention of diseases and disorders

- Dietary and nutritional services

- Health promotion services
- Rehabilitation services
- Health systems management services
- Those meeting the federal government's definition, such as HIM professionals

Allied health professionals are involved in every facet of care, including diagnostic and therapeutic procedures, education, counseling, and evaluation and management of care, all of which are directed at assisting the physician with patient care. Many allied health professionals are employed in an ancillary department of the hospital. Ancillary departments provide services that support the physician in the management of patient care. As health care delivery has advanced in sophisticated technology and specialization, the area of allied health has grown tremendously. There are more than 200 health care occupations in the United States, some of which are found in HIM, medical technology, respiratory therapy, occupational therapy, physical therapy, and nutritional therapy.

Although not true for HIM professionals, most allied health personnel function by order of physicians. In hospitals that are organized by departments, allied health professionals are employed in a specific department; in hospitals that are organized by function, allied health professionals may be cross-trained in several areas and employed in units that provide patient-focused care. The HIM professional as an allied health professional is described below, and others are discussed in the section on the organization of hospitals.

Health Information Management

With the technological advances in information management, the increased demands for patient data, and the push for cost containment, efficiency, and accessibility of health care, the area of HIM is rapidly growing. Health information managers and technicians are employed in numerous areas, including risk management, quality assurance, HIM departments, medical transcription, utilization review, reimbursement, and finance. They are responsible for maintaining health records in such places as acute and chronic health care facilities, public health departments, managed care settings, government agencies, peer review organizations, and insurance companies.

The manager functions in administration and management of health information systems, including paper and paperless information. A principal function of the health information manager is the planning and developing of information systems that support the mission and goals of the health care facility and that are in compliance with the regulatory and accrediting agencies.[40] Responsibilities include the following:

- Organizing, maintaining, and producing information
- Disseminating that information and knowledge to clients

In addition, the assurance of confidentiality and integrity of the information is a critical function of the health information manager.[40]

The technician is responsible for the following:

- Maintaining health information systems constant with the administrative and medical staff requirements and with internal and external regulations, including legal, ethical, and accreditation concerns
- Processing, compiling, maintaining, and reporting health information data
- Abstracting and coding clinical data.[40]

The manager has at least a baccalaureate degree in HIM and has successfully written the registration examination given by the AHIMA and is recognized as a registered record administrator. The technician has an associate degree and has completed the accreditation examination given by the AHIMA and is recognized as an accredited record technician.

Health Care Team Models for Care

Team Approach

Traditionally, health care is provided by a team approach. In this type of approach, the health care team is directed by a practitioner, with members of the team complimenting and supplementing each other's contributions.[1] The primary physician usually directs patient care, and the nursing staff is primarily responsible for managing the care, which involves many other health professionals. The makeup of the team depends on the patient's needs, the setting for health care, and the physician. For example, the health care team for a patient who is a resident in a long-term care facility consists of a primary care physician (perhaps a gerontologist), nursing staff (RN, LPN), a dietitian, a physical therapist, a recreation therapist, a nursing assistant, and a pharmacist. A patient in this setting is not likely to need a medical technologist, radiologist, nurse anesthetist, or surgeon.

With the team approach, the inpatient must be transported to different departments to receive many of the diagnostic and therapeutic procedures. For example, if the patient needs a radiograph of the chest, a nursing assistant or a radiology technician has to transport the patient to and from the radiology department.

Patient-Focused Care

Another, newer approach to health care delivery is patient-focused care (patient-centered practice). With patient-focused care, the primary goal is to provide care with the patient at the center. Advocates of patient-focused care claim that the approach reduces cost and increases patient-consumer satisfaction.[41] For example, much of the care the patient has received as a result of being transported to and from different hospital departments might have been provided at the patient's bedside. Patient-focused care requires that health care professionals be cross-trained so that fewer people are involved in patient care. For example, only two health care professionals or technicians may be responsible for patient care. A nurse and a technician are assigned to groups of patients with similar needs; these two persons provide most of the care, which may include drawing blood, administering intravenous fluid therapy, obtaining electrocardiograms, performing blood tests, and admitting the patient. All staff members are trained to provide basic comfort measures which include assisting with meals, baths, ambulation, and so on.[41]

Family-Focused Transitional Care

Another approach to health care delivery is described by Lippman and Deatrick, who advocate a family-focused transitional care for pediatric patients. This approach uses the concept of a clinical nurse specialist involving the family in providing care and "coordinating that care across the continuum from the hospital to the community and to the home."[42] The family-focused transitional care from hospital to community to home is applicable not only to pediatrics but to other areas as well, such as geriatrics, obstetrics, neonatal medicine, and patients with chronic debilitating diseases.

Nursing Care

Nursing care may be provided using different models, including primary nursing, patient-focused care, and team nursing. The term primary implies that one nurse is responsible for the management of care for each assigned patient. With primary nursing, the RN is responsible for the entire patient stay, 24 hours a day. The RN develops a written plan of care for each patient assignment. All other nurses who are providing care to this patient follow, update, and revise the plan of care as necessary.

FINANCING HEALTH CARE

Paying for health care services in the United States is a complex system that involves multiple payers and numerous mechanisms of payment. Payment methods may be direct pay or indirect pay. Direct pay is payment by the patient to the provider and is referred to as **self-pay, out-of-pocket,** or **direct pay.** Indirect pay involves payment by a third party on behalf of the patient. Indirect payers may be the government, insurance companies, managed care programs, or self-insured companies.

Insurance is a purchased contract (policy) in which the purchaser (insured) is protected from loss by the insurer's agreeing to reimburse for such loss. When the patient contracts with a health insurance company to provide health care coverage, payments for health care are considered indirect; in **coinsurance,** the insured is partially liable for the debt. Many people are employed by companies that offer health care insurance at a group rate; the company may finance its own insurance company (self-insured companies) or contract with an insurance company to provide coverage. Some employers (purchasers) may pay for the insurance in its entirety, some share the cost of premiums, and others merely negotiate the group rate and the employee bears the entire cost. Today, according to Seaver and Kramer, some health care providers are beginning to contract directly with employers to provide health care, eliminating the insurance carriers, which is directed at reducing cost.[43] Despite the expense, because there is no reduced group rate, some individuals purchase their own health insurance.

One of the largest nonprofit insurance companies in the United States is Blue Cross and Blue Shield of America (BCBS). BCBS is composed of Blue Cross, which is insurance that covers certain hospital services, and Blue Shield, which is insurance that covers certain physician services and other health care services. BCBS negotiates numerous health care contracts with employers, professional organizations or associations, schools, and individuals. The coverage, benefits, costs, deductibles, grace periods, and other policy specifications vary from group to group (see Terminology Common to Health Insurance Policies, next page).

Reimbursement

Reimbursement is critical to the livelihood of every health care facility and provider. In the United States, reimbursement for health care is a function of multiple payers, some of which are discussed in this section. The agreement between the third party payers and the providers as to what will be paid for and how much will be paid to the provider is called the **reimbursement for-**

Terminology Common to Health Insurance Policies	
Benefit	Amount of money paid for specific health care services or, in managed care, the health care services that will be provided or for which the provider will be paid
Beneficiary	One who is eligible to receive or is receiving benefits from an insurance policy or a managed care program
Benefit period	Time frame in which the insurance benefits are covered; varies from insurance policy to policy
Claim	Request for payment by the insured or the provider for services covered
Copayment	Type of cost-sharing in which the insured (subscriber) pays out-of-pocket a fixed amount for health care service
Coverage	Types of diseases, conditions, and diagnostic and therapeutic procedures for which the insurance policy will pay
Deductible	Amount of cost that the beneficiary must incur before the insurance will assume liability for the remaining cost
Exclusion	Specific conditions or hazards for which a health care policy will not grant benefit payments; often includes pre-existing conditions and experimental therapy
Fiscal intermediary	Contractor that manages the health care claims
Insurance	Purchased contract (policy) in which the purchaser (insured) is protected from loss by the insurer's agreeing to reimburse for such loss
Out-of-pocket costs	Moneys that the patient pays directly to the health care provider
Payer	Party who is financially responsible for reimbursement of health care cost
Premium	Payment required to maintain policy coverage; usually paid periodically
Pre-existing condition	Disease, injury, or condition identified as having occurred before a specific date
Reimbursement	Payment by a third party to a provider of health care
Rider	Policy amendment that either increases or decreases benefits
Policy	Written contract between insurance company and subscriber (insured) that specifies the coverage, benefits, exclusions, copayments, deductibles, benefit period, and so on
Subscriber	Person who elects to enroll or participate in managed care or purchase health care insurance
Third party payer	Party (insurance company, state or federal government, other) that is responsible for paying the provider on behalf of the insured (subscriber, patient, member) for health care services rendered

mula.[44] These formulas are quite complicated and differ according to what was negotiated by the provider and the third party.

Historically, payment for health care services has been by the **retrospective payment system**, which is a payment method in which the cost to provide the health care is figured after the health care was provided and based on the provider's statement of cost. The actual amount paid may be based on fee-for-service or on the usual, customary, and reasonable charges. **Fee-for-service** is a payment method in which the cost is based on the provider's estimate of the cost for services rendered. The **usual, customary, and reasonable charges** are based on the physician's usual charge for the service, the amount that physicians in the area usually charge for the same service, and whether the amount charged is reasonable for the service provided. In community or public health programs, the cost for care may be based on the patient's ability to pay, referred to as a **sliding scale fee**.

More recently, the method of reimbursing the physician depends on the agreement with the third party payer. "From a reimbursement standpoint, fee-for-service is decreasing as physician payment is increasingly becoming dictated by discounts, relative value scales and capitation."[45]

Under the retrospective payment system, a hospital is paid based on the number of days the patient needed care and the resources used during the course of treatment, such as medications, laboratory tests, and medical supplies.

In 1982, development of a mechanism for controlling the cost of the Medicare program was mandated by the Tax Equity and Fiscal Responsibility Act (TEFRA), Public Law 97-248. TEFRA set a limit on reimbursement for Medicare and required the development of a prospective payment system for Medicare reimbursement. Therefore, in 1983, an amendment to the SSA established the **prospective payment system,** a payment method in which the amount of payment is fixed in advance of services rendered; the rate is established annually by the HCFA. Reimbursement using the prospective payment system bases payment on the number of patient days and the resources that should be needed to care for a patient case. Under this system, the hospital reimbursement for Medicare patients is determined by a patient classification scheme called diagnosis related groups, and reimbursement for physician services is based on the resource-based relative value scale.

A third form of reimbursement, the capitation method, is common in managed care programs.[20] In the **capitation** method, a prepaid, fixed amount is paid to the provider for each person (per capita) served, regardless of how much or how often resources are used.

Government's Role as Payer

The bulk of the government's spending on health care goes to the Medicare and Medicaid programs. In 1965, the federal government spent $5.5 billion on health, whereas in 1991, the federal government spent $216.7 billion on Medicare and Medicaid alone.[10] As a result of the spiralling costs, the federal government is pressing for changes that will contain health care costs. A brief review of the Medicare and Medicaid programs is important in understanding the current state of affairs.

Medicare

As mentioned earlier, in 1965, the Social Security Act of 1935 was amended to establish Medicare (Title XVIII) and Medicaid (Title XIX). Medicare provides health insurance for elderly people and certain other groups, and Medicaid supports the states in paying for health care for the indigent. Because both Medicare and Medicaid are modeled after private insurance companies, much of the terminology is common to many insurance policies.

MEDICARE ELIGIBILITY, COVERAGE, AND BENEFITS. The Medicare program is designed to help pay health care costs for elderly people, based on their own or their spouses' employment, and for other groups, including people with permanent kidney damage and those receiving disability benefits for a minimum of 24 months.[8] The specific requirements for Medicare eligibility are published in the Medicare handbook, published annually by the DHHS.

The program consists of Part A and Part B, which cover different medical costs and are governed by different rules. Hospital insurance, called Part A, helps to pay for inpatient hospital care, inpatient care in a nursing facility, home health care, and hospice care.[8]

Part A basically covers hospital costs, which include semi-private room, meals, nursing service, medications, laboratory tests and radiology, intensive care, operating and recovery room, medical supplies, rehabilitation services, and preparatory services related to kidney transplantation.[8] Care provided while the beneficiary is in a nursing facility, at home, or in a hospice is also covered with some restrictions. The physician's fees are not covered by Part A, even though the beneficiary is hospitalized and receiving physician services.

Medicare medical insurance, Part B, is a voluntary insurance program designed to supplement the cost of inpatient and outpatient care that is not covered under Part A. Part B coverage includes the physician's fee for services such as diagnostic tests, medical and surgical services, radiography, durable medical equipment, ambulance service, home health, radiation therapy, and other outpatient services. **Durable medical equipment** is equipment such as wheelchairs, oxygen equipment, walkers, and other devices prescribed by the physician for use in the home.[8]

FINANCING OF MEDICARE. The Medicare program is administered by the HCFA of the DHHS. Financing of Part A is primarily by payroll tax, unless the beneficiary does not qualify for federal retirement benefits (social security); Part B is financed by federal appropriations with monthly premiums paid by the Medicare beneficiary.

The Medicare beneficiary is required to pay deductibles and **copayments** for health care services covered by Part A. In addition, the beneficiary pays monthly premiums, the deductible, and a percentage of the charges for Medicare Part B. A **deductible** is the cost that must be incurred by the patient beneficiary before the insurer assumes liability for the remaining charges.

REIMBURSEMENT UNDER MEDICARE. Hospitals, physicians, and other health care providers are reimbursed for services delivered to a Medicare beneficiary through a **fiscal intermediary.** The intermediary is an organization that has contracted to manage the processing of claims and payments to the providers for Medicare Part A, according to federal regulations. The federal government assigns local insurance companies or BCBS plans to act as intermediaries and operate under contract to process Medicare claims. The fiscal intermediaries vary within states and/or regional areas.

From 1966 to 1983, hospitals were paid by the retrospective payment system: Charges for inpatient services were submitted directly to the Medicare Part A fiscal intermediary and were paid based on the reasonable cost of providing the care. The hospital submitted reports that itemized the actual cost of health care services.

Beginning in 1983, reimbursement for Medicare patients became based on the prospective payment system. In this system, the reimbursement is established in advance of the coming fiscal year, regardless of the actual cost to provide the care.[20] If a particular case requires more than the average number of days in the hospital or consumes expensive hospital resources, the hospital may lose money on that patient. Conversely, patients who require fewer resources save the hospital money. Providers have to maintain quality and yet be careful not to order excessive tests or extend treatment beyond what is considered medically necessary by the HCFA.

Medicaid

Originally called the Medical Assistance Program, Medicaid was established by Title XIX of the Social Security Act. **Medicaid** is a joint program between the state governments and the federal government to provide health care to welfare recipients in the different states. Like other government programs, Medicaid has changed somewhat since its inception in 1965. This discussion is restricted to the program as it exists today.

Eligibility for coverage is determined by the individual states but must provide for welfare recipients, poor children under age 5 years, certain low-income pregnant women, and medically indigent people. The **medically indigent** are those whose incomes are above what would normally qualify for Medicaid, but their medical expenses are high enough to bring their adjusted income to the poverty level. A great deal of variability exists from state to state. Each state sets its own limits regarding income that is considered to be at poverty level. Although the states vary in coverage and eligibility, they must comply with the federal guidelines.

The federal government identifies certain essential services that Medicaid must provide. They are inpatient and outpatient hospital care, physician services, laboratory and radiology services, skilled nursing care for those over age 21, home health care, family planning services, and early and periodic screening, diagnosis, and treatment of individuals under age 21. Each state can choose to provide additional health care benefits, such as medical care services by licensed practitioners other than medical doctors, dental care, physical therapy, eyeglasses, and prescription drugs.

The federal government shares in the cost of the Medicaid program with each state. The percentage of cost-sharing varies based on the per capita (per person) income of the state. In addition, the states can set copayments and deductibles for the medically indigent and for the optional services for welfare recipients.

MEDICAID REIMBURSEMENT. Each state sets its own terms for Medicaid reimbursement to hospitals and health care providers. In some areas of the country, Medicaid recipients are encouraged to join an HMO or some other managed care plan.

Because of the variation in coverage and the fact that there is still a population that does not qualify for Medicaid and yet cannot afford or access health care, the program is under scrutiny. The federal government is pushing for universal health care coverage, and some states are looking at mandatory insurance benefits by employers.

Managed Care

The HIM professional needs to develop an understanding of managed care because it is a rapidly growing field with information needs of its own. According to Miller and Luft, there were 36 million subscribers to HMOs in 1991 compared with 9 million in 1980.[46] **Managed care** is a generic term for a payment system that is an alternative to health insurance and manages cost, quality, and access to health care.[47] The term managed care encompasses a continuum of practice arrangements, including HMOs, preferred provider organizations, and other alternative delivery systems. The characteristics of the various managed care programs are highly varied, some of which are discussed here. Subscribers to the plans prepay a fixed, periodic (usually monthly premium) payment and pay small copayments. Providers who agree to participate in the managed care plans may be salaried employees or be paid fee-for-service or by capitation, or the provider may negotiate a financial arrangement.

Health Maintenance Organizations

The oldest of the managed care plans is the HMO, which integrates health care delivery with insurance for health care. The health care services may be provided directly or by contract with other providers. The concept of prepaying a fixed amount per person (capitation) for health care services dates back to 1906, when a group of physicians offered health care services to a lumber company. The Western Clinic of Tacoma, Washington, offered the lumber company health care services for a fixed amount per capita.[48] One of the largest and best known of the HMOs is the Kaiser-Permanente in California, which is a nonprofit HMO that is hospital-based, employs full-time physicians, and provides comprehensive care.

There are basically four types of HMOs:

- Staff model
- Group model
- Network type
- Independent practice association

The staff model is an organization in which salaried physicians are employed by the HMO to provide care only for HMO subscribers. The group model contracts with a group of physicians to provide health care for subscribers. The network type of HMO contracts with a variety of providers to provide health care for subscribers; a physician's patient population may include both HMO and non-HMO patients. With the independent practice association, there exists an arrangement between the health plan and the health care providers that details the provision of services and the compensation for those services.[20] The patient population of the physician participating in such an association includes both HMO and non-HMO patients.

Basically, the HMO models feature the following characteristics:

- Subscribers voluntarily enroll in the plan.
- Providers voluntarily agree to participate in the plan.
- An explicit contractual responsibility for providing health care services is assumed by the HMO.
- A prefixed periodic payment is made by the subscriber to the HMO that is independent of utilization of health care services.
- The financial risk is borne by the HMO.

According to Merz, studies indicate that the traditional staff/group HMO does contain cost, delivers quality care, and satisfies the patient to the same degree as the traditional fee-for-service insurance.[49]

Preferred Provider Organizations

A **preferred provider organization** (PPO) is a network of physicians who enter into an agreement to provide health care services on a discounted fee schedule. Patients who subscribe to this plan may use nonparticipating physicians but are penalized by paying higher non-negotiated fees.

Point-of-Service Plan

This concept may be integrated in a number of different managed care plans. The **point-of-service** plan merely requires the patient to use a primary care physician as a gatekeeper. A **gatekeeper** refers to the primary care physician who participates in a comprehensive managed care plan and is responsible for all care provided to the managed care enrollee (patient). If a patient needs to see a specialist, the gatekeeper must make the referral. Patients who do not use the gatekeeper are charged higher fees or additional out-of-pocket fees.

TECHNOLOGY IN PATIENT CARE AND HEALTH INFORMATION

Advances in technology have had a tremendous impact on the delivery of health care, including improving the quality of and length of life; improving the efficiency of health care delivery; producing more accurate, timely, and reliable data; and creating larger data banks for research. Health care technology can be grouped into patient care technology and information technology.

Patient Care Technology

The advances in patient care technology have been tremendous and affect the quality, efficiency, and cost of health care delivery. Some patient conditions and diseases may be more appropriately managed using sophisticated technology, whereas others may necessitate more conventional methods.

Although sophisticated technology is initially expensive, it often reduces overall costs by shifting care from costly inpatient settings to outpatient settings and by enhancing early detection of disease, which minimizes costly complications and, in some cases, involves fewer resources on the part of the provider. On the other hand, some technologies have perhaps improved the quality of life but at a high price. For example, assisted-reproduction techniques, such as in vitro fertilization and gamete intrafallopian transfer, help women who are sterile to conceive. Not only are these procedures costly, but the outcome is often multiple births, which dramatically increases the hospital charges[50] as well as the neonatal and maternal risks for complications.

The following are examples of patient care technologies that have had a significant impact on health care delivery.

Fiberoptic Technology

Fiberoptic technology has drastically changed physicians' approach to the diagnosis and treatment of some internal conditions that previously required large incisions. By using a fiberoptic viewing device called an endoscope, a physician can visually examine an organ from within the body. The procedure can be used to identify abnormalities and to excise or obtain biopsy specimens of lesions or organs. Fiberoptics also allows abdominal surgery, including removal of the gallbladder and appendix, to be accomplished through a small incision while viewing the internal operative field on a video monitor. The procedure, laparoscopy, minimizes postoperative pain, shortens the recovery period, reduces scarring, is often performed in outpatient surgery, and is less expensive than the conventional laparotomy.

Laser Technology

The laser, a device that emits intense heat and radiation, is a safer, more efficient treatment modality for certain conditions as compared with therapy that involves surgical incisions. When combined with fiberoptics, the laser has numerous applications, including the destruction of abnormal growths or lesions, excision of cataracts, repair of detached retinas, and control of internal bleeding. Laser surgery often can be performed in outpatient surgical facilities, and recovery usually is shorter than for the more conventional surgical procedures.

Computed Tomography

Computed tomography (CT scan) is a diagnostic procedure that creates transverse images that detail the internal structures of the organ; the images appear as if one were viewing "slices" of the organ. A CT scan provides much more information with greater clarity and detail than the conventional radiograph meaning earlier and more accurate diagnosis.

Gamma Knife Stereotaxic Radiosurgery

One of the more recent developments in patient care technology is the gamma knife stereotaxic radiosurgery, which uses high, concentrated doses of radiation to destroy lesions, primarily in the brain. This procedure is precise in its destruction of tissue and appears to involve fewer risks and faster recovery than with former surgical procedures. As with other technology, the equipment (a 20-ton machine) is expensive at $4.5 million, which affects the accessibility and cost of health care.

Other Advances

Other advances include heart and lung transplantation, cochlear implantation for the hearing impaired, and self-regulating drug therapy.

Advances in technology continue to occur at a rapid rate and are too numerous to discuss. As an HIM professional, you should take every opportunity to keep abreast of patient care technologies.

Information Technology

Information technology has had and continues to have a tremendous impact on the organizational, financial, and operational areas of health care as well as supporting patient care areas. Like patient care technology, it is rapidly growing and changing the manner in which we manage information. The technology has improved the quality of data by producing or having the ability to produce legible, timely data from large databases with greater accuracy than could be achieved manually. According to Veale, "improved information access is the common and vital component of the various national healthcare reform programs proposed."[51] Improved information access is accomplished through the computer-based patient record (CPR) and other emerging technologies.

Today, pieces of the health record are in both paper and paperless format, which has created a fragmented CPR. Some examples that are in use are described below.

Computerized Laboratory Results

Results reporting systems are excellent examples of early applications of information technology. Without computers, the results of clinical tests, such as medical laboratory studies and blood gas analyses, must be manually written on slips of paper and individually posted in the health record. Reporting systems automate the clinical results and provide consistent, legible, and fast documentation. Just as important, such systems provide incremental results during the patient stay and provide a cumulative report.

Facsimile Machines

The facsimile (FAX) machine can transmit information from one location to another. The transmission may be within an organization or from one part of the world to another. The device scans a document and converts the image (text) to electronic impulses that travel over telephone lines. On receival by another FAX machine, the impulses are converted back to text. This equipment has dramatically improved communication among health care providers, third party payers, health care organizations, and medical suppliers and manufacturers and within multihospital systems. For example, with the FAX, one can consult with medical experts from around the world regarding a serious patient condition; communication, which occurs within minutes, is accurate and legible.

Point-of-Care Clinical Information Systems

Point-of-care clinical information systems (point-of-service information systems) allow caregivers to input data whenever and wherever necessary, which may be at the time of patient care. A popular point-of-care system not only allows the caregiver to document the course of care at the bedside but also enhances clinical decision making. Such systems, often hand-held computers, bring documentation close to the time of care and thus support accurate, timely reporting and patient-focused care.

Electronic Data Interchange

Electronic data interchange is the ability to edit, submit, and pay health care claims by way of electronic transfer. In 1991, the Workgroup on Electronic Data Interchange was commissioned by the secretary of DHHS to reduce the cost of health care administration by increasing the number of claims processed electronically. The goal was to identify ways to increase electronic interchange quickly and effectively. Preliminary savings for administrative costs were estimated at $4 to $10 billion. The extensive report, published in 1992, proposed dozens of actions the government could take to support electronic claims interchange.[52]

Other Information Technology

Although many pieces of the health record are computerized, there is no system that alone can automate the complete health record. The automation of the patient record creates new challenges, such as maintaining data integrity and security, formulating standards that facilitate exchange of information, and identifying and dealing with legal constraints.

Health care reform has brought about challenges to develop a "comprehensive health care delivery system that is based on demonstrated practice" and that contains cost, increases accessibility, and maintains quality.[53] Demonstrated practice depends on the information available and the ability to use that information. Ac-

cording to Alexandre, "information can support information-driven decision making in the delivery of health services to improve the quality of care while optimizing the use of health resources. The tool that offers the greatest promise in this regard is the electronic medical record."[54] There are numerous definitions for the **computer-based patient record** (CPR), but the most comprehensive and most appropriate at this time is all financial, administrative, and clinical information that pertains to patient care entered into the computer at the time service is provided. The proposals for health care reform envision a **point of service** in which clinical, administrative, and financial data will move electronically among all who need health information, including providers, payers, researchers, health plans, laboratories, nursing units, outpatient departments, and home health areas.

Institute of Medicine

To address some of the information concerns regarding computer-based patient records, the Institute of Medicine (IOM), a nonprofit organization serving in an advisory capacity to Congress, undertook a study. The major concerns that the Institute addressed were the "protection of confidentiality and privacy of personal health care data and the disclosure to the public of cost and quality information about institutions and clinicians."[55] One of the recommendations that came from the study was the creation in 1992 of the Computer-based Patient Record Institute (CPRI), which is charged with developing strategy that will support the development and adoption of the computer-based patient record in health care delivery systems.[56]

A report from the General Accounting Office identified the following ways in which the computer-based patient record can improve health care delivery:[57]

- Provides data that are more accessible, of better quality, versatile for display, and easier to retrieve—all of which support decision making

- Enhances outcomes research by capturing clinical data from large databases

- Improves hospitals' efficiency by reducing cost and enhancing staff productivity

In 1991, the General Accounting Office reported that the electronic health record reduced hospital costs by $600 per patient in a Veterans Affairs medical center because of the shorter length of stay.[57]

According to Dick and Steen, the following conditions support the concept and implementation of the CPR:[57]

- Increased demand for patient data

- Improved technology that is more powerful and affordable

- Acceptance of the computer as a valuable tool
- Need for records that manage large amounts of information that is transferable
- Automation seen as a necessity for health care reform

The integration of clinical data management into a common database allows the health care organization to develop strategies that support quality, control cost, and examine processes to improve efficiency.[56] The integration further supports the collaboration and coordination of efforts by all health care professionals.

Clinical information systems are critical to address the changing health care environment needs for containing costs, improving quality, and providing accessible health care, all of which are vital components of health care reform.[53] The immediate availability of legible data is, according to Alexandre, one of the greatest advantages of the computer-based patient record.[54]

Advances in information technology, especially the CPR, create exciting opportunities for the HIM professional to have an impact on the entire health care industry. Converting from the manual charting system to an automated documentation system that is fully integrated is difficult and presents numerous challenges, particularly in the areas of data security, integrity, and accessibility; standards for data interchange; outcomes research; and education. HIM professionals must be prepared for their role as experts in information management to educate others about the concept and applications of the computer-based patient record.[58]

CONCLUSION

A major dilemma for health care systems today is the balance between the business, the technological advances, and the social welfare goals. One also cannot ignore the concern for quality, cost, and access of care, which is affected by all aspects of health care delivery.

Moving into the year 2000, the hospital will continue to be a critical aspect of health care delivery. However, the hospital will probably "be controlled by coalitions of community interests: business interests, physicians, politicians, lobbyists." According to Kroph, the "local hospital is likely to retain its role as the major planner of health services in most communities. If demand for inpatient hospital services continues to decline, hospital planning probably will remain focused on creating services outside the hospital and making the remaining inpatient services attractive to patients and physicians."[7] Some of these services include home health care, adult day care, and outpatient surgery.

Major issues for health care systems in the 1990s continue to be providing high-quality care at a cost that is affordable as well as care that is accessible to all people and at a level that is satisfactory to United States citizens. HIM professionals will have numerous opportunities to affect the direction of health care by addressing issues of security and integrity of the paperless health record, practice standards, regulatory issues, and documentation that improves patient care quality. The growth in ambulatory care, long-term care, and home health care has brought to the forefront the information needs in these areas. HIM professionals are and will continue to be of vital importance to the information needs of every component of health care systems, but particularly the innovative programs that are emerging and the needs that the CPR movement has brought about.

Key Concepts

- Health care delivery systems in the areas of ambulatory care, home health care, and long-term care are rapidly growing and there is increasing need for the HIM professional to assist with the information needs of these areas.

- Increased regulations, with focus on cost containment, accessibility, and quality, have the potential to create a very complex health care delivery system resulting in new opportunities for HIM professionals.

- The technological advances in information management, the increased demands for patient data, and the push for cost containment, efficiency, and accessibility of health care has resulted in new challenges for the HIM professional.

- To function as an effective health care professional, the HIM professional must develop a good understanding of the organization and structure of the health care industry as a whole and the health care facilities comprising the industry.

- The information needs that are created by the CPR and other technologies present unique opportunities and challenges for HIM, such as regulatory issues, communication standards, data security, integrity, and ownership.

References

1. Snook DI: Hospitals: What they are and how they work, 2nd ed. Gaithersburg, MD: Aspen Publishers, 1992.
2. Hanken MA, Water KA (eds): Glossary of healthcare terms, rev ed. Chicago: American Health Information Management Association, 1994.
3. Ackerknecht EH: Medicine of ancient civilization. *In* Ackerknecht

EH (ed): A short history of medicine, 4th ed. Baltimore: Johns Hopkins Press, 1982, pp 21–26.

4. Stevens R: In sickness and in wealth: American hospitals in the twentieth century. New York: Basic Books, 1989.

5. Roberts JS, Coale JG, Redman RR: A history of the Joint Commission on Accreditation of Hospitals. JAMA 1987; 258:936–940.

6. Jonas S: Health manpower with an emphasis on physicians. In Kovner AR (ed): Health care delivery in the United States, 4th ed. New York: Springer, 1990, pp 50–86.

6a. Kovner AR: Governance and management. In Kovner AR (ed): Jonas's Health care delivery in the United States, 5th ed. New York, Springer, 1995.

6b. Kovner AR: Hospitals. In Kovner AR (ed): Jonas's Health care delivery in the United States, 5th ed. New York: Springer, 1995, p 180.

7. Kroph R: Planning for health services. In Kovner AR (ed): Health care delivery in the United States, 4th ed. New York: Springer, 1990, pp 324–351.

8. The Medicare 1994 Handbook. Baltimore: Health Care Financing Administration, 1994. U.S. Department of Health and Human Services publication HCFA 10050.

9. Healthy People 2000—National Health Promotion and Disease Prevention Objectives. Washington, D.C.: Public Health Service, 1991. U.S. Department of Health and Human Services publication PHS 91-50212.

10. Brecher C: Government's role in health care. In Kovner AR (ed): Jonas's health care delivery in the United States, 5th ed. New York: Springer, 1995, pp 322–347.

11. Office of Federal Register: The U.S. Government Manual. Washington, DC: US Government Printing Office, 1993, p 294.

12. What is a D.O.? Chicago: American Osteopathic Association, 1991.

13. Napolski PT, Rubin MS, Marshall-Cohen LA: Legislative and regulatory issues. In Youngberg BJ (ed): The risk manager's desk reference. Gaithersburg, MD: Aspen Publishers, 1993, pp 238–245.

14. 1995 Comprehensive accreditation manual for hospitals. Chicago: Joint Commission on Accreditation of Healthcare Organizations, 1994.

15. Standards manual and interpretive guidelines for organizations serving people with disabilities. Tucson: Commission on Accreditation of Rehabilitation Facilities, 1994.

16. AOA fact sheet. Chicago: American Osteopathic Association, 1993.

17. Rakich JS, Longest BB Jr, Darr K: Managing health services organizations, 3rd ed. Baltimore: Health Professions Press, 1992.

18. Burke M: New surgical technologies reshape hospital strategies. Hospitals, May 5, 1992, pp 30–42.

19. Lawrence RS, Jonas S: Ambulatory care. In Kovner AR (ed): Health care delivery in the United States, 4th ed. New York: Springer, 1990, pp 106–140.

20. Owenby D, Lambdin LA (eds): Encyclopedia of health reform terms. Knoxville: Fort Sanders Health System, 1993.

21. Goldstein AS: The Aspen dictionary of health care administration, Rockville, MD: Aspen Publishers, 1989.

22. What happens to physicians when hospitals merge, consolidate, and acquire? Medical Staff Briefing 1994;4(2):1–8.

23. Hudson T: Group practices without walls offer unique problems and possibilities. Hospitals and Health Networks, May 20, 1994, pp 52–55.

24. Banta DH: What is health care? In Kovner AR (ed): Health care delivery in the United States, 4th ed. New York: Springer, 1990, pp 8–30.

25. Richardson H: Long-term care. In Kovner AR (ed): Jonas's health care delivery in the United States, 5th ed. New York: Springer, 1995, pp 194–231.

26. Read S: Do formal controls always achieve control? The case of triage in accident and emergency departments. Health Services Management Research Feb 1994;7(1):31–41.

27. AHA guide to the health care field. Chicago: American Hospital Association, 1993.

28. Bartlett CA, Ghoshal S: Matrix management: Not a structure, a frame of mind. Business Review, July/August 1990, pp 138–145.

29. Taylor K: How feuding hospitals joined hands to serve their community [interview with S. Goodspeed]. Hospitals and Health Networks, December 20, 1993, p 10.

30. University of Alabama at Birmingham Master of Science in Health Information Management—Program Brochure, 1994.

31. Nursing facts: Advanced nursing practice. Washington, DC: American Nurses Association, PR-11 35M August 1993.

32. Nursing facts: Registered nurses: A distinctive health care profession. Washington, DC: American Nurses Association, PR-12 70M June 1994.

33. Shaughnessy PW, Bauman MK, Kramer AM: Measuring the quality of home health care. Caring 1990;9(2):4–6.

34. Allen JE: Key federal requirements for nursing facilities. New York: Springer, 1994.

35. Taylor TS: Hired hands. Hospitals and Health Networks, May 20, 1994, pp 58–62.

36. Deets HB: Healthcare costs: America can't afford to be sick. J AHIMA, Mar 1992;63(3):76–77.

37. Wilson FA, Neuhauser D: Health manpower. In Health services in the United States, 2nd ed. Cambridge, MA: Ballinger Publishing Co, 1987, p 61.

38. Purtillo R: The clinician. In Health professional and patient interaction, 4th ed. Philadelphia: WB Saunders Co, 1990.

39. Taber's Cyclopedic Medical Dictionary, 17th ed. Philadelphia: FA Davis, 1993.

40. Essentials for an accredited program for the health information technician and health information administrator. Chicago: American Health Information Management Association, 1995.

41. Townsend MB: Patient-focused care: Is it for your hospital? Nurs Management 1993;24(9):74–80.

42. Lippman TH, Deatrick JA: Enhancing specialist preparation for the next century. J Nurs Ed 1994;33(2):53–58.

43. Seaver DJ, Kramer SH: Direct contracting: The future of managed care. Healthcare Financial Management, August 1994, pp 21–28.

44. Medical staff organization management: Independent study program. Nashville: National Association of Medical Staff Services, 1993.

45. Robbins MM, Loudermilk RC: Lining up their shots. Hospitals and Health Networks, May 20, 1994, p 35.

46. Miller RH, Luft HS: Managed care: Past evidence and potential trends. Frontiers of Health Service Management, Spring 1993, pp 3–37.

47. McGuire JP: The growth of managed care. Healthcare Financial Management, August 1994, p 10.

48. Shouldice and Shouldice: Medical Group Practice and Health Maintenance Organizations, 1978.

49. Merz M: Managed care: The burden of a great potential. Frontiers of Health Service Management, Spring 1993, pp 39–42.

50. Callahan TL, Hall JE, Christiansen CL, et al: The economic impact of multiple-gestation pregnancies and the contribution of assisted-reproduction techniques to their incidence. N Engl J Med 1994;333i(4):244–249.

51. Veale FH: Optical imaging and the computer-based patient record: A step in the right direction? Healthcare Informatics, April 1994, p 24.

52. Workgroup for Electronic Data Interchange: Report to Secretary of U.S. Department of Health and Human Services. July 1992.

53. Andrew WF: Point of care systems. Topics in Health Information Management 1994;14(4):1–10.

54. Alexandre LM: Information technology as an enabler of health system reform. J Am Health Information Management Assoc 1994;65(7):36–40.

55. Lansky D: Getting the data—and the information—right: An interview with the IOM's Molla S. Donaldson. Joint Commission Journal on Quality Improvement 1994;20(4):208–214.

56. Shortliffe EH, Tang PC, Amatayakul MK, et al: Future vision and dissemination of computer-based patient records. *In* Ball MJ and Collen MF (eds): Computers in health care: Aspects of the Computer-based Patient Record. New York: Springer, 1992, p 273.

57. Dick RS and Steen EB: Introduction. *In Aspects of the computer-based patient record.* Washington, DC: National Academy Press, 1991: pp 1–15.

58. Morgan JD: The computer-based patient record challenges the health information management profession. J Am Health Information Management Assoc 1992;63(6):79–85.

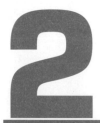

MILDRED P. ST. LEGER and MARY ALICE HANKEN

KEY WORDS

Accreditation
Accredited record technician
Board certified
Certification
Certified coding specialist
Certified record librarian
Conditions of Participation
Diagnosis related group
Fee-for-service
Information highway
Longitudinal record
Managed care
Medicaid
Medicare
Profession
Registered record administrator
Registered record librarian
Registration
Standardization movement
Tax Equity and Fiscal Responsibility Act

ABBREVIATIONS

AAMRL—American Association Medical Record Librarians
ACP—American College of Physicians
ACS—American College of Surgeons
AHA—American Hospital Association
AHIMA—American Health Information Management Association
AMA—American Medical Association
AMRA—American Medical Record Association

THE HEALTH INFORMATION MANAGEMENT PROFESSION

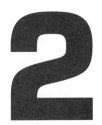

OBJECTIVES

- Define the key words.
- Compare and contrast early efforts to record medical information with today's patient record.
- Track the parallels between the development of health care in the United States and the development of the health record.
- Describe the influence of changes in the U.S. health care system on the health information management (HIM) profession.
- List the attributes of a profession and apply them to the HIM profession.
- Trace the development of the HIM profession.
- Describe the benefits of membership in a professional association.
- List and describe some of the roles of HIM professionals in today's health care environment.
- Identify major milestones in the HIM profession.
- Compare and contrast the purposes of the computer-based patient record with those of the patient record in the early 1900s.
- Describe the impact of information technology on the HIM profession.
- Identify the requirements for initial and continuing certification within the HIM profession.

This chapter examines early record keeping in health care and traces the beginning of the health information management (HIM) **profession** in the United States to its current status. The key professional association for HIM professionals in the United States, the American Health Information Management Association (AHIMA), is also discussed. The history of the profession is linked to the development of other health care organizations and to major landmarks in the health care system. These milestones are also explored. Although the roles of HIM professionals have matured and the variety of opportunities has increased in ways the early founders of the profession never imagined, one main thread binds the past to the future: *the goal of supporting quality patient care.*

HISTORICAL DEVELOPMENT OF THE HEALTH RECORD

Pre-1900

The value of recording clinical information about health care encounters has been recognized since prehistoric times. The methods used to record early attempts to treat disease are primitive and differ markedly from the computerized information systems now in use. The procedures and treatments of the past that were illustrated by crude drawings and, later, brief, one-line narratives in ledgers bear little resemblance to the complex treatments patients receive today.

Prehistoric cave paintings are thought to be the earliest accounts of treatment of the sick. The paintings depict skull trephination as well as the amputation of fingers and other parts of the extremities. Although these early patient records do not indicate the diagnosis that prompted the treatment, the cranial procedure may have been done to relieve some obvious malfunction or to release an evil spirit thought to be dominating the person. Amputations may have followed injury or infection or may reflect the administration of some sort of judgment as that in the Old Testament—"An eye for an eye and a tooth for a tooth."[1]

As civilizations developed, stone carvings were made in addition to drawings. The frequent appearance of serpents in the drawings and carvings is evidence of the belief of their importance to healing.[2]

The earliest hospitals were depicted as being vermin-infested places of filth and disease where patients who had no one to care for them at home were sent. Physicians were identified as priests, monks, and barbers. Early efforts to use dissection as a means to acquire knowledge are also well illustrated.[2]

In the United States, many early hospitals were established by religious groups or through private donations. They, too, were places where patients who had no one to care for them at home were sent or where patients went to die or be isolated from the healthy if they were infected with some contagious disease.

Methods to maintain patient records were slow to develop, and the earliest institutions used some abbreviated form. Many hospitals appear to have used a ledger to record at least minimum information about a patient—for example, name, address, date of birth, and major health problem.

The New York Hospital, established in 1771, did not begin recording patient clinical information until around 1790. Early medical records at Pennsylvania Hospital, established in Philadelphia in 1792 as the result of the leadership of Benjamin Franklin, included entries of the patient's name, address, and ailment. A number of entries were made in Franklin's handwriting. Charity Hospital in New Orleans entered its first medical records in large ledgers. Many of its earliest patients were seamen, and the terminology used reflects this nautical influence. Massachusetts General Hospital, established in 1821, maintained patient records from its beginning. These records were sufficiently comprehensive to enable the cataloging of diseases and operations.[3] One Virginia hospital, established in 1911, maintained its first clinical records in leather-bound volumes that contained between 50 and 100 patient records per volume. Each volume was labeled in gold-leaf lettering.

The use of ledgers for record keeping was popular in other businesses as well. They were used by banks, hotels, and other commercial enterprises. Many pioneer record keepers, such as Thomas Jefferson, George Washington, and Benjamin Franklin, used ledger-style recordings, so it is not surprising that the health care field initially adopted a similar system.

The ledger style of documenting can still be found in some emergency departments as the emergency "log." In the early days, this ledger, or log, contained all the information about an emergency visit. Now, individual patient records are created at the time of each visit. As hospitals computerize their patient information systems, the ledger data are accessible on the computer and, if needed, could be assembled into a document that resembles the emergency department log.

Post-1900

As the record-keeping process became more detailed and interest in learning from treatment experience increased, the minimal ledger entry was not sufficient. A record was created for each patient. Some hospitals filed the records of similar diseases or treatments together to help in this learning process. Others set up indexes to identify the diseases and treatments and associate them with particular patient records.

Early records, although brief, contained carefully handwritten entries. A hospital stay of 2 weeks might result in a six-page record. When typewriters became available, some portions of the patient record were typed, perhaps a brief operative report or the history and physical examination.

Most hospitals are moving toward a computerized patient record with the vision that someday paper records will no longer be necessary. Many, however, still have paper records or have microfilmed or scanned their paper records into alternative storage media to reduce the bulk for storage, and with the help of optical disk systems, the records are more readily accessible to users.

The early record keepers in hospitals looked beyond ledgers to find ways of making the individual patient record more accessible and useful by moving from ledgers to individual patient records. These records were organized into systems that allowed easier retrieval of a patient's record and the data within the document. Because health care has become more complex and the number of uses and users of the record have multiplied, the paper form of the record no longer meets the demands placed on it. For example, the paper record can only be in one place at one time, and the data, once entered into the record, cannot be manipulated to show trends or relations to other data.

New tools are available to help meet the increased demand for accessibility. The challenge is to rethink, once again, the patient record. It can now be a patient database that is linked to other data resources, such as the medical library. The patient database can be arranged in multiple forms—for example, a **longitudinal record** from birth to death or an in-depth view of how well a particular health problem is being managed. The records of many patients can be merged into a database to provide information on the outcome of particular treatments.

In the early hospitals, only a small circle of health care providers had access to patient records. The records were brief and maintained by the caregivers. Today's patient records have multiple uses, and many people have legitimate access to them. Because of the complexity of hospital treatment, more than 50 persons may access a given record to fulfill their duties. In paper form, the entire record is available to users. As records are computerized, it will be possible to limit access to portions of the data in the patient's database; for example, if a researcher only needs to know data about certain types of cases but does not need to identify an individual patient, then "disidentified" data can be shared with the researcher.

The **information highways** that are being built and the technologic possibilities for manipulating and accessing data are relevant to the systems for maintaining patient records. These systems allow caregivers who are in remote areas to be put in touch with colleagues for consultations and allow caregivers to easily look up articles that are pertinent to a given patient's problem. It also creates new uses for patient information, much of it good, some of it potentially harmful.

Privacy and confidentiality are major concerns in today's society. They are especially important in health care, where a person needs to be able to share intimate details of his or her history and illness to receive the best treatment. Therefore, each of us, as we help in designing and implementing the patient information systems of the future, needs to ask key questions and serve as advocates for appropriate use of patient information because the patient is not usually included in the decision about the system design.

Do we want to be able to link patient records with other databases? If so, which ones? Would it be wise to use an identifier that easily allows linkage to other, nonhealth databases? Can we structure access to a legitimate need to know? How can we protect the data in the system from intruders? Who will serve as the gatekeeper to the system for nonroutine uses? How will patient access be handled? These and many other questions will make the future interesting and challenging.

HEALTH CARE IN THE UNITED STATES AND THE DEVELOPMENT OF THE HEALTH CARE RECORD

Accreditation of Health Care Facilities

The most significant early influence on health records in the United States was the realization that to assess the quality of physician education and the resulting treatment provided to patients, those performing the assessment needed data. The primary data source was the patient record. In 1902, the American Hospital Association (AHA) included medical records as a topic for discussion at its annual meeting. In 1910, the Flexner Report (see Chapter 1) focused attention on the shortcomings of medical education. But the organization most keenly aware of the need for quality patient records was the American College of Surgeons (ACS).

To elevate the quality of surgery being performed in hospitals, the ACS established minimum standards and then began to survey hospitals to see if those standards were being met. In 1918, "only 89 of the 692 hospitals of 100 or more beds surveyed met the minimum standards."[4] The standards included specifications for the content of the patient's record and required that certain activities be documented within a specified time.

Members of the early voluntary hospital **accreditation** body were the ACS, the AHA, the American College of Physicians (ACP), the American Medical Association (AMA), and the Canadian Hospital Association. The Canadian Hospital Association withdrew from this body when Canada began its own accreditation program. The ACS provided leadership and funding for the accreditation activity for many years until the burden became too great. In 1952, the voluntary member organizations formed the Joint Commission on the Accreditation of Hospitals. Since then the accreditation activity has expanded beyond hospitals, and now the organization is called the Joint Commission on the Accreditation of Healthcare Organizations (JCAHO). The JCAHO accredits a large majority of hospitals and other health care organizations in the United States. All these organizations keep health records. In some settings, the records are called medical records and in others, patient, resident, or client records. The JCAHO plays a significant role in setting expectations for quality patient care as reflected in the documented patient record.

As computers become more the norm in hospitals, the JCAHO is attempting to change its methods of review. These new methods are also heavily information-dependent. At some point in the future, instead of patient records being reviewed on site, disidentified patient records that contain key data significant for quality comparisons with other hospitals could be submitted.

In addition to the health record, most health care facilities have other information that is important to the provision of quality care. A recent JCAHO standard on information management recognizes the value of information to the organization. This standard was developed with the participation of AHIMA representatives.[5]

Physician Certification

Physician specialty organizations developed in parallel with hospitals. To become **board certified**, physicians needed to meet certain criteria, which included documentation of the type and volume of cases in the specialty in which they sought **certification.** The patient record and many of the medical record department indexes helped physicians prepare for the certification process.

Insurance Payment for Health Care Services

Employers began to add benefits to workers' compensation packages in the 1950s and 1960s. One of these benefits was health insurance. Although the documentation requirements by insurance companies in the early years were not nearly as demanding as they are now, it was still necessary to document the care provided.

Licensing of Health Care Facilities

To set basic standards for facilities providing health care, the states began programs to license facilities. It is interesting to note the requirements for what constitutes a hospital. For example, in Washington State, the Washington Administrative Code defines the term "hospital" as

> any institution, place, building, or agency providing accommodations, facilities and services over a continuous period of twenty-four hours or more, for observation, diagnosis, or care of two or more individuals not related to the operator who are suffering from illness, injury, deformity, or abnormality, or from any other condition for which obstetrical, medical, or surgical services would be appropriate for care or diagnosis.

The code goes on to list what is not included in its definition of "hospital" and points out other areas of the code that pertain to specific care facilities, such as psychiatric hospitals, maternity homes, and nursing homes.[6]

Although many of the licensing codes focus heavily on the physical facility to assure safe surroundings, they also include sections on the basic requirements for a patient record and patient record system. Facilities accredited by the JCAHO's voluntary accreditation program may also need to meet state licensing requirements to be authorized to provide services. Ordinarily, state requirements are considered the basic minimum requirements, and the JCAHO would add a level or a step up in the quality ladder. Sometimes state licensing requirements are more specific than JCAHO standards; for example, the state may specify a retention period for patient records.

Professional Standards

The AHIMA, although not engaged in a licensing or voluntary accreditation program, does develop guidelines and standards for health records and health information systems. It also contributes to the standardization of data through its work with national standards organizations and by publishing documents such as the *Glossary of Healthcare Terms.* The AHIMA works closely with physician organizations, the AHA, and other groups that are interested in quality patient data and patient information systems.

Medicaid and Medicare

In 1965, Congress added provisions to the Social Security Act that created **Medicare** and **Medicaid** (see Chapter 1). This significant event resulted in the addition of regulations from the federal and state levels for health and medical records. Many of the basic JCAHO standards were incorporated into the regulations of these programs. Now, instead of voluntary standards, the regulations were part of the *Conditions of Participation.* Review programs were also required for participation. Each admission of a patient to the hospital was subject to review and potential denial of payment if the admission was judged, after the fact, to be unnecessary. The federal government set up a monitoring system for Medicare patients that contractually delegated the review of appropriate utilization of hospital resources and the review of the quality of patient care. Much of the review relied on the patient record for information. Medicaid programs are administered at the state level. Each state formulates its program and requirements on the basis of federal guidelines.

The Medicare and Medicaid programs also brought significantly more patients into the hospitals for care. The initial program was essentially a **fee-for-service** style of reimbursement. If a service was provided that Medicare had agreed to cover, a payment would be received at a discounted rate. The system encouraged more services to generate more payment. Fifteen years after its inception, the costs of the Medicare program were exceeding all expectations. The public as well as legislators were concerned about accelerating health care costs. In 1983, through the **Tax Equity and Fiscal Responsibility Act,** Congress enacted legislation that changed the method of reimbursement to hospitals for Medicare inpatient services. **Diagnosis related groups (DRGs)** were implemented and, essentially, the prices for these groups were predetermined. Once again, the health record was the source for the data justifying the payment for the DRG.

Technology

Technology is playing a role in the direct care offered to people. It adds many tools to the diagnostic, therapeutic, monitoring, and educational aspects of patient care. The results of using technology for care are documented in the patient record. Frequently, however, the actual scan or image is in a different location. As information technology matures, its capability is being brought to bear on the health record itself. Technology will provide tools for a totally new approach to the health record of the next century. It will allow data to be part of the record without forcing the data to paper, i.e., images, voice, sound. One view of the potential and capabilities of a future health record system is expressed in the Institute of Medicine's study on the computer-based patient record. The patient record of the future "will reside in a system specifically designed to support users by providing accessibility to complete and accurate data, alerts, reminders, clinical support systems, links to medical knowledge and other aids."[7] One recommendation of this study is that the "public and private sectors join in establishing a Computer-based Patient Record Institute [CPRI] to promote and facilitate development, implementation, and dissemination of the computer-based patient record."[7] The AHIMA supported the development of CPRI by housing the initial organization and lending one of its top executives to lead the formation of the organization. Among the groups that are members of the CPRI are the AMA, the American Nurses Association, the AHIMA, the ACP, American Medical Informatics Association, Motorola, Aetna Health Plans, Mayo Clinic, 3M Health Information Systems, and Kaiser Permanente.[8]

The AHIMA is also promoting the education of its members in implementing computer-based patient records and participating in the development of national standards to facilitate the implementation of computer-based patient records.

The story of the development of health care is strongly linked to the development of the health care record. As health care becomes more complex, so does the record of that care. As new patient care, payment, and technology changes are implemented, the health care record mirrors these changes. The one constant in the health care system is change. This will continue to provide many opportunities for HIM managers to meet the challenge of designing the health care record and health information systems of the future.

HEALTH CARE IN THE UNITED STATES AND THE CREATION OF THE HIM PROFESSION

The early efforts by the medical profession to upgrade the education of physicians and to evaluate the quality of care provided to patients have a direct link to the beginning of the HIM profession. The ACS's standardization program with its resultant voluntary accreditation standards for hospitals was the catalyst for organizing and educating people to support the informational needs of the accrediting bodies and medical educators. From early roles as custodian of the patient record, transcriber of operative reports, abstractor of data for reporting, and

organizer of clinical indexes has come what is today known as the profession of health information management.

Voluntary Standards and Regulations

Significant in the development of the profession is its ability to help hospitals and other health care orgnizations function effectively within multiple sets of voluntary standards and mandatory rules. For example, both accreditation standards and licensing regulations are based on recommendations of professionals in the health care field. When put in place, they represent the consensus of at least minimum performance to meet quality standards. However, regulations become outdated, and professionals need to actively recommend updating regulations. The JCAHO revises its standards annually. Although the entire set of standards does not change annually, the JCAHO is better able to respond to needed changes. Accreditation by the JCAHO has been an indication that a health care organization has achieved a level of quality beyond the basic requirements of licensing. For this reason, other organizations, such as third party payers and the federal government, have used JCAHO accreditation as a means of qualifying health care organizations for various programs or payment for services. For example, when Medicare was initiated in the mid-1960s, JCAHO-accredited hospitals were deemed to meet Medicare's *Conditions of Participation*.

HIM professionals are familiar with both licensing requirements and accreditation standards. Their knowledge and skill in designing and implementing systems have been valuable to health care organizations. As the basic licensing requirements and JCAHO standards evolved, so has the HIM profession.

Each type of health care facility has its own requirements and needs. Many types of external review commonly occur in the health care environment. For example, a children's psychiatric facility can be subject to state licensing, JCAHO accreditation, regional review by the county, and program review by funding sources.

JCAHO standards are designed to be a step above licensing requirements and are intended to foster high-quality care. They are stated in such a way as to encourage facilities to determine their own ways of meeting the standards. The standards typically state what the outcome should be but do not prescribe how it should be accomplished. This leaves each facility to design systems that first meet its own needs and then, in that process, meet JCAHO standards. Because the JCAHO constantly updates and interprets its standards, the HIM professionals involved in designing systems for JCAHO-accredited facilities both participate in and monitor this activity. Many HIM professionals serve as accreditation coordinators for their facilities. The most recent standards revision that HIM professionals helped to draft is the information management standard, which brings together and views as a whole information throughout a health care facility. HIM professionals believed that it was time to view a facility and its information systems in an integrated, rather than departmental, manner.[5]

Medicare and Medicaid

With the implementation of Medicare in the mid-1960s, HIM professionals were confronted with the federal government's requirements related to reimbursement. Governmental involvement in health care had been present in moderate measure, but with the coming of Medicare and Medicaid, the interaction between health care facilities and federal and state governments increased markedly.

Elderly people and people without resources for health care were now able to seek hospital services from any hospital in their community instead of from only the public hospital. Both Medicare and Medicaid require more information about a patient (e.g., need for hospital-level services, justification for care provided, description of diagnoses and procedures). Medicare requires a process called utilization review, which is designed to ensure that hospital facilities and other resources are being used appropriately. Medicare also requires assurance that patients are being given quality care; thus, what may have been a less formal activity for some hospitals was required. In addition, Medicare contracts with external review organizations to monitor utilization and quality care. All this activity brought new roles to HIM professionals as utilization review, quality assurance, and external review coordinators. These activities use patient data, which is the expertise of HIM professionals. Previous experience and expertise with JCAHO standards and licensing regulations made these activities natural roles for HIM professionals.

Malpractice

With the expectation of quality care, due perhaps to the shift from a strictly charity hospital to a business providing a service covered by insurance or paid for by the person receiving service, came lawsuits for malpractice. Now, in addition to being concerned about licensing, accreditation, and reimbursement, facilities had to factor in potential liability for services. This resulted in even more interest in licensing and accreditation standards, the quality of documentation in the patient record, and the use of facility policies and procedures as guides for providing patient care.

Tax Equity and Fiscal Responsibility Act

In 1983, a major wave of change equal to the initiation of Medicare hit the hospitals. The scene had been set by the increasing costs of health care and the search for a solution. Until that time, most health care reimbursement was based on a fee-for-service model. Although reimbursement was not always for the full fee charged, it was still a model that rewarded more service rather than less service. The Tax Equity and Fiscal Responsibility Act of 1983 altered the incentives in health care reimbursement for Medicare inpatient hospital care. Reimbursement would now be based on a fixed fee for a hospital stay, the fee established by the patient's diagnosis and procedure and known in advance of hospitalization. In fact, a hospital would receive the same payment for all patients with the same diagnosis and procedure. The system is frequently referred to as the DRG system. Several variables were part of the initial system; some of them were patient-based, such as age, complications, and comorbidities, whereas others were community-based, such as the location of the hospital in a rural or an urban setting, the local wage index, and participation in formal medical education programs. These variables provided some flexibility to more gradually introduce this major change.

The patient record is the primary resource document for reimbursement systems that use DRGs. Instead of focusing on how many days of care and the amount and type of services received, reimbursement is based on the patient's diagnosis and procedure. The 1983 DRG system essentially collapsed all payments for hospital care into fewer than 500 basic prices for hospital care. The underlying classification is built on the International Classification of Disease, 9th Edition, Clinical Modification (ICD-9-CM) coding system, which HIM professionals have been using for research, clinical, and administrative purposes since its adoption in the United States.[9] For the first time in the history of hospital reimbursement, clinical data received priority over billed charges. Many hospitals that had previously not linked their patient data systems with billing systems now began to redesign their systems and link these two components. HIM professionals were the key to making the new DRG system work.

Many other payers have since adapted the DRG system for reimbursement, and the initial system has been refined, expanded, and improved. This expansion has brought HIM professionals into the financial aspects of hospital operations. If patient information is insufficient for DRG assignment or the physician has not reviewed the diagnostic and procedure statement to be submitted for coding and billing, then the revenue is not billable. Bills must be submitted to receive payment for services.

Problems in this process can result in major cash flow delays for a hospital.

Technology

While Medicare in the mid-1960s and the DRG system in the 1980s were changing health care systems, the force of technology was working its own change in health care. Technologic developments brought patients to hospitals in increasing numbers. Technology is now enabling treatments on an outpatient basis that in the past were only performed in an inpatient setting. Hospitals and all other care sites (e.g., clinics, home health, long-term care) use technology. Through technology, physicians can do more preventive, therapeutic, and curative procedures. Technology also provides more sophisticated means for diagnosing, treating, and monitoring patients. Computers are used to design and manufacture products used in health care, such as prosthetics.

HIM professionals were affected by technology as well as the increased volume of patients and variety of health care settings in which services were delivered. The challenges include designing systems to document the application of technology to patient care and to information systems.

Technology is important in moving health care data from the basic paper-and-ink patient records of the early 1900s to the goal of computer-based patient records for the year 2000. Inherent in reaching that goal is moving beyond a view of departmental systems to a total rethinking of patient data and the possibilities of a computer-based system designed first for patient care and secondarily to report what is needed for billing. New tools are available to health information managers to help accomplish the goal of a computer-based patient record and other health information systems. Leadership is needed, however, to design effective systems to deliver quality care and to meet the needs of many users, including patients, physicians, nurses, physicians' assistants, occupational therapists, physical therapists, social workers, health care administrators, researchers, external reviewers, educators of health care practitioners, payers, governmental licensing agencies, JCAHO, health data organizations, and state agencies responsible for vital statistics and communicable disease.

Health Care Reform

Whether it is called health care reform or given some other title, scrutiny of the rising costs associated with health care and attempts to reorganize the system will continue. **Managed care**, in its various definitions, is considered an option for controlling health care costs in the future. If the United States were to move to a managed care system, think of the implications for health information systems. If all care was based on capitated systems, how would this change the information needs and structure of current billing systems? Of computer-based patient record systems?

DEVELOPMENT OF THE HIM PROFESSION

Formation of the Association

The HIM profession in the United States was created because of a need for accurate, complete data regarding the care and treatment of patients. Both the AMA and the AHA were founded in the mid-1800s (see Chapter 1). The goal of these organizations was to enhance the quality of care through improving medical education and improving the care provided in the hospital, respectively. The Flexner Report in 1910 indicated that major changes were needed in medical education. At about the same time, in 1912, the ACS wanted to recognize surgeons who were providing quality care. When the ACS turned to patient records to evaluate the quality of care, it found that the records were insufficient. Hospitals were also beginning to recognize the value of organized record-keeping systems. In 1912, a group of five women met at Massachusetts General Hospital to examine and study clinical records. A group of physicians, among them Dr. Harvey Cushing and Dr. Richard Cabot, encouraged these women to organize their efforts and work with the physicians to improve the quality of patient care documentation. The group began as the "Club of Record Clerks" and had as its objective to "evaluate the standards of clinical records in the hospital, dispensaries, or other distinctly medical institutions."[10] The ACS found as it tried to review physician candidates for membership in the college that the records of patient care were so poor that it was impossible to evaluate the care given. Therefore, improving the quality of patient records became a goal of the ASC's **standardization movement** of 1912.

An important leader in the hospital standardization movement was Dr. Malcolm MacEachern, director of hospital activities at the ACS. Recognizing the immediate need to bring about change in the quality of patient records, MacEachern invited medical record workers from the United States and Canada to attend a meeting of the Clinical Congress of the ACS. The program and exhibits at the meeting were devoted to subjects related to patient records. Grace Whiting Myers, Librarian Emeritus of Massachusetts General Hospital, was a member of the Club of Record Clerks and participated in organizing the medical record workers who attended the meeting. At the close of the program, Matthew W. Foley, editor of *Hospital Management,* delivered a strong challenge urging the organization of medical record workers. He reasoned that an organized approach would help to accomplish needed change and would benefit hospitals and the standard-setting efforts of the ACS as well.[11]

The medical record workers who attended that meeting (in Boston, October 8–12, 1928) began to organize, and on October 11, 1928, they formally initiated the Association of Record Librarians of North America (ARLNA). Grace Whiting Myers was elected the first president of this association, whose mission was "to elevate the standards of clinical records in hospital, dispensaries, or other distinctly medical institutions."[12]

The progress made by the ARLNA during its first year of existence was remarkable and a tribute to the vision and organizational ability of its founders. During the first annual meeting, held in Chicago in October 1929, a constitution and bylaws were adopted. Charter members numbered 53. The meetings were attended by representatives of the AHA, the ACS, and the AMA's Council on Medical Education. All joined in enthusiastic support of the new association and its mission. The representatives suggested that the group find a way of training workers for this new field.

By the close of this historic 1929 meeting of the association, the members had decided that one means of providing education and communication was through the quarterly publication of the *Bulletin of the Association of Record Librarians of North America.* The annual subscription price was set at $1.00. As soon as the national association was formed, local groups began to form to support the mission of the association and meet the needs of members.[13] In 1935, plans were initiated for formal affiliation of state and local record organizations with the national association. By 1938, the bylaws were amended to provide for the addition of this structure, and by 1939, 22 associations applied for affiliation.[13] In 1944, Canadian members formed their own association and the name of the U.S. association was changed to the American Association of Medical Record Librarians (AAMRL).[14]

The first executive office for the AAMRL opened with the help of the AHA in 1944. An increase in dues allowed the association to rent its own headquarters in 1946.[11] From a one-person office, the association staff has grown to a staff of more than 60 persons.

Membership that started with 53 charter members was reported at 4454 members in 1960 and more than 36,000 members in 1995.

Development of Formal Educational Programs

At the 1929 meeting of the ARLNA, a committee was formed to develop a course of study. This activity was led by Jesse Harned, who was later appointed to chair the committee that finalized a curriculum for the education of medical record librarians in 1932. The first schools for the education of medical record librarians were provisionally approved in 1934.[11]

In 1943, in an effort to achieve uniform standards in all schools, the ARLNA developed "Essentials of an Acceptable School for Medical Record Librarians." The "Essentials" have shaped the curriculum and structure of medical record and health information educational programs since that time.[11] The latest revision to the "Essentials" was approved by the 1994 House of Delegates of the AHIMA for submission to the national accrediting body for educational programs in health information management.

As noted earlier, education was recognized as a priority for the profession to grow and produce qualified members. As with many professions, members first learned in an apprentice model and then shifted to a formal educational model with an internship and other opportunities to learn in the health care setting.[11] Physicians, nurses, medical sonographers, and physical therapists all generally followed this developmental model. The profession of health information management is no different.

Early programs were primarily established in hospitals by pioneering professionals who gave their time and talent to educate others. These programs required from 2 to 4 years of college, and some required graduation from an approved nursing school. By 1952, 19 schools offered formal educational programs.[11] Growth has continued, and in 1995, there were 133 approved school programs for the preparation of health information technicians and 48 approved college and university programs offering baccalaureate and postbaccalaureate degrees in health information administration. A few universities are now offering graduate education in health information management.

In 1965, the AAMRL began to require candidates taking the certification examination for medical record librarian to have graduated from an accredited program. Until that time, it was possible for alternative methods to also qualify a candidate to take the certification examination.[15] In 1970, a baccalaureate degree was added to the requirements to write the certification examination.[4] During the 1960s and 1970s, hospital-based medical record librarian programs moved into 4-year college and university settings. Many programs also critically examined the needs of the community and the changes in the profession to substantially revise curriculum.

Although by 1950 formal educational programs for medical record librarians were established in a number of sites, the number of professionals graduating did not meet the needs of the hospitals. This led to the decision to train another level of personnel to aid the medical record librarian. In 1953, six schools for training medical record technicians were approved. These programs were 9 to 12 months in length and located in hospitals; no formal academic credit was granted. After completion of the program, the student was eligible to write an examination. Successful candidates were called **accredited record technicians** (ARTs).[15] In 1958, about 50 graduates per year were being produced by hospital-based technician programs. This was short of expectations and need. To help produce more trained support staff, the AAMRL created a correspondence course, which was in place by 1961. Initially, the correspondence course was not designed to prepare students to become medical record technicians.[16] However, the 1961 House of Delegates amended the bylaws to allow graduates of the correspondence course to take the medical record technician certification examination. The correspondence course was popular because students could remain on the job in health care settings while learning. Over time, this course has been revised and reorganized into modules that can be used for medical record technician preparation as well as by others who are interested in only a particular topic or module. Additional educational requirements, including college course requirements, were added to the program in 1976 in an effort to make the educational preparation of its graduates relatively comparable to that of graduates of a 2-year associate degree program. The program is now called the Independent Study Program for Medical Record Personnel.

Community colleges also took an interest in training medical record technicians, and by the mid-1960s, hospital-based training programs began to shift to community colleges. By 1969, 30 schools offered training for medical record technicians.

Although accredited programs are able to tailor their curriculum to meet the needs of their communities of interest, undergraduate programs must have as a goal the preparation of graduates who meet the basic competencies specified by the AHIMA. The competencies are based on periodic studies of entry-level graduates from approved educational programs and the expertise of knowledgeable professionals. Guidelines for course content are contained in the "Essentials." For example, the "Essentials" for an accredited program, as revised in 1994, lists the following as appropriate professional content areas for the baccalaureate level of health information administration:[17]

- Medical sciences, including language of medicine, structure and functions of the human body, and disease process
- Organization of the health care industry
- Systems and processes for collecting, maintaining, and disseminating health-related information

- Computer concepts and microcomputer applications
- Computer applications in health care
- Laws, regulations, ethics, and standards that affect the management of health information
- Management theory, principles, and practices
- Classifications, nomenclatures, and reimbursement systems
- Data analysis and presentation
- Systems analysis, systems design, and project management
- Clinical quality assessment and improvement
- Statistics, research, and evaluation methods

Accreditation of Educational Programs

Because of close ties with the AMA and because the AMA had a program for accreditation, it was natural to use these resources. From 1943 to 1994, the AHIMA (formerly AMRA and ARLNA) collaborated with the AMA in its accreditation of educational programs. The AMA's Council on Allied Health Education and Accreditation was a cooperative effort with several health-related professional associations. In 1994, with the recognition of a readiness for independence, a new accrediting body was formed by several health-related associations to continue this activity. The new group is called the Council on Accreditation of Allied Health Educational Programs (CAAHEP).

CERTIFICATION AND REGISTRATION PROGRAM

The early 1900s were formative years for physicians, hospitals, and health information management. The physicians had methods of credentialing members and recognizing those who provided quality care. Hospitals were undergoing accreditation against a set of standards to demonstrate the quality of care provided. Likewise, the ARLNA determined that it needed to set standards for its members. In 1933, the ARLNA organized a certifying body, the board of registration, and developed rules and regulations for **registration.** One qualification was that the candidate be "of the full age of 21 years, ethical and of good moral character".[18] Although there were requirements for registration, no formal examination was used. Essentially, those who knew the candidate helped to validate that the person met the requirements for registration.

Currently, the term "registered" is used to include the

concept of "certification." In 1978 the title registered record librarian (RRL) was changed to **registered record administrator** (RRA) in order to more accurately reflect the nature of the work done by members of the profession.* A person is deemed certified as an RRA by successfully passing a certification examination and successfully completing an approved educational program at either the baccalaureate or the postbaccalaureate level.[19] To some groups, registration simply means meeting basic qualifications to be placed on a list, or registry. For example, counselors in Washington State can become registered counselors by submitting the required application and fees. Some professions are licensed by states. The state license defines the scope of practice. Some health care professionals possess both a license and a credential.

Registered Record Librarian and Registered Record Administrator Credentials

By 1940, there were 809 **registered record librarians** (RRLs), with membership for all categories totaling 1064. The ARLNA recognized the importance of its certifying (registration) process. Therefore, the process was continually upgraded to reflect the responsibilities and education required to perform satisfactorily. Before 1952, people with 3 years' experience in the field could apply for registration or certification. After 1952, one had to have 4 to 6 years' experience in the field, an educational background equivalent to that required for admission to an approved school, and successfully write a national examination. In 1959, the House of Delegates of the AAMRL voted to end registration by means of experience. In 1962, it amended the bylaws to allow only graduates of approved schools to become RRLs. In 1970, a baccalaureate degree was added as a requirement for registration.[14] These requirements continue to be in place.[19]

Certified Record Librarian Credential

In 1954, a certification program was developed to recognize and honor the accomplishments of RRLs who had been employed in the field for at least 10 years and who had made substantial contributions to the profession. Again, the model for this program was probably the physician organizations, which had programs to recognize "fellows," physicians who had demonstrated their skills in caring for patients and their commitment to their profession.

Applicants for this special certification had to submit

a thesis of 3000 words as well as document their experience and contributions. After being approved, a person could use the designation **certified record librarian** (CRL) instead of RRL. In 1964, this program was discontinued. The program did not receive the support of the general membership, which thought that the use of another professional designation, CRL, detracted from the primary credential, RRL.[20]

Accredited Record Technician Credential

From the beginning of the technician educational programs in 1953, graduates were offered an examination to acquire the credential of ART. The requirements for the credential have changed since its beginning to upgrade the level and amount of college course work associated with the preparation. Community college programs offer a 2-year associate degree. The AHIMA independent study program combines a series of required learning modules with 30 semester hours of college courses.[19]

Certified Coding Specialist Credential

The most recent credential offered by the AHIMA is designed to recognize people with substantial on-the-job experience in ICD-9-CM and current procedural terminology (CPT) coding systems. This credentialing program was started in 1992. No formal course work is required at this time to take the national examination. People who successfully pass the national examination may use the designation **certified coding specialist** (CCS).

Coders are part of the team of trained staff who work closely with HIM managers. Their primary function is to assign diagnosis and procedure codes to clinical data. Accuracy in coding, which has always been important for research and administrative use, now has added importance because of its use for reimbursement.

The granting of the credential by the AHIMA is one way of helping to define standards for coding for workers who do not have the ART or RRA credential. Coding is included in the credentialing process for ARTs and RRAs.

Continuing Education Requirements

The value placed on lifelong learning was apparent in the early growth of the ARLNA. Mindful of the limitations of learning that relied heavily on apprenticeship and experience, the association began to sponsor institutes. The first institute was held in 1939.[11] Sponsorship of institutes, often weeklong educational sessions, be-

---

*Medical Record News, vol. 49, No. 5, p. 90, Oct 1978.

came part of the association's ongoing activities. In 1973, the House of Delegates adopted a continuing education requirement for RRAs and ARTs for the maintenance of certification. The initial implementation of the continuing education requirement occurred in 1975. Every 5-year cycle, RRAs were expected to complete 75 hours of continuing education and ARTs, 50 hours of continuing education. In 1978, the cycle was changed from 5 years to 2 years. The shorter cycle was easier to track and did not allow participants to put off acquiring continuing education. Currently, RRAs must complete 30 hours of continuing education within the 2-year cycle and ARTs must complete 20 hours.

The maintenance of certification guidelines adopted by the 1994 House of Delegates requires the completion of a specified number of hours of continuing education activities in certain topic areas.[21] Fifty per cent of continuing education must be earned in core content areas. The remaining 50 per cent may be earned in other topics related to health information management. The core content areas are as follows:

- Technology—applications of existing and emerging technologies for the collection of clinical data, the transformation of clinical data to useful health information, and the communication and protection of information

- Management — application of organizational management theory and practices as well as human resource management techniques to improve departmental adaptability, innovation, service quality, and operational efficiency

- Clinical data management—application of data analysis techniques to clinical databases to evaluate practice patterns, assess clinical outcomes, and assure cost-effectiveness of health care services

- Performance improvement—study of fundamental organizational changes and how they are functionally organized or how they deliver patient care, with special focus on the requisite changes made in health information systems and services

- External forces—knowledge of strategies that organizational and HIM professionals in particular have used to effectively address emerging legislative, regulatory, or other external party action that have the potential to significantly impact the collection and use of health data

- Clinical foundation—understanding of human anatomy and physiology, the nature of disease processes in humans, and the methods of diagnosis and treatment of acute and chronic medical conditions and diseases[21]

Naming the Profession and the Association

The discussion of the appropriate name for the profession and the professional association can be traced back to 1938. Although members were not satisfied in 1938 with the title medical record librarian, no acceptable alternatives were identified.[11] It took until 1970 for the AAMRL membership to agree to change the name of the association to the American Medical Record Association (AMRA). Subsequently, the medical record librarian title was dropped in favor of the title medical record administrator. Recently (1991), again in recognition of significant changes in the responsibilities of its members and the needs of the health care industry, the AMRA became the American Health Information Management Association (AHIMA). No decision has yet been reached regarding a change to the designated credential, although a number of suggestions have been discussed. Members currently use a wide variety of job titles to describe their work.

The AHIMA in the 1990s

Structure

The AHIMA has organized and at times reorganized to meet the needs of both its members and the health care communities it serves. Its current structure includes both a volunteer component and a staff component. Volunteers are organized at all levels within the AHIMA, from the board of directors to associations in every state, the District of Columbia, and Puerto Rico. The volunteer structure is responsible for setting the policies of the organization and for providing direction to a wide variety of essential AHIMA activities. In addition to the board of directors, other national-level activities include councils, committees, the Assembly on Education, sections, societies, task forces, and other groups as needed (Figure 2–1).

The AHIMA is a membership organization. Members elect the board of directors as well as members to the Council on Certification, the Council on Accreditation, and the nominating committee. The board then appoints other AHIMA members and, as appropriate, nonmembers to various councils and committees. The Assembly on Education and the sections and societies each have rules governing their operations, and the members of these groups elect their leaders.

The AHIMA headquarters is based in Chicago with a satellite office in Washington, D.C. Its executive director is hired by the board of directors. The executive director, the AHIMA's chief executive officer, and staff are responsible for carrying out the day-to-day operation of

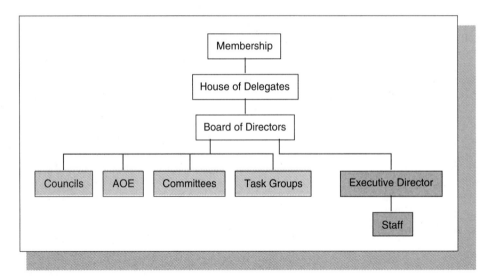

FIGURE 2–1. Organizational chart of the American Health Information Management Association volunteer structure.

the association. The executive director and the AHIMA staff are employees of the association. An important function of the board and the executive director is the overseeing of the association's assets. The assets and the budget of the association have grown over the years. In 1995, the assets of the association exceeded $16 million. The annual budgets of the AHIMA and its companion corporation, the Foundation of Record Education, combined are about $10 million.[22]

The structure of the staff organization changes as needed, but as of this writing, it includes the following functional areas:

• Business development
• Professional practice services
• Policy and research
• Marketing and creative services
• Membership and certification
• Human resources
• Volunteer development

Membership

The AHIMA offers membership in the categories of active, associate, student, corporate, inactive, and honorary. The membership structure allows anyone with an interest in health information management to join the association. Dues are assessed to all membership categories except honorary. Total membership in 1995 exceeded 36,000.

Mission

The mission of the AHIMA is a general statement that is used as the basis for prioritizing activities and making

resource decisions. In 1994, the association published a mission statement (see AHIMA's Mission Statement). As part of the AHIMA's ongoing strategic planning process, decisions regarding the use of resources are reviewed in perspective with the goals and initiatives of the association. The 1995 resources of AHIMA clustered around the following broad initiatives:

• Practice leadership: HIM practice and guidelines, alliances, health industry trends, information technology trends
• Education and professional development: Practitioners' roles and skills, leadership development, career management, formal education
• Building the association: Member services and communications, organization development, volunteer leadership development[21]

The Profession Defined

The purpose of the ARLNA in 1928 was "to elevate standards of clinical records in hospitals, dispensaries and other distinctly medical institutions." The 1994 mission statement of AHIMA begins by stating that "the American Health Information Management Association is committed to excellence in the management of health information for the benefit of patients and providers."[24] The mission statements, although years apart, are similar in the effort to implement standards of excellence in clinical data. The charter members were drawn together by a need to gain knowledge about their chosen work. Members of the profession in the 1990s still recognize the need to pursue lifelong learning in an ever-changing health care system to be effective professionals. The term "profession" may be defined as a group of people who adhere to the following criteria:

AHIMA's Mission Statement

The American Health Information Management Association is committed to excellence in the management of health information for the benefit of patients and providers. As the profession responsible for the management of health information, we serve our members and those who create and utilize health information by:

- Designing, implementing, and expanding programs that support and enhance the ability of those who work with health information
- Affecting government, educational, social, and business issues that impact the management and use of health information.[23]

The "Guiding Principles" which accompany the mission statement read:

We are committed to the:

- Creation and utilization of systems and standards to ensure quality health information
- Achievement of member excellence
- Development of a supportive environment and provision of resources to advance the profession
- Provision of the highest quality service to members and healthcare information users
- Investigation and application of new technology to advance the management of health information[23]

The mission and guiding principles are supported by a statement of values which reads:

We value

- The balance of patients' privacy rights and confidentiality of health information with legitimate uses of data
- The quality of health information as evidenced by its integrity, accuracy, consistency, reliability, and validity
- The quality of health information as evidenced by its impact on the quality of healthcare delivery[23]

The goals of the AHIMA, as adopted in 1994 as the Vision 2000 Statement, are:

- Be the profession responsible for the management of health information
- Provide the organizational infrastructure that champions the health information management initiative
- Design, implement, and expand educational programs that enhance the role of health information managers
- Achieve broad-based recognition and acceptance of the health information management role
- Achieve industry-wide acceptance of our leadership role in health information management[23]

- Possess specialized knowledge
- Define standards for the work they do
- Commit to lifelong learning to refresh and refine their knowledge
- Adopt standards of behavior for ethical conduct

The HIM profession has a body of knowledge and professional standards of practice. Its members have committed themselves to a continuing education program to maintain their credentials. In addition, members have adopted a code of ethics (see AHIMA Code of Ethics).

The code of ethics guides the practice of people who choose this profession. One of the tenets of the code is especially key to the role of the profession in working toward improved quality of patient care. It is the tenet that states, "The HIM professional refuses to participate

AHIMA Code of Ethics

Preamble
The health information management professional abides by a set of ethical principles developed to safeguard the public and to contribute within the scope of the profession to quality and efficiency in health care. This Code of Ethics, adopted by the members of the American Health Information Management Association, defines the standards of behavior which promote ethical conduct.

I. The Health Information Management Profession demonstrates behavior that reflects integrity, supports objectivity, and fosters trust in professional activities.

II. The Health Information Management Profession respects the dignity of each human being.

III. The Health Information Management Profession strives to improve personal competence and quality of services.

IV. The Health Information Management Professional represents truthfully and accurately professional credentials, education, and experience.

V. The Health Information Management Professional refuses to participate in illegal or unethical acts and also refuses to conceal the illegal, incompetent, or unethical acts of others.

VI. The Health Information Management Professional protects the confidentiality of primary and secondary health records as mandated by law, professional standards, and the employer's policies.

VII. The Health Information Management Professional promotes to others the tenets of confidentiality.

VIII. The Health Information Management Professional adheres to pertinent laws and regulations while advocating changes which serve the best interest of the public.

IX. The Health Information Management Professional encourages appropriate use of health record information and advocates policies and systems that advance the management of health records and health information.

X. The Health Information Management Professional recognizes and supports the Association's mission.

From Journal of the Am Health Information Management Assoc 1995; 66(1):69.

in illegal or unethical acts and also refuses to conceal the illegal, incompetent, or unethical acts of others."[25] Many HIM professionals are in positions where they are actively working as coordinators for quality improvement and quality assurance programs; other HIM professionals have access to detailed patient care data. Although health care practitioners strive to uphold high standards, this tenet of the code obliges certain actions if the HIM professional is aware of the illegal, incompetent, or unethical acts of others.

A second tenet is close to the activities of all HIM professionals. It holds the HIM professional responsible for protecting "the confidentiality of primary and secondary health records as mandated by law, professional standards, and the employer's policies."[25] Most HIM professionals are in positions in which confidential patient data are entrusted to them. HIM professionals extend this trust by educating staff within the facility and serving as patient advocates to protect the confidentiality of patient data.

A third tenet of interest states that the HIM professional will encourage "appropriate use of health record information and advocates policies and systems that advance the management of health records and health information." The first part of this tenet regarding "appropriate use" requires not only knowing and sometimes interpreting federal and state regulations, but also making many judgment calls as the demands for information increase and the capability of computer systems changes the control methods for information access. The latter part of the tenet speaks to the need to continue to look ahead and plan for the future in designing systems for managing health information.

The HIM profession offers its members many roles within the health care system. Periodically, studies are performed and panels are convened to update the description of the profession and the current roles of its members. In 1994, the House of Delegates adopted the following statement regarding the profession:

> Health information management is the profession that focuses on healthcare data and the management of healthcare information resources. The profession addresses the nature, structure, and translation of data into usable forms of information for the advancement of health and healthcare of individuals and populations.
> Health information professionals collect, integrate, and analyze primary and secondary healthcare data; disseminate information; and manage information resources related to research, planning, provision, and evaluation of healthcare services.[25]

The board of directors, in 1991, when reviewing the description of the profession, noted that HIM professionals were qualified through a unique combination of knowledges and skills that include the following:

- Health care databases and database systems
- Medical classification systems
- Flow of clinical information
- Relation of financial information to clinical data
- Uses and users of health care information, and
- Medicolegal issues and security systems[24]

The board also enumerated many of the uses of health information, including the following:

- For patient care, disease prevention, and health promotion
- For providers to evaluate the efficiency and effectiveness of care
- For reimbursement of health care services and analysis of alternative methods of coverage
- For developing public policy on health care, including regulation, legislation, accreditation, and health care reform
- For planning, research, decision support, and analysis[24]

Value of Health Information Management

Health information management professionals have for many years provided leadership in health information management. One of the major sources of health information is the patient record. The use of the data contained in the patient record has increased with the complexity of care and the complexity of the health care system. Health care no longer involves one physician, one nurse, one patient. Whether hospitalized or treated on an ambulatory basis, a patient is likely to encounter a variety of specialists. An increased number of caregivers and others rely on the patient record as a means of communication and as a source of data.

The patient record is a valuable source for individual patient treatment and for its potential in aggregating data for research. Much of the aggregate data that describe public health and illness have as their source the patient record. Published data on acquired immunodeficiency syndrome, sexually transmitted diseases, diseases caused by certain infections, and outbreaks of illness, such as *Escherichia coli,* rely on careful documentation in a source document. Health and disease issues are debated daily on television and in the newspaper. Hospital mortality rates are published as are reports of performance, good and bad, within the health care system. Some health plans give consumers information, sometimes referred to as "report cards," about health plans to help the consumer select a health plan.[26]

Changes in the use of the patient record have been pronounced in the area of reimbursement for care. First, third party payers have been requesting more and more data to pay claims. Second, the adoption of DRG methods of prospective payment, beginning with Medicare in 1983, focused attention on payment dependent on the diagnosis, which, after study, was determined to be the reason for admission, and any major procedures performed. Essentially, this resulted in fewer than 500 DRGs or "prices" for a hospital admission. HIM professionals played a pivotal role in making this system work for hospitals. Overseeing the use of patient data in planning, management, and research has long been the purview of health information managers. Reimbursement or prospective payment systems brought into sharp focus the need to merge patient data with the financial and billing systems in hospitals and other health care facilities.

Another major focus of the profession's contribution is on appropriate use of health information, which includes its leadership in the areas of privacy and confidentiality. The profession encourages members and others to find a balance between a person's rights and the needs of others for certain data.

HIM Roles in the Workplace

Today, members of the HIM profession are working in a wide variety of health care settings, governmental agencies, and managed care organizations. They are working wherever health information is collected, organized, and analyzed, including accounting firms, insurance companies, and research centers. As computerization of information progresses, an increasing number of professionals are involved in this process in the provider setting as well as the develop/vendor setting; i.e., HIM professionals are involved in development of software and systems in vendor environments, and some *are* vendors. Regional and national health information databases provide another challenge to HIM professionals. The skills and knowledge of HIM professionals are being used in an ever-widening circle for a greater variety of tasks. Many members are engaged in entrepreneurial ventures that demonstrate their ability to blend business knowledge with professional discipline. Although each person is free to select or develop a role that best fits his or her talents, there are a number of well-recognized roles in health information management, including the following:

- Manager
- Educator
- Consultant
- Entrepreneur
- Researcher
- Data analyst
- Accreditation coordinator
- Quality assurance coordinator
- Quality improvement coordinator
- Utilization management coordinator
- Systems analyst
- Systems developer
- Systems coordinator
- Database coordinator
- Medical staff coordinator
- Coder

CONCLUSION

Information technology brings new tools to the HIM professional. More is possible today than ever before. Health care is slower than other industries in investing in information systems, especially to support the clinical services it provides. Early initiatives beyond billing and accounting systems were directed more to single use rather than facilitywide or enterprisewide integrated systems. Technology is allowing the transfer and linkage of data well beyond the walls of a health care facility. It makes many things possible. It cannot be successful in accomplishing the goals and meeting the needs of the health care system, however, unless the data that it is able to transfer, manipulate, and aggregate are well defined, valid, and reliable.

As more data become available in electronic form, more potential uses and users will emerge. The capabilities of technology must be tempered with expertise as to appropriate uses of the data and legitimate users.

The commitment to accuracy, attention to detail, recognition of being part of the process of quality patient care, and skill in persuasion were attributes of the first medical record librarians. Doubtless there were physicians in the early 1900s who found documentation tedious and the support of someone skilled in the documentation process helpful. From the support given by the AMA, ACS, AHA, and other organizations to the development and continuance of the HIM profession, the value of the profession to the quality of health care is clear.

The pioneering professionals in medical record librarianship, now known as health information management, used the resources of the day to help create accurate records that documented patient care. Today's professionals have some of the same responsibilities but many more challenges as the value of health information and

Key Concepts

- The importance of recording clinical information is recognized from patient records maintained during early civilizations. The first U.S. hospitals used patient records, notable for their brevity when compared with the amount and variety of clinical data collected today. Diagnostic and treatment methods have been greatly expanded by developing technology resulting in the increase in the volume and complexity of information in the patient record.

- The American College of Surgeons influenced health records through its Hospital Standardization Movement in the early 1900s. The College recognized the value of clinical records in assessing the quality of physician education and treatment. Subsequently the Joint Commission on Accreditation of Health Care Organizations has continued to expand and shape the content of the patient record through voluntary accreditation. The initiation of federally funded Medicare and Medicaid in the mid-1960's prompted the involvement of Federal governmental agencies in patient record issues. In 1983, the Tax Equity and Fiscal Responsibility Act (TEFRA) became law, bringing prospective pricing to health care. The patient's record became pivotal in supporting and determining reimbursement to hospitals.

- Development of the health record and health care in the U.S. is concurrent as physicians, hospitals, early medical record professionals, and early regulatory agencies recognized the importance of the health record in evaluating patient care and developing reimbursement sources and payment systems.

- Computerization of the patient record enables access by multiple users, makes treatment protocols available to remote caregivers, and increases concerns for privacy and confidentiality. Protection of confidential information while facilitating legitimate use of a vast amount of information important to patient care remains a challenge now and for the future.

- The beginning of the medical record profession and the founding of its professional association, now known as AHIMA, is important in the dynamics of health information in the 1990s. The profession's focus from early times was the enhancement of patient care through better documentation. Early educational efforts are significant as they demonstrate an ongoing concern for quality preparation of health information professionals. The concept and importance of life-long learning were recognized in early efforts to provide workshops and other continuing education offerings for medical record practitioners. The Association established standards early on by its certification process. One mark of a profession is its code of ethics. AHIMA's Code of Ethics, simple and brief, is a useful guide to members' conduct.

References

1. Ancient Hebrew Levitical Law, Leviticus 24:29, 20 and Later Deuteronomic Code, Deuteronomy 19:20.
2. Bettman CC: Pictorial history of medicine. Springfield, IL: Charles C Thomas, 1979, p 16.
3. Huffman EK: Health information management, 10th ed. Berwyn, IL, Physicians' Record Co., p 3.
4. AMRA: The years of growth and development. Medical Record News 1978;50(1):66.
5. Accreditation manual for hospitals. Vol 1. Standards. Chicago: Joint Commission on Accreditation of Healthcare Organizations, 1994, pp 35–44.
6. Washington Administrative Code, Ch. 246–318, Hospitals, p 399.
7. Dick RS, Steen E (eds): The computer-based patient records: An essential technology. Washington, DC: National Academy Press, 1991.
8. Computer-Based Patient Record Institute. News release, 7/92.
9. Nomenclature and Classification Systems Module. Chicago: American Medical Record Association, 1987, p 13.4.21.
10. Bull Am Assoc Medical Record Librarians 1941;12(4):102.
11. AMRA: The first 20 years. Medical Record News 1978;49(4):70.
12. Bull Assoc Record Librarians North Am 1930;1(1).
13. Bull Assoc Record Librarians North Am 1939, p 14.
14. AMRA: The years of growth and development. Medical Record News 1978;49(5):84–90.
15. J Am Assoc Medical Record Librarians 1953; 49(5):79.
16. AMRA: The years of growth and development. Medical Record News 1979;50(1):83.
17. J Am Health Information Management Assoc 66(1):78.
18. Bull Am Assoc Medical Record Librarians 1941;12(4):102.
19. Standards for initial certification. Chicago: American Health Information Management Association, 1992.
20. AMRA, the years of growth and development. Med Record News 1978;49(5):85.
21. J Am Health Information Management Assoc 1995;66(2):62.
22. Interview with American Health Information Management Association Controller, 1995.
23. J Am Health Information Management Assoc 1994;65(11):60–62.
24. American Health Information Management Association, 1991.
25. J Am Health Information Management Assoc 1995;66(1):26,69,78.
26. Health Plan Employer Data Set 2.0. Washington, DC: National Committee for Quality Assurance, 1993.

Bibliography

Accreditation manual for hospitals. Chicago: Joint Commission on Accreditation of Healthcare Organizations, 1994.

Cofer J (ed): Health information management. Chicago: American Health Information Management Association, 1994. (Formerly Huffman: Medical Record Management, 10th ed.)

Donaldson MS, Lohr KN (eds): Health data in the information age: disclosure and privacy. Washington: National Academy Press, 1994.

Dose of history accompanies care at first hospital. Modern Healthcare, February 27, 1995, p 40.

Hanken MA, Waters KA (eds): Glossary of health care terms, 1994 ed. Chicago: American Health Information Management Assoc, 1994.

Hausam RR, Balas EA: Computerized medical records: Dream or reality? No Med 1993;90(10).

Maintenance, disclosure, and rediscolosure of health information. Chicago: American Health Information Management Assoc, 1993.

McKnight J: Hospitals and the health of their communities. Hospitals and Healthcare Networks, January 5, 1994, pp 40–41.

Professional practice standards for health information management services. Acute care. Chicago: American Health Information Management Association, 1992.

Schraffenberger LA: Practice bulletin, data security. J Am Medical Record Assoc 1987.

US Department of Health and Human Services: Conditions of participation. Washington, Social Security Administration, 6/17/86.

SECTION

II

HEALTH CARE DATA

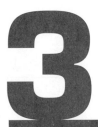

JEANETTE C. LINCK

KEY WORDS

Aggregate data
Capitation
Clinical data
Clinical data management
Data
Database
Database management system

Demographics
Fiscal intermediary
Information
Practice guidelines
Primary data
Providers
Secondary data
Socioeconomic data

ABBREVIATIONS

AHIMA—American Health Information Management Association
APA—American Psychiatric Association
ASTM—American Society of Testing and Materials
CARF—Commission on Accreditation of Rehabilitation Facilities
CPRI—Computer-Based Patient Record Institute
DHHS—Department of Health and Human Services
DRG—Diagnosis Related Group
HCFA—Health Care Financing Administration
HMO—Health maintenance organization
IOM—Institute of Medicine
JCAHO—Joint Commission on Accreditation of Healthcare Organizations
MDS—Minimum Data Set
NAHDO—National Association of Health Data Organizations
NCDB—National Cancer Data Bank
NCHS—National Center for Health Statistics
OBRA—Omnibus Reconciliation Act

PATENT AND HEALTH CARE DATA

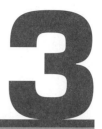

3

PRO—Peer review organization
RAI—Resident assessment instrument
UACDS—Uniform Ambulatory Care Data Set
UCDS—Uniform Clinical Data Set
UHDDS—Uniform Hospital Discharge Data Set

DEFINITIONS

Data—Data are things known or assumed; facts or figures from which conclusions can be drawn. The term data is a plural term and is used whenever more than one data element is described. Datum appropriately describes a single data element.

Information—Information is similar to data. It also includes the concept of information as data that can be stored in the computer.

Even in light of these definitions, the terms data and information should be distinguished. Data are not yet information but the raw facts and figures that are yet to be processed. When the processing is completed, the data become information. Information is data that have been manipulated in some way to make them valuable to the user.

TYPES OF DATA USED IN HEALTH CARE

Person-Specific Data

Socioeconomic Data

Socioeconomic data are those elements that describe the patient, such as the following:

- Name
- Address
- Date of birth
- Next of kin
- Race
- Sex
- Marital status
- Occupation

65

- Source of payment
- Ethnicity
- Education
- Employment

The term **demographics** is used in relationship to socioeconomic data. Demographics refers to the statistical and quantitative study of characteristics of human population.

Financial Data

Financial data refers to all types of business function elements that are required to be collected. They include billing and account data, such as charges and costs for all services received while in the facility.

Of particular significance is the expected payers (anticipated financial guarantor for services). These payers include Blue Cross, private insurance companies, Medicare or Medicaid or other governmental payers, worker's compensation, self-pay, and so on.

Patient Identification Data

Patient identification data include a personal identification number that is assigned to each patient within a health care setting. This number makes it possible to distinguish one patient from others receiving care within the facility. In addition to socioeconomic data, the admission and discharge dates of the patient are recorded. At the time of discharge, the disposition of the patient is identified (i.e., discharged to home or other health care facilities, left against advice, died).

A person's social security number may also be used to aid in identification. Except where required by law, people do not have to supply their social security numbers. The social security number is not recommended as the primary identifier for many reasons, including its ease in linkage to other, non–health care databases. However, a health care database that contains a social security number can be used to link to other approved health care data sets or to link data for health care research. The social security number can be encrypted and linked to meet the needs of researchers who want linked data but do not need to know an individual's identity.

Clinical Data

Clinical data are those elements related to the patient's health and treatment. Data are organized into a patient record that contains the following:

- History and physical examination
- Problem list

- Progress notes
- Physician's orders
- Operative reports
- Pathology reports
- Emergency services reports
- Nursing plans
- Social services evaluations
- Ancillary services reports
- Discharge summaries
- Other categories of reporting based on the provider and the services offered

The patient record is the primary source of clinical data and is used by health care practitioners, clinical support staff, and many other legitimate users. The data are collected and used for many purposes. One of the primary purposes is to support quality patient care.

During an inpatient hospitalization, all diagnoses that affect a patient's stay are collected. They include the principal diagnosis, which is the diagnosis chiefly responsible for the patient's being admitted to the facility, as well as other diagnoses that coexist at the time of admission, develop during the stay, or affect the treatment given and/or the length of stay.

In addition to diagnoses, procedural data are maintained. These data include all significant procedures. If more than one procedure is performed, one procedure is designated as principal. The principal procedure must be performed for definitive (not diagnostic) purposes or be necessary to manage a complication. In an outpatient or ambulatory care setting, health care practitioners also formulate a diagnostic statement and document services and procedures rendered to each patient. The general principle that patient care should be documented is consistent across all care settings, including mental health, long-term care, rehabilitation, occupational health, alcohol and drug abuse programs, and public health.

Clinical Data Management

Clinical data management involves all clinical data as maintained for direct care use by the health care provider and for peer review activities. Clinical data are used for performance monitoring, which uses performance indicators that affect the quality of products and services as well as the satisfaction of customers. "Customers" refers to individuals and departments both within the facility and external to it, such as the Joint Commission on Accreditation of Healthcare Organizations (JCAHO) and the health department. Clinical data are also used for research.

Individual patient, resident, or client data are collected as determined by the needs of the facility and external requirements and standards.

Aggregate Data

Aggregate data consist of a total or collection of data from the individual parts. These data, although drawn from individual records, are brought together and reported to identify trends. They also help the facility to see a "picture" of services given and identify problem areas that need correction or improvement and provide comparative statistical data. Although key people in a health care organization may have access to some databases that identify individual patients, residents, or clients, aggregate data, which is more readily accessible, serves many internal and external users. For example, it is important for an individual practitioner of care to know that his or her patient is a type II diabetic, but on a monthly, quarterly, or annual basis, a health maintenance organization (HMO) may want to know that it is serving 400 type II diabetics between ages 40 and 49.

IMPORTANT FACTORS IN DATA DEVELOPMENT AND USE

- Appropriateness—Data collected and information produced must be appropriate, meaning that data must relate to the overall needs and goals of the organization.

- Organization—Information generated must flow in an organized manner. Most areas in the health care delivery system contribute data to an organized and, one hopes, integrated information system. There *must* be standardization in data collection and information production to allow users to prepare accurate and reliable reports. Data should also be presented in a format that aids in assimilation of the information.

- Timeliness and availability—Departments that contribute data and information to the system need to know precisely what is expected and *when it is due*. These departments must know when reports are due back to them. In many instances, if information is not provided when it is needed, it need not be provided at all because it has lost its value to the organization. Many decisions are both time and data critical. Although each organization may define time in a different way, it is significant that decisions be made about how and when information must be provided to users.

- Accuracy and completeness—Accuracy refers to the correctness of the data. Without accurate and reliable data, it is difficult and often impossible to make the appropriate decisions. Because the immediate need for data may be paramount, sometimes it is necessary to sacrifice absolute accuracy and completeness when using supporting data.

- Cost-effectiveness—If the cost of collecting and disseminating the information far exceeds its value, there may be some question as to the real usefulness of the data.

DATA SETS AND DATABASES

Primary data are those obtained from the original data source. Good examples of primary data are the patient record and the daily census unit report. **Secondary data** are data sets derived from primary data, such as diagnostic and procedure indexes, cancer registries, and the JCAHO's Agenda for Change indicators.

Health care facilities, in addition to gathering data required for specific external reporting and review, must determine their own needs and collect the necessary data. In the past, health care facilities frequently collected clinical and financial data in the absence of integration between the systems. In fact, stand-alone laboratory, pharmacy, registration, billing, appointment scheduling, and order entry systems represent the early development of health information systems.

Information systems integration is essential to meet internal data needs as well as external needs such as reporting to the JCAHO, negotiating contracts in managed care systems, and meeting the needs of physicians in solo and group practices.

Data Sets

Data sets support and encourage the uniform collection and reporting of data. They have been developed for different health care settings and are used to categorize patient data using the following elements:

- Personal characteristics
- Services received
- Facilities used
- Medical staff specialties or units involved in care
- Source of payments for care

These data sets are intended to describe significant minimal data about patients, residents, or clients.

TABLE 3-1	DATA SETS
NAME	**PURPOSE**
Uniform Hospital Discharge Data Set	Uniform collection of data on inpatients; used by federal and state agencies
Uniform Ambulatory Core Data Set	Approve ability to compare data in ambulatory care settings
National Practitioner Data Bank	Data collected on malpractice payments and actions taken against physicians
Minimum Data Set for Long-Term Care	Comprehensive functional assessment of long-term care patients
National Cancer Data Bank	Designed to collect data on cancer patients and consolidate data from local registries
Uniform Clinical Data Set	Computerized data collection system used by peer review organizations
Hospital Discharge Databases	Hospital data collection systems to promote uniformity in collection and analytical techniques

Table 3–1 identifies some of the existing sets and differentiates them from one another. Chapter 4 discusses in more detail the elements contained in the data sets.

Uniform data sets permit the collection of specific data elements nationwide, making it possible to compare information about patients or residents relative to services received, personal characteristics, diagnostic or procedural information, medical staff specialties, and payment arrangements. It is important to remember, however, that although data may form the basis for patient care, additional factors are necessary for the delivery of that care.

Databases

A **database** is a collection of data that is related to a particular purpose. Therefore, the elements collected through a data set become a database. A **database management system** is a system that stores and retrieves information in the database.

In 1991, the Public Health Service branch of the U.S. Department of Health and Human Services (DHHS) produced a report titled *Healthy People 2000—National Health Promotion and Disease Prevention Objectives*. This report discusses the public health surveillance system that involves the collection, analysis, interpretation, dissemination, and use of health information. The surveillance and data systems provide information on morbidity, mortality, and disability from acute and chronic conditions. This information is used to interpret the health statistics of the population and to plan, implement, describe, and evaluate public health programs that control and prevent adverse health events. All data must be accurate, timely, available, and in a useful format.

Uniform Hospital Discharge Data Set

The Uniform Hospital Discharge Data Set (UHDDS) has been widely used for more than 20 years and is a minimum core of data for the collection of individual hospital discharge data for Medicare and Medicaid patients. Although the data set was promulgated at the federal level, it has been used as a standard in nonfederal and private sectors as well.

The UHDDS, as adopted in 1986, contains data elements for personal identification, date of birth, sex, race, ethnicity, residence, hospital identification, admission and discharge dates, physician identification, attending and operating physicians, diagnoses, procedures, disposition of patient, and expected payment source.

The UHDDS is being reviewed with a goal to improve the use of data for research and quality improvement. Included in this consideration is the addition of a unique identifier so that patients can be tracked no matter in what type of health care setting they are receiving care. Also, the number of secondary diagnoses and procedures collected will increase and neonatal identifiers will be included.

Uniform Ambulatory Care Data Set

The Uniform Ambulatory Care Data Set (UACDS) was approved in 1989 by the National Committee on Vital and Health Statistics. It was developed by the Subcommittee on Ambulatory Care Statistics and the DHHS Interagency Task Force.

Again, the purpose of this data set is to improve the capability to compare data by defining core data items. It is recommended for use in the records of all ambulatory care patients. Included are data elements related to personal identification, provider identification, and encounter data, specifically the patient's address, date of birth, sex, race, and ethnicity; the provider's address, type of practice, and profession; and the date and place of encounter, reason for encounter, diagnostic service, problem or diagnosis or assessment, therapeutic services, preventive services, disposition, expected principal source of payment, and total charges.

Minimum Data Set for Long-Term Care and Resident Assessment Protocols

When the Health Care Financing Administration (HCFA) eliminated the distinction between intermediate care and skilled-nursing facilities, it became necessary to fund all long-term care using a severity of illness (case mix) system. Case mix systems for reimbursement are valuable to government programs at both the state and the national level. They require accurate and up-to-date information. Initially, the type of data collected for long-term care was primarily financial. Because the administrators and owners of these facilities make all purchasing decisions, they were primarily interested in financial management. The Omnibus Reconciliation Act of 1987 (OBRA) shifted the focus from financial to clinical systems. OBRA regulations are intended to raise the standards in nursing facilities by shifting the emphasis to patient outcomes.

OBRA mandates comprehensive functional assessments of patients, using the Minimum Data Set (MDS) designed for long-term care. In addition, OBRA requires that attention be given to quality of care and quality of life. The statutory authority for the MDS and the Resident Assessment Instrument (RAI) is found in the Social Security Act, as amended by the OBRA. This act required the Secretary of the DHHS to specify a minimum data set of core elements to use in conducting comprehensive assessments; it further required the Secretary to designate one or more RAIs based on the MDS. The MDS forms the basis of the RAI.

The RAI requires a comprehensive assessment of each resident within 14 days of admission. A complete reassessment must be done at least once a year or after a significant change in the resident's condition. Federal requirements state that facilities must use an RAI that has been specified by the state. All state RAIs include at least HCFA's MDS, triggers, resident assessment protocols, and utilization guidelines. The resident's care plan must be evaluated and revised, if appropriate, each time an RAI comprehensive assessment is completed.

The RAI is composed of the MDS, guidelines, and assessment protocols. The MDS includes the following data:

* Resident background
* Daily pattern of activity
* Cognition
* Physical functioning
* Psychological status
* Health problems
* Specific body systems review

"Triggers," or signs and symptoms that attempt to prompt more thorough assessment, are built in. Triggers are specific resident responses for one or a combination of MDS items. The specific MDS response indicates that clinical factors are present that may or may not represent a problem. The final assessment is the basis for care planning.

ASTM E1384 Standard for the Content and Structure of the Computer-Based Patient Record

The American Society of Testing and Materials (ASTM) E1384 Standard for the Structure and Content of the Computer-Based Patient Record was developed through a consensus process. It is revised periodically by ASTM Subcommittee E31.19, which is responsible for vocabulary related to the computer-based patient record. It contains as one of its components a listing of potential data elements and their definitions. The data elements list is lengthy and designed to describe the potential breadth of the future patient record. Listings of both the recommended minimum content and the data elements not yet regularly incorporated into patient records are found in this Standard. The Standard recognizes that different users may need different views of the content of the record and that in a computer-based record system, the data elements can be presented in one view to an ophthalmologist and in a different view to the quality coordinator.

Uniform Clinical Data Set

The Uniform Clinical Data Set (UCDS) is under development by the HCFA. It is being tested by several peer review organizations (PROs). The data set requires detailed abstracting of a patient's medical history and treatment. The goal is to more readily identify cases that need physician review regarding the quality of care. In its current form, the UCDS is labor intensive. It does, however, provide a clinical database on a sample of Medicare patients. Until the UCDS can be cost-justified, it is not likely to be implemented. The HCFA and PROs appear to be refocusing their attention on studying the population of Medicare patients using the existing data available through Medicare and social security files. Once problems are identified and the existing databases are fully used, then the PROs may collect additional data using a focused study approach.

National Cancer Data Base

The National Cancer Data Base (NCDB) has grown out of a system for evaluating cancer patients developed by the American College of Surgeons (ACS). This program is designed to collect data on cancer patients and to consolidate data from local and regional registries. Data include cancer incidence, mortality, and survival. Using this data, it is possible to compare differences in cancer patients among racial and ethnic groups as well as between rural and urban groups.

From the analysis of the data, the National Cancer Data Bank publishes an Annual Review of Patient Care that describes treatment patterns for specific sites. Hospitals that participate in the program can get reports on their own performance.

In the past, there have been some concerns about the quality of data in the NCDB. Computer techniques now being used are addressing these concerns. Also, the NCDB has made a training program available to the National Tumor Registrars Association.

The NCDB provides valuable information on patterns of treatment. It is hoped that at least 80 per cent of all hospitals will eventually participate so that analysis of patient care will be truly representative.

National Practitioner Data Bank

Congress enacted legislation in 1986 to create the National Practitioner Data Bank (NPDB). The NPDB contains data on malpractice payments made and reports of actions taken against physicians, including license and privilege revocations. Reports can be made to state medical boards, hospitals, or professional societies. Hospitals are required to request a search to the NPDB before offering a physician staff membership.

This database began in 1990 and contains more than 18,000 reports, 85 per cent of which are of malpractice payments.

State-Level Hospital Discharge Databases

Because of the recognized need for data that are timely, accurate, reliable, and comparable for the population within a state, hospital databases have been developed in more than 30 states. The data collected and the requirements for reporting vary from state to state. Some discharge data systems are state-run systems, others are not. Some systems mandate participation by all hospitals in the state, others do not. Many states are cooperating and sharing information to begin to standardize this activity.

Hospital discharge data sets are the primary focus of the state-based data collections efforts. States use such tools as the Uniform Bill-92 (UB-92), the HCFA 1500 billing form for outpatient services, the UHDDS, and specially designed abstracts. The purpose of relying on billing forms to determine the data collected is to reduce the burden on the provider to supply the data. Therefore, systems that use data already being supplied for billing do not require an additional effort of data extraction by the providers. This may also mean that the state systems are not obtaining all the data they might want to collect for policy, planning, and research use.

One of the organizations that promotes uniformity in data collection and analytical techniques is the National Association of Health Data Organizations (NAHDO). The NAHDO membership includes about 100 organizations, including the American Health Information Management Association (AHIMA), as well as many individuals who are interested in the collection, dissemination, and public availability of quality data to support health care policy and research.

Registries

In addition to the data sets and databases described above, various registries have been developed and are continuing to develop nationally and statewide, including the following:

- Trauma registries
- International Implant Registry
- United Network of Organ Sharing
- Birth and death registries
- Cardiac registries
- Unique disease registries

These registries are designed to make information available to improve the quality of care and to measure the effectiveness of a specific component of the health care delivery system. Each registry has its own specific purpose, as implied by its title.

SOURCES OF DATA

There are many sources of data for the health care field. Some of these sources are within the health care setting (i.e., agency, hospital, clinic). Other sources are outside the immediate confines of a given health care setting (i.e., census data, statewide comparative data). The internal sources describe services provided and the infrastructure of the organization. Health care organizations have some of the same categories of data that would be expected in any organization (i.e., personnel, accounting, marketing, inventory, services provided). The category of primary interest for this discussion is services provided by the health care organization to patients, residents, or clients. The external data sources discussed also relate to the services component of the health care organization.

Within the health care organization, many individuals are both producers and users of data. We expect direct care providers to produce data, but a typical health care organization has many others who are also engaged in producing and using data. Because it is impossible to remember all the data generated by providing a service, the data are recorded on paper, by voice, in an image, or on a computer system.

Internal Data

The Patient, Client, or Resident

The patient, client, or resident is a primary source of data. The patient receiving the service is the source of information regarding personal medical history, family history, psychosocial history, demographic data, financial data, current illness, change in health status, compliance with recommended follow-up, medication used (prescription and nonprescription), personal health habits, satisfaction with care, and so on. The patient also provides data by contributing body fluids or tissue for analysis and by participating in various physical examinations and tests.

Most of the data are recorded by various staff of the health care organization, although some patient-recorded data is used in some settings. The data are frequently organized into reports to facilitate providing care or services. Some data are used to facilitate the payment process.

Direct Care Providers

Direct care providers (e.g., physicians, nurses, physical therapists) continue the development of the database on a patient. Physical examination, testing, and direct observation, for example, provide data about a patient's condition. Caregivers are also trained to ask questions to gather data. This information is usually assembled to formulate a plan for care.

As caregivers provide services, they record the service provided—for example, surgery or counseling. The report of the surgery or counseling session becomes part of the record to reflect the treatment provided. Caregivers also assess the patient's progress in treatment. If progress is not as anticipated, the plan is reviewed and may be revised.

All the data are assembled into various reports, including the following:

- Physical examination
- Consultation report
- Progress notes
- Flow sheets
- Physical therapy evaluation
- Nursing care plan
- Operative report
- Treatment plan
- Orders for treatment
- Medication administration reports

Caregivers are also the source of data regarding other factors related to providing services, such as how long it takes to provide a service, what resources are needed, and what could be improved in the care process.

In addition to caregivers who typically provide direct treatment services to the patient, there are ancillary personnel who may not be seen by a patient but who may generate data related to a patient's care or treatment. In a hospital or residential facility, ancillary personnel may work in the laboratory, the dietitian's office, or the blood bank. These service areas generate data that go directly into a patient's clinical record. Ancillary personnel are also a source of data on how to improve the service process.

Other Internal Sources

Other internal sources generate data related to an individual or a group, depending on the areas of activity and responsibility. The data generated are frequently structured to achieve the following goals:

- Assess the use of resources.
- Evaluate the quality of care.
- Encourage appropriate use of patient information.
- Improve the process of care.
- Monitor the revenue generated.
- Review expenses incurred in providing services.
- Account for payment received for services.

These activities are carried out in various ways, depending on the setting in which the service is provided. In a hospital or large clinic, staff are designated to be responsible for one or more of the functions listed above. Some facilities, for example, have a department assigned to carry out the utilization review or to review resource use. Another facility may make this part of a comprehensive health information management function.

General administrative activities that generate such data as staffing, planning, and inventory use can be combined with patient, resident, or client service data to take a better look at the organization and how well it functions.

The generation of useful-quality data by direct care providers, ancillary staff, and administrative staff is important in the direct service to individual patients, clients, and residents as well as the overall functioning of a health care organization.

External Data

External data are required by health care organizations. It is necessary to know your community and its needs. Most health care organizations are designed to serve a nearby geographic community. The exception might be a specialty center that serves a much wider region.

The following external data questions are often asked.

- What is the population of the community?
- Is the population increasing or decreasing?
- What is the age composition of the community?
- Which other health-related services are being provided by other health care organizations?
- What is the level of violence in the community?
- Which health status measures or indicators are in use?
- How does the community's immunization rate compare with that of other communities?
- How is care paid for in this community?
- Is the community well staffed by health care providers?
- How is quality care measured in the community?
- Are local, regional, or national standards for care available as a guide?
- Is there good continuity of care in the community, or are there major gaps in the process?
- Who are the main providers of care in the community?
- What is the organizational structure of the successful providers of care in the community?
- What are the trends in the delivery and payment of care?
- What data are available from external review sources regarding the performance of this facility or organization or staff?

The following discussion of potential external data sources is not exhaustive but provides a sample of national data sources. Communities and regions may also have data sources, such as a statewide database on hospital discharges, a state hospital association listing, and state registries for births and deaths.

American Osteopathic Association

The American Osteopathic Association (AOA) was founded in 1897 to promote public health and to maintain and improve high standards of education in osteopathic colleges. Their collection and dissemination of data are related to their role in the inspection and accreditation of colleges, hospitals, and specialty certification programs. They also collect data from physicians regarding the mandatory continuing education required of member physicians. In addition, the association compiles statistical data on the location of osteopathic physicians and the types of practices they have.

The AOA publishes an accreditation manual titled *Accreditation Requirements of the American Osteopathic Association*. This manual states the specific requirements for compliance and data collection.

American Medical Association

The American Medical Association (AMA) is the oldest and largest physician member organization. One of its primary roles is to disseminate scientific information to its members and to the public. The membership is kept informed of significant medical and health legislation at both the state and the national level, and the AMA represents the medical profession before Congress and other governmental agencies.

Data are necessary in the AMA's role in setting standards for medical schools, residency programs, and continuing education programs.

Practice guidelines have been developed that define practice parameters to help physicians make clinical decisions. By helping physicians determine what is appropriate medical care, these guidelines help to improve the quality of care. If the practice parameters are scientifically sound and clinically relevant, the AMA believes that they are the best means to ensure quality care.

Joint Commission on Accreditation of Health-care Organizations

The JCAHO includes members who represent the American College of Physicians, ACS, American Hospital Association (AHA), AMA, and the public. Its primary purpose is to establish standards and the conduct of accreditation surveys for hospitals, psychiatric facilities, substance abuse treatment facilities, organizations that provide services for the mentally retarded and developmentally disabled, long-term care facilities, hospices, and ambulatory and home care programs.

The JCAHO publishes individual manuals for different health care delivery systems. These manuals describe the standards and the data necessary for initial and continuing accreditation.

The JCAHO uses an indicator monitoring system to collect data. Quality indicators have been developed and tested for several areas of care, including obstetrics, anesthesia, cardiovascular disease, oncology, and trauma. The plan is to have accredited facilities submit detailed data to the JCAHO.

In 1994, the *Accreditation Manual for Hospitals* included a chapter on information management. This was done because the JCAHO believes that managing information resources is as important as managing a hospital's financial, human, and material resources. Areas addressed in the chapter include identifying information needs, design of the information management system, definition and capture of data, analysis and process of data into information, reporting of data, and use of data. AHIMA members helped to draft this new section.

The JCAHO, in emphasizing the requirements to document patient care, carefully details specific percentages of patient records that must comply with given standards. For example, an initial patient assessment must be found 100 per cent of the time, whereas other required documentation ranges from 91 to 100 per cent.

The information management chapter describes all the basic requirements for medical record documentation as well as systemwide information requirements. Other clinical service chapters provide information on specific record content. The JCAHO uses a tool called the "scoring guidelines" to determine compliance with published JCAHO standards.

The commission does not require a hospital to use computer technology to meet the information management standard. It does, however, indicate that integrated systems are essential. Hospitals need to gather and move data across departmental lines and be able to merge data where appropriate.

Health Care Financing Administration

The HCFA is a division of the DHHS. It has the responsibility for health care policy formulation and administers the Medicare and Medicaid programs.

In the early 1980s, the prospective payment system was established as the payment method for Medicare hospital services. This method, because it set a fixed price for a stay regardless of actual cost to the facility, played a major role in reducing hospital utilization.

The data supplied by hospitals to support the needs of the prospective payment system are essential to its effectiveness. The HCFA has compiled a major national database on Medicare patients. It is essentially a longitudinal summary record on Medicare patients. The HCFA, professional review organizations (PROs), and health care researchers are all able to use this database. For example, the HCFA reports statistical information related to its operations and periodically compares the expected versus the actual performance of providers.

American Psychiatric Association

The American Psychiatric Association (APA) was founded to further the study of the nature, treatment, and prevention of mental disorders. The organization assists in the formulation of programs to meet mental health needs and compiles and disseminates facts and figures about psychiatry. In addition, it furthers psychiatric education and research.

The APA publishes *The Diagnostic and Statistical Manual of Mental Disorders*. This statistical classification and glossary of mental disorders gives clear descriptions of diagnostic categories so that practitioners can diagnose, communicate, study, and treat mental disorders.

Commission on Accreditation of Rehabilitation Facilities

The Commission on Accreditation of Rehabilitation Facilities (CARF) is the standard-setting and accrediting authority for organizations that provide service to people with disabilities. The organization encourages the development of uniformly high standards of performance for all organizations that serve people with physical or emotional disabilities. It also surveys and accredits rehabilitation organizations and conducts research and educational activities related to standards for organizations that offer programs in comprehensive inpatient rehabilitation, spinal cord injury, chronic pain management, brain injury, outpatient rehabilitation, infant and early childhood development, vocational education, work adjustment, occupational skill training, job placement, work services, community living, psychosocial problems, alcoholism and other drug abuse, and community mental health.

An appointed 36-member board administers the accreditation program. CARF standards are published in the *Standards Manual for Rehabilitation Facilities*. CARF maintains information on accredited rehabilitation facilities.

American Hospital Association

The AHA is dedicated to promoting the welfare of the public through leadership and assistance to its members in the provision of better health services for all people. The organization carries out research and educational projects in areas such as health care administration, hospital economics, and community relations. It represents hospitals in national legislation; offers programs of institutional effectiveness review, technology assessment, and hospital administrative services to hospital personnel; conducts educational programs; and publishes topics of interest to hospitals. In addition, the AHA collects and analyzes data from hospitals. On an annual basis, the AHA conducts a survey of all hospitals and produces the *Guide to the Health Care Field*. It includes data related to organizational structure, facilities, services, bed use, financial status, personnel and medical staff, admissions, occupancy rates, and average daily census.

American College of Surgeons

The ACS was founded to improve the quality of care for surgical patients by evaluating the standards for surgical education and practice. It conducts programs to improve emergency care and hospital cancer programs. In addition, the ACS sponsors continuing education and self-assessment programs for surgeons.

The Commission on Cancer of the ACS has established standards for the approval of hospital tumor registries. Data collected in these registries are used to improve the management of cancer.

Agency for Health Care Policy and Research

The Agency for Health Care Policy and Research was established in 1989. One of its activities is the development of guidelines for the treatment of specific diseases and disorders. Clinical specialists from various practice locations participate in the development of guidelines on such topics as cataracts, benign prostatic hyperplasia, pain management, and sickle cell disease. In addition, the agency is funding medical effectiveness research. This research will, in turn, assist in the revision of the guidelines.

National Association for Ambulatory Care

The National Association for Ambulatory Care establishes standards for ambulatory care centers. Its goals are to provide lower-cost and more convenient outpatient medical care and to make the public aware of ambulatory care.

Peer Review Organizations

PROs were established through the Tax Equity and Fiscal Responsibility Act of 1982. They replaced the professional standards review organizations. The PROs monitor the activity of hospitals to verify the accuracy of diagnostic related groups (DRGs) submitted to the fiscal intermediary for reimbursement under the Medicare system. They also perform quality review and evaluate the effectiveness of the medical care provided. A variety of reviews are required in this monitoring responsibility, including admission review, day and cost outlier review, and DRG validation. The responsibilities require that data collected and disseminated be of high quality and produced on a timely basis. PROs engage in studies of the available data on their patient population to improve the quality of care. HCFA data are also available to the PROs.

National Center for Health Statistics

The National Center for Health Statistics (NCHS) is an agency of the DHHS that oversees the vital statistics data collection system in the United States. Vital statistics include birth, death, marriage, and divorce data. The department of health in each state is responsible for collecting the data. Data are then disseminated on a routine basis. The data are organized at the state level and transmitted to the federal level.

The NCHS prepares standard certificates for use in collecting the required data for live births and deaths and fetal deaths. These certificates help to standardize the data collected throughout the United States. The forms and the data collected may be modified by individual states to add data of interest at the state level. A number of states use electronic means to enter and transmit the data to the state registrar.

In addition to birth data, hospitals and funeral directors are required by law to report all deaths. The data collected permit the production of information that describes the incidence of death by age, sex, color, and so on as well as cause-specific information.

The NCHS collects data from all 50 states, the District of Columbia, Puerto Rico, the U.S. Virgin Islands, and Guam.

To gain information on the health of the population, sample surveys are used in which thousands of citizens participate. The National Health Interview Survey data are collected through personal household interviews. Other surveys include Adult Use of Tobacco, National Crime Survey, National Household Survey of Drug Abuse, and Linked Birth and Death Data Set.

Centers for Disease Control and Prevention

Although it is legally required that births and deaths be reported, only certain categories of morbidity data are required. The Centers for Disease Control and Prevention (CDC) of the PHS publishes the list of reportable diseases and receives the data collected by the states. The results are published in the CDC publication titled *Morbidity and Mortality Weekly Report*. Many diseases of significance in the United States are not included among those that must be reported. Penalties can be imposed on physicians for failure to report diseases on the required list. Physicians do not always report these conditions, however, because of the nature and implications of the reporting. For example, some physicians do not report venereal disease because they see it as an embarrassment to the patient.

Blue Cross and Blue Shield

Blue Cross and Blue Shield (BCBS) is a nationwide network of private nonprofit insurers that are locally based. This group is one of the largest insurers of hospital and medical and physician services in the United States. They serve as the **fiscal intermediary** in most states for the Medicare program.

TABLE 3-2 HEALTH CARE ORGANIZATIONS

NAME OF ORGANIZATION	PRIMARY PURPOSE	COLLECTION/DISSEMINATION OF DATA
American Osteopathic Association	High standards of education in osteopathic colleges; promote public health	Inspection/accreditation of colleges and hospitals for osteopathic physicians; requires physician continuing education; information available on location of physicians and type of practice
American Medical Association	Dissemination of scientific information to members and public; representation	Setting standards for medical schools; standards for residency programs; continuing education programs
Joint Commission on Accreditation of Healthcare Organizations	Establish standards; conduct surveys in all types of facilities	Use in preparation, conducting, and maintenance of survey process
Health Care Financing Administration	Federal agency division of Department of Health and Human Services responsible for health care policy	To determine compliance with prospective payment system requirements for Medicare/Medicaid
American Psychiatric Association	Further the study of the nature, treatment, and prevention of mental disorders	Compiles and disseminates facts and figures about psychiatry
Commission on Accreditation of Rehabilitation Facilities	Standard-setting and accrediting authority to organizations providing services to people with disabilities	Standard-setting; accreditation process; development of uniform standards
American Hospital Association	Promote welfare of the public in provision of better health services for all	Annual survey of all hospitals related to organizational structure, facilities, services, bed use, financial status, personnel, medical staff
American College of Surgeons	Promote quality care for surgical patients by evaluating standards for surgical education and practice	Data collected for tumor registries and used to improve management of cancer
Agency for Health Care Policy and Research	Branch of United States Public Health Service to support general health services research	Uses scientific base to develop practice guidelines
National Center for Health Statistics	Collection of births, deaths, marriages, divorce, national surveys	Vital statistics; data collection; dissemination to public; special and routine surveys
National Association of Ambulatory Care	Standards for care centers; provide lower cost and more convenient outpatient medical care	Data for standards on outpatient medical care centers
Centers for Disease Control	Collection of reportable disease information to protect public	Data on reportable morbidity and mortality publications
Peer review organizations	Verify accuracy of diagnostic related groups data for reimbursement	Data from admission review, day and cost outlier review, diagnostic related groups validation
Blue Cross/Blue Shield	Independent insurers that provide coverage for hospital and other services	Serves as fiscal intermediary for Medicare

In the early 1990s, the BCBS system included severity adjustment payments penalties that were probably the first reimbursement method to use quality as a factor. This severity of illness classification system is referred to as MedisGroups. Blue Cross is only one example of a third party payer that has a significant database on insured clients.

Table 3–2 is a quick reference table of the various health care organizations.

Managed Care

Although managed care may mean different things to different people, it is based on the principle of the provision of health care services after formal enrollment through one point where there is emphasis on prevention, accessibility, and comprehensive primary care, with reduced inappropriate use and costs. Managed care takes many forms and functions. There are multiple sources of data in managed care. The managed care environment has a great need for the exchange of information electronically because of the need to process claims, determine eligibility, preauthorize, conduct utilization review, manage services, and provide coordinated quality care.

Health Maintenance Organizations

The HMOs are an example of managed care. An HMO is responsible for providing comprehensive services for a prepaid fixed fee. Revenue is based on **capitation,** which means that there is an annual fee, intended to cover all services for the year, for each person enrolled in the HMO. This capitation fee is paid by the federal government for Medicare enrollees, the state for Medicaid patients, and employers or the enrollees themselves. The financial arrangement between enrollees and providers of service is not known to the members who pay their annual premium to the HMO. The HMO assumes all financial risk for services provided so the HMO must know and trust the providers. HMOs must be federally qualified or meet the definition a state has determined for HMOs. Nearly two thirds of all HMOs are for profit, but many of the largest are nonprofit (e.g., Kaiser Permanente, BCBS, Cigna).

Physician profiles for cost containment are developed by HMOs and insurers. Because they do not usually make adjustments for case mix differences, physicians with an unusually high number of chronically ill patients lose when the reimbursement system, like capitation, is based on averages. The Ambulatory Care Group Case Mix Management System is a software package that evaluates a physician in relation to the sickness of the patient population served. This system makes it possible to track the utilization of physicians in managed care settings. The system can look at the mix of patients and the severity of their conditions as treated over a period of time. The information then helps to determine the need for service.

Preferred Provider Organizations

Preferred provider organizations (PPOs) direct a volume of patients to a provider for a reduced fee. Data from the American Managed Care and Review Association indicated that in 1991, there were more than 800 PPOs covering people in 44 states. Most of the PPOs are for profit. PPOs are demonstrating that these organizations have been able to control costs and enhance quality.

Because of the nature of managed care, HMOs and PPOs try to get physicians to act in specific ways through financial and nonfinancial incentives. About one half of all managed care plans are using guidelines for productivity and clinical treatment. Current guidelines frequently relate to productivity data, such as how many patients are seen, how many tests are performed, and how many hospital days are used. Now the focus is shifting to quality of care. Major managed care systems are attempting to track compliance with process-of-care indicators and standards that involve such things as childhood immunizations, breast and cervical cancer screening, and rates of hospitalization (i.e., for children with asthma). The current focus is more on the "process" of care (i.e., "Was a mammogram done on all women between certain ages within the correct time window?").

The current primary source for these data is the patient bill. As more clinical data become available electronically and well defined for comparability, the system can better monitor the quality of care.

The National Commission on Quality Assurance in Washington, D.C., is actively working with the managed care groups to consistently define measures that can be applied to the process and quality of patient care. Because many health care facilities develop their own guidelines to collect and disseminate data on the process and quality of care, integrated information management systems are needed that cross departments, make record keeping easier, and notify physicians of applicable guidelines.

USE AND USERS OF DATA

Data are kept for various purposes and uses. Requests for data come from multiple sources. Each new day brings innovative requests for data, and decisions have to be made regarding the appropriate use of data.

Health Care Providers

The term health care **providers** is broad-based. It includes organizations that deliver health care services, such as hospitals, outpatient clinics, long-term care facilities, home care agencies, and hospices. Providers also can be individual practitioners, such as physicians, nurses, technicians, and other professional personnel. Data form the record of the provision of services. Health care providers use data to evaluate, monitor the use of resources, and get paid for services provided.

Communication and Continuity of Care

During the time the patient is receiving health care services, it is necessary for providers to maintain ongoing accuracy and a timely level of communication. No provider can be present 24 hours a day, and the recorded data are essential in the continuity of the care being given. Documentation makes it possible to assess this continuity.

This communication assists in supporting decisions made about the diagnosis and treatment of patients and in assessing and managing risk for individual patients. For example, it can remind providers of laboratory results and provide alerts regarding possible drug interactions.

If care is to be continued elsewhere, health information can be transferred to the new provider so care can resume immediately.

Reimbursement

Data are the basis of claims processing to pay for the services received. Payers include private insurance companies, HMOs, and fiscal intermediaries who process claims for Medicare and Medicaid. Because the purpose of health data is to document the course of illness and treatment, the data become the basis for determining the payment to be made. Although capitated care may change the current billing systems, payers still want to know the services provided for the dollar spent. Even if transaction-based bills as we know them today disappear, data will be needed to document services provided.

Billing data are currently the basis for reporting and managing costs of care.

Education

Within the health care setting, there are many people who are learning the skills of quality health care services delivery. They include physicians, nurses, mental health specialists, and ancillary service personnel. Data documentation assists these people in tying the theory learned in the classroom to the practical aspects of care.

Conferences and presentations about care already delivered are useful in training health care personnel. Data from the patient, resident, or client record are the basis for many educational programs and conferences that review treatment outcomes.

Quality of Care

It is essential that the delivery of health care be monitored retrospectively and continually. The basis for these reviews and the performance of quality assessment are the data recorded at the time care is given.

Utilization

Health care data include descriptions of care given and the justification for services. All organizational resources, including supplies, equipment, services, and providers, can be taken into consideration in utilization review. Criteria are available for some facets of the utilization review process, such as admission, continued stay, and discharge from an inpatient facility.

Compliance with Accreditation Standards

Review agencies require data that demonstrate compliance with accreditation standards for specific types of facilities. The data serve as evidence in assessing compliance with standards of care and in accrediting various health care organizations.

Research

Clinical research is a significant aspect of the improvement of care and assessment of the effectiveness of treatment, early disease detection, and improved methodology for future care.

Research may also study the cost-effectiveness of patient care, review patient outcomes, and assess the use of technology. Health services research and policy studies provide information regarding the health care system.

Planning

Data are the basis for supporting the ongoing need for services and the addition of new services by a health care organization. Health care delivery is a dynamic process that requires the evaluation of current needs and future demands for the individual provider and the community in general.

Payers

Health care data are used to substantiate the care given. Whatever is billed must be documented in the patient record. Payers for government insurance plans (i.e., Medicare and Medicaid) also actively monitor the appropriateness of the care and services given to a patient.

Social Users, Public Health Agencies, and Medical and Social Research

To protect and best serve the public in need of health services, agencies must be able to monitor the causes and prevalence of specific disease entities. Data are the basis for investigating the patterns of diseases and the effects of disease on the daily lives of individuals. As a result of the data, specific programs can be developed, assessed, and evaluated for a given community. Plans for future needs can be designed and implemented based on community data.

Employers

Health care data are used to evaluate and assess job-related conditions and injuries and to determine occupational hazards that may impede effective performance in the workplace.

Employers also use the data to determine the extent of employee disabilities and to improve working conditions.

Governmental Agencies

Governmental agencies at the local, state, and federal levels use health care data to determine the appropriate use of governmental financial resources for schools, health care facilities, and educational institutions. This review is done on an ongoing and retrospective basis. It is also important that an attempt be made to determine health care needs at all levels.

Judicial Process

Health care data are often the basis of evidence for the adjudication of both civil and criminal cases. The documentation supports the claims made by the individuals in a case and is often the only evidence available. In addition, data may aid in supporting the need for admission of the mentally ill for treatment.

Media

The media report data that are necessary for the public to know, such as health hazards, diseases that affect public health, and new developments in medical research.

Patients

Patients use their medical data to understand their health care and to become more active participants in maintaining or improving their health. Data can also be used in monitoring care when additional treatment is necessary. For example, patients with diabetes or hypertension can make a difference by actively participating

in controlling and monitoring their condition. Data are also used by patients to document the services received, to serve as proof of identity, and to verify billed services.

ORGANIZING AND PRESENTING INFORMATION

The presentation of information can take many forms and can use various media. The significant factor is that the information as produced is accurate, timely, and useful and increases the user's knowledge. Whether the system is manual or electronic, the data must be collected, manipulated, and then presented. Interpretation may be part of the presentation or the next step in the process.

Data originate from a source. This chapter has already included various sources of data, including individuals, such as the physician and patient, and organizations, such as the JCAHO. The data may be in the patient's record (a primary source) or in secondary locations (indexes or registers) that result from the data being drawn or abstracted from a primary source.

Manipulation and aggregation of data follow the collection of the data. At this point, the data are processed. This involves classifying, sorting, sequencing, merging, calculating, comparing, and so on. In a manual system, this may be paper-and-pencil worksheets or tallies. With electronic resources, application packages such as spreadsheets and databases make this task infinitely more manageable.

Presentation refers to provision of the output or information to the user. The presentation usually takes the form of various reports, tables, charts, and graphs used by individuals and groups at all levels within the health care delivery system.

Most health care organizations have some form of electronic database. This assists dramatically in the preparation and presentation of data. Once in electronic form, the data can be presented in a variety of ways.

System integration is essential to meeting the need for accuracy, timeliness, usefulness, and cost-efficiency of data in health care organizations.

Efforts to Organize and Standardize Data Systems

Workgroup on Electronic Data Interchange

In 1991, the Secretary of DHHS convened a group of leaders to discuss the administrative costs of health care.

The primary goal was to find a way to reduce the costs associated with the billing process. Even though standardized bills such as the UB-92 are used, payers are still able to set their own requirements for data needed to pay a bill. This results in a complex set of requirements unique to each payer that affect the billing form and frequently require providers to attach documents such as the operative report to the bill in order to be paid.

Participants in the workgroup recommended that all billings be done electronically. Bills can be sent from the providers to the payers in electronic form, reducing the paperwork and, one hopes, reducing the administrative costs of providing and paying for care. Payers need to reduce the volume of requests for additional data and attachments to make significant gains in reducing the costs associated with billing. As health care moves toward a capitated system, the purpose of the data will be to track the services provided rather than closely monitor the billed services against the plan's coverage.

Electronic Data Exchange

Groups working to create standards to facilitate the electronic exchange of data or messages in the health care field include ASTM, IEEE, X12N, HL7, and ACR-NEMA. These standards development organizations are working together on various aspects of the transfer of data. Both intrafacility and interfacility message standards are being developed cooperatively. In addition to "message" standards that facilitate the exchange of data, standards groups are working on data models, the content of the computer-based patient record, and data security. The American National Standards Institute (ANSI) serves as a coordinating body for United States standards. The ANSI does not develop standards, but it may encourage a standards organization to develop a needed standard, and standards groups from other countries look to ANSI to identify the United States standard on any given topic.

A few years ago, the standards group HL7, for Health Level 7, tackled the problem of multiple systems within an organization that did not "speak" to one another. Many health care organizations have existing systems that need to interface. Using the HL7 standard makes interface possible. As health care organizations request information from vendors on system capabilities, they also request information on their use of HL7 as a standard.

X12 standards are commonly used now for billing and related purposes, such as verification of coverage. X12N, the insurance subgroup, HL7, ASTM, IEEE, and ACR-NEMA are all cooperating in the development of standards for electronic data exchange.

AHIMA members participate in the voluntary standards process in HL7, ASTM, ANSI, and so on. The process is open, consensus-based, and structured to encourage participation from a variety of sources. Any interested person is welcome.

The Computer-Based Patient Record Institute (CPRI), an initiate of AHIMA, is organized for and dedicated to promoting the use of computer-based patient records. The work of this group assists health information management professionals in moving from the paper to the computerized health record. CPRI also encourages the development and implementation of standards for computer-based patient records.

QUALITY OF DATA

To assist in ensuring quality data, policies and procedures must be in place for each step in the process of data collection, manipulation, and dissemination. Because each step in the information processing cycle brings with it the possibility for error, properly developed procedures give direction to the actions of the individual in the data collection environment.

Quality standards need to be established for each aspect of the process and then evaluated for their reliability and validity. The standard, or measure, then becomes the means of ensuring that the performance is acceptable. The consequences of failure to meet the standard need to be promulgated and understood.

Data quality is essential in any system, whether it is manual or computerized. Errors can occur at data entry or in the manipulation, retrieval, and dissemination of data.

The following guidelines appeared in the *Journal of the American Medical Record Association* (now the *Journal of the American Health Information Management Association*) in February 1983. Written by Kathryn Sheehy, RRA, as part of a data quality action plan, they emphasize the importance of developing a method to plan and evaluate quality within an information system.

1. Analyze the information flow. Look for methods to improve timeliness.
2. Establish quality standards for the data collected.
3. Conduct in-service programs to train health care personnel and medical staff on data requirements, data definitions, and collection standards.
4. Conduct ongoing data quality monitors, using expert computer systems whenever possible.
5. Provide feedback based on performances and adherence to the data quality committee, hospital personnel, and medical staff.
6. Conduct ongoing educational programs on data quality.

Controls

Controls are important and should be in place throughout the cycle from data collection through dissemination. These controls need to be capable of detecting obvious errors, of locating errors, and of (at some point in time) correcting errors.

Checks on the validity of data can be built into the system. When only certain data values are valid, the validity check detects invalid data errors. For example, if the only valid values are 1, 2, 3, and 4, a value of 8 is quickly detected as an error. When entering coded data, error detection methods can determine that an entered code is incorrect or does not fit the definition. For example, if a field requires five digits and only four digits are entered, an error message is triggered.

Checks of reasonableness can also assist in error detection. Reasonableness might refer to the detection of an error in a value that is completely unreasonable in specific circumstances—for example, laboratory values so low that they would not result no matter who was being treated.

Error location refers to identifying locations in a system where errors might occur. For example, errors might happen during input, manipulation, and output. Once a location is identified, then the cause of the error can be found and addressed.

In recent years, the health care industry began studying and implementing the principles of total quality management. The major principles of this method are that everyone in the organization is committed and responsible for quality improvement and that quality is expressed in terms of the customer and the customer's needs. Everyone must believe that there is always room for improvement and that everyone is important in the improvement process. Motivation of employees is a key, and it becomes the responsibility of top management to be fully involved and committed to total quality management. This method is not an easy, quick fix; it is a way of approaching work that highly values quality work from each person in the organization. Quality is based on meeting the needs of the customer. If the needs of the customer are not met and the customer is not satisfied, then the benefits of a quality product are limited. Health care organizations have more than one customer. The primary customer is the patient.

CONFIDENTIALITY

Confidentiality of health information has always been a major concern of those involved with managing health information. The AHIMA has developed several position statements relative to confidentiality and privacy. These documents have clearly identified concerns and recommended policies and procedures for the protection of the patient's privacy. In December 1993, the following position statements were presented:

- Disclosure of health information
- Redisclosure of health information
- Disclosure of health information relating to adoption
- Disclosure of health information relating to alcohol and drug abuse

In the position statement titled "Issue: Disclosure of Health Information," the term confidential is defined as "any information that derives from a clinical relationship between patients and healthcare professionals. Confidential includes, but is not limited to, all clinical data and the patient's address on discharge."

Today, with the advent of multiple databases maintained in various health care settings, new challenges are presented to health information management (HIM) professionals, who must strive to develop systems that facilitate information flow and protect the confidentiality of the data.

The databases described in this chapter contain many data elements about patients, including patient identification data. Although many of the larger systems have security mechanisms, others are maintained in smaller systems like personal computers. Users are not always careful about protecting passwords.

Some data are maintained by organizations who are not legally bound by a specific law to protect the information. For example, the Medical Information Bureau is a for-profit organization that receives personal health data on individuals through its relation with member insurance companies.

Computer networks may also make it possible to access information directly. The current formal request, authorization, and disclosure process needs to be adapted to a computerized environment. As recently as early 1995, no comprehensive national legislation protected the confidentiality of patient health information. Although state laws do address this issue, they vary from comprehensive protection to limited protection. The AHIMA has developed model national legislation referred to as the Fair Health Information Act. The model legislation has been revised to address the concerns of a broad constituency and has sponsorship and support.

The increase in the use of technology and in the ease of information transfer for multiple uses without the need for human interaction raises new issues for health information management. In addition, there is increased and widespread access to information through the use of data networks. Some networks are local, others cover a wide area. The use of E-mail and Internet also poses new challenges. Examples of using "deleted" E-mail for audits and to settle lawsuits are emerging. Internet and E-mail, even when thought secure, are still showing signs of security breaches.

An Institute of Medicine (IOM) report in 1991 recommended the use of the computer-based patient record to improve care and the management of data, and in 1994, the Institute recognized the growing interest in the possibility of health data organizations serving as community health care information data brokers. The IOM also noted that the potential development of health data organizations should give added impetus for legislation such as the Fair Health Information Act. The information in health data organizations and networks will be accessible to a variety of users, including payers, providers, employers, and consumers.

All of these factors create concerns relative to the protection of confidentiality when information is in a more open communication environment. This responsibility begins with the health care providers and extends to all who have access to an individual's health information. Confidentiality must be an essential element in the design of systems, policies, and procedures. Users must be educated and committed to appropriate uses of information. Contracts with service organizations must recognize their responsibilities.

Internal measures might include limiting access by job classification and by requiring the use of individual passwords. Strictly enforced policies related to disclosure should be in place. Individuals should be permitted to access only the data they need to fulfill their responsibilities. The system should include the capability of tracking access of users. There should be a restriction on the use of data-copying functions and a plan to control viruses.

Computer security policies and procedures should include the requirement for written confidentiality statements by employees. The medical staff need to be educated regarding information system confidentiality and data security procedures.

AHIMA's position, as stated in the *Position Statement on the Disclosure of Health Information,* is as follows:

Health records (regardless of the media in which they are maintained) are the property of the healthcare provider, but the health information contained in the records belongs to the patient. Disclosure of health information must be done prudently to protect the patient's right to privacy.

Each healthcare facility must develop policies and procedures for disclosure of health information in accordance with federal and state laws. To assure consistent compliance with these policies and procedures, disclosure of health information should be made only by those appropriately trained and qualified to do so. AHIMA recommends that the responsibility for disclosure of health information be centralized under the direction of the facility's health information management professional. Employees responsible for information disclosure must be carefully trained and supervised to ensure their consistent compliance with the facility's policies.

PATIENT CARE

Today, health care delivery involves large networks of services, including hospitals, physicians' offices, and many types of ambulatory and home care services. This type of health care system requires integrated patient-centered information systems.

The patient-centered approach requires the planning of a system that brings together health care practitioners and community members who are involved with or concerned about health care. The patients' (customers') needs must be determined so that a system that meets their needs can be planned. Patients will probably be able to access information of all types from their home computers. In the future, it will probably be possible to make an appointment for care, review the potential adverse effects of the medication prescribed, and learn more about a disease by using a home computer. Information systems for prevention and patient care need to include the patient and be designed with patients in mind.

ROLE OF HEALTH INFORMATION MANAGEMENT

Every health care facility needs an HIM department or service that is prepared to provide appropriate systems and methods using the data that are important in patient care, administrative functions, planning for future needs, and focusing on quality care. The systems may be paper-based or computerized.

Decisions relative to patient care and financial reimbursement depend on the information in the patient, resident, or client record. Therefore, it is necessary that this information be complete and accurate.

The HIM professional is helping to lead the change from the paper-based record to the computerized HIM system. Clinical data management responsibilities are now paramount. Today's systems require the HIM professional to be knowledgeable about the needs of the clinical staff, patient accounts staff, financial managers, and others on the administrative team. Understanding health data collection, use, and interpretation fundamentals while also appreciating the importance of confidentiality allows the HIM professional to play a key role in the ongoing change process in health care.

Key Concepts

- Data are facts and figures from which conclusions can be drawn. There are a variety of data types. Primary medical data are original data resulting from patient care data whereas secondary data are data sets collected from the primary source and used for a variety of purposes.

- Data must be appropriate, organized, timely, accurate, and cost effective. While both clinical and financial data are collected by health care facilities, an essential aspect of this collection is the integration of data.

- Data sets have been developed to permit uniform collection and reporting. They categorize patients using such elements as personal characteristics, services received, facilities used, sources of payment.

- Data are collected for both internal and external purposes. The data collected must be of high quality and disseminated in a timely way. In addition, users need specific data to meet individual and organizational needs. Significant uses include communication and continuity of care, reimbursement, education, planning, quality/utilization of services.

- Since an essential aspect of data is quality, it is important that standards be established to assure this quality in either a manual or computerized system.

- The AHIMA has played a major role in the establishment of standards to protect the confidentiality of health care data. Position statements have been presented that identify concerns and recommended policies and procedures for the protection of a patient's privacy.

Bibliography

American Health Information Management Association: Position statement. Issue: Disclosure of health information. J Am Health Information Management Assoc 1993;64(12).

American Medical Record Association: Confidentiality of patient health information. A position statement. J Am Med Record Assoc 1985;5.

Barbetta MA: The implementation of a trauma registry in an acute care hospital. J Am Health Information Management Assoc 1992;63 (2): 50–54.

Bergman R: New system helps evaluate utilization. Hospitals and Health Networks, November 5, 1993, p 50.

Bock WH, Kane RL: Computerized clinical information for nursing homes: Selection criteria. Nursing Homes and Senior Citizen Care, May-June 1991, p 19.

Boester CM: What is this thing called managed care? J Am Health Information Management Assoc 1993;64(7):60–65.

Brandt M: Confidentiality today: Where do we stand? J Am Health Information Management Assoc 1993;62(12):59–61.

Bridgman S: HL7 looks beyond hospital walls. Computers in Healthcare, November 1992, p 13.

Broccolo BM, Fulton DK, Waller AA: The electronic future of health information: Strategies for copies with a brave new world. J Am Health Information Management Assoc 1993;64(12):38–40.

Burek DM: Encyclopedia of associations, 27th ed, vol 1, pt 2. Detroit: Gale Research, 1993.

Canright C, Arges G: Electronic data interchange. A guide for health care institutions. Chicago: American Hospital Association, 1993.

Cofer J: JCAHO focus on record content. Medical Record Briefing 1993;8(10):3–4.

Coley MB: Secondary data usage [editorial]. J Am Health Information Management Assoc 1992;63(4):31.

DePorter J: Hospital use of billing data for quality improvement. J Am Health Information Assoc 1992;63(4):46–48.

Epstein MH: Guest alliance: Use of state-level hospital discharge databases. J Am Health Information Management Assoc 1992; 63(4):32.

Fry JP, Young RW: The strategy control system. Healthcare Data Source Book. Chicago: American Hospital Association, 1992, pp 11–18.

Gallo JJ, Katz P, Levenson SA, et al: Can the new rules really improve nursing homes? Patient Care November 30, 1991, p 57.

Garfinkel L: The National Cancer Data Base: A cancer treatment resource. CA Cancer J Clin 1993;43:69.

Hard R, London J, Fischer W, et al: Three hospitals link clinical, financial data. Hospitals 1992;66:52.

Hudson T: Revolutionary aspects of regulations gives HMOs more latitude. Hospitals and Health Networks, November 5, 1993, p 54.

Huffman E: Information systems in health care. Medical record management, 9th ed. Berwyn, IL: Physicians Record Co, 1990, pp 579–582.

Kennedy BJ, Menk HR, Steele GD, et al: National Cancer Data Base: A clinical assessment of patients with cancer. CA Cancer J Clin 1992;69:276.

Kovner AR, Steven J: Population data for health and health care. In Health care delivery in the United States, 4th ed. New York: Springer, 1990, pp 35–44.

Lips E: HL7. J Am Health Information Management Assoc 1993;63 (8):45–46.

Mangano JJ: Utilization, quality, and risk management. In Health information management. Los Angeles: Practice Management Information Corp, 1993, pp 151–153.

McIlrath S: Next in Medicare Review—UCDS; PRO officials pushing for new data system. American Medical News, May 13, 1991, p 3.

Mullan F, Politzer RM, Lewis CT, et al: The National Practitioner Data Bank: Report from the first year. JAMA 1992;28:73.

Nichols DG: Millions to benefit from the Safe Medical Devices Act (SMDA) of 1990. J Am Health Information Management Assoc 1992;63(2):60–62.

Oberman L: Dishing the data: Joint Commission to detail performance of health facilities. American Medical News, June 14, 1992, p 2.

Palmer L: Moving toward electronic data interchange. For the Record 1993;6(7):6–8.

Sandrick K: Out in front—managed care helps push clinical guidelines forward. Hospitals 1993;67:30–31.

Schmitz H: Managing health care resources. Rockville, MD: Aspen Publishers, 1987.

Shackelford S: The importance of perceptions in successful implementation of total quality management. J Am Health Information Management Assoc 1993;64(3):73–75.

Simmons GE: The Uniform Clinical Data Set: An update. J Am Health Information Management Assoc 1992;63(4):51.

Skok R: Patient-centered information systems planning. J Am Health Information Management Assoc 1993;64(1):54–56.

Skurka M: Introduction. Health information management in hospitals. Chicago: American Hospital Association, 1994, pp 1–3.

VanMatre JG: The D*A*T approach to total quality management. J Am Health Information Management Assoc 1992;63(11):38–44.

Wear PK: Pam's packet: The computer-based patient record—secondary records and "what should you be doing?" J Am Health Information Management Assoc 1992;63(4):9.

Woodson TE: Integrated data management. J Am Health Information Management Assoc 1992;63(6):41–45.

4

MARY SPIVEY

KEY WORDS

Bottleneck	Encounter
Database	Graphical user interface
Data item encryption	(GUI)
Data set	Input device
Electronic data inter-	Input validation
change (EDI)	On-line

DATA COLLECTION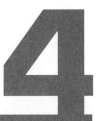

Practitioner   Transaction
Provider   Validity
Record   View
Scanning

ABBREVIATIONS

AAAHC—Accreditation Association for Ambulatory Health Care
AHIMA—American Health Information Management Association
AOA—American Osteopathic Association
ASTM—American Society for Testing and Materials
CARF—Commission on Accreditation of Rehabilitation Facilities
CPR—Computer-based patient record
EDI—Electronic data interchange
GUI—Graphical user interface
HCFA—Health Care Financing Administration
JCAHO—Joint Commission on Accreditation of Healthcare Organizations
LTCDS—Long Term Care Data Set
MDS—Minimum data set
MICR—Magnetic ink character reader
NCVHS—National Committee on Vital and Health Statistics
OCR—Optical character reader
PCP—Patient care plan
POMR—Problem-oriented medical record
PPR—Paper-based patient record
UACDS—Uniform Ambulatory Care Data Set
UHDDS—Uniform Hospital Discharge Data Set
UPIN—Universal personal identification number

OBJECTIVES

- Define key words.
- Identify the steps in the management decision-making process with particular attention to step two, the collection of data.
- Describe the users of health care data and the importance of addressing the needs of each.
- Discuss the importance of consistency and compatibility in data collection both within an institution and across the health care delivery system.
- Explain ASTM E 1384 and its relation to the computer-based patient record and data collection.
- Describe the concept of a universal personal identification number (UPIN) as the number that uniquely identifies the patient, provider, or practitioner, including encryption of the patient's UPIN.
- Identify the major minimum data sets, their scope, and special features.
- Identify the values and uses of uniform data sets.
- Explain the major data input technologies, including their applications, strengths, and weaknesses.
- Explain event and data validation checks and the use and value of each method.
- Describe the general principles of forms and views design.
- Identify the basic forms and format of the paper-based patient record.
- Compare and contrast the records for ambulatory care, acute care, long-term care and rehabilitation, home care, hospice, and mental health care.
- Describe the role of the health information manager in data collection.

The patient record is the centerpiece of the health care decision-making process. In either electronic or paper form, it contains the essential data, or raw facts and figures, related to the who, what, when, where, why, and how of patient care.

- Who is the patient and who is the provider?
- What services were provided and at what cost?
- When were the services provided?
- Where were the services provided?
- Why were the services provided, or what was the justification for services?
- How effective were the services, or what was the outcome?

Used in every setting in which care is provided, the patient record is the *essential* resource for clinical and administrative decisions.

Effective decision making proceeds through the following steps:

1. Problem identification
2. Data collection
3. Development of alternatives
4. Selection of the best alternative
5. Action
6. Follow-up and evaluation

Data collection is not an isolated function. It has a significant impact on both the efficiency and the effectiveness of the decision-making process. Well-defined and accurately collected data enhance the likelihood of an effective decision but do not guarantee it.

To be efficient, health information management (HIM) professionals must carefully consider the purposes for data collection and gather sufficient data items but no more than required. Significant costs are associated with data collection, including staff time for entry, review, and management as well as computer time and storage. Cost-effectiveness requires resistance of the more-is-better philosophy. The only reason to collect data is to satisfy an identified need for the retention, retrieval, and use of data. Once the essential data items are identified, it is generally agreed that data should be captured only once and used by all portions of the system that require knowledge of that particular data item.

DRIVING FORCES FOR DATA COLLECTION

There are several key uses for the patient record, including the following:

- Communication among **providers**
- Validation of accreditation and licensure decisions as well as legal actions
- Reimbursement for services and assessment of financial viability
- Education of professionals
- Evaluation of quality of care

Taken together, these uses should remind the health information manager that patient care is the fundamental purpose for committing resources to data collection and management. Health care providers enter data to document the care they have provided. They also refer to the care documented by others. This communication network reaches across a wide variety of care settings as well as throughout the patient's life span.

Accrediting and licensing agencies measure performance against standards. Accrediting bodies review for optimal achievable performance and include the Joint Commission on Accreditation of Healthcare Organizations (JCAHO), American Osteopathic Association (AOA), Accreditation Association for Ambulatory Health Care (AAAHC), and Commission on Accreditation of Rehabilitation Facilities (CARF). Licensure is a government function that focuses on minimal essential standards. Accrediting bodies and licensing agencies refer to the patient record to assess performance against their standards and regulations. Patients and providers who are involved in legal proceedings may require records to defend their claims or actions brought against them. The patient record is also an important resource for the facility's risk management program.

Federal agencies refer to the patient record to assess compliance with the *Conditions of Participation* (i.e., Medicare and Medicaid). Regulations and national recommendations detailing minimum **data sets** that are defined to promote consistent collection and reporting have a profound effect on data collection. They include the Uniform Hospital Discharge Data Set (UHDDS), Uniform Ambulatory Care Data Set (UACDS), and Long Term Care Data Set (LTCDS). Legislation is another source of content directives (i.e., advanced directives, patient rights acknowledgment). In addition to licensure, state agencies frequently require the collection of data, particularly data related to vital statistics and the reporting of communicable diseases. It is essential for the health information manager to stay abreast of legislative changes that impact data collection strategies.

Data collection is also part of the management of the health care facility, playing a role in utilization management, reimbursement, and assessment of financial viability. Continuing education and research rely on the patient record, as does the education of new professionals. Lastly, and supporting all the other uses, the evaluation of performance relies on the patient record as a core resource of continuous quality improvement.

The wide variety of uses for the patient record and related requirements provide the HIM manager with the challenge of collecting the necessary data to support and promote the efficiency and effectiveness on behalf of the patient, the provider, and the facility. Each of these constituencies benefits from the reliability and validity promoted by consistent definitions of data elements. Such definitions aid in facilitating data exchange and reducing misunderstandings. Standards are at the heart of a consistent data collection plan that supports the needs of individuals, organizations, and the health care delivery system at large.

Data Represent Health Care Activities

The data collected, organized, evaluated, and interpreted in health care are usually derived from a health care activity. Today's health care environment is filled with a wide variety of health care providers and **practitioners** who offer numerous services in an array of settings. The data associated with the health care process are documented to record what is happening in each environment. Some portions of the activity are administrative, some are clinical, and others are evaluative or analytic.

Often the data from like or similar activities are placed together (i.e., computer screen formats, paper forms). In the paper-based patient record (PPR), forms are created to allow documentation of similar activities on one form or a related series of forms. For example, inpatient nursing activities may be recorded in one section of the record on a series of related forms. As the activities of care and the methods for delivering care change, the forms are redesigned. Once recorded on paper, the data are static and cannot easily be reorganized or integrated with other data. Data entered using the computer screen format can be manipulated and reorganized.

If you conceptualize the data required to describe the activities of health care as data elements not tied to a paper form, you can begin to think of the patient data as a **database.** A database must be well organized and contain all the data elements necessary to describe the health care process. It is much more flexible in the ways data can be organized, reorganized, and retrieved to give various **views** of the data or to show trends. For example, the data, or view, needed by admitting staff is not the same view as that needed by the laboratory staff to carry out their responsibilities. A clinician may want to see the trend of blood glucose test results from the past 3 days mapped to insulin dose, meals, and activity. A database can extract and reorganize the data to provide this view both as raw data and as a graph.

Major effort is being invested in developing data models for health care. The natural result of these data models is the databases needed to describe and carry out health care activities. One of the major components is the computer-based patient record (CPR). This **record** in its final evolution is a sophisticated database. To help arrive at the CPR, those in the field must agree on definitions of terms and content. Although it is possible to create crosswalks between systems and to use alternate or alias terms, it is still essential that there is basic agreement on content definitions. For example, if HIM professionals are exchanging authorized data on a patient and the request is for "Medical Alerts—Allergy Section," then the data to be transferred should be retrievable and translatable into a message standard format, but most important, the *content must be any known allergies to medication, food, or other substances* for this patient.

The American Health Information Management Association (AHIMA) has published guides on the content of patient records and professional practice standards for a number of clinical settings. It also has supported the formal development of voluntary standards for CPRs by working with the American Society for Testing and Materials (ASTM), a national standards development body. The ASTM was formed more than 90 years ago to develop industrial standards. More recently, a section of ASTM has developed in health care informatics. Several committees are in place, including E 31.12 Computer-Based Patient Records, E 31.19 Vocabulary for CBPR Content and Structure, E 31.17 Privacy, Confidentiality and Access, E 31.19 Health Data Cards, and E 31.20 Authentication of Health Information.

An ASTM standard is a published guide that defines

and describes how business processes and/or data are to be managed consistently. The standard may specify how a computer application should be designed or how data elements are to be defined. Standards are also written as guides—for example, a guide for a software development process. Standards offer models for adoption and, in some cases, a specific blueprint to be followed.

As with JCAHO standards, ASTM standards are voluntary. They are developed through a consensus process and improved through feedback from users. Reviews are conducted frequently to verify the validity of published standards. In 1991, the ASTM published a standard (E 1384) as a guide to the content and format of a CPR. This standard was revised in 1995. It is presented in this text to help the reader conceptualize the patient record as a database within which all users would agree on data definitions. The data elements contained in the standard are based on research of the common data sets of interest in health care (e.g., UHDDS, UACDS) and on new or missing elements needed to fully describe the health record of a person over a lifetime. With universal content definitions, the content of data transferred between two facilities is clear, even if one of the facilities uses an alias term. An alias term would translate back into the formal term and definition. For example, if the formal term is "patient identifier (number)," a facility could choose to call the patient identifier a "medical record number." "Medical record number" would then be an alias term for "patient identifier." The electronic exchange of data, or **electronic data interchange (EDI),** at a meaningful content level requires the use of common data definitions.

Portions of ASTM standard E 1384 are presented for discussion. A current version of the full standard is available through ASTM (1916 Race Street, Philadelphia, PA 19103-1187).

Data Standards

The AHIMA has long been in the forefront of advocacy for the development and evolution of standards in record content, format, and nomenclature and in classification systems. It has continued this tradition by taking a leadership role in supporting the transition from the PPR to the CPR, including the recommendation of comprehensive federal legislation permitting the creation, authentication, and retention of health information in an electronic format. Specifically, the AHIMA has participated in developing the ASTM standards, which are specifically designed to facilitate the creation of electronic patient records. The ASTM, along with other standards organizations (HL7, IEEE, X12N, ACR-NEMA), is working to formulate standards for EDI.

ASTM standard E 1384 applies to all types of health

TABLE 4–1 PATIENT RECORD CONTENT STRUCTURE: DATA CATEGORIES, SEGMENTS, AND ENTITY RELATIONSHIPS

DATA	CATEGORY AND SEGMENTS	ENTITY
Administrative Data		
I	Demographics	Patient
II	Legal agreements	Patient
III	Financial information	Patient
IV	Provider/practitioner	Provider
Clinical Data: Problems/Diagnoses		
V	Problem list	Problem
Clinical Data: History		
VI	Immunization	Service instance
VII	Hazardous stressor exposure	Observation
VIII	Health history	Observation
Clinical Data: Assessments/Exams		
IX	Assessments	Observations
	* Patient-reported data	Observation
Clinical Data: Care/Treatment Plans		
X	Clinical orders	Orders
Clinical Data: Services		
XI	Diagnostic tests	Observations
XII	Medications	Service instance
XIII	Scheduled appts/events	Encounter
Administrative Data: Encounters		
XIV	a Administrative data	Patient
	* Encounter disposition	Encounter
Clinical Data: Encounters		
	b Chief complaint/diagnoses	Observation
	c Clinical course	Observation
	d Therapy procedures	Service instance

*These are new concepts and/or reordered data. Note that the clinical heart of the CPR is the core of the entities (Objects). The record segments that relate to these are shown.

care services, including those given in acute care hospitals, nursing homes, skilled nursing facilities, home health care, and specialty care environments as well as ambulatory care. (See Standard Guide for Description for Content and Structure of an Automated Primary Record of Care [E 1384].) The standard applies to both short-term contacts (e.g., emergency department services and emergency medical service units) and long-term contacts (e.g., primary care physicians and other health care providers with long-term patients).

The standard delineates the components and content of the patient record and includes definitions that conform to standard nomenclature. It is divided into segments that are grouped within or around an entity that organizes them into broad categories, such as patient, provider, problem, observation, and so forth. These broad groups are another way of depicting data in object-oriented systems design (Table 4–1).

*ASTM E1384 Content Guide for
Computer-Based Patient Record*

The following content is taken from the E1384 standard. To streamline and facilitate this presentation, the elements have been renumbered and limited descriptions provided. The complete standard and associated standards should be consulted if additional detail is needed.

SEGMENT 1: DEMOGRAPHICS

These are personal data elements, sufficient to identify the patient, collected from the patient or patient representative and not related to health status or services provided. Some elements may require updating at each encounter or episode and must satisfy various national standards and regulations, such as JCAHO Standards, *Conditions of Participation* for Medicare, UHDDS, UACDS, and LTCDS.

1.01 Name of patient

1.02 Multiple birth marker

1.030 Unique personal identification number (UPIN)

Permanent, unique number used by all providers and third party payers in conjunction with establishing and using the longitudinal record. It is used to link services for the patient across care systems.

1.031 Patient health record identification number. Patient number assigned by the provider as a unique unit number within that provider's system.

1.04 Patient's permanent address (mailing address)

1.05 Social security number

A pseudo social security number may be assigned if the patient does not have a number assigned by the Social Security Administration or does not authorize use of the social security number. Uses of the social security number are governed by law.

1.06 Date of birth

Age can be generated from date of birth; time can be included for neonates.

1.07 Place of birth

1.08 Sex

1.09 Race

1.10 Ethnic group

1.11 Religion

1.12 Marital status

Marital status of patient at start of care. *Never married* includes the annulment of a marriage. *Married* includes a common law marriage. *Separated* also applies to married people who are living apart because a spouse is institutionalized. *Widowed* applies to a person whose spouse has died and who has not re-married. *Divorced* means legally divorced and not re-married.

1.13 Educational level

The highest level in years within each major (primary, secondary, college, postbaccalaureate) educational system, irrespective of certifications achieved.

1.14 Occupation

1.15 Present employer's name

1.16 Mother's full name

1.17 Father's full name

1.18 Registration review date

Date when the registration record was reviewed by a responsible official for accuracy.

The data elements of the demographic segment characterize the patient. This segment is the root of the record; all other segments branch from it as required.

SEGMENT 2: LEGAL ELEMENTS

These data elements indicate legally binding directions or restraints on patient care, release of information, and disposal of body or body parts, or both, after death.

2.01 Consent to care acknowledgment

2.02 Date consent to care signed

2.03 Patient rights acknowledgment

2.04 Organ donor agreement

To include the donor patient's name (transplant recipient), donor patient's number (transplant recipient), recipient patient's number (transplant donor), and recipient patient's name (transplant donor).

2.05 Release of information authorization

2.06 Release of information purpose

2.07 Date of release of information authorization

2.08 Authorization for autopsy

This segment records the legal data that characterize the patient's agreements to care and caveats regarding that care or the disposal of his or her effects.

SEGMENT 3: FINANCIAL ELEMENTS

These are identifying data elements on all parties responsible for payment of patient health care services.

3.01 Primary payment source (may include address)

Responsible for the largest percentage of the patient's current bill.

3.02 Insurance group number

3.03 Insurance identification number

3.04 Medicare number

3.05 Medicaid number

3.06 Principal payment sponsor

Name of person who is responsible for the bill or whose insurance plan provides patient coverage.

3.07 Address of principal sponsor

This segment contains the references to the financial bodies that will cover the cost of care. It may be referred to from within the record, as during encounters or episodes. Such reference would eliminate the need for redundantly collecting this type of data during the visit.

SEGMENT 4: PROVIDER DATA

Identifying data on the primary organization, establishment, or practitioner responsible for the availability of health care services for this specific episode or encounter.

Practitioners are individuals who are licensed or certified to deliver care to patients, who had face-to-face contact with the patient, and who provided care based on independent judgment.

4.01 Provider's or practitioner's name

Name of the facility or practice submitting a bill; a business entity that furnishes health care. The name may be the same as that of the practitioner.

4.02 Provider's address

4.03 Provider type

Type of health care setting or practice type; includes sites of care as listed in Table 4–2.

4.04 Provider ID number

Numeric identifier used consistently. A unique number always associated with this provider. If the provider is a practitioner, the number for both provider and practitioner is the same. Provider number may need to be associated with numbers assigned by various payers: Medicare, Medicaid, Blue Cross/Blue Shield, federal tax number (assigned by federal government for tax-reporting purposes).

4.05 Practitioner's name (attending/referring/consulting/operating practitioner)

4.06 Practitioner's current role (e.g., primary, referring, consulting, operating)

Identifies the role practitioner plays with this patient.

4.07 Practitioner's profession

4.08 Practitioner's address

4.09 Practitioner's phone number

4.10 Practitioner's universal identification number (UPIN)

Universal numeric identifier used to link services for a practitioner across care systems. Each practitioner has a unique number that identifies him or her. The same number is used for the practitioner in all settings where he or she may practice.

TABLE 4–2 ASTM STANDARD E 1384 SITES OF CARE

Ambulance/Aid-Car	Hospital, Government
Ambulatory Surgery Facility, Free-Standing	Hospital, Outpatient Department
Ambulatory Surgery Facility, Hospital-Based	Hospital, Psychiatric
Birthing Center, Free-Standing	Hospital, Rehabilitation
	Hospital, Trauma Center Level 1
Birthing Center, Hospital-Based	Imaging Services Facility, Free-Standing
Clinic/Health Center, Comprehensive Outpatient Rehabilitation	Independent Laboratory
	Industrial Health/Occupational Health Center
Clinic/Health Center, Dental	Intermediate Care Facility
Clinic/Health Center, Free-Standing	Intermediate Care Facility—Mentally Retarded
Clinic/Health Center, Health Maintenance Organization	Mental Health Multiservice Organization
Clinic/Health Center, Outpatient Mental Health	Mental Health Partial Care Organization
Clinic/Health Center, Pain	Private Office, Group, Fee-for-Service
Clinic/Health Center, Rural	
Clinic/Health Center, Urgent Care Center, Walk-In, Free-Standing	Private Office, Group, Prepaid
	Private Office, Solo Practice
Clinic/Health Center, Vision	Residential Treatment Center, Emotionally Disturbed Children
Custodial Care Facility	
Day Care Center	Residential School
End-Stage Renal Disease Treatment Facility	Retirement Center
	School Clinic/Infirmary
Home Health	Sheltered Employment Workshop
Hospice, Free-Standing	
Hospital, Acute Care	Skilled Nursing Facility/Nursing Home
Hospital, Acute Care with Psychiatric Services	Special Education Program
Hospital, Burn Center	Substance Abuse Treatment Facility, Resident
Hospital, Cancer	
Hospital, Children's	Unlisted Facility
Hospital, Emergency Room	Vocational Rehabilitation Unit

4.11 Practitioner's license number

License identifying number and state for the license authorizing the practitioner to practice.

4.12 Practitioner's license state

This segment contains in one place the descriptive data about each provider or practitioner and may be referenced when recording data about the events of health care. Clinical segments are considered as accumulated data identified in the following segments.

SEGMENT 5: PROBLEM LIST

This segment contains a summary, an up-to-date list of clinically significant problems and diagnoses, health status events and factors—resolved and unresolved—of a patient's past and existing diagnoses, pathophysiologic states, potentially significant abnormal physical signs and laboratory findings, disabilities, stressor exposure, and unusual conditions. Social problems, psychiatric problems, risk factors, allergies, reactions to drugs or foods, behavioral problems, or other medical alerts may be included. The problem list is amended as more precise definitions of the problems become available.

5.01 Problem number

Identifier for this unique problem. For the present, it should be considered a sequential integer number.

5.02 Name of problem

5.03 Estimated date of problem onset

5.04 Date problem resolved

5.05 Current status (active versus inactive)

5.06 Problem subjective (textual synopsis of symptoms)

5.07 Problem objective (textual synopsis of examination)

5.08 Problem diagnosis (International Classification of Diseases, 9th Edition Clinical Modification [ICD-9-CM] codes)

Master list of all of a patient's problems diagnoses or ICD-9-CM–coded diagnoses. It may be referenced in presenting the diagnostic summary beginning each encounter or episode. All problems or diagnoses initially recorded in a specific encounter or episode are also entered in this master list.

5.09 Risk factors

Risk factors (medical alerts) that should be considered in the patient's health care and that should be known before any health services are implemented. These factors can be considered instances of a special type of patient problem and include allergies, contagious conditions, and adverse reactions to specified treatments.

The segment listing of this special problem type contains all alerting conditions that may adversely affect the patient when he or she is received for care. It may be duplicated on personal cards or devices for use in emergency situations. The medical alert section does not exist as a separate, defined segment. It is a subset of the problem list.

SEGMENT 6: IMMUNIZATION RECORD

Acquired (active or passive) or induced immunity or resistance to particular pathogens produced by deliberate exposure to antigens.

6.01 Name of immunization

6.02 Dates immunizations were given

This segment contains a chronologic list of all immunizations administered to the patient and their current status. This synopsis may also be copied to an emergency record to accompany medical alert data.

SEGMENT 7: EXPOSURE TO HAZARDOUS SUBSTANCES

The what, where, when, and how data on actual or potential exposure to all biologic, physical, or chemical agents that might be associated with adverse health effects are listed in this segment. This segment should provide data for epidemiologic studies to determine correlations of disease with exposure to environmental stressors.

7.01 Name of hazardous substance

7.02 Date of exposure

7.03 Date of exposure termination

Because of the potentially long latency period in exposure to stressor substances before the appearance of effects, the chronological record of exposure to hazardous chemical, physical, biologic, or radiologic stressors to the body, whether in the workplace or in some other environment, is contained in this segment.

SEGMENT 8: PATIENT MEDICAL OR DENTAL HISTORY—FAMILY/CUMULATIVE/MEDICAL

Synopsis of relevant natural family and patient history and signs that might aid practitioners in predicting or diagnosing illness or predicting the outcome of the patient's care, or both.

8.01 Prenatal and perinatal history problems

8.02 Illness summaries of immediate family (family history)

8.03 Patient's work history

8.04 Patient's medical or dental history

Includes social history, habits, and previous illness.

The historical record of previous signs and symptoms complements the problem list in itemizing, in an integral way, the manifestations of prior disease not documented in the problem list as well as characterizing those already present in that list.

SEGMENT 9: PHYSICAL EXAMINATION AND ASSESSMENT

Depending on the setting, this segment may include a physical examination and/or assessments by nursing, dietary, patient activity, social service, and therapy specialists. The assessments may be all-inclusive or may relate only to specific problems (i.e., particular body systems, dental, vision, mental health, communication). All data pertinent to prenatal and perinatal care, including monitoring during delivery, are included in a postdelivery examination and assessment. Details of the delivery are entered in the section that contains health factors of the neonate.

9.01 Date of history and physical examination/assessment

9.02 Height (most recent value, to include birth length)

9.03 Weight (most recent value)

9.04 Vital signs

9.05 Present health status

9.06 Review of systems

9.07 Findings

9.08 Text of history and examination/assessment

9.09 Functional independence measure

9.10 Assessment of nutritional status

9.11 Physical examination/assessment summary

9.12 Examiner or consultant recommendations (Table 4–3)

This segment records the observations of the practitioner during structured and systematic examinations and assessments of the patient during encounters or episodes. It includes objective observations and measurements that quantify attributes of each body system. These are the same body systems about which patient questions are asked during the history or review of systems. Such common categories allow characterization of expressed problems with observational evidence in explicit common terms and measures that, over time, allow practitioners to follow the course of illness and recovery. These observations complement the diagnostic terms described in the medication and encounter or episode segments.

TABLE 4–3 ASTM STANDARD E 1384, REVIEW OF SYSTEMS AND PHYSICAL EXAMINATION

REVIEW OF SYSTEMS

01. General appearance
02. Nutritional assessment status
03. Eyes
04. Ears
05. Nose
06. Throat
07. Neck
08. Thorax
09. Breasts
10. Lungs
11. Heart
12. Blood vessels
13. Blood/blood forming
14. Abdomen
15. Genitourinary
16. Vaginal
17. Musculoskeletal
18. Skin
19. Endocrine
20. Lymphatics
21. Neurologic
22. Behavioral assessment status
23. Disorientation or sensory impairment status, or both
24. Psychosocial assessment status
25. Basic functional assessment (self care)
26. Mobility assessment
27. Urinary/bowel continence
28. Dental status, and
29. Teeth

PHYSICAL EXAMINATION

01. General
02. Head/face
03. Eyes
04. Ears
05. Nose
06. Mouth/throat
07. Neck
08. Respiratory/lung
09. Cardiovascular
10. Gastrointestinal
11. Urinary
12. Genitoreproductive
13. Musculoskeletal
14. Skin
15. Endocrine
16. Lymphatics
17. Hematologic
18. Neurologic
19. Psychiatric, and
20. Dental

SEGMENT 10: ORDERS AND TREATMENT PLANS

This segment directs a patient's treatment and includes detailed data on the orders and treatment plans and compliance with diagnostic or therapeutic orders or treatment plans.

10.01 Date and time of order

10.02 Frequency of therapy or service

10.03 Duration of the order (including start and stop times)

10.04 Date and time of treatment plan execution

10.05 Plan of action/order/objective

Identify problem that occasioned this order/plan/objective.

10.06 Duration of therapy

10.07 Order confirmation received

10.08 Ordering practitioner's name

10.09 Action or service

Identify the action or service, providers, and the type and priority of the order.

10.10 Results

Data elements document the resulting data from the service or action, as appropriate.

10.11 Quality assurance group of data elements

This group of data elements documents events or outcomes that are exceptions to the routine process of care. These elements flag such events or outcomes so that they can be easily recognized for review. Their review is also documented in the quality assurance process/system to ensure that significant findings are not overlooked.

A clinical order is an action-oriented message describing an intervention in the health of a specific patient that is originated by or under the supervision of a specific physician or some other duly authorized practitioner. It draws on already captured data and links the action to a therapy-specific problem or diagnosis. The clinical order acts as a communication and coordinating mechanism for all the practitioners and ancillary professionals who may participate in the explicit and implicit actions set in motion by the order. A clinical order also has legal and quality assurance implications regarding responsibilities for the ordered intervention. The clinical order structure is complex and may be thought of as a network structure because of the relation between specific data elements within the clinical order and other data elements in the record.

SEGMENT 11: DIAGNOSTIC TESTS

Significant details of tests performed to aid the in diagnosis, management, and treatment of the patient. Documentation of results from the pathology and clinical laboratory, radiology, nuclear medicine, respiratory, and any other diagnostic examinations are included.

11.01 Name of test

11.02 Date and time test performed

11.03 Source facility identification

11.04 Findings, text, or measurement values with units

11.05 Date and time result reported

11.06 Name and credentials of practitioner performing diagnostic test

This segment contains the chronologic list of all diagnostic tests ordered and conducted on the patient. The attribute data about each such test reference the order, problem list, and appropriate physical examination, assessment, or medication segments that may relate to the monitoring of therapeutic interventions to either measure therapeutic effects or detect adverse effects.

SEGMENT 12: MEDICATION PROFILE

List of all long-term medications and significant details on all medications prescribed or administered, or both.

12.01 Date of prescription

12.02 Medication (generic or brand name)

12.03 Prescription number

12.04 Prescriber's name and credentials

12.05 Dose strength and unit

12.06 Dosage form

12.07 Route of administration

12.08 Interval

12.09 Total doses

12.10 Number of refills authorized

12.11 Dispensing person's name

12.12 Dispensing person's facility

12.13 Medication instructions

12.14 Medication notes

This segment contains data about the therapeutic chemical substances and treatments that have been prescribed as interventions in the disease process. All the attributes of the order described here are linked to this record by reference to the orders and treatment plans segment. Additional attributes provided by the pharmacist are also entered in the record, including adverse effects reported in the history segment or physical examination segment, or both. The problem list, which identifies the problem being treated, may also be referenced.

The segments that follow contain clinical data from multiple sources. These data may also be used to update the accumulative data segments. (See Segments 1–12.)

SEGMENT 13: SCHEDULED APPOINTMENTS

This segment includes a list of planned or scheduled appointments that implement the treatment plan. It includes the attributes or data that characterize the planned services and the locations and names of the practitioners who constitute the plan.

SEGMENT 14: ENCOUNTER OR EPISODE

Every **encounter** or episode included in the primary patient record in the course of a patient's lifetime is sequenced by means of a date and time. The subsections are organized to reflect the logical repetitions of care events that make up the continuing development of the patient record. Detail levels extend according to the specific care site. Hospitalizations and ambulatory visits are examples.

An encounter is a face-to-face session of the patient with a practitioner during which information about the patient's health status is exchanged. Under certain circumstances, telephone evaluations are also recorded. The encounter record captures the facts relating to the events that took place, whether they occur in an inpatient setting or an ambulatory care environment.

A. Administrative and Diagnostic Summary

Data elements clarifying time and date, location, type, and source of an encounter or episode as they differ from the information contained in previous segments. These should include the problem list, narrative, and coded descriptions of admitting and principal diagnoses as well as all other diagnoses that are a factor in the patient's care during the specific episode or encounter.

14a.01 Date and time of encounter commencement or admission episode

14a.02 Type of encounter or episode (e.g., visit, hospitalization, including facility name)

14a.03 Coded and narrative description of principal diagnosis or primary diagnoses in outpatient visits (at discharge)

Home health: principal diagnosis relates to the services rendered by the home health agency. If more than one diagnosis is treated concurrently, the diagnosis that represents the most acute condition and requires the most intensive services should be the principal diagnosis.

UHDDS: Conditions established after study to be chiefly responsible for occasioning the admission of the patient to the hospital (commencement of the episode). No symbols or abbreviations.

14a.04 Coded and narrative description of additional diagnoses

All conditions coexisting at the time of the episode that affect the treatment received or length of stay. A condition of sufficient significance to warrant inclusion for investigative medical studies. No symbols or abbreviations. Complications are additional diagnoses that describe conditions that arise after the beginning of the episode and that modify the course of the patient's illness or the medical care required. Also describes undesired result and/or misadventure in the medical care of the patient.

14a.05 Clinical resume or final progress note

This subsegment contains all the data that characterize the origin of the episode and the manner of arrival at the provider's facility, including the condition of the patient. It also summarizes the administrative and diagnostic conditions concerning the termination of treatment, excepting the disposition, which is contained in a later subsegment.

B. History of Present Illness

Medical or dental history of the patient, including chief complaint or reason the patient is seeking care. This includes a review of systems as appropriate to the individual case.

14b.01 Chief complaint or reason for visit

Reason for encounter or episode and the patient's complaints and symptoms that reflect his or her own perceptions of needs; the nature and duration of symptoms that caused the patient to seek medical attention, as stated in the patient's own words.

14b.02 Source of history (contact name)

Person who relates the patient's history to the practitioner.

14b.03 Review of systems

Summary of the systematic review of the status and functioning of the body's systems and regions (see Table 4–3).

C. Progress Notes and Clinical Course

Components that form an ongoing chronologic picture and analysis of the clinical course of the patient during an encounter or episode. This segment is applicable for any health care setting. These elements serve as a means of communication and interaction between members of a health care team. They may also occur as narratives or flow sheets.

14c.01 Date and time of clinical note

14c.02 Physician's progress notes

14c.03 Summary of inpatient monitoring

14c.04 Nursing and nonphysician notes

D. Therapies

Significant details on all preventive and/or therapeutic services performed at the time of the encounter or episode or scheduled to be performed before the next encounter or episode. This subsegment does not include any surgery performed in an operating room or that might be documented under later subsegments. Transfusions and physical, occupational, respiratory, rehabilitative, or mental health therapies are included.

14d.01 Name of therapy or preventive service type

14d.02 Date therapy commenced

14d.03 Date therapy finished

14d.04   Therapist's response assessment

Documentation of the patient's attitude toward the plan, including estimates of further therapeutic potential.

14d.05   Therapist's recommendations

Further plans for continued treatment and/or services, including an assessment of the patient's ability to improve and to what level.

These elements are recorded to characterize all the conditions of nonpharmacologic therapy and represent interdisciplinary therapy programs and results.

E.   Procedures

Significant data elements on all procedures performed in an operating room for diagnostic, exploratory, or definitive treatment purposes.

14e.01   Name and code of principal procedure

Principal procedure performed for definitive therapy rather than for diagnostic or exploratory purposes, or the procedure most related to the principal diagnosis. No symbols or abbreviations.

14e.02   Narrative description of the principal procedure

14e.03   Date and time of the principal procedure

14e.04   Name and code of additional significant procedures

14e.05   Narrative description of additional significant procedures

14e.06   Dates of additional significant procedures

14e.07   Findings (gross, microscopic, pathologic) of each procedure

14e.08   Organs explored

14e.09   Primary surgeon's name

14e.10   Assistant surgeon's name

14e.11   Preanesthesia assessment

14e.12   Type of anesthetic agent used

14e.13   Dosages of all anesthetic agents

14e.14   Anesthesiologist's name

14e.15   Current, regularly monitored vital signs

14e.16   Intravenous fluids given

14e.17   Specimens removed

14e.18   Postanesthesia assessment

14e.19   Complications (surgical misadventures, i.e., infections)

14e.20   Postoperative diagnosis

Determination of the case after operation.

This subsegment contains data that characterize those procedural events that accompany treatment of the patient, exclusive of laboratory phases of diagnostic procedures (recorded in segment 11).

F.   Disposition

Identifies the circumstances under which the patient terminated the encounter or episode and includes data about the length of stay, condition of patient on discharge, recommended treatment, and other information necessary for follow-up care.

14f.01   Date and time of discharge or death

14f.02   Type of discharge

14f.03   Total length of stay

14f.04   Disposition destination

14f.05   Referral and discharge patient instructions

14f.06   Autopsy or necropsy report (if authorized when disposition is "death")

This subsegment contains data that characterize the conditions under which the encounter or episode was completed and the arrangements for appropriate follow-up by either the current provider or other providers. It also contains information needed to maintain continuity of care over multiple encounters or several episodes.

G.   Charges

Charges represent billing for procedures and services rendered by the provider or practitioner and associates during the encounter or episode.

14g.01   Total charges

All charges for procedures and services rendered by the provider or his or her associates during or in conjunction with the episode. Includes procedures that occurred subsequent to the episode but ordered during the episode and facility fee if billed separately from the professional fee.

USER NEEDS

Understanding standards, rules, and regulations is a solid foundation for developing a quality health record.

Before one can be confident that a fully functioning record has been designed, it is essential to consider the specialized needs of all the users of the record. Discussion takes place in committees, including those described in JCAHO standards, and in other groups within the facility as well as with department heads and may include special interests from research to marketing. Understanding the flow of data and information throughout the health care facility ensures that computer views (or screens) and paper forms are designed to facilitate the collection of data elements. Training and practice in the design of computer views and paper forms as well as computer-based data capture techniques make the HIM professional a valuable management resource.

Data Item Encryption

It is appropriate at the close of this presentation of data items fundamental to the CPR to consider the important issue of **data item encryption.** The commitment of HIM managers to the protection of patient confidentiality raises the question of how to identify patients in order to retrieve and link their records. A patient identifier suitable for the CPR must possess the following characteristics:

- Uniqueness
- Unambiguity
- Controllability
- Verifiability
- Encryptability

Although this chapter does not address the legal or technical aspects of satisfying these criteria for a UPIN, it is worthwhile for those interested in data items to understand the concept of encryption. Encryption transforms data into a form that is effectively unintelligible to an unauthorized user. Authorized users, on the other hand, know how to re-create the original information through a process termed decryption. Taken together, encryption and decryption constitute cryptography. Encryption can also be effective in protecting data during transfer from one system to another, i.e., electronic transmission between a facility and a third party payer or between two providers. In addition to its important contribution to protecting patient identity, cryptography has an application in protecting selected sensitive data items, such as those obtained through genetic screening.

Data Entry Technology

Once the selection of data items has been completed, the method of data collection can be considered. Data can be entered into a patient record from various locations, using a wide array of technologies. Fixed locations include the professional's office, the patient's bedside, nursing stations, diagnostic centers, and clinical workrooms. Mobile locations can be almost anywhere, with data entered into hand-held devices. Technologies vary from pen-and-paper note taking to touch screens guiding a patient-entered history to EDI from such devices as electrocardiographic monitors. Regardless of the location or configuration of the workstation, all computer technologies include an **input device.** The data-processing cycle begins with data recorded in human language being converted into the electronic signals of machine language that the computer can then process.

A widely recognized goal is that data be captured only once and then made available to all users of that data item. Introducing steps between the primary user and data entry has the following disadvantages:

- Lack of accuracy caused by errors that occur as part of data transfer or transcription
- Lack of data availability caused by data entry **bottlenecks** or delays that may adversely effect patient management
- Lack of immediate feedback to providers for editing alerts and alarms and error checking
- Lack of availability of linked databases for assistance in the decision-making process

Although the HIM professional recognizes the value of direct data entry, organizations may require various technologies and personnel as they evolve in the direction of the CPR and address technologic, financial, legal, administrative, and attitudinal barriers to full implementation. Because of the differences in the devices used to enter data, they are divided, for convenience, into keyed entry or point-and-click devices, scanned entry devices, and other entry devices. An overview of portable and hand-held terminals that combine several of these technologies is also provided.

Keyed Entry Devices

Virtually all keyed entry devices feature a **graphical user interface (GUI)** that uses a Windows environment of icons and tool bars of pull-down menus. Data are entered directly on the terminal by providers, administrative staff, and, possibly, patients completing **on-line** questionnaires.

Keyboard and Mouse

The most common computer configuration is the terminal with an attached keyboard. Data items keyed into the system appear simultaneously on the display screen, allowing operators to see that they have entered the correct data. Data entry using a GUI is facilitated by the use of a mouse, a lightweight palm-sized device wired to the computer. A roller or sensor on the bottom of the mouse enables the user to move it across a flat surface. The system interprets the movement as an instruction to reposition the cursor telling the operator where the system is pointing. The mouse provides a fast and easy alternative to using the keyboard.

Light Pen

A light pen, which looks like an ordinary pen or pencil and functions similarly to a keyboard or mouse, is connected to the terminal by a wire. The point contains a small photosensitive element that resembles a small metal ball. This element performs the input when the tip touches the display screen and creates a change in electrical current, digitizing the data input. A light pen can also be used to select multiple-choice answers from a list shown on the display. Light pens are used for special applications and may be included in a system for the benefit of users who are uncomfortable with entering data by way of a keyboard.

Touch-Sensitive Screens

Touch-sensitive screens take the concept of pointing one step further by allowing the user to simply touch the screen with a finger to make a selection. Fingers are familiar, do not require installation, and are mostly maintenance-free. The touch screens do require special hardware, which is expensive but quite durable. The cost may be justified if users who are not trained on a system are asked to interact with it. Theme parks, resorts, and other service companies have successfully used touch screens to provide visitors with information. Data input directly by patients is one health care possibility that could save the time of high-salaried practitioners. As health care becomes more service-oriented, this technology may find a niche.

Graphics Tablet

A pen-like device called a stylus is used to record data on an electronic graphics tablet. The stylus allows a high degree of cursor control, and the tablet records the markings digitally for processing. This device is widely used by industries that require detailed drawings and is now appearing in pen-based, hand-held computers. Although cost is still a factor, their low maintenance, pen-like comfort, and ability to accept handwriting are pluses.

Scanned Entry

Direct keying of data is not always desirable because of accuracy and productivity limitations. It may be more practical to design the system so that the computer, through the use of document-oriented **scanning** technology, reads the data into memory. A familiar example are the universal product codes, or bar codes, that are printed on food package labels to capture data. Other common document devices are scanners, optical character readers (OCRs), magnetic ink character readers (MICRs), and marked sense readers. In the past, the most common input medium was cards in which machines had punched small holes. The holes in the cards could be read by a computer. The term "unit record processing" was used because each card was a record of data. Today, this method is obsolete.

Optical Scanners

Scanners enable the user to capture an image from a paper document and transmit it to the computer screen, where it can be inserted into an existing document or manipulated into a new image. For example, a black-and-white or color photograph identifying a patient can be scanned into the record along with descriptive text. This eliminates the need for pasting in the photograph or manually changing its size to fit, a task that can also be done using the computer. In addition, documents, including correspondence, can be digitized and added to the record. Once scanned into the system, they can be stored, transmitted over communication networks, or reprinted, including annotations or modifications made by users. Another major advantage of this technology is that several users can share the image at the same time. In veterinary health care, microchips with identification numbers that can be read by scanners have been implanted into pets.

Bar Code Readers

Bar code readers are similar to scanners in that they are dependent on a document—the bar code label. A series of black stripes in varying vertical patterns of wide and narrow bands identifies the item. The bars are read, or sensed, into the computer by a hand-held light pen (optical wand scanner) or a fixed optical scanner. The data are digitized and then processed by the computer. Bar codes have increased the efficiency and accuracy at the grocery store checkout and have helped package shipping companies track shipments. Examples of health care applications range from creating chiropractic reports by scanning appropriate phrases from a labeled chart to reading patient identification bands to tracking patient records. Bar codes take time to create, but their benefits include higher employee productivity, greater accuracy, and increasing availability of hand-held computers.

Optical Character Readers

Optical character readers sense data symbols that appear in predetermined locations on documents. Symbols can be in many forms—marks, bars, numbers, letters, special characters of certain fonts, and ordinary handwriting. Most OCRs use a scanning electronic light beam to detect these symbols, which are sensed as reflected light by the reader and digitized for the computer to process. Examples of uses include coding of documents for optical scanning, as illustrated in the next section, and patient-completed questionnaires. The necessity for handwritten characters to be in specific shapes has been a limitation to this technology. As systems become more sophisticated, the limitations on character shape are expected to decline. Advanced systems can also read thumbprints or signatures for comparison with previously stored records, providing positive user identification.

Mark-Sense Readers

Mark-sense readers are another method of scanned, document-oriented data input. Pre-established fields or positions on specially designed forms are blackened by a dark pencil to represent data. This method is probably most familiar to those who have taken standardized tests. Students taking multiple-choice, computer-graded examinations use lead pencils to mark or encode their answers. The completed mark-sense documents can then be processed by computer, the test analyzed, and grades given.

Magnetic Ink Character Readers

Closely related to the OCR is the MICR, which is designed to detect characters that are printed on documents in magnetic ink. The images set up a magnetic field in the machine that can be digitized for data input. The most common use of MICRs is in the banking industry for check processing. This technology is not commonly used in health care, although applications for it may be developed.

Other Entry Devices

Other technologies are also available that can supplement or replace keyed and scanned data collection.

Magnetic Strip

Magnetic strips are most familiar from automatic teller machine cards used to do banking transactions at remote terminals. Identifying data encoded onto a single magnetic bar on the back of the card can be read at any location. Health care has adopted this technology in the form of patient identification cards that contain basic demographic and insurance data. These cards have the advantages of being inexpensive, convenient to carry, and easy to use; the disadvantages are limited agreement on data definitions and a lack of compatible terminal locations. As the technology improves and readers become more standardized and available, the amount of data that can be encoded will increase, and cards may contain a microchip that can be updated. Inclusion of diagnoses, medications, allergies, and an entire patient record are future possibilities.

Voice Recognition

An increasing amount of work is being done to develop voice-input capabilities. Health care workers whose hands and/or eyes are otherwise occupied are likely to appreciate such capabilities. Wearing a small microphone or using a telephone handset, a radiologist can follow a checklist on a monitor; orally identify the patient, date, study, and characteristics of the image; and authenticate the report. The voice input is transmitted digitally directly to the computer. Voice may be the ultimate communication medium between people and machines; most of us have it and it is portable. Some systems can accept speaker-independent sound data, meaning that it can understand any user. This feature is hard to achieve because there is both interspeaker and intraspeaker variation. Most systems require that each user train the system to recognize his or her voice. Training involves repeating each "word" (sound of 2 seconds or less) the system will be expected to recognize about a dozen times. Currently, speaker-independent systems accept only a small vocabulary, making such specialties as emergency medicine and radiology the first to find success with this technology. Another limitation is the requirement to pause between words because units cannot as yet recognize continuous speech. Research has been improving accuracy to nearly 99 per cent. Increased worker productivity, significant cost savings, and substantial user appeal should combine to create many future applications.

Electronic Data Interchange

Electronic data interchange is at the heart of the CPR. Direct capture of digitized data at the point of care is the optimal beginning. The increase in products that collect data digitally helps to move this aspect toward reality. The next step is to transfer the data, ideally in native format, among computers. Until this type of transfer is routinely available, various scanning and file translations will continue to be used as intermediary steps. Also required are the continued development and implementation of hardware and software standards similar to the data item specifications in ASTM E 1384. This will facilitate the extensive manipulation of data originating from different sources and platforms required within the CPR. EDI at this level would realize one of the goals of the CPR—permitting views of all patient record data on a single workstation type, giving universal access to information. The most difficult data capture scenarios involve multimedia information management. The capture of full-motion video, video clips, diagnostic images, and associated voice annotation presents a substantial barrier to implementation. This is predominantly because of the immense quantity of data. Advances in standards, hardware, and software for input, storage, and output will eventually make a fully computer-based patient record a reality.

Portable and Hand-Held Terminals

A portable or hand-held terminal is used to transmit input and receive output, but most of the processing is done by a main computer elsewhere. By way of contrast, a portable microcomputer may complete the entire process. Today, the most popular portable and hand-held terminals combine keyboards, small TV-like or liquid crystal displays, and modems to establish computer connections by way of cellular telephone lines. Some also include a graphics tablet and bar code reader. Most units are lightweight and have internal storage units capable of holding the equivalent of several thousand characters of text. These units are especially useful for people whose job involves data gathering, such as health care practitioners. A user of one of these terminals can enter the data throughout the day and then dial the central computer by way of an ordinary or cellular telephone to periodically transmit and receive data. Point-of-care applications are well suited to this technology, including encounter data in clinic, home care, and emergency medical service locations. These terminals are also useful in obtaining attestation signatures, tracking supplies provided to patients, and recording responses to patient satisfaction surveys. They provide document security through write-once-read-many technology. The strengths of the portable or hand-held devices include convenience and the capability of nearly instant feedback on data capture, including validity checks and limited decision support at the point of care. Their weaknesses include the lack of the full spectrum of functions and the power of a fixed workstation. Innovations will surely improve capabilities and price, probably making the portable workstation a powerful and indispensable tool on a par with the stethoscope. Chapters 17 and 18 detail the technology and issues surrounding computers and health information systems.

Data Preparation Bottlenecks

Data input preparation is a major bottleneck in most data-processing operations. The buildup of a backlog usually occurs because data items cannot be prepared for input as fast as they can be read or accepted by the computer. In addition to data preparation delays, the time taken to prepare and verify each input document is costly. To reduce the data preparation bottleneck, a system design should meet the following criteria:

- Provide for direct entry of small amounts of data into the system as events occur

- Provide for automatic and immediate feedback for editing alerts and alarms and error checking

- Utilize documents that capture data at the source of the transaction in a form appropriate for subsequent scanning or entry into the system

In simplest terms, the computer's primary job is to process data. It does so to provide useful information. Our first duty as users who want to obtain that information is to make the needed data available for processing. Beyond the PPR, computer workstations vary in their support of some or all of the data entry methods described as well as in their portability, speed, memory, networking, communication capabilities, and price. The appropriate selection of the most efficient and effective combination of data collection technologies is a major responsibility of HIM professionals.

INPUT VALIDATION CHECKS

Validity is a characteristic of information that indicates that it is meaningful and relevant to the stated purpose. An important step in producing valid information is to assure the validity of the input. The familiar phrase "garbage in—garbage out" describes this concept in a humorous and memorable way. The source of errors varies from mistakes to attempts at making unauthorized data entries. Regardless of the source or the reason why the data are invalid, once processed, an invalid transaction has caused damage that may be difficult to repair. It is far better to avoid such problems in the first place by preventing an invalid transaction from occurring. There are two basic types of checks: event and data. The first check concentrates on the processing events to determine whether they are acceptable. The second helps locate errors in the content of data items or fields (see Input Validation Checks). Several relatively simple methods are available. All of them are appropriate for computer programming instructions or manual procedures. Although they are discussed separately, a well-designed **input validation** program should combine several of these approaches.

Input Validation Checks

Event Validation
- Transaction Validation
- Sequence Checks
- Batch Totals
- Audit Trail
- Duplicate Processing

Data Validation
- Format Checks
- Reasonableness Checks
- Check Digits

Event Validation Techniques

Event validation focuses on the activity of submitting data either manually or by computer. The checks look at the who, what, when, where, and why of these transactions. A **transaction** is an event that takes place during the routine course of business. It is usually entered into the computer for immediate processing whenever the activity that creates the data occurs. Computer systems process many types of transactions and millions of transactions per day. Transactions for a patient record may vary from admission orders to recording vital signs, from scheduling radiologic examinations to reporting laboratory results, from coding diagnoses to billing third party payers. The purposes of the transactions may also vary; some add records, some delete records, and some change the contents of selected data items in a specific record. In addition, some transactions originate at the computer site, whereas others come from remote locations. The mode may be batch or on-line. Many people or only a few people may have the authority to submit transactions for processing.

Transaction Validation

Transaction validation ensures that activities are acceptable, authorized, and legitimate and should confirm type, time, purpose, and authority. Type is a simple review of whether the system handles the transaction. Time may be an issue if an activity, such as the taking of the census, is time-specific. Transactions that are exceptions to these rules are invalid and rejected by the system. Purpose, or the reason for the transaction, is another consideration. For example, a transaction whose purpose is to correct a previous error may be valid and appropriately processed, whereas an attempt to delete historical records that are being kept for archival purposes may be unauthorized and, therefore, rejected. The location, site, or person who originates a processing activity may be a factor in determining transaction validity. An order may only be allowable if given by a physician. Transaction validation is such a basic way of controlling input that it may easily be overlooked.

Sequence Checks

Sequence checks are an effective technique when it is necessary to verify the processing of all transactions or documents and when order is important. The method simply assigns a number to each item or batch in sequence. During processing, review of the number sequence verifies that each transaction handling is both complete and in the correct order. This practice is common in the laboratory, where accession numbers control the flow of samples. Sequence numbers are also useful for individual events, such as billing numbers. Again, the computer can check for the billing number of each transaction. A break in the numbers may indicate the omission of one or more transactions.

Batch Totals

Batch totals ensure the processing of all items by adding numbers in a specific field in each transaction. The total is calculated before processing begins and the computer system accumulates another as processing occurs. Another application of batch totals is counting the number of records in the batch and then counting them again during individual processing. With either method, any discrepancy between the two totals indicates an error. Batch totals typically use fields of financial data. Records that do not include financial data use another field, such as an identification number. The term for this method is "hash total."

Audit Trail

An audit trail is most useful for a system in which data entry is from remote locations. This control technique traces stored data items back to the event that created, deleted, or modified them to contain their current values. To make this backtracking possible, the computer or operator maintains a log of each transaction processed. The log documents the location, date, and time of each transaction. Errors detected are traced back to their source, and events are reconstructed so that the problem can be located and the error corrected. The audit trail thus emphasizes being able to trace invalid data back to their origin and correcting them.

Duplicate Processing

Duplicate processing, or completely re-entering data, is an expensive strategy to use for input validation. Although seldom practical, it may be helpful to have two persons input data and compare results if there is reason to question the system's stability.

Data Validation Techniques

Whereas the event validation techniques look at the flow of transactions as quick and easy methods for validating data input, the data validation techniques focus on the content of the data items themselves.

Format Checks

Format checks are tests of field content to ensure that the data they contain are valid according to pre-established standards for item or field length, specifications, type specification, processing code, and so on. Length checks determine whether the number of characters or numbers in the field is correct. Type specification checks screen out any item that contains invalid numbers or characters before data entry. For example, a data item that contains an eight-digit social security number represents a length error because it is one digit short. If the field is to contain only numerical data, the use of hyphens or letters would represent a type specification error. Processing codes enable a program to first check a certain field in a record to determine the type of processing required. Checking the processing code prevents errors from entering files or databases.

Reasonableness Checks

Reasonableness checks are initial screening techniques that check items to ensure that the values fall within "reasonable values" before entering the system. Items screened in this way may not necessarily be errors, but they may be questionable enough to make reverification cost-effective. Checking both upper and lower limits is common. For example, a laboratory test frequently has a normal range with high and low limits. Alerts notify technicians when samples fall outside the range. Although they may not be errors, the values are still checked because they are outliers. This validation method is a quick and easy way to check data that requires no work before data entry. By using it, the most obvious errors can be detected.

Check Digits

Check digits use a different strategy than the techniques previously described. All the others compare data to a standard with which they should agree. Although it is easy and important to include an input validation program, such a program does not protect very well against certain types of errors in numerical data. For example, in numerical data entry, it is relatively easy to introduce four types of errors: transcription, transposition, omission, and insertion. Transcription errors are misinterpretations (i.e., mistakenly entering a "3" as an "8"). Transposition errors are number reversals (i.e., recording "25" instead of "52"). Such errors as well as omissions and insertions are both common and usually difficult to locate. They can, however, be detected by using an additional (check) digit at the end of the data item. The check digit itself has no value in processing other than to assure that the data are correct, as explained below.

There are many methods of deriving check digits; most use a formula applied to the original number. The result or remainder is then the check digit. If any error occurs that changes the base number or the check digit, the two will not agree. Because the computer can assign and compare check digits, the method is easy to use. One disadvantage of check digits is that they increase the item length, which sometimes leads to additional errors. Overall, this input validation process can be quite effective in preventing errors from entering files or databases, and it is particularly appropriate for patient identification numbers.

FORMS AND COMPUTER VIEWS DESIGN AND CONTROL

The design of paper forms and logical computer views is where content directives and technology meet. A complete program is an important component of health information management and involves both design and control. The design elements include the following:

- Selection of data elements
- User-friendly design
- Creation of a physical layout
- Production techniques

Control issues include the following:

- Identification of all forms and views
- Preservation of confidentiality
- Assurance of complete data capture
- Ongoing review and revision
- Cost control

When forms or views are well designed and controlled, they enhance technology by providing a smooth link in the communication process. This facilitates complete, accurate, and timely data and information while being almost transparent to the user. Regardless of the technology used, poorly designed forms or views can result in errors in data collection as well as incomplete and overlooked documentation and can waste human and computer time. As with data collection and technology, form or view design should emphasize the needs of users. When difficulties occur, they often represent conflict—real or imagined—among users. The need to resolve such conflict illustrates the importance of developing interpersonal as well as technical skills.

In determining and meeting user needs, it is the responsibility of each health care facility to develop its own forms or views. Accrediting and regulatory bodies such as the JCAHO and the Health Care Financing Administration (HCFA) and standards organizations such as ASTM do not recommend forms or views with which to collect the data elements they require or recommend, nor do professional organizations such as the American Hospital Association and the AHIMA. There are several valuable resources for suggestions, including the journals and newsletters noted in the references and professional colleagues in similar facilities. In addition to an informal exchange of ideas, in some areas, several facilities have formally joined together and adopted basic health record forms and views that are acceptable to the medical staffs of each facility. This saves the time of professionals who practice at more than one site and facilitates the paper or electronic interchange necessary to care for patients and carry out the business of each facility. It also allows for achieving administrative cost savings through bulk purchasing and reduced programming charges. Such strategies are also common in corporate facilities where core forms or views are designed for all the facilities and then local facilities design their own additions according to guidelines that have been provided.

Forms or Views Team

The management of forms or views is a collaborative process. Members of the forms or views team include the following:

- Health information management
- Information systems
- Materials management
- Patient care services
- Quality improvement
- Others as needed

The HIM professional plays a leadership role by providing knowledge of rules and regulations related to content directives, medical science, computer applications, and the flow of data throughout the facility and the health care delivery system. The forms or views design and control process also benefits from the involvement of an information systems manager who is responsible for computer input and output, a materials or purchasing manager who is responsible for inventory and ordering paper forms, a patient care professional who represents clinical needs, a quality improvement professional to provide input regarding forms or views created to address quality issues, and others as needed. The team's charge may be to work on administrative and patient information applications and to become involved in the selection of data collection technology. The team forwards its patient-related recommendations to the clinical information committee for approval and its administrative recommendations follow the organizational chain of command. Identification of the responsibilities of each team member as well as the flow of the process from request to implementation promotes the best results for the patients, the practitioners, and the facility.

General Design Principles

Forms and views share several key design principles whether they are intended for data input or output, for the PPR or the CPR. Designs should address the following basic considerations:

- Identification of user needs
- Purpose of the form or view
- Selection of appropriate data items and their sequencing
- Technology to be used, including an understanding of its strengths and weaknesses
- Use of standard terminology and abbreviations as well as development of a standard format
- Inclusion of instructions as necessary to ensure consistency in both data collection and data interpretation
- Value of keeping the form simple by omitting unnecessary items and streamlining designs

After the explanation of the general design principles that apply to both paper forms and computer views and their paper output, design differences between these two media are discussed.

Needs of Users

As with other areas of HIM practice, the needs of the user must be considered first. It is important to remember that users are not only the patient and providers, but the administrative, financial, and legal areas of the facility as well. External users collect data from many locations and the data are combined or **aggregated.** These may be local, state, and federal agencies and other planning and research groups. Collecting enough of the right type of data to satisfy this range of users means clearly defining the purpose of the form or view.

Purpose of the Form or View

Patient record forms serve many purposes. They standardize, identify and instruct, facilitate documentation and decision making, and promote consistency in data collection, reporting, and interpretation. Forms identify patients and practitioners and instruct them step by step in what data items to gather, where to obtain them, how to record them, and where they flow next. Good instructions, when followed, facilitate complete and accurate documentation, which is the foundation of effective decision making. History and physical forms provide a good example of these purposes. When standardized, all elements of the history, review of systems, and physical examination (as listed in the ASTM standard) are collected. Both the patient and the practitioner are identified with names and unique numbers either electronically or manually. The patient may follow a set of instructions on paper or computer to provide his or her medical history. The provider then follows a set of instructions when performing the review of systems and proceeding with the physical examination. The documentation thus collected is the foundation on which the patient and practitioner can make decisions and take action regarding lifestyle changes, diagnostic testing, medications, or other treatments. At the close of an encounter, a return appointment is frequently scheduled, which assigns responsibility to both the patient and the practitioner for follow-up. Thus, the history and physical form or view has structured the majority of the communication between the patient and the practitioner and will continue to communicate with other users as the need arises. Because forms and views are such central communication devices and serve so many purposes, a clear definition of purpose acts as a mission statement for the design team.

Selection and Sequencing of Items

This mission statement is then a point of reference for the selection of appropriate data items. It is helpful to construct a list or grid of items to ensure the collection of all essential items and the elimination of unnecessary or redundant items. Notes can be added to document the rationale for inclusion. Effective and efficient sequencing should follow the traditional pattern—from left to right and top to bottom—permitting a continuous operation whether reading, writing, or entering data on the computer. The flow should be logical and take into consideration the order of data collection or transfer. Record identifiers, or keys, that distinguish one record from another should be placed first. Once sequenced, grouping sets of related items helps structure the form or view. In addition, numbering items makes references to both items and instructions faster and easier.

Technology

Each of the data collection technologies previously described has unique form or view design considerations, and this impact should be considered throughout the systems design and implementation process. Specific design features differ for paper forms and computer views. Computer views require menus of alternatives to be developed and screen or window formats that may include spots to touch with a finger or light pen. Views can also be customized for more users than can paper forms, providing both the opportunities and the challenges of creating many times the number of paper options. Even with paper forms, the selection of a technology can impact formatting. For example, the selection of bar coding requires a design and location for the label; the selection of scanning technology benefits from machine-readable codes or titles and affects the selection of paper weight and color. Understanding the strengths

and weaknesses of the technology to be used adds to the likelihood of achieving a successful end product.

Standard Terminology, Abbreviations, and Format

Often large numbers of people use each form or view within an organization, and with the expansion of the CPR, this number increases. Effective communication, therefore, depends on the use of terminology that is understood by all. The use of standard terminology, where available, is recommended. For example, the ASTM definitions presented earlier and the data sets that follow provide standard definitions for commonly collected data items. Where standard definitions are not available, the form or view should supply the definition. Standard definitions are particularly important when using linked databases. Words, numbers, and abbreviations should be standardized as well. For example, as mentioned, users need to know whether hyphens should be included when entering social security numbers. They also need instructions on how many digits to use for the year of birth and how to enter coded data. Abbreviations have great appeal for health care providers because they save both reading time and entry time. Their major liability is misunderstanding. Caregivers depend on understanding the record to provide quality care. Administrative, legal, licensure, accreditation, and personal uses also depend on a clear understanding of the record. Any abbreviations permitted in the patient record should be understood by all. Another aspect of form or view design that promotes consistency is the development of a master format or template. The placement of data in the same sequence on similar forms or views with similar layouts facilitates rapid entry and retrieval.

Instructions

Instructions should briefly identify who should complete the data items and provide any additional guidance that is necessary. Computer views typically provide this information on introductory screens and as needed throughout data entry. Paper forms usually separate the instructions from the data entry spaces and place them at the top. The identification and distribution of copies also need to be specified. If the instructions need to be more extensive, they can be printed on the back, on a separate sheet, or in an administrative manual. If any of these alternatives are used, reference to the location of instructions should be made on the face of the form.

Simplification

With such a host of users, purposes, technologies, terms, and formats, it is easy to feel overwhelmed by the complexity. The last general consideration is to attempt to keep forms or views simple. Forms or views should be created only when there is an established need that is not being adequately handled by an existing form or view or when revision is impractical. The purpose of a form or view management program is to ensure that each tool has a desired purpose, that only necessary forms or views are maintained, and that all forms or views are documented and available. Simplification provides considerable savings in time, effort, and materials.

Paper Forms Design

In the continuing transition from the PPR to the CPR, the role of paper forms will change from primary data collection tools to intermediate aids for scanning technologies. Paper forms will also continue to have a role in providing computer output. This may be for release to patients or to providers who are less fully computerized or to provide reports within or among related facilities. As a guide to the design and technical aspects of preparing paper forms, discussion with a printer can provide basic information and help avoid costly mistakes. The development of a standardized guide, such as the one shown in Figure 4–1, will also help to ensure satisfactory results. The major segments of a paper form are the header and footer, introduction and instructions, and body and close. A guide, called a chart order, is also necessary to standardize the assembly sequence of the PPR.

Header and Footer

The title and any subtitle identify the form and typically are positioned at the top as a header. In facilities that bind their records at the top, it is easier to locate the title if it appears at the bottom. Forms for external use should include the facility name and perhaps a logo. Any code that is required for scanning technology should appear as part of the header. The footer contains information about the form, such as the control number, edition date, and page numbers or letters, usually at the left. This location enables reference information to be visible in most types of bindings and makes it easier to locate forms in the stock room. Forms that are multipage or printed on both sides should carry a footer on each page. This assists printing, completion, and insertion in the patient record. The edition date is particularly important in assuring the use of current forms and in the disposal of obsolete ones.

Introduction and Instructions

The introduction should explain the purpose of the form. The title is often sufficient, but sometimes patients and others outside the organization may need a subtitle and an additional explanation to understand the form's intent and complete it appropriately. The history form to be completed by the patient is one such example.

Body and Close

The body contains the main content of the form, and the close provides the space for authenticating or approving signatures. Design considerations include the data entry method, spacing, type styles, rules, and margins. Consideration of technology includes the data entry method for paper forms. Entries may be handwritten, computer-printed, or typed. OCR and bar codes should be considered along with the body because they provide direct data entry to the computer. Spacing provides an appropriate area to accommodate the data entry method. The amount of information a form can contain is significantly affected by spacing. For example, computer-printed or typewritten words require $\frac{1}{16}$″ vertical height, whereas handwritten words require $\frac{1}{3}$″. Type styles, or fonts, when well chosen, contribute to readability. Items of similar importance should be equal in size and type, and the overall number of fonts used should be low. Limiting the use of italics and boldface characters maintains the effect of emphasis. Style considerations may include the requirement to use a font identified with the name and logo of the organization.

Rules are vertical and/or horizontal lines that structure the form. They may vary in style but serve to divide the form into logical sections and to direct data entry length and location. If several people have areas to complete, the groups should be presented in the order of completion. Rules are often used to create either a line box or a ballot, or "X," box, as shown in Figure 4–1. Spacing must be provided, and vertical and horizontal rules should be aligned as much as possible. Titles should be located to the upper left of line boxes and immediately to the right of ballot boxes. Box entry is desirable because it is easier to follow visually, reduces the number of tab stops, and increases available space by as much as 25 per cent.

Rules that frame a section are called borders. Borders are preferable to screening or shading, which often causes indistinct electronic copies and transmissions. Some sections may be intentionally obscured or blacked out when, for confidentiality reasons, data items are not desired on every copy of a form. Borders around an entire form create a margin. Margins provide visual appeal as well as being important for printing. For example, a space of $\frac{3}{4}$″ maybe necessary for punched holes, and allowances may be needed for printing equipment. Discussing such specifications with a printer or the purchasing department is important in all aspects of form design.

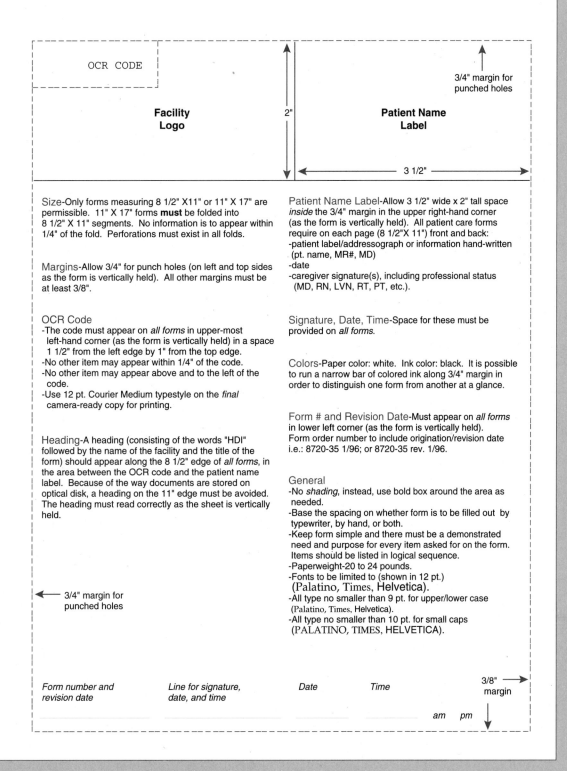

OCR CODE

**Facility
Logo**

2"

**Patient Name
Label**

3/4" margin for
punched holes

← 3 1/2" →

Size-Only forms measuring 8 1/2" X11" or 11" X 17" are permissible. 11" X 17" forms **must** be folded into 8 1/2" X 11" segments. No information is to appear within 1/4" of the fold. Perforations must exist in all folds.

Margins-Allow 3/4" for punch holes (on left and top sides as the form is vertically held). All other margins must be at least 3/8".

OCR Code
-The code must appear on *all forms* in upper-most left-hand corner (as the form is vertically held) in a space 1 1/2" from the left edge by 1" from the top edge.
-No other item may appear within 1/4" of the code.
-No other item may appear above and to the left of the code.
-Use 12 pt. Courier Medium typestyle on the *final* camera-ready copy for printing.

Heading-A heading (consisting of the words "HDI" followed by the name of the facility and the title of the form) should appear along the 8 1/2" edge of *all forms*, in the area between the OCR code and the patient name label. Because of the way documents are stored on optical disk, a heading on the 11" edge must be avoided. The heading must read correctly as the sheet is vertically held.

← 3/4" margin for
punched holes

Patient Name Label-Allow 3 1/2" wide x 2" tall space *inside* the 3/4" margin in the upper right-hand corner (as the form is vertically held). All patient care forms require on each page (8 1/2"X 11") front and back:
-patient label/addressograph or information hand-written (pt. name, MR#, MD)
-date
-caregiver signature(s), including professional status (MD, RN, LVN, RT, PT, etc.).

Signature, Date, Time-Space for these must be provided on *all forms*.

Colors-Paper color: white. Ink color: black. It is possible to run a narrow bar of colored ink along 3/4" margin in order to distinguish one form from another at a glance.

Form # and Revision Date-Must appear on *all forms* in lower left corner (as the form is vertically held). Form order number to include origination/revision date i.e.: 8720-35 1/96; or 8720-35 rev. 1/96.

General
-No *shading*, instead, use bold box around the area as needed.
-Base the spacing on whether form is to be filled out by typewriter, by hand, or both.
-Keep form simple and there must be a demonstrated need and purpose for every item asked for on the form. Items should be listed in logical sequence.
-Paperweight-20 to 24 pounds.
-Fonts to be limited to (shown in 12 pt.)
  (Palatino, Times, Helvetica).
-All type no smaller than 9 pt. for upper/lower case (Palatino, Times, Helvetica).
-All type no smaller than 10 pt. for small caps (PALATINO, TIMES, HELVETICA).

Form number and
revision date

Line for signature,
date, and time

Date

Time

3/8" →
margin

am   pm

FIGURE 4–1. Vertical forms guide.

Other Production Considerations

Beyond design guidelines, paper forms require some production considerations. The provision of margins for printing equipment is one example. Others include creating the master, physically building the form, and selecting the ink, carbonizing, and duplicating method. The master is the original from which the copies are produced. Masters may be designed and produced internally using desktop publishing software and a high-resolution laser printer. This approach is quick, easy, and cost-effective, particularly when photocopying is the method of duplication. When more elaborate and formal printing is needed, the master should be created by a professional typesetter. In either case, the master should be carefully proofed before reproduction. Physical building of the form refers to its size and special properties. Using standard-sized paper, such as $8\frac{1}{2}'' \times 11''$, keeps costs low and facilitates copying and filing. Double-sided forms should be carefully considered because of the need to turn them over when photocopying. Over-sized forms present similar special copying considerations because they require reduction.

Multipart forms require planning to provide sufficient copies and construction with carbon sheets, carbon spots, or NCR (no-carbon-required) paper. This packet of pages creates a forms set that is precollated and prefastened by a perforated stub. The advantages of multipart forms include standardization; having to write data only once, which reduces mistakes; and being able to provide quick, inexpensive copies. The disadvantages include the limited number of copies these forms can create. This is usually no more than 10, with fewer possible when the data are handwritten. Also, extra copies that are created and not used diminish any original savings and produce additional waste. Forms may be produced as individual form sets or as a continuous-feed strip. Forms may also be prepared as unit sets that are single forms glued along one edge to create a pad. Paper has many features, including weight grade, grain, and finish. These aspects combine to affect the form's suitability, durability, and permanence. The suitability reflects how easy the paper is to read and write on; durability measures how well a form stands up to handling; permanence reflects how long the paper lasts in hard copy. With the increasing use of scanning technologies, having paper with archival qualities is less important. What is extremely important is using a paper whose weight is suitable for use with copiers, facsimile machines, and scanning equipment. For electronic, environmental, and cost reasons, white paper is recommended. If color is necessary, a tinted border may be used. The ink should be a standard black because this type reproduces best and should meet scanning specifications. Again, color should be limited, although it may be appropriate for special applications, such as facility names and logos.

Duplicating methods include in-house preparation and commercial printing. In-house preparation entails the creation of the master and reproduction, most commonly by photocopying. Because this method is expensive, it is most suitable for a trial period or when only a small quantity of forms is needed. Offset printing can use the same in-house master and is more cost-effective for large quantities. Commercial printing uses a metal master, provides the best quality, and is more suitable for very large quantities. The commercial printer is also in the best position to provide value-added features, such as hole punching, perforating, collating, carbonizing, and prenumbering, which can be done in conjunction with the printing process.

Computer View Design

Computer views share the following general design features with paper forms:

- Needs of the user
- Purpose of the view
- Selection and sequencing of essential data items
- Standardization of terminology, abbreviations, and formats
- Provision of instructions
- Attention to simplification

There are profound differences as well. The CPR reaches far beyond the computerization of manual forms. The power of database management systems allows tremendous flexibility in the creation of views for data capture and data displays, including still and moving images and sound as well as text and graphs—all in living color. It is helpful to remember that standards such as those of ASTM are only a foundation from which to begin the data items selection process. Once captured, the data elements may be retrieved in new configurations to meet the needs of many different user groups. For example, a physician may want to view graphs that show the trends of laboratory data along with a menu of therapy options with costs, supported by a reference from a linked database. A social worker developing a discharge plan may select a summary of the patient's functional level, living arrangements, and insurance benefits to compare with services provided and prices charged by local home health care providers. This flexibility provides both the promise and the problems of designing computer views.

Computer Logic

In considering the data elements or fields within a database management system, the concept of format expands from a limited number of preprinted forms with standardized blocks of prescribed data elements to fields to be collected and retrieved in a multiplicity of ways, using computer logic. With all this flexibility, it is even more difficult to be sure that all items are collected. In addition to the general principle of creating a list or grid, the system requires development of controls and overrides. Controls are alerts and, possibly, stops that remind or require the user to complete particular fields, perhaps at particular times, such as entering a patient number. Overrides allow the option of bypassing the alert or stop, such as identifying an insurance carrier in an emergency, but may require that the item be captured later. Thus, views require consideration of computer logic in addition to the basics of good design.

On-Line System Interface

A person collecting data encounters computer logic at the boundary where users and computers meet on-line—the system interface. Good interface designs help make this interaction user-friendly while reducing errors. Windows is the most common interface format, in which each window can show information drawn from a different source. In some situations, systems can run separate applications in independent windows. Figure 4–2 shows such a GUI, with three windows overlaid one on top of the other as well as the icons and tool bar at the top. A well-designed interface allows the user to do the following:

- Initiate system actions, including data entry, editing, and retrieval as well as processing

- Navigate through the system in as natural a way as possible, avoiding tiresome or irritating routines

- Eliminate errors by avoiding a system interruption

Windows-style interfaces provide menus that pull down from choices shown on a tool bar at the top of the screen. A menu is an important component of a com-

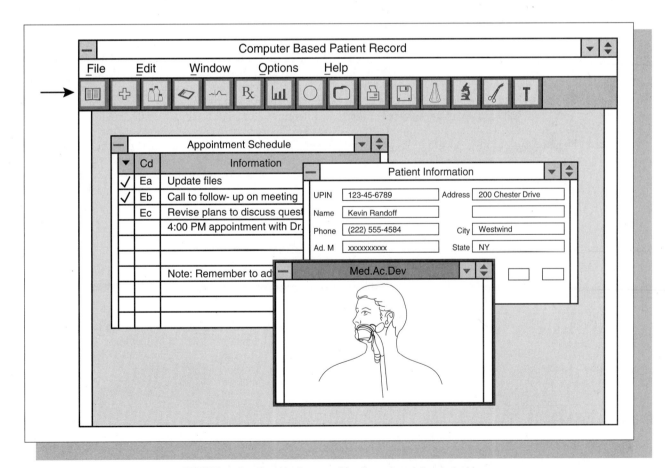

FIGURE 4–2. Graphical user guide. Arrow is pointing to tool bar.

TABLE 4–4 SAMPLE LIST OF ASTM E 1384-91 DATA ITEMS*

DATA ITEM	SIZE	TYPE†	SAVED	NOTES
Patient last name	20	X	Yes	
Patient first name	10	X	Yes	
Patient middle initial	01	X	Yes	
Patient UPIN	09	9	Yes	Item is record key
Date of birth	08	9	Yes	Ex: 11-13-1977
Sex	01	9	Yes	Code: 1 = male, 2 = female
Start date	08	9	Yes	Ex: 12-01-99, updated
Stop date	08	9	Yes	Ex: 12-31-99, updated

*Selected items for illustration only, not necessarily exact specifications
†Type codes: 9 = numeric, X = alphanumeric

puter view because it is central to ease of navigation. Therefore, a carefully constructed sequence of menus is part of a comprehensive design. Windows interfaces are not just used on personal computers, but on mainframe and minicomputer systems as well.

Record Content and Organization

For computer systems, grouping the data items to be used together in the application creates a logical record. The basic item list or grid must expand to include size and type specifications. Identifying which items are record keys (similar to the scanning OCR code) and which items must be saved is also helpful. The completed list becomes the record specifications (Table 4–4). Consideration of the physical file structure usually is unnecessary at this stage. Figure 4–3 shows one possible view of this data, called the master patient index. This index is often considered the most important resource in a health care facility, whether in paper or electronic format, because it is the link between the patient's name and the UPIN in a CPR or the unit record number in a PPR.

Other Display Features

In comparison to an $8\frac{1}{2}'' \times 11''$ sheet of paper, the computer page or view is the size of a 12″ television screen. The number of characters per line and of lines per view varies among terminals and software, some of which allow the user to change the size of the view. Typically, users can view the equivalent of one third of a page at a time. Consequently, this requires that more views be created to collect an equivalent amount of data. The advantages are that segments of a paper form completed by different practitioners can be separated for individual attention. The fact that the CPR completes part of the view with stored data is also a major advantage. Text displays can be customized with color from white characters on a black screen to more visually restful green or amber characters. Characters may be in different fonts and be bold, underlined, or in reverse video. Reverse video is the opposite of the traditional color pattern—for example, black characters on a white background instead of white characters on a black background. Color-coding text and menus can be helpful in distinguishing special features, such as instruc-

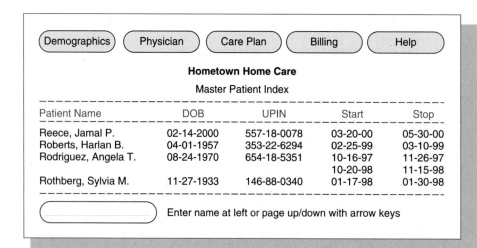

FIGURE 4–3. Sample master patient index view.

tions. Blinking may be added to characters or words to attract the user's attention, and scrolling moves the screen up or down a line or page at a time. As with paper forms, special features should be kept to a minimum to enhance their emphasis and simplify the view.

General Control Principles

Control issues include the following:

- Form or view identification
- Preservation of confidentiality
- Assurance of complete data capture
- Ongoing review and revision
- Cost control

Form or view identification is key to control. If the form or view does not have a name or number, reference to that form or view is subject to a great deal of misunderstanding. As mentioned, paper forms should contain a control number on each page, and computer views should be identified in the systems documentation. People who are uncomfortable in an electronic environment may cling to forms that they create themselves. Those who are computer literate may use desktop publishing software to create their own forms. In either case, keeping track of new additions is difficult, and inadequate or inaccurate documentation is likely. The creation of an open administrative atmosphere encourages users to bring their needs to the form or view management team. A similar situation exists with other software that allows users to customize their screens. Substantial advantages of this option are flexibility and its related user satisfaction. However, it is not without its disadvantages. The need to assure that all data elements are collected, that an audit trail of views is available for legal purposes, and that confidentiality is maintained requires that standardization programs, procedural guidelines, and input and output controls be developed.

Cost considerations are part of a control program and include selecting the most effective and efficient design, construction, and duplication methods for paper forms. For example, standard forms can be purchased from a publishing company as an alternative to coordinating forms design and production. Such forms are more expensive than photocopied forms but less expensive than custom printing. This approach eliminates the costs associated with the time and effort of design, but it also reduces the flexibility of custom features. A complete review of costs and benefits should be conducted before such a decision is made. In addition, purchasing and inventory need attention so that appropriate quantities are ordered and budget requirements are met.

Computer systems also have cost considerations. The paper output from the CPR system can vary from a simple printout of data entered to volumes of daily and summary reports. In all, the volume can easily exceed that generated in a PPR environment. It all can be programmed to happen automatically and can easily become overwhelming. But the computer program can also be changed. To control output as well as the information overload and its associated costs and confidentiality risks, the form or view management team must include the paper output within its scope of concerns. Happily, computer programs can be modified to address concerns such as these. Expenses are also incurred, however, when in-house or vendor programming is required.

Well-designed forms or views facilitate work by guiding the user through data entry, interpretation, and validation. They also contribute to the quantity and quality of work performed. An ongoing process of review and revision maximizes the benefits by clarifying ambiguities and collecting only necessary data items, which allows time to be devoted to other activities. Other chapters of this text explore the range of issues related to data analysis, evaluation, use, and access.

DATA NEEDS ACROSS THE HEALTH CARE CONTINUUM

Having explored the general concepts of data collection, we now investigate the specific applications along the health care continuum. As the health care delivery system has diversified, the number of providers and locations with which a patient will interact over a lifetime has multiplied. The following major areas of care are typically identified:

- Ambulatory care
- Acute care
- Home care (including hospice)
- Long-term care (including rehabilitation)
- Mental health care

Efforts such as those by the ASTM in standard E 1384 have taken on the challenge of establishing standard definitions for data elements to enhance the effectiveness and efficiency of EDI. This standard has been consciously designed to incorporate the requirements of various previously existing content directives, such as JCAHO standards; of government regulations, including the *Conditions of Participation* for Medicare; and minimum data sets (MDSs).

Minimum Data Sets

The purpose of all MDSs, as with E 1384, is to promote comparability and compatibility of data by using standard data items with uniform definitions. Although the data items are recommended as a common core, they do not constitute a complete record. In light of the data item definitions provided earlier, their presentation in the following sections has been abbreviated, and only special areas of interest have been highlighted. When applying any standard or data set, it is important to refer to the most recent edition. MDSs exist for ambulatory care, acute care, and long-term care. In situations where an MDS is not available, such as mental health, it is appropriate to use E 1384 and other data sets as guides.

General Forms and Views

As mentioned in the introduction to the preceding section, accrediting and regulatory bodies and professional organizations do not require or recommend particular forms or views. Although facilities are responsible for creating their own tools, it is not necessary to start from scratch. There are books, journals, newsletters, and vendor catalogs that offer examples, such as those listed in the bibliography for this chapter. Local professional organizations and networking with colleagues can also lead to valuable suggestions on what has worked well—and what has not. To provide a starting point, forms commonly included in the PPR are listed in Table 4–5 and described in the next section. Any differences in application are discussed under the appropriate care setting. Views meet the same needs but through their smaller, more flexible logical structure. A more complete understanding of the role of each form or view will develop through the balance of this chapter, related topics in other chapters, and through continuing professional education and experience.

Administrative Forms

REGISTRATION RECORD. Basic demographic and financial data are routinely collected on every patient in every care setting, except where not available. The data are collected before care is rendered and include sufficient items to positively identify the patient, such as name, address, date of birth, and next of kin as well as payment arrangements and a UPIN or patient identification number. Basic clinical data are also supplied on this form. The registration record is one of the most commonly computerized forms. It may also be called an identification sheet, face or summary sheet, or admission/discharge record.

CONSENT TO TREATMENT. All care settings must receive a consent for treatment from the patient or guardian. Special legal considerations exist in emergency situations. The body of the form contains a statement indicating that the patient agrees to receive basic, routine services, diagnostic procedures, and medical care. An additional statement explains that treatment outcomes cannot be guaranteed.

CONSENT TO RELEASE INFORMATION. The patient's signature on the consent to release information authorizes the exchange of medical information between the provider and other organizations. Most commonly, this specifies release of medical information compiled during the episode of care to third party payers. It may also permit the provider to request relevant health information from previous providers. This form is particularly appropriate to have translated into other languages. Verbal translation may also be necessary. It is generally understood that the provider has permission to release medical information for continuation of care. Confidentiality and legal considerations must be followed carefully in designing this form.

CONSENT TO SPECIAL PROCEDURES. A special consent is required to authorize any nonroutine diagnostic or therapeutic procedure before it is performed on the patient. For special consents to be valid, the physician must explain in lay terms the procedure named, the risks of having or refusing the procedure, available alternative procedures, and the likely outcome. Again, no guarantees are given. Signature by the patient or guardian confirms that the explanation has been given and understood and that the procedure has been agreed to. This form is particularly appropriate to have translated into other languages. Verbal translation may also be necessary. Both the *Conditions of Participation* and the JCAHO require that the medical staff bylaws, rules, and regulations address informed consent, including which procedures are covered. Consent must always be obtained, with the properly executed form on the chart before surgery. In emergencies, when consent is unavailable, the reason should be documented.

ADVANCED DIRECTIVES. Advanced directives give instructions regarding the patient's or guardian's wishes in special medical situations. The Patient Self-Determination Act, effective December 1991, requires that all patients be given written information about their rights under state laws so that they can make decisions concerning medical care, including their right to refuse or accept medical or surgical treatment. Also covered under the law is information regarding a patient's right to formulate advanced directives, such as living wills and durable powers of attorney for health care. Although the law requires that patients be informed, it does not require that the advanced directives be included in the chart. Patients are increasingly considering these options, discussing them with their family and personal advisers such as clergy and attorneys, and then executing the appropriate documents, and including appropriate information in the record.

TABLE 4-5 OVERVIEW OF COMMON PPR FORMS BY FREQUENCY AND MAJOR SITES OF CARE

FORM	ACUTE CARE	AMBULATORY CARE	LONG-TERM CARE	HOME HEALTH CARE	HOSPICE CARE	MENTAL HEALTH CARE
Administrative Forms						
Registration record	F	F	F	F	F	F
Consent to treatment	F	F	F	F	F	F
Consent to release information	F	F	F	F	F	F
Consent to special procedures	F	O	O	R	R	O
Advanced directives	F	F	F	F	F	F
Patient's rights acknowledgment	O	R	F	O	O	F
Attestation statement	F	M	M	M	M	M
Patient's legal status	R	M	O	M	M	F
Property/valuables list	F	R	F	R	O	O
Service agreement	M	M	M	F	F	M
Transfer/referral form	F	M	F	M	F	R
Birth certificate	F	O	M	O	R	R
Death certificate	O	O	F	O	F	R
Clinical Forms						
Registration record	F	F	F	F	F	F
Emergency record	M	F	M	M	M	M
Problem list	M	F	M	O	R	R
Medical history/review of systems	F	F	F	F	F	F
Psychiatric/psychologic history	R	R	R	R	R	F
Physical examination	F	F	F	F	F	F
Encounter record	M	F	M	M	M	M
Interdisciplinary patient care plan	R	R	F	F	O	F
Physician's orders	F	R	F	F	F	F
Progress notes	F	F	F	F	F	F
Consultation report	F	O	R	R	R	O
Discharge/interval summary	F	F	F	F	F	F
Operative Forms						
Anesthesia report	F	O	R	M	M	M
Recovery room record	F	O	R	M	M	M
Operative report	F	O	R	M	M	M
Pathology report	F	O	O	O	O	O
Obstetric Data						
Antepartum record	O	O	M	M	M	M
Labor and delivery record	O	O	M	M	M	M
Postpartum record	O	O	M	M	M	M
Neonatal Data						
Birth history	O	O	M	M	M	M
Neonatal identification	O	O	M	M	M	M
Neonatal physical examination	O	O	M	M	M	M
Neonatal progress notes	O	O	M	M	M	M
Nursing Forms						
Nursing notes	F	R	F	F	F	F
Graphic sheet	F	R	F	R	F	F
Medication sheet	F	R	F	R	F	F
Special care units	F	M	M	M	M	M
Ancillary Forms						
Electrocardiograph	F	F	F	F	F	F
Laboratory reports	F	F	F	F	F	F
Radiology/imaging reports	F	F	O	O	O	O
Radiation therapy	R	R	R	R	R	M
Therapeutic services (e.g., physical therapy, occupational therapy)	F	F	F	F	R	O
Case management/social service	F	F	F	F	F	F
Patient and/or family teaching and participation	O	O	O	O	O	O
Discharge or follow-up plan	F	R	O	O	M	O

F, frequent; O, occasionally; R, rarely; M, may never be seen in this record.

PATIENT RIGHTS ACKNOWLEDGMENT. This form lists the patient's rights while the patient is hospitalized. A patient must be informed of his or her rights at the time of admission, and there should be written evidence of this. A printed form containing rights may be signed by the patient and placed in the record as proof of the patient's being informed. If there are any changes in these rights, an updated copy should be signed and dated by the patient or guardian and added to the record.

PROPERTY AND VALUABLES LIST. An inventory of property and valuables brought by the patient should be created at the time of admission. Any items secured on the patient's behalf should be noted. Items such as visual aids, dentures, mobility devices, and prostheses are included, and the list is signed by the patient or a representative of the patient and a representative of the facility. Patients should be discouraged from retaining expensive, nonmedical items in their rooms.

BIRTH AND DEATH CERTIFICATES. State laws require the filing of vital records, including birth and death certificates. The forms and procedures vary by state, frequently in any event, copies are kept in the patient record.

Clinical Forms

REGISTRATION RECORD. The registration record may contain the attending physician's statement of diagnoses, intended procedures, and any allergies or sensitivities. A variation would be registration at a clinic, when only a chief complaint and allergies may be offered by the patient. Although not required, the inclusion of clinical data has many benefits. Any necessary third party authorization for services can be obtained, appropriate unit or room assignment can be made, and nursing care can begin. Standard terminology should be used and abbreviations and symbols avoided. The acute care admission/discharge record may also contain data on consultations and the disposition of the patient, including whether or not an autopsy was performed on a deceased patient.

MEDICAL HISTORY AND REVIEW OF SYSTEMS. The medical history, including a review of systems, forms the foundation for establishing a provisional diagnosis and developing a treatment plan. If the patient cannot reliably provide this important information, it should be obtained from the most knowledgeable available source. The source should be identified. As with other forms or views, standardization is important. An outline of the sequence of data items may be printed on the form or represented as fields to be completed on one or more

views. Computerization, with the options of alerts and alarms, makes it easier to assure that all essential data items have been captured. Whichever technology is used, the tone should be impartial and reflect the patient's statements. The components of the medical history consist of the chief complaint or a description of the symptoms that caused the patient to seek medical attention, the history of the present illness, past medical history, psychosocial or personal history, family history, and a review of systems (see E 1384, particularly Table 4–3). The JCAHO also requires that a developmental age evaluation and educational needs assessment be included when the patient is a child or adolescent. All symptoms (positive data) should be documented, and the term "normal" (or negative data) should be discouraged, except in summary statements. If the history is taken by someone other than the attending physician, such as a physician's assistant, nurse practitioner, intern, or medical student, it should be countersigned by the attending physician or a resident. If any of the information is in disagreement with the initial history, additions and/or corrections should be made before the form is signed. Some facilities, particularly those that provide acute care, require that the history and physical examination be completed within 24 hours. Their completion is also required before surgery can be performed.

PHYSICAL EXAMINATION. The physical examination adds objective data to the subjective data provided by the patient in the history. Together they provide the foundation from which the practitioner can establish a diagnosis and begin to develop a treatment plan. The examination should include all body systems (see Table 4–3) and consider the patient's age, sex, and symptoms. Any existing diagnostic data or physical findings are also included. A definitive diagnosis may not be possible, in which event a provisional (tentative) diagnosis may be used. If several diagnoses potentially fit the patient's clinical presentation, a list of these diagnoses is called a differential diagnosis. As with the medical history, the JCAHO requires a report of a comprehensive, current, physical assessment, usually within 24 hours and always before surgery is performed. In addition, a clinical impression and an intended course of action are required. Authentication and countersignatures are the same as for the history.

INTERDISCIPLINARY PATIENT CARE PLAN. Most care sites are required to have an interdisciplinary patient care plan (PCP). Exceptions are the physician's office or clinic and the acute care hospital, where the physician plan and other practitioners' plans are documented separately. The PCP is the foundation around which patient care is organized because it contains input from the unique perspective of each discipline involved. It includes an assessment, statement of goals, identification of specific activities or strategies to achieve those goals, and periodic assessment of goal attainment. The PCP is initiated when a patient is admitted or begins care and is periodically updated. The discipline responsible for implementing each part of the plan is identified. The PCP is reviewed and revised as often as the organization, regulatory agencies, and accrediting bodies require, when goals are achieved, or as the circumstances of the patient change. Changes in the PCP can easily be summarized at discharge. Because of its central role in planning and providing care, the PCP is a valuable tool in evaluating both individual patient care and overall organizational patient care performance.

PHYSICIAN'S ORDERS. Physicians communicate their plans for the patient by giving written or verbal orders or directions to the nursing staff and other practitioners. Orders are needed for any type of treatment or diagnostic procedure. Standing orders are a set of routine orders used for patients with a particular diagnosis or to prepare for or follow up a procedure. This type of order is discouraged, particularly with managed care, because all the actions may not be medically necessary for all patients. However, treatment guidelines and protocols that incorporate best practices for treating particular problems are being used. Orders based on these protocols provide a basic set of orders modified to address an individual patient's situation. Because they initiate actions, it is particularly important that all orders are dated and signed by the physician giving the order. The JCAHO requires that the medical staff bylaws, rules, and regulations address verbal orders and that such orders classified as being potentially hazardous to the patient be signed within 24 hours. With the exception of office visits, orders are needed for admission and discharge from facilities and for treatments such as radiation therapy. An admission order is written at the initiation of care, and a discharge order should be written on every patient when the physician determines that release is appropriate. The lack of a discharge order may indicate that the patient left against medical advice. If this situation occurs, the circumstances should be documented in the progress notes and discharge summary.

PROGRESS NOTES. Progress notes are interval statements that document the patient's illness and response to treatment as specifically as possible. Which practitioners write progress notes varies with the health care setting. For example, physicians write the majority of progress notes in their offices, and these notes are the focal point when patients are admitted for care. Because nurses coordinate and provide most of the patient care in home health, their notes are most prominent. In mental health, progress notes feature psychologist's documentation of counseling. Progress notes may be integrated, where all providers write sequentially on the same sheets, or they may be separated with physicians, nurses, and other providers writing separately, perhaps on custom-designed forms or views. Regardless of where the progress notes are located, any practitioner who writes such notes is responsible for recording observations about the patient's progress and response to treatment from the perspective of his or her profession. For example, physician progress notes for admitted patients should include an admission note, subsequent notes, and a final note. The admission note provides an overview of the patient at admission and adds any relevant information that is not included in the history and physical examination. The frequency of subsequent progress notes depends on the patient's condition as well as the site of care and its medical staff bylaws, rules, and regulations. Acute care notes are usually written daily, whereas long-term care notes may appropriately be written monthly. All treatments provided and the patient's response to each are to be included, as are any complications that the patient develops. When care of the patient is transferred from one physician to another, the physician releasing the patient should write a summary of the patient's course to that point. At the end of the admission, along with the discharge order, a final note is written stating the patient's general condition and instructions for patient activity, diet, and medications as well as any follow-up appointments. If the patient expires during the admission, the final notes describe the circumstances regarding the death, the findings, the cause of death, and whether or not an autopsy was performed.

CONSULTATION REPORT. A consultation report contains an opinion about a patient's condition by a practitioner other than the attending physician. Opinions may be sought from pharmacists, dietitians, physical and occupational therapists, dentists, other physicians, and so on. The opinion is based on a review of the patient record, an examination of the patient, and a conference with the attending physician. Many facilities, particularly in acute care, combine the request section, where the attending physician states the reason for consultation, with a space for the response, where the consultant details his or her findings and recommendations. Each signs his or her respective section.

The *Conditions of Participation* require that the medical staff bylaws, rules, and regulations address the status of consultants. To be considered a consultant, a practitioner must be well qualified by training, experience, and competence to give an opinion in the specialty in which the advice is sought. It is the responsibility of the attending physician to request a consultation. The categories of patients for which consultations must be requested are as follows:

- Patients who are not good medical or surgical risks

- Patients whose diagnoses are obscure
- Patients whose physicians have doubts as to the best therapeutic measure to be taken
- Patients who are involved in situations in which there is a question of criminal activity

In emergencies, exceptions may be made. The *Conditions* also state that routine procedures, such as radiologic studies, electrocardiograms, tissue examinations, and proctoscopic and cystoscopic procedures, are not normally considered to be consultations.

DISCHARGE AND INTERVAL SUMMARY. The discharge and interval summary, or clinical résumé, concisely reviews the patient's course. It is typically associated with admissions, but it may be provided in other care settings. The summary begins with the reason for admission and includes chronologic descriptions of significant findings from examinations and tests as well as procedures and therapies performed along with the patient's response. Details regarding discharge are also recorded, including the condition on discharge related to the condition on admission and instructions specifying medications, level of physical activity, diet, follow-up care, and patient teaching. Because the discharge summary is referred to frequently, standard terminology is essential and abbreviations as well as ambiguous terms such as "improved" should be diligently avoided. All relevant diagnoses established by the time of discharge and all operative procedures performed should be recorded in standard terminology that indicates topography and etiology as necessary. When final diagnoses and procedures are listed on more than one form, attention must be paid to their agreement. In special cases, a final progress note may substitute for a discharge summary. Patients admitted for less than 48 hours with minor problems, uncomplicated deliveries, and normal neonates are examples. The discharge summary should be written or dictated immediately after discharge.

Operative Forms

Data from each operative event are collected using a set of forms or views and are considered a unit. The consent for surgery and the pathology report are added to the forms described below.

ANESTHESIA REPORT. Patient procedures that require more than a local anesthetic also require an anesthesia report. Preoperative medication is recorded with time, concentration, and effect. The anesthetic agent is then documented, including the amount, route of administration, effect, and duration. The patient's condition throughout the procedure is described, including vital signs, blood loss, transfusions, and intravenous fluids given. The report should also describe any surgical ma-

nipulation that may affect anesthesia care, any complications during anesthesia, and any treatments that are unlikely to be documented elsewhere. The practitioner administering the anesthesia (either a nurse anesthetist or an anesthesiologist) records the data and signs the report.

Special anesthesia-specific notes are also required before and after surgery. The preanesthesia note, usually found in the progress notes, describes the planned procedure, the choice of anesthetic, and an examination of the patient. Also discussed are laboratory results, any drug history, any past or potential problems, and preanesthesia medications. The postanesthesia note may be in the progress notes, the recovery room record, or the anesthesia report. It documents the patient's condition, specifying the nature and extent of any complications. The postanesthesia note should be completed within 24 hours after surgery. Both notes are signed by the practitioner responsible for administering the anesthesia. The JCAHO requires at least one postanesthesia visit that describes the presence or absence of anesthesia-related complications. A visit is usually considered to occur apart from the operative or recovery area. Notes must specify time and date, with one occurring soon after surgery and another after the patient has completely recovered. The patient's condition may require additional visits. Although it is preferable that these notes be made by a physician or oral surgeon, any practitioner with pertinent comments regarding the patient's anesthesia care may add notes. If anesthesia personnel are unavailable to provide the documentation, the physician or dentist discharging the patient may complete the notes.

RECOVERY ROOM RECORD. The recovery room is designed to care for patients immediately after surgery or anesthesia. A separate form is usually used to record complete observation from the time the patient arrives in the recovery room until he or she leaves for the nursing unit or other destination. The JCAHO requires that this form include the patient's condition and level of consciousness when entering and leaving the unit; vital signs; status reports of infusions, surgical dressings, tubes, catheters, or drains; and any treatment provided in the unit. The postanesthesia note may be documented on this form and, depending on its design, may be signed by a physician, nurse, or both.

OPERATIVE REPORT. All patients who undergo surgery must have an operative report included in their record. The top portion provides identifying data, including the names of the surgeon and any assistants as well as the date, duration, and name of the procedure. A postoperative diagnosis is required. A preoperative diagnosis, which should be entered in the progress notes before surgery, is also desirable for easy comparison.

The body of the report contains a full description of the surgical approach, normal and abnormal findings, organs explored, procedures, ligatures, sutures, and the number of packs, drains, and sponges used. The condition of the patient at the conclusion of surgery completes the report, which is signed by the surgeon. The report should be written or dictated immediately after surgery and included in the record as soon as possible. If this is not possible, continuity of care can still be maintained by writing a timely and detailed operative note in the record.

PATHOLOGY REPORT. A pathology report documents tissue examinations that may be microscopic in addition to being macroscopic (gross). The tissue may have been removed from the patient during a specialized procedure, such as a biopsy, or during surgery. It may have been expelled, such as in an abortion, or be the entire body, as when an autopsy is performed. Occasionally objects, such as pennies, are submitted as well. As in a consultation, the tissue or object is identified, a clinical diagnosis provided, and an opinion requested. The pathologist examines the specimen and, at a minimum, writes a report describing its gross diagnostic features. A policy decision needs to be made regarding which specimens require only a gross examination and diagnosis. This decision may vary, depending on how and where the pathologist practices, but involves the medical staff in acute care. When a microscopic examination is performed, it is the basis for the diagnosis. The pathologist signs the report, and the original is included in the patient's record. When the report documents an autopsy, the pathologist summarizes the patient's illness and treatment followed by a detailed report of gross findings and an anatomic diagnosis at autopsy. An autopsy is a lengthy procedure, and as many as 60 days may pass before reports are completed. A provisional autopsy diagnosis should be recorded in the patient's record within 3 days. Both reports are also signed by the pathologist.

Obstetric Data

Another set of forms or views is collected for obstetric care. Again, any appropriate consent for surgery or associated pathology report is added to the forms described below. The American College of Obstetrics and Gynecology identifies the recommended content for these forms in its *Standards for Obstetric-Gynecologic Services*.

ANTEPARTUM RECORD. The antepartum or prenatal record begins in the office or clinic of the obstetrician or nurse midwife. Ideally started early in the pregnancy, the record includes a comprehensive history and physical examination as described previously, with particular attention to menstrual history, reproductive history including live births and abortions, a risk assessment, and attendance at any childbirth classes. Beyond routine laboratory tests, the blood group and Rh factor, rubella status, cervical cytology, and a syphilis screen should be checked. Women may choose to have their children at home, in a birthing center, or in a hospital. Whichever site is selected, a copy or abstract of current prenatal information should be available at the birthing site by at least the estimated 36th week of pregnancy. Arrangements should also be made for access to this information and to hospital care in case of an emergency in a birthing center or at home.

LABOR AND DELIVERY RECORD. This record tracks the patient from admission through delivery to the postpartum period. The antepartum record should be reviewed with attention to the special items described above. An evaluation is then made by the physician or nurse midwife, including an updated history or a complete history if there is no antepartum record, noting data on contractions, status of membranes, presence of significant bleeding, time and content of the patient's last intake of food or fluid, drug intake and allergies, choice of anesthesia, and plans to breast- or bottle-feed. The mother is monitored frequently, as is the child, using a fetal monitor. In the normal case, this is done by a nurse. At delivery, details regarding the mother are recorded, similar to those of a surgery. The neonate is also described, including his or her Apgar score (an infant rating system at 1 and 5 minutes after birth), sex, weight, length, onset of respiration, abnormalities, and treatment to the eyes. Any fetal monitoring strips are identified and annotated with relevant data and become part of the patient record.

POSTPARTUM RECORD. Postpartum data includes information about the condition of the mother after delivery. It may be a special form or included in the progress notes. In either case, attention is paid to assessing the lochia and condition of the breasts, fundus, and perineum as well as the usual postoperative status. Nursing staff continue this documentation as long as it is relevant.

Neonatal Data

The neonatal record includes the regular history, physical examination, and progress notes, with the addition of special identification data. The record for normal neonates is usually brief.

BIRTH HISTORY. This record may be shared with the mother's record, including pertinent history regarding pregnancy, any diseases, and delivery. The Apgar score, any prematurity or anomalies, and any problems that occur before transfer to the nursery are noted. Nurses and/or physicians sign the appropriate sections.

NEONATAL IDENTIFICATION. While the neonate is still in the delivery room, two identical bands are prepared noting the mother's number and the neonate's sex and time of birth. One band is placed on the mother and the other is placed on the neonate. A band number and identification form about the mother and neonate are also prepared. Both bands and forms should be checked by two responsible practitioners before the neonate leaves the delivery room. Footprinting and fingerprinting, if done, also require special forms. The nurse in charge of the delivery room is responsible for the identification process and signs the sheets along with any participating obstetrician.

NEONATAL PHYSICAL EXAMINATION. The neonatal physical examination repeats the birth data and concentrates on a detailed description of the neonate's appearance. The attending physician should examine the apparently normal neonate as soon as possible and before discharge. If the infant should remain in the hospital for additional days, additional notes are made. These notes are added to the infant's record and signed by the physician.

NEONATE PROGRESS NOTES. Neonates who remain in the hospital have progress notes added to the chart as well as other forms as needed. The American Academy of Pediatrics recommends frequent recording of vital signs until the neonate is stable (usually within 12 hours after birth). The JCAHO particularly requires that neonates who receive oxygen therapy should have the concentration recorded at intervals as written in the policies and procedures of the facility's nursery.

Nursing Forms

Although nurses document many forms within the record, the following forms are used exclusively by the nursing staff. The patient care plan is similar to the nursing assessment. Nurses should write conclusions in nursing diagnoses.

NURSING NOTES. Nurses may write nurses' notes or contribute to integrated progress notes. Regardless of the form, these notes describe the patient and his or her condition in objective, behavioral terms. Quantitative data are encouraged. The documentation begins with an admission note, including notification of the physician of the admission. Subsequent notes are written as needed and include nursing interventions and the patient's response. The documentation ends with a discharge note. If the patient should expire, a death note is written, including notification of the physician.

GRAPHIC SHEET. A graphic sheet is used to plot the patient's vital signs (temperature, pulse and respiratory rates, and blood pressure). Additional information may be noted, including weight and intake and output of fluids and solids. The frequency of entries depends on the patient's condition. One form usually provides space for six entries a day for several days, and additional sheets are added as needed. Nurses typically sign the form once and thereafter initial their entries.

MEDICATION SHEET. The medication sheet provides a detailed record of the medicines given orally, topically, or by injection, inhalation, and infusion. The date, time, name of drug, dose, and route of administration are included. If it is not possible to administer a scheduled dose, this is also noted and an explanation given in the nurses' notes. The practitioner giving the dose initials the entry.

SPECIAL CARE UNITS. Special units such as the intensive care unit and coronary care unit often have forms to suit their particular patient populations.

Ancillary Forms

Ancillary data are typically collected by practitioners other than physicians and nurses with the exception of patient and family teaching and case and staff conferences in which they may participate.

ELECTROCARDIOGRAPHIC REPORTS. The electrocardiograph records the electrical activity of the heart. The normal recording shows five waves, with the P wave indicating contraction of the atria followed by Q, R, S, and T waves, which relate to the contraction of the ventricles. Surface electrodes placed on the patient transmit impulses to the electrocardiograph. The electrocardiogram is the graphic tracing that plots these waves against time on a continuous paper roll or as a computer view. The report contains the cardiologist's signed interpretation and may include the tracing. When tracings are not provided, they are stored in the laboratory for reference.

LABORATORY REPORTS. Laboratory tests must be ordered by a physician and may include analysis or examination of blood, urine, stool, and other body substances. The medical laboratory may be within the facility or one that is used on a contractual basis. The laboratory usually provides the results of urinalysis and blood chemistry as well as hematology, microbiology, and serology reports. Tests should be completed and reported promptly. A report identifies the date, time, test, and results as well as reference values for the test's normal range. Reports are usually computer-generated and may be printed on standard-sized pages or on small slips designed to be taped on mounting sheets. Cumulative reports may be provided, which reduce the bulk of the chart. When blood banking is done, the American Association of Blood Banks has particular requirements detailed in its *Technical Manual*.

RADIOLOGY AND IMAGING REPORTS. Radiology reports describe diagnostic or therapeutic services. Diagnostic procedures include modalities such as radiography, nuclear medicine, computed tomography, magnetic resonance imaging, and ultrasonography, which create an image that can be visualized. On a form similar to that used for the consultation, the upper portion notes the attending physician's request for the study and specifies the area to be examined. A physician, usually a radiologist, dictates or writes a description of the image and adds an impression at the bottom of the form. Both physicians sign their respective sections. Films and computer images are stored in the department that produced them.

RADIATION THERAPY. Therapeutic radiology services more closely resemble the consultation process. They are major procedures that require a special consent. A treatment plan is written; each treatment is reported, including the amount of radiation given for each dose; and a summary is provided. The therapeutic radiologist signs each report.

THERAPEUTIC SERVICES. Therapies (e.g., physical, occupational, respiratory, speech, dietary) are initiated by a physician's order and include assessment and treatment plans designed to restore patient function. The therapist documents the services, including the patient's response, and signs the report or progress notes. Notes are objective and goal-oriented. The JCAHO has documentation requirements for each of these services, particularly as they relate to rehabilitative care. Evaluation and modification of the treatment plan is ongoing until the physician writes a discharge order, when a summary is prepared.

CASE MANAGEMENT AND SOCIAL SERVICE RECORD. Case management records collect data on the patient's background, social information, and problems identified by the patient, family, and case manager. The case manager has access to a great deal of sensitive personal information in addition to private medical information. The formal record includes a plan of action, progress notes, and a discharge note. One source of documentation guidelines is a book written by the Society of Social Work Directors of the American Hospital Association.

PATIENT AND FAMILY TEACHING AND PARTICIPATION. Evidence of patient and family teaching and understanding has become increasingly important as more treatments become available for patients and families to implement at home. Lifestyle changes are also appropriate topics for teaching. A wide variety of practitioners engage in patient and family teaching along the continuum of care. Regardless of the profession or the setting, the teaching and the redemonstration of understanding should be described. If any preprinted material is provided, it should also be noted and a copy kept on file in the HIM department if it should be needed to interpret the record. Some segments of health care require documentation of family participation in the planning, goal-setting, and carrying out of lifestyle changes, therapies, or other activities.

DISCHARGE AND FOLLOW-UP PLAN. A discharge plan is begun at the time of admission or initiation of services and gives a general assessment of plans to maintain continuity after this episode of care. This may represent transfer from acute care to long-term care, initiation of home health care, or provision of one or several available community services. Any agencies to be used should be identified. Social service often coordinates the plan, which includes both medical and financial arrangements and considers the family's needs as well as those of the patient.

Format Types

The organization of the PPR is referred to as its format. As with forms in general, there are no directives on which format to use. Facilities are free to design their own as long as the format chosen is standardized for all patients. There are three common formats: source-oriented, problem-oriented, and integrated.

Source-Oriented Medical Record

The most common PPR format is source-oriented, meaning that the record is organized into sections according to the practitioners who are the source of both the treatment and the data collection. Within each section, sheets are arranged in chronologic order, perhaps with some divisions by episodes of care. The sheet that defines the facility's standard sequence of pages to be followed in each record is called a "chart order." During admissions, the current episode is typically kept at the nursing unit in reverse chronologic order with the most recent materials on the top. The trend is to keep the record in this order rather than commit the staff time to reversing the chart. With implementation of the CPR, this will cease to be an issue. An advantage of standardized source-oriented records is the speed with which an individual sheet can be located. The major disadvantage is the lack of a clear picture of the patient's problems and how each department is contributing to their resolution.

Problem-Oriented Medical Record

The problem-oriented medical record (POMR) was developed by Dr. Lawrence L. Weed in the 1960s in response to the major deficiency in the source-oriented format—lack of a clear picture of the patient's problems. The POMR system focuses on the documentation of a logical, organized plan of clinical thought by practitioners. The system has four parts: a database, problem list, initial plan, and progress notes. The database was an early MDS similar to those in place today. The problem list is a dynamic document that titles, numbers, and dates problems and serves as a table of contents to the record. The problem is stated at the level of the physician's current understanding and modified as further data accumulate. Problems may be initial symptoms or well-defined diagnoses. The problems are past and present and social, financial, and demographic as well as medical. The initial plans describe what will be done to investigate or treat each problem. Plans refer to the problem number and can be of three types: the need to collect more decision-making information, therapy (e.g., medications, treatments), and patient education. Progress notes are written in a distinctive style with the acronym SOAP, which translates as follows:

> S = subjective, which records what the patient states is the problem
> O = objective, which records what the practitioner identifies through the history, physical examination, and diagnostic tests
> A = assessment, which combines the subjective and objective into a conclusion
> P = plan, or what approach is going to be taken to resolve the problem

SOAP notes are also numbered to correspond to the problems. The discharge summary is considered a special progress note.

Weed suggested that forms be designed to support the numbering and tracking of problems. He was also an early advocate of a team approach, encouraging all practitioners participating in the patient's care to document sequentially in the progress notes. Each practitioner would chart appropriate to his or her training, licensure, and understanding of the problem. The major advantage of the POMR is the way in which it creates a holistic picture of the patient and his or her care. Although it does not guarantee quality care, it provides an excellent communication and evaluation tool that highlights the thinking process. The major disadvantage is the time and commitment needed on the part of the practitioners to implement and maintain the system. With the exception of the SOAP style of progress notes, the system has not been widely accepted for use with the PPR. The POMR is well suited, however, to the CPR and is finding renewed support.

Integrated Medical Record

The integrated record is strictly chronologic without any divisions by source. This format keeps the episode of care clearly defined by date, which is an advantage when the flow of care is being considered. The major disadvantage is that information from the same source, such as laboratory data, is not easily compared. Some chart order arrangements integrate selected types of forms, such as progress notes, while keeping others, such as radiology reports, by source. Integrated progress notes resemble the team approach of the POMR, which provides a more holistic view of the patient. Physicians have also historically resisted charting alongside other professionals, believing that their notes need to be more prominent.

Ambulatory Care

Ambulatory care, or outpatient care, has emerged as the centerpiece of the U.S. health care delivery system. Physicians' offices and clinics are the most frequently used and most familiar care sites. Patients may be referred to other sites, including urgent care centers, diagnostic centers, freestanding surgery centers, and specialty care centers, for dialysis, physical therapy, and radiation therapy. Hospitals, in addition to providing acute inpatient care, offer the following types of ambulatory care:

- Ancillary services, such as laboratory and diagnostic imaging
- An organized outpatient department, which may include both primary care and specialty clinics
- Ambulatory surgery
- Emergency department

Multiple delivery sites and entry points for ambulatory care create unique operational challenges for hospitals. In addition, the definition of ambulatory care within a given facility is continually evolving as hospitals expand these services to keep pace with technologic advances.

Trends That Influence the Shift to Ambulatory Care

Four major trends since the mid-1980s have contributed to the shift away from acute inpatient care toward ambulatory care:

- Technology has provided the opportunity for many diagnostic tests, therapies, and surgeries to be done in the outpatient setting. Predictions for the year 2000 include expectations that 80 per cent of all surgical procedures will be done in ambulatory surgical centers.

- Government, third party payers, and business have provided reimbursement incentives, including prospective payment, to encourage the use of this more cost-effective segment of the delivery system. Another prediction for the turn of the century projects that 80 to 90 per cent of hospital revenues will come from ambulatory care.

- Managed care focuses on the primary care physician as the coordinator (or gatekeeper) of the patient's care, selecting other providers and care sites according to the patient's needs. Utilization of outpatient services is emphasized and often required to achieve the cost-saving objectives of managed care.

- Consumerism, which has increased since the mid-1960s, has also encouraged the expansion of this alternative to inpatient treatment primarily because of accessibility and convenience.

Data Needs

As we have seen, the root structure of the CPR, as defined in ASTM standard E 1384, is designed around a core header or demographic segment collected at the outset of care and updated as needed. This re-emphasizes the centrality of ambulatory care to both the data collection and patient care processes. The MDS that applies in this segment of the delivery system is the UACDS.

Uniform Ambulatory Care Data Set

The National Committee on Vital and Health Statistics (NCVHS) approved the UACDS in 1989. This data set was the product of a collaboration between its Subcommittee on Ambulatory Care Statistics and the Interagency Task Force of the U.S. Department of Health and Human Services (DHHS). The task force had been charged with surveying the data needs of the DHHS agencies while the subcommittee considered the applicability of the data set to the wider health care delivery system, including other agencies; private providers, practitioners, and payers; and researchers. Providers are encouraged to record all items in the individual patient's record, although some may be located in billing records. Where this is the case, the ability to link data from separate sources is an important requirement. The data set includes segments that describe the patient, the provider, and the encounter. Most items are required; some are optional. Detail of items is limited, given the E 1384 definitions stated previously. As with all MDSs, the most current edition should be consulted.

Segment 1: Patient Data Items

01. **Personal identification** (including name and number)

02. **Residence** (usual residence, full address, and zip code)

03. **Date of Birth** (month, day, and year)

04. **Sex**

05. **Race and ethnic background**

06. **Living arrangement and marital status** (optional)

The subcommittee and task force recognize that a person's social support system can be an important determinant of health status, access to health care services, and use of services. Frequently, marital status and/or living arrangements are used as surrogates for the social support system available to a patient. It is recommended that when this information is needed for program design, targeting of services, utilization and outcome studies, or other research and development purposes, the following definitions should be used for living arrangement and marital status. In terms of measurement of social support, the item on living arrangements will have greater utility than the item on marital status. The ultimate selection of items needs to be made on the basis of the context and purpose of the data collection.

Living Arrangement

a. Alone

b. With spouse (alternate: with spouse or unrelated partner)

c. With children

d. With parent or guardian

e. With relative other than spouse, children, or parents

f. With nonrelatives

g. Unknown

Multiple responses can be made to this item because of living arrangements that are a combination of spouse, children, parents, and nonrelatives. Longitudinal studies will have the opportunity to study transitions from one type of living arrangement or marital status to another.

SEGMENT 2: PROVIDER DATA ITEMS

An individual provider has been defined as a health care professional who delivers services or is professionally responsible for services delivered to a patient, who is exercising independent judgment in the care of the patient, and who is not under the immediate supervision of another health care professional. Note the difference between provider and practitioner as defined in E 1384. An encounter is defined as a professional contact between a patient and a provider during which services are delivered.

The following characteristics should be collected for the provider of record for each encounter. If a user decides to collect the additional provider data element, discussed above under definitions, for the provider who initiated the encounter (if different from the provider who delivered or was responsible for the services delivered), consideration also will have to be given to the necessary identification elements required for this item.

07. Provider identification (name and UPIN)

08. Location or address

09. Profession

This is the profession in which the provider is currently engaged and includes physicians (MDs and DOs), dentists (DDSs and DMDs), other licensed or certified health care professionals, and other health care providers. The speciality should be listed.

SEGMENT 3: ENCOUNTER DATA ITEMS

10. Date, place or site, and address of encounter, if different from item 08

a. Date of encounter: month, day, and year
b. Place or site of encounter (a list of 29 places of encounter are provided; examples include office, home, and hospital outpatient)
c. Address of facility where services were rendered when different from item 08

11. Patient's reason for encounter (optional)

Describe all conditions that require evaluation and/or treatment or management at the time of the encounter as designated by the provider. It is recommended that the standard coding convention for this purpose should be the widely used *International Classification of Diseases* and, if existent, its clinical modification (currently ICD-9-CM), with all codes available for use. This approach should accommodate the coding of symptoms, ill-defined conditions, and the problems when a firm diagnosis has not been established.

The condition that should be listed first is the diagnosis, problem, symptom, or reason for encounter shown in the patient record to be chiefly responsible for the ambulatory medical care services provided during the encounter. List additional codes that describe any coexisting conditions. Do not code diagnoses documented as "probable," "suspected," or "questionable," or "rule out" as if they were established. Rather, code the condition or symptom to the highest degree of certainty for that encounter.

13. Services

Describe all diagnostic services of any type, including history, physical examination, laboratory, radiography, and others that are performed pertinent to the patient's reasons for the encounter; all therapeutic services performed at the time of the encounter; and all preventive services and procedures performed at the time of the encounter. Also, describe to the extent possible the provision to the patient of drugs and biologicals, supplies, appliances, and equipment.

The diagnostic, therapeutic, and preventive services rendered in connection with the encounter should be captured where they are provided. The HCFA's Common Procedure Coding System (HCPCS), which is based on Current Procedural Terminology, 4th edition (CPT-4) for physician services and has been augmented for nonphysician services, is the most inclusive coding system for fostering uniformity in reporting these services.

14. Disposition

This is the provider's statement of the next step in the care of the patient. As many categories as apply should be reported. At a minimum, the following classification is suggested:

a. No follow-up planned
b. Follow-up planned
  (01) Return anticipated as necessary but not scheduled
  (02) Return to the current provider at a specific date
  (03) Telephone follow-up
  (04) Returned to referring provider
  (05) Referred to other individual provider
  (06) Referred to other provider for consultation
  (07) Referred to an adjunctive provider agency
  (08) Transferred to other individual provider

(09) Admit to acute care hospital

(10) Admit to residential health care facility

(11) Other

15. Patient's expected sources of payment

Related to E 1384, Segment 3, Financial. Eleven source categories are provided—for example, self-insured, insurance companies, workers' compensation, and government programs, including Medicare, Medicaid, and others.

a. Primary source

b. Secondary source

c. Other sources

d. Payment mechanism (related to this service)

(01) Fee for service

(02) Health maintenance organization/prepaid plan

(03) Unknown or unidentified

16. Total charges

List all charges for procedures and services rendered to the patient during this encounter. This includes a technical component or facility fee when billed separately from the professional component.

Special Forms and Views

In addition to the *Conditions of Participation* and JCAHO requirements, it is important to investigate any state regulations that specify record content.

PROBLEM LIST. Ambulatory care is the one setting in which the problem list from the POMR has found wide application. Symptoms and diagnoses are listed as Dr. Weed designed, with allergies, medications, significant surgeries, and perhaps any durable medical equipment that the provider has supplied.

ENCOUNTER RECORD. As defined in E 1384, an encounter is a professional contact between a patient and a provider during which services are delivered. The recording of ambulatory care encounters, with the exception of emergency care, is often done on a single form with minimum structure and used by all medical providers. Rubber stamps or stickers may be used to prompt for data items or serve as alerts. The *Conditions of Participation* for hospitals note the following standard when describing outpatient documentation: Enough information about the patient must be included to ensure continuity of care, including the following:

• Medical history

• Physical findings

• Laboratory and diagnostic test results

• Diagnosis

• Treatment record

The JCAHO has the following requirements:

• Identification

• Relevant history of the illness or injury and physical findings

• Diagnostic and therapeutic orders

• Clinical observations, including results of treatment

• Reports of procedures, tests, and results

• Diagnostic impression

• Patient disposition and any pertinent instructions given for follow-up care

• Immunization record

• Allergy history

• Growth charts for pediatric patients

• Referral information to and from agencies

In addition, procedures and outpatient surgeries must be documented in a manner similar to that described under General Forms and Views.

EMERGENCY RECORD. No form benefits more from efficient design than the emergency record. Data collection may begin with an ambulance service picking up the patient in the community. Vital signs, history of the present illness, monitoring of the patient's condition, and any procedures performed are documented. If the problem resolves or the patient expires, this is the complete record of care. If the patient is transferred to a hospital emergency department, a copy of this record may be attached or necessary information abstracted onto the hospital form. The *Conditions of Participation* for hospitals require the following data items:

• Identification

• History of the disease or injury

• Physical findings

• Laboratory and radiology reports, if needed

• Diagnosis

• Treatment

• Disposition of the case

The responsible physician signs the record. The JCAHO specifies that the following items be included:

- Identification
- Time and means of arrival
- History of present illness or injury
- Physical findings and vital signs
- Emergency care given before arrival
- Diagnostic and therapeutic orders
- Reports of procedures, tests, and results
- Clinical observations, including results of treatment
- Diagnostic impression
- Conclusion at the termination of treatment, including final disposition, patient's condition at discharge, and any instructions given to the patient or family for follow-up care
- Patient leaving against medical advice

Items are usually recorded on a single form divided into appropriate segments. A form is completed for each emergency encounter with the original kept by the provider. A copy may be sent to the patient's physician.

Issues in Data Collection

Maintaining continuity of care across multiple providers and practitioners delivering a wide scope of services is one of the most challenging aspects of ambulatory care. The potential for the CPR to transform this exchange of information into a true EDI will have profound advantages for providers, practitioners, and, particularly, patients. Because the record may develop over a long period of time, organization is important so that essential data can be located easily and not overlooked. All encounters, including those over the telephone or perhaps on-line, must be documented. Specificity is often a problem inherent to ambulatory care when diagnoses are in the process of being clarified. The evolution of reimbursement in ambulatory care toward a prospective payment system has required increasing detail in encounter records. Surgical reports have often omitted such items as length and size of lesions excised and wounds repaired; a description of the layers of fascia, muscle, and skin involved in a repair; wound debridement for major infections or contaminations; and complications encountered during or after a service.

Acute Care

Acute care, which is provided to hospital inpatients, has the longest history of regulation and accreditation. Hospitals may be small rural community facilities, large urban tertiary care centers, or designed to address the needs of specific patient populations. Acute care has been the focus of the early phases of the prospective payment system, which provided incentives to reduce the lengths of stay and contain costs. This mandate has been successful in achieving its goal, with inpatient acute care admissions continuing to decline. As we have just seen, ambulatory care has grown in response. Long-term and home health care have been impacted as well. Because of the resulting change in how patients receive their care, the severity of illness and intensity of service in acute care hospitals have increased. Because the length of stay in acute care sites is reduced, sicker patients are also being treated in long-term care and home health programs. Although acute care is facing many challenges, it has the advantage of being centralized, with a staff that is sophisticated and well controlled and that has a long history of documenting patient care.

Data Needs

Acute care hospitals function for three shifts, 7 days a week, every week of the year, and they collect a great deal of data. The *Conditions of Participation* detail the content of the inpatient record as does the JCAHO *Accreditation Manual for Hospitals*. Most of the basic forms described are included in the inpatient record and are designed to meet the requirements of the UHDDS.

Uniform Hospital Discharge Data Set

The UHDDS was promulgated by the secretary of the Department of Health, Education, and Welfare in 1974 as a minimum, common core of data on individual hospital discharges in the Medicare and Medicaid programs. As with other MDSs, the purpose was to improve uniformity and comparability of data. The UHDDS has undergone several revisions and is under the direction of the NCVHS of the DHHS. The UHDDS contains the 20 items listed below and is not segmented. Again, details are limited and the most current edition should be consulted.

01. **Personal identification** (UPIN)
02. **Date of birth** (month, day, and year)
03. **Sex**
04. **Race and ethnicity**
05. **Residence** (usual residence, full address and zip code—nine-digit zip code, if available)
06. **Hospital identification** (UPIN)

Three options are given for this institutional number, with the Medicare provider number as the recommended choice. The federal tax identification number or the American Hospital Association number is preferred to creating a new number.

07. Admission date (month, day, and year)

08. Type of admission (scheduled or unscheduled)

09. Discharge date (month, day, and year)

10. Attending physician identification (UPIN)

11. Operating physician identification (UPIN)

12. Principal diagnosis

The condition established after study to be chiefly responsible for occasioning the admission of the patient to the hospital for care.

13. Other diagnoses

All conditions that coexist at the time of admission or that develop subsequently that affect the treatment received and/or the length of stay. Diagnoses that relate to an earlier episode and that have no bearing on the current hospital stay are excluded.

14. Qualifier for other diagnoses

A qualifier is given for each diagnosis coded under "other diagnoses" to indicate whether the onset of the diagnosis preceded or followed admission to the hospital. The option "uncertain" is permitted.

15. External cause-of-injury code

Hospitals should complete this item whenever there is a diagnosis of an injury, poisoning, or adverse effect.

16. Birth weight of neonate

17. Procedures and dates

a. All significant procedures are to be reported. A significant procedure is one that (1) is surgical in nature, (2) carries a procedural risk, (3) carries an anesthetic risk, or (4) requires specialized training.
b. The date of each significant procedure must be reported.
c. When multiple procedures are reported, the principal procedure is designated. The principal procedure is one that was performed for defini-

tive treatment rather than one performed for diagnostic or exploratory purposes or was necessary to take care of a complication. If two procedures appear to be principal, then the one most related to the principal diagnosis is selected as the principal procedure.
d. The UPIN of the person performing the principal procedure must be reported.

18. Disposition of the patient

a. Discharged home (not to home health service)
b. Discharged to acute care hospital
c. Discharged to nursing facility
d. Discharged to home to be under the care of a home health service
e. Discharged to other health care facility
f. Left against medical advice
g. Alive, other; or alive, not stated
h. Died

19. Patient's expected source of payment

a. Primary source
b. Other source

20. Total charges

List all charges billed by the hospital for this hospitalization. Professional charges for individual patient care by physicians are excluded.

Special Forms and Views

Most acute care forms have been described previously, although, as mentioned, they are typically more elaborate than those for other sites of care. Of particular note are time frames related to the history and physical examination and the attestation form.

HISTORY AND PHYSICAL EXAMINATION. If a history and physical examination have been performed within a week before admission, such as in the office of a physician staff member, then a durable, legible copy of this report may be added to the record with any interval changes documented. When the patient is readmitted within 30 days for the same or a related problem, an interval history and physical examination may be completed if the original is readily available.

ATTESTATION STATEMENT. The attestation statement, a requirement of the Medicare prospective payment system, is signed by the attending physician and states: "I certify that the narrative description of the principal and secondary diagnosis and the major procedures performed are accurate and complete to the best of my knowledge." The attestation is typically included as part of a computer-generated record created with coded diagnostic and procedural data as well as related reimbursement information. Alternatively, it may appear on the registration (admission/discharge) record or may be on a separate form.

Issues in Data Collection

Acute care has the advantage of a long history of improving documentation and data collection. Stresses on data collection have increased since the implementation of the prospective payment system. Mandates to decrease lengths of stay have required that more data be collected before admission and that data be readily available to expedite treatment. Trends toward ambulatory and home care have resulted in admissions being limited to only the most severely ill patients receiving the most intensive services.

Long-Term Care

Integral to cost containment is the concern over the effect of the tremendous growth in the elderly population. The Bureau of the Census has projected a doubling of the 65-or-older age-group between 1980 and 2020 with an even more rapid increase in the 85-or-older age-group.

The reimbursement incentives that cause shorter lengths of stay in acute care facilities result in the discharge of patients with more complex problems to long-term care facilities.

Minimum Data Set for Nursing Home Resident Assessment and Care Screening

This MDS is under the direction of the NCVHS and shares the purpose of increasing uniformity and comparability of data. Implemented in the early 1990s, it was preceded by the *Long-Term Health Care Minimum Data Set* developed in 1980. The MDS contains 16 alphabetical sections, including options for each of the assessment items. These options are detailed and frequently lengthy and have not been included here. As with other MDSs, the current edition should be consulted.

SECTION A: IDENTIFICATION AND BACKGROUND INFORMATION
01. **Assessment date**
02. **Resident name**
03. **Social security number**
04. **Medicaid number** (if applicable)
05. **Medical record number**
06. **Reason for assessment**
07. **Current payment source**
08. **Responsibility/legal guardian**
09. **Advanced directives**
10. **Discharge planned within 3 months**
11. **Participation in assessment**
12. **Signatures**

SECTION B: COGNITIVE PATTERNS
01. **Comatose**
02. **Memory**
03. **Memory/recall ability**
04. **Cognitive skills for daily decision making**
05. **Indicators of delirium, periodic disordered thinking/awareness**
06. **Change in cognitive status**

SECTION C: COMMUNICATION AND HEARING PATTERNS
01. **Hearing**
02. **Communication devices or techniques**
03. **Modes of expression**
04. **Making self understood**
05. **Ability to understand others**
06. **Change in communication or hearing**

SECTION D: VISION PATTERNS
01. **Vision**
02. **Visual limitations or difficulties**
03. **Visual appliances**

SECTION E: PHYSICAL FUNCTIONING AND STRUCTURAL PROBLEMS

01. **Activities of daily living (ADL) and self-performance** (e.g., bed mobility, transfer, locomotion, dressing, eating, toilet use, and personal hygiene)

02. **ADL support provided**

03. **Bathing**

04. **Body control problems**

05. **Mobility appliances or devices**

06. **Task segmentation**

07. **ADL functional rehabilitation potential**

08. **Change in ADL function**

SECTION F: CONTINENCE IN PAST 14 DAYS

01. **Continence self-control categories** (bowel and bladder)

02. **Incontinence-related testing**

03. **Appliances and programs**

04. **Change in urinary continence**

SECTION G: PSYCHOSOCIAL WELL-BEING

01. **Sense of initiative or involvement**

02. **Unsettled relationships**

03. **Past roles**

SECTION H: MOOD AND BEHAVIOR PATTERNS

01. **Sad or anxious mood**

02. **Mood persistence**

03. **Problem behavior**

04. **Resident resists care**

05. **Behavior management program**

06. **Change in mood**

07. **Change in problem behavior**

SECTION I: ACTIVITY PURSUIT PATTERNS

01. **Time awake**

02. **Average time involved in activities**

03. **Preferred activity settings**

04. **General activity preferences** (adapted to resident's current abilities)

05. **Prefers more or different activities**

SECTION J: DISEASE DIAGNOSES

01. **Diseases** (narrative options provided in sections with "none of the above" available when none apply)

02. **Other current diagnoses and ICD-9-CM cdes**

SECTION K: HEALTH CONDITIONS

01. **Problem conditions** (within past 7 days, i.e., fever, constipation)

02. **Accidents**

03. **Stability of conditions**

SECTION L: ORAL PROBLEMS AND NUTRITIONAL STATUS

01. **Oral problems**

02. **Height and weight**

03. **Nutritional problems**

04. **Nutritional approaches**

SECTION M: ORAL DENTAL STATUS

01. **Oral status and disease prevention**

SECTION N: SKIN CONDITION

01. **Stasis ulcers**

02. **Pressure ulcers**

03. **Resolved or cured pressure ulcers**

04. **Skin problems and care**

SECTION O: MEDICATION USE

01. **Number of medications**

02. **New medications**

03. **Injections**

04. **Days the medication received**

05. **Previous medication results**

SECTION P: SPECIAL TREATMENTS AND PROCEDURES

01. **Special treatments and procedures**

02. **Abnormal laboratory values**

03. **Devices and restraints**

Special Forms and Views

The long-term care record is similar to the acute care record in that it is also an admission record. Differences include the size of the record, which typically needs to be thinned during the length of stay, and the emphasis on nursing care. Details of functional capacity, bowel and bladder habits, and medication interactions also take on prominence.

PHARMACY CONSULTATION. Because most elderly people take multiple medications, a pharmacy consultation is required to review for potential drug interactions, discrepancies in medications ordered versus those given, and any recommended changes. The consultation may appear on the physician's order sheet, in the progress notes, or on its own sheet, and should be documented monthly.

TRANSFER OR REFERRAL FORM. When a resident is admitted to a facility, a transfer form provided by the hospital, physician, or other facility should accompany the patient or follow immediately. The form facilitates the continuity of care and should include the following:

- Reason for admission
- Diagnosis
- Current medical information
- Rehabilitative potential

The physician should certify the level of care required and the anticipated length of stay. The form should also contain the following administrative data:

- Identification (resident's UPIN)
- Names of the transferring and receiving institutions
- Date of transfer
- Diagnoses
- Physician's and any nurses' report

When patients are routinely transferred between facilities, it is common to have a transfer agreement signed by both institutions. This formalizes and facilitates the ongoing exchange of information whenever patients move between the institutions. Transfers between long-term care facilities are also possible

Issues in Data Collection

Long-term care facilities have had to adjust to the extensive MDS. Many have computerized these data and have benefited from the alerts and alarms and the automatic generation of the PCP. The update intervals are also automatically identified. One particular difficulty in documenting long-term care is that the patient's status does not seem to change. Practitioners need to be encouraged to continuously be attentive to even small changes and reflect them in the patient's record.

Rehabilitation

Rehabilitation facilities vary widely in type from infant development to spinal cord injury, from chronic pain management to vocational evaluation. The range of services is equally extensive, from prosthetics to patient advocacy, from ADLs to audiology. Matching the patient's needs to the type of facility and its services is an important discharge planning function. When the facility has been selected, the patient is registered or admitted and oriented. During this screening process, the patient is assessed and the PCP developed. Any services that need to be referred are arranged.

The CARF has developed standards requiring that a single record be maintained for any patient and that it include the following:

- Identification data
- Pertinent history
- Diagnosis of disability
- Rehabilitation problems, goals, and prognosis
- Reports of assessments and individual program planning
- Reports from referring sources and service referrals
- Reports from outside consultations and laboratory, radiology, orthotic, and prosthetic services
- Designation of a manager for the patient's program
- Evidence of the patient's or family's participation in decision making
- Evaluation reports from each service
- Reports of staff conferences
- Patient's total program plan
- Plans from each service
- Signed and dated service and progress reports
- Correspondence pertinent to the patient
- Release forms
- Discharge report
- Follow-up reports

Issues in Data Collection

In rehabilitation, it is common for services to keep raw patient data, such as attendance, which are summarized for the record. Maintaining a comprehensive unit record must, therefore, be closely monitored for compliance with standards.

Home Health Care

Home health care describes services provided to the patient in his or her place of residence. Similar to ambulatory care, home health has been the recipient of both increased patient volume and regulatory attention as incentives have been provided to find alternatives to acute care. Advances in technology have added momentum to the home care movement with the availability of infusion for antibiotic therapy and chemotherapy, total parenteral nutrition, respiratory care (including ventilators), and other high-technology treatments. A nurse manager typically coordinates a case based on the attending physician's orders. Health care analysts predict that home care will become the hospital of the 21st century, which should see an increase in the number, regulation, and sophistication of home care agencies.

Regulations for home health care are more limited than for acute or long-term care and substantially follow the *Conditions of Participation* for Medicare-certified home health agencies. The focus is on collecting the following data to complete the standard HCFA forms:

- Home health certification and plan of treatment
- Medical update and patient information
- Plan of treatment
- Medical update and patient information addendum
- Home health agency intermediary medical information report

To be Medicare-certified, an agency must provide skilled nursing care and at least one of the following therapeutic services: physical, speech, or occupational therapy; medical social services; or home health aide services. The HCFA classifies home health agencies into the following categories:

- Hospital- or provider-based
- Proprietary
- Private nonprofit
- Government (state or local health and welfare departments)
- Voluntary nonprofit (Visiting Nurses Association)

The JCAHO has a standards manual for home care, and the National League for Nursing has an accreditation program. The National Homecaring Council represents and accredits agencies that provide homemaker and home health aid services and includes some record-keeping guidelines.

Minimum Data Set

There is no MDS for home care, although the assessment and screening for long-term care are appropriate to use in developing data items. A standard definition of a home care visit or length of stay has yet to be developed. For the purpose of Medicare reimbursement, each encounter with a health care practitioner is a visit; for example, if the nurse and the respiratory therapist both see the patient on the same day, two visits are counted.

Special Forms and Views

The home care record is similar to the ambulatory care record, although the interdisciplinary PCP is a central coordinating tool. A summary should be provided for the attending physician at least every 60 days. When the patient is discharged from a particular service, a service summary is written followed by an overall discharge summary at the termination of care. Most of the documentation is done by nurses and therapists. If the care is provided through a hospital, the home care record should be combined with the inpatient unit record.

SERVICE AGREEMENT. The patient or guardian should sign a service agreement that outlines the services to be provided, the times services are to be provided, the charges, and the parties responsible for payment.

Issues in Data Collection

One of the major challenges in home care is that a significant part of the record may remain in the home for documentation by practitioners representing various disciplines who provide care at intervals. Returning these portions of the record to the agency needs attention as one aspect of coordinating a team diverse in specialty and location. The record in the home should also contain the name of the agency, the people to contact along with their telephone numbers, patient and/or family instructions for care, a list of medications with potential adverse effects, and emergency instructions. The presence of this information in the home should be documented in the agency record. Training in patient record practices may also need special attention. Because the staff is not centralized, well-designed policies and procedures and initial orientation and follow-up sessions are important. Homemakers, companions, and family members may need to be instructed on how to record data.

Hospice

Hospice care provides supportive services for terminally ill patients, their families, and significant others. Psychosocial and spiritual support are central to this type of care, and only palliative medical attention is provided. In addition to the interdisciplinary team of health care providers, volunteers contribute in important ways to patient care. Hospice services are frequently provided in the home. A primary caregiver, who may be a relative or friend, is identified. Home care or an inpatient admission may occur for symptomatic management, but no life-prolonging measures are undertaken. Hospice is a philosophy of care more than a location. A unique feature of hospice care is that not only the patient but also the family or significant other are provided services. The family or significant other may receive aftercare for as long as 1 year after the death, depending on the need.

The following data are required by JCAHO hospice standards:

- Identification
- All pertinent diagnoses
- Prognosis
- Designation of an attending physician
- Designation of the family member or person to be contacted in the event of an emergency or death

An interdisciplinary PCP is the foundation of the record. Both a physical and a psychosocial assessment are required. The physical assessment describes functional capacity, acute or chronic pain, and other physical symptoms and their management. The psychosocial assessment of the patient as well as the family includes spiritual needs. As in other care settings, updating the PCP is ongoing. A review of the PCP is required every 30 days and must be documented. A summary of care is prepared and should include information on the coordination of transfer from the hospital to home care and when the patient expires. The Medicare *Conditions of Participation* closely follow the JCAHO standards. A specific addition relates to following the hospice PCP even when inpatient services are provided. Medicare reimburses hospices at four levels: routine home care, continuous home care, inpatient respite care, and general inpatient care. Data collected should justify the level of care provided. The National Hospice Organization is a resource for data collection guidelines.

Hospice is more specific in defining its episodes than home care. The first episode of care begins with the patient's or family's admission to the hospice program and ends when the patient is transferred or discharged or dies. This episode includes all services provided, regardless of the setting. The second episode of care begins with the patient's death and the transition of the family or significant other on the next day into bereavement care and ends when the survivors are discharged, perhaps as much as 1 year later.

Special Forms

If the hospice care is provided by a hospital or home care agency, the completed record should be filed with other records on the patient. Forms documenting spiritual needs and responses, pain assessment and management, and bereavement are particularly important in the hospice setting.

Issues in Data Collection

Similar to home care, hospice is a diverse team of people in various locations. Coordination and training are among the most important concerns.

Mental Health

Mental health provides psychological and psychiatric services to patients who may or may not have medical problems. Two unique features of mental health are the close monitoring of the patient's legal status and additional attention to confidentiality. Legal requirements must be carefully reviewed when both planning and managing patient information. Facilities may provide inpatient or outpatient care and can provide adult psychiatric, child and adolescent, and/or alcohol and substance abuse programs. These programs are all regulated by the *Conditions of Participation* and by the JCAHO in its *Consolidated Standards Manual*. There is no MDS, but data collection resembles patterns previously described for inpatient or outpatient care. A preliminary treatment plan is required on admission with an initial plan, based on a comprehensive assessment, completed within 72 hours.

Special Forms and Views

The previously explained forms and views apply to mental health care with some additions. The interdisciplinary PCP is reviewed during case conferences. Incident and accident reports are of particular importance. Issues of patients' rights receive particular attention in mental health care because of its restrictive nature. Patients and guardians must be informed of their rights, and whenever a patient's rights are denied, justification must be documented. When the reason for the denial is no longer present, rights must be restored.

ASSESSMENT. In addition to basic assessment features, the patient's legal status is assessed, and social, recreational, and vocational assessments are included. Complaints by others regarding the patient are added to the patient's comments.

SPECIAL ASSESSMENTS. When special treatments are considered, an assessment is required. Such treatments include seclusion, restraints, and electroconvulsive therapy.

PSYCHIATRIC HISTORY AND DIAGNOSIS REPORT. A separate report documenting the patient's psychiatric condition on admission is required. The patient's medical history and physical examination are also required.

RESTRAINT AND SECLUSION. When a patient is disruptive, the least restrictive attempts at control should be attempted first. If the patient continues to disrupt the therapeutic environment, seclusion may be considered. If this is unsuccessful, restraint is a further action that may be taken. Restraint and seclusion should only be used to protect the patient and others and to avoid damage to the facility. If either is chosen, the assessment with justification, implementation, monitoring, and termination of restraint or seclusion must be carefully documented. As mentioned, a physician must assess the patient and provide a clinical justification as well as attempt to manage the patient using less restrictive measures. An order is then written that is to last no longer than 24 hours. Staff are to monitor the patient every 15 minutes. If restraint or seclusion should be required in an emergency, trained staff may proceed, with a phone order from the physician for continuation. In any event, when restraint or seclusion is considered necessary for longer than 24 hours, the head of the professional staff should be informed and the case reviewed.

ELECTROCONVULSIVE AND OTHER THERAPY. Electroconvulsive therapy, psychosurgery, behavior modification using painful stimuli, and experimental treatment are other areas of mental health treatment in which extreme care must be exercised and documentation meticulously recorded. Special consents must be signed by the patient or guardian. Other therapies that may be used include therapeutic passes and behavior modification contracts. If either of these is used, any agreements with and response from the patient should be included in the record.

Issues in Data Collection

With the exception of medications ordered, mental health care is difficult to quantify and relies almost exclusively on narrative description. It is important that practitioners document as clearly as possible while continuing to be objective in their statements.

SUMMARY AND MANAGEMENT ISSUES

Health care decisions may make the difference between life and death for patients and between success and bankruptcy for providers. There is little room for error. Timely and accurate information is needed to make these decisions with the highest possible degree of confidence. A prerequisite to such quality information is quality data. Data items that are well selected, defined, and collected make efficient use of human and computer processing resources and produce valuable information. Awareness of the needs of users, the flow of data throughout the facility, and the health care delivery system, as well as standards and content directives, positions the HIM manager at the hub of the health care decision-making process.

There are a host of reasons why facilitating data collection and the transformation of data into information have value to an organization, but there may be problems as well. Knowledge—from information—is power. As systems are made increasingly accessible, people who previously had an information monopoly may oppose change. Others in the organization may fear the loss of their jobs. Some may be overwhelmed by the technology and conception of the wide scope of the CPR. Users may think that they have to compete to have their needs acknowledged. For these reasons and many others, HIM managers must develop interpersonal as well as information systems skills. The quality of data can be profoundly affected by fearful or angry users, and the potential positive outcomes may not be realized. Taking time to show genuine sensitivity to such concerns and to address them seriously will pay dividends at both the personal and the professional level. The following provides an example of facilitating data collection.

A major goal and advantage of the CPR is to have data captured only once and then be made available to all users of that data item. A closely associated goal is to have the data item entered by the primary user as close to the point of care as possible. It has been far easier to achieve consensus on the goal of entering data once than on the question of who should enter the data. Persuading physicians and other members of the patient care team to participate in data entry has been difficult because this has been historically viewed as a clerical task. An HIM manager may consider minimizing the need for practitioners to key data by using the point-and-click technology of a light pen or a mouse. The less keyboarding that is required, the less data entry resembles a clerical task. Even more persuasive is a voice recognition system. This offers two satisfiers—convenience and response time. Systems that respond in subsecond time frames for both data entry and retrieval find the highest positive reaction and encourage user participation. Another possible incentive would be to provide screens or reports that enhance physician practice management, perhaps linking records from multiple sites and again saving time. It is important for practitioners to see direct benefits from direct data entry into the CPR. Understanding user psychology helps the HIM manager to be an effective change agent.

A well-designed data collection program that is sensitive to the professional and personal needs of users is a challenging goal. It is not necessary to memorize the *Conditions of Participation,* the JCAHO manuals, ASTM E 1384, or MDSs. It is necessary to be aware of trends and the changes they bring and to know how and where to locate the resources you need. As the program develops, it is important to document the process and develop policies and procedures. They are invaluable aids both in remembering why decisions were made and by whom and in providing training to share the exciting future of health information management with others.

Key Concepts

- Sound decision making depends on having good data.

- Forces in data collection include communication among providers, accrediting and licensure requirements, reimbursement, legal interests, and evaluation of quality of care.

- Users include the patient as well as practitioners, providers, third party payers, agencies, and researchers.

- Cost-effectiveness includes resisting the more-is-better philosophy.

- The only reason to collect data is because there is an identified purpose for their retention, retrieval, and use.

- The *Conditions of Participation* for Medicare and the JCAHO standards have a profound impact on defining data items to be collected.

- ASTM E 1384 is designed to define the data items in a comprehensive CPR.

- The purpose of MDSs is to improve uniformity and comparability of data. They exist in ambulatory care, acute care, and long-term care.

- Once the essential data items are identified, it is generally agreed that data should be captured only once and be accessible to all portions of the system that use that particular data item.

- UPINs are used to identify the patient, practitioner, and provider.

- Confidentiality for the patient related to the inclusion of the social security number as a means of identification is a substantial concern regarding the CPR, and encryption is considered essential.

- Technology can provide for data collection to be keyed, pointed, scanned, or entered by voice or radio frequency.

- Data entry is a common bottleneck in the data processing cycle and should be monitored for delays.

- Input validation checks are of two types. Event validation includes transaction validation, sequence checks, batch totals, an audit trail, and duplicate processing. Data validation includes format checks, reasonableness checks, and check digits.

- Paper-based forms and computer views share many of the same design principles that consider the users; purpose; selection and sequencing of items; technology; standard terminology, abbreviations, and format; instructions; and simplicity.

- PPRs may be arranged in one of three formats: source-oriented, problem-oriented, or integrated.

- The POMR includes a database, problem list, initial plans, and progress notes in the SOAP format.

- The design, implementation, and management of forms and views are a collaborative process, including at least information systems, materials management, patient care services, and quality improvement.

- The health care delivery system includes ambulatory care, acute care, long-term care and rehabilitation, home care and hospice, and mental health care. All records share basic content and documentation characteristics. It is also important to be aware of variations for particular care settings.

- Data collection is not only a high-technology enterprise but a high touch one as well that must consider the personal reactions of people to the profound changes occurring in health care in general and health information management in particular.

Bibliography

American Society for Testing and Materials. E-1384: Standard guide for description for content and structure of an automated primary record of care. Philadelphia: American Society for Testing and Materials, current edition.

Ball, Marion J., and Morris F. Collen. Aspects of the computer-based patient record. Computers in Health Care Series edited by Kathryn J. Hannah and Marion J. Ball. New York: Springer-Verlag, 1992.

Commission on Accreditation of Rehabilitation Facilities. Standards manual for organizations serving people with disabilities. Tucson, AZ: Commission on Accreditation of Rehabilitation Facilities, current edition.

Department of Health and Human Services. Conditions of participation—Comprehensive outpatient rehabilitation facilities. Washington, DC: Code of Federal Regulations, Title 42, current edition.

Department of Health and Human Services. Conditions of participation—Hospice care. Washington, DC: Code of Federal Regulations, Title 42, current edition.

Department of Health and Human Services. Conditions of participation—Hospitals. Washington, DC: Code of Federal Regulations, Title 42, current edition.

Department of Health and Human Services. Conditions of participation—Skilled nursing facilities. Washington, DC: Code of Federal Regulations, Title 42, current edition.

Department of Health and Human Services. The uniform ambulatory care data set. Report of the National Committee on Vital and Health Statistics and Its Interagency Task Force in the Uniform Ambulatory Care Data Set, 1989.

Department of Health and Human Services. Long Term Health Care: Minimum Data Set. Report of the National Committee on Vital and Health Statistics, 1989.

Feste, Laura. Ambulatory care documentation. Chicago: American Health Information Management Association, 1993.

Glondys, Barbara A. Documentation requirements for the acute care record. Chicago: American Health Information Management Association, 1994.

Huffman, E. K. Health information management. 10th ed. Berwyn, IL: Physician's Record Company, 1993.

Joint Commission on Accreditation of Healthcare Organizations. Accreditation manual for home care. Chicago: Joint Commission on Accreditation of Healthcare Organizations, current edition.

Joint Commission on Accreditation of Healthcare Organizations. Accreditation manual for hospice facilities. Chicago: Joint Commission on Accreditation of Healthcare Organizations, current edition.

Joint Commission on Accreditation of Healthcare Organizations. Accreditation manual for hospitals. Chicago: Joint Commission on Accreditation of Healthcare Organizations, current edition.

Joint Commission on Accreditation of Healthcare Organizations. Accreditation manual for long term care facilities. Chicago: Joint Commission on Accreditation of Healthcare Organizations, current edition.

Joint Commission on Accreditation of Healthcare Organizations. Accreditation manual for mental health, chemical dependency, and mental retardation/developmental disabilities services. Chicago: Joint Commission on Accreditation of Healthcare Organizations, current edition.

Joint Commission on Accreditation of Healthcare Organizations. Ambulatory health care standards manual. Chicago: Joint Commission on Accreditation of Healthcare Organizations, current edition.

Lytle, Barbara V., J. Stephen Lytle, and Karen G. Youmans. Hand-held and pen-based computing: Empowering technology for the computer-based patient record. J Am Health Information Management Assoc 1993;64(9):68–72.

McLendon, Kelly. Electronic medical record systems as a basis for computer-based patient records. J Am Health Information Management Assoc 1993;64(9):50–55.

Senn, James A. Information systems in management. 4th ed. Belmont, CA: Wadsworth Publishing Co., 1990.

Shelly, Gary B., and Thomas J. Cashman. Computer fundamentals for an information age. Brea, CA: Anaheim Publishing Company, 1984.

Stewart, Margaret. Notes from the ambulatory care section. J Am Health Information Management Assoc 1993;64(6):22.

Topics in Health Record Management. Keyless data capture. Frederick, MD: Aspen Publishers, 1992.

Well designed paper forms speed automation. Medical Records Briefing, June 1993, 1, 3–4.

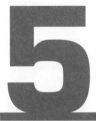

DONNA J. WILDE

KEY WORDS

Accessibility of data
Alphanumeric data
Authentication
Categorical text/categorical data
Clinical pertinence documentation
Completeness of data
Confidentiality of data
Current
Data integrity
Data redundancy
Data steward
Database
Database management system
Delinquent record
File management system/flat file system

Key field
Legality of data
Legibility of recorded data
Meaning
Parallel processing
Password
Point-of-care documentation
Quality assessment and improvement
Quantitative analysis
Quantitative data
Reliability of data
Security of data
Timeliness, currency of data
Validity of data

DATA QUALITY

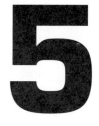

5

OBJECTIVES

- Discuss the importance of data quality.
- Identify the role of the health information management (HIM) professional as it relates to data quality.
- Identify and define characteristics of data quality.
- Identify sources of patient clinical information, and describe potential quality problems related to the collection and recording of that data.
- Differentiate between retrospective record completion and point-of-service documentation.
- Apply and evaluate an information system database structure and model; design a personal computer relational database software HIM application.
- Write documents related to an HIM system or application, including policies, procedures, instructions, and data dictionary.
- Conduct quality assessment or clinical pertinence review studies of patient record documentation.
- Evaluate the quality of data and the clinical documentation system in an alternative care setting; recommend changes.
- Evaluate the quality of statistical reports; prepare statistical reports using computer spreadsheet, graphics, and statistical software programs.
- Participate in the development of a facility information systems plan.
- Apply professional practice standards for HIM services.

IMPORTANCE OF DATA QUALITY

Health information management (HIM) professionals have always been concerned about the quality of information in both primary and secondary health records and have used various methods to help ensure the accuracy and completeness of these records. Data quality activities have been a priority for the health information manager because of the many users and uses of the data; these functions have had a sharper focus with the advent of computerized patient records. However, the model has changed from assuring data quality through documentation audits and retrospective completion of missing reports to designing systems that assure data quality at the point of service and then monitoring the effectiveness of these systems.

There are many individuals and groups who rely on health data and who demand quality in the data collected, analyzed, interpreted, and reported, including the following:

- Physicians, nurses, and other clinicians who are treating the patient, who use the record as a primary means of communication among themselves

- Physicians or other health care providers at the follow-up facility or agency to which the patient is transferred after discharge, who rely on the data for continuing care

- Third party payers, who need the data to reimburse for care rendered

- Nursing staff, who review and evaluate the data to develop critical pathways outlining important nursing interventions in the care of patients

- Attorneys and the courts, who use the records as documentary evidence of a patient's course of treatment to protect the legal interests of the patient, health care providers, treating facility, and the public

- The National Physician Data Bank, which uses secondary health care data to assure that only qualified physicians practice medicine

- State health departments, which use information related to vital statistics, disease incidence and prevalence, reports of child and adult abuse, and so on to provide aggregate data for public policy development and for intervention in individual situations as needed

- Quality assessment and improvement committees, which use the information as a basis for analysis, study, and evaluation of the quality of care given to the patient

- Researchers, who analyze and interpret data to determine causes, prevention methods, and treatment for diseases and disabilities

- Administrators, who analyze financial and patient case mix information for business planning and marketing activities

- Accrediting, licensing, and certifying agencies, who review patient records to provide public assurance that quality health care is being provided

- Federal government, which uses the information to develop health care policy and service

ROLE OF THE HIM PROFESSIONAL IN DATA QUALITY

The HIM professional directs or actively participates in all phases related to the collection, storing, retrieval, analysis, evaluation, and dissemination of health data. Figure 5–1 provides a description of the profession, drafted by the 1994 American Health Information Management Association's (AHIMA's) Health Information Management Curriculum Project Group Leaders, which is now incorporated into the *Essentials for an Accredited Educational Program for the Health Information Technician and Health Information Administrator*.[1] One crucial role for the HIM professional is to assure that all these activities provide accurate and quality data to the user of the

Health information management is the profession that focuses on health care data and the management of health care information resources. The profession addresses the nature, structure, and translation of data into usable forms of information for the advancement of health and health care of individuals and populations.

Health information management professionals collect, integrate, and analyze primary and secondary health care data, disseminate information, and manage information resources related to the research, planning, provision, and evaluation of health care services.

FIGURE 5–1. Description of the health information management profession. (From Essentials for an accredited educational program for the health information technician and health information administrator. Chicago: American Health Information Management Association, 1994, p 7.)

information. The HIM professional has roles in the following groups:

- Within the health care organization
- With individuals, groups, or agencies external to the organization
- Within the HIM profession itself

Johns discusses the paradigm shift of the activities of HIM professionals from the traditional role of managing the physical medical record to managing the data.[2] This change will be implemented in incremental phases over time as the information base changes from paper to computerized data.

Professional Domains

Roles Within the Health Care Organization

Because problems related to data quality can occur in all phases of the health care organization's manual or automated health information systems, the HIM professional performs the following functions:

- Works with the appropriate people to design the data model for the HIM system, whether it is manual, automated, or a combination of both

- Develops, reviews, evaluates, or modifies databases, structures, and systems to capture accurate, complete, timely, and useful health data

- Participates in developing and modifying the organization's data dictionary

- Evaluates and recommends changes to improve the efficiency of the health information system to avoid duplication of effort and, possibly, data inconsistencies

- Develops systems to assure data access to authorized internal and external users when and where needed

- Works with the appropriate people to design, implement, and monitor security systems to prevent unauthorized access, misuse, or corruption of data

- Develops backup methods to assure data recovery after intentional or unintentional loss

- Develops and implements continuous data quality validation activities

- Analyzes, interprets, and prepares reports based on the data and disseminates as appropriate

- Actively brokers data; educates others on what data are available, where to locate the data, and how to access, use, analyze, and interpret the data

- Develops clear, complete written policies, procedures, and other documentation related to data collection, analysis, evaluation, and dissemination
- Provides education and training to those who collect, retrieve, analyze, evaluate, and disseminate the data

External Roles

The AHIMA is playing an active role in health care reform activities on the national level. AHIMA members also need to be active at the local level as states reform their own health care delivery systems. Traditionally, HIM professionals have protected patient confidentiality; now they also need to assist policymakers and implementers in designing data systems and data standards and in developing public policy and methods to meet the National Health Promotion and Disease Prevention Objectives outlined by the U.S. Department of Health and Human Services in its *Healthy People 2000* summary report.[3] The report recognizes that information is needed from all states and territories and from many sources in local communities, such as funeral directors, medical examiners, coroners, and hospitals. It supports the concept of the need for surveillance and data systems for guiding public health into the 21st century. Figure 5–2 shows the official objective related to information systems.

HIM managers need to work with vendors, health departments, community health agencies, and others to develop systems for data collection beyond one admission at a facility. Systems to collect and report data for entire episodes of care are needed to track patient problems and status as the patient moves from one health care setting to another. Refinement and implementation of the lifelong (longitudinal) primary record of care will allow appropriate centralized data input and access by all health care providers over the life of the patient. HIM professionals must continue to develop this record.

HIM professionals also interact with attorneys, courts, third party payers, external health care providers, and others for the release of data for continuity of care, legal, and reimbursement purposes. Efficient and accurate authorized data transfer must take place when and where needed.

Roles Within the Profession

HIM professionals need to educate, research, write, lobby, and take other leadership roles to promote and improve the profession.

CHARACTERISTICS OF DATA QUALITY

Definition

The term "quality" has several meanings, according to the dictionary. The following definitions are especially pertinent to the HIM professional:

- A degree of excellence of a thing
- A required character or property that belongs to a thing's essential nature

The expression "data quality" suggests the correctness of data. When reference is made to the "qualities of data," however, the characteristics or attributes that make up data or factual information are implied (see Characteristics of Data Quality). Both concepts are integral in the development of health information systems and the subsequent monitoring of data to assure that the information produced is accurate and dependable.

Attributes of Data Quality

Correctness, Validity

Correctness or **validity of data** refers to the preciseness or accuracy of data. The data represent what was intended or defined by their official source, are objective or unbiased, and comply with known standards. For example, the patient's address in the database is what the patient says it is; the patient's vital signs stored in the database are what were originally recorded; the diagnostic code complies with the requirements of the International Classification of Disease, 9th edition, Clinical Modification (ICD-9-CM) coding standards. When applicable, only permitted or valid values for a data item

---

> **To improve surveillance and data systems, by the year 2000 . . .**
>
> **22.1 Develop and implement common health status indicators for use by Federal/State/local health agencies**
>
> Other objectives target creation of data sources to track the year 2000 objectives; expanded State-based activity to track the progress of the population toward the year 2000 objectives; improvement of related data for blacks, Hispanics, American Indians and Alaska Natives, Asian Americans, and people with disabilities; improvement of information transfer capabilities among Federal, State, and local agencies; and more speedy processing of survey and surveillance data.

FIGURE 5–2. Objective of the Department of Health and Human Services. (From U.S. Department of Health and Human Services, Public Health Service: Healthy People 2000: National health promotion and disease prevention objectives. Boston: Jones & Bartlett, 1992, p 79.)

Characteristics of Data Quality

- **Correctness, Validity:** The numbers, characters, or symbols stored, processed, and displayed are exact and conform to known standards. The data represent what was intended by their original source. The data are supported by objective truth or generally accepted authority.
- **Reliability:** The data yield the same results on repeated collection, processing, storing, and display of information in the same database; the data are consistent when entered into two or more databases.
- **Completeness:** All required data are present in the information system.
- **Legibility:** The data are decipherable or readable.
- **Currency:** The data are recorded at or near the time of the event or observation.
- **Timeliness:** The length of time is minimized between an event or observation that produces data and when the data are available to those who need the information.
- **Meaning:** The data convey understandable information; are consistent when naming or describing the same findings or treatment; and are relevant and useful to the provider, patient, health care institution, and public.
- **Accessibility:** The data are available to authorized people when and where needed.

---

are allowed. For example, if numbers from 15 to 85 are the only valid values or characters for a field, the values 5, 86, or D7 are invalid.

The concept of validity has several dimensions but begins with the soundness or correctness of data collection and the input of data into the database. Data for the health care facility are obtained in various ways from many sources. Patients and families are interviewed by physicians and other health care providers, and the information that is obtained may or may not be complete or accurate, depending on the provider's interviewing ability, the existence of patient-provider language barriers, the patient's physical health and emotional or mental health state at the time, and the provider's recording skills.

Other sources of data include historical records that provide information related to past illnesses and treatment. The accuracy of current data may be compromised if prior records are not available when needed.

In addition to interviewing the patient, physicians and other providers make observations, provide diagnostic and therapeutic treatment, assess patient problems, and evaluate results of therapy. This information is recorded on paper or computer; quality depends on the accuracy of the observation, the treatment skills of the providers, and the faithful recording of the observations and events. Data quality may be compromised if any of the following occur:

- Paper records are not available on which to record in a manual system.
- Dictation equipment is not working properly or located in inaccessible areas, which inhibits the clinician from dictating at the time of the event or observation.
- Transcription of the information is inaccurate or delayed and not available for health care providers when needed.

- Problems exist with other computer data entry devices, such as equipment failure, lack of sufficient devices at appropriate treatment areas, and lack of provider training in the proper use of the devices.

Other sources of patient information include computer data from diagnostic equipment, such as that used in the laboratory and the radiology department; on-line patient monitors, such as those used in the intensive care or coronary care unit; and other automated equipment used by pharmacy and other ancillary department personnel. Accuracy relies on the dependability of software, equipment, and communications media during the electronic transfer of information to the main clinical database.

Another dimension to be considered in the concept of validity is that the data conform to identified record content requirements, such as those for state or national licensure or certification, or to accreditation standards. Data must also meet national and international standards for patient data structure and data interchange, including those for registration–admission, discharge, and transfer (R–ADT) systems, content and organization of primary care records, and automated longitudinal records.

Reliability

Reliability of data implies that the data are consistent, no matter how many times the same data are collected and entered into the system or into multiple systems.

Examples of health record content inconsistencies include those related to the documentation of diagnoses found in several areas of a patient's record, such as the admitting diagnosis, the impression on physical examination, the diagnosis found on operative and pathology reports, and the principal and secondary diagnoses documented at the time of discharge. Some of these inconsistencies are legitimate because they incorporate the results of tests and other findings not available at the time of earlier documentation of diagnoses; the record also indicates diagnostic variations that reflect changes in the patient's status. Some inconsistencies, however, may reflect errors on the part of the practitioner responsible for documenting the diagnostic assessment. For example, a patient record may include an operative report for an appendectomy, but the final diagnosis may indicate that the patient had pneumonia and no secondary diagnoses. Another illustration of documentation inconsistency is a nursing admission assessment that indicates that a patient is deaf, but the physical examination completed by the physician does not document the fact that the patient's hearing is compromised. Another case is one in which the nursing staff recorded a temperature spike for several days, the laboratory report shows an increased white blood cell count, but no physician documentation is present regarding these signs. Another type of consistency problem relates to the individual diagnoses provided by the physician related to a series of outpatient visits for treatment and follow-up for the same condition. An example is one in which the physician documents skin cyst as the diagnosis for the first visit. On the second visit, the physician indicates abscess and on the third, skin infection. The diagnosis for a fourth visit is skin lesion, and at a subsequent visit, the patient had "an open wound of the skin."

Reliability also depends on different but simultaneous transactions showing the same data. For example, the pharmacy prescription and outpatient visit registration transactions should simultaneously show the same name, birthdate, and so on for the same person.

Other factors that impact the reliability of health data are problems related to data sharing when the same data item is used by many application systems and users. In a shared data environment, the same data item may be updated by more than one application or organizational unit. For example, the patient's address can be updated by both the R–ADT system and the tumor registry module. Procedures need to be developed to assure that data modifications replace old data and that obsolete data do not replace current data.

Difficulties can also occur when data are electronically transferred from one database to another. In addition to the quality of the transmission media and the software, problems related to the downloading and uploading of data to and from a main database can occur if these functions are not performed consistently or correctly. For example, information may be downloaded from the clinical database to a personal computer for a quality improvement or other study and be manipulated, changed, and analyzed locally. A new report is generated, based on this revised information, and dissemi-

nated to the appropriate people. The new information may or may not be uploaded to the main database, depending on facility policy, the capability of the automated system, and follow-through of the analyst. Consequently, the data may be inconsistent between two systems or reports. Figure 5–3 shows this exchange of data.

HIM professionals may be a source of problems related to data reliability when they code and/or abstract patient records and enter the data into the computer. Reliability depends on their coding and abstracting abilities and the completeness of the source data at the time of these activities.

Another major problem occurs in facilities that have differing, nonintegrated computerized applications used by various departments. These applications are either existing specialized programs directly available from a vendor or those developed by staff using a generic relational database or file management program on their own personal computers or local area networks. Because the applications are not integrated, the same data are entered repeatedly in the various programs; this overlap of data is known as **data redundancy.** Employee time is wasted in entering redundant data, and storage space is used unnecessarily. More important, however, is that frequently there are contradictions in the data, especially over time, as one file is updated but the other is not, or two persons entering the same data in two different programs may make errors, leading to data inconsistency. Because database field requirements often differ among programs, data entry at the time of collection is usually incompatible, even though the data entry operator keys the data correctly. For example, the number of characters allowed in a field for patient last name may be less for one program than for another, or a field for patient diagnosis may be in narrative text in one program and in coded form in another. Figure 5–4 shows

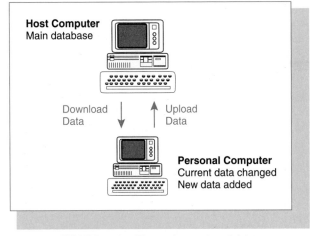

FIGURE 5–3. Electronic transfer of data.

EXAMPLES OF FILE MANAGEMENT SYSTEMS

Duplicate Systems Entering Redundant Data In Incompatible Format.

OPERATING ROOM LOG - Entered by Operating Room Staff on its own personal computer

Date Surg	Patient Name	Patient Number	Surgeon	Assist. Surgeon	Operation	Preop Diagnosis	Postop Diagn.	Start Time	End Time	Anes Type	Anes-thetist	Units Blood
9/2/93	Smith, P.	12345	Wilson	Jones	Appendectomy	Appendicit	Same	0730	0815	Gen	Brown	0
9/2/93	Green, M.	67890	White	Ames	R. Rad. Mastect	AdenoCa	Same	0800	0945	Gen	Moore	2
9/3/93	Mason, V.	38475	Warren		Bx Skin, R. Leg	Melanoma?	Nevus	1100	1130	Loc		0

ANESTHESIA LOG - Entered by Anesthesia Department Staff on its own personal computer

Date Anes	Patient Name	Patient Number	Anes-thetist	Surgeon	Operation	Start Anes	End Anes	Total Anes	Start Oper	End Oper	Total Oper	Preop Med	Anesthes Given
9/2/93	Smith, P.	12345	Brown	Wilson	Appy	0715	0810	55	0730	0815	45	x	yyyyy
9/2/93	Green, M.	67890	Moore	Ames	Rad. Mast.	0740	0940	120	0800	0945	105	r	lyqp
9/3/93	Mason, V.	38475	Wilson	Wilson	Bx. skin							x	xyl

OPERATION INDEX - Entered by Health Information Management Staff on its own personal computer

Date Disch	Patient Number	Age	Sex	LOS	Proced Code	Diagnoses Codes					Surgeon	Attending Physician
9/4/93	12345	32	M	3	47.0	541	492.8				Wilson	Wilson
9/10/93	67890	41	F	9	85.43	174.9	729.0	564.1	287.5		Ames	Moran
9/3/93	38475	19	F	1	86.3	448.1					Wilson	Wilson

FIGURE 5–4. Examples of file management systems.

the quality problems that could occur in a nonintegrated system of separate department databases.

Completeness

Completeness of data in a manual or computerized patient record is critical not only to provide good patient care but also to meet regulatory, legal, and reimbursement requirements. Facility administrators and public policymakers also rely on valid, reliable, and complete data. Individual facility and state or national standards must be developed and followed to assure uniformity in record content.

The health record must adequately reflect the following:

- Problems
- Diagnoses
- Clinical history
- Diagnostic tests
- Care and treatment
- Rationale for treatment
- Results of treatment
- Patient's status

In addition, for each item of information, all required data items must be present. For example, an address is logically composed of four data items—street, city, state, zip code. If any one data item of address is present, then all four must be present.

In addition to identifying required content, user-friendly data capture methods, incorporating the latest technology, should be available to ensure efficiency and completeness in data recording. Examples include dictation and transcription, the use of a mouse to "point and click" data selections, touch screens, and computer voice recognition.

Legibility

The **legibility of recorded data** is critical to its use. Handwriting is difficult to read, not only on a paper record but also in microfilm, photocopy, or optical disk formats. Transcribed or printed information is easier to read and is a much more efficient form of data collection.

A problem also occurs in both paper and computerized patient records if undecipherable codes or symbols are used or there is inconsistency in the use and meaning of abbreviations among practitioners.

Currency and Timeliness

Data must be **current,** or contemporaneous, recorded at or near the time of the event or observation. *Signatures or other forms of authentication recorded several weeks after an order is written have questionable legal value. A patient history and physical examination that are recorded several months after patient discharge lose their clinical usefulness and create potential data accuracy problems.* Because care and treatment depend on accurate, current data, an essential component of data quality is the timeliness of the documentation or data entry.

Meaning, Usefulness

The Institute of Medicine (IOM) indicates that another element of data quality is that the data have **meaning** for users, that the information is pertinent and useful. The IOM states:

Effective retrieval and use of information from patient records depend on consistency in naming or describing the same findings, clinical problems, procedures, drugs, and other data within a single patient record, across many patient records in a single record system, or in other systems that contain data relevant to the understanding and treatment of patient problems. Communication among practitioners can be aided by a common clinical data dictionary and a clinical coding system that are interchangeable [with] any clinical data common to different specialists or professions but specific enough to describe the detailed data unique to a profession or specialty.[4]

Legibility and appropriate use of standardized abbreviations also improve the meaning and usefulness of the record. The record has meaning if the use of standard terminology related to describing findings or treatment is consistent, if it meets the content and format needs of the health care practitioners at the facility or agency, and if it is relevant to its intended purposes.

The meaning and usefulness of the record has increased with the computer-based patient record, especially since it has helped with clinical decision making in the treatment of patients. Glondys indicates that

The CPR (computer-based patient record) can assist in, and in some instances guide, the process of clinical problem solving by providing clinicians with decision analysis tools, clinical reminders, prognostic risk assessment, and other clinical aids.

Medical decision making has traditionally been considered a scientific, as well as intuitive, process. In recent years, however, formal methods for decision making have been applied to medical problem-solving and computer-assisted medical decision making has gained wider acceptance. For example, computers can be used to interpret ventilatory status based on blood gas re-

ports. In addition, computers can be used to alert physicians, nurses, or pharmacists when a medication may be contraindicated. Computers can also be used to provide physicians guidance using patient treatment protocols.

The CPR will analyze data as it is collected and provide feedback, alerts, reminders, clinical support and links to medical knowledge to physicians.[5]

The meaning and usefulness of information are often obscured because of the sheer volume of detail provided, which discourages review and interpretation of the data by the health care provider. An example is in the area of nursing documentation in the acute care setting where studies have shown that 70 to 80 per cent of the documentation provides information on what is right or normal with the patient rather than information relative to what is wrong with the patient. Physicians may avoid reviewing the documentation because of the time needed to read, analyze, and interpret the data. The previous health record paradigm was "if it wasn't documented, it wasn't done." Consequently, lengthy nursing documentation resulted. The new concept should be "if it wasn't documented, it was done." In other words, the paradigm needs to be changed to allow for development and recording in the patient's record of a planned treatment protocol and expected outcomes for that patient. Documentation by exception would be established, which would indicate variances from the planned treatment or expected outcomes and the reasons for the discrepancies.

The true meaning of statistical reports based on patient record content depends on commonly accepted definitions of terms and uniform formulas for descriptive statistics based on these terms. This principle is the basis for the development of the Glossary of Healthcare Terms, published by the AHIMA.[6]

In addition to too much data in a patient record, problems can occur within secondary reports, especially when computer printouts and reports provide a large amount of data but no useful information. For example, long computer lists of patients seen each day or lengthy lists of other transactions in the physician's office are not valuable to the physician unless the data are converted to useful information. In a capitated managed care environment, bar graphs comparing the number of unique or unduplicated patients seen by the physician during the month and the total number of patient visits (duplicated counts) could be quite useful to the physician and administration because in a capitated payment environment, revenue is based on the number of unique patients rather than the number of visits. Comparison with national averages, such as those provided by the Medical Group Management Association, can assist in determining whether the number of initial and follow-up visits are appropriate; that is, will the activity volume

---

CASE STUDY

Requests for Paper Record Post-Discharge General Hospital

Monday	•	John Jones is discharged after treatment for a leg injury. Paper record remains on nursing unit for record completion by nursing staff.
Tuesday	•	HIM department receives record to assemble forms, code, and abstract. Important for the billing office to have codes as soon as possible after discharge.
	•	Record needed by Orthopedic Clinic for scheduled outpatient visit. Physician does not release record because it is needed for clinic visit documentation which he or she will do later.
	•	Radiology requests record for review prior to MRI examination scheduled for 1 hour after conclusion of Orthopedic Clinic visit. Record remains in Orthopedic Clinic and is unavailable to others.
Wednesday	•	Record needed for Physical Therapy Department visit.
	•	Radiologist has requested review of the patient's record related to the MRI examination taken yesterday.
	•	Staff from Orthopedic Clinic say they returned the record to the HIM Department earlier in the day, although the record has not yet arrived.
	•	Record is received by the HIM Department two hours after the scheduled Physical Therapy visit. Record, which is sent to Radiology, is not returned by the end of the day.
Thursday	•	Record is needed for second follow-up visit to Orthopedic Clinic.
	•	Record is needed for second Physical Therapy visit.
	•	Social Service Department requests record to assist patient in arranging needed community services in the home.
	•	Record that was sent to Radiology yesterday is retained by Radiology until the end of today.

FIGURE 5–5. Case study requests for paper record post discharge.

provide increased revenue while lowering costs and yet assure quality of care? The number of unique or unduplicated patients treated classified according to age, gender, zip code, payer, and diagnoses can also be useful indicators of the case mix in the practice.

Accessibility

The **accessibility of data** to an authorized user when and where the data are needed is an essential component of data quality. Paper record systems present major problems related to data availability. In this type of record system, if one person only needs access to the data, employee time is needed to request the record, prepare outguide or record transfer forms, find and retrieve the record folders, and send the record to the user. This may take from several minutes to several days for the requested record to arrive. Another major disadvantage of a paper record system is when more than one user needs a patient's record at or near the same time. This often occurs during the first few days post discharge of a patient from the facility. Figure 5–5 shows the demand for a patient record by many people within a short time frame. In one hospital, tumor registry personnel are 23rd on the requester priority list, which means that it may take several months to obtain the

record for abstracting and follow-up activities. If a transcriptionist needs information from the record to complete a dictated report, the patient information is frequently not available.

Numerous accessibility problems in a paper record system occur in home health agencies, when the patient is in the home and the original paper record must remain in the office. The record is either inaccessible to the clinicians during patient care in the home or data redundancy and confidentiality problems arise when duplicate records are maintained by the nurses and therapists treating the patient. The advantages of an automated health record include its instant accessibility and the capability of its being reviewed by more than one user at the same time. The location of computer terminals and printers used by physicians and other health care providers while interviewing, examining, or treating patients is an important consideration related to data accessibility. Scarcity of computer workstations or improper location of terminals also impedes the practice of health care and affects data quality.

Another aspect of accessibility is the ability to receive summary data when needed. For example, monthly statistical reports that are to be reviewed by the board of trustees of a health facility should not be received 1 week after the meeting.

Confidentiality and Security

Confidentiality of data and **security of data** to prevent unauthorized access, misuse, corruption, or loss of data are also attributes of data quality. Manual or automated systems must be developed and monitored to safeguard the record against intentional or accidental unauthorized access to or modifications of primary and secondary health data. The **data steward** is a person to whom a facility has given the responsibility and authority to protect and control access to specific data items or databases. Although the data steward has the authority to deny access to data, she or he also has a responsibility to grant access to others for legitimate facility use and to promote data sharing throughout the organization. *Data stewards should take an active role in advising others on the appropriate use of the data under their stewardship. The HIM manager should be the steward for all the clinical data item sets.*

Legality

Legality of data is an attribute of data quality that relates to the concept that information must be documented, authenticated, corrected, and/or stored in a format that is consistent with the requirements of law or regulation. Documentation requirements in a paper system include the following:

- Use of ink, done contemporaneously with the event or observation and with errors corrected legally
- Entries dated and authenticated by the person making the observation or providing the treatment

State laws vary regarding the legal aspects of computerized records in the creation and authentication of entries. Laws and regulations also differ regarding the length of time records must be maintained and which storage media are permitted (i.e., paper, microfilm, optical or other computer or electronic disks or tapes).

Because all these factors influence the accuracy of data, the chances for error are high (see Factors Influencing Data Accuracy). The HIM manager must develop systems, write policies and procedures, provide training, and monitor data quality to assist in assuring accurate and timely data to all those who rely on the information.

METHODS TO ENSURE DATA QUALITY

The accuracy of data depends on the manual or computer information system design for collecting, recording, storing, processing, accessing, and displaying data as well as the ability and follow-through of the people involved in each phase of these activities. One of the crucial methods to ensure the accuracy of data is to develop systems that ensure accuracy and timeliness of documentation at the point of care, to monitor its output, and to take appropriate corrective action when needed.

Before discussing methods to develop quality data at the point of service, it is helpful to review the concepts of record content review and retrospective record completion activities related to that content because historically, that process was one of the primary methods to obtain missing data and authentications. It was also the basis for the Joint Commission on Accreditation of Healthcare Organization (JCAHO) record of deficiency standards (see JCAHO Type I Recommendations).

Factors Influencing Data Accuracy

- Correctness and completeness of the original source data
- Correct entry of that data onto paper or into the computer database at the point of service
- Appropriate database structure, based on internal and external standards
- Correct computer programming to obtain, process, and report the data
- Dependability of computer data transfer, including quality of communications media and transmission standards
- Presence of approved procedures regarding additions or modifications of data when the same database is shared by others or in facilities with nonintegrated systems
- Reliability of storage media and backup systems
- Accuracy of coded data
- Adequate security systems to safeguard the data
- The HIM professional's skills in research, computer data query, and statistical reports

---

JCAHO Type I Recommendations

Too many delinquent records may cause the hospital to receive a Type I Recommendation which must be resolved in order to retain accreditation. These guidelines indicate that any of the following would give the institution a Type I Recommendation:

- The number of delinquent records is greater than 50% of the average number of discharged patients for a month.
- The number of medical records delinquent due to the absence of a medical history and physical examination exceeds 9, or 2% of the average monthly discharges, whichever is greater.
- The number of medical records delinquent due to the absence of an operative report exceeds 9, or 2% of the average monthly operative procedures, whichever is greater.

From Joint Commission on Accreditation of Healthcare Organizations: Accreditation manual for hospitals 1994, scoring guidelines. Chicago: JCAHO, 1993, sec 2, p 13.

Record Content Review and Retrospective Completion

The review of patient records for documentation accuracy and completeness has always been a functional role of the HIM department staff in all types of health care facilities. This review has been needed because of the variety of sources of patient record information and the large number of entries made by different people in the patient's record on a daily basis. If the health care provider has a busy day or if internal systems for assuring the presence of required content or authentications are not adequate, documentation may be inadvertently omitted or inaccurate.

The thoroughness and methodology of this evaluation have evolved over time in an attempt to meet licensure, certification, and accreditation standards for completion and timeliness of documentation. In the past, the HIM department in an inpatient or a home health setting used a traditional approach and performed a detailed review, or **quantitative analysis,** of all predischarge or postdischarge patient records for the presence of required reports and **authentications** and then obtained the signature or reports retrospectively, often weeks or months after the event. Although the quality of the data within the reports was not evaluated, the analyses did help to assure the eventual presence of authentications and categories of data required by standard-setting agencies. The usefulness and legal value of these very late reports and signatures, however, was doubtful.

In the traditional retrospective data collection process, after the patient's paper record has been received in the HIM department on discharge, clerical staff assemble the record forms in a prescribed order and then review all records for missing authentications and reports. Although categories of information reviewed vary with each facility, those typically checked include the following:

- Listings of principal and secondary diagnoses on discharge
- Presence of discharge summaries, history, physical reports, and operative or procedure reports

In addition, forms are checked to see if there is correct patient identification on every page (front and back) and if all physician reports, progress notes, and orders are authenticated by the appropriate resident or attending physician. Some facilities may review for the presence of other reports and authorizations. Documentation review may be performed at the nursing unit while the patient is still active. If the record is incomplete, a deficiency slip is prepared by the analyst that itemizes missing documentation or signatures (Figure 5–6). Pages are flagged with colored tabs at the location of missing signatures, and appropriate HIM department procedures are followed to obtain these from the physician.

The method to assist physicians in record completion after patient discharge varies by facility and includes either a manual or a computer system of physician notification, record location tracking, and administrative reporting. One copy of the deficiency slip usually is attached to the record. The incomplete record is either placed in a designated record completion area or interfiled in the main record storage area.

If the retrospective completion process is in use at the facility, it usually has a requirement that physicians complete reports and records according to the time frame specified in the medical staff bylaws, based on licensure or accreditation standards in effect at the time. When an incomplete record has not been finished within the time specified in the bylaws, it is termed a **delinquent record.** Most hospitals have some type of physician sanction when delinquent records exist. Some may impose fines based on the number of delinquent records. Others may temporarily place a physician on a suspension or no admissions list until delinquent records are completed. In this instance, physicians may not admit patients or arrange surgery on unscheduled patients unless authorization is received from the chief of staff or designated hospital administrator.

Because of the seriousness of the sanctions for both the physician and the hospital, it is extremely important that the retrospective completion process be reviewed to determine if it should continue. The HIM professional should take the lead in encouraging the facility to discontinue the process because this is not a value-added activity related to quality data, and it is an expensive activity for the facility. If the medical staff, hospital administration, and legal counsel deem it important to continue this process, then policies and procedures need

DOCTOR _____	DOCTOR _____	DOCTOR _____
SIGNATURES MISSING	SIGNATURES MISSING	SIGNATURES MISSING
_____ History	_____ History	_____ History
_____ Physical	_____ Physical	_____ Physical
_____ Consultation	_____ Consultation	_____ Consultation
_____ Operative report	_____ Operative report	_____ Operative report
_____ Discharge summary	_____ Discharge summary	_____ Discharge summary
_____ X-ray report	_____ X-ray report	_____ X-ray report
_____ Doctors' progress notes	_____ Doctors' progress notes	_____ Doctors' progress notes
_____ Doctors' orders	_____ Doctors' orders	_____ Doctors' orders
Other (specify)	Other (specify)	Other (specify)
MISSING REPORTS	MISSING REPORTS	MISSING REPORTS
_____ Diagnoses/Procedures	_____ Diagnoses/Procedures	_____ Diagnoses/Procedures
_____ History	_____ History	_____ History
_____ Physical	_____ Physical	_____ Physical
_____ Consultation report	_____ Consultation report	_____ Consultation report
_____ Operative report	_____ Operative report	_____ Operative report
_____ Discharge summary	_____ Discharge summary	_____ Discharge summary
_____ Doctors' orders	_____ Doctors' orders	_____ Doctors' orders
Other (specify)	Other (specify)	Other (specify)

PATIENT
CHART NUMBER
DISCHARGE DATE

FIGURE 5–6. Deficiency slip.

to be carefully developed. For example, if the procedure for obtaining signatures retrospectively is to continue, then the review should be done on a predischarge basis to obtain the signatures as close to data entry as possible. Only those orders that the medical staff consider potentially hazardous to the patient as outlined in the medical staff's rules and regulations should be checked for authentication. Only key reports should be monitored to determine if they are present with follow-up as appropriate. They include the history and physical examination, operative reports, pathology reports, radiology reports, and discharge summary. Even though these reports may be received after patient discharge and are of questionable value to the hospital at that point, they are still helpful to follow-up facilities that are treating the patient because they rely on the data in these reports. The reports would be more valuable, however, if they were sent to them at the time of patient transfer to the facility or organization.

Point-of-Care Documentation

Data entry into the patient's record at the time and location of service is called **point-of-care documentation.** It is most effective when automated systems replace handwritten documentation. This documentation can occur through the use of terminals or other data input devices located in such places as patient examination rooms, diagnostic and therapeutic treatment rooms, individual patient rooms at bedside, and physician offices and at nursing stations. Systems should be developed to assure that the data capture is timely, accurate, and efficient because it is the foundation for the computer-based patient record. Data quality is enhanced through the use of system documentation prompts, built-in edits, menus, screen instructions, and so on. This concept is supported by the AHIMA in its May 1994 *Position Statement,* as follows:

> To adequately support patient care, clinical information must be available at the point of care for clinical decision-making. Healthcare practitioners should record their findings at the point of care or within 24 hours of an encounter. If second party intervention is required such as transcription of dictated information, processes should be in place for prompt completion and transmission of the information to the patient's record. This should be done as soon as possible but in no more than 24 hours after the encounter.
>
> Retrospective documentation does not add value to patient care. Healthcare reform and the development of a computer-based patient record challenge healthcare professionals to rethink old practices and raise the standards to improve patient care. The timeliness of documentation is a critical issue we must address.[7]

As record formats move from paper to computer-based, the use of traditional methods for analysis of documented records for completeness and accuracy will automatically change at the same time and will support the concept of assuring data quality at the point of collection. For example, manual reviews for the presence of authentication of physician orders will be eliminated because the physician must identify himself or herself at the time of access to the computer. *Strict log on/log off controls, however, will need to be followed, so that the person who logged on to the system at that terminal, before the current user, logs off properly to avoid "authenticating" the latter user's order by mistake.*
Computer alerts may be developed regarding the absence of required reports (e.g., history and physical ex-

amination) beyond a specified time frame after admission, and a message could be sent to the physician's E-mail. This might encourage the physician to dictate the report within the recommended 24 hours.

The paradigm must change from "quantitative analysis" and retrospective completion to "qualitative analysis" of data. It must also assure that the automated information systems design provides for an adequate database structure that meets the information requirements of standard-setting agencies and the facility, data quality at the point of collection, and integrated data-sharing capabilities as well as accurate analysis, evaluation, and reporting of data.

The AHIMA is working with other organizations, including the Health Care Financing Administration (HCFA) and the JCAHO, regarding authentication and authorship of data items entered into the patient's record. In addition, these groups are developing standards to assure quality content in the medical record during patient care and to eliminate retrospective record completion.

DESIGN OF SYSTEMS TO ENSURE DATA QUALITY FOR PATIENT RECORDS AND SECONDARY REPORTS

Database Structure and Model

Data quality in any information system, whether it is for a computer-based patient record or a specific database application for a department (e.g., master patient index or a correspondence log on a personal computer), begins at the database design phase. It is important to review all relevant legal and regulatory information requirements for the system or application and to determine additional needs pertinent to the facility or department in which the database will be housed because a model will be developed for it. A data model is a plan or pattern for an information system, including database structure and content as well as methods to input, store, retrieve, analyze, and display data (see Activities Related to Data Model Design).

Types of Data

Several types or categories of data are identified for each field in the **database.** The name or category for that field varies somewhat by program but usually includes all or some of the following. It is important that the field be properly categorized in the computer program to assist in data reliability.

The first type is **quantitative data,** or data that provide some type of measurement information, such as the following:

Activities Related to Data Model Design

- Developing the list of data items and field types
- Creating coding schemes for categorical data fields
- Establishing edits for appropriate data fields
- Selecting the type of data management software program to use
- Developing relational tables or entities that incorporate redundant (key) and nonredundant data fields
- Determining who will enter and/or modify data and who will have database query rights
- Establishing passwords for fields, tables, records, files, applications, and structure
- Designing screen formats for complete, efficient data capture
- Designing ad hoc and routine reports or data query abilities for authorized users
- Developing policy regarding data backup procedures, storage media, and data retention time lines
- Preparing a data dictionary and written policies

- Monitor readings
- Laboratory test results
- Results of calculations (e.g., age can be automatically calculated by the computer by subtracting the date of admission from the birth date)
- Dollar amounts for care

It is important not only to enter data correctly into the field at the point of data but also to categorize the field correctly at the database design phase and to program the formulas for calculating information correctly.

Another type is **categorical text** or **categorical data,** in which subjects or events are classified or labeled by name or number, such as the following:

- Patient identification information (e.g., last name, first name, address)
- Coded information (e.g., ICD-9-CM, CPT, disposition codes)

Even though a number may be used in this field (e.g., in a disposition coding scheme for an abstract system, #1 means discharged home, alive and #2 means transferred to a nursing home on an abstract system), it is still considered categorical data rather than quantitative data if no arithmetical calculations can be performed with the data. The data are called **alphanumeric data** when the codes include numbers, letters, and/or symbolic characters.

To have reliable data, the field must be correctly categorized, one must have a good coding scheme developed for the application (see related discussion below), and the individual case must be coded accurately and entered into the computer correctly by HIM department personnel.

Another field data type is that for narrative information that is difficult or impossible to code (e.g., progress notes, history, comment field on an abstract). Other synonymous terms that might be used are memo or note fields and textual data. The number of characters allowed in this type of field varies by computer system. In large mainframe systems, this is not a problem, but in personal computer database systems, a narrative or memo field is usually limited in terms of numbers of characters allowed in the field and is an item that should be reviewed before purchase of the software.

There are usually date fields for activities (e.g., date of discharge) and time fields to show hour and/or minutes that an event occurred (e.g., time of admission). Some software packages have a logic field for yes or no entries. Examples are "Has the patient been admitted to this hospital before—yes or no?" and "Has the patient signed an authorization to release information—yes or no?"

Computer Coding Design

Many text or categorical fields in a database are those in which the data are coded in some way. Examples are disease and operation codes, disposition codes, codes for reimbursement sources, severity codes, and extent of metastasis. Fox and colleagues provide an excellent resource for a discussion on these guidelines.[8] Fuller and O'Gara discuss these concepts more fully when describing a database design for a utilization management application.[9] Lee describes using personal computer database software to design a quantitative review and active caseload list in a community health center for mental health, developmental disability, and substance abuse services.[10] Basic principles include the following recommendations:

- *There must be no confusion regarding how to categorize data elements or fields.* The more precise the data elements, the less training time and fewer written instructions are needed. For example, data that are easy to classify are the patient's sex and disposition at discharge. Data that are difficult to classify include stage of

Sample Coding Designs for Disposition at Discharge

Hospital A	Hospital B
1=Alive, home	1=Alive, to home
2=Alive, transferred to other facility	2=Alive, to nursing home
3=Expired	3=Alive, to home health
	4=Alive, to mental health
	5=Alive, to hospice
	6=Alive, to another acute care hospital
	7=Alive, to inpatient rehab
	8=Expired

FIGURE 5–7. Sample coding designs for disposition at discharge.

cancer at diagnosis and influence of environmental factors on the patient's ability to recover. Complex abstracting requires additional education of the abstractor.

- *The codes should be as specific and detailed as necessary.* Review the two sets of coding schemes in Figure 5–7 for disposition of patient at discharge. Although Hospital A's data are somewhat helpful, Hospital B's data would provide much more useful information to physicians, hospitals, and public policymakers.

- *The coding scheme must include all possibilities.* In the Hospital B example in Figure 5–7, the list is detailed but does not include a code for outpatient services. Add a code for "other" if there is a probability that the classification does not include all possibilities.

- *The scheme should allow the information to be classified into only one category, not more than one.* In the Hospital B example, it would be difficult to determine which code would be used if the patient went to a home health hospice program or a home health mental health program. If there is the chance that the patient could be classified into more than one category, the codes should be expanded or instructions should be written to guide the coder into the correct category for those situations.

- *Code numbers or letters should be self-explanatory* when possible (e.g., I = in situ, L = localized, R = regional, D = distant for stage of cancer at diagnosis) or *preprinted on data input forms.*

- *The space allotted in the field should be wide enough to adequately provide information without the need to truncate or remove part of the data at* the end of a field. Many abstracting systems do not allow sufficient space for patient last name, especially hyphenated names such as "Williamson-Browning." If the field is not wide enough, "Williamson-Br" might appear as the last name, which can cause confusion. Another problem includes lack of foresight for future expansion needs for a field. For example, many abstract systems had five spaces reserved for the zip code field. Now, 10 spaces are needed (including a space for the dash). Another example might be if a facility has eight physicians on staff and each physician is assigned a one-space number for his or her identification code. If more physicians are added to the staff, extra space will be needed or alpha characters must be assigned in addition to numbers.

- *The amount of space used must not be unnecessarily large* to avoid wasted computer storage space, data entry errors, and time loss in data entry. Review the reimbursement category codes for Nursing Home A and Nursing Home B in Figure 5–8. Nursing Home B's system is much more practical.

- *It varies among programs whether the data in the fields must be an exact width.* For example, if the disposition code field has two spaces reserved, must the abstractor use both spaces and enter a leading zero for a one-digit code (e.g., 08)? Or can the data entry operator just enter one digit in the first space and leave the second space blank? If the system allows, it is best to avoid the use of leading zeros to increase speed of data entry and to minimize data entry errors.

Development of Edit and Validation Checks

Edits or rules should be developed for data format and reasonableness consisting of conditions that must be satisfied for the data to be added to the database, along with a message that will be displayed if the data entry does not satisfy the condition. In some instances, the

Nursing Home A	Nursing Home B
Med = Medicare	M = Medicare
Mcd = Medicaid	C = Medicaid
BlCr = Blue Cross	B = Blue Cross
PvtIns = Private Insurance	P = Private Insurance

FIGURE 5–8. Sample coding designs for reimbursement source.

computer does not allow an entry to be added if it fails the edit. In other instances, a warning is provided for the data entry operator to verify the accuracy of the information before entry. One example is that each patient must have a unique number because it is the key indexing or sorting field. Another example is that the patient number must fall within a certain range of numbers or the computer does not allow the data entry operator to move to the next field or to save the data. A laboratory value must fall within a certain range of numbers or a validity check must be done. McDonald and Barnett provide an example of a computer check that "can verify that values have the correct mathematical relationship (for example, white-blood-cell differential counts [reported as percentages] must sum to 100)."[11] Other edits include format requirements, such as the use of hyphens, dashes, or leading zeros. Data consistency checks could include a rule that the date of admission must be the same as or earlier than the date of discharge. The date of birth must be earlier than the date of admission (except for newborns). Consistency edits can be developed to compare fields (e.g., a male patient cannot receive a pregnancy diagnostic code). Other input validation checks, such as sequence checks, batch totals, audit trails, duplicate processing, and check digits, also assist in providing quality data at the point of entry into the system.

Selection of Appropriate Type of Data Management Software

Each facility has a number of databases in addition to those related to patient clinical data, including information regarding physician admitting privileges and credentialing, accounting, financial analysis, purchasing and inventory, personnel and payroll, administrative, and marketing. They may or may not be able to be linked, allowing automated access by several programs. There are three generally recognized systems for database

management software programs that are selected by information systems department personnel. They are as follows:

- Hierarchical database
- Network database
- Relational database

The HIM professional frequently develops and uses personal computer applications in addition to the facility's main database to provide the ability to meet other information requirements. These applications may include the following:

- Tracking the release of information
- Physician's incomplete record system
- Master patient index
- Abstracting system for an alternative care setting

In addition, the capability usually exists in which specific information from the main database can be downloaded into a department personal computer database application program for analysis and reporting. The person designing the personal computer application can select either a file management or a relational database management software program. There are advantages and disadvantages to each program type (Table 5–1).

FILE MANAGEMENT SYSTEM. A **file management system** is a program to manage the files of one application. This is also called a **flat file system,** or a "one-table" system. If this type is used and if many individual file management programs are set up within a department or organization, they do not interface, and thus, data redundancy, data inconsistency, wasted storage space, and inefficient use of employee data entry time occur. The information in each field is usually not set up or recorded in the same way, so automatic integration is not possible. Examples of personal computer file management programs are Professional File or those

TABLE 5–1 COMPARISON OF FILE MANAGEMENT AND DATABASE MANAGEMENT SOFTWARE

ATTRIBUTE/FEATURE MANAGEMENT	FILE MANAGEMENT	DATABASE
Software cost	Less	More
Time needed to learn	Less	More
Difficulty of application development	Less	More
Time needed to develop application	Less	More
Risk of data redundancy*	More	Less
Risk of data inconsistency*	More	Less
Data storage space required*	More	Less
Employee data entry time*	More	Less
Time needed for data editing in fields when the same information appears in many rows	More	Less
Number of fields available	Less	More
Ability to produce sophisticated reports	Less	More

* If more than one file management program is used with similar information.

available with spreadsheet programs. Assume that you want to have an automated master patient index using a file management software program and that you need fields for both patient and attending physician demographics because you also want to track physician activity at your facility by patient. You would need to set up the fields for each patient as follows: patient's name, address, telephone number, dates of admission and discharge, name of attending physician, physician address, physician telephone number, and physician specialty. You would need to enter the attending physician's name, address, telephone, and specialty for *each* patient at the time of registration. If the physician's address changes, *all the rows of all the patients* who had that person as an attending physician would need to be edited. Another disadvantage to a file management system is that the number of available fields for an application frequently are more limited than in a database management program and less sophisticated reports are possible. The advantages of a file management system are that the software is generally less expensive, quickly learned, and relatively easy to use in setting up an application.

DATABASE MANAGEMENT SYSTEM. A **database management system** is a computer software program that processes information, either storing it in or retrieving it from a database. The concept of linking, or "relational" tables of associated or similar data items that access one or more databases, makes data entry, data updating, and data query easier and more efficient than in a file management program. Examples of personal computer relational database software packages are the latest versions of dBase, R:Base, Access, and Paradox. If we use the master patient index example mentioned above, two relational tables would be developed instead of one, as in the file management system, with the following fields:

PATIENT TABLE	PHYSICIAN TABLE	
Record number	Physician number	←
Last name	Last name	
First name	First name	
Street address	Street address	
City, state	City, state	Relational
Zip	Zip	link
Telephone number	Telephone number	
Birth date	Specialty	
Date of admission		
Date of discharge		
Physician number ←		

Data for the physician's table are entered only once, at the time of system setup, or when a new physician receives admitting privileges. Thereafter, when individual patients are added to the master patient index, the physician code number is the only field related to infor-

mation about the attending physician that needs to be entered by the operator. The physician code number is considered a **key field** because it is needed to link the physician demographic information with the patient information. Thereafter, if the physician should change his or her address, the physician table would be updated only once, and all patients with that physician code number who are listed in the master patient index would have the physician address information updated simultaneously.

A table can be used in more than one application; for example, you might want to set up a correspondence log with two more tables. One table might be the patient table from the master patient index. The second table might be called a release table, which the following illustrates:

PATIENT TABLE		RELEASE TABLE
Record number ←———————→		Record number
Last name	Relational	Date request received
First name	link	Name of requester
Street address		Address of requester
City, state		Date information sent
Zip		Amount billed
Telephone number		Amount received, etc.
Birth date		
Date of admission		
Date of discharge		
Physician number		

Because the two tables are linked, only one redundant data field is needed—patient number. The need to enter patient last name and first name and other patient demographics for the automated correspondence log would be eliminated. Individual software programs vary as to whether one must use all the fields identified in the patient table for the correspondence log or just those fields that would be most useful for that application. Because the fields are linked, no extra space is needed to store the patient table information in the correspondence log application. The only redundant field to be stored is the record number, the linked field. As a result, the data redundancy and inconsistency found in file management programs are eliminated if a relational database management software program is used, less storage space is needed, and data entry time is reduced. Updating information is relatively simple if the program is designed correctly, and there is usually the capability to design field edits to assist in reducing data entry errors. Hundreds or thousands of fields are available for a personal computer system (file management systems are usually more limited). More sophisticated reports can be developed on either a routine or an ad hoc basis compared with a file management system (see Components of a Good Personal Computer Database System).

Components of a Good Personal Computer Database System

- Is user friendly with good use of menus and/or system prompts
- Allows a large number of fields and tables as well as varieties of types of fields (e.g., numerical, text, long memo fields, date, time, calculated)
- Is limited only by the size of the computer storage media
- Permits creation of custom forms and reports
- Allows the design of menus
- Permits the establishment of rules or built-in edits
- Allows the user to edit the program or structure over time without losing data
- Grants importing of data already stored on disk by a different program (e.g., spreadsheet or word processing) or in a different database
- Allows the user to add, delete, and change data as required
- Permits the user to sort records and selectively retrieve data on an ad hoc basis *easily*. It should use the *Structured query Language* (SQL) for this purpose.
- Allows the user to maintain security, e.g., use passwords on the full database, selected fields, or selected patients or entities.

Database management system software is more expensive to purchase than software for a file management program, and it takes time to learn the database system and develop the application programs. If it is not used correctly, data quality can be a serious problem.

Data Collection

As described in detail elsewhere, data collection is based on a needs analysis of internally and externally required data. The data model includes methods to assure that the data needed for patient care and other purposes are obtained accurately and consistently, primarily at the point of service. Another important consideration relating to data collection is the development of screen data input forms. They should be designed in a style that aids in data quality and data entry efficiency by staff. Custom screen forms allow the capability to do the following:

- Organize the data entry fields in logical format
- Include field edits
- Include passwords to add, delete, or modify data
- Allow simultaneous entry or updating into many tables at one time
- Include brief instructions on the screens or provide more lengthy help screens
- Make the screens attractive through the use of color, lines, borders, and so on
- Use default values in a field to eliminate the need to key repeated data between entries (e.g., date field could be automatically set up to add today's date without the need to key the characters)

- Allow automatic sequential numbering (e.g., accession register numbers)
- Show data on the screen from a different table when the key field is entered (e.g., for the master patient index screen form, when the person enters the physician number, the physician's name, address, and so on can automatically appear on the screen
- Develop or customize menus or submenus to add, delete, or change data

Report Accuracy

The dependability of manually prepared or computer-generated reports is based on several factors. They are the accuracy of the database software program, adequacy of the database field structure, reliability of the integration of information from different databases within the facility (data consistency), completeness and accuracy of the source documents or information, report-writing capabilities of the computer program, design of the report, and expertise of the person preparing the reports.

Manually prepared and computer-generated reports must be reviewed for accuracy of data when first generated and when revised. Among other items, the HIM professional should audit the computer reports for accuracy of statistical totals or the computed fields to determine whether formulas were entered correctly into the data field. For example, in one commercial home health computer system, the denominator for the average length of service in a computed field was the number of patients admitted, rather than the number of patients discharged, which led to inaccurate data. One can compare the new report with previous manual reports to see if the data are comparable. One can perform **parallel**

processing during the first several months; that is, continue the old system at the same time you are implementing the new system and compare the results.

Computer reports can be either routine or ad hoc, on-line or printed on paper or other media. The reports, both statistical tables and graphics, can be generated not only from the facility's main database but also from various personal computer software programs, such as spreadsheets, some word processing programs, file management software, database management software, graphics programs such as Harvard Graphics, and statistical packages such as the Statistical Package for the Social Sciences. *Automated programs for the development and analysis of statistical tables and graphs are preferred over manually developed and calculated reports to promote quality of data content and display.* Some facilities have the capability of downloading information from the mainframe to an intelligent terminal for data manipulation, analysis, and separate reporting. Because of the volume of data available, it is important that the reports be uncluttered, understandable, accurate, timely, and useful.

A facilitywide database and report inventory should be done, and an analysis of the results should be conducted by an appropriate group, such as a facility information resource management committee. Performing this inventory is helpful not only in planning new reports or applications but also in identifying duplications and streamlining data acquisition and reporting. One clinician may be unaware of another's use of the same data. It may be that the staff in the facility's finance department, the quality assessment and improvement (QAI) manager, the utilization review manager, the case mix manager, the nursing director, and the chief of staff may be unaware that they are all collecting and processing the same body of information for generally the same purposes. The inventory can help in developing good report-generating systems, facilitate the development of data quality control procedures, and help managers, other hospital planners, and researchers to know what data are available when requesting statistical or other reports. Policy needs to be developed relating to which individual or committee should be authorized to determine which reports should be *routinely* generated, by whom, how they should be distributed, and their frequency. Useless reports should be eliminated, duplications of reports should be omitted (or combined with similar reports), and manual reports should be avoided if computer-generated reports are available.

Testing Database Program Design

After the main database structure is defined, the input screens are developed, and the reports are programmed, it is important to test the system, using simulated data to determine whether there are system or software errors, or "bugs." It is also important to test software received from commercial vendors to determine whether there are database structure or system design errors that could result in poor data quality.

Backup and Data Retention

Even though you may treat your storage media with care, they can be damaged accidentally or on purpose and files can be inadvertently changed or erased. Portable media, such as floppy disks and tapes, can be mislaid or stolen. Making backup copies limits the amount of information that is lost if something goes wrong, an important data quality consideration. Backups can be made of individual files, floppy disks, or hard disk directories or subdirectories as well as entire databases. *It is important to test the "restore" capabilities of the system to assure that they work.* One home health agency lost 6 months of data because of a system crash. The agency was unable to restore data that had been backed up because the original backup instructions had been incorrectly written by the vendor. Backup media should be safely stored in a different location—preferably a different building—than the originals. If a building or department is damaged by fire, flood, or some other disaster, it is important that the backup media not be destroyed at the same time as the originals.

It is also important to determine the archival quality of storage media and the environmental conditions under which they should be stored. Will information stored on floppy disks be there 10 years after it is initially copied to the disk? Will backup cassette tapes still have the information when you need them 15 years later? Will information stored on a floppy disk be corrupted if the disk is placed on a car dashboard in 95° weather or placed next to a magnetic field, such as near a telephone?

Paper records must also be preserved from accidental loss due to theft, fire, or flood, a consideration often overlooked when archiving old records.

When determining the length of time to keep original records or backup data—another data quality consideration—laws and regulations as well as the needs of the facility need to be reviewed. The decision needs to be made by administration based on recommendations from the HIM professional. Facility legal counsel and members of the appropriate medical staff or institutional information coordinating committees should be consulted.

In a related backup issue, some facilities have redundant backup storage capability for dictated reports not yet transcribed to reduce the possibility of lost dictation during equipment malfunction.

Data Security Procedures

Complete and accurate information, also known as **data integrity,** can also be compromised if good security measures are not set up. We need to protect the data not only from unauthorized disclosure of confidential information but also from unauthorized modifications or destruction. Schechter discusses these security problems as they relate to data integrity as well as data quality problems related to an integrated database system that lacks control over who is allowed to add, change, or delete data and that is used by many departments.[12]

PASSWORD PROTECTION. Most database management systems allow the application designer to establish **password** protection, which is important not only for controlling disclosure of information but also for protecting the data from being improperly modified. Several different levels of password protection can be established. A master password that precludes anyone except authorized users from modifying the basic database structure can be set up. Passwords for individual applications, files, records, or data fields can also be set up; some may allow a user to read and modify data, whereas another type may allow read-only capabilities. For example, a payroll database would not allow access to information about employee salaries except to supervisors and authorized employees in the personnel department, payroll office, and business office. Specified employees in the personnel department would have both read and write permission for the payroll database, whereas the password for supervisors and authorized personnel in the payroll and business offices would have read-only permissions. They would not be able to add or change salary information. The password for other authorized staff might allow access to all employee payroll data except for salary information (see General Rules for Passwords).

COMPUTER AUDIT TRAILS. Computer audit trails should be reviewed frequently to determine possible problems related to breach of confidentiality or security. A first violation may be recorded only by the systems security office or on the audit trail because most users can be expected to make isolated mistakes. If a second attempt is made to enter an invalid code or access an unauthorized file, the system should react immediately by locking the terminal immediately from further access. Only the system security officer should be authorized to reopen the terminal. Employees and others should be disciplined immediately if unauthorized nonaccidental breaches are discovered, including verbal or written warnings or termination of employment.

AUTOMATIC CALL-BACK SECURITY MEASURES. Use automatic call-back security measures when appropriate. In this instance, a person at a remote station on a wide area network dials the host computer and, when prompted, enters a log-on name and password, requests access, and hangs up. The host terminal verifies the password against the log-on name and the terminal location. If all appears satisfactory, the host computer automatically dials the remote terminal and allows access.

VIRUS DETECTOR SOFTWARE. Virus detector software should be used routinely to locate and eliminate hidden unlawful computer instructions to delete or corrupt data. The facility must develop and strictly enforce policies regarding downloading of data from outside computers or services (i.e., games from electronic bulletin boards). These data often have computer viruses in them.

PHYSICAL PROTECTION OF HARDWARE. Physical protection of computer hardware must be assured. The organization's main or host computers should be maintained in a locked room with authorized access only. No signs indicating that this is the facility's computer center should appear on doorways. Screens that portray sensitive information should be directed away from public view.

There may be some areas in which only limited access or limited function terminals should be located. This restriction ensures that terminals receive only those transmissions programmed for them and that users can access only those data files that need to be there. For example, terminals on the nursing unit would be able to access most patient files but would not be able to access the business office database.

Reports, disks, associated written procedures, and other documentation should be stored in locked cabinets or drawers. There have been numerous instances of theft of floppy disks in unlocked locations. Expensive terminals should be bolted to desks or secured in such a way that easy access and transport are avoided. Instances have been reported in which people have used ladders in hallways outside locked doors, allowing them easy access to ceiling tiles. They then climbed the ladders, moved the ceiling tiles aside, crawled through the opening, and jumped down into the adjacent room where computer hardware or floppy disks were available. They unlocked the door from the inside and removed the hardware and software. Although this activity can be easily seen in a busy hospital location, it can prove to be a problem in a small facility or agency that closes at the end of the day.

Computers must be protected against smoke, water damage, humidity, volcanic dust, earthquakes, and other

---

General Rules for Passwords

- Each person must have his or her own unique password.
- Password sharing should not be allowed.
- The system should not have a feature to automatically assign passwords; this should be done by only one authorized person.
- Passwords should be changed frequently.
- A password should be somewhat complex—not a person's name or birthday, too few letters or numbers, or a word that is easy to figure out (e.g., "record" or "health"). The password should be 8 to 12 characters in length and should include a combination of upper- and lower-case letters as well as numbers or symbols. One must be careful not to choose a password that is too complex or it might be forgotten. If it is too easy, someone could figure it out within a short time using computer algorithms or other methodology.

---

environmental problems. Eating or drinking should not be allowed at computer workstations. The computer must also be protected against power failure or voltage reductions through the use of surge protectors, antistatic mats, and other devices.

Diskless workstations should be used, when appropriate, which makes copying data onto personal diskettes or using personal diskettes for computer games impossible.

Recovery procedures and downtime procedures need to be developed. Does there need to be a backup generator that would allow an orderly shutdown of the entire system during times of power outages? If the main computer is down, does the facility have a plan for recording transactions on paper or using a personal computer with floppy disks? When a computer is back on line, is there a procedure for updating the transactions that occurred during the downtime?

CONFIDENTIALITY POLICIES AND PROCEDURES. Policies and procedures related to confidentiality of data must be clearly written and provided to all health care organization employees and members of the medical staff. It is recommended that employees read and sign an "Oath of Confidentiality" that outlines the policies and procedures that must be followed as well as the sanctions for lack of follow-through.

Documentation to Support the Database

Policies and procedures need to be developed and written to support all aspects of the manual or automated information system as well as assist in assuring data quality. Detailed instructions and training manuals need to be developed for data entry onto paper forms or screens and for report generation, backups, and so on. Brief instructions or "cheat sheets" that provide summary instructions applicable to his or her job should be prepared for each user. These instruction sheets should be developed by the HIM professional, so that they are consistent and accurate among the employees who perform the same computer activity. A data dictionary should be developed and updated regularly that gives the following information for each data element:

- Description of the field
- Origin of the data
- Edits or rules that apply to that field
- Type and width of field
- Security levels applicable to that field
- Description of codes used (if any)
- Applications or reports that use the data element

Training

Education and training sessions should be provided to those who are to enter data into the system as well as those who need to use the applications. Written material should be available during the training sessions, and instruction should take place in an area where the trainees can have hands-on practice at the terminal. Simulated data should be available on which to practice, and the trainees should be allowed to practice on their own outside the formal training sessions.

DATA QUALITY MONITORING METHODS AND SOLUTIONS

If the database system is developed to allow for data quality capture and reporting and if point-of-care systems are designed to capture data correctly, the next step is to monitor data in patient records and secondary reporting systems to determine possible quality problems so that corrective action can be taken when necessary.

Quality Assessment and Improvement Study of Patient Record Documentation

One method to evaluate data quality is to do a QAI study of paper or computerized patient records that assesses the presence of reports and authentications as well as the quality of the information documented in the entries. The purpose is not to obtain data retrospectively but to monitor the adequacy of current systems and make changes in the information system when needed.

Quantitative Analysis

Performing a quantitative analysis means ensuring that the following has been done:

- Patient identification on the front and back of every paper form or screen is correct.

- All necessary authorizations or consents are present and signed or authenticated by the patient or legal representative, including those for general agreement, specific procedures, photographs, experimental treatment, advance directives, and autopsy.

- Documented principal diagnosis on discharge, secondary diagnoses, and procedures are present in the appropriate form or location within the record. This information is completed and authenticated by the physician or authorized clinician.

- Discharge summary is present, when required, and authenticated.

- History and physical report are present, documented within the time frame required by appropriate regulations, and authenticated as appropriate.

- Consultation report is present and authenticated when a consultation request appears in the listing of physician or practitioner orders.

- All diagnostic tests ordered by the physician or practitioner are present and authenticated by comparing physician orders, financial bill, and the test reports documented in the patient's health record.

- An admitting progress note, a discharge progress note, and an appropriate number of notes (frequency depends on the type of case or health care agency) documented by physicians or clinicians throughout the patient's care process.

- Each physician or practitioner order entered into the record is authenticated. An admitting and a discharge physician or practitioner order is present. Orders are present for all consultations, diagnostic tests, and procedures when these reports are found in the record.

- Operative, procedure, or therapy reports are present and authenticated when orders, consent forms, or other documentation in the record indicates that they were performed.

- A pathology report is present and authenticated when the operative report indicates that tissue was removed.

- Preoperative, operative, and postoperative anesthesia reports are present and authenticated.

- Nursing or ancillary health professionals' reports and notes are present and authenticated.

- Reports required for patients treated in specialized units, such as those for patients receiving care in the obstetrics unit, neonatal nursery, or mental health or rehabilitation units, are present and authenticated.

- Preliminary and final autopsy reports on patients who have expired at the facility are present and authenticated.

The amount of detailed checking varies by facility according to the nature of the QAI study, type of health care agency, and facility policy.

Legal Analysis

A legal analysis consists of checking for the following:

- Entries are documented in ink if a paper record or recorded on other legally recognized media, such as microfilm or a disk. The entries are legible and timely.

- If gaps in documentation appear on handwritten pages, such as progress notes, orders, or nurses' notes, a line is drawn through this area to prevent future tampering.

- Entries are authenticated by the person who made the observation or who conducted the test or treatment.

- If regulations, standards, or hospital policy require an attending physician to complete a report and if the report is written by a resident, the report should reflect authentication by both persons. Examples are physical examinations, consultations, and operative reports.

- Errors in documentation are corrected in a legal manner. For paper records, a single line is drawn through the error, the phrase "error in entry" or synonymous words are written, the new information is inserted, and the corrected entry is dated and authenticated by the person making the change. For computerized records, a procedure needs to be present, by means of audit trails or some other method, to demonstrate corrected entries, and the procedure should be reviewed.

- No misfiled documents are present.

Qualitative Analysis

A qualitative analysis involves checking for the following:

- Review for obvious documentation inconsistencies related to diagnoses found on admission forms, physical examination, operative and pathology reports, care plans, and discharge summary.

- Analyze the record to determine whether documentation written by various health care providers on one patient reflects consistency.

- Compare the patient's pharmacy drug profile with the medication administration record to determine consistency.

- Review an inpatient record to determine whether it reflects the general location of the patient at all times or if serious time gaps exist. Times noted on nursing documentation indicating when the patient left the unit and returned to it can be used as the reference point for this type of study.

- Determine whether the patient record reflects the progression of care, including the symptoms, diagnoses, tests, treatments, reasons for the treatments, results, patient education, location of patient after discharge, and follow-up plans.

- Interview the patient and/or family. Review recorded patient demographic information and medical history with the patient at several hours or days after admission to determine completeness and accuracy. A patient or family may be too physically ill or mentally confused at admission to provide valid data.

- Compare written instructions to the patient that are documented in the record with the patient's or family's understanding of those instructions. Ask the patient or family to repeat instructions to verify consistency.

- Review for other documentation as determined by the individual facility.

The results are presented to the appropriate medical or clinical staff committee for appropriate follow-up.

Special Concerns of Alternative Care Settings

The HIM professional needs to design a flexible approach in assuring data quality that considers the type of health care facility, its data requirements, level of technology available, type of health care providers who are the major sources of documentation, types of common documentation problems, and results related to missing documentation (e.g., loss of revenue). Whether or not retrospective documentation should occur is a decision to be made by the facility administrator, medical staff or medical director, and legal counsel with advice from the HIM professional. However, accuracy of documentation at the point of care should be emphasized.

Ambulatory Care

An outpatient clinic or a physician's office has similar but different data requirements and documentation practices for records than does an acute care hospital. A QAI approach for documentation review may be more appropriate than an ongoing daily record review on all patient visits. Feste provides an excellent discussion related to this process in the outpatient setting and has a sample QAI form that could be used[13] (Figure 5–9). Many outpatient surgical centers use the same manual or automated systems to monitor data quality as do acute inpatient facilities.

A major problem related to accessibility and completeness of data in the ambulatory care setting, especially in large clinics, is the availability of the patient's record at the time of the visit. The record frequently is needed by several physicians and ancillary departments, such as radiology, because the patient may be treated by more than one clinic provider on the same day. Also, the patient may be treated during a series of appointments that are scheduled for consecutive days or for several days during 1 week. Computerized patient records can solve the accessibility problem. If the facility uses paper records, then systems need to be developed to allow access to the record at the appropriate time for all who need it. This includes record availability for scheduled appointments, unscheduled visits, patient telephone calls, prescription renewals, and so on. Reviews of record retrieval times in paper record systems are essential. The use of technology to assist in record location tracking, such as bar code systems, is critical as the patient's record moves to different locations on the same day.

Deficiency Analysis

Medical Record Number _____

Primary Care Physician _____

	Present	Absent	Not Applicable	Specify
General Documentation Requirements				
The medical record contains patient identification data.				
Significant diagnosis/symptom/surgeries are entered on the summary list.				
Current and past medications are entered on the medication sheet.				
Medical record entries are dated and signed by practitioner name and profession.				
Medical record entries are legible to clinical personnel.				
Presence or absence of allergies is documented in a prominent and uniform location.				
Every patient visit includes documentation of: -chief complaint/purpose of visit -history and physical consistent with chief complaint -diagnosis or impression -treatment -patient disposition, referral, instructions -signature of practitioner				
Immunization record includes: -date -vaccine manufacturer name and lot number				
Diagnostic Reports				
Test results are filed in sequential order. All test results initialed and dated by practitioner.				
The medical record contains evidence of informed consent prior to performance of any invasive procedure.				
Preanesthesia Evaluation				
The preanesthesia evaluation is recorded prior to surgery.				
The preanesthesia evaluation includes documentation of: -review of patient's medical history -previous anesthetic experiences -current medications -date and signature of anesthesiologist				

FIGURE 5–9. Deficiency analysis. (From Feste LK: Ambulatory care documentation. Chicago: American Medical Record Association, 1989, pp 16–17.)

Illustration continued on following page

	Present	Absent	Not Applicable	Specify
Anesthesia Record				
The anesthesia record includes documentation of: -anesthesia type and method of administration -regular monitoring of vital signs -date and signature of anesthesiologist				
Postanesthesia Record				
Postanesthesia record includes documentation of: -time based monitoring of vital signs and level of consciousness -status of surgical dressing -status of tubes -date and signature of discharging practitioner				
Operative Records				
Appropriate history and physical are part of the medical record prior to surgery.				
The operative report includes documentation of: -preoperative diagnosis -postoperative diagnosis -findings -technique used -specimens removed -primary surgeon and assistants -date and signature of surgeon				
The medical record includes documentation of post-operative instructions given to the patient.				
The pathology report is filed in the medical record.				

FIGURE 5–9 *Continued*

Stopwatch studies of physician outpatient clinic activities during the day have shown that 50 per cent of the physician's time is spent on activities related to patient interviews, examinations, and procedures and 50 per cent of the time is spent reviewing records, documenting records, dictation, and x-ray film review and on other "housekeeping" activities. It is critical for the HIM professional to evaluate current practices of the physician, review the clinic office system and organizational structure, and modify the information system to help improve physician efficiency and allow more patient appointments to occur during the day, an important revenue consideration. For example, one clinic found that if a physician documented in the visit note what he or she planned to do at the patient's next visit, the nurses or medical assistants could review the record the day before the next appointment and would know how to prepare the examination or treatment room for that visit and what supplies were needed for that encounter. En-

couraging the physician to document orders rather than give verbal orders decreases the chance for error by the office staff. Physicians may resort to verbal orders because documentation time may be excessive. The HIM professional should identify the nature of the problem, evaluate the current system, and find solutions to the problem. Improved efficiency of documentation of orders might be accomplished by using simple check-off paper forms or by having physicians input data directly into the computer using such equipment as a touch screen or pen-based device.

Even though the ambulatory care setting may have current records in electronic format, systems should be in place to assure timely access to archived historical records that are in paper or microfilm format.

Surveys of or focused interviews with physicians and the clinic staff can determine their satisfaction with the current system, their ideas, their needs, how they would like to use computers in their practice, the type of computer training they would like, and their satisfaction with transcription and other systems.

Home Health Care

Home health records pose special problems related to record documentation systems, and until such patient records are computerized, these problems will continue because the patient is not located at the health care facility when treatment is rendered. Figure 5–10 shows a flow chart of documentation received on home health patients at a typical agency. Initial referring information is obtained by telephone or facsimile (fax) from the transferring health care facility or physician. Copies of the referring facility's history and physical report, discharge summary, and transfer form are critical at this point. A clinician is assigned to the patient, and the referring information must be available to the nurse or therapist before the first home visit. The clinician verifies demographic and reimbursement information with the patient on the first visit, and signed patient consent-for-care forms are obtained. Subsequent information is recorded in the patient's home, clinician's car or home, agency office, or other location by the clinician. The documentation includes the following:

- Assessments
- Plans of treatment
- Progress notes (one note per visit is required)
- Clinician discharge summary

This information is brought to the agency's HIM department at a later time (often several days later) for incorporation into the patient record. The original patient record must not leave the office to avoid the possibility of tampering or loss and so that it is available for others who need access to the record, such as other clinicians involved in the case and clinical supervisors. Therefore, the nurse or therapist relies on copies of original records that are maintained at home or in the car, preferably in a locked briefcase when not stored at the clinician's office desk. The nurse or therapist may not visit the office every day, which may create problems in terms of record access and updating of the original record by the clinician. *Paper record systems in home health agencies not only pose systems problems but also have the potential to create major problems related to loss of confidentiality.*

Designing a method of documentation review for a paper record system is difficult at best. Miller has written an excellent discussion on client record review guidelines and procedures.[14] The first review should be done within 10 days of patient admission to the home health agency. The record should be reviewed for the following:

- Receipt of information from transferring facilities

- Correct and complete referral information
- Presence and authentication of assessment documents by all professional disciplines involved in the case
- Plans of treatment and other reports
- Signed consent-for-care forms from the patient

Every 30 to 60 days while the patient is still active and again at discharge the record should be reviewed to make sure the following are present:

- Team case conference notes
- Updated and signed plans of treatment and orders from physicians
- Home health aide supervisory visit notes by a nurse or therapist
- Clinician discharge summary and other reports
- Authenticated progress notes for each visit made by the clinician

Third party payers require a progress note for each visit billed. If the note is not present, the agency could lose revenue for that visit. This last item is difficult to review because the patient usually is not visited every day. Therefore, a method needs to be devised to match the date of each billed visit with the presence of a progress note. In many agencies, this is a complex problem because thousands of patient visits may be made each month. Many agencies have daily or weekly individual employee service records, sometimes referred to as "itineraries," on which the clinician documents each patient visit (Figure 5–11). This form is sent to the business office, which uses it as the data source for billing third party payers as well as an employee time card. Many agencies require that the clinician attach the individual progress notes to these handwritten service records and bring them to the HIM department. The HIM department staff record the receipt of these progress notes by comparing them with each visit noted on the service record. They follow through on missing documentation with the clinician before the final monthly bill is submitted to the third party payer by the business office. Other agencies bill directly from the progress notes and do no further checking. Some agencies perform random review only, comparing bills with patient records to assess accuracy. A paper clinical record system is cumbersome for home health agencies, not only for the clinicians but also for the HIM department staff. To assure data quality, it is imperative that the HIM professional understand and evaluate the agency's current system of data collection and make changes as necessary.

Paperless records in the form of optical disk or electronic medical record systems streamline the home health agency's data collection, record access, and data

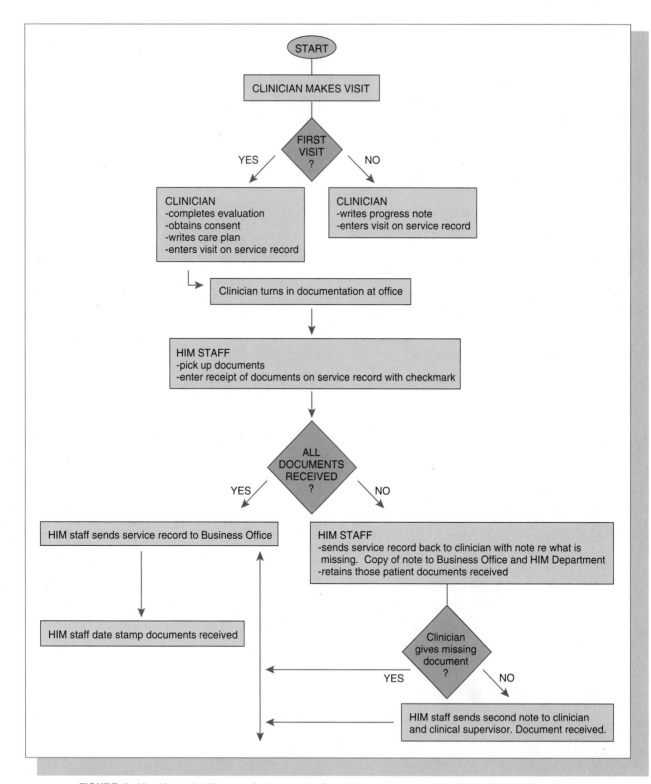

FIGURE 5-10. Home health care documentation flow chart, manual system. (From Feste LK: Ambulatory care documentation. Chicago: American Medical Record Association, 1989, pp 16–17.)

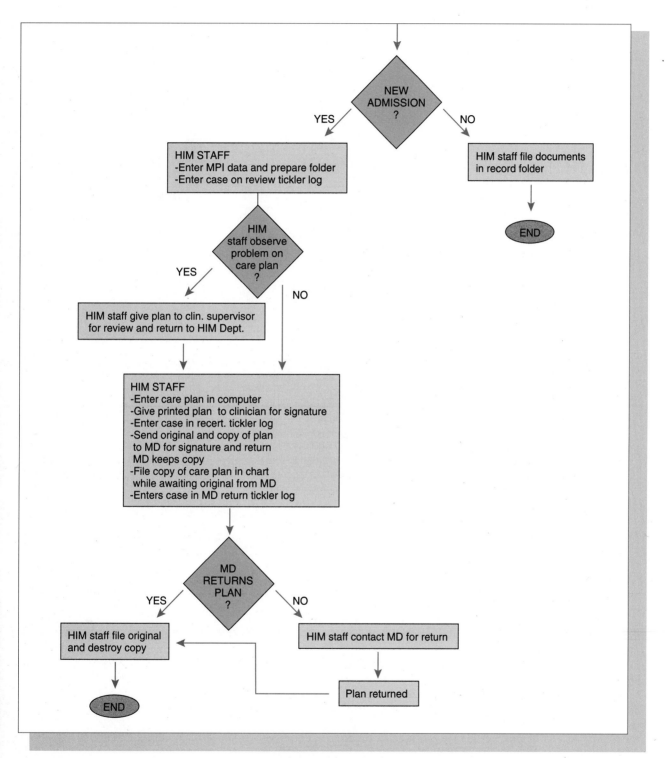

FIGURE 5-10 *Continued*

Employee: _____		Date: _____		
Patients visited	Travel Time	Visit Time	Type of Visit	Miles

HOURS			TIME CARD	
Visits			Regular hours	
Travel			Overtime hours	
Patient office time			Holiday	
Meetings			Vacation	
Other (specify)			Sick leave	
TOTAL			Mileage	
			Parking/Toll	
Employee Signature _____			Pager	
Supervisor Signature_____				
Date _____				

FIGURE 5–11. Employee service record.

quality procedures. Documentation at point of care through the use of laptop computers, hand-held or pen-based computers, voice recognition, or other devices that is electronically transferred to the office using a modem assures timely data and immediate accessibility to all. Charges for each visit are automatically generated, and consistency between the two databases (clinical and financial) is assured. Figure 5–12 shows an example of a revised home health documentation flow chart used by an agency that has an ideal computerized system. In this scenario, it is interesting to note the absence of an HIM department role in the clerical processing and monitoring of data collection. The HIM professional's role, then, is to help design the systems, monitor the quality or accuracy of the information, and assist with

other activities related to quality assessment and improvement of patient care. Because of the excessive use of wide area networks in such a system, it is critical that the HIM professional work with information systems department personnel and clinical staff to develop strict confidentiality and security policies and procedures and to perform frequent audit trail checks to detect unauthorized access to patient information. It is important to set parameters regarding database query and documentation when using laptop computers, so that they are done in a private, secure location and not in areas such as restaurants and public parks. Once a clinician is no longer involved in the care and treatment of a specific patient, he or she should no longer have password access to the database on that patient.

Long-Term Care

Long-term care records are created for patients or residents who stay at a nursing facility for months or years. Because documentation requirements vary significantly from acute inpatient settings, many of the traditional acute care inpatient record documentation review systems need to be modified to meet the needs of the long-term care industry. Quantitative and qualitative reviews are usually done within 1 to 2 days after admission, then periodically at least every 30 to 60 days, and again at discharge. Appendix A at the end of this chapter provides forms and instructions for long-term care documentation reviews developed by Marilyn Noe, RRA, a long-term care consultant at the North Pacific Data

---

Criteria for Documentation of Residents with Skin at Risk or Pressure Sores

1. Assessment present on admission

2. Skin assessment completed

3. Problem on problem list

4. Problem on care plan

5. If developed in facility, has the physician been notified?

6. Are there physician orders for treatment?

7. Are treatments administered at specified intervals?

8. Are weekly assessments and progress documented?

Criteria developed by Marilyn Noe, RRA, Long-term Care Consultant, North Pacific Data Service, Bellevue, Washington.

Criteria for Documentation of Weights of Residents

1. Problem and goal on care plan

2. Weighing frequency on care plan

3. Weighing frequency on nursing assistant care flow sheets

4. Weights recorded according to schedule

5. Discrepancies in weights and unplanned gain or loss have evidence of follow-up

6. Physician notified, when necessary; documented in progress notes

7. Consultation with dietitian

Criteria developed by Marilyn Noe, RRA, Long-term Care Consultant, North Pacific Data Service, Bellevue, Washington.

Service, Bellevue, Washington. These forms consist of an admission data review criteria form, a health record review reporting form, and medication or treatment documentation reviews. Written procedures for form completion are also provided. Quality assessment and assurance worksheet forms can also be developed to check documentation for specific topics. Also see criteria developed by Noe for QAI documentation reviews (see Criteria for Documentation of Residents with Skin at Risk or Pressure Sores and Criteria for Documentation of Weights of Residents).

The excellent examples shown in Appendix A can be used by HIM professionals working in various long-term care settings and can be easily adapted to review documentation in computer-based patient record systems.

Hospice

Hospice records usually reflect the characteristics of the facility or agency that maintains the hospice program, often use the same or similar forms of the facility as a whole, and use many of the same record completion review procedures. Many hospices are affiliated with home health agencies or long-term care facilities and reflect those systems. Miller provides forms, record content requirements, and procedures unique to hospice programs.[15]

Managed Care Environments

As managed care environments increase, particular attention is being paid to the development and use of a common computer database for all inpatient, home care, physician offices, and clinics that are integral to a specific managed care group. The innovative concept of having just one location provide all health information services for all care sites of a managed care group is proving to be an efficient and accurate method to capture, store, monitor, analyze, evaluate, and disseminate data related to patient care delivered at various sites for one episode of care. Cost and other financial data can be integrated with the clinical database, which assists in analyzing and interpreting aggregate data relative to short- and long-term costs in various categories, such as by problem, by provider, or by patient age. It also is the basis for the development of a longitudinal record for patients in that managed care group.

Medical Staff Activities Related to Data Quality

Medical Record Committee

Responsibility for the timeliness and accuracy of patient records is shared by the individual physician and

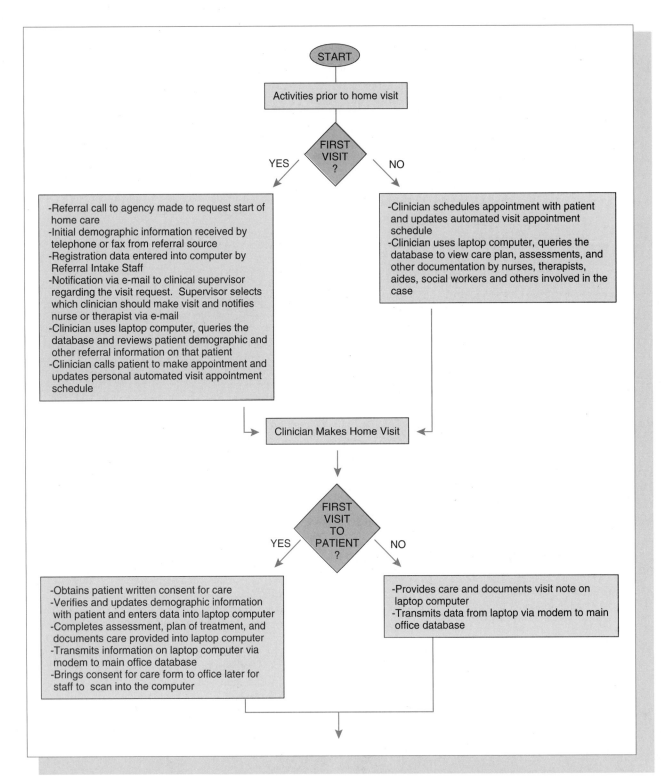

FIGURE 5–12. Home health care documentation flow chart, computer system.

Illustration continued on following page

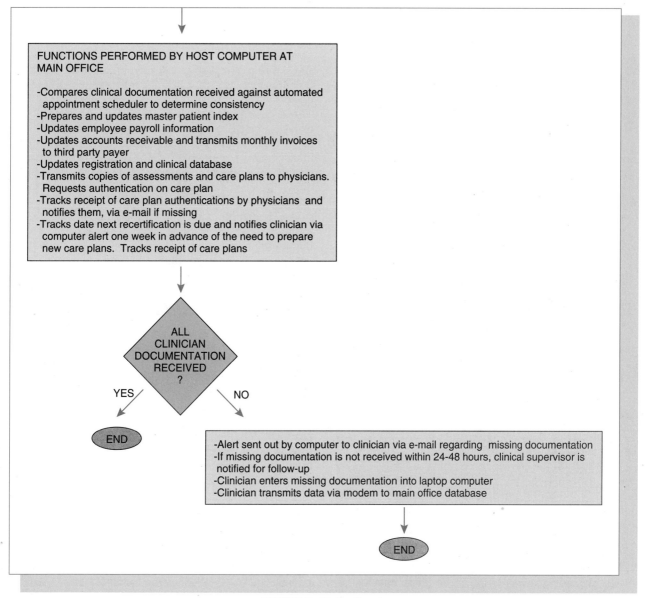

FUNCTIONS PERFORMED BY HOST COMPUTER AT MAIN OFFICE

-Compares clinical documentation received against automated appointment scheduler to determine consistency
-Prepares and updates master patient index
-Updates employee payroll information
-Updates accounts receivable and transmits monthly invoices to third party payer
-Updates registration and clinical database
-Transmits copies of assessments and care plans to physicians. Requests authentication on care plan
-Tracks receipt of care plan authentications by physicians and notifies them, via e-mail if missing
-Tracks date next recertification is due and notifies clinician via computer alert one week in advance of the need to prepare new care plans. Tracks receipt of care plans

ALL CLINICIAN DOCUMENTATION RECEIVED ?

YES

NO

END

-Alert sent out by computer to clinician via e-mail regarding missing documentation
-If missing documentation is not received within 24-48 hours, clinical supervisor is notified for follow-up
-Clinician enters missing documentation into laptop computer
-Clinician transmits data via modem to main office database

END

FIGURE 5–12 *Continued*

mittee members, who are representatives of the medical staff, administration, HIM department, nursing, and other departments or services, develop policies relating to analysis of patient records for documentation deficiencies, including items to review, frequency, and types of penalties for incomplete reports. The committee also coordinates activities with clinical staff departments and other medical staff groups related to clinical documentation, such as QAI committees and credentialing committees. If no separate medical record committee exists, these functions are carried out by other medical staff committees. Relevant documentation policies developed by the medical record committee, such as loss of admitting privileges for incomplete records, are adopted by the medical staff as a whole and incorporated into medical staff regulations.

Clinical Pertinence Reviews

JCAHO states that medical records should be reviewed "at least quarterly" and indicates that the medical staff, nursing, HIM department, administrative personnel, and other services perform the review.[16] The standards further specify that "the review determines that each medical record, or a representative sample of records, reflects the diagnosis, diagnostic test results, therapy, the patient's condition and in-hospital progress, and the patient's condition at discharge."

Lewis describes her facility's clinical pertinence review process, which meets JCAHO requirements.[17] In describing the process at her hospital, Lewis indicates that a review for **clinical pertinence documentation** refers to the "completeness, adequacy, appropriateness, accuracy, and quality of documentation rather than to the quality of clinical care." A detailed documentation review of a representative sample (5 per cent) of the health records is completed by her hospital's HIM staff, physician reviewers, and nursing staff. HIM personnel review the record for the presence of specified content within reports. For example, the operative report for each surgery is reviewed to determine the presence of a description of the findings, technical approach used, specimens removed, preoperative diagnosis, postoperative diagnosis, surgical indications, estimated blood loss, and detailed description of the procedure performed. Other reports in the record that are reviewed for the presence of content by the HIM staff include the history and physical examination, anesthesia report, discharge summary, consultations, and progress notes.

Lewis further describes the review by the physicians, which relates to the quality of specified content.[17] For example, they read and indicate whether the history and physical examination are adequate to meet JCAHO requirements, whether the discharge summary has adequate medical information to provide continuity of care, whether progress notes adequately reflect the patient's course in the hospital and are sufficient to permit continuity of care, and so on. Nursing staff review adequacy of nursing documentation.

Simple check-off review forms have been developed for record analysis. The completed evaluation forms are reviewed by the HIM professional, summarized in report format, and presented to the medical record committee for review and action.

Indicator Monitoring Program

The ability to perform accurate health record reviews for the quality of patient care is impacted by the accuracy and completeness of the documentation describing the patient's health history, diagnostic and therapeutic care, examination and test results, and patient status. For example, one type of hospital clinical care evaluation process required by JCAHO includes the development and use of an indicator monitoring program,[16] the subsequent reporting of results to JCAHO, and the use of JCAHO feedback reports for hospital benchmarking and performance improvement activities. Careful planning is needed to develop a data collection system to meet these requirements. The success of this system depends on the presence of required information in the health record. As an example, JCAHO describes an indicator focus for oncology as "availability of data for diagnosis and staging." The indicator (numerator) for that

focus includes "surgical pathology consultation reports (pathology reports) containing histological type, tumor size, status of margins, appropriate lymph node examination, assessment of invasion or extension as indicated, and AJCC/pTN classification for patients with resection for primary cancer of the lung, colon/rectum, or female breast." Another JCAHO oncology indicator focus is the "use of tests critical to diagnosis, prognosis, and clinical management." The indicator (numerator) is "female patients with invasive primary breast cancer undergoing initial biopsy or resection of a tumor larger than 1 centimeter in greatest dimension who have presence of estrogen receptor diagnostic analysis results in the medical record." It is critical that staff who perform QAI studies and those who report results of indicator monitoring work jointly with the HIM professional to design the information collection process for the study and refer documentation problems to the appropriate medical staff committee and HIM professional for resolution.

Data Quality in Statistical Reports

Standardization of Statistical Terms and Formulas

Manually generated or computer-generated statistical reports based on patient data must also be accurate and timely to meet the needs of the institution and public. The *Glossary of Healthcare Terms* should be used as a basis for definition of terms and formulas.[6] Figures on routine or ad hoc reports should be monitored and evaluated to determine if they are accurate and complete.

Face Validity

Face validity means evaluation of data to see whether the information is logical and if the results appear accurate on the surface. It is a quick method to identify possible quality problems. For example, is it logical to have 3000 patients discharged in 1 month in a 100-bed hospital? This would mean that 100 patients a day (or all the patients in the hospital) would need to be discharged every day. Is this reasonable? Is it logical to have an average length of stay of 53 days in a primary care acute hospital? Could the decimal have been omitted? Should it be 5.3 days? If the death rate for obstetric patients is reported as 15 per cent, could the decimal have been omitted, or could the formula for calculation of the percentage have been in error?

Report Comparisons

Comparison of selected data that appear in two or more reports often can reveal consistency problems. Two types of reports that are often developed or reviewed for accuracy by the HIM department are those related to the census and those that describe the professional activities of the medical staff done at the time of patient discharge, commonly called the "discharge analysis." The census report, usually automated, prepared by the admitting office personnel from information received from the nursing and other units includes names and room locations of patients admitted, discharged, and transferred that day as well as a listing in alphabetical order and in room and bed number order of all patients who occupied a bed at the census-taking hour, usually at the end of the day. HIM personnel review daily and monthly census reports to verify data completeness and accuracy. If a good census admission, discharge, and transfer (ADT) reporting system is in place, only random reviews are needed. If frequent problems occur, this verification is done more frequently, typically on a daily basis. Various census reports are compared to assure consistency. For example, if a patient is listed as discharged from the hospital that day on the ADT list, he or she should not be listed as occupying a bed at the end of the day in another report. If a patient is transferred from one room or bed to another according to the ADT list, the patient's correct location should appear in the bed occupancy report at the end of the day.

The discharge analysis reports relating to the professional activities of physicians are usually calculated based on records of patients discharged. These records can be manually prepared, be an outcome of an abstracting system, or be automatically available as an outcome of a point-of-care automated patient record. Consistency of data between related reports should be reviewed. For example, does the number of monthly discharges on the discharge analysis report agree with the number of discharges on the monthly census report? Does the number of deaths reported on the discharge analysis report agree with the information found in the death register? Averages and percentages reported should be verified periodically to assure that correct data fields and formulas are used.

Appropriateness of Statistical Reports

When data are interpreted, one must be careful in analyzing and displaying data. Are totals and formulas appropriate? For example, is the mean average length of stay in a hospice appropriate when most of the patients stay 5 to 10 days but a few patients who stay 1 to 2 years distort the mean? Is the mode or the median a better average to use to portray the typical length of time in the program? Or do you eliminate cases that are 2 or more standard deviations beyond the mean? Do you have a large enough sample for valid comparisons? In small facilities, a detailed analysis of discharge patients may not be a good idea. Simple totals and basic averages and percentages may be enough. Are you re-

porting unduplicated and unique cases or duplicated cases in your reports? Unduplicated and unique figures count a patient only once, no matter how many times he or she is readmitted. Duplicated counts, for example, in the discharge analysis include the number of discharge *occurrences,* rather than the number of *patients* discharged because many of these patients may have been in the facility one or more times before this episode of care during the same reporting period. In other words, if you were to report that 50 patients with cerebrovascular accident were discharged from your hospital during the month but one half of them were readmitted for the same condition, are you telling the correct story? You may need to footnote your report to indicate the basis of your figures. The purpose of the report needs to be reviewed to determine which of the two counts is appropriate. If an unduplicated count is needed, your system needs to be designed to track these cases.

Inter-rater and Intra-rater Reliability Studies

Inter-rater reliability studies are good methods to verify consistency of data when two or more persons capture or manipulate the same data. This is a common tool to evaluate the quality of data entry, coding, and abstracting by HIM personnel. A random or other sample of records is reviewed by another person, who then codes and abstracts the same cases. The original codes or abstracts are then made available and compared. If discrepancies occur, the cause is determined. The number of data elements reviewed and the number of correct data elements coded and abstracted are totaled. The percentage correct is then calculated. For example, if 40 records with 50 data elements each (total 2000) were coded or abstracted and 1931 elements were deemed correct, a 96.6 per cent accuracy rate is then reported. Accuracy norms and standards are established for each institution. If the coder or abstractor does not meet the norm, appropriate retraining or other steps are taken to help the coder improve his or her skills. Some hospitals contract with external proprietary companies to send their HIM professionals to recode or abstract the facility's records. Results are reviewed with HIM management and other administrative staff for appropriate follow-through. Intra-rater reliability studies use essentially the same process, but in this case, the same coder or abstractor recodes and reabstracts a sample of records he or she did previously and they are compared to determine consistency.

Coding Quality

A variety of coding "audits" quality reviews are described by Kost and others.[18] They include quarterly retrospective coding reviews by coding supervisors on a random number of cases, concurrent audits on problem diagnostic related group (DRG) cases before Medicare billing, retrospective coding audits on cases identified on the Medicare remittance advices where assigned DRGs appear inappropriate based on length of stay for that DRG, and so on.

FACILITY STRUCTURE THAT ENCOURAGES DATA QUALITY

JCAHO Information Management Standards

The JCAHO in its *Accreditation Manual for Hospitals*[16] recognizes the need to combine information management requirements into one chapter in an effort to promote coordination of activities that relate to the acquisition, analysis, and reporting of information within the health care facility.

The JCAHO standards require the following:

- Institutionwide planning and design of information management processes
- Confidentiality, security, and integrity of information
- Uniform data definitions and methods of data capture
- Education and training in principles of information management by decision makers as well as those who generate, collect, and analyze data and information
- Timely, accurate transmission of data in standardized formats when possible
- Integration and reporting of data with linkages of patient care and non–patient care data across departments and care modes over time
- Detailed list of patient-specific data
- Aggregate data from the entire institution
- Incorporation of knowledge-based information, including the library, formulary, and poison control information into the information management systems plan
- Contributions to and use of external reference databases

The AHIMA actively participated in the development of this JCAHO standard.

Information Resources Management Committee

Although many health care facilities have an information resources management committee (also called man-agement information system committee, health information systems committee, or data quality council) to coordinate automation activities, not all are truly successful because of the lack of adequate leadership, competition between departments, lack of a mission, and so on. The JCAHO requires coordination of activities, and its information management standard can help to focus more centralized planning within a facility. The HIM and information system departments must work closely together to meet the JCAHO information management standards. A chief information officer (CIO) may be an added management position in the future in those health facilities that do not have adequate leadership. The information resources management committee, with the assistance of the CIO, can help with hardware and software selections, approve systems to ensure the quality of computer data input activities, assure the inventory of facility databases and the preparation of data dictionaries, approve the frequency and distribution of computer reports, and approve systems to assure report accuracy.

Facility Information Systems Plan

The information resources management committee can also help design the data quality assessment plan required by the JCAHO. Appendix B describes JCAHO documentation review criteria to be incorporated into such a plan.[19]

APPLYING PROFESSIONAL PRACTICE STANDARDS FOR HIM SERVICES

The quality of health care data relies on excellence of data collection at the time of service, the information system model design and implementation, data monitoring and evaluation, and the services provided by or under the direction of the HIM professional. In addition to ongoing assessment of the quality of health data, continuous monitoring and evaluation of the quality of HIM services, based on practice standards, must be essential activities in all health care or non–health care organizations that have these services. The *Professional Practice Standards for Health Information Management Services* of the AHIMA is an excellent tool that provides a structured model of standards, guidelines, and measures of quality and quantity.[20] Figure 5–13 outlines the construction of the practice standards. The standards manual indicates that the evaluation checklists can be used as a self-evaluation of the individual HIM professional, internal review completed by a committee or HIM service, peer review by an external HIM professional, or external review by several managers within the facility.

Seven major areas of professional practice for managing patient care information in a health information service have been identified and a standard articulated for each. These areas include:

1. Content of the Patient Record
2. Patient Care Data
3. Confidentiality
4. Health Information Management
5. Storage and Retrieval
6. Management and Supervision
7. External Requirements and Standards
8. Quality Assessment/ Improvement Systems

Within each major area, the standard is presented in a systematic format moving from a broad guiding principle and its rationale to component functions and measures of quality for organizing and managing these component functions. Finally, self-evaluation tools are presented along with a bibliography of relevant resources. The diagram below illustrates the construction of the Practice Standards:

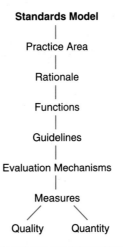

Standards Model
|
Practice Area
|
Rationale
|
Functions
|
Guidelines
|
Evaluation Mechanisms
|
Measures
/   \
Quality   Quantity

FIGURE 5–13. Construction of the practice standards. (From Professional Practice Standards for Health Information Management Services. Chicago: American Health Information Management Association, 1992, p 6.)

Once the evaluation is complete, the HIM professional must analyze any variations, determine the cause of problem areas, and develop and implement a plan of action to correct the deficiencies.

Key Concepts

• Because of the wide use of health care data for many purposes, it is crucial that data be accurate, complete, reliable, legible, accessible to authorized users, and secure from misuse, corruption, and loss.

• The HIM professional directs or participates actively in all phases related to collecting, storing, retrieving, analyzing, evaluating, and disseminating health data.

• Data for the patient record are collected in various ways from many sources. Data quality relies on accurate receipt and recording of this information at the point of service.

• Data integrity also relies on appropriate database structure, reliable hardware and software, data and transmission standards, reliable storage media and backup processes, accuracy of coded data, computer data query proficiency, skills in data analysis and interpretation, and report-generation abilities.

• Quality of data in paper and computer-based patient records must be monitored and evaluated. Systems for these reviews must be flexible to reflect facility size and type of care rendered.

- Post discharge or retrospective data completion activities for current patients beyond 24 to 48 hours have doubtful value. Systems should emphasize completeness and accuracy at the time care is rendered.

- Database and report inventories and controls assist in timely, accurate data.

- The information management structure at the facility can assist in data quality and information management efficiencies. Aids include the presence of a CIO position and information resource management or data quality control committee and definition of data responsibilities between and among departments. The HIM professional is a logical choice for clinical data coordinator for the institution.

- Continuous monitoring and evaluation of the quality of HIM services, based on practice standards, must be essential activities in all organizations that have these services.

References

1. Essentials for an accredited educational program for the health information technician and health information administrator. Chicago: American Health Information Management Association, 1994, p 7.
2. Johns L: Information management: A shifting paradigm for medical record professionals? J Am Health Information Management Assoc 1991;62(8):55–63.
3. U.S. Department of Health and Human Services, Public Health Service: Healthy People 2000: National health promotion and disease prevention objectives. Boston: Jones & Bartlett, 1992, p 79.
4. Dick RS, Steen EB (eds): The Computer-based Patient Record. Washington, DC: National Academy Press, 1991, pp 41–42.
5. Glondys BA: Documentation requirements for the acute care patient record, 3rd ed. Chicago: American Health Information Management Association, 1993, p 275.
6. Glossary of healthcare terms, rev ed. Chicago: American Health Information Management Association, 1994.
7. American Health Information Management Association: Position statement. Issue: Documentation timeliness. Chicago: May 1994.
8. Fox LA, Anderson RJ, Joseph ML: Data dynamics: Meeting the challenge of the information age. Chicago: American Medical Record Association, 1988, Chap 3.
9. Fuller S, O'Gara SA: Techniques for dataset design: A utilization management system model. Top Health Record Management 1992;12(4):8–16.
10. Lee FW: Using database software for quantitative review and active caseload lists in a community health setting. Top Health Record Management 1992;13(1):35–44.
11. McDonald CJ, Barnett GO: Medical record systems. In Shortliffe EH, Perreault LE (eds): Medical informatics, computer applications in health care. Reading, MA: Addison-Wesley, 1990, p 189.
12. Schechter KS: Conversion issues and data integrity: A consultant's perspective. Top Health Record Management 1988; 9(2):62–69.
13. Feste LK: Ambulatory care documentation. Chicago: American Medical Record Association, 1989, pp 13–19.
14. Miller SC: Documentation for home health care. Chicago: American Medical Record Association, 1986, Chap 1.
15. Miller SC: A medical record handbook for hospice programs, 2nd ed. Chicago: American Medical Record Association, 1987, Chap 1.
16. Accreditation Manual for Hospitals. Chicago: Joint Commission on Accreditation of Healthcare Organizations, 1993, sec 2.
17. Lewis KS: Medical record review for clinical pertinence. Top Health Record Management 1991;12(1):52–59.
18. Kost B, Muller PE, Smith AM: Coding and abstracting. In Mangano JJ (ed): Health information management. Los Angeles: Practice Management Information Corp, 1993, pp 91–93.
19. Grzybowski DM: The transition from signature to authorship. J Am Health Information Management Assoc 1993;64(9):90.
20. Professional Practice Standards for Health Information Management Services. Chicago: American Health Information Management Association, 1992, p 6.

Appendix A

Long-Term Care Documentation Review Forms and Instructions

HEALTH RECORD PROCEDURES

ADMISSION PROCEDURES

Admission Audit Review Procedure

PURPOSE

1. To ensure that all data required for admission and immediately following are obtained/completed in a timely manner.

2. To provide a monitoring system to document timely gathering of needed data, identify deficient areas, provide a system of notification to responsible individuals, provide follow-up monitoring for completion of deficiencies, and provide a reporting mechanism for a Quality Assurance program.

RESPONSIBLE STAFF:

Health Information Manager or other designee.

PROCEDURE

1. Utilize the *Admission Data Review Criteria* Form (form 2-16) as the guideline and affirmation tool.

2. In the space provided at the top of the page, enter the month, year, and starting and ending dates (usually the 1st through the 31st).

3. Enter the resident's name, admission (admit) date, and room number in the spaces provided.

4. Reviews are completed as listed below utilizing the following Key: Y = yes, the item is present and complete; N = no, the item/form is missing or is present but blank; N/A = not applicable, does not apply to this resident; I = incomplete, item/form is present, has been started but has not been completed. Pencil should be used to record "N" or "I" to facilitate update.

First Review is completed on the first workday following admission.

1. Items 1 through 23 are reviewed.

2. Each document/form is monitored for criteria listed on the *Admission Data Review Criteria* form. Enter Y, N, N/A, or I as appropriate.

Note: Once an item has been indicated as "met", it is considered to be complete and additional reviews for the item are no longer necessary for this time period.

3. When any of the criteria for an item are not met, "N" or "I" is placed in the column and deficiencies listed on the *Health Record Review Worksheet* (procedure follows).

Second Review is completed on the 14th day following admission.

1. Items 24 through 31 are reviewed plus any items in 1 through 23 marked as "N" or "I".

2. Follow procedures 2 through 3 listed in "First Review" above.

Third Review is completed on the 21st day unless all criteria have already been met.

1. Items 32 through 34 are reviewed plus any items in 1 through 31 marked as "N" or "I".

2. Follow procedures 2 through 3 as listed under First Review above.

Once all items have been marked "Y" or "N/A", the record is considered complete for Admission Review Purposes. NOTE: The facility may have additional criteria that must be met that are not listed here. It is the responsibility of the Health Information Manager to assure these items are also met.

Notification of deficiencies

1. Any item marked with "N" or "I" is listed on the Health Record Review Worksheet and a photo copy given to each responsible individual for follow-up.

2. To notify those responsible for and track needed completion of noted deficiencies, the Review Worksheet is used. (See Procedure for Review Worksheet.)

3. All items on the form should be completed by the 21st day following admission of the resident to the facility with the following possible exceptions:

    a. Any form which may have been sent out to a physician for an authenticating signature might not be returned to the facility within 7 days.

    b. Advance Directives and CPR Decision if family and resident decisions are not readily available.

Admission Data Criteria Review Form

Resident Name: _____ Admission #: _____ Room #: _____

Admission Date: _____ Audit Completion Date: _____ Auditor: _____

ADMISSION DATA REVIEW CRITERIA	1st Review Date:_____				2nd Review Date:_____				3rd Review Date:_____				COMMENTS
	Yes	No	N/A	Met	Yes	No	N/A	Met	Yes	No	N/A	Met	
1. Nursing Facility Identification Screen													
2. Identification & Summary													
3. Admission Agreement													
4. CPR Decision/Advance Directives													
5. Legal Guardian/MDPOA/POA/Surrogate													
6. Personal Possessions/Clothing List													
7. Physician's Orders													
8. 2-Step PPD Ordered or Refusal Justified													
9. Nurse's Admitting Progress Note													
10. Alert Charting Initiated													
11. Nursing Assessment Initiated													
12. Skin Assessment													
13. Initial Nursing Orders for NAC's													
14. Vital Signs and Weights Record													
15. Intake & Output													
16. Tray (Meal) Monitor													
17. Problem List Initiated													
18. Care Plan Initiated													
19. Diagnoses Update List Initiated													
20. Admission Transfer Form													
21. History & Physical													
22. Hospital Discharge Summary*													
23. Medicare Certification													
24. PPD 1st Step Started and Results Documented													
25. Nursing Assessment Completed													
26. Activities Assessment													
27. Social History & Assessment													
28. Nutritional Assessment													
29. Minimum Data Set (MDS)													
30. Triggers & RAPS													
31. Medicare First Recertification Completed													
32. Comprehensive Plan of Care													
33. Discharge Plan													
34. PPD 2nd Step/Chest X-ray Completed and Documented													

* Developed by Marilyn Noe, RRA, Long-term Care Consultant, North Pacific Data Service, Bellevue, Washington.

Admission Data Review Criteria

The items listed on the "Admission Data Review Criteria" form are considered indicators, several of many components of a complete health record that can be monitored and evaluated during the Admission Review. Each item is to be completed and in the health record within the specified number of days following admission of the resident to the nursing facility.

The following items are criteria by which each indicator is measured. Criteria are based on Federal and State Regulations and facility policy.

Items 1 through 23 must be in the health record at the time of admission. Those items with an asterisk may be missing on admission but must be obtained as soon as possible.

1. Nursing Facility Identification Screen
   a. Are all identification data complete, accurate, and legible?
   b. Have all appropriate sections been completed?
   c. Is there the signature and title of the individual completing the form?
   d. Is the date of completion entered?
2. Identification and Summary (Face Sheet)
   a. Are all identification data complete, accurate, and legible?
   b. Are there any blank spaces?
   c. Is there an alternate physician, dentist?
   d. Is a funeral home named with area code and telephone number?
3. Admission Agreement
   a. Does each section have all the necessary signatures?
   b. Is each signature identified: i.e., resident, legal guardian, Power of Attorney (POA), designated surrogate?
   c. Are dates and times of signatures indicated?
   d. Is the form filed in the appropriate section of the health record?
4. Cardiopulmonary resuscitation (CPR) Decision/Advance Directives*
   a. Is a form in the record?
   b. Has it been completed appropriately, dated and signed?
   c. Has a "CPR status" been established?
   d. Has the "CPR status" been identified on physician orders and chart cover?
5. Legal Guardian/MDPOA/POA/Designated Surrogate*
   a. If the resident has a Legal Guardian, are copies of the papers on the health record?
   b. If someone has Durable (for health care) Power of Attorney, are copies of the papers maintained in the health record?
   c. If someone has only Power of Attorney, did the resident sign the Consent for Treatment and Release of Information portion of the Admission Agreement?
   d. The Attending Physician needs to determine whether the resident is capable of understanding his or her rights. If not, did the physician give medical reasons why and specify who will be acting in behalf of the resident (designated surrogate decision-maker) RCW 7.70.065?
6. Personal Possessions - Clothing List
   a. Has the form been completed?
   b. Has it been signed and dated by the resident or responsible party?
   c. Has it been signed and dated by a facility employee?
7. Physician's Orders
   a. Are physician's orders present at time of admission of the resident?
   b. Are admitting orders confirmed with the physician?
   c. Are the following orders available on admission as appropriate?
      1) Diet
      2) Medications
      3) Treatments
      4) Lab and X-ray
      5) Consultation and treatment by therapists
      6) Consultation and treatment by other physicians
      7) Activity level
      8) Mobility
      9) CPR Status
      10) PPD
      11) Vaccinations
      12) Level of Care Certification
      13) Other
8. 2 Step PPD Ordered or Refused and Justified
   a. Is there an order for a 2 Step PPD (Tuberculosis Test)?
   b. If physician refused, is there justification documented?
9. Nurse's Admission Progress Note
   a. An admitting progress note is written by the admitting nurse at the time of admission.
   b. Content of the note includes: Date and time of admission; age and sex of the resident; admitted from; mode of transportation; accompanied by; mental status (alert, cheerful, sad, etc.); general condition; presence of appliances, when applicable; placement (bed, chair, etc.); when physician was called, diagnoses and orders confirmed; medications and diet ordered; any other pertinent information.

10. Alert Charting
    a. Initiated on admission and continued for a minimum of 72 hours following admission unless the resident's condition warrants, or
    b. If the resident is a Medicare beneficiary, for the duration of the covered period.

11. Nursing Assessment Initiated
    a. Has the Assessment been started by the admitting nurse?
    b. Has the Skin Assessment portion been completed with any unusual findings marked?
    c. Have identified problems been added to the Problem List and Care Plan?

12. Skin Assessment
    a. Has the assessment been completed?
    b. Is it dated and signed by the nurse?
    c. If there is an identified skin problem, is it on the problem list?
    d. Is it on the care plan?

13. Initial Nursing Orders for CNA's
    a. Have initial nursing orders been written and implemented?
    b. Are additional orders written and/or orders revised as needed and at the time of the first care conference?

14. Vital Signs and Weights
    a. Have the admitting height and weight been recorded on the Nursing Assessment?
    b. Have the admitting height and weight been recorded on the Vital Signs and Weights Form?
    c. Have admitting vital signs been recorded on the flow sheet (q shift × 72 hrs)?

15. Intake and Output
    a. Has the I and O flow sheet been implemented?
    b. Are data collected for a minimum of 72 hours following admission?
    c. If needed, has data collection continued beyond 72 hours?

16. Tray (Meal) Monitor
    a. Is food consumption documented for each meal a minimum of 72 hours?
    b. If there are nutrition related problems, is the monitor continued beyond 72 hours?
    c. Is the need for food consumption monitoring included as a care plan approach?
    d. Are offerings and consumption of replacements entered in space provided?
    e. Are offerings and consumption of supplements entered in space provided?

17. Problem List Initiated
    a. Has the Problem List been started?
    b. Do the Problem Titles agree with those listed on the Care Plan?

18. Care Plan Initiated
    a. Must be started on the day of admission
    b. Should list problems related to the reasons for admission

19. Diagnoses Update List Initiated
    a. Are the current admitting diagnoses recorded?
    b. Do the admitting diagnoses agree with those found on the Transfer, Form, History and Physical, Hospital Discharge Summary, or other authenticated source?

20. Admission Transfer Form
    a. Is the form in the record?
    b. Is the form signed by a physician if resident is admitted from a hospital?
    c. Is it signed by the nurse completing the form?
    d. If missing, has it been requested from the transferring facility?

21. History and Physical
    a. Is there a History and Physical Examination Report on admission, i.e., a copy of the hospital History and Physical (check Discharge Summary), from the physician's office, or written in this facility?
    b. Is it signed or authenticated by the physician who wrote it?

22. Discharge Summary*
    a. Is a copy of the hospital Discharge Summary present?
    b. Is it signed or authenticated by the physician who wrote it?

23. Medicare Certification
    a. Is the initial Medicare Certification checked on the physician-signed Transfer Form or
    b. The Medicare Certification Form signed at the time of admission?

Item 24 must be started and documented in the health record within 72 hours following admission.

24. PPD 1st Step Completed and Documented
    a. Has the 1st step been taken within 3 days following admission?
    b. Have the results been documented?

Items 25 through 31 must be completed within the 14 days of admission with the MDS ready for transmittal to the State.

25. Nursing Assessment Completed
    a. Have all sections been completed by the admitting nurse?
    b. Did the nurse sign and date the form?
    c. Are problems identified using nursing diagnoses (non-medical)?
    d. Are all identified problems on the Problem List?

26. Activities Assessment
    a. Has the assessment been completed within 7 days of admission?
    b. Has the assessment been dated and signed?
    c. Have problems been identified and incorporated on care plan?
27. Social History and Assessment
    a. Has the Social History and Assessment been completed, dated and signed?
    b. Was it completed within 14 days of admission?
    c. Have identified problems, goals and approaches been added to the care plan?
28. Nutritional Assessment (by dietitian)
    a. Was the assessment completed within 14 days of admission?
    b. Was there telephone consultation with dietitian if needed?
    c. Has phone consultation been documented in progress notes?
    d. Is there documented follow-through based on dietitian recommendations?
29. Minimum Data Set (MDS)
    a. Has the MDS been completed?
    b. If any assessment data was missing within the first 14 days, has it been entered and dated on the assessment form on or before the 21st day following admission?
    c. Is the form ready for transmittal to the State?
30. Triggers and RAPS
    a. Have the Triggers been figured?
    b. Have Resident Assessment Protocols for each triggered item been completed and documented?
    c. Has the RAP Summary been completed?
31. Medicare First Recertification
    a. Has the first Recertification been signed, dated, and justified by a physician on or before the 14th day, if applicable?
    b. Is the Certification and Recertification Form filed in the appropriate section of the health record?

Items 32 through 34 must be completed and in the health record within 21 days following admission.
32. Comprehensive Plan of Care
    a. Must be completed within 7 days following completion of the Initial Assessment (no later than the 21st day following admission)
    b. Does it include all problems identified on each assessment?
    c. Are goals measurable and related to problems?
    d. Do approaches relate to goals?
    e. Have any refusals for treatment been included, i.e., Advance Directives?

33. Discharge Plan
    a. Is the Discharge Plan included as part of the Comprehensive Plan of Care?
    b. If there are plans to discharge the resident within the next three months is this reflected?
    c. Are there approaches related to preparation for discharge?
    d. If there are no plans to discharge in the next three months, is there a plan to reassess in three months?
34. PPD 2nd Step/Chest X-ray Ordered, Completed, Documented
    a. Has the 2nd step been given within 1 to 3 weeks following first test?
    b. Have the results been documented in the record?
    c. If an X-ray was required, has it been completed and results recorded in the record?
    d. If the X-ray was positive, has the problem been included in the Care Plan?

HEALTH RECORD PROCEDURES

ADMISSION PROCEDURES

Health Record Review Worksheet Procedure

PURPOSE

To provide a means of documenting deficiencies found in the health record, to notify the responsible staff, to monitor for completion/correction of deficiencies, to provide a mechanism for reporting Quality Assurance Program activities.

RESPONSIBLE STAFF:

Health Information Manager or other designee.

PROCEDURE:

Utilizing the "Review Worksheet"
1. Completion of form:
    a. Enter name of resident whose record contains deficiency.
    b. Resident's Room #.
    c. Name of responsible staff
    d. Identify the deficiency in the area marked "findings."
    e. Enter the date deficiency is to be corrected/completed by in space "date due."
2. Upon completion of the review:
    a. Photocopy the "original" Review Worksheet and maintain in a file by "date due."
    b. Cut the copy of the Review Worksheet into individual sections - creating individual deficiency notices.

HEALTH RECORD REVIEW WORKSHEET

Review: _____ Date: _____ Page: _____

Resident:		Room #:
Staff:	Date Due:	Completed:
Findings:		

Resident:		Room #:
Staff:	Date Due:	Completed:
Findings:		

Resident:		Room #:
Staff:	Date Due:	Completed:
Findings:		

Resident:		Room #:
Staff:	Date Due:	Completed:
Findings:		

Resident:		Room #:
Staff:	Date Due:	Completed:
Findings:		

Signature of Auditor: _____ Date: _____

Based on a design by Marilyn Noe, RRA, North Pacific Data Service, Bellevue, Washington.

c. Give the deficiency notices to the appropriate individual(s) or Director of Nursing, whichever is appropriate.

NOTE: This will depend on the procedures to be followed for the particular review. Some reviews may require the notices be given to the Director of Nursing Service for direction of follow-through. Other reviews may indicate the deficiency notices be given directly to the individual responsible for the deficiency and a copy of the entire Review Worksheet given to the supervisor.

3. Completion/correction of deficiencies:
   a. Each deficiency must be completed/corrected by the responsible individual within the time frames indicated on the "deficiency notice" in the "date due" section.
   b. Upon completion/correction of the deficiency, the individual must enter the following under "completed":
      1) Date completed
      2) Initials
      3) The completed deficiency notice is then returned to the Health Record Box at the nursing station.

4. The *Health Information Manager* marks the "original" Review Worksheet to indicate the deficiency notice has been returned.
   a. To make certain deficiencies have been corrected/completed, periodic spot checks should be completed to assure accuracy of information received.
   b. If deficiencies remain incomplete, it is necessary to re-notify the responsible individual and the supervisor, DNS, and Administrator, utilizing the above procedure.

5. At the end of the specified review period, a report of Quality Assurance Activity is completed and submitted to the Administrator, Director of Nursing Service, and Quality Assurance Coordinator. Utilize the designated Quality Assurance Report Form as a method of reporting and maintaining files on Health Record Service Quality Assurance Program participation.

MEDICATION/TREATMENT DOCUMENTATION REVIEW

PURPOSE:
Review Medication or Treatment Administration Records for charting omissions during the medication or treatment pass, to identify PRN medications or treatments not charted appropriately, to identify orders transcribed onto or discontinued from the flow sheet following established procedures, to identify nurses who do not complete the signature legend on each MAR or TAR on which their initials appear, and to identify possible medication errors.

TO COMPLETE THE FORM, STARTING AT THE TOP:

A. Enter the Date the review is completed, Page number of the review form, wing, floor, or station at which the review is taking place.

IDENTIFY EACH RECORD REVIEWED:

B. ROOM & BED #: Enter data for each resident's record reviewed.
C. RESIDENT'S NAME: Last name of resident whose record is being reviewed.
D. ORDER:
   a. Enter "CTD" (current to date) if no omissions or errors are found for the resident's record.
   b. Name of medication/treatment with omission or error.
E. DATE: Date of charting omission.
F. TIME: Time of missing charting.
G. Check the appropriate box(es) for type of missing information:
   1. Routine not charted (may require Incident Report)
   2. PRN not charted on back of page
   3. PRN results not charted on back of page
   4. PRN not charted on front
   5. New order not initialed in order box
   6. New order not dated in order box
   7. Dc'd order not signed (initialed)
   8. Dc'd order not dated
   9. Circled initials on front not explained on back
   10. Nurse's initials not identified
   11. Resident identification incomplete at bottom of page
   12. Possible administration error.
H. At the bottom of the page space is provided to total the number of records reviewed, the number "current to date," the number with charting omissions "INC", and the number of omissions, citations per category G.1. through G.12. above.

Medications and Treatments not charted by the end of the shift may require completion of an Incident Report or Medication Error Form by the responsible nurse.

Document developed by Marilyn Noe, RRA, North Pacific Data Service, Bellevue, Washington.

MEDICATION DOCUMENTATION REVIEW   DATE: _____ Page: _____
FACILITY: _____ WING: _____ TIME START: _____

1. Routine order not charted	7. Dc'd order not signed			
2. PRN not charted on back	8. Dc'd order not dated		**CTD - current to date**	
3. PRN results not charted on back	9. Circled initials not explained		**No omissions noted**	
4. PRN not charted on front	10. Nurse's initials not identified			
5. New order not initialed in order box	11. Resident identification incomplete			
6. New order not dated	12. Possible administration error			

Room	Resident	Order	Date	Time	1	2	3	4	5	6	7	8	9	10	11	12
Reviewed: _____ CTD: _____ INC: _____																

Review Completed by: _____

Developed by Marilyn Noe, RRA, North Pacific Data Service, Bellevue, Washington.

Appendix B

Recommended Joint Commission Documentation Review Criteria

1. Each department within a hospital must have a quality assessment plan in place to monitor the accuracy, timeliness of documentation, and corrective action plan.

2. The results of documentation monitoring and/or clinical pertinence reviews must be reviewed in appropriate quality assessment committees, with interdisciplinary input, and reflected in clinical staff evaluations and in the Medical Staff Credentialing processes.

3. There must be qualified personnel with appropriate education, credentials, or competency levels performing all tasks of documentation and documentation reviews.

4. The overall content of the record must be sufficient enough to provide for continuity of care as a primary goal.

5. Basic documentation elements (do not have to be in a specific place, report, or form) include

    A. Evidence of patient informed consent

    B. Evidence of patient education, including understanding of instructions for care

    C. Diagnoses and procedures

    D. Pertinent history

    E. Observations, assessments (includes consultations), and plans

    F. Diagnostic data

    G. Therapeutic data, including orders and medications

    H. Evidence of authorship and action audit trial for all documentation, retrievable in chronologic manner.

6. UHDDS-Demographic Data Elements.

Purpose: to control demographic accuracy for statistical and reimbursement purposes.

Controls

    A. Facility must have a policy and mechanism in place to identify and correct data discrepancies (such as checking for duplicate numbers in the master patient index)

    B. Secondary indices and associated registers or data collection systems must be routinely reviewed for accuracy and prevention of duplicates

    C. Wherever possible, data fields must be compatible with ASTM data sets.

7. Other General Documentation Monitoring Guidelines:

    A. Reviews must be designed using interdisciplinary input with a focus on
      - problem cases
      - high-volume cases
      - sampling across all cases

    B. Each department responsible for producing entries in the permanent medical record (paper or computer-based) must maintain a policy regarding timeliness and methods of data distribution.

    C. Where equipment is used to produce documentation, a policy must be in place to allow for
      - demonstrated equipment operational standards
      - documentation output quality (paper and ink quality, format, standardization, and retention)

    D. Evidence of morbidity/mortality (outcome) measurement or indicators possibly including:
      - External database comparisons
      - Cost and quality variances measurements
      - Not vendor driven

    E. All documentation should be supported by appropriate confidentiality and security controls and guidelines.

    F. Health Information Management/Transcription/QA must show clinical pertinent policies and examples of documentation reviews, if applicable.

    G. Evidence of policies relating to data correction, revisions, and editing.

From Grzybowski DM: The transition from signature to authorship. J Am Health Information Management Assoc 1993;64(9):90.

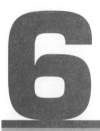

LYNN KUEHN and MARGARET STEWART

KEY WORDS

Access time
Accession register
Active record
Alphabetic identification
Cache memory
Color coding
Computer output microfiche (COM)
Computer output to laser disk (COLD)
Cross-reference
Destruction letter
Electronic data interchange (EDI)
Encounter
Exchange time
File guide
File server
Inactive record
Jukebox
Magnification ratio
Master patient index (MPI)
Microfiche
Microfilm jacket
Microfilm reader
Microform
Numeric identification
Open architecture
Open system
Optical character recognition (OCR)
Outcard
Outguide
Pay-back period
Proprietary system
Purge
Record tracking
Reduction ratio
Requisition
Retention period
Roll microfilm
Scanner
Serial numbering
Serial-unit numbering
Small computer system interface (SCSI)
Statute of limitations
Symbology
Terminal digit filing
Thin
Transfer notice
Uninterruptable power supply (UPS)
Unit numbering
Unit record
Write once read many (WORM)

ABBREVIATIONS

CAR—Computer-Assisted retrieval
COLD—Computer output to laser disk
COM—Computer output microfiche

DATA ACCESS AND RETENTION

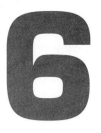

CPR—Computer-based patient record
DPI—Dots per inch
EDI—Electronic data interchange
LAN—Local area network
MPI—Master patient index
OCR—Optical character recognition
SCSI—Small computer system interface
UPS—Uninterruptable power supply
WORM—Write once read many

OBJECTIVES

- Define key words.
- Discuss the various numbering systems for health information.
- Compare and contrast the filing options for the paper record.
- Compare and contrast microfilming of records versus commercial storage and identify when each method is desirable.
- Identify key milestones in a file conversion.
- Identify considerations important to the selection of file folders.
- Describe the benefits of color coding to any of the filing methodologies.
- Describe how an automated record-tracking system can be developed and implemented.
- Identify how bar code technology interacts with an automated record-tracking system.
- Explain how the statute of limitations pertains to record retention.
- Identify the different microform options available when designing a micrographics storage and retrieval system.
- List the necessary components of an optical imaging system and the various cost factors involved in implementing an optical imaging system.
- Identify possible steps in the implementation of an optical imaging system.
- Describe why electronic storage of data is a prerequisite to the successful implementation of the computer-based patient record.
- Examine a current storage and retrieval system and determine alternative solutions to solve identified problems.
- Prepare strategies for planning and implementing solutions to information systems problems.

Health care is information-dependent and cannot efficiently be provided without information regarding the patient's past and current condition. Various systems are necessary to assure that the information is available where and when it is needed for patient care at a reasonable cost.

This chapter describes various ways that patients' health information can be accessed and retained. The discussion begins with paper record and progresses with technology to microforms, optical imaging, and electronic data interchange.

The role of the health information management (HIM) professional is to evaluate past and current methods as well as current and future needs and to select the best system to meet these needs. This may involve converting to new filing methods or filing media, maintaining current systems more efficiently, or making decisions regarding the destruction of nonuseful material.

The HIM professional's knowledge of information management consists of more than information systems concerning the formal patient record. Information management knowledge can easily be applied to other areas as well, such as radiology film storage, personnel information, and administrative records. No other field of study within the health care arena provides information management background, although each discipline maintains patient health care records. Wise facility managers utilize the HIM professional as an in-house consultant to these other areas to improve overall facility efficiency. Therefore, the concepts covered in this chapter present ways of accessing and retaining information, regardless of the scope, size, or shape of the information or storage media involved.

ACCESS AND RETENTION OF PAPER-BASED RECORDS

Most health care facilities maintain most of their patient information in a paper-based format. The first portion of this chapter discusses maintenance of this format of patient record and methods of identifying the record.

Record Identification

Alphabetic Identification

Identifying the record by patient name, called **alphabetic identification,** is the most basic identification system used in health care. Although it sounds simple, the system can be more difficult to maintain than it appears.

When maintaining an alphabetic identification system, the correct patient name is the vital piece of information. All patient names must be spelled accurately, both first and last, to be sure that the record can be located in the future. All name changes must be indicated on the patient record folder, creating a **cross-reference** for the previous location in the file. Alphabetic identification systems can be maintained without separate **master patient index (MPI)** because the records themselves form a large patient index. If a separate index is used, cross-referencing of name changes must also be completed in the index, requiring extra work.

An advantage of the alphabetic identification system is that the record can be located using information obtained directly from the patient. The disadvantage of the system is the complex spelling of many names within our population. In addition, not everyone knows instinctively how to file names alphabetically. To achieve the consistency needed for successful future retrieval, the record maintenance staff must be taught the filing rules adopted by the facility and reference them while completing their work.

Numeric Identification

An alternate method of identification is to use a number to identify the patient record, called **numeric identification.** Assigning a number to a patient record requires the use of the **MPI,** which contains a minimum of the patient name and patient identification number. Additional data elements to be included in this index are covered later. In the manual version of this identification system, the MPI cards are filed alphabetically and referenced to find the patient identification number. In an automated format, a computerized database serves as the MPI. The computer file is searched for the required name or a similar combination of letters. The correct name is determined, and the associated identification number is displayed on the computer screen.

The manual version of this method has some of the same problems as the alphabetic filing of the patient records themselves. The computerized version provides the added advantages of allowing access to the identification number by multiple users at one time and consistently sorting the database the same way for each user. The computer also provides the flexibility of producing reports in both alphabetic and numeric order for reference.

METHODS OF NUMBERING. A number identification system can be designed in several ways. Serial, unit, and the hybrid method called serial-unit are discussed here.

Serial Numbering. **Serial numbering** is a system of number assignment in which a patient receives a number for each encounter at the facility. The patient could have multiple numbers, which all require entry onto the manual index card or maintenance in the computerized database. This method is time-consuming and makes computer database space difficult to allocate, especially in a facility with a high volume of encounters. This method also has a higher supply cost because each encounter at the facility requires the use of a new file folder. Each new folder is filed in a different location, requiring the searching of multiple locations to retrieve one patient's entire record, a time-consuming process. Serial numbering can be used effectively when the patient return rate is low or the population served is transient.

Unit Numbering. To avoid the extra effort of assigning a new number for each encounter and the searching of multiple locations for record folders, the unit numbering system was developed. In the **unit numbering system,** each patient receives an identification number at the first encounter and retains that number throughout all contacts with the facility. This numbering system allows a facility to easily create a **unit record** for the patient, filed all in one location in the file.[1] Labor costs are reduced because the number is entered into the MPI only once, and supply costs are lower because the same folder is being used for all the encounters.

Technically, any number could be chosen as the unit number identifier, but most facilities prefer to assign numbers sequentially, starting with the number 1. Some facilities, such as those that are government-sponsored, have chosen to use the social security number as the unique patient identifier and ask the patient to provide it. In this system, any patient without a social security number receives a pseudonumber, or fake number, as the identifier until a number is permanently assigned.

A variation of the unit numbering system is the assignment of a number to a family rather than to an individual. This numbering system is common in community health centers that treat a family as a unit. This allows for common identification of a family unit, even if the family members have different last names. If this method is chosen, consideration must be given to assigning each family member his or her own identifier as an additional number and giving the person his or her own folder.

Serial-Unit Numbering. In an attempt to combine the ease of number assignment from serial numbering and the unit record concept from unit numbering, the **serial-unit numbering** method was developed. Numbers

TABLE 6-1 NUMBERING SYSTEMS

SYSTEM	NUMBER ASSIGNMENT	FILING CONCEPTS
Serial numbering	A new number is assigned for each encounter.	Each record is filed separately using the number that has been assigned for that visit.
Unit numbering	One number is assigned at the first encounter and used for all future encounters.	The record is filed using the unit number.
Serial-unit numbering	A new number is assigned for each encounter.	The record containing each number is brought forward and filed together using the newest number assigned.

are assigned serially, but as each new encounter takes place, all the former records are brought forward to the most recently assigned record number and filed as a unit.

Table 6–1 shows a comparison of these three numbering systems. In the future, the concept of a unique (unit) identifier for each patient will become more attractive. Some form of unique identifier can provide the common link between all the information contained in the multiple computerized databases of information maintained on individual patients.

Filing Equipment

Making a decision about how to store patient records and other record-related material is a situation that all HIM professionals face at some point in their career.

Although sales personnel are trained to assist in the decision-making process, it is helpful to know the advantages and disadvantages of the different types of storage equipment before the process begins. Table 6–2 compares the available types of storage equipment according to physical description, strengths, weaknesses, and facility types where they are best suited. Figure 6–1 shows an aerial view of open shelves and compressible units.

The Occupational Health and Safety Administration (OSHA) requires that certain minimum allowances be made for aisles and spaces between equipment. OSHA requires that main aisles leading out of a room or to a fire exit be a minimum of 5 feet wide and that secondary aisles, such as between shelving units, be a minimum of 3 feet wide. These minimums are set to provide adequate work space for all workers as well as access to exits.

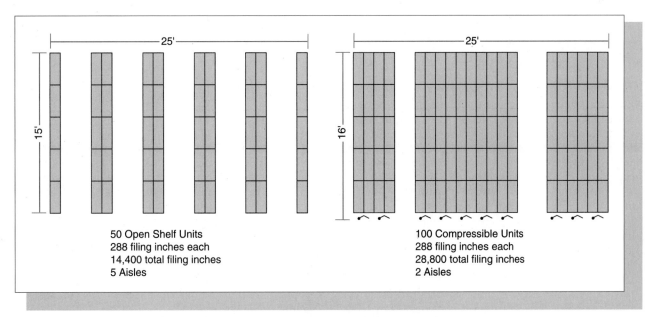

25'

15'

50 Open Shelf Units
288 filing inches each
14,400 total filing inches
5 Aisles

25'

16'

100 Compressible Units
288 filing inches each
28,800 total filing inches
2 Aisles

FIGURE 6–1. Aerial view of open-shelf and compressible units.

TABLE 6–2 COMPARISON OF DIFFERENT TYPES OF STORAGE EQUIPMENT

EQUIPMENT	PHYSICAL DESCRIPTION	STRENGTHS	WEAKNESSES	FACILITY BEST SUITED FOR
Filing cabinets	3 to 5 drawers, vertical or lateral arrangement	Can be purchased as a fireproof cabinet Can be purchased with locks Protects records from the environment	Requires dedicated aisle space Difficult and time-consuming to open each drawer Can only open one drawer at a time	Small facilities Dirty environments High fire dangers Low file activity requiring high security
Open-shelf files	5 to 8 shelves with full access to the front (similar to bookshelves)	Easy access to any part of the shelves and multiple shelves at a time Can accommodate multiple workers at one time	Requires a 36-inch dedicated aisle between shelving units Records open to the environment	High-volume files with multiple file maintenance workers Relatively clean environments with sufficient space for aisles Works well in a clinic facility for active records and in hospitals for outpatient records
Motorized revolving units	Shelves move around central spine like a Ferris wheel with records carried on bucket shelves; run by a motor	Little aisle space needed All work is at one height level Records can be covered and locked	Must be carefully loaded and unloaded in a balanced manner or it will not run Motor or power failure causes record unavailability High initial cost, maintenance contract costs	Limited space with low file activity and one primary file maintenance worker Dirty environments
Compressible units	Open-shelf files that move in parallel lines to form an aisle opening Motor-assisted movement or hand-cranked	Saves space of unused aisles Easy access to shelf currently opened to the aisle One dedicated aisle required	Time needed to locate where the access aisle is needed and open the mechanism to the aisle Limited number of aisles Mechanical failure causes record unavailability Maintenance contract costs	Limited space with low to medium file activity and two to three file maintenance workers Works well in a hospital facility for inpatient records and/or inactive records

Filing Cabinets

Vertical filing cabinets are the traditional type of drawer files seen in many offices. They vary in height, width, depth, and number of drawers. These cabinets are specifically constructed to hold cards, letter files, and legal files, or they can be constructed as a combination of card file drawers and larger-size drawers.

Lateral filing cabinets are also available. The file drawers in a lateral filing cabinet open from the long side, and the entire cabinet resembles a chest of drawers. Because these cabinets have drawers that are not deep, they are well suited to narrow spaces, such as along walls or as room dividers.

Both vertical and lateral filing cabinets are available with two to five drawers and can be purchased with special fireproof wall and drawer construction or locks.

They protect records from the environment, but considerable effort is required to open each drawer when filing or retrieving a record.

Open-Shelf Files

Open-shelf files resemble bookshelves and provide ready access to records without having to open any drawers. They are available with five to eight shelves per section and are usually adjustable to accommodate different heights of folders. Adjustable shelf dividers help support the file folders on the shelves. The files require a dedicated 36-inch aisle and leave records open to the environment. Open-shelf files are the storage equipment of choice for high-volume file rooms that have multiple people requiring simultaneous access to the shelves, such as in clinics.

Motorized Revolving Units

The motorized revolving file contains 16 shelves that revolve around a central spine like a Ferris wheel. The records are placed on a shelf similar to an open shelf or on a bucket shelf in a lateral file. Files must be loaded or unloaded from the machine in a balanced manner, just as passengers are alternately loaded onto and off of a Ferris wheel. If the load is unbalanced, the machine will stop to avoid damaging the internal mechanism. These files are best suited to small facilities in which record retrieval is limited and performed by one person, such as solo physician or dental practices.

Compressible Units

These movable-aisle systems, or compressible units, are similar to open-shelf files but are mounted on tracks secured to the floor. The shelf units move on the tracks, and the operator opens the file at the appropriate place to create the aisle where needed. They are available in both manual and motor-assisted models. This type of file saves considerable floor space, but access to files is limited because only one or two aisles can be created at a time. Compressible units are best suited to files with low to medium file activity with only a few people working in the files at one time. They may solve some space issues for health information departments.

Space Management

Centralized and Decentralized Files

Facilities can use a centralized or a decentralized filing method. In **centralized** files, there is a single location for all records created throughout the facility. This centralized file location is staffed by specialized personnel who provide records that have been requested by authorized users.

In the **decentralized** filing method, parts of the record are filed in different locations in the facility. Outpatient and emergency departments frequently file their records in their own departments. In clinic facilities, decentralized records may be created when specialty departments maintain their own records. Table 6–3 describes the advantages and disadvantages of the centralized and decentralized record management alternatives.

Filing Methodologies

Designing a numbering and filing system within a facility is a large responsibility, and the decisions can impact other functions in the facility. Understanding

TABLE 6–3 COMPARISON OF CENTRALIZED AND DECENTRALIZED RECORD MANAGEMENT ALTERNATIVES

CENTRALIZED FILES	DECENTRALIZED FILES
Overall supply costs are lower.	Supply costs from storage equipment and multiple folders are increased.
High level of security with record control is easy to maintain.	Record control is more difficult to maintain.
Standardized procedures for file maintenance can be developed.	File format can be flexible to meet the unique needs of the patient and providers.
Specialized staff can be used, trained to perform file maintenance as their primary duty.	File maintenance staff are harder to train consistently, and file maintenance may be a low priority for staff with other duties.
Consistent supervision is available for file maintenance staff.	Supervision is provided by department staff in the area where the records are located.

each of the options is important. Although the term "filing" does not connote a high degree of professionalism, the efficient management of files in any format is an important asset to a facility provided by an HIM professional.

Alphabetic Filing

HOW TO USE. An alphabetic identification system and the alphabetic filing method must be used together. The alphabetic filing method starts with last names that begin with A and continues through all the names, ending with Z. Patient records with identical last names use the first name and then the middle initial to determine the exact filing order. When first names are a single initial or no middle initial is given, the rule of nothing before something is used to determine filing order. Each name (last, first, middle) or the corresponding initial is treated as a group when filing. A single-initial name is the shortest name possible and would be filed first. The file would look like this:

Henri, Martha
Henry, J
Henry, J T
Henry, John T
Henry, Judy
Henry, Judy R

Specific alphabetic filing rules are shown in the chart Alphabetic Filing Rules.

Alphabetic Filing Rules

1. Place the last name first and then the first name followed by the middle name or initial, using strict alphabetical order.

2. If there are two or more identical last name and first name combinations, use the middle initial to determine the order. If the middle initial is the same or no middle initial is given, use the birth date, filing the oldest patient first.

3. Names with prefixes (O', D', Mc, Mac, Von, etc.) are filed as if there was no apostrophe or space (O'Dell is O'-D-E-L-L). The apostrophe should be typed as one character when entering information into a database.

4. Hyphenated names are filed as if there was no hyphen (Smith-Jones is S-M-I-T-H-J-O-N-E-S). The hyphen should *not* be included when entering information into a database.

5. If an initial is given instead of a first or middle name, use the "nothing before something" rule to file J T Henry before John T Henry. Periods should not be entered as characters when entering information into a database.

6. Do not abbreviate names in alphabetic filing. However, if the name is abbreviated, file it as it is spelled (Wm is W-M).

7. Do not include seniority designations (Sr, Jr) or titles (MD, PhD) in alphabetic filing. If found, do not use in determining filing order.

Modified from Johnson M, Kallaus W: Records management. Cincinnati, Southwestern Publishing Co., 1982.

Names that contain nonalphabetic characters, capitals, or spaces, such as O'Dell, McCallum, and Van Braun, often cause variations in filing accuracy. Each facility should maintain consistency in filing by deciding how special filing situations are to be handled, documenting the correct order, and referencing the documentation as the filing process is completed.

SPACE PLANNING. Letters of the alphabet appear in any given volume of records with an average frequency. These frequencies can be used to predict the percentage of file space that should be allowed for each letter of the alphabet (see Frequency Distribution of the Alphabet).

FILE GUIDES. **File guides** are used to aid in the filing process. These guides list the letter of the alphabet and any vowel subdivisions within the main letter category, such as Da, De, Di, Do, Du, all within the main letter category of D.

BENEFITS AND CONSIDERATIONS. Alphabetic filing

Frequency Distribution of the Alphabet	
A-3.00%	M- 9.50%
B-9.38%	N- 1.85%
C-7.18%	O- 1.52%
D-4.84%	P- 4.93%
E-1.87%	Q- .17%
F-3.72%	R- 5.05%
G-5.05%	S-10.20%
H-7.38%	T- 3.37%
I- .38%	U- .24%
J-2.59%	V- 1.24%
K-4.24%	W- 6.31%
L-4.85%	X,Y,Z- 1.14%

Reference is from Table from Waters KR, Murphy GF: Medical Records in Health Information. Germantown, MD, Aspen Systems Corp, 1979, pp. 449–450.

systems work well for facilities with less than 5000 records, a stable patient population, and little or no computerization. It may not work well in an ethnically homogeneous area in which last names are frequently repeated.

Straight Numeric Filing

HOW TO USE. Facilities with more than 5000 records, frequently changing populations, or that have become computerized usually assign numbers to their patients. They may choose to file their records in straight numerical or sequential order, a basic system that starts with a record of the lowest number value and ends with a record of the highest number value. New records are always added at the end of the number series, concentrating most of the filing activity in one area of the file. Accountability for filing accuracy is harder to track when most of the record maintenance staff is focused in one area of the files.

FILE GUIDES. File guides are used in this system to help the eye determine the change in digits. If the folders are thick, file guides should be placed every 100 records. If the folders are thin, one guide for every 1000 records may be sufficient.

SPACE PLANNING. To plan space adequately for a straight numeric filing system, consideration should be given to thinking of the file room as a circle. As **inactive records** are removed from the lower-numbered areas, these areas can be consolidated forward, creating additional room for the end of the number series to grow into. This method is far easier than moving the entire contents of the file area back to the starting point whenever the end of the number series has come to the end of the filing space. Inactive records are also discussed under record management later in this chapter.

Terminal Digit Filing

HOW TO USE. The terminal digit filing methodology is based on a patient identification number that is divided into three parts. Most facilities use a minimum of six digits (filling any unused digits on the left for numbers lower than 100000 with zeros), and other facilities use the terminal digit method with numbers as large as the nine-digit social security number.

For purposes of this example, a standard six-digit number is used.

12	34	56
Tertiary digits	Secondary digits	Primary (or terminal) digits

The number is read from left to right for identification purposes and from right to left (from the terminal end) for terminal digit filing purposes. To understand the filing concepts, it is best to first visualize the file layout in a terminal digit system. If the file room has 100 sections of filing equipment, each would contain the records labeled with one of the 100 possible primary digit combinations (from 00 to 99). Using the example above, the 56 section would be further visually subdivided into 100 possible locations for records. Record number 12-34-56 would be in the 34th subdivision (secondary digits of 34), or about one third of the way into primary section 56. Within the 34th subdivision, records are filed in straight numeric order by the tertiary digits. In this example, the record is number 12, following record 11, and preceding record 13. File sections 56 and 57 would look like this:

```
11-34-56
12-34-56
13-34-56 . . . to 99-34-56, with the next folder
           being
00-35-56
01-35-56 . . . until 99-99-56 is reached, with the
           next folder being
00-00-57
01-00-57 and so on.
```

The steps in finding record 12-34-56 are:

1. Go to Section 56.
2. Within Section 56, go to the subdivision of 34's.
3. The record is the 12th record in subdivision 34 if all records are present.

The same concepts used in our monetary system of 100 pennies in a $1 bill and 100 dollar bills in a Benjamin Franklin $100 bill apply here. In this system, the pennies are records.

FILE GUIDES. File guides are used to mark primary digit sections in small files. In larger files, each group of 10 secondary digits are guided, in addition to the primary digit sections. Space planning is the easiest in a terminal digit system. Because new numbers assigned sequentially are evenly distributed among all 100 filing sections, the file grows evenly. Time has shown that records become inactive at a relatively even rate of distribution, allowing the file to increase or decrease evenly in size.

SPACE PLANNING. To determine the size of each primary section in a new file area, calculate the available inches of filing space by measuring the lengths of the actual shelves or drawers available. Divide the total number of inches of filing space by 100. The result is the number of inches of filing space to allow for each primary digit combination. Remember to start allocating space for number 00, not 01. This may leave considerable space between primary sections but saves the time of shifting the records later as the file grows. Filing units should be purchased in multiples of 5, such as 5 units (or cabinets), 25 units, 50 units, or 100 units, if space permits. This allows each terminal digit number to reside in an area of a filing unit. If 50 units of storage space are purchased, two terminal digit numbers are placed in that shelving unit or cabinet. Table 6–4 compares the advantages and disadvantages of straight numeric filing and terminal digit filing.

Master Patient Index

The MPI is the key to locating the patient record in a numeric identification system. It identifies all patients who have been treated by the facility and lists the number associated with the name. The index can be maintained manually or as part of a computerized system. In either case, the MPI should be maintained permanently.[1]

The MPI should contain enough demographic data to readily identify the patient and his or her record. The minimum content of the MPI includes the following:

- Full name (last, first, and middle)
- Patient identification number(s)
- Date of birth

TABLE 6–4 CHARACTERISTICS OF STRAIGHT NUMERIC FILING AND TERMINAL DIGIT FILING

STRAIGHT NUMERIC	SAMPLE ORDER	TERMINAL DIGIT	SAMPLE ORDER
Training period is short.	29160	Training period is slightly longer.	24-29-04
File grows at the end of the number series, requiring backshifting.	30158 101412 107412	File grows evenly throughout 100 sections—no backshifting required.	25-29-04 10-14-12 49-32-12
Inactive records are pulled from one general area.	107643 107644 123456	Inactive records are purged evenly throughout the 100 sections.	10-74-12 10-76-43 10-76-44
File staff is "bunched" in the highest numbers, causing less accountability for filing accuracy.	242904 252904 493212	Work is evenly distributed throughout the 100 sections, causing accountability for accuracy in that section.	12-34-56 03-01-58 02-91-60
Number is dealt with as a whole, causing mental fatigue, transpositions, and misfiles.		Number is dealt with in two-digit pairs, easing mental fatigue and causing fewer transpositions and misfiles.	

It is highly recommended that additional information be maintained, if possible. This additional information is as follows:

- Sex
- Social security number (voluntary data)
- Dates of admission and discharge (or encounter)

If multiple facilities are serviced through one index, such as a multihospital system, the index should indicate the facility in which the admission or encounter occurred.

A manual index is maintained using the alphabetic filing rules (see Alphabetic Filing Rules), keeping in mind the need for consistency in filing. Computerized indexes must have the same consistency in data entry. Database software is not intelligent. It only retrieves what it is given. Therefore, names with special characters or spaces must be entered in the same manner each time to be retrieved when needed.

Hyphenated names are retrieved differently than the same two names combined without a hyphen. Also, prefix names entered without a space (such as McDonald) are retrieved separately from those entered with a space (Mc Donald). When assigning numbers in a unit numbering system, these database retrieval problems can cause the patient to be incorrectly assigned an additional number.

New MPIs should be entered consistently, and ongoing indexes should be verified for possible problems with inconsistent data entry. Figure 6–2 shows a sample MPI screen for a facility that uses unit numbering.

Records Management Issues

File Folders

Until the day that all records are computerized, the folder that contains patient information is important for anyone who has responsibility for the record. Many facilities may still use the paper patient record as a historical document well into the future. This will be true until the transfer of all data to computers has taken place. For this reason, it is important to be aware of the difference choosing the right folder can make. All these considerations also apply to the management of other records, such as radiology films. Consideration in folder size and design are as follows:

- Standard folders for patient records are $9\frac{1}{2}$ inches high and $12\frac{1}{4}$ inches wide.
- Reinforced top and side panels are important when records have a high rate of retrieval from the file.
- Folder bottoms should be scored (manufactured with indented lines that assist in creating straight folds) to allow the folder to accommodate a patient record of average size for the facility. Consider the average number of pages per discharged record, the number of annual outpatient **encounters**,[2] or both when estimating the average record size. Also consider

---

Name: Smith, John James   MR#: 12-34-56

DOB: 03-03-1936   SS#: 294-55-3235*

Sex: M

Dates of Admission: 01-10-84   Discharge: 01-15-84
                    06-05-91   06-07-91
                    10-20-94   10-26-94

* Social Security numbers are obtained voluntarily from patients

FIGURE 6–2. Master patient index screen.

whether the facility provides any services that
are long term in nature (e.g., oncology, dialysis)
or creates especially large records from documenting complex care, such as neonatal intensive care records. High-volume ambulatory
practices can also produce a large amount of
paper documentation.

- The weight of the folder should be appropriate
for the expected rate of use, with the understanding that heavier folders cost proportionately more. The two standard weights are 11-
point and 14-point, with 14-point being the
heaviest and most durable. To determine the
correct weight, consider the following:
  —The specific retention period of the paper
    record
  —The average number of times the folder will
    be removed from the shelf in its lifetime of
    use (the wear-and-tear factor)
  If the wear-and-tear factor is low or the **retention period** for the paper folder is projected to
  be short (2 to 3 years), then the 11-point folder
  is adequate. If the paper record is expected to
  be used for 3 or more years, then the 14-point
  folder is a wiser investment.
- Folders can be purchased with or without fasteners, and the fasteners can be applied in
various positions within the folder to aid in
organizing the data to best meet the facility's
needs.

Color Coding

Using **color coding** to designate certain letters or
digits helps to prevent misfiles and aids in rapid storage
and retrieval. Color can also provide an easy way to
distribute workload and make sorting of folders much
easier.

Different colored folders can be used to designate
changes in primary digits of a terminal digit system.
Color bars can be preprinted on the folder or added
using adhesive labels, designating letters or digits. The
color bars may have both a color designation and a
position designation. If either the color or the position
on the folder is incorrect when it is placed in the file, it
indicates a misfile.

Record Security

Patient records should be stored in an area or a room
that can be locked to prevent inadvertent loss, tampering, or other unauthorized use. The area can be secured
with either the traditional lock-and-key method or a
computerized access panel that operates by activating
the correct key combination. The computerized access
panel has the advantage of easily being updated with a

new code if a security problem is noted, rather than
attempting to locate all the physical keys.

Storage of Inactive Records

Records are **active** when the last discharge or encounter date is within 3 to 5 years of the current date.[1]
Active records are stored in a location commonly referred to as the active files. Activity is determined by the
frequency of encounters by the typical patient and the
amount of filing space that is conveniently located.
Records that no longer meet the active record criteria
are **inactive**. Inactive records do not need to be as
readily available but do need to be accessible when
needed.

ALTERNATE LOCATION. When considering how to
store inactive records that are no longer in high demand, two options are available without changing the
records to another format or media. One option is to
store records in a duplicate filing system located in
another area of the facility. Another option is to use the
services of a commercial storage company.

Commercial Storage. Commercial storage companies store different types of records but may specialize
in highly confidential records, such as legal or patient
records. As a minimum, the commercial storage company should have the following:

- Confidentiality policies and statements signed
by their employees
- Acceptable references from health care facilities
- Insurance coverage for loss, damage, personal
injury, and workers' compensation
- Record return guarantee and/or fax capability
- Reasonable retrieval fees
- No surrender fee (cost to remove all the records
from storage)
- Quality control in both storage and retrieval
methods

Other items to be included in contract discussions
with commercial storage companies are the "hidden," or
seldom thought of, questions, such as the following:

- Who pulls the files from the current storage
system (who pays for it)?
- Who completes the list of what is to be stored
(who pays for it)?
- Exactly when does the custody of the record
change over to the storage company (whose insurance is paying for it)?
- What are the billing terms (yearly, monthly, as
used)?

Each possible storage company should be screened to evaluate its overall costs and services provided. Investigate other alternatives discussed in this chapter when developing a long-term storage and retrieval system. Calculate the costs for all options over a minimum of 10 years to provide adequate comparison of the costs.

File System Conversion

Existing alphabetic and straight numeric filing methods often do not meet the future needs of growing facilities. Increased filing efficiency is usually sought by converting existing systems to numeric identification and the terminal digit filing method. The thought of conversion sounds intimidating but does not need to be if thorough planning takes place. Conversion concepts can apply to moving the contents of a department or file room to a new location (see Conversion Checklist).

PLANNING PROCESS. Make as many changes as possible before the actual conversion. If the files are being converted from an alphabetic arrangement to a straight numeric or terminal digit arrangement, they need to have numbers assigned to them and an index needs to be created. If a computer system is already in use, a patient number field needs to be available to store the numbers. Either assign the numbers and enter them into the computer or have the computer complete the number assignment process.

Before converting the filing systems, the following steps should be taken:

1. Change to new folders.
2. Apply color-coding or other labels to ease the resorting process during the conversion.
3. Purge the files not being converted, so that the fewest records possible will need to be moved.

Schedule the conversion during an off-peak time for the facility, such as during the slower summer months. The move should be scheduled for a weekend from Friday at 5:00 PM to Monday at 8:00 AM.[2] Trial tests should be made with a small number of records to determine the time it takes to complete each phase of the conversion work, with an average time per unit of work being multiplied by the estimated number of work units to be completed. Allow for 10 per cent fatigue time when converting patient record folders and 15 per cent fatigue time when converting radiology film jackets. (Radiology film jackets are much larger and far heavier than patient record folders.) Schedule enough workers to complete the conversion based on the number of hours available and the average times calculated from the trial tests.

Develop a visual display of the project timelines. Post the chart in a prominent place in the department, and educate all staff members of their role in adhering to the

Conversion Checklist

1. _____ Take "before" pictures.

2. _____ Develop a chart of project timelines and post it.

3. _____ Purge the records if all are not to be converted.

4. _____ Assign numbers to records, if necessary, and create an index.

5. _____ Apply color coding and/or bar code labels, if necessary.

6. _____ Schedule an actual conversion date.

7. _____ Hold a project meeting with the staff.

8. _____ Complete test trials to determine average times.

9. _____ Complete an estimated count of the records to be converted.

10. _____ Calculate staff needs and obtain staffing commitments.

11. _____ Assign team leaders, project teams, and duties.

12. _____ Hold a project meeting with the staff.

13. _____ Train the staff in the terminal digit system; take "field trips" as necessary.

14. _____ Take "halfway" pictures (with color-coded labels out of order).

15. _____ Alert and train the medical staff about conversion.

16. _____ Hold a project meeting with the staff to establish ground rules for the conversion weekend.

17. _____ Order food for breaks and meals and tables and carts for sorting.

18. _____ Determine and label new terminal digit section placement in the file.

19. _____ Organize the chart return day for 1 day before conversion.

20. _____ Locate a secure area, with keys, for personal belongings.

21. _____ Receive delivery of tables and carts.

22. _____ Actual conversion takes place.

23. _____ Take "after" pictures (with labels in order).

24. _____ Send thank-you notes.

25. _____ Hold an open house party.

conversion timeline. Hold as many preparatory meetings as necessary to make the staff feel comfortable with the conversion.[2] Take "before" pictures of the file room area before the conversion starts.

Train all staff to a working comfort level. Give the theory behind terminal digit filing, train employees in its use, and have the employees practice the new methods.[3] If possible, ask the file folder vendor to help provide a small mock file room for practice purposes. Check the work of each employee to determine her or his understanding of the new system. Also, educate the remainder of the facility staff and the medical staff about the changes that will be taking place in the department to increase their understanding.[3] Answer their questions, reassure them that service will not be interrupted during the conversion, and enlist their cooperation during the conversion time period.

Have sufficient staff and supplies available for the conversion. Use department staff and supplement them with other workers as necessary. Order folding tables for sorting and transportation carts from a rental company or borrow them from another facility.[3]

CONVERSION PROCESS. There are four project phases in the conversion, each requiring a team leader assignment:

1. Transportation of the records to the sort area and back to file
2. Rough-sort into 10 terminal digit sections (e.g., 00-09, 10-19)
3. Secondary-sort into 00, 01, 02, and so on
4. Fine-sort into strict terminal digit order on the file shelves

Begin the conversion by removing records from the areas prelabeled as section 00 and section 50. Remove an equal number of records from the areas that will hold each terminal digit section. This minimizes the number of records that needs to be off the shelves at any given time and provides a place to put records as soon as they are sorted. Team 1 transports the records to the sort area and back to the file. Team 2 rough-sorts the records onto sorting tables (or boxes on chairs), and Team 3 does an intermediate sort into 00, 01, 02, and so on. To minimize back injury from lifting, avoid placing records on the floor or lower than waist height. Use carts to transport all records.

When sufficient records are available in any given primary section where shelving is available, Team 1 transports the records back to the shelving area and places them on the appropriate shelf. Team 4 then fine-sorts the records into strict terminal digit order. Continue this process until all records have been rough-sorted and returned to the file in their primary section. At that time, Teams 2 and 3 become fine-sorters with

Team 4 and Team 1 assists in any shifting of files necessary within primary sections.

Teams should be scheduled in 8-hour shifts, all taking breaks and lunches together.[3] The facility food service or outside catering service should prepare meals and breaks for the team staff. A secured, lockable area where personal belongings can be stored should be provided.[2] Throughout the process, expect the unexpected and adjust plans as necessary.

When the process is complete, take "after" pictures of the finished product. Tell of your success, and hold an open house for the facility.[2] Don't forget to sent thank-you notes to all participants.

Record Tracking

Regardless of how records are filed within the facility, one of the biggest concerns is knowing where the record is when it is needed. For a record management system to be efficient, there must be some method of tracking the current location of a patient record.

Manual Record-Tracking Systems

Manual **record-tracking** systems are the most common, using **outguides** and **requisitions** as their basic tools.

OUTGUIDES. An **outguide** is a plastic folder used in place of the record when the record has been removed from the files. It can be thought of as a placeholder. Outguides usually contain two separate see-through pockets, one to hold the requisition slip and one to hold any loose papers to be filed in the record that accumulate while the record is out of file.

REQUISITIONS. A **requisition** is somewhat like an IOU. It is an acknowledgment that someone has taken a record and intends to return it.[4] Figure 6–3 shows a typical patient record requisition slip. Part 1 of the requisition slip is placed in the outguide as the record is removed from the file. Parts 2 and 3 travel with the record as a routing slip. Part 2 can be used by the requester as a **transfer notice** if the requester forwards the record to another location. Notification of a record transfer is important to obtain but can be especially difficult to obtain in a manual system. The notices are usually 3 × 5-inch slips that can easily be lost in transit. The transfer notices that do make their way to the file area should be given a higher priority than the retrieval of records. By filing the transfer notices first, it assures that the most current location for every record is known before retrieval is attempted.

Manual record-tracking systems should also be able to determine when the record has been **purged**, or

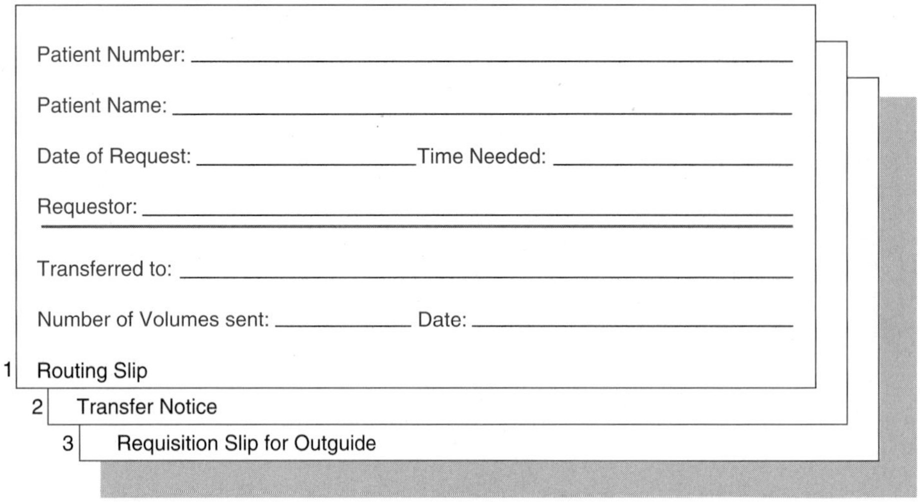

Patient Number: _____

Patient Name: _____

Date of Request: _____Time Needed: _____

Requestor: _____

Transferred to: _____

Number of Volumes sent: _____ Date: _____

1 | Routing Slip

2 | Transfer Notice

3 | Requisition Slip for Outguide

FIGURE 6–3. Requisition slip.

thinned, from the active files and either moved to an alternate storage site or converted to another medium, such as microforms or optical disks, discussed in this chapter. **Outcards** listing the new location or medium should be used for this purpose.[4] An outcard differs from an outguide in that outcards are usually cardboard to allow the patient name and record number to be written directly on them. Outcards stay in the file permanently to tell the new location of the paper record or the new medium it has been transferred to.

RECORD RETRIEVAL STEPS. The steps in retrieving a record in a manual system are as follows:

1. Receive the request for a record.
2. Verify the name and number of the record.
3. Place the requisition slip in an outguide.
4. Locate the record on the shelf.
5. Put the outguide on the shelf and remove the record.
6. Forward the record to the requester.

When the record returns, refile it on the shelf and remove the outguide.

Color coding can also be applied to the use of outguides. Two common methods of color coding outguides are assigning colors for specific request reasons or assigning colors to a specific retrieval time period. Using unique colors for different request reasons alerts the staff to immediately check another location, such as the release of information area or the physicians' incomplete area.

When assigning colors to a specific retrieval period, some departments use a different colored outguide every week on a 4-week rotating cycle. As a new week begins, the outguides from the past 4 weeks (four different colors) are counted. All outguides older than 3 weeks are checked and updated with the new location. This provides a constant file review process for records out of file longer than 4 weeks. Other similar plans can be used to track records according to specific facility needs.

A sufficient supply of outguides is important to a record-tracking system. Past activity levels can help determine the quantity of outguides to have on hand. Be sure that the outguide pockets are large enough to accommodate both the requisition slip and any loose papers. Filing loose papers into the outguide allows the staff to forward information to a requester if the record is unavailable and allows the record to be updated immediately when it returns to the file.

Although these manual system procedures have been used for years, this tracking system is not without certain disadvantages, including the following:

- Time lags in updating record locations[5]
- Excessive time needed to file transfer notices to keep record locations current
- Illegibility of many handwritten requests[5]
- Difficulty in prioritizing workload
- High frustration levels of staff whose work is crisis-oriented[5]
- Dissatisfaction about service by record requesters

Automated Record-Tracking Systems

SOFTWARE CONSIDERATIONS. Automated record-tracking systems were developed to address the concerns listed above. An automated record-tracking system is a database that stores the current and past locations of the record. The automated system is similar to inventory control software that is used in manufacturing to track parts. Just because the system is automated, does not mean that outguides and requisition slips are forgotten. Outguides still aid in the refiling process and hold loose papers. Requisition slips identify the name and number associated with the outguide. However, once the record is retrieved, the outguide is no longer considered the source of information on the record location. The tracking system holds the information about all record requests and transfers.

The tracking system is often linked to other facility systems to avoid duplication of effort. For example, linking the tracking database to the MPI eliminates the need for this second database to contain large amounts of patient demographic information. It is also efficient to link the record-tracking database to a patient scheduling system to allow automatic transfer of requests for appointment records. Linking the system to a record-deficiency system gives an added advantage of knowing which records need to be returned for completion.

Having an on-line request-for-records feature speeds the request process and produces legible requisitions with complete and accurate information with each printing. This feature also allows the tracking software to prioritize the requests according to date and time of need and whether the request is for direct patient care. This feature significantly decreases the need for telephone requests for records and frees the staff to spend time retrieving records rather than answering the telephone. Impact printers are usually used for printing requisitions and are placed in the file area near where the records are located (see Features of an Automated Record-Tracking System).

An automated record-tracking system should be able to produce both management reports and statistical reports (see Software Requirements of an Automated Record-Tracking System).

Software Requirements of an Automated Record-Tracking System

Dictionary-driven, User-definable
- Reasons for requests
- Out-of-file locations

Reporting Capabilities

Management Reports
- Appointment listings
- Unsatisfied requests listings
- Location listings (for use during downtime)
- Overdue listings by user-defined time frames
- Out-of-file listings by location
- Inactive record listings by alternate storage site or media
- Individual record activity listing (for search purposes)

Statistical Reports
- Total scheduled appointments and percentage satisfied
- Total walk-in appointments and percentage satisfied
- Total stat requests and percentage satisfied
- Total requests for each out-of-file location and percentage satisfied
- Grand total of all requests and percentage satisfied
- Total records refiled
- Total records retrieved from inactive storage or other media

---

Features of an Automated Record-Tracking System

- On-line requesting of records, individually or in batch
- Prioritizing of requests done by the software
- On-line inquiry, both current and historical, from every system terminal
- Tracking of multiple volumes of the same record
- Tracking of multiple file room locations
- Updating of system done in real time
- Support of bar code technology, both hand-held and portable
- Support of keyboard data entry of patient identification number or name
- Operation in a user-friendly environment
- Alerts staff when a returned record has been requested during its absence

---

DATA ENTRY CAPABILITIES. Automated systems work extremely well when integrated with bar code technology to speed the data entry process. Bar code labels can be applied to existing folders in preparation for converting to a bar code system or as an enhancement to a current record-tracking system to increase productivity.

Bar codes have been used in health care for many years. The Health Industry Bar Code Council was formed in 1984 and approved a particular bar code symbology specifically for use in health care, code 39. The **symbology** of a bar code means the way the lines and spaces in a bar code are arranged. Code 39 was selected for its variable length, accuracy, and flexibility.[9] Materials Management, Radiology, and Food Service all use the same standard bar code to track supplies, radiology films, and meals, respectively.

The bar code symbology for record folders contains at least two pieces of information, the patient number and the volume number of the record. If other information is needed, it is usually retrieved by on-line access to the MPI or other database.

When a bar code is read, the software receives the

characters as if they were entered by way of the keyboard and processes the information the same way. This is the same process used in a grocery store scanner that reads the universal product codes (UPC) from canned and packaged products. If the UPC is unreadable, the cashier enters the number on the keypad.

HARDWARE NEEDS. Hardware requirements for the system are laser printers, placed where new records are generated, and a variety of bar code reader devices, depending on the quantity of records to be scanned. Programmable color laser printers can be purchased that can print a strip label for the side of the folder that contains the patient's name and identification number, the bar code, and the color-code bars. This method assures that each record is labeled uniformly and that the labeling process is completed with the least amount of hardware and supplies.

Bar code scanners are available in two types: contact and noncontact.[9] A contact scanner is sometimes referred to as a light pen or wand and must come in contact with the bar code to read its contents. Noncontact scanners can be hand-held or fixed. Department store cashiers frequently use hand-held scanning "guns" to read product labels. Fixed scanners read labels that are passed over or under them, such as grocery store scanners.

Even with all the automated assistance, the ultimate success or failure of an automated record-tracking system still depends on proper training, commitment of all staff to use it consistently, and the system's ease of use.

It is important to understand that even though health information management continues to move closer to the true computer-based patient record (CPR), record tracking will not become obsolete for many years. The entering of all data contained in previous paper records would be an extremely costly project, and therefore, these records need to be tracked until they are no longer useful or the vast majority of historical information is entered into the CPR.

Application in Use: University of Texas—James W. Aston Ambulatory Care Center

The University of Texas Southwestern Medical Center, at its James W. Aston Ambulatory Care Center in Dallas, saw 550 patients per day during 1992. The Medical Record Department processed 114,000 requests for records that year.[6] Because of the academic setting, the records move throughout all the facilities, and the Medical Record Department estimated that about 50 per cent of the medical records were out of the file at any point in time. The facility did not have a policy prohibiting the removal of records from the facility or a policy on timely return of records.

The center has continued to grow since it was established in 1984, and it became obvious to the administrative staff that the manual record-tracking system in place could not keep up with current volume, much less future growth. It was decided that two areas needed attention. They were firm policies on the return of records to file and the proper tracking of files throughout the facility.

A task force of representatives from the medical records, information systems, and administrative departments met to discuss these issues and decided to purchase and implement a software package that was available from the current mainframe computer system vendor. All current mainframe users would have access to the system through their existing terminals, and regular system security would be applied as before, including user names and passwords.

The system that was chosen uses "dictionaries," or data tables, used by the system to provide consistency of data. These dictionaries were developed before implementation to standardize requester names, locations, and request reasons for reporting purposes. New requesters, locations, and reasons could be added as future needs developed.

Before implementation, two projects needed to be completed in the Medical Records Department. The first was the converting of records from the old social security numbering system to a new six-digit terminal digit numbering system, with a number being automatically assigned by the accounts receivable system. Only records that had activity in the prior 13 months were converted. All others were converted when patients returned for appointments.

The second major project was the application of the bar code labels used with this system. These labels contained the patient's social security number and the new computer-assigned number and were applied to all converted charts.

When the system was implemented, the facility started using the on-line requesting system for records. It also used the reports and statistics produced by the system for management of the department and monitoring of the chart return policy that was implemented. The new system was able to track record volumes and handle multiple home locations of different file rooms for the staff.

Because of implementation of the system, the medical record job functions and job descriptions changed. Staff was added to the department and service was greatly improved. Record retrieval time averaged 15 minutes and retrieval percentages were at 99 per cent of all requested records after implementation of the automated record-tracking system.

Application in Use: University of Iowa Hospitals and Clinics

The University of Iowa Hospitals and Clinics is a combined health care system in Iowa City whose Medical Record Department processed more than 600,000 patient record requests in 1989, the year they implemented an automated record-tracking system using bar code technology.[8] The previous tracking method was a standard manual system using index cards and outguides. The manual system could not keep up with increasing volumes and demands from users. Workload volume increased by 24 per cent but the size and staffing of the department did not.

A facilitywide committee structure was put in place to investigate the problem, and the committee eventually decided to design its own automated record-tracking system especially for the University of Iowa. The Management Engineering Division helped to collect data about department activities and volumes. The Training Division assisted in the hands-on training of 600 staff members once the system was ready to implement.

The Medical Record Department staff placed bar code labels on each patient record not in storage. Each record that was out of file had the location indicated in the computer. All records without a location in the computer were assigned to the storage location. The Medical Record Department started using the system first, and all areas of the facility gradually began using the system over a 2-month period.

The bar code labels were printed on sheets by a laser printer and used code 39 symbology. The University of Iowa decided not to put the patient number on the bar code label but rather to preprint other numbers on the label and let the computer "associate" the two numbers in the database.

Any computer terminal in the facility can be used to access the system by authorized users to determine record locations and update the system on record transfers. The system also displays frame and reel locations for records stored on roll microfilm. The same system security previously in use controls access to the system.

On-line requesting of records is available, with the system alerting the requester if the record is already signed out of file, either to the requester or to another party. Requesters then contact the other party to make arrangements for retrieving the record. This on-line request system reduced telephone calls by 83 per cent within 2 months after installation. The overall satisfaction rate for record requests went from 82 per cent to 93 per cent in the same 2 months.

The system also produces the basic management reports and statistics expected from an automated system. It has helped to significantly improve the quality of medical record services provided to the staff at the University of Iowa Hospitals and Clinics.

These are excellent examples of how the functions involved in access and retention records can have a substantial impact on the efficient delivery of health care.

Record Retention

HIM professionals are frequently asked questions about how long to keep patient records. There is no universal answer to the question. Several factors need to be considered.

State Statutes and Regulations

State law provides the most concrete guidance on retention. The state law can be referenced individually or obtained from *Healthcare Records: A Practical Legal Guide,* written by Jonathan Tomes[10] and published by the Healthcare Financial Management Association. Tomes details what constitutes a record and what the retention laws are in each state. The **statute of limitations** in each state should be considered specifically when determining a retention policy. The statute of limitations determines the period of time in which a legal action can be brought against a facility for injury, improper care, or breech of contract.[1] The statute of limitations begins at the time of the event or at the age of majority if the patient was treated as a minor.

Facility Needs

Institutional policy is another source to be considered. Because the facility maintains the record for the benefit of the patient, the physician, and the health care facility, it is the responsibility of the facility to keep the record for the use of all three parties.[11] Facilities usually require that records of admissions and all encounters be kept in some form indefinitely. Although this is the best policy, it may not be possible from a financial or space standpoint for every facility.

A facility should also consider the rate of patient re-admission and the level of commitment to research and education in the final decision on retention. A facility with a high re-admission rate will find its own records extremely valuable in the future care of the patient. Longitudinal studies conducted in research facilities are difficult to complete if short retention periods are chosen for patient records.

Retention Schedule

If destruction is determined to be the only option, a minimum retention schedule should be as follows:

- If the patient was over the age of majority when treated—10 years

- If the patient was a minor when treated—10 years past the age of majority

This retention schedule should be observed except when otherwise directed or prohibited by state statute, ordinance, regulation, or law. The following information should be retained permanently in some format, even if the remainder is destroyed:

- Dates of admission, discharge, and encounters
- Physician names
- Diagnoses and procedures
- History and physical reports
- Operative and pathology report
- Discharge summaries[1]

Destruction of records should take place only after approval by the facility administration, facility attorney, malpractice liability insurance carrier, and the board of directors. Complete details of all records destroyed must be kept indefinitely. A manifest including all patient record numbers and patient names should be created as the records are purged, or removed from the files. The destruction process, either by shredding or by incineration, should take place in the presence of two witnesses who both sign a **destruction letter** that has the complete manifest as a referenced attachment.

Facility Closure

Special considerations are necessary regarding record retention when a facility closes, either by sale or by dissolution of a physician practice. The two major considerations are protecting the confidentiality of patient information and assuring that authorized parties have access to the information as provided by law.[12]

If the facility is sold to another provider of health care services, the records are usually considered an asset of the sale because they provide a considerable marketing advantage to the new owner. If the buyer is not a health care provider, records should not be considered assets of the sale and other arrangements should be made. To assure that patients are aware of what is happening to their information, a series of notices should be published in local newspapers informing interested parties of the new location of the records. The facility can then contract with another health care provider, the facility attorney, or a commercial storage company to assume responsibility for the records and provide information to authorized requesters in the future. As a last option, the state department of health may assume responsibility for the records. In any case, every effort should be made to assure that all records are complete as of the date of transfer.

ACCESS AND RETENTION OF IMAGE-BASED RECORDS

Micrographics

The most traditional and well-known option for image-based record storage is micrographics. Micrographics is the formal name for the process of creating miniature pictures on film. It is commonly referred to as microfilm. Micrographics were first used commercially by the banking industry in the 1920s as a solution to the growing volume of canceled checks banks needed to store.[4] The microfilming process has been used for years in health care for the storage of patient records, and many facilities routinely microfilm their inactive records after a certain period. Microfilmed images are small negative photographs of the original documents that cannot be read with the unaided human eye. They must be magnified for viewing by specialized reading devices.

Microforms

Facilities have several micrographics options to choose from when planning a storage and retrieval program. The generic word for any micrographics format is a **microform.** Choosing the correct microform for the project requires knowledge of four key facts about the project:

1. The type and amount of information to be microfilmed, including age and present format
2. The frequency at which the material will require updating
3. The amount of access needed for patient care and other uses
4. The budget available for the microfilm conversion project

The various microforms are discussed here in relation to these four key facts.

ROLL MICROFILM. **Roll microfilm** is a continuous film strip, similar in appearance to movie film, that holds several thousand document pages, depending on the reduction ratio used when the documents were filmed.[4] The **reduction ratio** refers to reducing an image in size by the amount stated in the ratio. A standard ratio for patient records is 24X, or 24-to-1, meaning that the image is 1/24th the size of the original.[4]

In a patient record environment, several patient records are normally stored on a roll of film. Patient records must be complete when filmed because roll microfilm cannot be updated. Documents must also be in a consistent order when filmed to make future retrieval possible. Roll microfilm is similar in concept to the serial numbering and filing methodology. Multiple records on the same patient can be found on various rolls of film if the patient returns several times over the years. Bringing these records together for current patient care purposes is difficult unless paper copies are made and used for reference. Therefore, roll microfilm is usually only a choice for extremely old records or records of deceased patients that will never need updating. It also works well with the serial filing methodology.

JACKET MICROFILM.   Roll film can be converted to different packaging to provide the ability to update it. This can be done by cutting the film and placing it into microfilm jackets. **Microfilm jackets** are 4×6 holders that have channels, or narrow sleeves, formed by fusing together two panels of transparent material. A strip of roll microfilm can be inserted into this channel. Each jacket can hold about 70 document pages, depending on the reduction ratio used when the documents were filmed.

When microfilm jackets are used for patient record storage, each of the jackets is a patient record, maintaining the unit record concept. Records of subsequent admissions or encounters can be added to the channels as they become inactive and are filmed. The jackets are labeled, or indexed, with the patient name and identification number and normally filed by the same method used for the original paper-based records in that facility. Jackets can be purchased with different color strips on the top edge to provide the same color-coding scheme used in the active files.

MICROFICHE.   **Microfiche** is a copy of a microfilm jacket made on a special 4×6 sheet of polyester film (Mylar). Copies of microfilm are useful because many facilities do not remove the microfilm jacket from the file for routine use. Instead, they make microfiche copies to circulate for patient care and provider use, protecting the original from loss or damage. These microfiche copies can be destroyed when no longer needed. Microfiche can also be used as the primary source document in the facility if the original microfilm jackets are stored away from the facility for safekeeping.

Microfiche copies can be added to a paper record folder in a pocket to keep the unit record intact if the patient returns to the facility. These copies can also be added to active record folders for those patients whose active record is too large or cumbersome to deal with in a paper format in the active file. This means that facilities with patients who return consistently and frequently can film older portions of the record and file microfiche copies in the paper folder to use less space in the active

files. This can be done without changing the retention schedule of the active file.

Microfiche can also be filmed directly from the source document. This eliminates the need for cutting the roll film and inserting it into jackets. Indexing of the jackets is also eliminated because the indexing is created by the camera when the images are filmed. Microfiche can be filmed at $24\times$, $42\times$, or $48\times$. Using a larger reduction ratio can save considerable money over the jacket method that contains 70 images per jacket filmed at $24\times$.

COMPUTER-ASSISTED RETRIEVAL—ROLL MICROFILM. Microfilm needs to be created differently to be used in a computer-assisted retrieval (CAR) system. When the microfilm is created, the images are numbered. In its most simplistic form, the images are cataloged by patient name, patient identification number, roll number, and frame number. These roll and frame numbers are entered into the MPI or another database specially designed for this purpose. In a more advanced form, the database can contain more data than may be required by a particular application. In any CAR system, when a particular patient's records are requested, the roll and frame numbers are retrieved from the index and the roll is located. The roll is searched until the appropriate frames are found.[4] Some reader-printers automatically locate the frame number desired if it is entered on a keypad by counting the images that pass an internal scanner.

COMPUTER-ASSISTED RETRIEVAL—JACKET MICRO-FILM.   The same concepts can be applied to jacket film in a CAR-jacket system. Sequentially numbered film frames are loaded into sequentially numbered jackets. The MPI or other database records the jacket and frame numbers of each patient's film. The needed jackets are retrieved as the patient's record is requested.

Table 6–5 describes micrographics options frequently chosen in health care. Table 6–6 describes the advantages and disadvantages of these options.

COMPUTER OUTPUT MICROFICHE.   Another micrographics option used in health care is **computer output microfiche (COM)**. COM allows large amounts of electronically stored data to be placed on microfilm quickly. In COM, the computer displays data on a special screen connected to a microfilm camera called a recorder. The recorder films the screen, reduces the image in size, and places the image directly onto a Mylar microfiche sheet. As more screens are filmed, they are added to the microfiche until it is full, usually 240 images at $48\times$. This process continues until the entire computer file has been copied to film.[4]

This technology is applicable to the filming of in-

TABLE 6-5 MICROGRAPHICS OPTIONS IN HEALTH CARE

ROLL MICROFILM	CAR-ROLL MICROFILM	MICROFILM JACKETS	CAR-JACKET MICROFILM
Description: Continuous film containing about 2400 images Multiple patients can be found per roll. It can be used well with extremely old records or records of deceased patients.	*Description:* Continuous film containing prenumbered images Database references the patient by roll and frame number. Multiple patients can be found per roll. It eliminates the disadvantage of roll film's inability to be updated.	*Description:* 4 × 6 holders containing up to 70 images cut from continuous roll film Film is held in channels. All channels may not be used if the record has few pages. There is a single patient per jacket. It can be used well in facilities with a high patient return rate or when a unit is vital to patient care.	*Description:* 4 × 6 holders containing about 70 images cut from continuous roll film Film is held in channels. All channels are completely filed with prenumbered images. Database is used to reference the patient by jacket and frame number.

dexes, such as the MPI and the Diagnostic Index. Microfiche copies can then be used as a backup source for locating patient numbers or data if the computer is unavailable. This process can be accomplished 20 times faster than the creation of a computer printout and eliminates the steps of filming the printout, developing the film, and loading the microfilm jacket. Considerable savings can be realized by using this completely automated process.

Other micrographics options that are available but seldom, if ever, used in health care are aperture cards, roll cartridges, and roll cassettes. Aperture cards are used mainly to hold film copies of large documents, such as architectural drawings. Roll cartridges and cas-

TABLE 6-6 ADVANTAGES AND DISADVANTAGES OF MICROGRAPHICS OPTIONS

FACTOR	ROLL MICROFILM	CAR-ROLL MICROFILM	MICROFILM JACKETS	CAR-JACKET MICROFILM
Cost	Least expensive method	More expensive than roll film because of database of roll and frame number	Most expensive method because of indexing and loading of jackets	May be as expensive as microfilm jackets because of jacket loading and database of jacket and frame number
Security	Images cannot be misfiled on the roll, but entire rolls may be misfiled or lost.	Image cannot be misfiled on the roll, but entire rolls may be misfiled or lost.	Jackets can be color-coded and filed in a miniature version of the paper system	Jackets can be misfiled because they are numbered sequentially and usually are not color-coded.
Unit record	Difficult to create without converting to paper Difficult to perform longitudinal studies	Difficult to create without converting to paper; easier to create than with regular roll film Difficult to perform longitudinal studies but easier than with regular roll film	Automatically created Easy to perform longitudinal studies Microfilm or a copy can be placed in a new paper folder for later use	Difficult to create without converting to paper Difficult to perform longitudinal studies
Access	Film cannot be used for court or patient care without converting to paper because of multiple patients on roll	Film cannot be used for court or patient care without converting to paper because of multiple patients on film	Copies of film can be taken to court or given to patient care areas because there is only one patient on film.	Film cannot be used for court or patient care without converting to paper because of multiple patients on film.
Ability to update	Cannot be updated as a unit; record must be complete when filmed	Cannot be updated as a unit but database directs the user to additional records on a different roll	Additional records updated into space available in an open channel or additional jackets used	Cannot be updated as a unit but database directs the user to additional records on a different jacket
Ability to partial film	Cannot film an older portion of an active record	Can film an older portion of an active record, but it must be converted to paper for use	Can film an older portion of an active record and place the microfilm or a copy in the paper folder	Can film an older portion of an active record, but it must be converted to paper for use

settes are other ways to package roll film to protect the film surface. Roll film in this format is still unable to be updated. Cartridges or cassettes may be used in file systems where files are frequently referenced.

Equipment

STORAGE EQUIPMENT. Jackets are commonly stored in filing cabinets specifically made for microfilm, having shallow but sturdy drawers. A 10-drawer microfilm cabinet is especially efficient for creating a miniature terminal digit file with microfilm. The cabinet drawers should be managed using the same tools discussed in connection with paper-based records, such as file guides for determining file location, outguides to mark the place of removed film, and requisition slips if original film is removed from the files.

REPRODUCTION EQUIPMENT. Microfilm images must be read using a **microfilm reader.** A reader, also called a viewer, is a projection box that magnifies the image, passes light through it, and displays it on a screen. Readers can be combined with the reproduction capabilities of a copy machine to form a reader-printer combination. This allows the displayed image to be copied onto paper for use again as a paper record. It is best to have readers and reader-printers that display a full-page image, making viewing easier. Smaller viewers can be used when a large space is unavailable, but staff may find them more difficult to use.

Readers and reader-printers are constructed to accommodate one format of microform, although they can be purchased with combination adapters to allow them to view both roll and jacket film. This saves a considerable amount of space and money. The magnification ratio of the reader or reader-printer must be matched to the reduction ratio used when the film was created. The **magnification ratio** is the inverse of the reduction ratio.

DUPLICATION EQUIPMENT. A duplicator for microfilm creates a copy of the film with adequate clarity for use as if it was the original film. Entire rolls can be duplicated or jackets can be duplicated as microfiche. Duplication of film can be done for many reasons. Facilities may choose to use duplicated copies to circulate instead of the originals or to satisfy multiple requests received for the same record at the same time. Duplicate of microfilm jackets can also be sent to another facility that uses the same micrographics format if a request for the record has been received.

Legal Considerations

It is important to realize that microfilm is legal in the United States. Federal legislation was passed in 1951, in the form of Public Law 129, that allows microfilm as primary evidence in court. If necessary, the facility must be able to prove that the original record was destroyed by producing the destruction letter and manifest for the court. Public Law 129 supersedes any state law to the contrary.

Cost Analysis

Storing paper records in a storage room or with a commercial storage company seems like an economical alternative to having crowded active files. The reality is, however, that converting the records to another medium may have a **pay-back period** (the time in which a project saves enough money to pay for itself) that is less than suspected.

Table 6–7 shows a sample cost analysis for a paper-based system and a microfilm jacket system over the same 10-year period. After the initial investment year, the microfilm system expenses remain constant throughout the next 9 years. The paper-based system begins to have modest increases in retrieval costs and has tremendous increases in storage space and shelving costs for the 10-year period. The microfilm system actually pays for itself somewhere in the middle of the 6th year. The system will pay for itself even faster if the storage space is at the facility and can be converted into revenue-producing patient care space.

When converting to microfilm, an initial decision must be made about which portions of the record will be filmed. The easiest choice is to film the entire contents of the record. However, for purposes of economy, the record may be purged of certain items not important to ongoing patient care. Some examples of unnecessary items are belongings lists and detailed data that are summarized elsewhere in the record. Also, photocopies of records received from other facilities, such as documents from previous hospitalizations, need not be filmed. These records are retained by the originator of the documents.

During this initial decision-making phase, test films should be created to determine the best method for filming "difficult" documents, such as documents on colored paper and documents where resolution is vital, like electrocardiograms. Once the extent of the project has been identified and exact methods to be used are determined, the remaining decision is regarding how the work will be performed, either in-house or by a contracted microfilm service bureau.

IN-HOUSE MICROFILM PROCESSING. Microfilming records at the facility requires a large investment in equipment as well as a new body of knowledge and a new set of skills about the use and maintenance of the equipment. A description of the equipment needed and an overview of the process are included here to provide the background information necessary in deciding

TABLE 6-7 SAMPLE COST ANALYSIS*

YEAR	PAPER-BASED SYSTEM					MICROFILM IMAGE-BASED SYSTEM					
	No. of Records to Store	Retrieval Costs	Storage/ Shelving Costs	Yearly Costs	Cumulative Costs	Records to Film	Film Costs	Equip- ment	Upkeep Costs	Yearly Cost	Cumulative Cost
1	70,000	$ 9,450	$11,880	$21,330	$ 21,330	70,000	$50,974	$7,000	$2,100	$60,074	$ 60,074
2	83,000	$ 9,750	$ 8,880	$18,630	$ 39,960	13,000	$10,241	$1,300	$2,100	$13,641	$ 73,715
3	96,000	$10,050	$ 9,800	$19,850	$ 59,810	13,000	$10,241	$1,000	$2,100	$13,341	$ 87,056
4	109,000	$10,350	$10,800	$21,150	$ 80,960	13,000	$10,241		$2,200	$12,441	$ 99,497
5	122,000	$10,650	$11,880	$22,530	$103,490	13,000	$10,241		$2,300	$12,541	$112,038
6	135,000	$10,950	$12,880	$23,830	$127,320	13,000	$10,241		$2,400	$12,641	$124,679
7	148,000	$11,250	$13,880	$25,130	$152,450	13,000	$10,241		$2,500	$12,741	$137,420
8	161,000	$11,550	$14,880	$26,430	$178,880	13,000	$10,241	$1,000	$2,600	$13,841	$151,261
9	174,000	$11,850	$15,880	$27,730	$206,610	13,000	$10,241		$2,700	$12,941	$164,202
10	187,000	$12,150	$16,880	$29,030	$235,640	13,000	$10,241		$2,800	$13,041	$177,243
Total					$235,640						$177,243

* Assumes no inflation.

whether to complete the work in-house or write an outside contract.

The pieces of equipment used in the process are a camera, a film developer, and, for a jacket system, a typewriter and a jacket loader, or inserter. An in-house microfilm program requires at least one microfilm camera of a type best suited for the records to be filmed. Microfilm cameras are large pieces of photographic equipment that are able to reduce the size of the photograph as the image is recorded. These cameras require periodic maintenance, usually under a maintenance contract with a qualified service vendor.

The three types of cameras are rotary, planetary, and step-and-repeat. The rotary camera is the least expensive to use to produce microfilm images. It produces a lower-quality image because the paper source document is moving rapidly past the camera lens as the photograph is being taken. This camera is appropriate for standard-sized documents and can also be used for continuous documents, such as monitor strips and electrocardiograms. It is not appropriate for irregular-sized documents or shingled copies where one sheet has multiple other sheets taped or stapled to it.

The planetary camera is more expensive to use in creating microfilm images because each paper document must be individually placed on the glass plate for the photography process. This camera is used when high-quality images are required, when fragile documents are being filmed, or when documents require special positioning for filming. Either camera can be equipped with

an automatic eye to sense color and density changes on the paper source document.

A step-and-repeat camera is used only for creating microfiche. It films directly onto 4 × 6 Mylar sheets of film.

No matter which camera is used for the process, documents must be prepared ahead of time to speed the filming process. The steps included in the preparatory process are as follows:

1. Create an eye-readable target sheet, printed in large print, for the record. It contains the patient's name and identification number and is used as the first image to identify the record that is to follow. Additional targets can be made to identify individual admissions or encounters.
2. Remove staples and fasteners from all sheets of the record.
3. Verify all sheets for correct name, correct location in the record, and eligibility for filming within the retention schedule.
4. Repair any damaged sheets.
5. Unmount any sheets mounted with tape to another sheet.
6. Make an entry for the record on a microfilm control log. The control log follows the record through the filming process and eventually becomes the manifest attached to the destruction letter to verify that the record was filmed and then destroyed.

Once the pictures have been captured on the film, the

film needs to be developed. Some in-house operations choose to send the film elsewhere for developing rather than buy a developing machine and the chemicals required for the process. The roll film is usually checked for image clarity by the developer.

Developed film can remain as a roll if the micrographics program uses that format. If jackets have been chosen, a supply of jackets, a typewriter, and a jacket loader (or inserter) are required. Jackets are indexed on the top strip with the identifying information, including a volume number, by the use of the typewriter. Rather than indicating volume 1 of 3, jackets no. 1 and no. 2 would be coded with 1 + and 2 +, respectively. Jacket no. 3 would be coded with only a 3, indicating that it is the last jacket in the series. If other images are added later and jacket no. 4 is required, a plus sign (+) would be added to jacket no. 3's code.

Jackets are loaded by using an inserter to cut the roll film to the appropriate length and feed it into the jacket channels. Loaded jackets should be checked to assure that images are clear, straight, and loaded correctly, with the contents matching the indexing.

CONTRACTED MICROFILM SERVICE BUREAUS. Because most facilities do not have the volume necessary to support the purchase of a camera, a developer, and a jacket loader, they choose to engage the services of a microfilm vendor, or service bureau. The service bureau performs microfilm conversions for multiple customers in large volume and can justify the cost of the many pieces of equipment needed for the process.

Microfilm service bureaus price their services by the cost per 1000 images, based on the specific service requirements that the customer outlines. Requesting certain procedures or methods may increase the price. It is wise to ask the vendor what the least expensive method would be in comparison to the method designed by the facility. Most vendors who routinely convert patient records to microfilm have a "standard" method that they are equipped to offer at an economical price. Choosing the standard plan may reduce the cost significantly.

Table 6–8 shows a sample evaluation matrix used to determine the best vendor for a conversion to a jacket microfilm system for 70,000 records with 1,200,000 images. An estimated 15 per cent of the 70,000 patients would have records that are more than 70 images, therefore requiring a second jacket. The total number of jackets projected for this system is 80,000. The prices range from $25.81 to $31.03 per 1000 images of completed microfilm, excluding the jacket cost. As Table

TABLE 6–8 SAMPLE EVALUATION MATRIX-CONTRACT MICROFILM SERVICES

Criteria and Weight		VENDOR #1			VENDOR #2			VENDOR #3		
		Rating		Results	Rating		Results	Rating		Results
Cost/1000 images	5	Excellent ($25.81)($30,974)	5	25	Very good ($29.75)($35,700)	4	20	Good ($31.03)($37,236)	3	15
Cost/4 × 6 jacket	5	Excellent ($0.25)($20,000)	5	25	Excellent ($0.25)($20,000)	5	25	Excellent ($0.25)($20,000)	5	25
Control sheet production	4	Excellent (done by vendor N/C)	5	20	Good (facility not required to do but not done by vendor)	3	12	Fair (facility required to do)	2	8
Record pull	4	Excellent (done by vendor N/C)	5	20	Excellent (done by vendor N/C)	5	20	Fair (facility must do)	2	8
Jacket color selection	3	Excellent (all colors matched)	5	15	Fair (off by two colors)	2	6	Excellent (all colors matched)	5	15
Storage after filming	2	Excellent (6 months)	5	10	Excellent (6 months)	5	10	Good (2 months)	3	6
Emergency returns	2	Excellent (1 hour N/C)	5	10	Very good (fax N/C)	4	8	Very good (2 hours N/C)	4	8
Payment schedule control	2	Excellent (requests honored)	5	10	Good (100 working days)	3	6	Good (vendor preference)	3	6
Total				135			107			91

5, excellent; 4, very good; 3, good; 2, fair; 1, poor.

6–8 shows, price was not the only factor considered in determining the vendor. The evaluation matrix was used to rate all the important factors.

This evaluation matrix can be applied to any situation in which a decision needs to be made between two or more alternative systems, vendors, or methods as candidates. The steps in building an evaluation matrix are as follows:

1. Determine the items most important to the success of the project. Use these items as evaluation criteria.
2. Weight each criterion on a scale of 1 to 5 regarding how critical these items are to the overall success of the project.
3. Place the name of each candidate at the top of a column. Assign a rating to each candidate for each criterion, using a 1-to-5 scale with excellent being rated 5 and poor being rated 1.
4. Multiply the weight times the rating score to determine the results.
5. Total the results scores for each candidate to select the best possible choice.

A matrix similar to the one in Table 6–8 helps to show how the decision was made. It also provides a large amount of information to final decision makers regarding which items were evaluated and the results of the evaluation.

With the top candidate identified, the contracting process can proceed. Each evaluation criterion should be detailed in the contract to assure that the expected results are agreed on. Other items to include in the contract are confidentiality provisions; quality expectations, including retakes at no charge; and the details of the destruction schedule and process.

Many vendors also include an addendum to the contract that details how roll film will be labeled or jackets will be indexed and any special image requirements determined during the test phase. All aspects of the conversion should be detailed in the contract to avoid future disagreements between the facility and the vendor.

Although microfilm may seem like an older technology, it is still frequently used to solve many storage and retrieval problems that do not require more advanced technology as a solution. Facilities that have an active and stable population, such as health maintenance organizations, may not have large volumes of inactive records. They do have large active files that cause active storage requirements to grow continually. Microfilm provides a solution to the active storage space problem through the use of microfilm jackets. Older portions of active records are filmed by a contracted microfilm service bureau and placed in jackets. These jackets are labeled with the patient name and identification number and can be color-coded using the same method used for the paper record. The jacket or jackets are placed inside the paper folder and are available for use by the patient care staff if they are needed.

Using microfilm in this manner does not require the purchase of storage cabinets or a microfilm duplicator. It requires the purchase of readers to be conveniently located in the patient care areas and at least one reader-printer for creating paper copies. This method converts inactive paper stored on the active shelf into microfilm, creating new and available space while maintaining a unit record system usable for patient care. It also provides a method for the facility to try a micrographics program on a limited scale without a major purchase of equipment.

Application in Use: Kurten Medical Group in Racine, Wisconsin

When the newly hired Director of Information Services and the Health Information Supervisor at Kurten Medical Group, both HIM professionals, surveyed the active and inactive files, they found some disturbing situations. They had no overall storage and retrieval plan in place for the future and had not documented past practices.

The 114,000 active records were stored in 11 motorized revolving file units that were more than 10 years old. They required frequent servicing, sometimes weekly, from a company 30 miles away. The maintenance agreements on some of these units were not being offered for renewal the coming year. The 19,000 filing inches in these motorized units were overcrowded and difficult for the growing staff of 14 to access. These active records were in color-coded folders, using a 10-color system, and filed using the terminal digit method. The only problem with the folder was a typed label that was hard to read. Because of inadequate file space, the records were purged to inactive storage after 13 months of inactivity.

There were 81,000 inactive records from 1979 to 1988 kept in a large storage room about 100 feet from the main Health Information Department. These records had numbers, but many had been indexed manually and this manual index was no longer available. The records had not been entered into the facility's first computer in 1982. Therefore, all inactive records had been filed alphabetically since the late 1970s. An additional 5000 records from the early 1970s had been microfilmed and placed in microfilm jackets, all with a red stripe. These jackets were also filed alphabetically for the same reason. A group of inactive records from 1975 to 1978 were destroyed. Later requests for information from these records prompted multiple patient complaints.

All inactive records, both paper and microfilm, were labeled with the patient's name, date of birth, and record number. No numbers had ever been duplicated, and new patients were still receiving unit numbers from the same continuous number series, approaching 25-00-00 at that time.

Kurten Medical Group had recently purchased a new mainframe computer and software for on-line requesting of records, automated record tracking, and bar code label production. This health information software module was ready for installation when the department could accommodate it. The facility had been using the manual outguide and requisition method up to that time. All the past practice information was obtained from interviewing long-term employees, from investigation, and from calculations done by the director and supervisor because no storage and retrieval plan could be found.

The HIM professionals began working on a storage and retrieval plan to improve the information system and allow implementation of the automated record-tracking system that was available. Their plan involved replacing the motorized units with open-shelf files, microfilming the inactive records into a jacket format, and applying the bar code labels to all active records.

Later the same year, administrative approval was obtained and a microfilm service bureau with sufficient storage space to accommodate 81,000 records was located. The service contract was written for a color-coded jacket system. Jackets were chosen because of the previous 5000 records filmed using the jacket method and the need to place the jacket microfilm into a new paper folder if the patient returned to the clinic. In addition, the jacket method allowed them to film older portions of large active records and, therefore, control the space used in the active files. The records in the storage room were emptied into boxes and picked up by the service bureau with the microfilm conversion process starting immediately.

The next weekend, as many of 114,000 active records as possible were moved from the motorized files into the temporary Health Information Department set up in the storage room down the hall. This storage room was the department's home for the next 2 weeks. The remainder of the records were stored in the employee lounge and other non–patient care areas on large, rented four-tier carts. A moving company was secured to disassemble the motorized revolving files and remove the used parts. The motorized units were not replaced because of the increased size of the active files and the number of file workers who needed to access the records simultaneously. In addition, no funds were available to replace all 11 units. Instead, additional filing inches were gained by reconfiguring the same space using open-shelf filing at far less cost. The overall filing space was increased to 21,024 inches.

The removal of the motorized units, replacement of worn flooring, upgrading of the lighting, and painting of the walls took 7 weekdays. The new open-shelf filing units were installed on the 8th and 9th weekdays. On the weekend, the records were returned to their new file shelves, leaving the storage room available for other use. The 30-physician clinic continued to operate at full capacity during the conversion, and patient care was not compromised.

Next, the 10-drawer microfilm cabinet arrived for the miniature, color-coded terminal digit system, along with the reader-printer and the readers. Microfilm started arriving shortly after that. During available time periods, the reception staff checked returning film and old film for the presence of a computer record on the patient. If none was found, the patient's name, date of birth, and record number were entered as a minimal database entry, along with a record-tracking location of "microfilm" in the new automated record-tracking software. If the jacket color was wrong (all old jackets were red), new jackets were retyped and reloaded into the correct color. Finally the film was all filed in terminal digit order into the microfilm cabinet.

During the same time, the HIM professional team was building requester location and reason files in the record-tracking software and were training all facility staff in the use of the automated record-tracking software. The Health Information Department staff was applying bar code labels, which contained the patient's name, date of birth, and record number in large print, to the front of all active records. When the label application was complete, all records out of file were recorded to their requester location and all others kept the default location of "In File."

Less than 6 months from the implementation of the plan, Kurten Medical Group's Health Information Department was using its new storage and retrieval system, with decreased costs, adequate space, and increased morale.

Application in Use: New York Hospital–Cornell Medical Center in New York City

Fetal heart monitor strips are an unusual size and provide a unique storage problem. New York Hospital–Cornell Medical Center used microfilm jackets to store their fetal heart monitor strips as part of the patient record in a smaller, more convenient form. Each microfilm jacket holds 7.64 hours of fetal monitoring records filmed with a $20\times$ reduction ratio.[13]

The monitor strips are filmed on a special continuous-feed camera, similar to a rotary camera. The film is then cut and loaded into microfilm jackets. These jackets can be stored with the paper record throughout its active shelf life and then form the first microfilm jacket if the record is converted to jacket film later.

This facility also used microfilm for storing prescription records, requiring permanent storage. This technology is also applicable to continuous electrocardiographic tracings from stress test machines, electroencephalogram tracings, and polysomnography tracings.

Optical Image Processing

One of the fastest growing areas of technology in the market of health information is optical imaging. This is the method of digitizing documentation on a laser disk. To understand the technology, the components of an optical disk system, methods of data entry and conversions, and implementation strategies are discussed in this section. Table 6–9 describes the optical image processing system components and their major attributes.

System Components

SCANNER. The first component is the **scanner**. This instrument transforms the images on paper into digital images. Dots called bit-maps are created in the same pattern as the dots in the paper image, much like today's fax technology. The scanner itself looks like a copier, with an automatic document feeder, a flatbed, or both. Scanner quality is rated in pixels per inch (PPI). The higher the PPI, the higher the resolution and the clearer the document. The image can be scanned at 200 to 400 PPI, with 200 to 300 PPI being the average resolution. Most scanners only read in paper-based images, but some special scanners can read in microfilm images.[14]

The HIM professional should be aware of the speed at which a scanner is able to scan documents into the system. Scanner speed is rated in pages per minute (PPM), with 90 to 140 PPM signifying a fast rating. When considering a scanner purchase, actual speed should be determined using sample forms from the current files. The speed of the scanner determines, in large part, the labor involved in placing documents in the system because work can only proceed as fast as the scanner can go. The scanner should be equipped with an image enhancement feature that adjusts the density and contrast of an image automatically. This eliminates the need to stop the scanner to manually adjust these settings.

SCANNING WORKSTATION. The scanning workstation is normally a microcomputer or minicomputer that performs the function of compressing the bit-map that has been created by the scanner. Compression is required because the scanned bit-map data are too large to store

TABLE 6-9 OPTICAL IMAGE PROCESSING SYSTEM COMPONENTS		
SYSTEM COMPONENTS	**USE**	**IDENTIFYING ITEMS**
Scanner	Digitizes images	Speed in pages per minute (PPM) and quality in pixels per inch (PPI) Should have image enhancement to automatically adjust density and contrast
Workstation, scanning or retrieval (CPU, video display, keyboard, and optional mouse)	Compresses digitized images Runs database software for indexing	CPU speed in megahertz Video refresh rate in hertz Video quality in dots per inch Bandwidth in megahertz
Optical character scanning devices (OCR/ bar codes)	Indexes automatically by reading special characters or codes	Resolution quality in dots per inch (DPI)
File server	Retrieves images for users on the system	Proprietary systems PC-based systems UNIX-based systems
Magnetic disk	Stores images temporarily before they are moved to permanent storage	Storage capacity in megabytes Access time in milliseconds
Optical disk platter	Stores images permanently	Storage capacity in gigabytes
Jukebox	Holds and retrieves optical disks as they are requested	Exchange time in seconds Access time in milliseconds
Cache memory	Stores packets of information temporarily between workstation and file server	Storage capacity in megabytes
Printer	Reproduces digitized/stored images to paper copies	Speed in pages per minute Quality in dots per inch

in the scanned format. The bit-maps are compressed to about 1/20th of the raw size for eventual storage on the optical disk.

The scanning workstation is also responsible for the indexing of images. The index is in a database format and allows the documents in the optical system to be retrieved easily. The information can be indexed by patient name, medical record number, or other identifying information. For example, portions of the record may be indexed separately, such as the discharge summary and operative report. Some facilities regularly index the physician number, diagnosis codes, and procedure codes associated with the encounter. This indexing step can be valuable if there is a need to locate a particular report quickly rather than having to search through the entire record. The disadvantage to the complex indexing is the time consumed in completing the process. For maximum efficiency and flexibility, the scanning workstation should be able to run other software, such as word processing or desktop publishing, in addition to the optical disk database software.[15]

OPTICAL CHARACTER SCANNING DEVICES. Indexing is a portion of the system setup that requires careful attention and consideration. It is the other major factor that determines the overall labor costs of placing documents in the system. However, there are ways that documents can be indexed other than manually. **Optical character recognition (OCR)** and bar coding of documents are some automated options that help decrease the cost of indexing.

These indexing methods recognize codes on a document in a standard position and create the indexing from these codes. Documents must be redesigned into standard formats that are readable by the equipment for this indexing method to be effective.

FILE SERVER. The **file server** takes requests for images stored in the system, prioritizes them, and, subsequently, sends them to the requester. A minicomputer or a mainframe computer may be used as the file server. The file server acts as the data storage component of the system and literally "serves" the other components of the system, providing them with the data that is needed when requested.

The file server should be able to directly connect the scanner to it by the use of a **small computer system interface (SCSI),** pronounced "Scuzzy." A SCSI port is a parallel interface for high-speed access to peripheral devices such as scanners and disk drives.[16] Connecting a scanner directly to the server, rather than going through a workstation, can speed the scanning process dramatically. The direct connection can be used only if an automatic indexing function using OCR or bar codes is

used. Without automatic indexing, the workstation keyboard is required to create the indexing.

MAGNETIC DISK. Information is stored on a magnetic disk until it is copied onto the permanent optical disk. This allows the re-scanning of images that are of poor quality or otherwise incorrect before the image becomes permanent. The magnetic disk can also accept data from other facility systems using **electronic data interchange (EDI).**

EDI is a computer-to-computer exchange of information based on communication standards written by the American National Standards Institute (ANSI). These standards allow information to be exchanged between electronic media such as magnetic disks, tapes, and computer networks. The goal of EDI is the paperless trading of information in a readily understandable format. The receiving system does not have to translate any information if it has been transmitted using the ANSI standard format.

EDI enables other industries to become automated, as in the banking industry's widespread use of automated teller machines. EDI makes these transactions possible. The same process allows transcribed documents from a word processing system or results from laboratory equipment to be automatically entered into the optical system, either in place of a paper copy or in addition to it. The automatic transfer of data to optical disk is similar in theory to COM, in which computerized data is transformed to image-based data for use or storage. This technology is called **COLD,** or **computer output to laser disk.**

OPTICAL DISK PLATTERS. The optical disk is encased in plastic and resembles a 3.5-inch floppy disk. The image is burned into the disk's surface by using a laser beam and is also read using a laser. The surface of the optical disk is similar to a music compact disk and can store a large amount of information. The laser technology uses light to record data in a more tightly packed form than that used by the magnetic read/write heads of a conventional drive.

One type of laser technology is called **WORM (write once read many)** because it stores the data in a permanent capacity and does not allow the user to alter the documents. The document is written once and can be read as many times as necessary from the disk. WORM technology is preferred for health information storage because data cannot be misfiled, accidentally erased, or altered.

The disks are available in different sizes and are capable of holding varying amounts of data. The typical sizes are 5¼ inches, 12 inches, and 14 inches. A single-density 5¼-inch platter can hold about 940 megabytes of information, whereas a 12-inch platter can hold between

2 and 3.2 gigabytes (billions of bytes) of information (3.2 gigabytes of information is equal to about 100,000 [8½ × 11] pages of stored information). A double-density platter can increase the storage capacity to twice that volume.[14] The highest-capacity disk commercially available is a 14-inch platter. Double-density 14-inch platters can hold about 10 gigabytes of data. A disadvantage of the 12-inch format is the lack of standards among vendors, which affects the compatibility of disks. The 14-inch platter is the format for which ANSI standards are being developed.

Another type of laser technology is rewritable magneto-optical platters. Although this rewritable technology does not provide unalterable images that guarantee permanence, it does provide the ability to use optical technology for working documents. For example, a nursing graphic record of a hospitalization may need updating multiple times during a patient's stay. Rewritable technology would allow the document to be changed until the patient was discharged. The document could then be written to WORM technology for permanent storage.

Optical disks are written using a disk drive that resembles a magnetic disk drive. If the facility determines that both WORM and rewritable technology are required, multifunctional drives that accommodate both technologies are available.

JUKEBOX. The **jukebox** holds and retrieves the individual disks as they are requested, much like a music record jukebox. With the record jukebox, the listener selects the record he or she wants to hear and the internal mechanism of the jukebox retrieves the record and plays it. The optical disk system jukebox works the same way. Each box or cabinet holds multiple disks and is capable of high-speed retrieval. In some configurations, jukeboxes are linked together which allows for even greater storage capacity.

The amount of time it takes the jukebox to locate the disk and retrieve it is called the **exchange time.** The exchange time is rated in the number of seconds it takes to complete the process. Users may consider 30 seconds the longest acceptable exchange time, with 20 seconds being optimal. Once the disk is placed in the disk drive, the appropriate image must be located for display on the terminal screen. The time it takes for this process to be completed is called **access time.** Access time is rated in milliseconds because access is an electronic process, in comparison to exchange, which is a mechanical process.

Fragmented WORM platters, or disks on which multiple images from the same record have been written to different areas of the platter or even different optical platters, can increase the access time of the system. Fragmentation can be corrected by rewriting all the images on the platter into the correct sequence on a different platter. This process is similar to defragmenting a magnetic hard drive if it was rewritten to a new hard drive. Although defragmenting platters speeds access, it makes the old platter unusable and can be an expensive process.

RETRIEVAL WORKSTATION. Once the system is operational, users must have a retrieval workstation to access records that are stored within the system. The most common equipment used for this workstation is the minicomputer. Many of the minicomputers in use today in health care facilities can easily be converted to retrieval stations. The size of the monitor and the resolution of the images vary, depending on the user's needs. The standard monitor has a resolution of 150 dots per inch (DPI), but some monitors can display a much higher resolution. Image resolution requirements are determined by the users' needs, with radiographic film images requiring the highest resolution available.

CACHE MEMORY. An extremely important capability of the workstation is the caching of images.[14] **Cache** (pronounced "cash") **memory** is memory within the magnetic disk on the workstation. When a request is received by the file server, as many images as possible are copied onto the local magnetic disk. Future requests for images that were copied are handled rapidly because the images have been temporarily stored locally on the workstation magnetic disk. Some cache systems attempt to anticipate future data requirements by transferring the data from the optical disk into the cache even if it has not been formally requested.

Caching is done in optical disk systems for two reasons. The first is a reduction in the time it takes to page through the record because the record, in total, is stored on the disk. Therefore, the user would not have to request each page of a record from the file server individually. This capability creates the second reason: Fewer requests are sent to the file server, which decreases access time for all users on the system. Optical systems with caching are, therefore, faster and more efficient.

DATABASE SOFTWARE. One of the most important components of any system is the imaging system software. This part of the system determines the practicality and appropriateness of the system to your environment. As with other software, there are proprietary systems and open, or public domain, systems. **A proprietary system** is owned or copyrighted by an individual or a business and is available for use only through purchase or by permission of the owner. These systems allow for no modification by the user and are specifically written for a particular hardware configuration. In **open systems,** the specifications are made public to encourage third party vendors to develop add-on products for them. These systems are designed to incorporate all kinds of devices, regardless of the manufacturer or model, that can use the same communications facilities and protocols.

PRINTERS. All optical systems must have at least one output device. High-quality laser printers are used to reproduce images that have previously been stored or scanned onto the optical disk. For fastest reproduction speed, printers should be connected directly to the file server.

UNINTERRUPTABLE POWER SUPPLY. Another necessary item is an **uninterruptable power supply (UPS)** or battery to keep the system running during a power failure and to protect it from the power surge associated with power outages. All major pieces of equipment in the optical system should be connected to the UPS, including at least one printer, to assure that vital patient records are continuously available.

FAX TECHNOLOGY. As an optional component, an optical disk system can be combined with a facsimile, or fax, as an additional output device that allows images to be sent to another location over telephone lines.[15] The fax sends images directly from the server rather than routing them to the workstation for printing and then conventional faxing.

System Benefits and Advantages

SPACE SAVINGS. The simplest and easiest to implement use of an optical imaging system is to utilize it as a storage system to replace inactive paper-based records. Although this provides a great space savings, similar to the space saved by the use of micrographics, it does not utilize the technology of optical imaging to the fullest extent.

PRODUCTIVITY GAINS. An optical disk system can dramatically decrease the amount of time spent moving records from one location to another. The tasks of retrieving, assembling, transporting, and filing paper-based records are eliminated. Telephone calls to initiate record searches and requests to copy records on the photocopy machine are also eliminated. By deleting these paper-based steps from the records management process and replacing them with an automated retrieval system such as optical imaging, the facility realizes several important advantages.

One advantage is 24-hour access to records by authorized users without clerical staff assistance at a considerable reduction in retrieval time. There are also no lost or misplaced documents to be searched for and the documents maintain their long-term quality for future use. An additional advantage is the opportunity to use available work hours to complete other tasks, such as monitoring documentation patterns and performing quality studies.

INCREASED USE OF COMPUTER TECHNOLOGY. The use of optical imaging technology encourages the use of computer technology. To retrieve an image, the user must use a workstation, and the workstation displays a familiar-looking document, much like the paper document that has always been used. This familiarity allows the user to easily accept the optical images that are computer-generated, such as laboratory values and transcription output. The optical system helps prepare the user for future information technologies that are completely computer-based.

MULTIUSER ACCESS. One of the greatest benefits of an optical imaging system is that is offers multiuser access to the same information—something that neither paper-based nor microfilmed records can provide. With an optical disk system, many people can view the same information at the same time because each is viewing a copy of the image. Coders, abstractors, and correspondence clerks can all be viewing the record at the same time, providing greater efficiency by eliminating the waiting time for the record before they can perform their functions. A physician treating a patient in the Emergency Department can view the same record from the patient's recent visit to the hospital at the same time as administrative users are viewing it. This has a positive impact on the quality of care that can be provided.

ON-LINE AVAILABILITY OF INFORMATION. An optical imaging system can create an on-line medical record for patients as they are admitted. The system can incorporate data from different sources as it is created electronically at multiple points in the hospital (e.g., Admissions, Laboratory, Radiology). The data are compiled into one record, maintained digitally during hospitalization, and viewed by many users while the patient is being treated. The images remain on magnetic media throughout the completion process and then are moved to an optical disk once the record is complete. The images are stored as a group to one platter, speeding future retrieval time considerably.

Nurses' notes can be stored on separate platters that can be removed from the jukebox in a shorter amount of time than the remainder of the record. The notes could be maintained in a remote jukebox with a much longer exchange time and would not take up space in the jukebox, providing the fastest on-line response time.

SYSTEM SECURITY AND CONTROL. System security is maintained because optical images stored in the system must be viewed at a viewing station. Access to viewing stations can be controlled by the same system security measures that are now used on mainframes. This use of access control makes the optical imaging system more secure than any paper-based or microfilm system could ever be. Paper records and microfilm can easily be removed from the facility by an unethical user. Images stored on the optical disk must be printed to allow their removal from the facility, but even then, the permanent image cannot be removed from the optical disk.

User-specific retrieval of information can be implemented to increase security. Clerks can receive only the portions of the record that are required for their assigned duties. Physicians can view only cases that their facility numbers have been associated with. A physician's billing staff can only view demographics and insurance data and only on those patients whose records carry the physician's facility number. Other user-specific retrieval specifications can be developed to increase security.

DATABASE RETRIEVAL. The optical imaging software can perform database searches for specific information that may have been indexed. If the diagnosis and procedure codes were indexed, the imaging software can form the MPI, disease index, operative index, and physician index that were traditionally done manually or in an abstracting system. After performing a database search for a specific diagnosis, the software displays the list of patients with that diagnosis and can cache their records for immediate review.

Evaluating System Requirements

Once the need for an alternative solution to a storage and retrieval system has been recognized, obtain approval from the appropriate level of authority in the facility to evaluate possible alternatives. Without this prior approval, considerable time and effort may be expended needlessly. Full commitment later usually depends on prior approval to begin the investigation process.

ANALYZE PROBLEMS AND CONCEPTUALIZE SOLUTIONS. As system requirements are being determined, the current problems must be analyzed and appropriate solutions conceptualized. All proposed automated systems must resolve the major problems identified in the current system, not merely add costs.[17] If the proposed system can solve problems without creating long-term additional ones, then the system should be developed in detail, including the following:

- Identifying new or different tasks to be completed in the new system
- Determining the current volume of work and the projected volume of each task to be completed in the new system

- Determining whether the skill levels of the staff need to be adjusted to a higher or lower level in the new system
- Developing productivity targets
- Identifying tasks that could be completed during off-hours
- Interviewing potential system users in the facility to obtain their view of the current system, its problems, and their future needs
- Designing a diagram of the processes in the new system for explanation and training purposes
- Determining equipment needs and specifications

IDENTIFY POTENTIAL VENDORS. Once the system concept has been developed and equipment needs are known, locate a minimum of three vendors who are capable of providing the equipment required, the system integration, and the long-term service needed. System integration is the process of combining all the necessary hardware and software into a system that functions according to the system design. The successful vendor should be able to provide a system with sufficient size and capacity, including expansion capability. The vendor must also provide training and system support, have an exceptional service record, and quote a competitive price on all equipment and services.

Open architecture is the best choice, in most cases, to assure that the system can be integrated from the best possible products that provide the best speed and processing capabilities. The opposite of open architecture is a proprietary system that only uses equipment designed and manufactured by a certain vendor. Open architecture protects the facility's investment against possible vendor bankruptcy or complete closure. It also allows individual pieces of equipment to be exchanged as rapidly as technology advances, not only as rapidly as one vendor makes upgrades. It does carry the risk that one weak piece of equipment could adversely affect the entire system design.[18] This risk can be minimized by thorough investigation of all equipment choices.

Optimal specifications should be set for all equipment required for the system, using speed and processing capabilities as the identifiers. Any equipment that does not meet the optimal specifications should not be considered. If the optimal specifications cannot be met or are met only to a minimum as the equipment is being evaluated, the equipment will probably be obsolete before the installation takes place.

Interview references and visit other health care installations completed by the vendors being considered. Ask the users and the selection committee at the reference facility if they would use the same vendor again and how they could have proceeded differently.

COST/BENEFIT ESTIMATES. The purchase price of an optical disk system can be difficult to justify for many facilities. Although the price of technology has been decreasing over the years, the prices can still seem exorbitant to budgetary decision makers. Cost justification of a system must begin by determining the costs involved with the current system. Both paper-based record costs and micrographics costs need to be included if both are being replaced.

Use the same approach described in Table 6–7 for the comparison of paper-based records and microfilm systems. The cost justification could even involve a comparison of all three systems over a 10-year period, assuming no inflation. Rather than listing the savings of the systems involved, list the costs associated with the process in the system that uses it. For example, if 50,000 fewer photocopies will be made monthly with the optical system, list the cost of 50,000 copies under the paper-based system that uses them. Also include the cost of replacing the photocopier as it becomes no longer usable. If the same 50,000 copies are replaced by 35,000 retrievals on a retrieval workstation and 15,000 prints on the optical system printer, list the cost of 15,000 prints under the optical system. The number of retrieval workstations needed for the system should be calculated but accounted for in the system configuration and overall purchase price of the system. Ongoing costs as well as one-time costs should be included. This cost-based method allows direct comparison of costs for each system.

Direct Costs. Direct costs to include in the analysis are as follows:

- *Photocopy supply costs.* Include the cost per copy times the number of copies made per month in each system.

- *Storage and supply costs.* Include file folders, fasteners, dividers, boxes, warehouse and/or facility space, and shelving costs.

- *Microfilm and supply costs.* Include service bureau charges, film, jackets, equipment, and supplies.

- *Labor costs.* The labor costs involved with all tasks associated with each system can be determined by multiplying the volume of each task times the time it takes to complete the task times the average hourly wage of the staff, including benefits. For example, one record retrieval $\times$ .016 hours $\times$ $10.00 per hour = $0.16.

- *Outside service costs.* Include courier services between facility locations and/or physicians' offices.

Indirect Costs. Attempt to quantify indirect costs, such as the loss of interest income when bills are de-layed in a paper-based system. The faster the bill is delivered to the payer, using efficient methods, the faster the facility is paid and has use of the money to meet commitments and earn interest. The fax feature also speeds the answering of requests for information from third party payers and outside review agencies. The facility Financial Department is able to provide estimates in this area.

Offsetting Revenue. The Financial Department may also be able to provide estimates about revenue that can be produced as a result of installing an optical disk system. Revenue produced by the sale of equipment or the conversion of space should be included. The revenue produced from the eventual sale of unneeded shelving and microfilm readers, reader-printers, and cabinets should be applied to help offset the cost of the optical system. Remember that some equipment may still be needed to maintain the old system as long as the old system is still functional.

Other revenue can be produced when vacated storage space is converted to space for revenue-producing patient care activities. For example, if a facility is interested in establishing a cardiac catheterization unit but cannot find the needed space, transferring paper-based records to an optical system may provide the needed space. If the only factor stopping the development of a profitable catheterization unit is space, the conversion of paper-based records to an optical system will produce savings that can be used to compensate for the purchase price of the optical system.

Optical disk system space itself produces revenue if it is rented to physicians. The physician's office staff can use communication software to access the optical disk system from their office and store their patient records on the system. This practice strengthens the facility-physician bond by providing physicians with an affordable way to use technology they may be unable to afford individually.

UNQUANTIFIABLE BENEFITS. There are benefits associated with any system that are unquantifiable. They should be listed along with the actual cost figures for each system. The benefits and advantages of the optical system that are listed in this chapter should be included as well as improved patient and medical staff satisfaction that can be obtained by installing an efficient system.

OBTAINING COMMITMENT AND PURCHASE AGREEMENT. Prepare a detailed proposal for approval by the budgetary decision makers, usually the Board of Directors of the facility. Include the following major items in the information given to the Board of Directors for review.

- *System diagram.* This diagram is an overview in pictures, using whatever method is normally used in the facility. Use enough detail to make it understandable but not so much that it is overwhelming. Test the diagram with a knowledgeable person who has not been previously exposed to the discussion of the system to be sure that person can understand the system flow.

- *System summary.* This is a written, descriptive overview of the system, sometimes called an executive summary, that explains the system concepts. It identifies the current system and the problems associated with it as well as the proposed system and how it addresses or eliminates these problems. It also includes a description of the hardware needs by areas of the facility.

- *Financial summary.* This is the cost/benefit analysis and may be similar to the one presented in Table 6–7. It should list which system components are to be purchased, which are to be leased or rented, and the purchase timetable.

- *Vendor comparison and references.* This is a listing of the final vendor selection criteria and may be similar to the one presented in Table 6–8. A written summary of the reference checks and installation visits performed should be included.

- *Implementation plan and schedule.* This is a calendar or chart displaying the phases of the implementation with projected timelines, including implementation teams. It should be realistic from both the workflow aspect and the financial aspect.

Be prepared to give a presentation, if it is required, to defend the analysis and assure the approval of the project. There will undoubtedly be questions that even the best documentation cannot answer. If the documentation and presentation are well prepared, the necessary commitment for purchase and installation will be given.

Implementation Strategies

PHASING IN THE NEW SYSTEM. There is no perfect or universal method for phasing in a new optical imaging system. Some sources suggest that the initial place to start is the outpatient area or emergency department of the hospital, continuing with old records instead of microfilm, converting records immediately after discharge, and, finally, on-line patient records at admission.[14]

Others suggest that the new system could be initiated by scanning discharged charts the day after discharge, continuing with hardware installation to the entire facility and interfacing to current electronic systems.[19] Regardless of where the implementation starts, forms should be redesigned to include bar codes for automatic

indexing as soon as possible. The bar codes should be placed in the exact same location on every form and provide sufficient information to identify the patient, the form type, and the date of the documentation contained on the page.

No matter how intense the planning, implementation is never easy. Strong commitment from facility administration and pretesting of all hardware and software before live conversion go a long way toward providing smooth implementation.

All medical staff should be trained in the use of the new system as soon as the final configured system with actual documentation is available. Their office staff should also be trained thoroughly because the medical staff look to them for support when change is happening rapidly. Training the office staff also provides motivation for the physician's office to rent space on the system and further increase the physician's comfort level with the technology.

REDEFINING JOBS AND SKILLS. The introduction of an optical imaging system will result in the need for internal change in the Health Information Department more than in any other department of the facility. The department staff needs to learn as much as possible about their new technology before it is implemented and should help in the redesign of their job functions. Positions will probably not be eliminated with the initial implementation of optical imaging. In an attempt to reduce their fears, employees should be reassured that staffing will be changed but not eliminated. Any eventual staffing decreases that might be realized can be handled through transfers, formal retraining, or attrition.

New position titles will evolve to replace the familiar "file clerk" and "assembler." Titles decided on at the University of Cincinnati Hospital during that facility's job redesign were Image Processing Specialist, Information Processing Specialist, and Record Processing Specialist.[20] The Image Processing Specialist position handles record preparation and scanning. The Information Processing Specialist position handles record completion, release of information, and coordination of input from other sources. The Record Processing Specialist position handles hard-copy reproduction and other record management activities.

Legal Considerations

Each state can specify whether business records reproduced by a particular medium are admissable as evidence but not all have addressed the issue of optical imaging. Even fewer have directly addressed the admissibility of optical images of medical information.

When states address business records as evidence, the Federal Rules of Evidence, Rule 803(6) of the Uniform Rules of Evidence, or the Uniform Photographic Copies of Business and Public Records Act is used as their basis. Facility legal counsel should be consulted for an opinion if the state statutes are unavailable or unclear.

Application in Use: Doyne Hospital in Milwaukee, Wisconsin

John Doyne Hospital in Milwaukee, Wisconsin, uses optical imaging technology in its Department of Radiology.[21] This hospital is a 550-bed teaching tertiary care facility, having an affiliation with the Medical College of Wisconsin. The system uses a fiberoptic network to link two computed tomography scanners and one magnetic resonance imaging unit to two electronic imaging display stations and two referring clinician display stations. The system is called the Picture Archiving and Communication System (PACS).

PACS allows the radiologists to monitor studies that occur throughout the department, report study results quickly, and send images and reports to referring clinicians in a timely manner. Display stations have 19-inch monitors with a 1000-line display (1280 horizontally and 1026 vertically) and a bandwidth of 78 MHz. The display can accommodate from 1 to 16 images per screen, depending on the size of the image. PACS is menu-driven and mouse-activated, and the system is interfaced to the transcription system and an electronic signature software package.

Application in Use: San Jose Medical Center in San Jose, California

The San Jose Medical Center implemented an optical imaging system after 6 months of planning.[21] A team approach was used for developing operational plans and project timelines involving hardware, software, implementation, training, transitions, document flow, and Information Systems Department technical support.

San Jose Medical Center made system decisions to maintain hardware independence by using open architecture, to choose systems that were easy to use, and to implement a system that had a 3-year payback period. The center decided on a PC–local area network (LAN)–based system so that staff could use their existing computer skills. The software choice was a Windows-based application to provide speed in the learning process.

The implementation plan was designed to assure that patient care was not disrupted, that the medical staff was comfortable with the transition, and that the implementation could be done with no additional Health Information Department staff. The transition took place in stages, with newborn patient records entering the system first on July 6, 1991. These records were chosen because of their low volume and low usage, which afforded a "safe" place to start. The Emergency Department was next and provided high visibility for the

successful new system. Ambulatory surgery, maternity care, outpatient, and pediatric records followed in that order. The project was completed in July 1993.

Physicians have responded well and complete their records by one of three methods at San Jose Medical Center. They use autoauthentication during dictation, sign on-line with an electronic stylus (or pen), or sign the hard copy during the patient's stay.

The Health Information Department staff have responded well to the system implementation because it has reduced the frustrations associated with the paper-based system. Three new job titles have been created: Document Preparation/Scan Clerk, Image Processing Technician, and Supervisor, Document Image Processing. These positions have been assumed by current staff; no additional staff has been required.

The medical center realized $116,000 in accounts receivable improvement (getting the bill paid faster) and generated $100,000 in revenue from in-house fulfillment of release of information requests, a previously contracted service that generated no revenue. The medical center has also realized its goals of improving patient care, instituting universal and parallel access to patient records, increasing revenue, and decreasing costs. It learned a few things along the way and recommends that forms be analyzed for size and printing options, staff be pre-educated on the system, job skills be analyzed for position reassignments, and space allocation for the equipment be preplanned. It also recommends celebrating successes and completed milestones as they occur because the implementation process is long and can occur over several years.

ACCESS AND RETENTION OF ELECTRONIC INFORMATION

Integrating Automated Clinical Functions

When patient records are needed for review, one alternative to using the paper record is to have the information displayed on a computer terminal. There are several advantages to this method. The data can be presented in a quick and efficient manner. The requester does not have to wait for someone to deliver a record. There is no worry about losing papers from a computerized record, and with communications software, the results of laboratory or other ancillary testing can be immediately available. Computerized systems increase the availability and immediate accessibility of patient information.

The full computer-based patient record (CPR) is discussed in detail in Chapter 17. Many facilities do not have the full CPR but have computerized significant portions of patient information. Common portions that have already been computerized are the patient registration or admission/discharge/transfer system, the administrative function of financial management, laboratory tests, diagnostic imaging, pharmacy, and medical word processing. The documentation made by physicians, nurses, and therapists at the time the patient is treated (point of care) is the documentation least frequently computerized because it presents the biggest challenge.

With the advent of hand-held computer terminals, pen-based data entry into computers, voice recognition, and unthought of other methods, point-of-care documentation will become easier to capture electronically. When this technology becomes more readily available, economical, and tested, facilities will then be able to combine all the electronic information into one system and begin to build the fully functional CPR with all its characteristics.

To help their facilities in the development of effective electronic storage and retrieval of information, HIM professionals should familiarize themselves with information storage methods, understand communication methods used between computers, keep up to date on current technology, and be able to visualize information flow and start to develop long-term plans or strategies for implementing computerization in the facility.

Application in Use: Regenstrief Medical Record System in Indianapolis, Indiana

The Regenstrief project is the work of a group of physicians in Indiana who thought that a standard paper record, although difficult to maintain and keep track of, could not "audit" itself in a way that a computer record possibly could.[22] Their efforts are worthy of serious attention by HIM professionals who understand the challenges of managing patient information.

HISTORY AND OBJECTIVES. The project began in 1972 with the Regenstrief Health Center Diabetes Clinic, part of Wishard Memorial Hospital in Indiana. The number of patients to be entered into the system when it began was 35. The first task to be accomplished was to capture data concerning the patient, such as diagnoses, test results, and medications. The second task was to develop programs based on the data that would organize and interpret it in ways that would be useful. It had initially been thought that designing and creating monitors, reminders, and meaningful reports would be the heart of the work. The developers of the system soon discovered that the input (capturing the data) was the most difficult part of the process.

The Regenstrief system has grown tremendously and now contains information on more than 500,000 patients (more than 70 million encounters) at three hospitals at Indiana University as well as 30 clinics and other health care sites in Indiana. The objectives of getting the

data organized, displayed, and producing reminders for the clinicians have been met to a remarkable degree. The task of inputting the data into the computer in a timely, efficient manner is the task that still receives the most attention.

SPECIFICS OF THE SYSTEM. The Regenstrief system uses hardware ranging from desktop personal computers to large-scale mainframes from the Digital Equipment Corporation (DEC). The large computers can be clustered together to provide a multiprocessing environment that serves thousands of on-line users. The system uses a relational database. In this type of database, relationships between files are strictly logical, through matching numbers or names. Ad hoc reporting is facilitated in a relational database. The programs for the system are written in a language proprietary to DEC computers.

The facilities connected in the system are Wishard Memorial Hospital and Clinics (400 beds), Roudebush Veterans Administration Medical Center and Clinics (400 beds), Indiana University Hospital and Riley Hospital Combined (6000 beds), 5 public health clinics, 2 neighborhood clinics, and 19 freestanding clinics. The hospitals within the system are independently managed and geographically separate. Although each hospital has a dedicated computer, the computers are all housed in the Wishard Memorial Hospital. They are connected to the outlying hospitals by fiberoptic cable links. A fiberoptic cable carries light rather than electricity and is made of a thin fiber of glass. Large amounts of data can be transferred by way of a single fiberoptic cable. While authorized users are physically seated at a terminal in one institution, they can obtain information about a patient at another institution. A 960-character-per-second telephone communication cable links outlying clinics with the computers at Wishard Memorial Hospital. Each clinic is capable of having 8 to 16 terminals and 2 laser printers served by the line.

DATA INPUT. As mentioned earlier, the designers and users of the system have discovered that data input can be difficult. The consistency of the data obtained varies, based on the conditions at the institution and the practices of the clinicians. The system allows capture of data in three ways: (1) electronic capture of data through interfaces, (2) data entry from special forms, and (3) direct physician entry.

Electronic Capture of Data. For computers to communicate, or interface, two tasks must be undertaken. First, programs must be written to translate representation of data in one system into a representation compatible with the other system. Second, the terminology that is used by the different ancillary services must be translated into terms that can be understood by both the different computer systems and the users. The way data is coded into a billing system may be quite different than the way it is understood by a clinician. To alleviate this problem, there needs to be a mapping process of one department's coded data to the actual patient record codes. For the Regenstrief project, the designers developed a common dictionary definition that could easily be understood by all facilities.

Within the system, the use of electronic data capture and transmission is common. There are interfaces to bedside terminals to capture vital signs for both inpatients and outpatients. Also, there are interfaces to 18 other systems: 3 patient registration, 3 laboratory, 3 pharmacy, 2 appointment scheduling, 2 medical word processing, and 5 billing systems.

With medical word processing, the reports are frequently typed without a mandatory patient identification number. There is a computer check that must be done to validate whether the information is correct. With ancillary services, this often is automatically printed out by the computer, so that there is no doubt that the patient number and date are correct. With the departments of radiology, nuclear medicine, and surgical pathology, the information is entered into the computer directly, so that the information is validated at the point of entry.

Forms and Manual Entry. In most computer systems, free text is not accepted but rather must be represented as codes. For programs in the Regenstrief system, certain terms have been programmed into the system, allowing a technician to enter a term and have the code be automatically assigned. When a report is displayed or printed, the actual term is used rather than the computer code.

Forms, created by a word processor, have a printed format that allows for easy data entry (check-off or fill in the blank). A corresponding input form is created on the computer screen in the same format as the paper forms and allows the data entry clerk to enter the information into the computer easily. The Regenstrief project has found that using this method to code and enter the encounter forms for patients can reduce the number of personnel in such areas as quality assurance, utilization review, and abstracting.

Physician Entry. In a computer system, just as in a paper system, physicians are more eager to retrieve information than to write or dictate it. For the most part, the paper forms are interpreted and coded by personnel other than the physician and entered into the system. There are promising signs in Indiana, however, and physicians are beginning to enter many notes, orders, and problem lists directly into the computer.

The system began with the entry of physician orders, rather than notes. This decision was made for several reasons. The orders have a more uniform structure and a potential to shape practice patterns by providing computer feedback on the orders. When a physician enters an order into the system, the value of computerization

can immediately be realized. Edits can be built into the system that alert the clinician to risks for certain patients and error checks that provide a preventive quality control measure. Also, the cost of the treatment or medication can be displayed for the physician to take into consideration when ordering. The system also helps the physician refine the orders. When a general panel or test is ordered, the computer can ask the physician to be more specific and, therefore, cost-effective.

The personal computers used by the physicians are linked to the mainframe computer for entering the orders. By using the computer screen, the physician has access to the *American Hospital Formulary,* the *Scientific American's Textbook of Medicine,* and flowsheets or graphs concerning the patient. Also, some reminders for the physician to keep in mind when prescribing a specific drug or treatment appear on the screen as orders are entered. For example, there are prerequisite requirements for a premenopausal woman to undergo a pregnancy test before having an abdominal computer tomographic scan. There are also reminders for the physician concerning when follow-up tests or preventive measures are due, based on the patient's condition and rules that have been defined by physicians in the care protocols.

Another feature of the system is that it provides pocket cards for the house staff to use when making rounds in the hospital. The cards are reduced, laser-printed versions of what the ordering system has stored for each patient and are reproduced so that two "pages" of information fit on an $8\frac{1}{2} \times 11$ sheet of paper. They can be folded and carried in the physician's pocket and have proved to be quite popular.

REPORTS AND OUTPUT OF THE SYSTEM. The system produces reports that can be printed out and placed in the patient's paper record. The encounter form is the most commonly used form. It includes a listing of the patient's diagnoses. The physician is asked to cross out the diagnoses that no longer apply and circle the diagnosis that led to this encounter. This helps in identifying the correct diagnosis for billing purposes.

Certain sections of the form are tailored for the different types of specialties and patients. For example, different items are captured for internal medicine patients that are not applicable in the perinatal clinic. The forms are completed by a nurse or physician and entered into the computer by a technician at a later time.

The physician can also write free text in a large write-in area. With free text, however, there are currently no resources to invest in transcription of notes; therefore, it is not entered in the computer.

The bottom area of the form is where the clinic orders are written. The system may print out certain orders for specific patients or alert the physician with messages and reminders about what may need to be ordered or discontinued. They may differ by specialty.

Certain sites within the system have electronic access to the patient's prescription history, and a second page of the encounter form is a list of medications for the patient from all sites. The form is used as a prescription form for the encounter, and the physician can reorder medications by simply documenting the amount of the drug to dispense next to the name of the drug on the form.

The system can also produce a discharge summary or abstract of the patient's current conditions. Each of the clinics can determine the variables that will be part of their particular abstract.

Another feature of the system is to produce flowsheets that summarize the patient's status and findings (i.e., test results). These flowsheets can be placed in the patient's record. A new flowsheet is printed for each encounter. The new flowsheet is filed in the record and the old one is discarded, helping to assure that the information is current.

TERMINAL VIEWING OF INFORMATION. One of the greatest advantages of the system is that any of the users can access the patient information that is stored on the computer, using one of the more than 100 computer terminals located throughout the facilities. Any printed output can be viewed. For example, if a physician wants to review a patient's serum levels in reference to the reaction from diuretic treatment, he or she could simply type in "diuretics, electrolytes" at the point where the system asks the user for variables of interest. The computer would then display a flowsheet that shows the daily doses of the patient's diuretics and the corresponding electrolyte values for those time frames.

The physician can also view radiology reports, cytology reports, discharge summaries, the patient's past and future appointments, and prescriptions on any computer terminal.

ADMINISTRATIVE SERVICES. The Regenstrief medical record system helps with the functions of appointment scheduling, patient registration, management reporting, and collection of data for billing. Within the appointment system, there are ways in which the computer can assist in the appointment-making process. For example, if a patient needs to see a number of physicians on the same day, the system can schedule it so that all the appointments can be made without inconvenience or overlap in time.

The designers of the Regenstrief system have learned many things over the years of developing their system. They advise that future systems should be more flexible in allowing both structured data and free text. Free text is very understandable to users and could be directly entered by the clinician. They also advise that check digits should be used on the patient numbers, registration numbers, and providers' numbers. These digits can

prevent misfiles of patient data and duplicate patient registration numbers. The designers highly recommend building the computerized system in stages, accomplishing the easiest tasks first, such as electronic data transfer. They do not recommend trying to capture data recorded in script by clinicians but rather advocate the use of technicians to enter information written by clinicians. Once the physicians are convinced that the computer is their ally and see what it can do for them, then their habits will change and they will become more willing to comply.

Key Concepts

- Paper-based records are the most common records found in health care today, although it is widely recognized that paper is not the best media for all situations. Image-based records and electronically stored information are two alternatives.

- Records are identified by two methods, alphabetic identification and numeric identification. Alphabetic identification uses the patient's name as the identifier for the record, and numeric identification uses a number, either supplied by the patient or assigned by the facility.

- Paper records are stored in different types of equipment. Filing cabinets work well for small files, compressible files work well for medium and moderately active files, and open-shelf files work well for large, active files.

- Filing systems can be either centralized or decentralized and use one of the three common filing methodologies: alphabetic filing, straight numeric filing, or terminal digit filing.

- File folders for paper records should be chosen after considering the size of the average record, the usage rate of the record, and the type of filing equipment used to store the record. Filing efficiency can be enhanced by choosing colored folders or by adding color coding to a plain folder.

- Manual record-tracking systems use outguides, requisitions, and transfer notices as their primary tools. Outguides mark the spot where a record was removed; requisitions list the patient identifiers and requester; transfer notices alert the file personnel that a record has been moved to a new location.

- Automated record-tracking systems hold the requisition and transfer information in a database. They allow computerized requesting of records and on-line inquiry regarding the current record location.

- Paper-based systems require large amounts of storage space. As records become less actively used, the format or media is often changed to reduce the storage space they require. Imaged-based systems, such as micrographics and optical imaging, are considered an acceptable alternative.

- Micrographics programs offer the different micro-form options of roll microfilm, jacket microfilm, microfiche, CAR-roll microfilm, and CAR-jacket microfilm. Computer output microfilm can also be used to store computer output in a miniaturized form.

- Facilities must choose between completing the microfilming process in-house and using a contracted microfilm service bureau. In-house microfilming requires the purchase of a camera, developer, and jacket loader as well as management of the staff to complete the process. A service bureau charges for its work at a negotiated price per 1000 images of film.

- An optical imaging system uses special disk platters that are written and read by a laser beam. Other system components include a scanner, workstation, file server, jukebox, and printer.

- An optical imaging system can be costly, but the cost can be justified by considering the space savings, productivity gains, multiuser access, on-line availability of information, and increased system security.

- The legality of optical imaging records as admissible evidence in court is determined differently in each state, and opinions should be obtained from the facility attorney.

- The electronic storage and retrieval of information such as laboratory results and medical word processing are the preliminary steps necessary in the evolution to the computer-based patient record.

References

1. Skurka M: Health information management in hospitals: Principles and organization for health record services. Chicago, American Hospital Publishing, 1994.
2. Estep B, Kirk R: Relocating a medical record department: "A moving experience." J Am Med Record Assoc 1986;57(6):22.
3. Bertrand M: Moving a medical record department: A case study. Topics in Health Record Management 1985;6(2):65.
4. Johnson M, Kallaus W: Records management. Cincinnati, Southwestern Publishing Co., 1982.
5. Allen B, Barr C: The impact of automated medical record tracking systems on the ability to reduce staff —a research study. J Am Health Information Management Assoc 1993;64(9):74.
6. Glass B, Mitchell S: The ambulatory care medical record: An administrative nightmare. J Med Group Management 1992; 39(5):60.
7. Majerowicz A: Selection and implementation of a bar code–based record management system in ambulatory care. J Am Med Records Assoc 1990;61(5):29.
8. Platz K, Thoman D, Craft T: Making tracks at the University of Iowa Hospitals and Clinics: Design and implementation of a bar coded medical records tracking system. J Am Med Records Assoc 1990;61(9):45.
9. Lach J, Longe K: Bar coding and the medical record manager. J Am Med Records Assoc 1987;58(11):24.
10. Tomes J: Healthcare records: A practical legal guide. Dubuque, IA, Kendall Hunt Publishing Company for the Health Care Financial Management Association, 1990.
11. American Hospital Association: Preservation of medical records in health care institutions. Chicago, AHA Institutional Practices Committee, 1990.
12. Position Statement Issue: Protecting patient information after a closure. Chicago, American Health Information Management Association, 1994.
13. Lauersen N, Hochberg H, George M: Microfilm storage of fetal monitoring records: A practical solution. Obstet Gynecol 1978;51(5):632.
14. McLendon K: Optical disk imaging—tomorrow's technology today for medical records. J Am Med Records Assoc 1990;61(2):32.
15. Sjogren K: The technical evolution of document image processing. J Am Health Information Management Assoc 1993; 64(4):70.
16. Spencer D: Webster's New World Dictionary of computer terms, 4th ed. New York, Simon & Schuster, 1992.
17. Kahl K, Casey D: How to evaluate and implement office automation. J Am Med Records Assoc 1984;55(8):20.
18. Little E: Starting up an imaging system: Lessons learned. J Am Health Information Management Assoc 1993;64(4):61.
19. Barbetta M: Optical imaging system implementation: Our experience. J Am Health Information Management Assoc 1993; 64(4):54.
20. Mahoney M, Doupnik A: Health information department reorganization resulting from the implementation of optical imaging. J Am Health Information Management Assoc 1993;64(4):56.
21. Kohn D: Optical technology demonstrates benefits. Computers in Health Care 1991;12(5):22–26.
22. McDonald C, Tierney W, Overhage J, et al: The Regenstrief medical record system: 20 years of experience in hospitals, clinics, and neighborhood health centers. MD Computing 1992;9(4):206.

7

ELIZABETH D. BOWMAN

KEY WORDS

Ambulatory Patient Groups
Attestation
Case mix systems
Classification
Coding
Comorbidity
Complication
Cooperating Parties
Diagnosis Related Groups (DRGs)
Encoder
Grouper
ICD-9-CM Coordination and Maintenance Committee
Index
Nomenclature
Operating room procedure
Principal diagnosis
Resource Based Relative Value Scale (RBRVS)
Severity of Illness System
Significant procedure
Unbundling
Uniform Hospital Discharge Data Set (UHDDS)

ABBREVIATIONS

APG—Ambulatory Patient Groups
CPT—*Current Procedural Terminology*
DRG—Diagnosis Related Groups
DSM—*Diagnostic and Statistical Manual*
HCFA—Health Care Financing Administration
HCPCS—*HCFA Common Procedure Coding System*
ICD-9-CM—*International Classification of Diseases, Ninth Revision, Clinical Modification*
ICD-O—*International Classification of Diseases, Oncology*
NCHS—National Center for Health Statistics
NHDS—National Hospital Discharge Survey
PRO—Peer Review Organization
RBRVS—Resource-Based Relative Value Scale

CODING AND CLASSIFICATION SYSTEMS

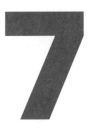

7

SNDO—Standard Nomenclature of Diseases and Operations

SNOMED—Systematized Nomenclature of Human and Veterinary Medicine

SNOP—Systematized Nomenclature of Pathology

UB-92—Uniform Bill, 1992

UHDDS—Uniform Hospital Discharge Data Set

OBJECTIVES

After reading this chapter, the reader should be able to:
- Define key words.
- Identify the abbreviations commonly used in coding and classification.
- Discuss the purpose of coding.
- Identify the major coding systems currently in use.
- Describe the system used to keep ICD-9-CM and CPT updated.
- Outline the process by which records are coded in both the inpatient and the ambulatory setting.
- Summarize the factors that affect coding for reimbursement.
- Explain the PRO review process.
- Differentiate between the types of encoders and give the advantages and disadvantages of each type.
- Determine ethical problems that coders might face and suggest methods of dealing with them.
- Discuss the factors that constitute quality data and how to determine whether data is of adequate quality.
- Categorize the factors that must be considered in hiring, training, and retaining coding personnel.
- Distinguish between concurrent and retrospective coding and give the advantages and disadvantages of each method.
- Describe the services provided by contract coding and DRG review companies and discuss the issues involved in choosing to use such services.
- List coding systems, other than ICD-9-CM and CPT, that are in use in facilities currently.
- Compare the systems that facilities use in case mix and severity of illness determinations.
- Examine the factors that influence a facility's selection of a classification system.

DEFINITION OF CODING

Coding is classifying data and assigning a representation for that data. In abstracting, for example, numbers may be used to code the patient's sex, such as 1 = female, 2 = male, 3 = unknown. This chapter discusses the concept of coding diagnoses and procedures, called clinical coding. When the numbers are assigned for diagnoses and procedures, codes are used from either a nomenclature or a classification system.

Nomenclature System

A **nomenclature** is a systematic listing of proper names. A list of the Latin names of flowers, for example, is a nomenclature. A disease nomenclature is a listing of the proper name for each disease, and each disease is given its own code number. Parkinson's disease, parkinsonian syndrome, and paralysis agitans are different names for the same disease. A nomenclature, however, might indicate that the proper name for this disease is parkinsonian syndrome. An example of a nomenclature currently used is the *Systematized Nomenclature of Human and Veterinary Medicine*.

Classification System

Classification is the grouping together of similar items. A classification of cereals, for example, might group together all cereals into certain types, such as oat, rice, wheat, or a combination of grains. It would be helpful for a cereal company, in planning a new product, to know whether more people eat wheat cereal than eat rice cereal. In a **classification** of diseases and operations, similar diseases and operations are grouped together under a single code. A common example of a classification of diagnoses and procedures is the *International Classification of Diseases, Ninth Revision, Clinical Modification* (ICD-9-CM). In that system, code 537.89 —Other Specified Disorders of Stomach and Duodenum, for example, includes such varied conditions as gastric or duodenal prolapse or rupture, intestinal metaplasia of gastric mucosa, and passive congestion of the stomach. In looking at health care policy, it might be useful to see which groups of diseases are causing the most illness or death.

Attempts have been made to name and classify diseases and operations for centuries, and many methods have been used. Hippocrates was known to have classified diseases according to the part of the body they affected or according to some analogy he saw between disease types.[1] In the early 20th century in the United States, nomenclatures were often developed for use in a particular hospital. Bellevue Hospital in New York City and Massachusetts General Hospital in Boston both developed nomenclatures that were then adopted by other hospitals.[1] Having hospital-specific nomenclatures, however, made it difficult to compare information on diseases and operations across the country. The *Standard Classified Nomenclature of Diseases,* later known as the *Standard Nomenclature of Diseases and Operations* (SNDO), was developed to solve this problem. It classified diseases according to their topography (site) and etiology (cause). SNDO was the predominant coding system until the 1950s and 1960s. By that time, the classification of diseases using only two factors was thought to be too simplistic for increasing medical knowledge.

During the late 1940s and into the 1960s, hospitals began to use the *International Classification of Diseases* for coding. This system was derived from the Bertillon Classification adopted in 1891 that classified causes of deaths.[1] It has been revised about every 10 years since 1891. A revision is first done by the World Health Organization (WHO) for use throughout the world. Often this WHO version does not completely meet the needs for coding in the United States because it emphasizes more acute, infective processes seen in underdeveloped countries rather than the chronic diseases, such as arteriosclerosis and hypertension, so prevalent in the United States. For that reason, it is modified for use in the United States. ICD-9-CM is the modification of the WHO revision called ICD-9. ICD-9 is used in the United States for coding death certificates, but ICD-9-CM is used in health facilities such as hospitals and clinics.

Physicians' office coding sprung from a need for an easy, uniform, and accurate way for physicians to report their services to third party payers. *Current Procedural Terminology* (CPT) was developed in the 1960s to meet that need.

PURPOSES OF CODING

Coding is performed for a variety of reasons. A primary reason is to permit retrieval of information according to diagnosis or procedure. If a physician requests a list of patients who have had a myocardial infarction, the health information management department must have a way to find these patients. Coding allows these cases to be retrieved because all patients who have had a myocardial infarction are assigned the same code number. The code numbers are then entered into a computer database and can be easily retrieved. Entering the information as a code number makes entering and retrieving the information easier than entering the verbal statement of the diagnosis or procedure. This is because a standardized number is assigned regardless of what terminology the physician uses for the diagnosis or procedure. Such varied terminology as influenza, flu, and La grippe would all have the same code number, 487.1. Health professionals may want to retrieve information on diagnoses and procedures to do research on a particular disease or operation or to perform quality assessment studies.

Under current payment methods, coding is also an important part of reimbursement. Medicare, for example, pays the hospital based on the **Diagnosis Related Group (DRG)**. The main factor that determines which DRG is assigned for the patient is the code number to indicate the reason the patient entered the hospital.

CODING SYSTEMS IN USE

International Classification of Diseases, Ninth Revision, Clinical Modification

The most common coding system used to code hospital inpatients is the ICD-9-CM. Although ICD is usually revised every 10 years, ICD-9-CM was published in 1979 and has not yet been totally revised. It is believed that the 10th revision will not appear before the year 2000. ICD-9-CM has required many updates since 1979 to keep it current with changing medical practice.

The responsibility for keeping ICD-9-CM accurate and up to date is shared by two federal agencies. The National Center for Health Statistics (NCHS) is responsible for changes to the disease classification, and the Health Care Financing Administration (HCFA) is responsible for changes to the procedure classification. To help them in this process, an advisory committee, the **ICD-9-CM Coordination and Maintenance Committee,** has been established. It consists of ICD-9-CM users from the federal government, such as the Veterans Affairs Hospitals and the Indian Health Service, but provides an open forum for anyone interested in changing the classification system. Changes are published each fall to become effective on October 1. Revisions often include provision for additional detail in coding diagnoses. One change, for example, allowed coders to identify the episode of care for patients with myocardial infarctions. Other changes provide codes for new conditions, such as human immunodeficiency virus infections, and new procedures.

Two other organizations, along with NCHS and HCFA, make up the **Cooperating Parties** for ICD-9-

CM. The first is the American Hospital Association, which maintains the Central Office on ICD-9-CM. The Central Office answers ICD-9-CM coding questions and publishes the *Coding Clinic,* a newsletter that provides official coding advice. The second organization is the American Health Information Management Association (AHIMA). It develops a certification examination that experienced coders can take to become credentialed Certified Coding Specialists. AHIMA also includes the Council on Coding and Classification, which is made up of volunteer members who provide leadership for the Association in the area of coding (see Cooperating Parties for ICD-9-CM). They develop coding guidelines and deal with issues related to coding. As part of AHIMA, there is also the Society for Clinical Coding, a membership organization for people interested in coding.

HCFA Common Procedure Coding System

Another widely used coding system is the *HCFA Common Procedure Coding System* (HCPCS), which consists of three levels of codes:

Level 1 *Current Procedural Terminology*
Level 2 National codes
Level 3 Local codes

Level 1 codes, CPT, were developed in the 1960s by the American Medical Association (AMA) for physician coding, and physicians' offices continue to use it to report their services. When HCPCS was developed, the already-existing CPT codes became the basis of the system. In addition, Level 2 national codes were developed by HCFA for procedures needed for the national reimbursement systems, such as Medicare and Medicaid, but local codes not covered by CPT and Level 3 were developed by the fiscal intermediaries (the companies responsible for processing bills for Medicare) for proce-

dures not provided a code in levels 1 and 2 but seen and reported on the local level. CPT codes are strictly for physicians' services, so the codes in Levels 2 and 3 were needed to include items like dental care and ambulance service. Level 2 and Level 3 codes can be distinguished from Level 1 CPT codes because they are alphanumeric, whereas CPT codes are strictly numeric.

A new version of CPT is published every year. The AMA has a CPT editorial panel that is responsible for the yearly revision of the CPT codes. It consists of 14 physician members—10 from the AMA and 1 each from the Blue Cross and Blue Shield Association, the Health Insurance Association of America, the HCFA, and the American Hospital Association.[2] Two advisory committees also provide input into this process. The first is the CPT Advisory Committee, composed of 60 physicians, and the second is the Health Care Professionals Advisory Committee, consisting of allied health professionals and professionals with limited license.[2] Changes include deletion of codes for procedures that are no longer done and inclusion of codes for new procedures or methods of performing surgery. The AMA also publishes *CPT Assistant,* a newsletter that provides coding advice on using the CPT system. The Level 2 national HCPCS codes are updated by HCFA, and the Level 3 local codes are updated by each fiscal intermediary for the area they serve (see Organizations Responsible for Maintaining HCPCS). HCFA reviews the local codes periodically to see if some of them need to move from Level 3 to Level 2 because they are becoming generally reported on the national level.

Currently, ICD-9-CM procedure codes are used for inpatients and HCPCS/CPT procedure codes are used for patients seen in the ambulatory setting. The National Committee on Vital and Health Statistics is evaluating the factors to be considered in developing a new procedure coding system that would replace both the ICD-9-CM procedure codes and the CPT codes.[3] Having a uniform procedure coding system would alleviate the confusion over which system to use in which setting.

Cooperating Parties for ICD-9-CM	
Organization	Responsibility
• National Center for Health Statistics	• Maintaining the disease classification
• Health Care Financing Administration	• Maintaining the procedure classification
• American Hospital Association	• Central Office on ICD-9-CM • Coding Clinic
• American Health Information Management Association	• Coder certification • Education • Council on Coding and Classification

Organizations Responsible for Maintaining HCPCS

HCPCS Level	Responsible Organization
Level 1 CPT	American Medical Association CPT Editorial Panel CPT Advisory Committee Health Care Professionals Advisory Committee
Level 2 National Codes	Health Care Financing Administration
Level 3 Local Codes	Local fiscal intermediary or carrier

INPATIENT CODING PROCESS
(FIGURE 7–1)

The procedure followed in coding varies from facility to facility. Coding should, however, always begin with a thorough review of the patient's record. It is important for the coder to obtain an overall picture of the patient's problems and the care received. Sometimes the record that the coder reviews is complete and contains all documentation, including a discharge summary. Often, however, the record is incomplete. The coder must select the conditions and/or procedures to code from the available documentation in the record. In that process, the coder is guided by the physician's diagnosis and procedure statement, if available, as well as by symptoms, medications, and other treatments that may point

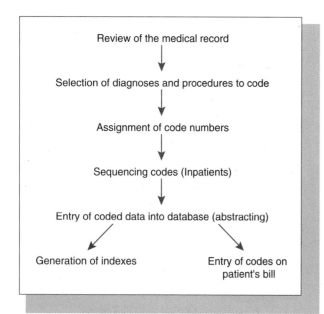

FIGURE 7–1. The coding process.

to diagnoses or procedures that have been missed and additional information about the diagnoses or procedures identified by the physician. In coding pneumonia, for example, the coder may check the culture and sensitivity report to determine the infectious agent that has caused the pneumonia. If the coder makes changes in the physician's diagnosis and procedure statement, the physician's approval should be obtained. Once the diagnoses and procedures have been determined, code numbers are assigned.

The coder's job is not finished at this point. The codes have to be sequenced. Diagnoses are sequenced based on the **Uniform Hospital Discharge Data Set (UHDDS)** definitions. The coder must first select the **principal diagnosis.** According to UHDDS, the principal diagnosis is the reason, after study, that caused the patient to enter the hospital. If a patient comes into the hospital with the chief complaint of upper right quadrant pain and then is diagnosed as having cholecystitis, the principal diagnosis is cholecystitis. It is not necessarily the most serious problem that the patient has. The patient with cholecystitis might fall out of bed and break a hip while in the hospital, and although a serious problem, it is not the reason the patient entered the hospital and is not the principal diagnosis. The principal diagnosis code should be listed first followed by any other diagnosis codes. All **significant procedures** should be coded and listed. The UHDDS defines a significant procedure as one that is surgical in nature, or carries a procedural risk, or carries an anesthetic risk, or requires special training. Each hospital should develop guidelines on what procedures should be coded.

If the coder encounters problems in assigning codes or determining the principal diagnosis, the physician responsible for the case should be consulted for assistance.

Once the codes have been assigned and sequenced, they must be entered into the computer. This step is part of a process called abstracting. In abstracting, pertinent information about the patient is entered into the computer. In some facilities, this is done directly into the terminal. In other facilities, a paper abstract is prepared first (Figure 7–2), and then the information is entered into the computer. Part of the information entered about the patient includes the properly sequenced codes for diagnoses and procedures. The codes are therefore part of a database that includes all discharged patients, and from this database a variety of reports can be generated. The reports that are produced from coded data include a disease **index** (see Disease Index), which lists all cases in disease code number order, and an operation index, which lists all procedures in procedure code number order. The codes must also be placed on the patient's bill. In some cases, the computer automatically sends the codes to another computer program to be entered on the patient's bill. If no such method is

HEALTH INFORMATION MANAGEMENT ABSTRACT

1. Last Name _____ First Name _____ Middle Initial _____

2. Medical Record Number _____

3. Birthdate _____

4. Age _____

5. Race _____ (W-White, B-Black)

6. Sex _____ (M-Male, F-Female)

7. Street Address _____

8. City _____ State _____ Zip Code _____

9. Admission Date _____

10. Discharge Date _____

11. Attending Physician Number _____

12. Service _____

13. Principal Diagnosis _____

14. Other Diagnoses _____

15. Principal Procedure _____

16. Procedure Date _____

17. Other Procedures _____

18. Procedure Dates _____

19. Operating Physician Number _____

20. Death _____ (1-Died, 2-Discharged Alive)

21. Autopsy _____ (1-Yes, 2-No)

22. DRG _____

23. MDC _____

24. Emergency Room _____ (1-Yes, 2-No)

25. Physical Therapy _____ (1-Yes, 2-No)

26. Consultation _____ (1-Yes, 2-No)

FIGURE 7–2. Abstract form.

Disease Index			
Diagnosis	MR#	Age	Sex
008.8	0796	32	2
070.9	0730	24	2
162.9	0016	66	2
	0027	72	1
216.3	1933	31	1
220	1990	28	2
250.40	1081	80	1
366.9	0664	64	2
410.81	0533	51	1
414.0	0427	54	2
	0700	46	1
	1219	46	2
427.81	0547	66	2
463	0620	16	1
474.0	0412	7	1
481	0505	60	1
482.8	1321	90	1
486	0609	46	2
	0639	23	2
550.11	0596	87	1
550.90	0807	16	1
	1243	40	1
560.39	1788	75	2
562.11	1174	41	1
565.0	0515	49	2
574.10	0476	51	2
	1380	59	2
592.1	0403	28	2
	0455	28	1
	0528	30	1
607.84	1292	48	1
634.91	0060	29	2
	0592	29	2
645.01	0061	39	2
669.51	1047	30	2
722.10	0710	40	1
823.82	0458	94	2
846.0	0770	55	2
901.41	1417	29	1
998.8	1511	46	1

available in the hospital, a list of the coded information is sent to the business office to be entered on the bill.

CODING FOR REIMBURSEMENT

There are many important reasons for coding, including retrieval of information for patient care, planning, and facility management as well as reimbursement. When coding for reimbursement, the coder must become aware that the code becomes a communication mechanism between the provider of the care and the insurer or other third party payer. The coder must, therefore, become familiar with the reimbursement system to communicate accurately.

Historically, inpatient care was paid for on a per diem basis. The hospital received a certain payment for each day of basic care, which included the cost of room, board, and nursing services. Each additional service, such as radiography, laboratory tests, and medications, was paid for separately, over and above the basic per diem rate. Another method of reimbursement is called prospective payment. Under the prospective payment system, the facility is paid a flat rate for the stay that is set prospectively, or before the patient is even hospitalized. For example, if you are having a deck built onto your house, there are two ways you can pay for it. You can pay the workers by the day along with a separate amount for materials, such as lumber and stain. The second method is to pay the workers a flat amount for the total job. Under the first method, the workers might have an incentive to take a long time to complete the work and to use more expensive materials. The second method would provide an incentive to get the job done as quickly as possible with the most reasonable cost of materials. It was thought that prospective payment methods in health care would provide similar incentives for hospitals to provide the most efficient and effective care possible, thus cutting the patient's length of stay and unnecessary expenses.

In the early 1980s, the federal government chose to pay for care to Medicare inpatients using a prospective payment system based on DRGs. Some states and other third party payers have also switched to DRG payment. Since a classification is a system that divides patients into groups based on diagnostic and procedural information, DRGs are, therefore, another classification system. In this case the groups are based on use of resources. Under this system, the codes for each patient are entered into a computer program called a **grouper.** The basic method used by the grouper is first to divide the patients into large groups called Major Diagnostic Categories, which are based on the body system affected in the principal diagnosis. Next the grouper determines whether this is a medical DRG or a surgical DRG by looking at the procedure codes and looking for **operating room (OR) procedure** codes. When DRGs were developed, it was decided that medical cases would be separated from surgical cases based on whether the patient had a procedure in the OR. Which operations were done in the OR could vary from facility to facility, so all procedure codes were reviewed to determine whether or not they would be considered OR procedures. A list of OR procedure codes was then produced.[4] Finally, the grouper looks for complications and comorbidities. **Complications** are conditions that arise during a patient's hospitalization and are expected to increase the length of stay by 1 day for 75 per cent of patients. A **comorbidity** is a condition the patient had, in addition to the principal diagnosis, when entering the hospital and that is expected to increase the length of stay by 1 day for 75 per cent of patients. Cases in which the patient had a complication or comorbidity are usually reimbursed at a rate higher than that for cases in which the patient did not have a complication or comorbidity. Although this is the basic method by which DRGs are assigned, there are many other factors that may affect the assignment of individual DRGs, such as patient age and discharge status.

EFFECT OF THE DRG REIMBURSEMENT SYSTEM ON THE CODING PROCESS

Basic coding principles should be followed regardless of who is paying the bill. The coder must, however, be aware of how the codes affect reimbursement.

- First, because the DRG assignment depends on the selection of the principal diagnosis, the coder must be careful in reviewing the patient record and assigning the principal diagnosis code.
- Next, coders must be certain to identify all OR procedures because they affect DRG assignment also and because surgical DRGs usually pay more than do related medical DRGs.
- Finally, complications and comorbidities must be identified because in many cases, their presence increases reimbursement to the hospital.

Most code books have the OR procedures and the complications and comorbidities marked or color-coded to help the coder. An updated list of OR procedures and complications and comorbidities is also printed yearly in the *Federal Register*. Factors other than principal diagnosis, complications and comorbidities, and OR procedures may affect individual DRGs. The coder must, therefore, be familiar with the DRG system.

Formerly, the attending physician was required to sign an **attestation** statement for Medicare cases before the claim could be submitted. When the DRG system was developed, HCFA wanted the physician, not the coder, to determine the principal diagnosis as well as other diagnoses and procedures that affect DRG assignment. The attestation form was developed to ensure that this happened. In September 1995, as a part of regulatory reform in the Medicare program, HCFA published the final rule eliminating the physician attestation form for Medicare cases. As of July 11, 1995, Medicare no longer required physicians to sign the form to process Medicare hospital claims.

CHAMPUS claims still need attestation by the physician. For CHAMPUS cases, the physician must affirm the selection of the principal diagnosis, the secondary diagnoses, and the procedures performed through the following statement:

> I certify that the narrative descriptions of the principal and secondary diagnoses and the major procedures performed are accurate and complete to the best of my knowledge.

According to Medicare reimbursement regulations, the physician must sign an acknowledgment statement when becoming a member of the medical staff, which contains the following:

> **Notice to Physicians:** Medicare payment to hospitals is based in part on each patient's principal and secondary diagnoses and the major procedures performed on the patient, as attested to by the patient's attending physician by virtue of his or her signature in the medical

---

FIGURE 7–3. Attestation form.

DRG 198 Cholecystectomy without common duct exploration without cc

HCFA wt. 0.8757

Principal Diagnosis

574.00 Calculus of gallbladder with acute cholecystitis, without mention of obstruction

Principal Procedure

51.23 Laparoscopic cholecystectomy

I certify that the narrative descriptions of the principal and secondary diagnoses and the major procedures performed are accurate and complete to the best of my knowledge.

Physician
Signature _____   Date _____

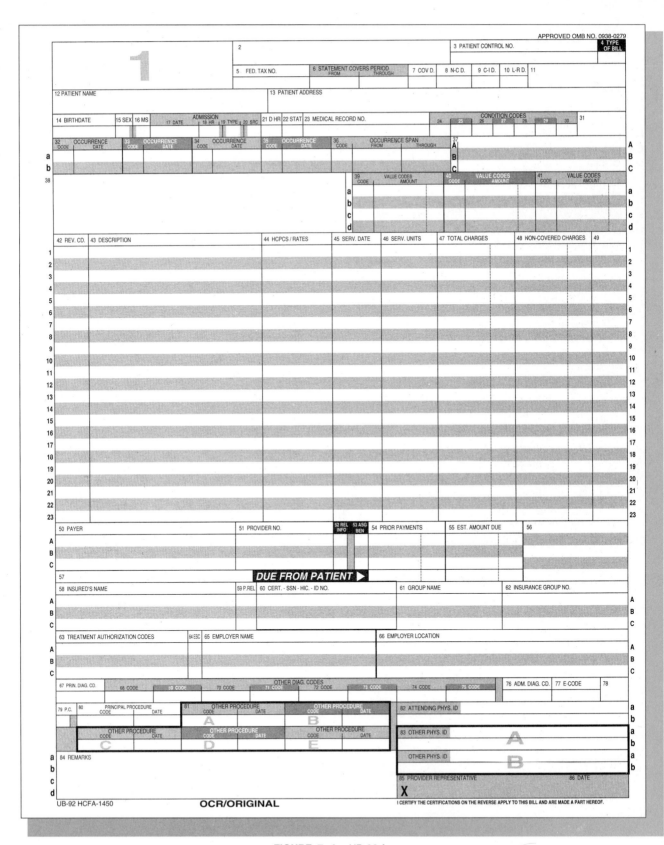

FIGURE 7–4. UB-92 form.

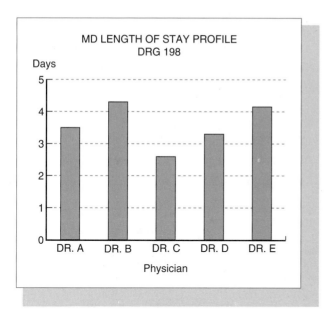

FIGURE 7–5. Physician profile.

record. Anyone who misrepresents, falsifies, or conceals essential information required for payment of Federal funds, may be subject to fine, imprisonment, or civil penalty under applicable federal laws.[5]

The purpose of this statement is to assure that the physician is aware of the serious consequences of misconduct in reporting diagnoses and procedures.

The government requires that Medicare bills be submitted on a form called the UB-92, which is a uniform billing form (Figure 7–4). This form allows space for the submission of nine diagnosis codes and six procedure codes. If a patient has more than nine diagnoses or six procedures, the coder must be certain that the codes that affect reimbursement, such as complications and comorbidities and OR procedure codes, are included in the available space on the form.

Hospitals often develop reports to help them monitor their DRGs. One such report is a physician profile, in which a physician can compare the cost of treating his or her patients and the patients' average length of stay for each DRG with the cost of treating and average length of stay of other physicians' patients (Figure 7–5). There may also be reports that examine hospital costs per DRG or use of ancillary services by DRG.

Health information management departments frequently get accounts receivable lists showing cases that have not yet been paid because the codes are not available. Since the list indicates the amount of money not paid because the bill has not been sent, extra effort can be made to find those records that are holding up large amounts of money and facilitate the coding.

The remittance advice can also be used to monitor the coding done for DRGs. A remittance advice is the statement received from the fiscal intermediary indicating the amount the hospital was paid. These statements should be monitored to see that the DRG determined by the fiscal intermediary for payment is the same one that the hospital determined during the coding process. If it is not, the source of the discrepancy should be investigated. Sometimes the problem is simply a clerical error with code numbers transposed or resequenced rather than a coding error.

CODING OUTPATIENT OR AMBULATORY CARE RECORDS

For ambulatory care, diagnoses are reported with ICD-9-CM and procedures, with HCPCS, including CPT-4, national, and local codes (Figure 7–6). The record must be reviewed and codes selected for diagnoses and procedures. The codes should be sequenced with the code reflecting the most significant problem related to the visit or encounter first.[6] Coders in ambulatory settings must be sure, however, that there is a diagnosis for each procedure reported. Coding guidelines for ambulatory care have been developed and differ

FIGURE 7–6. Coding systems used in health care facilities.

TYPE OF FACILITY	CODING SYSTEM USED	
Hospital Inpatients	ICD-9-CM for Diagnoses and Procedures	
Hospital Ambulatory Surgery	ICD-9-CM	Diagnoses
	HCPCS/CPT	Procedures
Physicians, Offices	ICD-9-CM	Diagnoses
	HCPCS/CPT	Procedures

from inpatient guidelines in some areas, so ambulatory care coders must be aware of these guidelines when assigning codes. Inpatient coders, for example, are directed to code suspected conditions as confirmed. When coding chest pain with a suspected myocardial infarction, myocardial infarction would be coded. In the ambulatory setting, coders are to assign codes to the highest level of certainty. When a patient presents with a cough that the physician suspects may be pneumonia, only the cough would be coded until a diagnosis of pneumonia has been established.

Ambulatory care coding is done almost exclusively for reimbursement as a mechanism for the provider to communicate the services provided to the payer, although some ambulatory centers do maintain internal databases on diagnoses and procedures. The traditional method of payment for ambulatory care was fee-for-service, in which patients paid for the visit and for each service received. When DRGs were implemented in the hospital, many patients who were formerly seen as inpatients were shifted to the outpatient setting to avoid the restrictions of the inpatient prospective payment system. Methods to control costs in the outpatient setting have, therefore, now been implemented. All these methods use coded data as a basis for payment.

In the Medicare payment system for ambulatory surgery, the CPT codes have been divided into groups called ASC (which stands for ambulatory surgery centers) payment groups, and payment rates are set for each group. The *Federal Register* publishes a yearly listing of the HCPCS/CPT codes along with the group and payment rate for each. These rates are then used in a formula to determine reimbursement.

Physician office coding is used in the **Resource Based Relative Value Scale (RBRVS)** system, a payment method used by the federal government to reimburse physicians for Medicare patients. In a relative value system, services are priced in relation to a reference or standard service. RBRVS uses a standard service with a relative value of 1.00, so that under this system, a service with a relative value of 2.10 is 2.1 times more valuable than the standard.[7] Each HCPCS/CPT code is given a relative value, and all the codes and their relative values are printed in the *Federal Register* annually. These relative value units represent three components:

- Physician work
- Practice expense
- Malpractice insurance expense

To compute the physician's payment, the relative value unit is adjusted for the geographic area in which the service was given and is multiplied by a conversion factor that is a monetary amount set annually by the federal government.[7] If the incorrect HCPCS/CPT code is assigned, the payment will be inaccurate too.

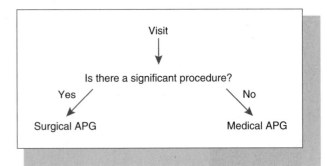

FIGURE 7-7. Assignment of Ambulatory Patient Groups.

Because DRGs caused a shift to the less regulated ambulatory care setting, Congress also mandated that the HCFA develop a prospective payment system for all of ambulatory care rather than only ambulatory surgery and physician payment. This system is based on **Ambulatory Patient Groups (APGs).** Like DRGs, APGs are assigned with a grouper program that looks at the patient's ICD-9-CM diagnosis, CPT procedure codes, age, sex, and visit disposition. Patients are divided into either a surgical APG or a medical APG based on whether or not the patient has a CPT procedure code. Surgical APGs are based on the CPT procedure code. If the patient does not have a CPT procedure code, a medical APG is assigned based on the ICD-9-CM diagnosis code (Figure 7–7). Unlike DRGs, where a patient is assigned to only one group, the ambulatory patient may be assigned to more than one APG. In that instance, the case must undergo a process called bundling to determine a single payment. Ambulatory coders must be certain that their coding is accurate and complete to ensure proper reimbursement under this system.

IMPACT OF COMPUTERS ON THE CODING PROCESS

Computer products called **encoders** are available to help in the coding process. There are basically two types of encoders. The first uses a branching logic system. The coder first enters the main term from the diagnosis or procedure and is then guided through a series of questions resulting in a code assignment. The second type of encoder is more like an automated codebook with the screen looking like the actual alphabetical index and tabular list. Coders who are more experienced usually prefer the automated codebook encoder because it uses their current coding skills. Coders also believe that they can code more quickly with the automated codebook, rather than having to work through all the questions in a branching logic system. In turn, most less experienced coders prefer the branching logic system because it guides them through the selection of a code. Encoders are available for both ICD-9-CM and HCPCS/CPT.

In addition to providing code numbers, encoders usually include other products. Most are integrated with a grouper that provides the DRG. They often incorporate prompts to help the coder optimize coding—for example, suggesting that the coder look for items that cause the patient to be grouped to a higher-paying DRG, such as complications and comorbidities and OR procedures.

ETHICAL PROBLEMS IN CODING

Because codes are used for reimbursement, sometimes coders face dilemmas about coding correctly versus coding to maximize reimbursement for the facility. AHIMA has developed "Standards of Ethical Coding" (see chart) to guide coders in making coding decisions.

The first point in the standards requires that coders thoroughly review the entire medical record before assigning the proper code. Such a thorough review is necessary to assure that all pertinent diagnoses and pro-

cedures have been coded as well as that the correct principal diagnosis has been selected.

As standard 2 says, the selection of the principal diagnosis and principal procedure must follow UHDDS guidelines. It would be unethical to change the principal diagnosis to the diagnosis that consumed the most resources and received the most reimbursement rather than the diagnosis that caused the patient to be admitted, as required by the UHDDS.

The primary factor in standard 3 is that coders must ensure that the patient record substantiates the choice of codes and the choice of the principal diagnosis. The main purpose of coding is to numerically reflect the content of the record, and this purpose is not met if the codes do not accurately reflect record content.

Standard 4 emphasizes to the manager that skilled coders must be hired and provided with the resources to produce quality coding. A common problem relating to standard 5 is that encoders print out the verbal description of the code assigned by the encoder rather than the physician's actual diagnostic statement. It may say, for example, other polyp of sinus, which is the

---

Standards of Ethical Coding

In this era of payment based on diagnostic and procedural coding, the professional ethics of medical record coders continues to be challenged. The following standards for ethical coding developed by the AHIMA Council on Coding and Classification are offered to guide the coder in this process.

1. Diagnoses that are present on admission or diagnoses and procedures that occur during the current encounter are to be abstracted after a thorough review of the entire medical record. Those diagnoses not applicable to the current encounter should not be abstracted. Also, diagnoses that would not be abstracted if they did not influence payment should not be included.

2. Selection of the principal diagnosis and principal procedure, along with other diagnoses and procedures, must meet the definition of the Uniform Hospital Discharge Data Set (UHDDS).

3. Assessment must be made of the documentation in the chart to assure that it is adequate and appropriate to support the diagnoses and procedures selected to be abstracted.

4. Medical record coders should use their skills, their knowledge of ICD-9-CM and CPT, and any available resources to select diagnostic and procedural codes.

5. Medical record coders should not change codes or narratives of codes so that the meanings are misrepresented. Nor should diagnoses or procedures be included or excluded because the payment will be affected. Statistical clinical data is an important result of coding, and maintaining a quality database should be a conscientious goal.

6. Physicians should be consulted for clarification when they enter conflicting or ambiguous documentation in the chart.

7. The medical record coder is a member of the healthcare team, and, as such, should assist physicians who are unfamiliar with ICD-9-CM, CPT, or DRG methodology by suggesting resequencing or inclusion of diagnoses or procedures when needed to more accurately reflect the occurrence of events during the encounter.

8. The medical record coder is expected to strive for the optimal payment to which the facility is legally entitled, but it is unethical and illegal to maximize payment by means that contradict regulatory guidelines.

The Official Coding Guidelines, published by the Cooperating Parties (American Hospital Association, American Health Information Management Association, Health Care Financing Administration, and National Center for Health Statistics), should be followed in all facilities regardless of payment source.

Reprinted with permission from the *Journal of the American Health Information Management Association*, July 1992, Vol. 63, No. 7, p. 27.

verbal description of code 471.8, rather than maxillary polyp, which was the physician's diagnosis and is grouped with other conditions under code 471.8. The code descriptions can be modified in the encoder, and it is the coder's responsibility to ensure that the verbal description reflects the physician's actual diagnosis.

As outlined in standards 6 and 7, coders have a responsibility to consult with the physician if the documentation in the chart is conflicting or ambiguous or if the physician needs assistance about proper definitions and guidelines. It is important for coders to develop a relationship with the medical staff in which they are seen as helping to ensure the most accurate database for the hospital as well as the most appropriate reimbursement. Many hospitals help physicians' offices in assigning codes for physician billing and can use this assistance as a means of enlisting the physicians' help.

Many ethical dilemmas can arise for standard 8. Using HCPCS/CPT, it would be unethical to code several separate CPT codes for a service (called **unbundling**) when one inclusive code is available.[9] When assigning codes for repair of a laceration, for example, it would not be correct to assign separate codes for cleaning the laceration, sewing it up, and applying a bandage instead of the single code for repair of a laceration. Coders should remember that, as professionals, they have an obligation to follow established coding rules and regulations and code only what is documented in the record. Coding is done for many purposes, not just reimbursement, and should provide quality data for all these purposes.

QUALITY OF CODED DATA

Outside agencies monitor the accuracy of coding because it impacts the amount that the physician or the facility is paid in a coding-based reimbursement system such as DRGs. The insurance company or fiscal intermediary reviews the patient's bill for coding errors. For Medicare cases, the intermediary puts it through the Medicare code editor, which is a computer program that looks for inconsistencies such as age and sex conflicts (e.g., a man having a hysterectomy), invalid diagnosis and procedure codes, invalid fourth or fifth digits, E codes that appear as the principal diagnosis, manifestation codes that appear as the principal diagnosis, V codes that are unacceptable as the principal diagnosis, and questionable admissions.[10] Most encoders include the Medicare code editors for both inpatients and outpatients. Many of this type of error can be corrected before the bill is sent.

The government also contracts with agencies called Peer Review Organizations (PROs) to review Medicare cases. Because Medicare cases are paid based on the codes selected, the government checks the accuracy of coding as a way to be sure that the amount paid is correct. The coding is monitored by the PRO through a process called DRG validation. In this process, the reviewers from the PRO check inpatient records to see whether the principal diagnosis, secondary diagnoses, and procedures listed are valid, coded accurately, sequenced according to the UHDDS definitions, and reported accurately on the UB-92. The PRO may change the principal diagnosis, delete diagnoses that were not verified by the content of the patient record, or add diagnoses that would affect the DRG assignment. The patient's discharge disposition (where he or she went on discharge, such as whether the patient was discharged alive or dead or if he or she was discharged home or to a skilled nursing facility) is also verified[11] (See Items Checked in PRO DRG Validation Process).

PROs review care in settings other than hospital inpatients. Ambulatory surgery cases are reviewed. If a patient is readmitted to the hospital within a short period, the PRO reviews the intervening care between the two hospitalizations, regardless of the site of the care.

Hospitals and other facilities also do internal monitoring of coding accuracy. Their focus in this internal monitoring is to assure the accuracy of coding for retrieval, research, and planning as well as for reimbursement. It is important that the coded data provided by the health information management department be accurate. Because coded data in disease and operation indexes provide a way of retrieving records by diagnosis and procedure, inaccurately coded records cannot be retrieved. Codes provided for bills must also be reviewed so that the physician or the facility is appropriately reimbursed for the patient's care.

Elements of Quality Coding

Several elements must be evaluated in looking at the quality of coded data:

- Reliability
- Validity
- Completeness
- Timeliness

Reliability

Reliability refers to measuring the degree to which something yields the same results in repeated attempts.[12] For example, several different coders using the same record should assign the same codes. A single coder,

Items Checked in PRO DRG Validation Process

- Accuracy of sequencing of diagnoses
- Accuracy of coding of principal diagnosis, secondary diagnoses, and procedures
- Accuracy of codes on UB-92
- Discharge disposition

coding the same diagnosis, should assign the same diagnosis codes in comparable patient records.

Validity

In coding, validity is the degree to which the codes accurately reflect the patient's diagnoses and procedures.[12] Coding that indicates that a patient broke the radius when the femur was actually the bone that was broken would be a validity problem.

Completeness

A record cannot be said to be coded in a quality manner if the codes do not reflect all the patient's diagnoses and procedures that apply to this encounter or admission.[12]

Timeliness

A record can be coded reliably, validly, and completely, but if it is not coded in a timely manner, the record is not available for billing or retrieval.

CAUSES OF ERRORS IN CODING

Many studies have been done to determine the accuracy of coded data and the sources of error. The Institute of Medicine has conducted several studies, including one that looked at the reliability of data in the National Hospital Discharge Survey (NHDS).[13] It found a poor reliability of the coded data studied.[13]

Factors that cause coding errors include the following:

- Failure to review entire record
- Selection of incorrect principal diagnosis
- Selection of incorrect code
- Coding diagnoses or procedures not validated by the content of the record
- Errors in entry of codes into database or on the bill

Failure to Review Entire Record

A major source of error in the Institute of Medicine study was found to be coding from the statement of discharge diagnoses and procedures, usually found on the face sheet, rather than from a thorough review of the entire record.[13] Part of the problem may be that coding often is done on incomplete records. The coder may not have the discharge summary, culture and sensitivity reports, and pathology reports that are necessary to code completely and accurately. If incomplete records are coded, the facility should have a procedure for ensuring that those records are reviewed when complete documentation has been received.

Selection of Incorrect Principal Diagnosis

Other sources of error arise from the physician's selection of an incorrect principal diagnosis on the face sheet.[14] Physicians are not always familiar with the UHDDS definition of principal diagnosis and sometimes select the patient's most serious problem or the underlying cause of the disease rather than the principal diagnosis that caused the patient to be admitted to the hospital.

Coders may also have a difficult time determining the correct principal diagnosis in some cases. Sometimes there is not a single condition that caused the patient's hospitalization.[15] In contrast, sometimes the patient has multiple conditions, none of which alone would require hospitalization but taken together do. In both these instances, the coder should consult with the attending physician to get the truest possible understanding of the case.[15]

Selection of Incorrect Code

Sometimes the problem is not in sequencing but actually in miscoding the diagnoses and procedures.

Coding Diagnoses or Procedures Not Validated by Record Content

The error may also arise from including codes for diagnoses which should not be coded or excluding diagnosis and procedure codes for items which should have been included.[16]

Clerical Errors in Database or on Bill

Finally, errors may result from clerical mistakes.[14] For example, a correct code may be incorrectly entered into the abstracted database.

IMPROVING THE QUALITY OF CODING

Several steps can be taken to improve the quality of coded data.

Developing Coding Policies

One of the most important steps is the development of coding policies for each facility. Coding policies establish guidelines to be followed in the coding process and are important in the assurance of reliability among coders in a facility (see Items to Be Included in a Coding Policy). If all coders are following the same guidelines, they have a better chance of coding consistently with the other coders in the department.

Coders need to know what to do about conflicting documentation in the patient record.[17] If the diagnosis states that the patient broke his or her left leg and the radiology report indicates that the right leg was broken, the attending physician should be consulted. Also, coders should be directed on what to do if they cannot find a code for diagnoses and procedures in the record.[17] Steps to take in reviewing the patient record are an important inclusion as well.[17] Coders might be directed, for example, to check the emergency department report for additional information for assigning E codes in the case of an accident or to read the history in abortion cases to determine whether it was a spontaneous or an induced abortion. Some codes in ICD-9-CM are optional, such as morphology codes and outcome of delivery codes, and the policy should identify which of these codes are used by the facility. The UHDDS definitions for principal diagnosis, other diagnoses, and significant procedures should also be included. Coders should participate in the process of developing the guidelines so that problems they have encountered in the past can be addressed in the policy.

Items to Be Included in a Coding Policy

- Instructions on what to do about conflicting documentation
- Instructions on what to do when a code cannot be found
- Directions for reviewing the record
- Use of optional codes (e.g., outcome of delivery, M codes)
- List of UHDDS definitions
- Directions for keeping books updated
- Use of reference materials (e.g., *Coding Clinic*)
- Requirements for abstracting

Quality Assessment Studies

A second method to improve coding quality is to do quality assessment studies on the coding done in the facility. One method that can be used is the reabstracting method in which records are recoded. The codes are then compared with the codes originally assigned. This reabstracting can be done by the coder, a process that is called intrarater reliability. Intrarater reliability deals with whether the coder is consistent in assigning codes. Interrater reliability is tested if someone other than the original coder does the reabstracting. In this case, the reliability among the coders is checked. It is important that a large enough sample of records be reabstracted to provide reliable and valid results. A sample size of at least 30 to 50 is usually required.[16] A defined period of time should also be set. Reabstracting is helpful in determining how accurate a coder is, detecting individual instances of incorrect coding, and determining reliability problems among coders.

To determine patterns of inaccuracies—for example, difficulties in areas such as coding cardiovascular cases or pregnancies—using criteria for particular areas can be helpful. In looking at pregnancies, an example of a criterion would be that code 650 for a normal case should never be coded with any other code from the pregnancy chapter. To look at patterns of coding, it is often more helpful to apply the criteria to the diagnosis and operation indexes rather than looking at individual records. In the indexes, for example, all cases that involve code 650 could quickly be scanned to see if they meet the criterion listed above.

Whatever type of monitoring is done, it should be maintained on an ongoing basis. When errors are found, the source of the error should be identified and communicated to the coders. Educational sessions may be needed to correct a problem. If the problem is one of reliability among coders, sometimes the solution is for the coders to decide which is the one best way to code a type of diagnosis or procedure that has been a problem.

Documentation Guidelines

Physician documentation is also an issue in looking at data quality. Sometimes coding errors occur because of poor documentation in the medical record. One method to improve physician documentation is to provide the medical staff with documentation guidelines that outline what should be included in the patient record. Education on the correct UHDDS definition for principal diagnosis may also be helpful. Many health information management departments address documentation problems by providing physicians with specific instances in which improved documentation would improve coding, such as listing the organism (e.g., pneumococcus) causing pneumonia.

CONSIDERATIONS IN HIRING CODERS

Quality coding requires well-trained and knowledgeable coders. There are several sources where coders can be found. First, some facilities hire only credentialed coders, meaning those who are registered record administrators (RRAs), accredited record technicians (ARTs), or clinical coding specialists (CCSs). An advantage of hiring RRAs and ARTs is that the supervisor knows that they have received basic coding instruction in their educational programs, although this training is usually at an entry level. CCSs are experienced coders who have passed the credentialing examination provided by the AHIMA. This examination tests coders at the advanced level in both ICD-9-CM and HCPCS/CPT. Noncredentialed experienced coders may also be hired. It is necessary to determine whether such coders have the training and experience to be accurate coders in your facility. A noncredentialed coder who has been trained and worked in a physician's office, for example, may only be familiar with the coding in the area of that physician's specialty, such as cardiology.

Another source of coders may be employees within the health information management department. They have the advantage of being familiar with the facility's records, particularly if they have been serving as abstractors or record processors. It is necessary that they receive training in anatomy and physiology, medical terminology, disease processes, and the content of the record before they undergo training in coding.

Another issue in hiring is whether to test coding applicants. Any test developed for this purpose must meet the Equal Employment Opportunity Commission's guidelines. The facility must be able to show that the test reflects performance required on the job. The coding supervisor who makes up such a test should, for example, be certain that the diagnoses and procedures included are representative of those typically coded in the facility. If a cutoff score is used, it must be used consistently for all applicants and must be reasonable. Most facilities keep a list of their most common diagnoses and procedures, and this list would be helpful in determining cases to be included in the test. Some facilities have applicants code actual records rather than isolated diagnoses and procedures because they believe that coding records is a more accurate reflection of the performance required on the job. Facilities must also keep annual records that include the following:[18]

- Number of applicants by sex, race, and national origin
- Selection procedures used

- Number of persons hired, promoted, and terminated for each job

Records kept on the tests are required to show that the test causes no adverse impact that "is defined as discrimination based on sex, age, race, color, creed, national origin, and handicap."[18]

Another helpful guide in the hiring process is a job description for the coder. It should include all the responsibilities of the coder, such as review of the record, coding of diagnoses and procedures by indicated coding systems, use of the encoder/grouper, reporting of productivity, and participation in quality assessment studies.

DETERMINING THE NUMBER OF CODERS NEEDED

A common formula used in deciding on the number of coders needed is as follows:

$$\frac{\text{Coding time per record} \times \text{number of discharges for the period}}{\text{Number of hours worked per coder for the time period}}$$

Therefore, if it is determined that it takes 15 minutes (.25 hours) to code a record, there are 900 discharges per month, and the coders each will work 150 hours per month (with time allowed for lunch, breaks, and so on), the calculation .25 × 900/150 would indicate that 1.5 coders are needed to handle this workload.

TRAINING CODERS

Once a coder has been hired, a training process must begin. The length and content of training depend on the skills and experience of the person hired. If departmental personnel inexperienced in coding are hired, it is necessary for them to receive basic coding instruction that can be obtained through workshops, self-study modules, and computer-based training programs. Current coders can also be used as mentors and trainers for new coders. All coders new to the facility, whether experienced or not, should review the facility's coding guidelines as well as pertinent issues of *Coding Clinic* and *CPT Assistant*. A system of giving the coder increasing responsibility usually is used in the training process. Coders often begin by coding outpatient records, which are shorter and less complex than inpatient records. Next they may be given inpatient records in which the codes do not impact reimbursement. Finally, the coder is allowed to code records in which coding does impact reimbursement, such as Medicare cases. All newly hired coders should be monitored for a period of time until their coding meets the facility's quality and quantity requirements.

RETENTION OF CODERS

Coders are in short supply, as can easily be seen by looking at any listing of job openings. Managers may find that just as a coder becomes thoroughly trained at the facility, he or she is attracted by a better job offer. When facility employees are trained on the job as coders, it is a good idea to require them to work at the facility for a defined period of time after their training.

To retain coders, some facilities pay their coders on an incentive system. Under such a system, the best and most efficient coders receive additional pay for their superior work. A base number of records usually is established per day, and a coder who codes more records than this base number receives additional pay for each additional record. Such an incentive pay system should be developed with the facility's personnel department to ensure that the system comes within their pay guidelines. Other inducements for coders can include providing continuing education opportunities for credentialed coders, who are required to complete a certain number of continuing education hours to maintain their credential. This may involve sending coders to outside workshops or providing in-service opportunities within the facility. Some hospitals and other facilities offer college tuition reimbursement and may pay professional dues in organizations such as the AHIMA and the Society for Clinical Coding. Coders should be encouraged to look at benefits as well as salary when assessing other job offers. Providing a quiet environment conducive to work can help in keeping coders satisfied with their work setting. Other incentives could include flexible work schedules, which cost no more for the facility but provide the employees with the opportunity to set their hours within certain restrictions. Possibilities for advancement may also offer incentives for coders to stay in a particular position.

CODING RESOURCES

In addition to properly training and motivating coders, facilities need to provide them with adequate resources to code accurately. The first resource that coders need is up-to-date codebooks or encoders. As indicated previously, ICD-9-CM and HCPCS/CPT are updated at least annually, and coders must have current books, encoders, and groupers to code accurately. Basic reference books, such as medical dictionaries, a basic medical science text, a basic drug list, and an anatomy and physiology text, should be available to help coders interpret the patient record. Every facility using ICD-9-CM and CPT should have *Coding Clinic* and *CPT Assistant* to provide coding advice. Some facilities even test their coders over the latest issues of these publications to assure that they have been read and understood.

Sometimes the PRO distributes communications, called transmittals, that affect the coding process. These transmittals should be made available to coders as soon as they are received. Coders also need information on the reimbursement systems that affect coding in their facilities as well as any changes in these systems, such as in the uniform bill (UB-92) or the DRG system. Finally, each coder should have a copy of the facility's coding guidelines.

USE OF CONTRACT CODING AND DRG REVIEW SERVICES

When health information management departments have difficulty filling coding positions or fall behind in coding, they sometimes contract with outside companies to do coding in the facility. Other companies specialize in reviewing the accuracy of coding and DRG assignment to help facilities optimize their reimbursement. There are many factors to consider in selecting such companies. The first consideration should be the qualifications of the coders assigned. They should be required to have at least as much training and experience as the coders in the facility. Another question should be whether the contract coders and reviewers work full time for the company or do the contract coding in addition to another job. The facility needs the coder to be able to concentrate on the job to be done.

When contract coders are used, an orientation process should take place in which they are given the facility's coding guidelines and become familiar with the patient record. Their work should be reviewed for errors, and productivity data should be maintained. When DRG review is done, another issue is whether the review occurs before the submission of the bill or afterward. If the review comes after the bill has been submitted, a revised bill must be sent. This takes time and may result in PRO review of the case. Reviewers should also be willing to train coders and provide feedback on methods the facility can use to optimize the coding. If this step is not done, the facility will be constantly dependent on the outside reviewers to catch and correct coding errors.

MEASURING CODING PRODUCTIVITY

In looking at the productivity of coders, both quality and quantity must be considered. A quality level of 95 per cent or better usually is established. As far as quantity, hospitals vary in the specificity of the productivity standards they use. In some cases, it is as simple as saying that all the records for a week must be coded before leaving on Friday. Standards often are developed regarding the number of records that must be coded per

	MON	TUES	WED	THUR	FRI
Name: _____ Date: _____					
INPATIENT					
NON-MEDICARE					
Short Stay					
Long Stay >30 days Trauma >15 days					
MEDICARE					
Short Stay					
Long Stay >30 days Trauma >15 days					
Review					
OUTPATIENT					
Amb. Surgery					
Clinic					
ER					
Lab/Laser/Other					
Hours Worked					
Inservice/Meetings					

Points=Standard Time for type of record x number of records coded

SUBTOTAL POINTS _____

TOTAL HOURS CODING _____

AVG/DAY PRODUCTIVITY _____

FIGURE 7–8. Coder productivity sheet.

day, and this standard commonly varies by type of record, with inpatient records taking longer to code than outpatient records and inpatient Medicare cases taking longer than non-Medicare cases. Departments usually look at actual performance over a period of time to determine these standards. It is important that the standards developed are realistic (Figure 7–8).

CONCURRENT VERSUS RETROSPECTIVE CODING

Another issue is whether records should be coded concurrently (while the patient is still hospitalized) or retrospectively (after discharge). Concurrent coding is done during the patient's hospitalization and often includes the assignment of a working DRG. The record is reviewed throughout the patient's stay so that a final code can be assigned immediately at discharge. This process may be done by coders from the health information management department who are assigned to work on the nurses' station to perform concurrent coding. In other cases, concurrent coding is done by utilization review personnel during their review of the record and sometimes is performed by ward clerks who have been trained to code. An advantage of concurrent coding is how quickly the codes are available for the bill. Because concurrent coding usually is done on the nursing unit, the coder can have greater contact with the physician involved, thus improving the quality of the coding as well as the timeliness of attestation completion. The coder can also work with the physician on documentation problems during the documentation process rather than later in the completion process. Problems that have occurred with concurrent coding have included the need for more coding personnel to cover all the nursing units. If utilization review personnel or ward clerks are used to code, it is often difficult to find someone to adequately perform the multiple duties required in such positions in addition to coding. Often in such cases, too, the health information management department will code the record again after discharge to check the coding done by the non–health information management department coders, which is a duplication of time and effort. Working DRGs have also been found to be misleading at times because the understanding of a patient's case can change drastically between the times of admission and discharge.

Coding after discharge is more common. In some departments, coding is the first activity done to the record, whereas in others, the record is assembled, checked for deficiencies, and/or abstracted before it is coded. The advantages of coding after discharge include the use of the existing workforce within the health information management department and an avoidance of duplication with the concurrent coding process. It is also easier to supervise coders who are all physically located in one place rather than spread out throughout the hospital. The codes, however, are not available in as timely a manner as with concurrent coding. Coders also do not have the regular contact with physicians that enables the concurrent coder to improve the physician's documentation as well as the coding. (See Advantages and Disadvantages of Concurrent Coding Versus Coding After Discharge.)

SPECIALIZATION OF CODERS

Many coders specialize in either inpatient or outpatient coding. Some facilities have gone beyond this basic division and have coders specialize by service, such as cardiology, cancer, or trauma. The advantages to such specialization include the coder's ability to become an expert in certain diagnoses and procedures. It is much easier to become familiar with the factors that affect the DRGs for a limited number of cases than to become familiar with the factors that affect the DRGs for all cases. Coders who specialize can also become acquainted with the physicians in their specialty more easily than with the medical staff as a whole. A coder is, therefore, more likely to consult the attending physician regarding coding questions. A problem with coder specialization is the possibility of a poor distribution of work among the coders if certain specialties have a heavier volume of cases during a time period. Coders may also lose their knowledge in areas of coding outside their specialty, which makes it difficult to provide adequate coding services during times when coders are absent because of vacations or illness (see Advantages and Disadvantages of Coder Specialization).

OTHER CODING AND CLASSIFICATION SYSTEMS

There are a variety of coding and classification systems other than ICD-9-CM and HCPCS/CPT.

Advantages and Disadvantages of Concurrent Coding Versus Coding After Discharge

Advantages

Concurrent Coding
- Quick availability of codes for billing
- Greater contact with physicians, leading to better documentation and more accurate coding

Coding After Discharge
- Avoidance of duplication between floor personnel coding and health information management department coding
- Ease of supervising coders in one physical location

Disadvantages

- Difficulty of professionals with other job duties to find time to code
- Repetition of coding process after discharge
- Misleading nature of working DRGs

- Coding not as timely
- Less contact with physicians

Advantages and Disadvantages of Coder Specialization

Advantages
- Added expertise in assigned speciality
- Greater ease in becoming acquainted with physicians in the specialty leading to greater consultation

Disadvantages
- Possible poor distribution of work
- Loss of knowledge in areas outside of specialty leading to problems providing coverage in case of absence

Diagnostic and Statistical Manual of Mental Disorders

This system is used in mental health settings and includes definitions and diagnostic criteria for mental disorders in addition to code numbers for the diagnoses. Developed by the American Psychiatric Association, this system is derived from ICD and the structure of the codes is, therefore, similar. Some codes, however, include six digits rather than the maximum of five used in ICD-9-CM. The *Diagnostic and Statistical Manual of Mental Disorders, 4th ed.* (DSM-IV) is used by mental health professionals to assign a diagnosis as well as by health information management professionals to assign a code. It is used in psychiatric hospitals, community mental health centers, developmental disability (mental retardation) centers, and mental health units in hospitals.

International Classification of Diseases for Oncology

Another classification system derived from ICD is the *International Classification of Diseases for Oncology* (ICD-O). This system is used to classify neoplasms according to their site, behavior, and morphology. It is developed by the WHO and is commonly used in tumor registries. The site or topography codes come from the malignant neoplasm codes in ICD-9, and the morphology codes are identical to those in ICD-9. Each neoplasm receives a site code that begins with T and a morphology code that begins with M.

Systematized Nomenclature of Human and Veterinary Medicine International

A third system is not related to ICD. It is the *Systematized Nomenclature of Human and Veterinary Medicine International* (SNOMED), which was developed by the College of American Pathologists. It provides preferred medical terms in 11 modules, including topography; morphology; function; living organisms; chemicals, drugs, and biologic products, including pharmaceutical manufacturers; physical agents, activities, and forces; occupation; social context; disease/diagnosis; procedures; and general linkage-modifier. Coding a diagnosis may involve codes from one or more of the modules. Otitis media, for example, includes a topography code for the middle ear and a morphology code for infection (T-XY300, M-40000), whereas a code for urinary tract infection due to *Pseudomonas* consists of a disease code for the urinary tract infection and an etiology code for the *Pseudomonas* (D-6501, E-2300). SNOMED was originally developed to aid in the computerization of diseases and operative information. With the increased interest in computer-based patient records, interest in using SNOMED has been revived.

SNOMED was developed from an earlier system, the *Systematized Nomenclature of Pathology* (SNOP), also developed by the College of American Pathologists. SNOP had only four axes—topography, morphology, etiology, and function—and was developed for use in the pathology department. It is still used by some tumor registries but has not been updated recently.

Other methods are used to classify patients that do not involve codes. Some of these are **case mix systems,** which attempt to classify patients according to a common characteristic. Others are **severity of illness systems,** which attempt to judge the severity of the patient's illness.

DRGs are one case mix classification system. When they were developed, a criticism was that they did not consider the severity of the patient's illness. It was thought that more severely ill patients require more resources to treat, and therefore, a case mix system used to divide cases into groups for payment purposes should consider severity of illness as a factor in assigning these groups. A new system called Refined DRGs has been developed to deal with this problem. The complications and comorbidities were "assigned a specific severity classification depending on its expected effect on resource use."[19] This refinement has improved the prediction of costs based on this grouping.

Another revision of the DRG system is the New York grouper, which has added DRGs to make the system more applicable for all payers. Medicare DRGs were developed using only Medicare data and so do not reflect diseases and conditions uncommon in the Medicare population. The New York grouper also provides an improved capability to predict cost.[19]

Disease staging is a severity measurement system that was an outgrowth of the methodology used in cancer staging systems. It uses ICD-9-CM codes and divides patients into one of four severity levels from stage I, in which the patient has no complications, to stage IV, in which the patient dies. It uses UHDDS data set items, which are available from the discharge abstract.

Patient Management Categories is a severity system

based on the diagnoses and procedures from the UB-92, age, and sex. It is not dependent on the sequence of the codes, which is an improvement over DRGs, where errors in selection of the principal diagnosis can lead to errors in the DRG assignment. Patient Management Categories are combined with patient management paths that outline efficient care and cost weights.[20]

The Computerized Severity of Illness Index adds a sixth digit to the ICD-9-CM code. This severity digit is assigned based on disease signs and symptoms, vital signs, and radiology and physical findings.[20]

In the ATLAS system, formerly called the Medical Illness Severity Grouping System (MedisGroups), patients are assigned to a severity level based on factors called key clinical findings from the history and physical, laboratory, radiology, and other areas of the record. These factors must be abstracted from the patient's record. The patient's diagnosis is *not* a factor.

Acute Physiology and Chronic Health Evaluation (APACHE) was developed as an intensive care unit severity measurement. It uses 12 physiologic measures, such as serum potassium level and white blood count, and then makes adjustments based on age, previous health status, and reason for admission to determine the score. Like ATLAS/MedisGroups, the diagnosis is not used in the APACHE system.

FACTORS TO CONSIDER IN CHOOSING A CLASSIFICATION SYSTEM

Needs of the Facility

The most important factor in choosing a classification is considering the needs of the facility. If extensive research is done, a classification system that groups diseases together under one code may result in too many records being pulled. Looking for cases of laryngeal abscess, for example, would result in pulling cases assigned code 478.79 in ICD-9-CM. This code is also assigned for necrosis of the larynx, obstruction of the larynx, ulcer of the larynx, and many other conditions. Once the cases coded 478.79 have been retrieved, there is still a lengthy process to look through the cases to determine which are laryngeal abscess. Facilities often offer unique services that must be considered in selecting a classification system. A hospital that specializes in oncology might, for example, select a system that provides a more thorough classification of neoplasms.

Requirements of the Reimbursement System

Because coded data are now used in reimbursement methods, another primary factor must be which coding system is required for the reimbursement system. Most third parties require diagnostic information coded in ICD-9-CM, for example. If a facility chooses a different coding system for its internal use, it would still have to code cases with ICD-9-CM for reimbursement purposes. Such duplication of effort would be expensive and time-consuming.

User's Needs for Coded Data

Coded data on diseases and operations also form an important database that is used in the hospital for planning and research purposes. These needs of administration and other users within the facility must be considered when selecting a coding system. Coded data on the number of potentially terminal illnesses treated in the hospital, such as acquired immunodeficiency syndrome and cancer, might, for example, be used to determine and defend the need for a hospice service. Researchers could use such a database to retrieve data to assess the effectiveness of certain operations in treating a particular disease.

Ease of Obtaining Data for a Severity of Illness System—UB-92 Versus Additional Data

In choosing severity of illness systems, the source of the data and the ease of obtaining it must be of prime consideration. Some systems, like Patient Management Categories and Disease Staging, use the existing data from the UB-92 and do not require further abstracting of data from the record. Other systems, like ATLAS/MedisGroups, require that the record be abstracted to determine the severity levels. For such systems, additional personnel are needed to provide the data.

Some states mandate the use of a particular severity of illness system. Pennsylvania, for example, requires the use of ATLAS/MedisGroups, and Ohio specifies Refined DRGs. Such state requirements have a strong bearing on the use of a severity system.

How severity of illness systems are to be used by the professionals in the hospital should be another factor to consider. It is futile to provide data that does not meet the needs of the professionals requesting it.

Reliability and Validity of the Data Obtained

The reliability and validity of the data used are also factors. It is much easier and quicker to use a system that takes data from the UB-92. If that data is not accurate, however, the resulting classification will be flawed.

FUTURE OF CODING

Some professionals believe that in the future, coding will be done automatically by the computer. It might in fact be unnecessary to code patient records if the computer-based record acts as a large database from which any element can be retrieved. Coders and the coding function will change to include coding-related activities such as verification of the accuracy and completeness of computer-assigned codes as well as retrieval of coded data from the database. In the meantime, coders perform a necessary function that enables health information management departments to provide a needed service.

Key Concepts

- Clinical coding is assigning a number to diagnoses and procedures for retrieval, research, and reimbursement purposes.

- ICD-9-CM and HCPCS/CPT are the primary coding systems in use currently.

- The coding process involves steps that include review of the record, selection of items to code, assignment of the code, sequencing of the codes, abstracting, entry of the code on the bill, and storage and retrieval of the coded data in the database.

- When coding for reimbursement, coders must be aware of how the codes affect reimbursement and then assure the accuracy and completeness of the data provided.

- Encoders assist in the coding and DRG assignment process.

- Because the codes affect reimbursement, coders may be faced with an ethical dilemma between coding accurately and coding to maximize the amount the facility is paid. This dilemma should be solved by coding as accurately as possible the diagnoses and procedures verified by the content of the patient record.

- The quality of coded data must be assessed, and steps must be taken to assure the quality of coding.

- In hiring coders, facilities must determine the qualifications required, whether to use tests in the hiring process, how many coders to hire, how to train them, and how to retain them.

- Facilities have an obligation to provide coders with resources needed to assure accurate coding.

- Records may be coded either concurrently (while the patient is in the hospital) or after the patient's discharge.

- Many factors should be used to determine whether or not a contract coding or DRG review organization should be used.

- Many coding and classification systems other than ICD-9-CM and HCPCS/CPT are used in facilities throughout the United States.

References

1. Kennedy J, Kossman CE: Nomenclatures in medicine. Bull Med Libr Assoc 1973;61:239.
2. Hasenberg M: A glimpse into the CPT process. J Am Health Information Management Assoc 1993;64:24.
3. Hays BC: Classification updates. J Am Health Information Management Assoc 1994;65:16.
4. Averill RF: Development. In Fetter RB, Brand DA, Gamache D (eds): DRGs: Their design and development. Ann Arbor, MI, Health Administration Press, 1991.
5. Federal Register, 49(no. 171), August 31, 1984, 34759.
6. Finnegan R: Coding notes. J Am Med Record Assoc 1988;59:26.
7. Grimaldi PL: Medicare physician fees overhauled. Health Progress, 1992;73:32.
8. Fox LA: An ethical dilemma: Coding medical records for reimbursement. J Am Health Information Management Assoc 1992;63:35.
9. Holloway J: Professional ethics in today's reimbursement oriented coding environment. Newsletter of the California Medical Record Association, August 1990.
10. Tucker J: The coder's desk reference. Chicago: Care Communications, 1985.
11. Murphy-Muth SM: Medical records in a changing environment. Rockville, MD: Aspen, 1987.
12. Finnegan R: Data quality and DRGs. Chicago: American Medical Record Association, 1983.
13. Institute of Medicine: Reliability of national discharge survey data: Report of a study/Institute of Medicine. Washington, DC: National Academy of Sciences, 1980.
14. Waterstraat FL, Barlow J, Newman F: Diagnostic coding quality and its impact on healthcare reimbursement. J Am Med Record Assoc 1990;61:55.
15. Connell FA, Blide LA, Hanken MA: Ambiguities in the selection of the principal diagnosis: Impact on data quality, hospital statistics and DRGs. J Am Med Record Assoc 1984;55:18.
16. The imperative for coding accuracy. Coding Clinic 1989;6:7.
17. Currie MS: Clinical data quality: Impact on revenue. J Am Med Record Assoc 1985;56:27.
18. Benjamin CD, Baum B: Testing coding skills as a pre-employment screening process. J Am Health Information Management Assoc 1993;64:63.
19. Metzler S: Refined DRGs: An add-on system identifying groups of patients with similar resource usage profiles. J Am Med Record Assoc 1990;61:34.
20. Arbitman DB: Severity of illness measures: Can they work for us? Computers in Healthcare, June 1989.

SECTION
III

DATA MANAGEMENT AND USE

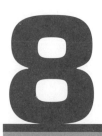

SUE WATKINS

REGISTRIES 8

OBJECTIVES

- Define key words.
- Explain the overall purpose of disease, implant, and
    equipment registries.
- Define the overall organization of the cancer registry
    model.
- List case identification sources.
- Describe and develop data collection methods.
- State important uses of registry data.

Registries are established for various disease and health problems and with differing goals and objectives. The need to create data banks as a **surveillance** mechanism for specific disease processes or incidence, to monitor the impact of using medical devices, and to assess the health issues surrounding the exposure to hazardous substances has led to the design and implementation of numerous registries. The mission, design, size, use of technology, and regulatory bodies vary with each type of registry. Examples of some of the most widely encountered registries include those for cancer, trauma, heart disease, acquired immunodeficiency syndrome (AIDS), diabetes mellitus, kidney disease, birth defects, liver disease, hazardous substances, and medical implants.

Cancer registries are described in this chapter in more detail than other registries because they are the most common type of registry the reader will encounter. They are located in hospitals of all sizes and in every region of the country. In addition, most states have central cancer registries. Understanding the fundamentals of cancer registries provides the reader with an excellent foundation for developing other types of registries. Information on some of the other, more common disease registries encountered by health information management (HIM) professionals are also provided later in the chapter.

HISTORY AND DEVELOPMENT OF CANCER REGISTRIES

The collection, retrieval, and analysis of cancer data by cancer registries have long been accepted as essential by physicians and epidemiologists concerned with assessing cancer **incidence**, treatment, and end results.

Hospital-based cancer registries or their equivalents have existed in the United States for many decades. Reports on cancer experience were issued in the late 1800s from such institutions as the American Oncologic Hospital in Philadelphia, the General Memorial Hospital in New York City, the Johns Hopkins Hospital in Baltimore, and Charity Hospital in New Orleans.[1] In the 1920s, the American College of Surgeons (ACS) asked its members to submit information on living patients with bone cancer. Subsequent requests were made later in the same decade for data collection on cancer of the cervix, breast, mouth and tongue, colon, and thyroid. In

1930, the ACS's Commission on Cancer developed standards for hospital cancer clinics and began surveying facilities. By 1937, there were 240 approved cancer clinics, but it was not until 1956 that a cancer registry providing lifelong follow-up of cancer patients became a requirement for an approved cancer program.[2]

The first *central registry* was established in Connecticut when a group of New Haven physicians began compiling data that showed a steady increase in the cancer rates in their community. The physicians proceeded to start cancer clinics in their hospitals and to maintain uniform records. The Connecticut Medical Society formed a Tumor Study Committee and was instrumental in getting legislation passed that created the Division of Cancer and Other Chronic Diseases in 1935. In 1941, statewide cancer surveillance began when a team from the division visited each hospital and abstracted data from the records of all patients with cancer for the period 1935 through 1940.[2]

The National Cancer Act of 1971 mandated the collection, analysis, and dissemination of data for use in the prevention, diagnosis, and treatment of cancer. This mandate led to the establishment of the Surveillance, Epidemiology, and End Results (SEER) Program, an ongoing project of the National Cancer Institute (NCI). The SEER Program operates *population-based cancer registries* in various geographic areas of the country covering about 13 per cent of the U.S. population. The selection of demographic areas is based primarily on the areas' epidemiologically significant subgroups to provide a sampling of the U.S. population. Trends in cancer incidence, mortality, and patient survival in the United States are derived from this database.[3]

With the passage of the Cancer Registries Amendment Act (Public Law 102-515) in 1992, a national program of population-based cancer registries came into being. Funding of $16.83 million was allocated by Congress for 1994 to be used to set up statewide registries in states where none existed and to enhance existing registries.

Today, there are more than 2000 hospital-based cancer registries and a large majority of states have population-based registries. The categories of cancer registries are generally defined as hospital- or population-based.[2]

Hospital Cancer Registries

The primary goal of hospital-based cancer registries is to improve patient care. The cancer registry provides a system for monitoring all types of cancer diagnosed or treated in an institution. The data collected are used for the following:

* To make certain that optimal care is provided for patients with cancer

* To compare the institution's morbidity and survival rates with regional and national statistics

* To determine the need for professional and public education programs

* To allocate resources[4]

Hospital-based registries may be in single- or multi-institution settings, military hospitals, managed care programs, or freestanding treatment facilities. The patient care–oriented goal usually dictates the type of data collected. Data items collected routinely include patient identification and demographic information, cancer diagnosis, treatment rendered, prognostic factors, and outcome.

Hospitals are not required by law to operate cancer registries. When a hospital-based registry is associated with a population-based registry, the latter often supports and facilitates the hospital's efforts, becoming the major source of its data. Support from the population-based registry may consist of analyzing data, generating reports that allow for comparison of data, providing data collection software, assisting in quality-control activities, and providing professional training to the hospital cancer registry staff.

The Commission on Cancer of the ACS has operated a voluntary system of approval for cancer programs since 1932. The goal of the approvals program is to decrease the morbidity and mortality of patients with cancer. Standards have been developed for approval of cancer programs. The major components of an approved cancer program are as follows:

* Cancer committee

* Cancer conferences

* Patient care evaluation

* A cancer registry

Most hospital-based cancer registries operate in accordance with the standards defined by the Commission on Cancer.[4] In 1995, there were more than 1300 approved hospital cancer programs in the United States.[5]

Population-Based Registries

Conceptually, there are three types of **population-based cancer registries**. They are as follows:

* Incidence only

* Cancer control

* Research

Most incidence-only registries are operated by a government health agency and designed to determine cancer rates and trends in a defined population. Monitoring cancer incidence is legislatively mandated in most states. The mandate usually outlines the duties of the registry system and the data to be collected, targets the sources from which data are to be obtained, details the confidentiality policies of the system, provides protection from any liability, and, in many states, defines the penalties for noncompliance. Data collected are typically limited to patient and cancer identification. There is generally no need for treatment or outcome data.

Cancer control population-based registries serve a broader function, often combining incidence, patient care, and end results reporting with various other research and cancer control activities, such as cancer screening and smoking cessation programs. Their data set is often the same as that of their reporting hospitals, including treatment and outcome data as well as incidence-only information.

Many research-oriented registries are operated by universities to conduct epidemiologic research focused on **etiology**. Research requirements commonly include rapid case ascertainment, so that patients can be identified and contacted as soon as possible after diagnosis. Research data are typically defined and collected on a project-specific basis by an ad hoc mechanism of chart review, patient contact, or some other special procedure. For example, a study of the incidence of cancer in twins may include sibling identification, chart review of a twin with cancer, and patient and family interviews. Another study may be conducted to determine the risk factors of women under age 30 with breast cancer (a population with a low incidence of this disease).

Conversely, a cancer-control type of registry is operated primarily to support the targeting and evaluation of control programs, such as cancer screening for early detection and education. The registry may be limited to specific types of cancer for which distinctive intervention strategies have been established. The data collected are limited to what is needed for an intervention strategy or to evaluate the intervention effect. Data are used to assess areas of high risk, plan education programs, and focus resources aimed at reducing or eliminating the incidence of cancer. Information is shared with public officials and health care providers and often published in medical and research journals.

Many population-based registries are, in effect, combinations of all three types. The legislative mandate and funding sources normally dictate the effort expended in any one particular area—incidence monitoring, research, or cancer control.[2]

HOSPITAL CANCER REGISTRY MODEL

The hospital cancer registry model is described in this section to provide HIM professionals with an overview of registry operations. In many instances, other disease registries have patterned their operation and data collection methods after the cancer registry prototype. Examples of materials and resources used by different disease registries and other comparisons are presented later in this chapter.

The following components are vital for developing and operating the hospital cancer registry:

- Database
- Lifetime follow-up of the cancer patient
- Quality control
- Patient care evaluation
- Use of registry data
- Confidentiality
- Staffing

Database Development and Management

The goal of the hospital cancer registry is to collect data on every patient with cancer, to maintain the data in an organized manner, and to make the data readily available for use by the medical staff and others interested in the morbidity and mortality of cancer patients. To accomplish these goals, guidelines for casefinding, abstracting, and quality control measures to ensure accuracy of the data have been defined by the ACS.[4] These guidelines address the following criteria:

- Reference date
- Case eligibility
- Patient eligibility
- Patient index
- Casefinding
- Accession register
- Abstracting
- Coding
- Staging
- Primary site file
- Quality control

Reference Date

The **reference date** is the beginning date of data collection. It is established as January 1 of a given year. Every eligible case first seen at the hospital on or after this date must be included in the cancer registry.[4]

Case Eligibility

A reportable list must be developed that includes all the types of cases that are to be included and those that are to be excluded in the database. The best source for developing a reportable list is the *International Classification of Diseases for Oncology, Second Edition* (ICD-O-2).[6] The ACS requires all tumors with a behavior code of two or higher, indicating an in situ or a malignant tumor in the ICD-O-2, to be included for approved cancer programs.[4] The medical staff frequently requests that other cases be included (i.e., nonmalignant meningiomas, villous adenomas of the colon, benign liver tumors). Subject to approval of the cancer committee, these requests should be granted whenever possible.

Patient Eligibility

All inpatients and outpatients diagnosed (clinically or histologically) and/or treated for active disease on or after the reference date of the registry are eligible for inclusion in the database. This includes patients who were diagnosed and are being treated at the hospital, patients who were diagnosed elsewhere and are receiving all or part of their first course of therapy or whose therapy was planned at hospital, and patients who were diagnosed at the hospital and are receiving all of their first course of therapy elsewhere. Patients who were diagnosed at autopsy are also included.

Patients who are seen only for consultation to confirm a diagnosis or treatment plan are ineligible. Also excluded are patients who receive transient care while on vacation: patients who are admitted to a designated hospice or home care service or for terminal supportive care, patients with active cancer who are admitted for other medical conditions, patients with a past history of cancer who have no current evidence of the disease, and patients with precancerous conditions.[4,6]

Patient Index

The patient index is similar to the master patient index used by HIM departments. In cancer registries, the patient index is a permanent alphabetical file that, in a manual system, contains one card for each patient, living or deceased, entered into the database. The purpose of the patient index is to identify patients who have been entered into the registry database. Both primary and secondary cancers are listed on the same card. The following data are recorded in the patient index:

- Patient name
- Sex
- Primary sites of cancer, including laterality for paired sites, such as breast, when applicable
- Histology
- Date of diagnosis
- Accession number
- Sequence number
- Date of birth
- Date of death
- Patient record numbers

Other, optional information may be recorded, such as address, telephone number, primary payer, and employer. The patient index may also be maintained in a computer database. In that case the same information must be included, and the file must be an alphabetical printout. An on-screen listing is acceptable as long as printouts with all the data elements in natural language are generated. An example of a standard patient index card is shown in Figure 8–1.

Casefinding

The ability to identify every reportable case of cancer is essential to the success of a cancer registry system.[6] The primary casefinding sources are the pathology and HIM departments as well as the radiation therapy and other outpatient departments, where applicable.

PATHOLOGY DEPARTMENT. The pathology department is the primary source of identification of cases to be included in the database. All the pathology reports, including the surgical, autopsy, bone marrow, hematology, and cytology reports, are reviewed by cancer registry personnel who are knowledgeable in reporting requirements. Photocopies of reportable cases are provided by the pathology department for use by the registry staff.

HEALTH INFORMATION SERVICES. The second most common source for casefinding is the disease index. A copy of the disease index is generally furnished to the registry for use in case identification. Although most cases seen at the hospital have a positive pathology report, some types of cancer may be diagnosed in the physician's office and then the patient is admitted for treatment (i.e., leukemia and lymphoma cases).

RADIATION THERAPY AND OTHER OUTPATIENT DEPARTMENTS. Most patients seen in radiation therapy and other outpatient departments may never be included in the registry database without appropriate casefinding procedures established to identify them. These departments usually keep a log of patients treated. A review of this log on a regular basis ensures inclusion of these cases.

Accession Register

The **accession register** is a permanent log of all the cases entered into the database. The objectives of the

Patient Name	Medical Record Number	Accession Number

Address (Street, City, State, Zip Code)	Phone Number

Date of Birth	Age	Sex	Race	Social Security Number

Relative or Friend (Name, Address, Phone Number)

Date of Diagnosis	Place of Diagnosis (Hospital, City, State)	Physician(s)

Primary Site	Histology

First Course of Treatment

Date of Death	Cause of Death	Place of Death	Autopsy

CANCER REGISTRY PATIENT INDEX CARD

Front Side Of Cancer Registry Patient Index Card

Admit Date	Medical Record Number	Site/Histology Code(s)	Physician(s)

CANCER REGISTRY PATIENT INDEX CARD

Back Side Of Cancer Registry Patient Index Card

FIGURE 8–1. Patient index card.

accession register are to assess the annual caseload and to provide each patient with a registry identification number. This register is also used to monitor casefinding, assess workload, and verify data in other files.

The accession register is an annual sequential listing. Every case entered into the registry is assigned a unique accession number, preceded by the **accession year**, the year the case is entered into the database. For example, the first case in 1994 would be assigned the number 94-0001, the second case would be 94-0002, and so forth. A two-digit number is usually added to indicate the number of primary cancers the patient has. A patient with one primary cancer would have a number such as 94-0001/00 (the /00 indicates that this patient has only one known neoplasm). If the patient has two primaries (i.e., prostate and colon), the sequence of primary numbers assigned would be 01 and 02, as shown in Figure 8–2 (94-0004/01 and 94-0004/02). The sequence number indicates the number of primaries a patient has had, regardless of where the patient was diagnosed and/or treated for each of the primary sites of cancer. Only one accession number is assigned to a patient. A patient who is first seen at the hospital in 1994 for colon cancer but who has a history of breast cancer would receive a 94 accession number with a sequence number of /02, indicating that this is the second primary for this patient, as shown in Figure 8–2 under the name Mother Goose. Figure 8–2 also reflects an entry for a patient who was first seen in 1993 with a reportable cancer, assigned an accession number, and who was then diagnosed at the same facility in 1994 with a second primary (Christie, A). Because this patient already had an accession number, a new number was not assigned. Rather, the second primary was given a sequence number of 02 and entered into the accession register as the third case for 1994. (Note that accession number 94-0003 was never used.)

The accession register commonly is maintained in a binder or notebook that is divided by accession year. The following data are recorded:

- Accession number
- Sequence number
- Patient's name
- Primary site
- Date of diagnosis

Other data often recorded are histology, medical record number, and vital status. In an automated system, an on-screen display or computer printout in natural language may be used (Figure 8–3).

Administratively, cancer registry managers, the cancer committee, and hospital management who oversee the cancer registry can use the accession register to monitor productivity. Cases should only be accessioned when abstracted. A review of the accession register should provide data useful in evaluating the currency of abstracting and data collection.

Abstracting

Abstracts are prepared for every case that is eligible for inclusion in the database. The information recorded on the abstract form is obtained from the patient's hospital record. **Abstracting** provides a succinct summary that characterizes the patient, disease process, extent of disease, treatment, and outcome. The Commission on Cancer, for approved cancer programs, allows a maximum delay in abstracting of 6 months from the date of initial discharge.

The abstract generated may be handwritten, typed, or computerized. The form or system used must be adequate to permit recording of all relevant data in a logical and uniform manner. Abstracting guidelines are provided in the *Self Instructional Manual for Tumor Regis-*

ACCESSION REGISTER				
Account Number	**Patient's Name**	**Primary**	**Site**	**Date of Diagnosis**
94-0001/00	Christopher, St.	Liver	C22	01/02/94
94-0002/02	Goose, Mother	Colon	C18	01/03/94
93-0345/02	Christie, A.	Lung	C34	01/03/94
94-0004/01	Doe, John	Prostate	C61	01/04/94
94-0004/02	Doe, John	Colon	C18	01/04/94
94-0006/00	Washington, M.	Breast	C50	01/04/94

FIGURE 8–2. Accession register.

DATE: 09/27/93 * * * * * * * * C/NET * * * * * * * * PAGE:1
Sample Database Accession List for 1987 Cases
Accession Number List
CTR
Selection Criteria:
ACCYR: 87

ACCESN	DATE ADMIT	NAME	MR#	SITE	DATE DX	SEX	CLASS
750029/02	05/06/87	Small, Weeneeta	4033	C549	05/06/87	2	1
770280/02	11/26/87	Woolworths, Deepart	4278	C809	11/26/87	2	1
780334/02	07/28/87	Gwellyn, Llewellyn	4132	C180	07/28/87	1	1
800269/02	08/30/87	Spinner, Web	4165	C241	08/30/87	1	1
810117/02	06/28/87	Gonzalez, Victorian	4087	C519	06/28/87	2	1
810142/02	04/02/87	Frazier, Antonia	3996	C343	04/02/87	2	1
810417/02	05/18/87	Human, Halfway	4036	C775	05/18/87	1	1
820205/02	06/27/87	Souse, Egbert	4085	C809	06/27/87	1	1
830323/02	09/15/87	Samarkand, Robert	4678	C679	06/15/87	1	3
870004/00	01/05/87	Travels, Gullivers	3915	C679	01/05/87	1	1
870011/00	01/11/87	Tuffy, Fluffy	3913	C421	01/11/87	2	1
870013/00	01/14/87	Grass, Leavesof	3925	C421	01/14/87	1	1
870015/00	01/11/87	Upstart, Crow	3911	C320	01/11/87	1	1
870018/00	01/24/87	Mackey, Lackey	3924	C672	01/18/87	2	0
870019/01	01/26/87	White, Snow	3921	C250	01/26/87	2	1
870021/00	01/27/87	Sharper, Vision	3916	C421	01/27/87	1	1
870022/00	01/27/87	King, Offools	3928	C349	01/27/87	1	1
870023/00	01/28/87	Farley, Ranger	3919	C770	01/28/87	1	1
870024/00	01/28/87	Worn, Tired	3926	C421	01/28/87	2	1
870030/00	02/02/87	Lopalong, Hopalong	3940	C349	02/02/87	2	1
870032/00	02/04/87	Nohera, Yuhera	3933	C672	02/04/87	1	1
870034/00	02/10/87	Maine, Harbor	3948	C343	02/10/87	1	1
870042/00	02/17/87	Feasable, Fairly	3946	C187	02/17/87	1	1
870047/00	02/24/87	Wright, Rong	3942	C341	02/23/87	2	2
870049/00	02/26/87	Trucker, Joe	3939	C209	02/26/87	1	1
870060/00	03/09/87	Jenkins, Box	3981	C259	03/09/87	2	1
870063/00	03/11/87	Moor, Glynnis	3963	C421	03/11/87	2	1
870066/00	03/15/87	Wight, Isla	3965	C209	03/09/87	2	2
870069/00	03/17/87	Intrance, Constant	3980	C250	03/17/87	2	1
870071/00	03/18/87	Record, Broken	3979	C341	03/18/87	2	1
870074/00	03/19/87	Purl, Knit	3975	C778	03/19/87	1	1
870075/00	03/22/87	Allen, Adams	3970	C165	03/22/87	1	1
870084/00	03/30/87	Shall, Wee	3974	C051	02/15/87	1	2
870085/00	03/30/87	Simian, Chimpy	3977	C258	03/30/87	1	1
870090/00	04/04/87	Shark, Jawsey	4007	C342	03/22/87	2	2
870092/00	04/05/87	Frankenstein, Frank	3999	C696	03/17/87	1	2
870098/00	04/12/87	Schotzy, Snoopy	4015	C343	04/07/87	1	0
870104/00	04/14/87	Meyers, Oscar	4008	C341	03/30/87	1	2
870106/00	04/18/87	Lowing, Cowabunga	4009	C549	03/15/87	2	2
870107/00	04/19/87	Lisp, Iva	4003	C187	04/19/87	2	1
870109/02	04/20/87	Zion, Bryce	3993	C619	04/20/87	1	1
870110/00	04/29/87	Stanley, Livingston	4021	C619	04/20/87	1	1
870112/00	04/21/87	Nshirley, Laverne	4017	C549	04/21/87	2	1
870114/00	04/22/87	Randy, Dandy	4012	C259	04/22/87	1	1
870115/00	04/23/87	Peck, Hunt	4018	C659	04/23/87	1	5
870116/00	04/23/87	Greene, Kelley	4019	C187	04/23/87	1	1
870117/00	04/23/87	Swallow, Flicker	4020	C341	04/23/87	1	0
870120/01	05/01/87	Parnassus, Harry	4071	C649	05/01/87	1	1

FIGURE 8–3. Computer-generated accession register.

trars, *SEER Program, Book 5,*[7] and the *Registry Operations and Data Standards (ROADS), Commission on Cancer, American College of Surgeons, 1990.*[8] In addition, many state and regional registries have established abstracting requirements. The amount of data collected is dictated by the Commission on Cancer for approved cancer programs, a central registry, policies established by the cancer committee, and the limitations inherent to a specific computer software system (see Commission on Cancer Data Set). A sample abstract is shown in Figure 8–4.

Coding

The coding scheme traditionally used by cancer registries is the ICD-O-2, published by the World Health Organization. This coding scheme is recommended by the Commission on Cancer[4] and is used by the National Cancer Registrars Association, Inc., in its annual certification examination.

The ICD-O-2 represents a more detailed extension of the *International Classification of Diseases, Tenth Edition* (ICD-10-CM) chapter on neoplasms. ICD-O-2 permits coding of all neoplasms to include **topography, morphology, grading,** and **differentiation**.[6]

Staging

The extent of the spread of disease is recorded for every case entered into the registry database. The stage at the time of initial diagnosis and treatment is documented. Numerous staging systems have been developed for use by the medical community. Some are site-specific (e.g., Dukes A-D Stage Grouping for Colorectal Cancer) or system specific (e.g., International Federation of Gynecology and Obstetrics [FIGO] classification for gynecologic sites). Others are general and may be applied to almost all sites.

Historically, the staging system most commonly used was developed in 1977 by the SEER Program of the NCI, *Self Instructional Manual for Tumor Registrars, Book 6,* or the *Summary Staging Guide.* This system is used to stage cases as in situ, localized, regional spread to lymph nodes or adjacent tissue, or distant spread to lymph nodes in other areas of the body, or distant sites.

In addition, the Commission on Cancer requires that all sites, excluding pediatric tumors, must be staged using the current edition of the *American Joint Committee on Cancer (AJCC) Manual for Staging of Cancer.*[4,9] Registries have the option of using either the AJCC staging scheme for pediatric tumors or nationally accepted protocol staging systems. In the AJCC staging system, the extent of disease is categorized according to tumor size (T), lymph node involvement (N), and metastases (M). Frequently referred to as the TNM system, it brings together information on staging of cancer at various anatomic sites in cooperation with the TNM Committee of the International Union Against Cancer. The proper classification and staging of cancer allow physicians to determine appropriate treatment, evaluate results of case management, and compare outcome with worldwide statistics reported from various institutions on a local, regional, state, and national basis.

Although the TNM system was designed for use by physicians, in some hospitals staging is done by the registry staff.[6,10] A working knowledge of both the SEER and the AJCC staging systems is necessary. The National Cancer Registrars Association, Inc., includes both staging systems in its national certification examination.

Primary Site File

The primary site, or abstract file is a permanent file that contains a paper abstract of every case entered into the data system. A separate abstract is prepared and maintained for every primary neoplasm a patient has. Abstracts are filed alphabetically by primary site under the year accessioned. Abstracts of living and deceased patients are filed together. This filing system is designed to provide rapid retrieval of cases of a specific site of cancer for studies, audits, and reports; that is, all the cases of colon cancer accessioned during a specific year are filed alphabetically under "colon."

In an automated setting, the primary site printout by year may be used in place of paper abstract files. The computerized registry system must be able to print hard copies of abstracts in natural language.

Quality Control

The usefulness of the data collected by a registry depends on the quality of the data. Quality control procedures are important to assure the completeness, accuracy, and timeliness of the data collected. The Commission on Cancer places accountability for quality control of registry data with the cancer committee because it is responsible for the overall supervision of the cancer registry.[4]

Quality control procedures vary. In some hospitals, a physician member of the cancer committee serves as the medical adviser to the cancer registry and assumes responsibility for reviewing abstracts of cases entered into the database. Other hospitals rotate this duty among different providers. The percentage of cases reviewed differ with the caseload. The Commission on Cancer recommends a random review of at least 10 per cent of all accessioned cases. Cases are selected by the reviewer from the accession register. Care is taken to include cases from all primary sites.

It is the policy of many registries to perform visual inspection on 100 per cent of their cases. In large regis-

Commission on Cancer Data Set

Required[1]

Institution ID Number
Accession Number
Sequence Number
Year First Seen For This Primary
   (Accession Year)
Medical Record Number
Social Security Number
Name (Last, First, Middle)
Address at Diagnosis (Street, City,
   State, Zip, County, Telephone)
Current Address (Street, City, State,
   Zip, Telephone)
Date of Birth
Race
Spanish Origin
Sex
Following Physician
Primary Surgeon
Primary Payor at Diagnosis
Abstracted By
Class of Case
Date of Initial Diagnosis
Primary Site
Laterality
Histology
Grade/differentiation
Diagnostic Confirmation
Size of Tumor
Regional Nodes Examined
Regional Nodes Positive
AJCC Clinical T, N, M, Suffix/prefix,
   Group*
AJCC Pathological T, N, M, Suffix/
   prefix, Group*
AJCC Other T, N, M, Suffix/prefix,
   Basis, Group*
Pediatric Stage**
TNM Edition
Physician Staged
First Course of Therapy
   Surgery
   Date of Surgery
   Surgical Approach
   Residual Tumor Following De-
      finitive Surgery
   Radiation Therapy
   Date Radiation Therapy Started
   Chemotherapy
   Date Chemotherapy Started
   Hormone Therapy
   Date Hormone Therapy Started
   Immunotherapy
   Date Immunotherapy Started
   Other Therapy

Date of First Recurrence
Type of First Recurrence
Date of Last Contact
Vital Status
Cancer Status
Follow-up Source
* Only one required
** Required for Pediatric Cases in
   absence of AJCC staging

Supplementary[2]

Social Security Suffix
Title
Maiden Name
Alias
Census Tract
Census Coding System
Age at Diagnosis
Physician 3
Physician 4
Physician 5
Institution Referred From
Institution Referred To
Date of Admission
Date of Discharge
Tumor Marker 1
Tumor Marker 2
Presentation at Cancer Conference
Referral to Support Services
SEER EOD
   Extension
   Lymph nodes
   Site of Distant Metastasis 1
   Site of Distant Metastasis 2
   Site of Distant Metastasis 3
General Summary Stage
Reason No
   Surgery
   Radiation Therapy
   Chemotherapy
   Hormone Therapy
Reconstructive Surgery
Radiation Therapy Detail
   Regional Dose (cGy)
   Number Treatments
   Elapsed Treatment Time (days)
   Volume
   Location
   Intent of Treatment
   Regional Treatment Modality
Chemotherapy Detail
   item 1
   item 2
   item 3
   item 4

Summary of Treatment at This
   Facility
Participation in Protocol
Date Other Recurrence
Type Other Recurrence
Second (third/fourth/etc.) Course for
   Recurrence or Progression
   Date each modality
   Treatment type (surgery,
      radiation, etc.)
Next Follow-up Source
Cause of Death

Optional[3]

User-defined:

County Current Address
Place of Birth
Patient History of Other Cancer 1
Patient History of Other Cancer 2
Primary Occupation
Family History of Cancer
Tobacco Use History
Alcohol Use History
Inpatient/outpatient Status
Date First Biopsy
Screening Date
Screening Result
Protocol Eligibility
Site(s) of Recurrence
Following Registry
Unusual Follow-up Method

Delete:

Marital Status at Diagnosis
Reporting Source
ICD-9-CM Revision Number
Radiation to CNS
Radiation/Surgery Sequence
Autopsy
Quality of Survival

Under Evaluation for Future
   Refinement:

Symptoms
Complications
Quality of Life

---

[1] Required for Commission-approved cancer programs.
[2] Considered integral to the operation of an outcome-based registry, but not required for Commission-approved cancer programs.
[3] May be useful to individual or central registries; not required for Commission-approved cancer programs.
Used with permission of the Cancer Department, Commission on Cancer, American College of Surgeons, Chicago.

Diagnosis | Hospital | Acc yr | Accession No | Doc No | Reg No

Cluster No | Admission Date

PATIENT IDENTIFICATION

Last | First | Middle

Medical Record No | Type Reporting Source | Phone

Address At Diagnosis | County of Residence

Marital Status | Race | Sex | Age | Date of Birth

Place Of Birth | Maiden

Social Security No | Religion | Alias

Hospital Referred From | Hospital Referred To

Diagnosis Date | Admission Date | Discharge Date | Place of Diagnosis

PHYSICIANS

Class of Case | Attending (Cancer) | Other

Referring | Other

Primary Surgeon | Following

Occupation Industry

TUMOR DATA

Laterality | DX Confirmation | ER: | PR:

Summary Stage | EOD: | Size | Extension | Lymph Nodes

No. Nodes Positive/Examined | TNM Edition | TNM Coder

AJCC Stage: | TNM Basis | T | N | M | AJCC Summary Stage

Sites of Distant Metastasis: | 1 | 2 | 3 | Residual Tumor

DIAGNOSTIC PROCEDURES

Physical Exam

X-rays/Scans

Scopes

Laboratory Tests

Operative Findings

Path/Autopsy (Gross & Micro)

TREATMENT

Surgery

Radiation

Chemotherapy

Hormone

Immunotherapy

Other

First Course/This Hospital | Site-Surg | Reason No | Radiation | Rad CNS | Rad Seq | Payer 1

Chemo | Hormone | Immuno | Other | Source of Casefinding

Subsequent Treatment | Payer 2

REMARKS

Fdx:

Date Last Contact | Vital Status | Tumor Status | Follow-Up Source

Dc File No | Cause of Death | Place of Death

Date 1st Entered | Date Completed | Abst Id | Date Printed | Coding Proc | Tum Rec No

Confidential Report of Neoplasm | California Tumor Registry | California Public Health Foundation

CCR 002 (6/92)

FIGURE 8–4. Abstract.

tries, a review or reabstracting of a portion of the cases by another member of the registry staff ensures consistent recording and interpretation of information. In the latter instance, the two abstracts are compared and discrepancies are noted and discussed.[6]

Computerized registries have the advantages of computer edits and computer-assisted coding. Registry staff must not rely solely on the computer for quality control because there is no way for the computer to read the documentation to determine completeness, accuracy, and support for the coded data.

Quality control activities should be well documented. A form may be implemented to record the abstracts reviewed, suggestions and corrections, reviewer, and review date. An example of such a form is shown in Figure 8–5. Another option is for the registry staff to make copies of case abstracts and then have the reviewer write his or her comments directly on the abstract copy. The reviewer then initials and dates the abstract. The abstracts are kept in a quality control file.

Patient Follow-Up

To ensure continued medical surveillance and to provide meaningful outcome data, the ACS requires annual **follow-up** information on every patient with a diagnosis of cancer for approved cancer programs. The objective of monitoring these patients on an annual basis is to document recurrence of disease, early diagnosis of new or subsequent cancers, assessment of treatment outcomes, and the institution of preventative measures. Length of survival is documented and mortality rates are calculated through this lifetime surveillance. Another goal of patient follow-up is to assure that the patient continues to see a physician at least once a year. Early detection of recurrence or spread of disease is usually essential to a favorable prognosis.[6]

Successful follow-up is defined as documented contact with the patient through his or her physician, re-admission to the hospital, a clinic visit, response to a follow-up letter by the patient or a relative or friend of the patient, or another registry. A 90 per cent successful follow-up rate is the target for cancer programs approved by the Commission on Cancer. A follow-up rate of 80 per cent of living patients is encouraged. Follow-up is based on the date of last contact. Cases are considered "lost to follow-up" by the Commission on Cancer if no patient contact has been made within the past 15 months.[4]

Follow-Up File

The objective of the follow-up file is to identify patients who are due for annual follow-up. In a manual system, a rotating dual tickler file consisting of two sets of monthly file guides and a follow-up card for every living patient is required. It is considered a temporary file because the cards are used only while patients are alive. One set of cards is used for filing the cards of patients who are due for follow-up; the other set is used for cards of patients who are not due for follow-up until the ensuing year.

One card is maintained for each patient, regardless of the number of primary malignant neoplasms the patient has. The following patient information is recorded on the follow-up card (Figure 8–6):

- Name
- Address
- Telephone number
- Social security number
- Date of birth
- Age
- Sex
- Primary site(s) of cancer

FIGURE 8–5. Quality control log.

Accession #	Site	Summary Stage	AJCC Stage

Primary Site Correct? Yes __ No __ Correct Site:
Summary Stage Correct? Yes __ No __ Correct Summary Stage:
AJCC Stage Correct? Yes __ No __ Correct AJCC Stage:
Suggestions/Corrections:

Reviewer: _____   Date: _____

Patient Name		Date of Birth	Social Security Number	Accession Number	Date Admitted

Address (Street, City, State, Zip Code)	Phone Number

Primary Site	Histology

Follow-Up Source	Date	Source #	Letter No.		Phone	Date of Last Contact	Date	Source #	Letter No.		Phone	Date of Last Contact
1												
2												
3												
4												

CANCER REGISTRY FOLLOW-UP CARD

Front Side Of Cancer Registry Follow-Up Card

Follow-Up Source	Date	Source #	Letter No.		Phone	Date of Last Contact	Date	Source #	Letter No.		Phone	Date of Last Contact
5												
6												
7												
8												
9												
10												
11												

CANCER REGISTRY FOLLOW UP CARD

Back Side Of Cancer Registry Follow-Up Card

FIGURE 8–6. Follow-up file card.

- Accession number
- Medical record number
- Follow-up sources
- Date of last contact
- Source of last contact

A computerized control document may be used in place of a tickler file as long as it contains the same data fields as the manual card system. Monthly lists of patients due for follow-up are generated. The names of patients who are lost to follow-up (past due) must appear on a delinquent list until follow-up is obtained. A report of the rate of successful follow-up should be available as a printout or on-screen.

Specific policies pertaining to follow-up and the procedures used by the registry to obtain follow-up data must be established by each hospital.[6] Policies must be instituted for contacting patients directly when contact through their physicians is not feasible. The following additional policies and procedures are required:

- The use of the word cancer or its synonyms when answering the telephone or in patient correspondence
- When requests are received for physician referrals
- Request for an opinion of a diagnostic workup or treatment modalities[6]

Follow-Up Forms and Letters

There are numerous follow-up forms and letters that are used to monitor the morbidity and mortality status of the cancer patient. Descriptions of the various documents that could be used to obtain follow-up information follow.

POSTHOSPITAL TREATMENT SUMMARIES. Forms are used to solicit information pertaining to the first course of treatment therapy that may have been given after patient discharge (Figure 8–7). These forms are not sent out on every patient but only when additional treatment is planned or suspected. They are usually generated when a case is abstracted and are sent directly to the physician.

PHYSICIAN FOLLOW-UP LETTERS. The primary source of follow-up information is the patient's physician. The physician is the most qualified judge of the patient's condition; he or she can report accurately on cancer status, spread or recurrence of disease, new primaries, and the patient's quality of life. Receipt of a follow-up letter often serves as a reminder that the patient is due for an annual check-up (Figure 8–8).

PATIENT LETTER. Sometimes the patient's physician loses contact with the patient and has no current follow-up information. When permitted, the registry staff contacts the patient directly (Figure 8–9).

THIRD PARTY LETTER. Occasionally the registry staff finds it necessary to contact a relative or friend of the patient to obtain follow-up information (Figure 8–10).

Resources used by cancer registries in locating patients who are no longer in contact with their physicians and who have moved leaving no forwarding address are numerous and vary from state to state. This situation places the registrar working on follow-up in a role resembling that of a detective. Friends and relatives are an excellent resource, but they are not always listed in the patient's record. Fortunately other resources are available, such as the following:

- State department of vital statistics or vital records
- Department of motor vehicles
- Central (population-based) registries
- County voter registration and property tax records
- Street address and phone directories
- Religious organizations
- Employers
- Home Care Financing Administration (Medicare)
- Newspaper obituaries

Discretion must be exercised when using these sources of follow-up, particularly with employers.[6]

Space, Equipment, and Supplies

In developing and maintaining a hospital cancer registry, consideration must be given to the space requirements, equipment needs, and supplies that are often unique to registry operations.[6]

Space

Space requirements for a cancer registry include the following:

- A quiet setting conducive to abstracting, confidential follow-up activities, and preparation of statistical reports
- Access to patient records
- Convenient and adequate accommodations for physicians to review cancer data
- Place for data files and computer hardware

POST HOSPITAL TREATMENT

Re: _____

Birthdate: _____

Diagnosis: _____

Dear Doctor _____ :

In cancer data collection, it is imperative that we obtain ALL treatment information. In order to complete this case, will you please provide the CANCER REGISTRY with the following information. Thank you for your courtesies.

Sincerely,

Cancer Registry Services

1. Diagnosis:

Place: _____

Date: _____

2. Treatment PRIOR to admission:

Type: _____

Date: _____

3. Treatment POST discharge:
   RADIATION THERAPY:

Facility: _____

Start Date: _____

Site: _____

cGy/Fractions/Days: _____
(i.e. 5040/28/42)

   CHEMOTHERAPY:

Facility: _____

Start Date: _____

Drugs: _____

   OTHERS: (Hormones/Immunotherapy/Other):

Facility: _____

Start Date: _____

Type: _____

4. Date of Last Contact:
   Tumor/Patient Status Free: _____   Not Free: _____   Alive: _____   Dead: _____

5. Patient Referred to: Name: _____

Street: _____

City: _____

State: _____ Zip: _____

FIGURE 8–7. Posthospital treatment summary.

Dear Doctor _____ :

An important part of the Cancer Program at Community Memorial Hospital is to assure that all of our registered cancer cases receive continuing medical follow-up care. Annual follow-up is conducted by the Cancer Registry and provides statistical information of survival data at yearly intervals as required by the American College of Surgeons. Please record the latest information you have concerning the patient's condition as requested on this form. Thank you for your assistance.

Cancer Registry
Community Memorial Hospital

PATIENT _____ DATE OF BIRTH _____

ADDRESS _____ DATE OF ADMIT _____

DIAGNOSIS _____ DATE OF LAST CONTACT _____

- -

LAST FOLLOW-UP DATE _____

ADDITIONAL THERAPY

MEDICAL EXAM _____ OTHER _____ DATE _____

FREE _____ NOT FREE _____ MODALITY _____

QUALITY OF SURVIVAL

1. Normal Activity = 0 _____

2. Symptomatic and ambulatory = 1 _____

3. Ambulatory more than 50%, occasionally needs assistance = 2 _____

4. Ambulatory less than 50%, nursing care needed = 3 _____

5. Bedridden, may require hospitalization = 4 _____

DEATH INFORMATION

Date of Death _____ Place _____ Autopsy: ____ Yes ____ No

COMMENTS AND OTHER SOURCES FOR FOLLOW-UP_____

_____

Signed _____ , M.D.

FIGURE 8–8. Physician follow-up letter.

The Community Memorial Hospital has a continuing interest in the progress of its former patients. We would like to know how you are feeling now.

If you wish, you may write your answers on the bottom of this letter, answering the few questions listed.

A pre-addressed, postage paid envelope is enclosed for your convenience. Thank you for your assistance.

Sincerely,

Cancer Registry
- -

How are you feeling now (please feel free to use the reverse side)? _____
_____
_____
Have you had any treatment for the condition for which you were seen here? _____
_____

Who is your present doctor? _____
What is his address? _____
What is your current occupation? _____
Work status: working _____ not working _____ unable to work _____ retired _____
Who (not husband or wife) will always know your address?
Name: _____ Relationship: _____
Address: _____ Telephone No: _____
Is there anything else you would like to add? _____
Your present address: _____
Telephone No: _____

FIGURE 8–9. Patient follow-up letter.

The number of staff working in the registry at any given time may vary and is a factor in determining the amount of space and equipment required. The nature of the work performed in the registry is such that the traditional 9-to-5 hours are not necessary. Flexible hours and staggered shifts may be considered. The size and age of the cancer database must also be considered when determining the space required for the cancer registry. A new registry does not need the abstract storage space that an older registry requires; however, long-term projections for space needs must be considered. The mode of operation and the amount of technology used also impact the required space allocation.

Equipment

Equipment needs are similar to those of the HIM departments. In addition to traditional office furniture, the following equipment is needed:

- Separate telephone line(s) or extension
- Computer hardware and work stations
- Lateral or vertical file cabinet(s) for the primary site file (three to four drawers per 300 to 500 annual caseload)
- Computer printout files, two to four card files for patient index and follow-up cards with a capacity of 1000 cards each
- Storage space for reference materials, telephone books, and supplies

Supplies

The following supplies are unique to the registry:

- Printed follow-up forms
- Pre-addressed return envelopes for follow-up

CANCER REGISTRY
January 4, 1996

RE:
RELATIONSHIP: Daughter

Dear Ms _____ :

Will you please take a few minutes of your time to help us. The person listed above has been admitted to our Registry at Community Memorial Hospital for lifetime follow-up, and we have been unable to contact him or her.

May we ask your help in furnishing the information requested below and returning this letter to us in the enclosed envelope.

Present Address:
    Street Address _____
    City _____ State _____ Zip _____

Present Condition:
    Apparently well _____ Not well _____

If deceased, please give:
    Date of death _____ Place of death _____

If known, name and address of physician:
_____
_____
_____

Thank you for your assistance in this matter.

Sincerely,

Cancer Registry

FIGURE 8–10. Third party follow-up letter.

- Request log
- Accession register
- Patient index
- Follow-up cards

Automation

As noted earlier in this chapter, the integration of computers in cancer registry activities is common. Cancer registry software emerged in the mid-1980s and is available for both hospital- and population-based registries. At the 1993 Annual Conference of the Registrars Association, 25 software providers had been identified by the ACS, in addition to the software available from the ACS itself.[13] A 1993 study conducted by the ACS showed that more than 80 per cent of hospitals with approved hospital cancer programs were computerized. Features included in basic software programs are easy-to-use menus, abstracting screens, on-line help functions, automatic coding and editing, accession register, master patient index and follow-up files, statistical analysis (cross tabulations, summary analysis, and survival analysis by life-table or actuarial method), report writing, and customized follow-up letters and other follow-up routines. The data collection component encompasses the data items required by the Commission on

Cancer for approved hospital programs. Optional data fields might include hospital-specific, financial, and Joint Commission on Accreditation of Healthcare Organizations (JCAHO) clinical indicators. Other features available from some vendors consist of multiple-user networks, hospital mainframe interface, expanded statistical applications, and graphics. Some hospital software vendors maintain national databases that contain aggregate data submitted by their users. A Tumor Registry Software Checklist presented at the 1993 annual meeting of the National Cancer Registrars Association, Inc., can be used by hospitals to evaluate cancer registry software (Figure 8–11).

Computers are an integral part of central registry operations. Many central registries have found it beneficial to provide and support software for a micro-based system suitable for a hospital cancer registry and interfaced with the central registry system. In some states, the electronic reporting of cancer data by hospitals is included in the legislation. The advantage to the hospital is that the central registry often provides the software, user support, training, quality control of data, hospital incidence reports, and comparison data. The central registry is assured of computer-readable data that has passed an initial set of edit checks and meets pre-established reporting requirements. Hospitals submit their data electronically or by mail. Some central registries receive hard copy abstracts that require data entry by staff at the registry. Hospital cancer registries seeking approval by the ACS need to verify that the software provided by the central registry meets the requirements for approval. Many population-based registries are interested only in capturing incidence data, and the software may not include all the data items required.

The North American Association of Central Cancer Registries, Inc. (NAACCR), has developed a national standard for data exchange. The NAACCR Record Layout provides a common standard record layout that can be used for electronic exchange of data.[14] The NAACCR Record Layout has been used by the ACS Commission on Cancer National Database Call for Data, which includes data from more than 500 hospitals in 1990 and 1992, and the NAACCR National Call for Data, which received information from 30 central registries in 1990 and 1992.

Confidentiality and Release of Information

Confidentiality policies and procedures are required in all phases of cancer registry operations for the following purposes:

- To protect the privacy of the individual patient
- To protect the privacy of the facilities and physicians reporting the cases
- To provide public assurance that the data will not be abused
- To abide by any confidentiality protecting legislation or administrative rule(s) that may apply

Hospital cancer registries have been established to monitor and evaluate patient care and the incidence of the disease. Other registries have been established to comply with mandated state legislation or regulation or have been implemented to meet the needs of the hospital and/or the community. Regardless of the purpose, confidentiality must be maintained. Studies using cancer registry data should include aggregate data only, with all patient identifiers removed. Physician identifiers must be disclosed with caution and with permission. Every cancer registry has a responsibility to protect its data from unauthorized access or release.

Policies and Procedures

Policies in general are established by hospital administration and apply to all departments.[4,6] The ACS requires the cancer committee to serve a policy-advisory role in approved cancer programs and the cancer registry to maintain a complete up-to-date procedure manual that documents each phase of its operation. Policies established by the cancer committee must comply with those of the hospital. Examples of policies set by the cancer committee include the following:

- Contacting patients directly for follow-up when the physician has not seen the patient
- Evaluating the quality of care of the cancer patient and making recommendations for improvement
- Making certain that consultative services are available to patients with cancer

Policies are also established by the cancer registry, usually under the direction and approval of the cancer committee. Examples of these policies include the overall objectives of the cancer program, issues of confidentiality, and access to registry data.

Procedures detail the specific tasks required to implement the policies and objectives of the cancer program and indicate who is responsible for performing the work. The procedure manual should include the following:

- Cancer committee composition
- Casefinding procedures
- Case eligibility criteria
- Reportable and nonreportable lists
- Filing systems

This checklist can be used to evaluate tumor registry software

Functional and Technical Requirements	Commission on Cancer Requirements	Software _____
Overall software		
Menu-driven		
User-friendly		
Network capability (single or multiple users, one or several locations)		
Case identification		
Suspense file/system	●	
Interface with other data bases (pathology, disease index, outpatient visit/charge file) to assist in casefinding		
Flags for special populations, eg, cancer screening		
Combined with master patient file		
Patient Data Collection		
Data sets		
Commission on Cancer	●	
State registry		
SEER		
Hospital specific		
Other data items,such as JCAHO clinical indicators, financial		
English text space		
Data entry		
Capability to add/change/delete cases		
Retention of follow-up information		
Ease in changing previously entered materials		
Assistance in coding		
Duplicate record detection	●	
Verification of data entry	●	
Edit checks (valid codes and interfield/relational edits)		
Editing of new data and changed data		
Help screens to assist in coding		
Reporting		
Flexibility in selecting data elements	●	
Interface with any "canned," ad hoc report, or follow-up listing		
Accurate and useful reports	●	
Reports displayed on screen as well as printed		
User-designed reports		
Statistical analysis (cross tabulations, summary analysis, & survival analysis by life-table or actuarial method)	●	
Administrative reports (printouts and on-screen displays)		
Alphabetic patient listing (patient index file)	●	
Numerical listing of patients (accession register)	●	
Abstract or case summary	●	
Primary site list by year (abstract file)	●	
Suspense list (file)	●	
Staff productivity report (cases abstracted, follow-up posted, suspense cases added, etc, by each staff member)		
Other reports		

● Required, ▭ Preferred

Source: Suzanna Hoyler, CTR, Washington Hospital Center, Washington, D.C. 1993 NTRA Annual Meeting, 5/6/93

FIGURE 8–11. Tumor registry software checklist.

- Accessioning of cases
- Patient index
- Coding schemes and staging systems used
- Data elements and abstracting procedures
- Patient follow-up
- Patient care evaluation
- Reporting practices
- Quality control procedures
- Tumor board and cancer conferences
- Job descriptions
- Hospital and cancer program organizational charts

The procedure manual should document each phase of the cancer program and be approved by the cancer committee. It should be written in a format that provides clear, step-by-step instructions for completing each task. Each time a procedure is changed or changes are made in staging systems or coding schemes, the manual must be revised. An annual review and update of the policies and procedures provides the documentation needed for a well-functioning cancer program.

Use of Cancer Registry Data

Cancer registry data are used for **patient care evaluation** studies, cancer conferences, administrative reports, and marketing. Hospitals with ACS-approved cancer programs are required to publish and distribute an annual report. Approved cancer programs are also required to document the use of cancer registry data through the use of a request log.[4]

Annual Report

The annual report reflects the quality and comprehensiveness of the cancer program. It provides the hospital with a forum in which to highlight the goals and accomplishments of the cancer program and can be an excellent public relations tool.[12] The content requirements are quite specific, entailing a narrative by the cancer committee or one of its members. They are as follows:

- Description of the goals, achievements, and activities of the overall cancer program
- Report of the cancer registry activities
- Statistical summary of cancer data for the calendar year
- In-depth statistical report on at least one major site, complete with survival analysis and narrative critique

- State, regional, and national data comparison
- Narrative interpretation of patient care evaluation studies, including findings and actions taken[4]

Published by November 1 of the next cancer data calendar year, the annual report is distributed to the medical staff and administration. Other internal and external distributions are determined by the hospital.

Patient Care Evaluation

The purpose of the hospital cancer data system is to collect and maintain information on every patient with cancer from the initial date of diagnosis and/or treatment until death. The information collected furnishes the medical staff with data that enables them to see the results of their diagnostic and therapeutic efforts and provides them with the tools to improve cancer patient care.

To evaluate the adequacy of care given to this patient population, a meaningful review of the hospital's performance through quality assurance studies is necessary. Comparison of local experience with regional and national data provides insight on whether the care given at the hospital meets or exceeds that given elsewhere.

The Commission on Cancer of the ACS has specific patient care evaluation requirements for hospitals seeking approval of their cancer programs. A minimum of two studies must be conducted each year. One of the studies must include a survival analysis. Comparison with regional and national data is also required. The Commission on Cancer does not prescribe a format for the studies but does require a written description of the audit system and methodology used. The studies may be done in conjunction with other in-house quality assurance activities, through participation on the Commission on Cancer's nationwide patterns of care studies, or in site-specific problem-oriented audits. Patient management guidelines and cancer protocol studies such as those instituted by the Southwest Oncology Group also provide a means for evaluating patient care. The hospital's cancer committee is required to review the study criteria and outcome, make recommendations where appropriate, and ensure that the recommendations are implemented. Coordination with other hospital quality assurance activities is appropriate.[11] Two checklists were developed for use by cancer registries in patient care evaluation studies and in-house audits (Figures 8–12 and 8–13).

Two patterns-of-care studies are conducted each year by the Commission on Cancer, one short-term (process) and one long-term (outcome). Participation in these studies is voluntary and does not effect the approval status of the cancer program. The following are included in the format:

1. Select study topic and objective(s) _____
2. Draft criteria _____
3. Present topic, objective(s), and criteria to Cancer Committee for approval _____
4.* Identify eligible cases _____
5. Obtain patient records _____
6.* Abstract study data _____
7. Ratify criteria _____
8. Review cases failing to meet performance standards _____
9. Analyze audit findings, identify problems _____
10. Formulate recommendations for corrective action _____
11. Prepare presentation for Cancer Committee _____
12. Present completed audit to Cancer Committee _____
13. Present audit findings to appropriate committees and sections _____
14. Re-evaluate _____

*Tasks usually performed by cancer registry staff

FIGURE 8–12. Patient care evaluation: In-house audit checklist. Used with permission of the National Cancer Registrars Association, Inc.

- Study site
- Scope of the patients to be included
- Study objective
- Criteria for data retrieval

Study forms are completed for eligible cases and sent to the ACS. Study findings are sent to all participating hospitals so that they may compare their cancer care on a national basis.[4]

Administrative Reports

Cancer data are a valuable resource for administration who use the information to assess the following:

- Service areas
- Target populations
- Patterns of referral
- Need for increasing or decreasing services

1. Review study objectives _____
2. Recommend to Cancer Committee one of the following: _____
   a) participate
   b) participate and expand into an in-house audit
   c) non-participation (no further action needed)
3.* Identify eligible cases _____
4.* Duplicate abstracting forms _____
5. Obtain patient records _____
6.* Abstract study data _____
7. Review abstracted data for accuracy and completeness _____
8. Submit data to American College of Surgeons _____
9. Review and analyze study results to identify variations from national standards _____
10. Prepare presentation for Cancer Committee _____
11. Make presentation to Cancer Committee _____
12. Make further action as requested by Cancer Committee _____

*Tasks usually performed by cancer registry staff

FIGURE 8–13. American College of Surgeons: Patterns of care checklist. Used with permission of the National Cancer Registrars Association, Inc.

The data are also used as documentation for regulating agencies, cost containment and financial planning, and for physician recruitment. Cancer admissions that fluctuate, variations in the type of cancer cases seen at the hospital, an increase or a decrease in diagnostic services and treatment modalities used, and changes in referral patterns would all be of interest to the administration.[6]

Cancer Conferences

Cases presented at cancer conferences can be compared with the hospital's overall experience and with regional and national data to evaluate morbidity and mortality. Similar cases may be used to assess the effectiveness of diagnostic and therapeutic efforts.

Marketing

Marketing and dissemination of cancer data are integral roles for the HIM professional. Maintaining visibility for cancer program services is vital to the success of the program. Newsletters, brochures, and other promotional materials should be directed to the medical staff, patients, family members, other health care professionals, health insurance providers, and community agencies. Each potential user should be reminded on a regular basis of the data and services available. The marketing of the cancer data and/or cancer program must tie into the hospital's overall strategic plan or business improvement plan. The cancer registry staff should work with the hospital's public relations or marketing department to promote the activities and accomplishments of the cancer program.

Request Log or File

Requests for data are documented in a request log or file. The use of the database is vital to monitor the cancer experience at the hospital, analyze patient morbidity and survival, track the effectiveness of treatment modalities, and assess trends in the cancer patient population as well as for professional education. The request log or file should contain the following information (Figure 8–14):

- Date of request
- Use of the data
- Topic of reports and time period covered
- Report parameters or variables
- Name(s) of person(s) requesting data
- Purpose or use of data
- Final disposition of data

Staffing

Administratively, the hospital cancer registry staff usually report to hospital administration, quality assurance, or HIM managers. When the registry is a component of a hospital cancer program, the staff is responsible to the cancer committee and the medical staff in addition to the administrative department to which they report.

The cancer registry staff perform a wide variety of administrative and technical duties that reflect many similarities to the HIM profession. The National Cancer Registrars Association, Inc., offers a national certification examination. Candidates who successfully sit for the examination are awarded the Certified Tumor Registrar (CTR) credential. The cancer registry staff requirements depend on the size and sophistication of the program and the goals of the cancer program. A wide range of positions may be needed, from highly specialized technicians, such as a follow-up clerk/secretary/assistant, to administrators.[10]

The technical expertise required of the staff responsible for data collection is such that the ACS recommends that the registry staff include at least one CTR.[4] Some state registries require that the hospital and central registry data collection be staffed with all CTRs. The *Registry Staffing Manual, 1989*,[10] published jointly by the National Cancer Registrars Association, Inc., and the ACS Commission on Cancer, defines two categories for registry professionals: technicians and administrators (see Activities of Cancer Registry Technician and Activities of Cancer Registry Manager).

Activities of Cancer Registry Technician

- Processes, maintains, compiles, and reports health information data for research, quality assurance, facility planning, marketing
- Abstracts and codes clinical data using appropriate classification systems
- Obtains long-term follow-up data
- Analyzes health records according to published governmental or institutional standards

---

National Cancer Registrars Association, Inc., Mundelein, IL. Used with permission.

The following activities should be considered when estimating cancer registry staffing needs:

- Casefinding
- Abstracting
- Follow-up
- Patient care evaluation and other studies

REQUEST FOR CANCER REGISTRY DATA

Data Requested:
  Please specify the type of data desired, e.g. primary site, histology, time period, variables such as age, sex, race, and stage. (Example: All 1990 lung cancer cases, small cell carcinoma, males ages 40-59, staged with regional node extension-would like to see first course of treatment given.)

Purpose/Intended Use of Data:

Date Data Needed:

Name of Person(s) Requesting Data:

Data Requested:

FIGURE 8–14. Request log.

Activities of Cancer Registry Manager

- Plans and develops cancer-related data collection systems that meet the standards of accrediting and disease-reporting agencies
- Designs cancer-related data collection systems appropriate for various sizes and types of health care facilities
- Manages human, financial, and physical resources of the registry
- Participates in medical staff and institution activities, including quality assurance and research
- Serves as an advocate for privacy and confidentiality of health information
- Plans and offers in-service educational programs for health care personnel

National Cancer Registrars Association, Inc., Mundelein, IL. Used with permission.

- Report preparation
- Cancer committee and cancer conference support and meeting or conference attendance
- Clerical (filing, chart retrieval)
- Quality control
- Fiscal planning
- Cancer prevention and control
- Continuing education

The *Registry Staffing Manual, 1989* provides formulas that are useful in calculating staffing needs.

APPROVED CANCER PROGRAM

As stated earlier, there are four major components of a cancer program that is approved by the Commission on Cancer. Two of them—the cancer registry, including follow-up and quality control, and patient care evaluations—have already been discussed. The other two components are the cancer committee and cancer conferences.

Cancer Committee

The cancer committee is the policymaking body of the cancer program. Leadership is a chief ingredient necessary for an effective cancer program. "The committee is responsible for planning, initiating, stimulating, and assessing all cancer-related activities in the institution."[4] According to the ACS, committee composition must include representatives from the medical staff involved in the care of patients with cancer, such as delegates from surgery, medical oncology, radiation oncology, diagnostic radiology, and pathology. Hospitals without their own radiation therapy department must have a referral agreement with a treatment facility to provide this therapy. Other disciplines such as internal medicine, pediatrics, and family practice should be part of the committee, if appropriate. Required nonphysician members are representatives from administration, nursing, social services, quality assurance, and cancer registry. Additional representatives from the pharmacy, nutrition, rehabilitation, and clergy staff may also be included.

The cancer committee must meet at least quarterly to achieve the following goals:

- Make certain that patient-oriented, prospective cancer conferences are held that include all the major sites of cancer during the course of a year.

- Ensure that consultative services are available for patients with cancer.

- Evaluate the quality of care.

- Actively supervise the cancer registry.

- Publish and distribute an annual report.

In addition to serving as active members of the committee, cancer registry personnel frequently serve as staff to the cancer committee.[6,10] It is often the cancer registrar who monitors committee activities to ensure compliance with the ACS-approved cancer program requirements. Keeping the committee informed of the contributions and time restrictions paramount to the production of the annual report, presenting suggestions for patient care evaluation studies, and enlisting their help in quality control efforts are just a few of the responsibilities the registry staff assumes.

Cancer Conferences (Tumor Boards)

Cancer conferences are held to provide consultative services to cancer patients and to educate the medical staff in current diagnostic and therapeutic modalities. The Commission on Cancer has found that "prospective, patient-oriented, multidisciplinary cancer conferences can improve the care of patients with cancer in an institution."[4] To achieve the goal of providing consultative services, multidisciplinary attendance and participation in the conference are required. Case presentations must include all major sites of cancer seen at the institution during the year. The frequency of conferences (weekly or monthly) depends on the category of cancer program approved by the Commission on Cancer. Categories designated by the ACS include Comprehensive Cancer Program, Teaching Hospital Cancer Program, Community Hospital Comprehensive Category, Community Hospital Cancer Program, Hospital Associate Cancer Program, Special Cancer Program, Integrated Cancer Program, and Freestanding Cancer Center Program.

Cancer registry personnel often serve as staff for the cancer conference activities.[6,10] In this role, they may perform the following duties:

- Assist the chairperson in scheduling cases.

- Arrange for the attending physician or a designee to present the case.

- Notify members of the medical staff of the cases to be presented.

- Obtain case protocols.

- Tabulate registry data pertinent to the cases being presented.

- Make the meeting room arrangements including setup, audiovisual equipment, and refreshments.

Documentation

Documentation of both the cancer committee and the cancer conference activities is required. Minutes of the cancer committee must be recorded and maintained as required by the JCAHO. The medical staff secretary usually records the minutes for the cancer committee, as is done for other medical staff committees. In some institutions, a member of the registry staff is charged with this responsibility.[6,10] Members in attendance and committee action are documented.

The documentation of cancer conferences should include the conference date, medical disciplines represented, and the cases discussed. A copy of the meeting notice, a sign-in sheet with disciplines noted, and copies of case protocols may be used to document the conference. Case protocols are summaries of the cases, including a brief description of the patient's history, pertinent physical and clinical findings, and the treatment given to date. Case protocols are usually prepared or dictated by the attending physician and distributed for reference at the conference.[6] Patient names are usually not documented on the case protocols or meeting notices to maintain patient confidentiality.

NATIONAL CANCER REGISTRARS ASSOCIATION, INC.

Founded in 1974, the National Cancer Registrars Association, Inc. (NCRA; formerly the National Tumor Registrars Association) is composed of people who are involved in central and hospital-based cancer registries, including cancer registrars, physicians, hospital administrators, HIM professionals, epidemiologists, data managers, and health care planners who maintain ongoing records of the cancer patients' history, diagnosis, therapy, and outcome. The purposes of the NCRA are as follows:

- To promote research and education in cancer registry administration and practice
- To improve service to cancer patients
- To establish standards of education and provide a standardized course of study for cancer registrars
- To raise the level of knowledge and performance of cancer registrars through continuing education
- To disseminate information regarding current activities, research, and trends in the cancer field
- To initiate and participate in programs to improve and standardize the compilation of cancer-related data

In 1983, the NCRA offered its first annual national certification examination. The association sponsors an annual national meeting and regional workshops and seminars that provide continuing education programs to help members maintain certification and offer educational assistance for new registrars. The NCRA publishes a journal, *The Abstract;* a newsletter, *The Connection;* an annual membership roster; brochures; and educational material. Because many HIM professionals work with or in cancer registries, the president of NCRA annually appoints an active member to serve as an official liaison to the American Health Information Management Association.

The following sections address a variety of registries. Although these registries share some similarities with the cancer registry model, each has unique characteristics.

AIDS REGISTRIES

Since it was first described in 1981, AIDS has had a major impact on the health care industry both in the United States and in other countries. Numerous hospital- and population-based registries have been established. Monitoring trends in reported AIDS cases reveal how the AIDS epidemic has spread in different patient populations. The AIDS morbidity data play a key role in many human immunodeficiency virus (HIV)-related funding, program, and policy decisions.[15]

Database Management

The goals of the AIDS registry are as follows:

- To identify and collect data on every patient with AIDS
- To maintain the data in an organized manner
- To make the data readily available for use by the medical staff, hospital administration, state health agencies, and the Centers for Disease Control and Prevention (CDC)

Case Eligibility

AIDS is a manifestation of HIV infection that is characterized by the presence of one or more diseases or conditions as defined by the CDC. The surveillance case definition includes all HIV-infected people with CD4+ T-lymphocyte counts of less than 200 cells/microliter or a CD4+ percentage less than 14. There are 26 clinical conditions that are considered to be indicators of AIDS and to be reportable.[16] These conditions are listed on the Aids Adult Confidentiality Form shown in Figure 8–15.

Casefinding

AIDS cases are identified using all the sources listed for cancer registries plus other sources in which AIDS patients may have been seen or treated, including such departments as respiratory therapy, laboratory, pharmacy, and nuclear medicine. The hospital's infection control nurse, the county AIDS surveillance office, and community AIDS agencies are other casefinding resources.

NOTE: HIV infection without an AIDS Defining Condition is NOT reportable in California

Patient's Name: _____ Phone No.: ( ) _____
(Last, First, M.I.)

Address: _____ City: _____ County: _____ State: _____ Zip Code: _____

RETURN TO STATE/LOCAL HEALTH DEPARTMENT — *Patient identifier information is not transmitted to CDC!* —

U.S. DEPARTMENT OF HEALTH & HUMAN SERVICES
Public Health Service

ADULT HIV/AIDS CONFIDENTIAL CASE REPORT
(Patients ≥13 years of age at time of diagnosis)

CDC
CENTERS FOR DISEASE CONTROL AND PREVENTION

II. HEALTH DEPARTMENT USE ONLY

Form Approved OMB No. 0920-0009

DATE FORM COMPLETED:
Mo. Day Yr.

REPORT SOURCE:

SOUNDEX CODE:

REPORT STATUS:
1 New Report
2 Update

REPORTING HEALTH DEPARTMENT:
State: _____
City/County: _____

State Patient No.:
City/County Patient No.:

III. DEMOGRAPHIC INFORMATION

DIAGNOSTIC STATUS AT REPORT (check one):
1 HIV Infection (not AIDS)
2 AIDS

AGE AT DIAGNOSIS:
Years
Years

DATE OF BIRTH:
Mo. Day Yr.

CURRENT STATUS:
Alive Dead Unk.
1 2 9

DATE OF DEATH:
Mo. Day Yr.

STATE/TERRITORY OF DEATH:
_____

SEX:
1 Male
2 Female

RACE/ETHNICITY:
1 White (not Hispanic)
4 Asian/Pacific Islander
2 Black (not Hispanic)
5 American Indian/Alaska Native
3 Hispanic
9 Not Specified

COUNTRY OF BIRTH:
1 U.S. 7 U.S. Dependencies and Possessions (including Puerto Rico)
(specify): _____
8 Other (specify): _____ 9 Unknown

RESIDENCE AT DIAGNOSIS:
City: _____ County: _____ State/Country: _____ Zip Code: _____

IV. FACILITY OF DIAGNOSIS

Facility Name _____

City _____

State/Country _____

FACILITY SETTING (check one)
1 Public   2 Private   3 Federal
9 Unknown

FACILITY TYPE (check one)
01 Physician, HMO   31 Hospital, Inpatient
88 Other (specify): _____

This report is authorized by law (Sections 304 and 306 of the Public Health Service Act, 42 USC 242b and 242k). Response in this case is voluntary for federal government purposes, but may be mandatory under state and local statutes. Your cooperation is necessary for the understanding and control of HIV/AIDS. Information in the surveillance system that would permit identification of any individual on whom a record is maintained, is collected with a guarantee that it will be held in confidence, will be used only for the purposes stated in the assurance on file at the local health department, and will not otherwise be disclosed or released without the consent of the individual in accordance with Section 308(d) of the Public Health Service Act (42 USC 242m).

V. PATIENT HISTORY

AFTER 1977 AND PRECEDING THE FIRST POSITIVE HIV ANTIBODY TEST OR AIDS DIAGNOSIS, THIS PATIENT HAD (Respond to **ALL** Categories):

	Yes	No	Unk.
• Sex with male	1	0	9
• Sex with female	1	0	9
• Injected nonprescription drugs	1	0	9
• Received clotting factor for hemophilia/coagulation disorder	1	0	9

Specify disorder: 1 Factor VIII (Hemophilia A)   2 Factor IX (Hemophilia B)   8 Other (specify): _____

• *HETEROSEXUAL* relations with any of the following:

	Yes	No	Unk.
• Intravenous/injection drug user	1	0	9
• Bisexual male	1	0	9
• Person with hemophilia/coagulation disorder	1	0	9
• Transfusion recipient with documented HIV infection	1	0	9
• Transplant recipient with documented HIV infection	1	0	9
• Person with AIDS or documented HIV infection, risk not specified	1	0	9
• Received transfusion of blood/blood components (other than clotting factor)	1	0	9

First (Mo. Yr.)   Last (Mo. Yr.)

	Yes	No	Unk.
• Received transplant of tissue/organs or artificial insemination	1	0	9
• Worked in a health-care or clinical laboratory setting	1	0	9

(specify occupation): _____

VI. LABORATORY DATA

1. HIV ANTIBODY TESTS AT DIAGNOSIS:
(Indicate first test)

	Pos	Neg	Ind	Not Done	TEST DATE Mo.	Yr.
• HIV–1 EIA	1	0	–	9		
• HIV–1/HIV–2 combination EIA	1	0	–	9		
• HIV–1 Western blot/IFA	1	0	8	9		
• Other HIV antibody test (specify):	1	0	8	9		
• HIV–2 EIA	1	0	–	9		
• HIV–2 Western blot	1	0	8	9		

2. POSITIVE HIV DETECTION TEST: (Record earliest test)

	Mo.	Yr.
• HIV culture		
• HIV antigen test		
• HIV PCR, DNA or RNA probe		
• Other (specify): _____		

• Date of last documented negative HIV test (specify type): _____   Mo. Yr.

• If HIV laboratory tests were not documented, is HIV diagnosis documented by a physician?
Yes No Unk.
1 0 9

If yes, provide date of documentation by physician.   Mo. Yr.

3. IMMUNOLOGIC LAB TESTS:

AT OR CLOSEST TO CURRENT DIAGNOSTIC STATUS   Mo. Yr.
• CD4 Count _____ , _____ cells/μL
• CD4 Percent _____ %

First <200 μL or <14%   Mo. Yr.
• CD4 Count _____ , _____ cells/μL
• CD4 Percent _____ %

CDC 50.42A   REV. 07-93   (Page 1 of 2)   — ADULT HIV/AIDS CONFIDENTIAL CASE REPORT —

FIGURE 8–15.   AIDS case report.

Physician's Name: _____ Phone No.: (___) _____ Medical Record No. _____

(Last, First, M.I.)

Hospital/Facility: _____ Person Completing Form: _____ Phone No.: (___) _____

– Physician identifier information is not transmitted to CDC! –

VIII. CLINICAL STATUS

| CLINICAL RECORD REVIEWED: | Yes [1] No [0] | ENTER DATE PATIENT WAS DIAGNOSED AS: | Asymptomatic (including acute retroviral syndrome and persistent generalized lymphadenopathy): | Mo. [ ] Yr. [ ] | Symptomatic (not AIDS) : | Mo. [ ] Yr. [ ] |

AIDS INDICATOR DISEASES	Initial Diagnosis Def. / Pres.	Initial Date Mo. / Yr.	AIDS INDICATOR DISEASES	Initial Diagnosis Def. / Pres.	Initial Date Mo. / Yr.
Candidiasis, bronchi, trachea, or lungs	[1] NA	[ ][ ]	Lymphoma, Burkitt's (or equivalent term)	[1] NA	[ ][ ]
Candidiasis, esophageal	[1] [2]	[ ][ ]	Lymphoma, immunoblastic (or equivalent term)	[1] NA	[ ][ ]
Carcinoma, invasive cervical	[1] NA	[ ][ ]	Lymphoma, primary in brain	[1] NA	[ ][ ]
Coccidioidomycosis, disseminated or extrapulmonary	[1] NA	[ ][ ]	*Mycobacterium avium* complex or *M.kansasii,* disseminated or extrapulmonary	[1] [2]	[ ][ ]
Cryptococcosis, extrapulmonary	[1] NA	[ ][ ]	*M. tuberculosis,* pulmonary*	[1] [2]	[ ][ ]
Cryptosporidiosis, chronic intestinal (>1 mo. duration)	[1] NA	[ ][ ]	*M. tuberculosis,* disseminated or extrapulmonary*	[1] [2]	[ ][ ]
Cytomegalovirus disease (other than in liver, spleen, or nodes)	[1] NA	[ ][ ]	*Mycobacterium,* of other species or unidentified species, disseminated or extrapulmonary	[1] [2]	[ ][ ]
Cytomegalovirus retinitis (with loss of vision)	[1] [2]	[ ][ ]	*Pneumocystis carinii* pneumonia	[1] [2]	[ ][ ]
HIV encephalopathy	[1] NA	[ ][ ]	Pneumonia, recurrent, in 12 mo. period	[1] [2]	[ ][ ]
Herpes simplex: chronic ulcer(s) (>1 mo. duration); or bronchitis, pneumonitis or esophagitis	[1] NA	[ ][ ]	Progressive multifocal leukoencephalopathy	[1] NA	[ ][ ]
Histoplasmosis, disseminated or extrapulmonary	[1] NA	[ ][ ]	Salmonella septicemia, recurrent	[1] NA	[ ][ ]
Isosporiasis, chronic intestinal (>1 mo. duration)	[1] NA	[ ][ ]	Toxoplasmosis of brain	[1] [2]	[ ][ ]
Kaposi's sarcoma	[1] [2]	[ ][ ]	Wasting syndrome due to HIV	[1] NA	[ ][ ]

Def. = definitive diagnosis   Pres. = presumptive diagnosis   * RVCT CASE NO.: [ ][ ][ ][ ][ ][ ][ ]

• If HIV tests were not positive or were not done, does this patient have an immunodeficiency that would disqualify him/her from the AIDS case definition?   [1] Yes   [0] No   [9] Unknown

IX. TREATMENT/SERVICES REFERRALS

Has this patient been informed of his/her HIV infection? [1] Yes [0] No [9] Unk.

This patient's partners will be notified about their HIV exposure and counseled by:
[1] Health department   [2] Physician/provider   [3] Patient   [9] Unknown

This patient is receiving or has been referred for:

	Yes	No	NA	Unk.
• HIV related medical services	[1]	[0]	–	[9]
• Substance abuse treatment services	[1]	[0]	[8]	[9]

This patient received or is receiving:

	Yes	No	Unk.
• Anti-retroviral therapy	[1]	[0]	[9]
• PCP prophylaxis	[1]	[0]	[9]

This patient has been enrolled at:

Clinical Trial	Clinic
[1] NIH-sponsored	[1] HRSA-sponsored
[2] Other	[2] Other
[3] None	[3] None
[9] Unknown	[9] Unknown

This patient's medical treatment is <u>primarily</u> reimbursed by:
[1] Medicaid   [2] Private insurance/HMO
[3] No coverage   [4] Other Public Funding
[7] Clinical trial/ government program   [9] Unknown

FOR WOMEN:
• This patient is receiving or has been referred for gynecological or obstetrical services: .... [1] Yes [0] No [9] Unknown
• Is this patient currently pregnant? .... [1] Yes [0] No [9] Unknown
• Has this patient delivered live-born infants? .... [1] Yes (if delivered after 1977, provide birth information [0] No [9] Unknown below for the most recent birth)

CHILD'S DATE OF BIRTH: Mo. Day Yr.	Hospital of Birth: _____	Child's Soundex:	Child's State Patient No.
[ ][ ] [ ][ ] [ ][ ]	City: _____ State: _____	[ ][ ][ ][ ]	[ ][ ][ ][ ][ ][ ][ ][ ][ ]

X. COMMENTS: _____

_____

_____

Public burden for this collection of information is estimated to average 10 minutes per response. Send comments regarding this burden estimate or any other aspect of this collection of information, including suggestions for reducing this burden to PHS Reports Clearance Officer; ATTN: PRA; Hubert H. Humphrey Bg, Rm 721-B; 200 Independence Ave., SW; Washington, DC 20201, and to the Office of Management and Budget; Paperwork Reduction Project (0920-0009); Washington, DC 20503. – DO NOT MAIL CASE REPORT FORMS TO THESE ADDRESSES –

CDC 50.42A   REV. 07-93 (Page 2 of 2)   – ADULT HIV/AIDS CONFIDENTIAL CASE REPORT –   ☆ U.S. GOVERNMENT PRINTING OFFICE: 1993—534-375

Abstracting

The CDC has developed a case reporting model for use in collecting data on AIDS cases. The following data elements should be included:

- Basic patient demographic information
- Risk factors pertinent to HIV and AIDS, such as sexual orientation, intravenous drug history, and blood transfusions
- Presence or absence of AIDS indicator diseases
- Laboratory tests

Hospital-based AIDS registries also collect information on diagnostic test results and treatment.

Coding

The coding system used by AIDS registries is the *International Classification of Diseases, Ninth Edition* (ICD-9-CM). Codes 042.0 through 044.9 human immunodeficiency virus are the common codes. Codes used for cross reference are 279.19 and 795.8.

Staging

Two staging systems are commonly used for staging AIDS cases: the CDC classification and the Walter Reed Army Institute of Research system, with the CDC system being the one most widely used by AIDS registries. The CDC classification system was revised in 1993 along with the definition of AIDS. The main clinical categories in the CDC system are as follows (Figure 8–16):

- A—Asymptomatic acute (primary) HIV, or persistent generalized lymphadenopathy (PGL)
- B—Symptomatic, not A or C conditions
- C—AIDS-indicator conditions

Automation

Hospital-based registries use software that is developed in-house or through a cancer registry system reformatted to meet the specific data collection needs of an AIDS registry. Population-based registries use mainframe programs to store and analyze the data. Data collection forms are submitted by health departments to state AIDS registries or to the CDC for the development of a national AIDS database.

Uses of AIDS Registry Data

Hospital-based AIDS registries analyze the data and monitor trends in their patient population to provide

	CLINICAL CATEGORIES		
CD4 + T-Cell Categories	(A) Asymptomatic Acute (Primary) HIV or PGL†	(B) Symptomatic, Not (A) or (C) Conditions∮	(C) AIDS-Indicator Conditions¶
(1) ≥ 500μL	A1	B1	C1
(2) 200-499/μL	A2	B2	C2
(3) < 200μL AIDS-Indicator T-Cell Count	A3	B3	C3

1993 Revised Classification System for HIV Infection and Expanded AIDS Surveillance Case Definition for Adolescents and Adults*

*Persons with AIDS indicator conditions (Category C) as well as those with CD4+ lymphocyte counts<200/μL (Categories A3 or B3) will be reportable as AIDS cases in the United States and Territories, effective January 1, 1993.

†PGL = persistent generalized lymphadenopathy. Clinical Category A includes acute (primary) HIV infection.

∮For a list of possible conditions, see original CDC document.

¶Category C includes the clinical conditions listed in the AIDS surveillance definition in Appendix B of the original CDC document.

FIGURE 8–16. Centers for Disease Control HIV/AIDS classification system.

administrators with tools to allocate valuable resources. Because of the 1993 change in the CDC classification system and revised AIDS definition, people are being reported earlier in the course of their HIV infection and, therefore, are living with AIDS for a longer period of time.[16] AIDS registry data make valuable information available to the medical staff, which ensures that the clinical care needed by these patients is provided. The population-based AIDS registry monitors incidence data to provide estimates of the prevalence of HIV infection for health care planning purposes. States use the data for allocation of funds to local consortia for care and treatment services and for public education.[17] Many states have laws that govern the reporting of AIDS cases, especially to a state agency, which in turn is responsible for tracking AIDS patients.

BIRTH DEFECTS REGISTRIES

Birth defects are the leading cause of infant mortality in the United States, and genetic diseases account for about one half of pediatric hospital admissions.[18] In addition, birth defects are the fifth leading cause of years of potential life lost and contribute substantially to childhood morbidity and long-term disability. Major birth defects are diagnosed in 3 to 4 per cent of infants in their first year of life.[19]

Population-based birth registries have operated since the 1920s, with the earliest being in the state of New Jersey. In the early years, birth registries strictly used vital records to identify malformations. Birth defects surveillance systems are characterized as either active or passive case ascertainment systems.

Active surveillance systems use trained staff to identify cases in all hospitals, clinics, or other medical facilities through systematic review of patient records, surgery records, disease indexes, pathology reports, vital records, and hospital logs (obstetric, newborn nursery, neonatal intensive care unit, postmortem) or by interviewing health professionals who may be knowledgeable about diagnosed cases. The information is recorded on standard forms designed for the program.

The first active case ascertainment system, the Metropolitan Atlanta Congenital Defects Program (MACDP) was implemented in 1967 by the CDC. State and regional birth defect registries are modeled after the Atlanta registry.

Passive case ascertainment systems rely on reports submitted by hospitals, clinics, or other facilities, supplemented with data from vital statistics. In some states, staff submit reports voluntarily, but in general, reporting requirements are established by state legislation. One example of a passive surveillance system is the national

Birth Defects Monitoring Program. Newborn hospital discharge summaries are obtained from data tapes, and investigators have no opportunity to review the rest of the patient record.

Active systems identify almost all cases of birth defects, whereas passive systems miss 10 to 30 per cent of all cases, depending on the number of sources. In 1992, seven states had active case ascertainment systems providing data on about 700,000 births. An additional 18 states had passive case ascertainment systems.

Database Management

The goal of a birth defects registry is indicated by the type of case ascertainment system (active versus passive) it is operating.

Case Eligibility

Case eligibility may vary among active and passive registries.[19] The MACDP criteria include cases in which the infant has a serious or major structural defect that can adversely affect health and development and cases of live-born infants and stillbirths, 20 weeks' gestation or more, 500 grams or more. Pregnancies with birth defects prenatally diagnosed and terminated before 20 weeks' gestation are ascertained whenever possible, but because of incomplete ascertainment, the records are kept as separate data.

Classification and Coding

In 70 to 80 per cent of cases, birth defects occur as isolated defects. Attempts are being made to classify infants with multiple birth defects according to biologically meaningful categories to assist in identifying etiologic and pathogenetic mechanisms. Birth defects can also be classified as major or minor; major birth defects are those that affect survival, require substantial medical care, or result in marked physiologic or psychological impairment.

The ICD-9-CM lists most birth defects within the range of 740.0 to 759.9. Some registries use a modified British Paediatric Association *Classification of Diseases, 1977,* six-digit code that is more detailed than the ICD-9-CM codes.

Abstracting

The data collected for birth defects surveillance precisely describe all birth defects. Included are the following:

- Syndrome identification by geneticists or **dysmorphologists**
- Demographic data
- Pregnancy history
- Birth-related data
- Cytogenetic and laboratory data
- Family history
- Etiologic information

A set of core data items has been defined by the CDC and is reflected on the Reproductive Outcomes Case Record (Figure 8–17).

Quality Control

To evaluate the completeness and accuracy of data collection, reabstracting procedures similar to those used by cancer registries are often followed. The linkage of computerized discharge summary indexes with prenatal records is another quality control procedure that is used. The abstracts are reviewed by clinical geneticists or dysmorphologists who evaluate them for accuracy and completeness of the diagnosis as well as for defect coding.[20]

Uses of Birth Defects Registry Data

The analysis of birth defects surveillance data allows health care planners and epidemiologists to monitor the differing birth defect rates in different areas as well as changes in the rates. The data are monitored by statistically evaluating the difference between observed and expected numbers of specific defects or defect combinations for a specified time in a deprived area. Comparisons may lead to the identification of clusters of birth defects. Investigation of such clusters may yield useful etiologic information. The goal of many birth defects registries is to provide health care providers and policymakers with information necessary to plan, develop, and implement strategies for the treatment and prevention of serious congenital malformations.[21]

Because individual birth defects are rare, researchers have difficulty in obtaining enough cases for etiologic studies. Few national databases are available on the occurrence of birth defects. Data for population-based state systems are an important source of information to improve knowledge and understanding of birth defects and to further prevention and intervention.

At one time, the CDC funded some state and regional birth defects registries. More recently, funding has been restricted to providing monies to conduct special studies. In the early 1990s, the birth defects branch of the CDC fostered the collaboration of 17 states (accounting for 25 per cent of the total U.S. population) with population-based birth defects surveillance systems and published a report of the incidence and descriptive epidemiology of spina bifida and Down syndrome.[19]

DIABETES REGISTRIES

The detection and management of diabetes can result in significant improvement in health and morbidity. Population-based registries provide an excellent foundation for family studies of autoimmune disease. Registries provide accurate information regarding the incidence of disease in the general population.[22] Monitoring diabetes at a regional, state, or national level is critical to identify where diabetes is the greatest problem so that resources can be allocated for primary and secondary prevention. Moreover, it is necessary to evaluate the effect of prevention programs. Diabetes registries surveillance data are used for the following purposes:

- To identify high-risk groups
- To target intervention programs
- To evaluate disease prevention and control activities
- To establish an infrastructure for community-sponsored disease prevention programs[23]

The following types of diabetes registries are used to cover the diabetic patient population:

- Juvenile diabetes
- Adult diabetes
- Insulin-dependent diabetes mellitus (IDDM; type 1)
- Non–insulin-dependent diabetes mellitus (NIDDM; type 2)
- Maternal diabetes
- Pharmacy-based

Complications of diabetes include severe eye disease (e.g., blindness), amputations of the lower extremities, and end-stage renal disease. Diabetes also places the patient at an increased risk for cardiovascular disease. IDDM aggregates in families. Cumulative risk estimates for first-degree relatives range from 3 to 6 per cent by age 30 compared with less than 1 per cent for the general population. Other autoimmune diseases, such as rheumatoid arthritis and autoimmune thyroid disease, are also frequently observed in IDDM families.[22] NIDDM is almost 10 times more common than IDDM. Increased life expectancy, along with changes in life habits, has resulted in an increasing prevalence of NIDDM in many geographic areas.[24] Pregnant women with diabetes are at

U.S. DEPARTMENT OF HEALTH AND HUMAN SERVICES
Public Health Service
Centers for Disease Control and Prevention (CDC)
Atlanta Georgia 30093

(1-) ROCR

REPRODUCTIVE OUTCOMES CASE RECORD

CDC
FORM APPROVED
OMB No. 0920-0010
EXP. DATE 12/92

STATE (5-) __ __

I.D. No. (7-) __ __ __ __ __ __ __

INFORMATION RECORDED: Mo   Da   Yr

INITIALS (13-) __ __ __   DATE (16-) __ __ __ __ __ __   HOSP (22-) __ __ __ __

PATIENT NAME: (26-) LAST FIRST MIDDLE

MOTHER'S NAME: (50-) LAST FIRST MIDDLE

AGE AT BIRTH (74-) __ __

RESIDENCE AT BIRTH (76-)

FATHER'S NAME: (108-) LAST FIRST MIDDLE

AGE AT BIRTH (132-) __ __

CITY (134-)

COUNTY (150-) __ __ __

ZIP (153-) __ __ __ __ __

CENSUS TRACT (158-) __ __ __ __ __ __

HOME PHONE (164-) __ __ __ / __ __ __ __ __ __ __

MOTHER'S BIRTH DATE (174-) __ __ __ __ __ __ (MDY)

MOTHER'S SSN (180-) __ __ __ __ __ __ __ __ __

FATHER'S BIRTH DATE (189-) __ __ __ __ __ __ (MDY)

FATHER'S SSN (195-) __ __ __ __ __ __ __ __ __

MOTHER'S RACIAL OR ETHNIC GROUP (204)
☐ 1 WHITE, NOT HISP   ☐ 3 HISPANIC
☐ 2 BLACK, NOT HISP   ☐ 4 AMERICAN INDIAN OR ALASKAN NATIVE
☐ 5 ASIAN OR PACIFIC ISLANDER
☐ 9 NOT STATED

PENDING (206)   ☐ 1 YES   ☐ 2 NO

	DX CODE	DIAGNOSIS
SEX (214) ☐ 1 MALE ☐ 2 FEMALE ☐ 3 AMBIGUOUS ☐ 9 NOT STATED	(258-) __ __ __ • __ __ __	
PLURALITY (215) ☐ 1 SINGLE ☐ 2 TWIN ☐ 3 OTHER MULTIPLE BIRTH ☐ 9 NOT STATED	(264-) __ __ __ • __ __ __	
OUTCOME OF DELIVERY (216) ☐ 1 LIVE BORN ☐ 2 STILL BORN ☐ 3 INDUCED AB ☐ 9 NOT STATED	(270-) __ __ __ • __ __ __	
CO-TWIN SEX (217) ☐ 1 MALE ☐ 2 FEMALE ☐ 3 AMBIGUOUS ☐ 9 NOT STATED	(278-) __ __ __ • __ __ __	
CO-TWIN CONCORDANCE (218) ☐ 1 CO-TWIN NORMAL ☐ 2 CO-TWIN WITH SAME DEFECT ☐ 3 CO-TWIN WITH OTHER DEFECT ☐ 9 NOT STATED	(282-) __ __ __ • __ __ __	
CO-TWIN LB/SB (219) ☐ 1 CO-TWIN LB ☐ 2 CO-TWIN STILL BORN ☐ 9 NOT STATED	(288-) __ __ __ • __ __ __	

APGAR SCORE   1 MIN (220-) __ __   5 MIN (222-) __ __

DATE OF BIRTH   Mo   Da   Yr   (224-) __ __ __ __ __ __

BIRTH WEIGHT
(230-) __ __ __ __ GRAMS
OR
(234-) __ __ LBS. __ __ OZS.

HOSPITAL OR PLACE OF FIRST DIAGNOSIS
(238-) __ __ __ __

DATE OF FIRST DIAGNOSIS   Mo   Da   Yr
(242-) __ __ __ __ __ __

HEAD CIRCUMFERENCE   (251-) ☐ 1 CM
(248-) __ __ • __   ☐ 2 IN

LENGTH   (255-) ☐ 1 CM
(252-) __ • __ __   ☐ 2 IN

MOTHER"S HEMATOCRIT (256-) __ __ __

GEST. AGE BY NEONATAL EXAM   (294-) __ __ WKS

DUBOWITZ EXAM (296)
☐ 1 YES   ☐ 3 NOT APPLICABLE
☐ 2 NO   ☐ 9 NOT STATED

ULTRASOUND DATE   Mo   Da   Yr
(297-) __ __ __ __ __

ULTRASOUND DATING (303-) __ __ WKS

DATE OF   Mo   Da   Yr
LMP (305-) __ __ __ __ __
EDC (311-) __ __ __ __ __

SYNDROME (317-) __ __ __ __ __ __

CYTOGENETICS: (323)
☐ 1 NORMAL   ☐ 4 NOT DONE
☐ 2 ABNORMAL   ☐ 9 NOT STATED
☐ 3 PENDING

LABORATORY (324-) __ __ __ __

DIAGNOSIS (328-) __ __ __ __ __ __

TO BE INTERVIEWED (334)   ☐ 1 YES   ☐ 2 NO

ACTION CODE (335)   ☐ 1 ORIG.   ☐ 3 CORR.   ☐ 2 CONT.   ☐ 4 DELE

(SEE REVERSE)

CDC 84.1A REV. 11-92

The Centers for Disease Control is authorized to collect this information including the Social Security number (if applicable), under provisions of the Public Health Service Act 301 (42 U.S.C. 241). Supplying the information is voluntary, and there is no penalty for not providing it. The data will be used to increase understanding or disease patterns, develop prevention and control programs, and communicate new knowledge to the health community. Data will become part of CDC Privacy Act system 09-20-01 36, "Epidemiologic Studies and Surveillance of Disease Programs" and may be disclosed to appropriate State or local public health departments and cooperating medical authorities to deal with conditions of public health significance; to private contractors assisting CDC in analyzing and refining records; to researchers under certain limited circumstances to conduct further investigations; to organizations to carry out studies and reviews on behalf of HHS; to the Department of Justice for litigation purposes, and to a congressional office assisting individuals in obtaining their records. An accounting of such disclosures that have been made by CDC will be made available to the subject individual upon request. Except for these and other permissible

FIGURE 8-17. Reproductive outcomes case record.

a higher risk for complications and congenital malformations in their offspring than are pregnant women without diabetes.

One of the first childhood diabetes registries was established in 1979 in Allegheny County, Pennsylvania, as a collaborative effort between the Children's Hospital of Pittsburgh, the department of epidemiology at the University of Pittsburgh, and the HIM professionals at the hospitals both inside the county and in neighboring areas. The Children's Hospital has collected data on patients under age 20 years since 1950, whereas the Allegheny County Diabetes Incidence Registry has collected data on patients under age 19 years since 1979. This registry has served as a model for diabetes registries worldwide, and the University of Pittsburgh has been designated as a World Health Organization Collaborating Center for Diabetes Registries and Training.[25]

The following three diabetes registries have been developed by the North Dakota Department of Health and Consolidated Laboratories:

- Type 1 surveillance program established in 1979 in a cooperative effort with the University of North Dakota School of Medicine
- Maternal Diabetes Reporting System in cooperation with family planning agencies and physicians, nurses, and dietitians from private health care agencies
- Pharmacy-based diabetes registry established in a cooperative effort with the North Dakota State Board of Pharmacy[23]

The type 1 surveillance program targets identification of newly diagnosed type 1 diabetics under age 30 years. A network of sentinel reporting sites was established with nurses and physicians treating newly diagnosed type 1 diabetics. Registry information is collected monthly and updated annually.

The Maternal Diabetes Reporting System is a voluntary system that identifies women with pre-existing and gestational diabetes. Data report cards are used by physicians, nurses, and dietitians from private health care agencies to collect tracking information on pregnancy status and patient needs (Figure 8–18). The information is then provided to five regional pregnancy counseling centers, and patients are contacted directly to determine pregnancy assistance needs.

The pharmacy-based diabetes registry identifies patients who are taking prescription medications for diabetes (insulin and oral agents). Pharmacy data cards are completed by the patient to collect demographic and medical data (Figure 8–19). Diabetics visit pharmacies up to six times more frequently than they visit physician offices. Patients who request diabetic medications complete the reporting cards while waiting for their prescriptions. The cards also include informed consent. This system provides multiple opportunities to collect and update patient information. Completed cards are submitted to the registry by the pharmacies monthly.[23,26]

Database Management

Database management for diabetes registries includes defining the patient population and case eligibility, casefinding, abstracting, and coding.

Case Eligibility

To determine case eligibility status, a definition of the segment of the diabetic population to be included must be established: IDDM, NIDDM, gestational diabetes, juvenile onset, or adult onset.

Casefinding

Casefinding sources include hospital admission and discharge logs, pharmacy records, dietary records, emergency logs, and physician surveillance and reporting.

Abstracting

Data are obtained by reviewing hospital patient records and data reporting forms submitted by physicians and pharmacies. Data variables include patient demographics, diagnoses, reasons for admission, treatment, attending physician, complications, and length of stay (Figures 8–20 and 8–21).

Coding

The ICD-9-CM is used to code diabetes mellitus, its types, and its manifestations.

Automation

No uniform software system is used by all diabetes registries. Software is usually designed by and for the registry and tailored to meet its needs. The Indian Health Service, an agency of the U.S. Public Health Service, encourages each of its clinics and hospitals to maintain a diabetes registry. (Native Americans and Inuits suffer one of the highest known prevalence rates of type 2 diabetes.) Although the registries may be maintained in a manual or computer format, integration

NORTH DAKOTA DIABETES REPORT
DEPARTMENT OF HEALTH AND CONSOLIDATED LABORATORIES
SFN 13999 (7-87)

Complete Both Sides of Card

NAME OF PATIENT			SEX	DATE OF BIRTH
MAILING ADDRESS	CITY	STATE	ZIP CODE	COUNTY

RACE: ☐ WHITE, ☐ NATIVE AMERICAN, ☐ BLACK, ☐ HISPANIC, ☐OTHER (Specify)

Does the State Health Department have permission to send the patient litetrature regarding diabetes? ☐ YES ☐ NO

ATTENDING PHYSICIAN		PHONE NO.
MAILING ADDRESS	CITY	STATE	ZIP CODE

Complete report on both sides of this card -- then mail to:

NORTH DAKOTA STATE DEPARTMENT OF HEALTH AND CONSOLIDATED LABORATORIES
Division of Disease Control
State Capitol
Bismarck, ND 58505

FOR CONSULTATION IN COMPLETING REPORT CALL 224-2378 OR 1-800-472-2180

TYPE OF DIABETES: ☐ TYPE I   ☐ TYPE II   ☐ GESTATIONAL

PRESCRIBED TREATMENT: ☐ INSULIN   ☐ ORAL AGENTS   ☐ DIET ALONE   ☐ NONE

COMPLETE THIS SECTION OF CARD ONLY FOR PREGNANT DIABETICS

Approximate date patient was diagnosed with diabetes	Anticipated Delivery Date	Previous Number of Pregnancies	Previous Pregnancies With Diagnosed Diabetes

PATIENT HAS RECEIVED: ☐ PRE-CONCEPTION DIABETES AND PREGNANCY COUNSELING

☐ POST-CONCEPTION DIABETES AND PREGNANCY COUNSELING

☐ NO DIABETES AND PREGNANCY COUNSELING

PROVIDER OF COUNSELING	Approximate Date of Counseling
REPORTED BY	REPORT DATE

FIGURE 8–18. North Dakota maternal diabetes case report card.

DIABETES REGISTRY
STATE DEPARTMENT OF HEALTH AND CONSOLIDATED LABORATORIES
DIVISION OF DISEASE CONTROL
SFN 17190 (3-90)

COMPLETE FORM AND RETURN TO:

SDHCL
Division of Disease Control
600 E. Boulevard Avenue
Bismarck, ND 58505

Name (First, Middle Initial, Last)

Address	City	State	Zip Code

County	Date of Birth (M/D/Y)	Telephone No.	Sex
			☐ Male - 1 ☐ Female - 2

Primary Physician (First, Middle, Last)	Name of Pharmacy	Last Eye Exam ☐ 1 Year Ago
		☐ 2 Years Ago ☐ 3 Years or More

Race
☐ White - 1
☐ Black - 2
☐ Other (Specify) - 5
☐ Native American - 3
☐ Hispanic - 4

Type of Diabetes
☐ Type 1 Juvenile Onset - 1
☐ Type 2 Adult Onset - 2
☐ Gestational - 3

Age Diabetes Was Diagnosed

No. of Years You've Been a Diabetic

Treatment
☐ Insulin - 1
☐ Oral Agents (Pills) - 2
☐ Diet Alone - 3

Have you ever received treatment for any of the following (Check all that apply)
☐ High Blood Pressure - 1   ☐ Eye Disease - 3   ☐ Heart Disease - 5
☐ Kidney Disease - 2   ☐ Circulation Disorders (Hands, Feet, Legs) - 4

I hereby authorize you to release information contained in this report, or in a similar report maintained in your records, to the North Dakota State Department of Health and Consolidated Laboratories for statistical purposes. I also authorize the department or its agents to use this information to maintain contact with me for the purpose of providing health care and information concerning programs involving the diagnosis, treatment and care of diabetes and associated complications and diseases.

_____
Signature of Patient

_____
Date

_____
Signature of Witness

_____
Date

FIGURE 8–19. Diabetes registry pharmacy report card.

of the diabetes registry with the hospital clinical information system is recommended.[27]

The pharmacy-based diabetes registry in North Dakota stores the data in a mainframe computer. The information on the cards submitted by the pharmacists is entered into the computer system by patient name, address, zip code, and attending physician and is cross-referenced by age and other factors. Duplicates are eliminated through name and birth date matching.

Follow-Up

A follow-up of patients with diabetes is conducted every 2 years by the Allegheny County (Pennsylvania) Diabetes Incidence Registry to determine patient survival status.[25] Registry data are used in North Dakota to track patients with complications to ensure that treatment is provided. This follow-up information is used to demonstrate the effectiveness of screening and prevention programs.[23]

Uses of Diabetes Registry Data

The complications of diabetes can be prevented with early diagnosis and treatment. Diabetes registries improve our understanding of disease determinants and are an important component to the success of programs designed to prevent the complications of diabetes. Multiple local, state, national, and international studies are conducted using the diabetes registry data. Blood testing for risk markers and other family members who are converters to diabetes, parents and offspring, multiple siblings, and first-degree onset of diabetes in immediate family members are examples of such studies. International studies include the DiaMond (Diabetes Mondiale), a World Health Organization multinational project for childhood diabetes. The objectives of this effort are as follows:

• To monitor the international patterns of IDDM incidence to the year 2000

• To provide a uniform basis for standardized studies of risk factors for IDDM

MEDICAL RECORD ABSTRACT OF PATIENT HISTORY FOR JUVENILE DIABETES MELLITUS

Hospital Code ( ) Data Collector _____ Date _____ Data File Code (   )

Case ID _____ Family ID _____ Onset record: Yes ____ No ____

Name: _____ Maiden: _____

Address: _____

City: _____ Zip: _____

County: _____ Township: _____

Parent/Guardian: _____ Telephone Number: _____

Birthdate: _____

Date of Diagnosis and Place: _____

Race: _____ Sex: _____ Age: _____

Characteristics (symptoms, infections, stress, etc.) at or recently before onset of JDM:

_____

_____

_____

_____

_____

_____ Insulin dose at discharge: _____

Family History of Diabetes: _____

_____

Medical Record Number: _____

Referring Physician: _____

Attending Physician: _____

Family Structure (CHP only) and Comments:

FIGURE 8–20. Juvenile diabetes abstract form.

JOD: Epidemiology & Etiology
Registry and/or Children's Hospital Files
Patient Entry/Update

Form No. $\boxed{O}\boxed{1}\boxed{O}\boxed{1}$ Case ID $\boxed{}\boxed{}\boxed{}$

Data File Code: $\boxed{}$
  1-Rgs/2-CHP/3-Both

Group: HPR-1, NR-2, $\boxed{}$
P-3, NDM-4, RE-5
HPDM-6, REG-7,
NONDM-8

Family ID $\boxed{}\boxed{}\boxed{}\boxed{}\boxed{}\boxed{}\boxed{}$

Date of Birth: $\boxed{}\boxed{}\boxed{}\boxed{}\boxed{}\boxed{}$ Date of Diagnosis: $\boxed{}\boxed{}\boxed{}\boxed{}\boxed{}\boxed{}$ Age at Diagnosis: $\boxed{}\boxed{}$

Race: 1-White, 2-Black, 3-Oriental, 4-Biracial, 5-Other, 9-Unknown $\boxed{}$

Sex: 1-Male, 2-Female, 9-Unknown $\boxed{}$

Residence Code: 1-Allegheny Co., 2-Not Alleg. Co., 9-Unknown $\boxed{}$

Hospital/Physician Code of this record: $\boxed{}\boxed{}$

Data Collection Date_____ Data Collector_____

Case Name: Blank-Unknown

Last_____

First_____ M.I._____

Case Address (when diagnosed):   Blank-Unknown

House No.: _____

Street _____

County _____ Twp. _____ ZIP Code _____

Census Tract: (Cole's Directory) $\boxed{}\boxed{}\boxed{}\boxed{}$

Socio-Economic Rating   (Cole's Directory) $\boxed{}$
1-High, 2-Med High, 3-Med, 4-Med Low, 5-Low, 9-Unknown

FIGURE 8–21. Diabetes data collection/entry form.

- To assess the mortality associated with the disease
- To evaluate health care (e.g., insulin availability) and health economics associated with diabetes
- To develop training programs for diabetes research

Many population-based diabetes registries are participating in this important study.[28]

IMPLANT REGISTRIES

In 1988, the International Implant Registry was started by the Medic Alert Foundation, a nonprofit emergency alerting organization. The main objectives of the registry are to track patients so that their whereabouts are known and to facilitate timely, accurate communication between manufacturers, health care providers, and patients.[29]

Millions of patients have medical devices implanted in or on their bodies. They include pacemakers, heart valves, artificial joints, lenses, defibrillators, breasts, and other prostheses. Although these medical devices have improved the quality of life for many people and have saved the lives of countless others, numerous safety alerts and voluntary manufacturer recalls have beeen issued for these devices. These safety alerts and recalls have raised procedural questions with life-threatening implications: Who is responsible for notifying the patients? Through the International Implant Registry, physicians are notified when important safety information needs to be communicated. If the physician cannot be contacted, patients are notified directly to contact their physicians or the manufacturers of their devices. The Safe Medical Devices Act of 1990 became effective in November 1991. This law requires manufacturers to register and track certain implantable medical devices and to notify medical recipients of important safety information. It also requires hospitals, ambulatory surgical facilities, nursing facilities, and outpatient diagnostic or treatment facilities, other than physicians' offices, to file reports with the Food and Drug Administration and/or device manufacturers when there is a probability that a device caused or contributed to a death, serious illness, or serious injury.[30] Hospitals may choose to keep internal implant registries to identify patients and answer manufacturer recall or other research questions. Maintaining this information in a retrievable mode facilitates current and future requests for data on these patients.

ORGAN TRANSPLANT REGISTRIES

The first successful organ transplant operations were not performed until 1954. Thanks to medical advance-ments, today's technology makes transplantation a recognized and an accepted mode of treatment for patients with organ failure. The success of transplantation and the scarcity of organs have raised many ethical, legal, and economic issues.[31]

The National Organ Transplant Act (NOTA, Public Law 98-507) was passed by Congress in 1984. The NOTA called for a national task force on organ transplantation that was charged with conducting an in-depth study of transplantation and making recommendations about medical, ethical, legal, economic, and social issues pertaining to human transplantation. In 1986, the task force recommended the establishment and operation of a national scientific registry. In October 1986 the Human Resources and Services Administration awarded the contract for the scientific registry to the United Network for Organ Sharing (UNOS).[32] The primary goals of the UNOS are as follows:

- To provide a fair and equitable distribution of organs to all available waiting transplant recipients
- To improve the effectiveness of organ procurement to decrease wastage of organs by improving the system for sharing renal and extrarenal organs
- To assure quality control by collection, analysis, and publication of data on organ donation, procurement, and transplantation[33]

UNOS members include transplant centers, independent procurement organizations, tissue-typing laboratories, consortia, public members, and voluntary health and professional associations.

In addition, the NOTA provided for the establishment of a national Organ Procurement and Transplantation Network. The network collects information on all transplant candidates registered on the UNOS waiting list and on all organ donors. The scientific registry collects data on all organ recipients from the time of transplantation until last graft failure and/or patient death.

To place a patient on the waiting list, the transplant center submits a form that contains such patient information as address, race, ethnicity, education level, cause of organ failure, and number of previous transplants as well as whether or not the patient's name appears on any other lists. All UNOS member institutions and organizations involved in organ procurement, tissue typing, and organ transplantation are required to submit comprehensive data concerning transplant activities. The UNOS subcontracts with four organ-specific registries (kidney, liver, pancreas, and heart/lung) to collect transplant and follow-up data on organ recipients. Each registry maintains its own database besides collecting UNOS data.

Database Management

UNOS hospital-based organ transplant registries are designed to improve patient care, increase the efficient use of scarce lifesaving organs, and provide data for scientific studies.[31] Transplant recipient data are submitted to subcontractor registries on forms developed by the UNOS in collaboration with subcontractors and members. Each registry sends data on compatible diskettes in a format specified by the UNOS. Copies of recipient forms are also sent to the UNOS for storage and serve as a full backup of the data collected by subcontracting registries. The UNOS uses a mainframe computer system to store and analyze the data. The computer and various software programs are accessible to transplant programs, organ procurement organizations, and tissue-typing laboratories throughout the United States.

Quality Assurance

Extensive visual and computerized checks on data entered into the computer are performed by the quality assurance department at UNOS. Quality assurance reviews of the data forms submitted by subcontracting registries are performed, and incomplete or incorrect forms are returned to the reporting facilities for correction. Discrepancies among forms submitted on the same patient between UNOS and subcontractors must be resolved.

Training

The quality assurance department at UNOS provides training for data coordinators and related personnel in the use of the data collection forms and offers assistance to members when they have questions or concerns about reporting requirements.

TRAUMA REGISTRIES

Trauma is the leading cause of death for people under age 50. It kills more people between ages 1 and 34 than all other causes combined. Injuries cost the general public billions of dollars a year in direct and indirect costs.[34]

The goal of a trauma system is to decrease morbidity and mortality by assuring the rapid delivery of an injured person to a medical facility that is prepared to provide optimal medical evaluation and care. The following are major components of a trauma system:

- Emergency response ability
- Official designation as a trauma center, which mandates the operation of a trauma registry
- Triage criteria for determining which patients are likely to require the special services of a trauma center
- Oversight agency to evaluate the integration of these resources[35]

Decisions directed at improving trauma care must be based on a complete understanding of the causes, treatment, and outcomes of injury.[36]

Trauma registries may be hospital- or population-based. The implementation of state and local trauma registries parallels the establishment of trauma systems nationwide. The state of Illinois implemented the first statewide trauma registry in 1971. The mission of the registry was to collect data on all patients who were admitted to the state's designated trauma centers. The data were used for improving prehospital and hospital care, providing descriptive and analytic epidemiology, and evaluating and managing the program statewide. The Illinois Trauma Registry served as the model for all future trauma registries.[35]

One of the first hospital-based trauma registries was implemented at Allegheny General Hospital in Pittsburgh, Pennsylvania, in 1981. The data collected are used by the medical staff and administration to evaluate the trauma population admitted to the facility, a tertiary care hospital in a metropolitan area.[37]

In the mid-1980s, the ACS Committee on Trauma made a recommendation for the development of a computerized trauma registry to monitor the effectiveness of these systems. The process and outcome indicators defined by the ACS cover the full range of trauma care phases from prehospital care through hospital discharge (see Suggested American College of Surgeons' Audit Filters).

Database Management

The goal of a trauma registry is to identify and collect data on every eligible trauma patient.

Case Eligibility

Triage criteria are established to ascertain which patients require the special services provided at a trauma center. The standard criteria include a set of anatomic, physiologic, or cause of injury descriptors known to place patients at high risk for severe injury. The Committee on Trauma recommends the following case criteria for inclusion in a trauma registry:

Suggested American College of Surgeons' Audit Filters

1. Ambulance scene time 20 minutes.

2. Absence of ambulance report on medical record for patient transported by prehospital EMS personnel.

3. Patient with a Glasgow Coma Scale of less than 13 who does not receive a computed tomography (CT) scan of the head within two hours of arrival at the hospital.

4. Absence of sequential neurologic documentation on emergency department record of trauma patients with a diagnosis of skull fracture, intracranial injury, or spinal cord injury.

5. Absence of hourly chart documentation for any trauma patient beginning with arrival in emergency department, including time spent in radiology, up to admission to the operating room or ICU; death; or transfer to another hospital.

6. Comatose trauma patient leaving emergency department before mechanical airway is established.

7. Patient seen in emergency department and admitted to the hospital within 72 hours of initial evaluation.

8. Any patient sustaining a gunshot wound to the abdomen who is managed nonoperatively.

9. Patients requiring laparotomy, which is not performed within two hours of arrival at emergency department.

10. Patients with epidural or subdural brain hematoma receiving craniotomy more than four hours after arrival at emergency department, excluding those performed for intracranial pressure (ICP) monitoring.

11. Patients transferred to another health care facility after spending six hours in the initial hospital.

12. Interval of more than eight hours between arrival and treatment of blunt compound tibial fracture or open laceration of joint.

13. Abdominal, thoracic, vascular, or cranial surgery performed more than 24 hours after arrival.

14. Unplanned return to the operating room within 48 hours of initial procedure.

15. Trauma patient admitted to hospital under care of admitting or attending physician who is not a surgeon.

16. Patient with diagnosis at discharge of cervical spine injury not indicated in admission diagnosis.

Adapted from Committee on Trauma: Resources for optimal care of the injured patient. Chicago: American College of Surgeons, 1993.

- ICD-9-CM injury code between 800 and 959.9
- Admission to the hospital for more than 48 hours
- Admission to an operating room or intensive care unit
- Death in the hospital emergency room[36]

Casefinding

Casefinding is performed by reviewing emergency department logs, admitting face sheets, patient records, and the disease indexes—injury codes 800-959.9 and E codes listed in the ICD-9-CM.

Abstracting[36,38]

Data variables collected include the following:
- Patient-specific and demographic information
- Place of accident
- Cause of injury (E code)
- Site of injury
- Condition of patient at the scene of the accident
- Transport modality
- Prehospital interventions
- Vital signs on admission
- Consciousness status
- Blood transfusions
- Procedures and treatment
- Total days in the intensive care unit
- Complications
- Discharge recommendations

Coding

The ICD-9-CM is used to assign the diagnosis and procedure codes.

Injury Scales

Both the Abbreviated Injury Scale scores and the Injury Severity Scale scores are routinely documented. The Glasgow Coma Scale is required by the ACS Trauma Registry on admission to the emergency department.[39]

Automation

Trauma registries have used a variety of data collection methods, ranging from manual to computerized databases using modified hospital mainframe programs to microcomputer systems. The ACS maintains that most hospitals can expect to see between 1000 and 4000 trauma patients annually. Similar to cancer registries, paper-based manual systems are rapidly becoming obsolete.

The National Trauma Registry of the ACS released software for use by hospitals with trauma registries in 1993. Data from trauma cases are entered on personal computer–based software at participating trauma centers. The information reflects the following:

- Type of injury
- Management of the patient's medical condition
- Course of treatment
- Patient outcome

Data are submitted to the ACS in response to requests for inclusion in its national database and are used to establish a national standard for trauma registries to improve efforts to prevent injury as well as to evaluate the cost and effectiveness of trauma treatment.[39]

Individual hospitals use the software to compile and analyze data that pertain to their own trauma experience. The software is also available for state registries or as a local area network.

Some states have developed software for use by hospitals. The state of Illinois has developed software and distributes it free of charge to all Illinois trauma centers.[40]

Quality Control

Accuracy and completeness of data are important to ensure data integrity. The value of registry data is directly related to the validity of the data collected. To ensure data validity, the ACS Committee on Trauma recommends a systematic quality control sampling of 5 to 10 per cent of all trauma cases for an annual review of data quality.[36]

Key Concepts

- Registry data are used as a surveillance mechanism for specific disease processes or incidence, to monitor the impact of using medical devices, and to assess the health issues surrounding exposures to hazardous substances. The need for such information has led to the development and implementation of numerous registries.

- Registries vary in mission, design, size, use of technology, and regulations.

- Registries, regardless of the type, track patient referral patterns, assess care through follow-up and quality assessment activities, provide data for administrative planning of valuable resources and for marketing of hospital programs, and provide data from local, state, and national agencies that impact the development of health policies.

- Regardless of the type of registry established, the patient record is a primary source of information.

- HIM departments play a significant role in facilitating access to the data sources required for the development of the registry database.

- Disease and health-related registries are frequently hospital-based and often come under the supervision of the HIM manager. In many cases, the registry is staffed by HIM professionals.

- Understanding the purpose of disease registries and how they impact the medical community are important concepts for HIM professionals to recognize.

- Health care reform should increase the need for additional disease registries to monitor disease and the quality of patient care provided as well as the need for qualified HIM professionals who can design, implement, and manage disease registries.

References

1. Zippen C, Feingold M: Service role of the hospital tumour registry in the U.S.A. *In* Parkin DM, Wagner G, Muir C (eds): The role of the registry in cancer control. IARC Scientific Publications No. 66, International Agency for Research on Cancer, Lyon, France, 1985, pp 121–131.
2. Menck HR, Smart CR (eds): Central cancer registries: Design, management and use. Bethesda, MD: American Association of Central Cancer Registries, 1994.
3. Cancer statistics review, 1973–1987. NIH Publication No. 90-2789, Institute Division of Cancer Prevention and Control Surveillance Program. Bethesda, MD: U.S. Department of Health and Human Services, 1990.
4. Cancer program manual, 1991. Chicago: American College of Surgeons, Commission on Cancer, 1991.
5. Kraybill WG (ed): News from the Commission on Cancer, vol 4, no. 2. Chicago: American College of Surgeons, 1993.
6. Watkins S (ed): Tumor registry management manual, 4th ed. Santa Barbara, CA: Tumor Registrars Association of California, 1992.
7. Shambaugh E (ed): Self-instructional manual for tumor registrars, Book 5. SEER Program, Biometry Branch. DHEW Publication No. (NIH) 77-1263. Bethesda, MD: National Cancer Institute, 1977.
8. Data acquisition manual, rev ed. Chicago: American College of Surgeons, Commission on Cancer, 1990.
9. American Joint Committee on Cancer: Manual for staging of cancer, 4th ed. Philadelphia: JB Lippincott Co, 1992.
10. National Tumor Registrars Association, Inc, and American College of Surgeons, Commission on Cancer: Registry staffing manual. Mundelein, IL: National Tumor Registrars Association, 1989.

11. Watkins S, Scarlett P: Patient care evaluation . . . A hospital cancer program component. Mundelein, IL: National Tumor Registrars Association, 1988.

12. Creech C, Scarlett P, Watkins S: Guidelines for preparing a hospital cancer program annual report, 2nd ed. Oakland, CA: American Cancer Society, 1986.

13. Software Providers. List distributed at the 1993 annual meeting, National Tumor Registrars Association, Inc., Mundelein, IL.

14. AACCR National Standard for Cancer Data Exchange, Record Description. Bethesda, MD: American Association of Central Cancer Registries, 1993.

15. California HIV/AIDS Update, Office of AIDS, vol 6, no 1. Recent trends in reported AIDS cases in California. Sacramento: Department of Health Services, 1993.

16. San Francisco Epidemiologic Bulletin, vol 9, no 1. 1993 revision of the HIV infection classification system and the AIDS surveillance definition. San Francisco: Department of Public Health, 1993.

17. Towarick CC: Developing an AIDS registry: From vision to reality. *In* The abstract, vol 19, no 2. Mundelein, IL: National Tumor Registrars Association, Inc., 1993.

18. Cordero JF: Registries of birth defects and genetic diseases. Medical Genetics 1992; 39(1):65.

19. Lyndberg MC, Edmonds LD: Surveillance of defects program: Surveillance of birth defects. *In* Halpern W, Baker EL, Monson RR (eds): Public health surveillance. New York: Van Nostrand Reinhold, 1992, pp 157–177.

20. Khoury MJ, Edmonds LD: Metropolitan Atlanta congenital defects program: Twenty-five years of birth defects surveillance at the Centers for Disease Control. Paper presentation. Italian Association for Study of Malformations, International Symposium. December 1992.

21. Murray AL: 1988–1990 North Carolina birth defects registry report, no 74. Raleigh: State Center for Health and Environmental Statistics, 1993.

22. Dorman JS: Use of diabetes registries to identify at-risk family members. Paper presentation. Multi-purpose diabetes registries: Innovation in research and practice, Berkeley, CA, June 1993.

23. Schaubert DS: Role of registries in diabetes prevention and control: A perspective from North Dakota. Paper presentation. Multi-purpose diabetes registries: Innovation in research and practice, Berkeley, CA, June 1993.

24. Bruno G: Application of capture-recapture methodology, an approach to diabetes registries. Paper presentation. Multi-purpose diabetes registries: Innovation in research and practice, Berkeley, CA, June 1993.

25. Pittsburgh IDDM Registry Group: Insulin-dependent diabetes mellitus: Applications of health records for understanding etiology. Top Health Record Management 1990;11(2):25–33.

26. Kelly EK (ed): First of its kind: Diabetes registry is pharmacy-based. Adv Health Information Professionals 1993;3(15):11.

27. Mayfield J: Diabetes registration within the U.S. Indian Health Service. Paper presentation. Multi-purpose diabetes registries: Innovation in research and practice, Berkeley, CA, June 1993.

28. LaPorte RE, Tuomilehto J, King H: WHO multinational project for childhood diabetes. Diabetes Care 1990;13(10).

29. Nichols DG: Millions benefit from the Safe Medical Devices Act (SMDA) of 1990. J Am Health Information Management Association 1992;63(2):60–62.

30. Bryant LE: Health law: Medical record implications of the Safe Medical Devices Act of 1990. J Am Health Information Management Association 1992;63(2):17–18.

31. Hearington DK, Ettner BJ, Breen T, White R: National Scientific Registry of Organ Transplantation: Data needs and uses. Top Health Record Management 1990;11(2):1–12.

32. Devney MF: UNOS: United Network of Organ Sharing: The link between organ donors and organ recipients. J Am Health Information Management Association 1992;63(2):63–65.

33. Annual Report of the U.S. Scientific Registry for Organ Transplantation and the Organ Procurement and Transplantation Network, Richmond, VA, 1990.

34. Forrester CB, McMinn DL: Anatomy of a statewide trauma registry. Top Health Information Management 1990; 11(2):34–42.

35. Morabito DJ, Proctor SM, May CM: Overview of trauma registries. Am Health Information Management Association 1992;63(2):39–44.

36. Trauma registry. *In* Resources for optimal care of the injured patient: 1993. Chicago: Committee on Trauma, American College of Surgeons, 1993, Chap 17.

37. Ackerman MA, Peterson FV, Manni PJ, Young JC: Evolution of a hospital-based trauma registry. Top Health Information Management 1990;11(2):49–58.

38. Ehlinger K, Gardner MJ, Nakayama DK: The trauma registry: An administrative and clinical tool. Top Health Information Management 1990;11(2):43–48.

39. News from the American College of Surgeons: National Trauma Registry is initiated by the American College of Surgeons. Press release, Chicago, March 1993.

40. Kelly CK: Trauma registries track injuries. Adv Health Information Professionals 1993;3(15):17.

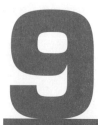

VALERIE J.M. WATZLAF

KEY WORDS

Autopsy rate	Morbidity rates
Bar graph	Mortality rates
Case-control retrospective study	Nominal data
	Odds ratio
Census statistics	Ordinal data
Clinical trial	Pie chart
Coefficient of variation	Prevalence rate
Community trial	Prospective/cohort/incidence study
Confounding variables	
Continuous data	Range
Cross-sectional prevalence study	Relative risk (RR)
	Reliability
Direct method of age adjustment	Sample size
	Sensitivity
Discrete data	Specificity
Frequency distribution	Standard deviation
Frequency polygon	Standardized mortality ratio (SMR)
Histogram	
Incidence rate	Tests of significance
Life table analysis	Validity
Mean	Variance
Median	Vital statistics
Mode	

RESEARCH, STATISTICS, AND EPIDEMIOLOGY

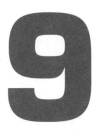

ABBREVIATIONS

FN—False negatives
FP—False positives
gr—gram
IR—Incidence rate
IRB—Institutional review board
NI—Nosocomial infections
r—correlation coefficient
RR—Relative risk
SMR—Standardized mortality ratio
TN—True negatives
TP—True positives
χ^2—Chi square

OBJECTIVES

- Define Key Words.
- Evaluate health care statistics, including mortality and morbidity rates, autopsy rates, measures of central tendency, and dispersion, and determine the most appropriate use of these health care statistics in health information management.
- Organize data generated from health care statistics into appropriate categories, including nominal, ordinal, discrete, and continuous.
- Display data generated from health care statistics using the most appropriate tables, graphs, and figures, including frequency tables, bar graphs, histograms, Pareto diagrams, pie charts, and frequency polygons.
- Explain the steps necessary for designing a research proposal or study.
- Given a specific hypothesis, design a research proposal to test the hypothesis.
- Given an explanation of different research study designs, state the advantages and disadvantages of each and the health care statistics that should be used or generated from each design.
- Explain how each research study design can be used in health information management.
- Given examples of research studies conducted in health care settings, detect and describe the different types of biases that occur within these research studies.
- Determine the most effective methods to use to test validity and reliability.
- Demonstrate knowledge of the most applicable computer software to use when applying health care statistics and research study design principles.

Now more than ever, health care data are being collected to serve many purposes. One primary purpose is to establish health care statistics to compare trends in incidence of disease, quality and outcome of care, and management of health information departments; another primary purpose is to conduct epidemiologic research. Data can be manipulated in many ways to demonstrate one result or another. Health information management (HIM) professionals need a broad base of knowledge to determine what data elements should be used and when data are being analyzed appropriately and inappropriately. To do this, an understanding of health care and vital and public health statistics is needed. Furthermore, knowledge in statistical analysis as well as research methods is necessary, so that HIM professionals are the forerunners in data analysis and research design.

Because HIM professionals oversee a vast array of health data, it is imperative that the interpretation of the analysis and results of health care data start with them. For example, reports generated from the Health Care Financing Administration (HCFA) mortality data, Medisgroup data, cancer registry data, and quality assessment studies, all include statistical values that must be understood by HIM professionals in order to provide the entire health care profession with an accurate and consistent analysis of that information.

This chapter explains basic and advanced health care statistics that are used in the health care field. The definition, formula, and calculation of each health care statistic are given. Examples of how each of the statistics is used are also provided. Steps in designing a research proposal or study, different research designs, and methods to display data are also discussed with examples.

OVERVIEW OF RESEARCH, STATISTICS, AND DATA PRESENTATION

The health care facility generates health care data continuously. The HIM professional's goal is to properly collect, organize, display, and interpret health care data to meet the needs of the users. The users can be internal, such as the patient, medical staff, nursing staff, and physical, occupational, and speech therapists, or external, such as state and federal regulatory agencies, the Joint Commission on Accreditation of Healthcare Facilities, and insurance companies. No matter who the user be, the goal of the HIM professional remains the same: to meet the user's needs while complying with the standards of the health care facility. To accomplish this goal, the HIM professional should be familiar with methods used to calculate specific types of statistics. Knowledge of the differences in rates, ratios, proportions, and percentages is necessary to evaluate mortality, autopsy, and morbidity rates as well as census and vital statistics.

Organizing and displaying health care data are necessary. Nominal, ordinal, continuous, and discrete data are different and, therefore, should have different statistical tests performed and different methods used to display data. Measures of central tendency (mean, median, mode) and dispersion (variance and standard deviation) as well as tests of significance are used when data are displayed in tables and graphs. Tables and graphs of health care data usually originate from a research study. Familiarity with research study protocol, including formulating a hypothesis, reviewing and analyzing the literature, developing specific aims, determining the significance of the research, and defining the methodology to include how the data will be collected and analyzed, is necessary for the HIM professional. Once the steps of the research design are well formulated and understood, then the data, statistics, and data display are easier to interpret.

Familiarity with the different types of research study designs is necessary to determine if the health care data generated from a research study are accurate and appropriate. The different research study designs to be examined are the descriptive study, analytic study, and experimental study. Each of these study designs should be used when analyzing different ideas or hypotheses.

HIM professionals should recognize that every research study produces some degree of bias or error. This may be due to sampling variability, methods of data collection, or confounding variables.

This chapter introduces the reader to research, statistical analysis, and data presentation. HIM professionals who are actively involved in analysis, interpretation, and complex research study design should take additional coursework in these areas as well as work closely with a statistician and epidemiologist.

ROLE OF THE HIM PROFESSIONAL

The HIM professional should assume the lead in recommending and using appropriate research study designs, research study protocols, and statistical tests that guarantee improvement in the analysis, use, and dissemination of health care data. The HIM professional fills many diversified roles and responsibilities. They may include manager of a cancer registry, director of quality assessment and improvement and utilization management, or director of health information systems.

In each of these roles, understanding and applying the methods used to collect, analyze, display, interpret, and disseminate data are essential. Responsibilities undertaken in these roles may vary from person to person. For example, the manager of a cancer registry may play a clearly visible role in cancer research study design and analysis as well as interpretation of the data; the director of quality assessment and improvement and utilization management may play a key role in organizing and displaying quality-related data so that the information is understood by members of the medical staff; the director of health information systems may determine the appropriate databases to use when analyzing cost and length of stay data.

The HIM professional may assume other managerial roles in which statistics are used to assess productivity in coding, transcription, correspondence, and chart analysis. The HIM professional should have sufficient knowledge and skills to do the following:

- Collect quality health data.
- Develop appropriate research study designs.
- Analyze results of the research.
- Develop, generate, and interpret health care statistical reports.

HEALTH CARE STATISTICS

Vital Statistics

Vital statistics include data collected from vital events in our lives, such as births and adoptions, marriages and divorces, and deaths and fetal deaths. Birth, death, and fetal death certificates are familiar reports to HIM professionals. Although each state can determine the format and content of its certificates, the National Center for Health Statistics (NCHS) recommends standard forms that most states have adopted. The purpose of the NCHS standard forms is to have a national uniform reporting system of vital statistics. These standard forms are revised periodically. They are normally completed within the HIM department, and a copy of the birth or death certificate is kept in the medical record. A copy of the fetal death certificate is kept in the mother's medical record. The attending physician is responsible for the completion of birth, death, and fetal death certificates. The accurate completion of these certificates is supervised by the HIM department. Once the certificate is complete, the original is sent to the local registrar, who keeps a copy and forwards the original to the state registrar. During each of these stages, the certificate is checked by the registrar to make sure it is complete. Individuals can obtain from the state registrar certified copies of birth, death, and fetal death certificates. Each state sends tapes of birth and death statistics to the NCHS. The death statistics are then compiled onto the National Death Index. The death index is used for research purposes by epidemiologists and other workers involved in health care research.[1] The natality or birth statistics are compiled onto the monthly vital statistics reports, and the data tapes are available for research purposes also.

Refer to your state health data center or division of vital statistics to receive state-specific information on preparing and registering vital records.

Rates, Ratios, Proportions, and Percentages

A rate is defined as the number of people with a specific characteristic divided by the total number of people. It is also thought of as the number of times an event *did* occur compared with the number of times it *could* have occurred.

A rate contains two major elements: a numerator and a denominator. The numerator is the number of times an event *did* occur. The number of events under study or the numerator alone conveys little information. However, when the numerator is compared with the denominator or the population of people in which the event *could* have occurred, a rate is determined. The results of a quality assessment study showed that 20 patients with diabetes suffered a stroke while taking a certain medication. What does this tell you? Should this medication be discontinued in this population? The data provided here include only the numerator. To compute a rate, the denominator is needed. For this example, you need to know the total number of patients with diabetes who are taking the medication. This particular example included a sample size of 1000 patients. The rate is 20 in 1000, or 2 in 100.

A rate is normally expressed in the following manner: 20 in 1000; 2 in 100; 1 in 100,000, 10 in 1,000,000, and so on. A proportion and a ratio are similar to a rate. A proportion is normally expressed as a fraction—$\frac{20}{1000}$, $\frac{2}{100}$, $\frac{1}{100,000}$, $\frac{10}{1,000,000}$, and so on. A ratio is a comparison of one thing to another, such as births to deaths, marriages to divorces. A ratio is expressed as 20:1000, 2:100, 1:100,000, 10:1,000,000, and so on. The ability to pay debts can also be expressed as a ratio. For example, if one has $3 million in available cash if needed and $1.5 million in debts, the ratio is expressed as $3 million:$1.5 million; this ratio shows that the amount of dollars available if needed is twice as much as the amount of dollars owed.

A percentage is based on a whole divided into 100 parts. A fraction, such as $\frac{1}{5}$, may be expressed as a percentage by first converting the fraction into a decimal by dividing the numerator, 1, by the denominator, 5, to obtain .20. The decimal is then converted into a percentage by multiplying the decimal by 100, which can be accomplished by moving the decimal point two places to the right, and affixing a percent sign. The result is 20 per cent.

Table 9–1 summarizes examples of rates, proportions, ratios, and percentages.[2,3]

Once percentages are calculated, they can be compared across different subgroups, as seen in Table 9–2. This table concisely shows differences among different geographic areas for the percentage of elderly people by age categories. It even allows a glance toward the future by projecting percentages for the years 2010 and 2025. By comparing percentages among different areas, it can be seen that Europe has the highest percentage of population aged 65 or over (13.7 per cent in 1990) and that it should remain the world leader for at least the next three decades. North America and Oceania also have relatively high percentages of elderly people, which are projected to increase substantially from 1990 to 2025.[4]

Mortality Rates

Mortality rates are computed because they demonstrate an outcome that may be related to the quality of the health care provided. There are many types of mortality rates. Table 9–3 provides the definition and formula for the most commonly used mortality rates.[2,3]

TABLE 9–1 EXAMPLES OF RATIOS, PROPORTIONS, PERCENTAGES, AND RATES			
RATIO	PROPORTION	PERCENTAGE	RATE (PER 100,000)
1:100	1/100 = 0.01	1.0	1,000 in 100,000
3:10,000	3/10,000 = 0.0003	0.03	30 in 100,000
250:100,000	250/100,000 = 0.0025	0.25	250 in 100,000

TABLE 9–2 PERCENTAGE OF ELDERLY BY AGE: 1990–2025				
REGION	**YEAR**	**65 YEARS AND OVER**	**75 YEARS AND OVER**	**80 YEARS AND OVER**
Europe*	1990	13.7	6.1	3.2
	2010	17.5	8.4	4.9
	2025	22.4	10.8	6.4
North America	1990	12.6	5.3	2.8
	2010	14.0	6.5	4.0
	2025	20.1	8.5	4.6
Oceania	1990	9.3	3.6	1.8
	2010	11.0	4.8	2.8
	2025	15.0	6.6	3.6
Asia[1]	1990	4.8	1.5	0.6
	2010	6.8	2.5	1.2
	2025	10.0	3.6	1.8
Latin America/Caribbean	1990	4.6	1.6	0.8
	2010	6.4	2.6	1.2
	2025	9.4	3.6	1.8
Near East/North Africa	1990	3.8	1.2	0.5
	2010	4.6	1.6	0.8
	2025	6.4	2.2	1.1
Sub-Saharan Africa	1990	2.7	0.7	0.3
	2010	2.9	0.8	0.3
	2025	3.4	1.0	0.4

* Data excludes the former Soviet Union.
Source: U.S. Bureau of the Census: Center for International Research, International Data Base on Aging.

Gross Death Rate

The gross death rate is a crude death rate because it does not consider such factors as age, sex, race, and severity of illness. Controversy surrounding its usefulness has occurred because it does not take into account the factors above, which also play an important part in death rates. As long as the HIM professional is aware that other factors influence this rate and that they have not been taken into account in the calculation, the gross death rate can prove to be a quick, useful means to analyze mortality.

EXAMPLE

The discharge analysis report of Anywhere Health Care Facility shows 752 discharges (including deaths) for October 1995. Twelve deaths were also shown in the report.

Gross death rate: $\dfrac{12 \times 100}{752}$

= 1.60 per cent

This means that 1.60 per cent of total discharges from Anywhere Health Care Facility during October 1995 ended in death, or that the gross percentage of deaths, or the hospital death rate, for October was 1.60 per cent.

Net Death Rate

The net death rate, or institutional death rate, is different from the gross death rate because it does not include deaths that occurred less than 48 hours after admittance to the health care facility. The net death rate is useful because it provides a more realistic account of patient deaths. For example, a 90-year-old patient arrives at the emergency department with shortness of breath, chest pain, and arrhythmia. After being evaluated, the patient is admitted, and it is determined that the patient has suffered a severe myocardial infarction.

EXAMPLE

Inpatient deaths at Anywhere Health Care Facility for 1995 totaled 50. Inpatient deaths that occurred less than 48 hours after admittance to the facility totaled 15. Total discharges (including deaths) were 15,546.

Net death rate: $\dfrac{(50 - 15) \times 100}{15,546 - 15}$

= 0.23 per cent

This means that 0.23 per cent (less than 1 per cent) of the deaths of discharges for 1995 occurred more than 48 hours after admittance to the health care facility, or that the net percentage of deaths or net death rate for 1995 was 0.23 per cent.

TABLE 9–3 MORTALITY RATES

MORTALITY RATES	FORMULA
Gross death rate (hospital death rate)	$$\frac{\text{Total number of inpatient deaths for the period} \times 100}{\text{Total number of discharges (including deaths) for the period}}$$
Net death rate	$$\frac{\text{Total number of inpatient deaths} - \text{inpatient deaths} < 48 \text{ hours} \times 100}{\text{Total discharges (including deaths)} - \text{deaths} < 48 \text{ hours}}$$
Anesthesia death rate	$$\frac{\text{Total number of anesthetic deaths for the period} \times 100}{\text{Total number of anesthetics administered for the period}}$$
Postoperative death rate	$$\frac{\text{Total number of deaths (within 10 days of surgery)} \times 100}{\text{Total number of patients who received surgery for the period}}$$
Maternal death rate	$$\frac{\text{Total number of deaths of obstetric patients} \times 100}{\text{Total number of discharges (including deaths) of obstetric patients}}$$
Neonatal mortality rate (death of neonate within the first 27 days, 23 hours, and 59 minutes of life)	$$\frac{\text{Total number of neonatal deaths (born in hospital) within 27 days, 23 hours, and 59 minutes of life for a period} \times 100}{\text{Total number of neonatal discharges (including deaths) for the period}}$$
Fetal death rate a. Early fetal death (abortion) rate < 20 weeks' gestation or 500 gr or less	a. $$\frac{\text{Total number of fetal deaths that occurred} < 20 \text{ weeks' gestation or 500 gr or less for a period} \times 100}{\text{Total number of births (including fetal deaths} < 20 \text{ weeks' gestation or 500 gr or less) for the period}}$$
b. Intermediate fetal death ≥ 20 weeks' gestation or 501–1000 gr	b. $$\frac{\text{Total number of fetal deaths that occurred} \geq 20 \text{ weeks' gestation or 501–1000 gr for a period} \times 100}{\text{Total number of births (including fetal deaths} \geq 20 \text{ weeks' gestation or 501–1000 gr) for the period}}$$
c. Late fetal death (stillborn) ≥ 28 weeks' gestation or over 1001 gr	c. $$\frac{\text{Total number of fetal deaths that occurred} \geq 28 \text{ weeks' gestation or over 1001 gr for a period} \times 100}{\text{Total number of births (including fetal deaths} \geq 28 \text{ weeks' gestation or over 1001 gr) for the period}}$$
Infant mortality rate (death at any time from moment of birth to the 1st year of life)	$$\frac{\text{Total number of deaths of infants (within 1st year of life) born in hospital for a period} \times 100}{\text{Total number of infants discharged (including infant deaths) for the period}}$$

About 24 hours later, the patient goes into cardiac arrest and dies. This particular death would be included in the gross death rate but not the net death rate because it occurred less than 48 hours after admission. Sometimes net death rates are requested by reporting agencies, but their use is limited when measuring the quality of care because they do not take into consideration other risk factors.

Anesthesia Death Rate

The anesthesia death rate can also be referred to as a cause-specific death rate because the death is determined to be due to a specific cause (i.e., an anesthetic

EXAMPLE

Anywhere Health Care Facility performed 492 surgical procedures during November and administered 452 anesthetics. Deaths resulting from the administration of an anesthetic totaled two for the month.

Anesthetic death rate: $$\frac{2 \times 100}{452}$$

$$= 0.44 \text{ per cent}$$

This means that 0.44 per cent (less than 1 per cent) of anesthetics administered resulted in a patient's death, or that the anesthetic death rate for November was 0.44 per cent.

agent). This rate determines the number of deaths that are due to the administration of anesthetics for a specified period. If the anesthetic death rate is higher than in previous periods, a focused evaluation may be necessary to determine why this is so.

Postoperative Death Rate

The postoperative death rate may be considered a cause-specific death rate as well. This death rate determines the number of patients who die within 10 days of surgery divided by the number of patients who underwent surgery for the period; therefore, it determines the number of deaths that may have resulted from surgical complications. In both the anesthesia and the postoperative death rates, other risk factors, such as age, sex, race, and severity of illness, are not considered. Therefore, if it is found that these rates are higher in certain periods than in others, specific evaluations are necessary to determine if the death is truly due to the anesthesia or surgery or to other risk factors.

EXAMPLE

> Surgery was performed on 492 patients in the Anywhere Health Care Facility during November, and 27 of those patients died within 10 days of surgery.
>
> Postoperative death rate: $\dfrac{27 \times 100}{492}$
>
> $= 5.49$ per cent or 5.5 per cent
>
> This means that 5.5 per cent of those patients who underwent surgery died within 10 days of the procedure, or that the postoperative death rate for November was 5.5 per cent.

Maternal Death Rate

Death rates are further categorized into type of service or department, such as the maternal death rate. A ma-

EXAMPLE

> Anywhere Health Care Facility had a total of 752 discharges for October, including 120 obstetric discharges and 1 obstetric death.
>
> Maternal death rate: $\dfrac{1 \times 100}{120}$
>
> $= 0.83$ per cent or 0.8 per cent
>
> This means that 0.8 per cent (less than 1 per cent) of obstetric patients discharged during October died, or that the maternal death rate for October was 0.8 per cent.

ternal death results from causes associated with pregnancy or its management but not from accidental or incidental causes unrelated to the pregnancy. The maternal death rate determines the number of obstetric deaths divided by the number of obstetric discharges. Again, like all the rates described previously, it does not consider any other risk factors. The maternal death rate is useful because maternal deaths are rare. Therefore, if there is even one maternal death in a period, it is necessary to examine the cause of death in more detail.

Neonatal and Infant Death Rates

Neonatal and infant death rates are computed to examine deaths of the neonate and infant at different stages. Fetal death rates examine differences in the rate of early, intermediate, and late fetal deaths. The definition of early, intermediate, and late fetal deaths may vary from state to state.

EXAMPLE

> Anywhere Health Care Facility developed the following discharge analysis report for 1995. A segment of the report shows the following:
>
> | | |
> |---|---:|
> | Live births | 127 |
> | Neonatal discharges | 115 |
> | Neonatal deaths (before 28 days) | 2 |
> | Infant discharges | 50 |
> | Infant deaths (before 1 yr and at or after 28 days) | 5 |
> | Fetal deaths (at or after 20 weeks' gestation) | 13 |
>
> Neonatal mortality rate: $\dfrac{2 \times 100}{115 + 2}$
>
> $= 1.71$ per cent or 1.7 per cent

> This means that 1.7 per cent of the neonates discharged died, or that the neonatal mortality rate for 1995 was 1.7 per cent.
>
> *Note:* Because the intermediate fetal death rate is most commonly used, an example of that rate is given.

> Intermediate fetal death rate: $\dfrac{13 \times 100}{127 + 13}$
>
> $= 9.29$ per cent or 9.3 per cent

> This means that intermediate fetal deaths made up 9.3 per cent of live births (excluding those live births at or before 20 weeks' gestation), or that the intermediate fetal death rate for 1995 was 9.3 per cent.

Infant mortality rate:
$$\frac{5 \times 100}{50 + 5}$$
$$= 9.09 \text{ per cent or}$$
$$9.1 \text{ per cent}$$

This means that 9.1 per cent of infants discharged died, or that the infant mortality rate for 1995 was 9.1 per cent.

Using and Examining Mortality Rates

There are many ways in which mortality statistics and trends in mortality are used and examined. When examining trends in mortality, one should consider the possible reasons that differences in mortality occur. Mortality trends could be influenced by three variables: time, place, and person. Changes over time include the following:

- Revisions in the rules for International Classification of Disease (ICD) coding of death certificates
- Improvements in medical technology
- Earlier detection and diagnosis of disease

In relation to place, the following factors influence mortality trends:

- Changes in the environment
- International differences in medical technology
- Diagnostic practices of physicians

Finally, the following characteristics of groups of people can also influence mortality:

- Age
- Sex
- Race
- Ethnicity
- Social habits (diet, smoking, alcohol intake)
- Genetic background
- Emotional and mental characteristics

All of the above must be taken into consideration when examining mortality trends within the health care facility or across health care facilities in relation to the quality of care provided.[5]

When one is examining mortality within a specific population, as in the gross and net death rates, it is important to show age-specific rates or to age adjust. Mortality rates are routinely adjusted for age because it is the most important influence in relation to death. As one ages, there is greater likelihood that one will die. Age-specific rates can be used, but it becomes difficult to make comparisons of data with four or more age levels or categories. Therefore, age adjustment is performed. Statistically, age adjustment removes the difference in composition with respect to age.[1]

There are two methods that can be used to do age adjustment. One is the **direct method of age adjustment,** and the other is the indirect method of age adjustment, or **standardized mortality ratio (SMR).** The calculations for these two methods are shown in Table 9–4.

TABLE 9–4   AGE-ADJUSTMENT METHODS

DIRECT METHOD	FORMULA	
Age-adjusted death rate (A)	= $\dfrac{\text{Total expected number of deaths at population A's rates}}{\text{Total standard population}}$	× Constant
Age-adjusted death rate (B)	= $\dfrac{\text{Total expected number of deaths at population B's rates}}{\text{Total standard population}}$	× Constant
Compare age-adjusted death rates for population A and B.		

INDIRECT METHOD	FORMULA
SMR for population A	= $\dfrac{\text{Observed deaths in population A}}{\text{Expected deaths in population A at standard rates}}$
SMR for population B	= $\dfrac{\text{Observed deaths in population B}}{\text{Expected deaths in population B at standard rates}}$
Compare the two SMRs for population A and B.	

SMR, standardized mortality ratio.

HOSPITAL	COMMENTS	NUMBER OF PATIENTS	*AVERAGE ADMISSION SEVERITY SCORE	AGE 65 AND OVER (%)	DEATHS			MEDICALLY UNSTABLE DURING FIRST WEEK MAJOR MORBIDITY			AVERAGE STAY (DAYS)	AVERAGE CHARGE ($)
					Actual Number	Expected Number	Statistical Rating	Actual Number	Expected Number	Statistical Rating		
1		268	2.5	85.1	23	21.03		35	25.12	—	7.9	15,420
2	✔	412	2.4	87.1	30	33.08		61	36.66	—	9.2	8,149
3		201	2.2	87.1	17	12.16		9	14.52		9.4	7,645
4		208	2.6	64.4	8	16.56	+	24	21.52		7.7	15,669
5		471	2.5	89.0	40	40.31		40	44.18		8.3	8,193
6		90	2.6	78.9	9	7.49		12	9.35		9.0	14,766
7	✔	347	2.3	81.3	36	22.31	— .	24	27.78		8.9	12,099
8		291	2.1	90.0	20	18.15		20	20.97		8.7	9,180
9		255	2.3	82.0	11	17.04		18	21.09		6.4	6,292
10		477	2.2	85.5	32	29.55		32	36.78		8.4	12,039

TABLE 9-5 DRG 127 HEART FAILURE AND SHOCK

Hospital Effectiveness Report, Pennsylvania Health Care Cost Containment Council. Reporting Period January 1–December 31, 1991.

The direct method uses a standard population and applies the age-specific rates available for each population. One then determines the expected number of deaths in the standard population. To use the direct method of age adjustment, age-specific rates must be available for both populations and the number of deaths per age category should be at least 5. The indirect method, or SMR, is used more often and can be used without age-specific rates and when the number of deaths per age category is small or less than 5. Standard rates are then applied to the populations being compared to calculate the expected number of deaths, which are compared with the observed number of deaths.[6]

Because the SMR is used in most national and state-wide mortality reports, it is the method that is explained in more detail here. For example, in Table 9–5, hospitals across a state are examined for death rates due to Diagnostic Related Group (DRG) 127—Heart Failure and Shock. The actual or observed number of deaths in the hospital is compared to the expected number of deaths. The expected number of deaths is taken from a comparative national database adjusted for age and patient severity for each DRG. Table 9–5 shows a sample of those hospitals that treated patients with the DRG 127 and the actual and expected number of deaths. An SMR of 1 means that the number of observed deaths and the number of expected deaths are equal, and therefore, the mortality rate is equal to what is expected from national norms. An SMR of less than 1 means that the observed deaths are lower than the expected deaths and, therefore, a lower mortality rate than is expected from national norms. An SMR of greater than 1 means that the observed deaths are greater than the expected deaths and, therefore, a higher mortality rate than is expected from national norms. For hospital #1, an SMR of 1.09 ($\frac{23}{21.03}$) means that the hospital had a 9 per cent higher mortality rate for DRG 127 than is expected from national norms. For hospital #4, an SMR of 0.48 ($\frac{8}{16.56}$) means that the hospital had a 52 per cent lower mortality for DRG 127 than is expected from national norms. The statistical rating column displayed in Table 9–5 is covered later in this chapter in the discussion on tests of significance.

Autopsy Rates

Autopsy rates are computed so that the health care facility can determine the proportion of deaths in which an autopsy was performed. This enables the facility to examine why they may be seeing a higher or lower autopsy rate from one month to another. Autopsies are

TABLE 9–6 AUTOPSY RATES

AUTOPSY RATE	FORMULA
Gross autopsy rate (ratio of inpatient autopsies to inpatient deaths)	Total number of inpatient autopsies for a given period × 100
	Total inpatient deaths for the period
Net autopsy rate	Total inpatient autopsies for a given period × 100
	Total number of inpatient deaths − unautopsied coroners' cases
Hospital autopsy rate (adjusted)	Total hospital autopsies for a given period × 100
	Number of deaths of hospital patients whose bodies are available for hospital autopsy

Gross Autopsy Rate

$$(10 \times 100)/52 = 19.23 \text{ per cent} = 19.2 \text{ per cent}$$

This means that 19.2 per cent of the hospital inpatients who died during January received an autopsy, or that the gross autopsy rate was 19.2 per cent.

Net Autopsy Rate

$$(10 \times 100)/(52 - 2) = 20 \text{ per cent}$$

This means that 20 per cent of the hospital inpatients who died during January received an autopsy within the hospital, or that the net autopsy rate was 20 per cent.

Hospital Autopsy Rate (Adjusted)

$$(13 \times 100)/52 - (2 \text{ coroner cases})$$
$$+ (2 \text{ outpatients}) + (2 \text{ home care patients})$$
$$= 54 = 24.07 = 24.1 \text{ per cent}$$

This means that 24.1 per cent of all health care patients who died in January (inpatients, outpatients, and home care patients) received an autopsy within the hospital, or that the adjusted hospital autopsy rate was 24.1 per cent.

performed to determine the cause of death, to better understand the disease process, or to collect tissue samples, as in patients with Alzheimer's disease. Autopsy rates can be further broken down to show the gross autopsy rate, or the rate of autopsies performed on total inpatient deaths; the net autopsy rate, or the rate of autopsies performed on inpatient deaths, excluding unautopsied coroner cases; and the adjusted hospital autopsy rate, or the autopsy rate performed on all deaths of hospital patients whose bodies are available or brought to the hospital for autopsy (those *not* removed by coroners, medical examiners, and so on). Autopsies may be performed on deaths of inpatients, outpatients, home care patients, skilled nursing care residents, patients who died at home, previous patients, and so on. Table 9–6 presents the most commonly used autopsy rates.[3]

EXAMPLE

Anywhere Health Care Facility developed the following report regarding discharges, deaths, and autopsies during January 1995.

JANUARY 1995	HOSPITAL STATISTICS
Discharges (including deaths)	1000
Total deaths	56
Inpatient (including two coroner cases)	52
Outpatient	2
Home care	2
Autopsies	13
Inpatient	10
Outpatient	1
Home care	2

Morbidity Rates

Morbidity rates can include complication rates, such as community-acquired, hospital-acquired or nosocomial, and postoperative infection rates. It can also include comorbidity rates and the prevalence and incidence rates of disease.

Hospitals use each of these rates to study the types of disease or conditions that are present within the health care facility as well as to examine the quality of care provided by the facility. These rates can aid health care facilities when planning specific health care services and programs. Table 9–7 provides a summary of the more common morbidity rates and the formula used to compute them.[3]

Complication rates normally include infection rates and are computed so that the health care facility can determine when they developed and, therefore, how they may be prevented. A nosocomial, or hospital-acquired, infection rate includes those infections that occur longer than 72 hours after admission.[7] Health care

TABLE 9–7 MORBIDITY RATES

DEFINITION	FORMULA
Complication (condition that occurs during the hospital stay that extends the length of stay by at least 1 day in 75% of cases)	$$\frac{\text{Total number of complications for a given period} \times 100}{\text{Total number of discharges for a given period}}$$
Nosocomial infection rate (infection that occurs > 72 hours after admission into the hospital)	$$\frac{\text{Total number of infections that occur} > 72 \text{ hours after admission for a given period} \times 100}{\text{Total number of discharges for a given period}}$$
Postoperative infection rate	$$\frac{\text{Total number of postoperative infections for a given period} \times 100}{\text{Total number of surgical operations performed}}$$
Community-acquired infection rate (infection that occurs in the community or < 72 hours of admission)	$$\frac{\text{Total number of community-acquired infections that occur} < 72 \text{ hours of admission for a given period} \times 100}{\text{Total number of discharges for a given period}}$$
Total infection rate (includes both nosocomial and community-acquired infections)	$$\frac{\text{Total number of community-acquired infections and nosocomial infections for a given period} \times 100}{\text{Total number of discharges for a given period}}$$
Comorbidity (pre-existing condition that will, because of its presence with a principal diagnosis, increase the length of stay by at least 1 day in 75% of cases)	$$\frac{\text{Total number of comorbidities for a given period} \times 100}{\text{Total number of discharges for a given period}}$$
Prevalence (number of people with a specific disease at a specified period of time; number of existing cases of disease)	$$\frac{\text{Number of existing cases of disease present in a population at specified time period} \times 1000}{\text{Number of people in the population at the specified time period}}$$
Incidence (number of people who develop a disease during a specified time period; number of new cases of disease)	$$\frac{\text{Number of new cases of a disease occuring in a population during a specified time period} \times 1000}{\text{Number of people in the population at the specified time period}}$$

facilities may be more interested in this rate because it may show infections that occur as a result of the care that is provided in the health care facility. Further analysis of the nosocomial infection rate may show that other risk factors, such as age, compromising conditions such as cancer, and the use of chemotherapy treatment, as well as the overall severity of the disease, may make an individual patient more susceptible to infection. Therefore, as with several of the mortality rates, other factors play a part in the development of the nosocomial infection. The postoperative infection is a nosocomial infection and is normally calculated to pinpoint how the infection may have developed. Postoperative infection rates are important to examine because the health care facility can determine which infections occur after surgery and are probably due to the surgical procedure. It is also important to distinguish between nosocomial and community-acquired infections because community-acquired infections typically are present less than 72 hours before admission to the health care facility. Health care

facilities may be interested in this rate because it demonstrates those infections that the patient probably had before admission to the facility. If the facility finds that their community-acquired infection rate is high, they may need to develop communitywide prevention programs, such as administering a vaccine for pneumonia. It is beneficial for health care facilities to analyze their total infection rate (both nosocomial and community-acquired infections) to determine the additional cost, length of stay, and overall effect the infections have on the quality of care provided to the patient.

Comorbidities are pre-existing conditions, such as diabetes, hypertension, and osteoporosis. It is important to analyze the comorbidity rate because comorbidities can increase the length of stay as well as affect the outcome of care provided. Comorbidities include some of the other risk factors that affect mortality and morbidity rates.

The example on the following page shows morbidity data for Anywhere Health Care Facility during March 1995.

EXAMPLE

ANYWHERE HEALTH CARE FACILITY	MARCH 1995 STATISTICS
Discharges (including deaths)	2000
Surgical operations	1543
Number of comorbidities	238
Number of complications	120
Nosocomial infections (includes post-operative infections)	22
Postoperative infections	8
Community-acquired infections	30

Complication Rate

$$(120 \times 100)/2000 = 6.0 \text{ per cent}$$

This means that 6.0 per cent of all discharges for March had at least one complication, or that the complication rate for March was 6.0 per cent.

Nosocomial Infection Rate

$$(22 \times 100)/2000 = 1.1 \text{ per cent}$$

This means that 1.1 per cent of all discharges for March had a nosocomial or hospital-acquired infection, or the nosocomial or hospital-acquired infection rate for March was 1.1 per cent.

Postoperative Infection Rate

$$(8 \times 100)/1543 = 0.52 \text{ per cent}$$

This means that 0.5 per cent of all surgical operations performed during March developed a postoperative infection, or the postoperative infection rate for March was 0.5 per cent.

Community-Acquired Infection Rate

$$(30 \times 100)/2000 = 1.5 \text{ per cent}$$

This means that 1.5 per cent of all discharges for March had a community-acquired infection, or that the community-acquired infection rate for March was 1.5 per cent.

Total Infection Rate

$$(52 \times 100)/2000 = 2.6 \text{ per cent}$$

This means that 2.6 per cent of all discharges for March had an infection, or that the total infection rate for March was 2.6 per cent.

Comorbidity Rate

$$(238 \times 100)/2000 = 11.9 \text{ per cent}$$

This means that 11.9 per cent of all discharges for March had at least one comorbidity, or that the comorbidity rate for March was 11.9 per cent.

Prevalence and incidence rates are determined to examine the frequency of specific types of disease, such as cancer, acquired immunodeficiency syndrome (AIDS), and heart disease. Prevalence means the number of *existing* cases of disease, whereas incidence refers to the number of *new* cases of disease.

The **prevalence rate** is the number of existing cases of a disease in a specified time period divided by the population at that time. The quotient is then multiplied by a constant, such as 1000, 100,000, and so on

EXAMPLE

In a community of elderly people, the number of women alive with osteoporosis in 1993 is 3593. The population of women in this community is 100,000.

$$\text{Prevalence rate} = \frac{3,593}{100,000} \times 1000$$
$$= 35.93, \text{ or } 36 \text{ osteoporosis cases per } 1000 \text{ women in this community}$$

The **incidence rate** is the number of newly reported cases of a disease in a specified time period divided by

EXAMPLE

In the same elderly community, the number of new cases of osteoporosis reported in 1994 is 1113 and the population of women in the community at that time is 100,000.

$$\text{Incidence rate} = \frac{1113}{100,000} \times 1000$$
$$= 11.13, \text{ or } 11 \text{ new osteoporosis cases per } 1000 \text{ women in this community}$$

the population in a specified time period. The quotient is then multiplied by a constant such as 1000, 100,000, and so on.

Prevalence and incidence rates of specific diseases that are prominent within a particular region or state should be analyzed by the HIM professional to effectively manage health care services. National sources of morbidity data include the National Health Survey. Originated in 1956, this survey is performed annually on a representative sample of 40,000 persons. Many subprograms are part of the National Health Survey, such as the National Discharge Survey, National Ambulatory and Medical Care Survey, and National Nursing Home Survey. Results of these surveys include incidence and prevalence rates of disease for specific geographic areas, length of hospital stays, cause of hospitalizations, and use of ambulatory care services.[1] The HIM professional should be aware that this information exists and can be used in conjunction with other morbidity rates to further ana-

lyze the distribution and effectiveness of health care services.

Characteristics similar to those that influence trends in mortality also influence trends in morbidity—time, place, person. For example, infectious diseases tend to occur more often at specific times of the year. The place of employment or geographic location can also increase susceptibility to disease. Age can increase infectious diseases, such as measles and chickenpox in the young. Sex can influence morbidity trends with differences in coronary artery disease for men and women. Race also influences morbidity trends with hypertension being more prevalent in African-Americans.[5]

Census Statistics

Ratios, percentages, and averages related to the length of stay, occupancy, bed turnover, and total number of

TABLE 9-8 CENSUS STATISTICS	
DEFINITION	**FORMULA**
Daily inpatient census (number of inpatients present at census-taking time plus any inpatients who were both admitted and discharged after the census-taking time the previous day)	Formula is presented as the definition.
Inpatient service day (unit of measure including services received by one inpatient in one 24-hour period. Synonyms: patient day, inpatient day, census day, bed occupancy day)	Formula is presented as the definition.
Inpatient bed count (number of available inpatient beds [occupied and vacant] on any given day. *Note:* Not all beds are included in the inpatient bed count. These include beds in examination rooms, therapy, labor rooms, and recovery rooms as well as bassinets. Beds set up for temporary use are not included.)	Formula is presented as the definition.
Average daily inpatient census (average number of inpatients in a facility for a given period of time)	Total number of inpatient service days for a period ——————————————————— Total number of days in that period
Length of stay (for an inpatient; number of calendar days from admission to discharge)	Duration of hospitalization for one inpatient: Day of admission is not counted unless it is the day of discharge and/or the day of discharge is not counted unless it is the day of admission. Either method is correct if done consistently.
Average length of stay (average length of stay of inpatients discharged during a specified period)	Total inpatient service days ——————————————————— Total number of discharges (includes deaths)
Inpatient bed occupancy ratio (proportion of inpatient beds occupied, defined as the ratio of inpatient service days to inpatient bed count days in the specified period. Synonyms: percentage of occupancy, occupancy percentage)	Total inpatient service days or discharge days × 100 ——————————————————— Total inpatient bed count × number of days in the period
Bed turnover rate (number of times a bed, on the average, changes occupants during a given period of time)	Direct formula: Number of discharges (including deaths) for a period ——————————————————— Average bed count during the period Indirect formula: Occupancy rate × number of days in period ——————————————————— Average length of stay

patients present at a specified time within the institution can be useful to health care administrators and HIM professionals. Such data can be used for the following purposes:

- To evaluate the current status of the health care facility
- To plan for future health care events
- To determine why differences in, for example, length of stay are seen between patient units

The **census statistics** are extremely useful in the overall analysis of how much, how long, and by whom the health care facility is being used. Table 9–8 provides the formulas for the common census statistics.[3]

EXAMPLE

A 500-bed health care facility, during the month of June (30 days), had a total of 3600 discharges (including deaths) and a total of 14,647 inpatient service days.

The total number of discharges from the oncology department was 1322, and the total number of hospital days for those discharged patients was 10,576. Patient A was admitted on June 18 and died the same day. Patient B was admitted on June 18 and discharged on June 19. Patient C was admitted on June 19 and discharged on June 25. Patient D was admitted on June 25 and discharged August 8.

Inpatient Bed Occupancy Ratio (Percentage of Occupancy)

(14,647 × 100)/500 (beds) × 30 (no. of days in June)
= 97.6 per cent

This means that 97.6 per cent of the available beds were occupied, or that the inpatient bed occupancy ratio was about 14,647:15,000, or that the percentage of occupancy was 97.6 per cent.

Average Daily Inpatient Census

14,647/30 (no. of days in June) = 488

This means that the average number of inpatients during June was 488, or that the average daily inpatient census for June was 488.

Average Length of Stay

14,647/3600 = 4.1 days

This means that patients stayed in the health care facility an average of 4.1 days during June, or that the average length of stay for June was 4.1.

Average Length of Stay for Oncology Department

10,576/1322 = 8.0 days

This means that patients in the oncology department stayed an average of 8.0 days during June, or that the average length of stay for the oncology department for June was 8 days. One can then compare the oncology department average length of stay (8 days) with the overall facility length of stay (4 days) and determine why the oncology department length of stay doubles the facility length of stay.

Patient A Length of Stay: 1 day
Patient B Length of Stay: 1 day
Patient C Length of Stay: 6 days
Patient D Length of Stay: 44 days

Each of the individual patient lengths of stay are self-explanatory but can be used to compare one to another, especially if the patients received the same services or were from the same department.

Bed Turnover Rate

Direct: $\frac{3600}{500} = 7.2$

Indirect: $= \frac{97.6 \text{ per cent} \times 30}{4.1}$
(average length of stay for June)

$= \frac{(0.976) \times 30}{4.1}$
(average length of stay for June)

$= 7.1$

This means that during June, each of the hospital's 500 beds changed patients about 7.2 times using the direct method and 7.1 times using the indirect method—a small difference between the two methods.

ORGANIZING AND DISPLAYING THE DATA[8]

Types of Data

Before deciding how to display data, it is important to know that different types of data should be displayed in different ways. Variables or data can be collected and organized into the following categories:

- Nominal
- Ordinal
- Discrete
- Continuous

Nominal Data

Nominal data, also called categorical or qualitative data, include numerical values assigned to categories, such as the sex and race of the subjects in a research study. It is easier to analyze or categorize the data if it is given a numerical code. For example, a female category would be coded as "0" and a male category coded as "1". Employment status could be coded "10" = employed and "9" = unemployed, and so on.

Ordinal or Ranked Data

Ordinal data are rankings according to some criterion. Severity of illness scores used in Medisgroup data are ordinal or ranked data:

0 = no or minimal risk of vital organ failure
1 = low risk of vital organ failure
2 = moderate risk of vital organ failure
3 = high risk of vital organ failure
4 = a presence of vital organ failure

Ordinal data can also include responses relative to questionnaires or interviews:

1 = strongly disagree
2 = disagree
3 = neutral
4 = agree
5 = strongly agree

Discrete Data

Discrete data are numerical values in which the number has meaning and usually assumes whole numbers, such as the number of medications a person is taking, the number of children in a family, or the number of records that are coded.

Continuous Data

Continuous data can assume an infinite number of possible values, and the number has meaning. Examples include weight, blood pressure, pulse rate, and costs or charges.

Types of Data Display

Many methods are used to effectively display data. Some methods of particular value to the HIM professional are the frequency distribution tables, bar graphs, pie charts, histograms, frequency polygons, and Pareto diagrams.

Frequency Distribution

The **frequency distribution** allows nominal, ordinal, and continuous data to be grouped into specific categories and the total number of observations in each category to be recorded. Percentages represent relative frequencies and are often used for comparison within the table. The frequency table should be self-explanatory and not show too much data so that the table is uninterpretable. The table should be clearly labeled, the total sample size displayed, and units of measurement included. When intervals are used, the number of intervals should be no less than 5 and no more than 20, of equal width, and the endpoints of the intervals should not overlap. Tables 9–9 through 9–12 are examples of frequency tables for nominal, ordinal, continuous, and discrete data, respectively.

Bar Graph

Bar graphs are used to present nominal, ordinal, discrete, and continuous data. The discrete categories are shown on the horizontal, or x, axis and the frequency is shown on the vertical, or y, axis. The purpose of the bar graph is to show the frequency for each variable. Each bar graph's vertical scale must begin at zero so that the heights of the bars are proportional to the frequencies. Figure 9–1 is an example of a bar graph using the data in Table 9–9. Other types of bar graphs are those shown in Figures 9–2 and 9–3. These graphs are still considered bar graphs but incorporate a line over the bars to show the total number of cases of measles (see Figure 9–2). Also, Figure 9–3 shows incidence of measles by age from 1988 to 1990 by using a stacked bar graph.

Pie Chart

A **pie chart** is effective in displaying nominal, ordinal, and continuous. It is constructed by drawing a circle, 360°, and dividing that circle into sections that correspond to the frequency in each category. For example, if the relative frequency is 15 per cent, then the slice of pie should be (.15) × (360°), or 54°. Figure 9–4 is an example of a pie chart using the data in Table 9–9.

Histogram

The **histogram** is used to present a frequency distribution with continuous-interval data. It is similar to a bar graph, but the horizontal axis of the histogram usually includes continuous-interval categories rather than

TABLE 9-9 FREQUENCY TABLE—NOMINAL DATA. PRINCIPAL HEALTH INSURANCE COVERAGE BY SEX

HEALTH INSURANCE	MALE n = 50 NO. (%)	FEMALE n = 50 NO. (%)	TOTAL n = 100 NO. (%)
Medicare	13 (26)	25 (50)	38 (38)
Medicaid	2 (4)	6 (12)	8 (8)
Blue Cross	25 (50)	10 (20)	35 (35)
Commercial	9 (18)	6 (12)	15 (15)
Other	1 (2)	3 (6)	4 (4)
Totals	50 (100)	50 (100)	100 (100)

Watzlaf VJM, Abdelhak M: Descriptive statistics. J Am Medical Record Assoc 1989;60(9):37–41. Reprinted with permission from American Health Information Management Association.

TABLE 9-11 FREQUENCY TABLE—CONTINUOUS INTERVAL DATA. 152 INPATIENTS IN A LARGE TEACHING HOSPITAL

TOTAL CHARGES ($)	FREQUENCY	RELATIVE FREQUENCY (%)
0–4,999	62	40.8
5,000–9,999	46	30.3
10,000–14,999	25	16.5
15,000–19,999	7	4.6
20,000–24,999	5	3.3
25,000–29,999	4	2.6
30,000–34,999	0	0
35,000–39,999	0	0
40,000–44,999	0	0
45,000–49,999	3	2.0

Watzlaf VJM, Abdelhak M: Descriptive statistics. J Am Medical Record Assoc 1989;60(9):37–41. Reprinted with permission from American Health Information Management Association.

the discrete categories used in the bar graph. For equal class intervals, the heights of the bars correspond to the frequency in each category, but the area of the bar is also important because it is proportional to the total frequency. Figure 9–5 is an example of a histogram using data in Table 9–11.

Frequency Polygon

The **frequency polygon** is another method used to present a frequency distribution with continuous-interval data. It is constructed by joining the midpoints of the top of each bar with a straight line. The area under the polygon is equal to the area of the bars in the histogram and proportional to the total frequency. The frequency polygon is effective when comparing two or more data sets. Figure 9–6 is an example of a frequency polygon

using data in Table 9–11. Figure 9–7 is an example of a frequency polygon comparing two data sets.

The reader may find variations of these data presentation methods. For example, statistical process control, which is used in the quality improvement process, uses many of the graphs and figures displayed previously but may change them slightly or call them different things. For example, the Pareto diagram is similar to the bar graph and the histogram and is used to order causes or problems from the most to the least significant. The Pareto diagram takes its name from the Pareto principle, which states that a few causes account for most of the effect. This was first established by economist Vilfredo Pareto, and so the chart was named after him. Compare the Pareto diagram in Figure 9–8 with a bar chart and histogram.[9,10]

TABLE 9-10 FREQUENCY TABLE—RANKED ORDINAL DATA. STUDENT PERCEPTIONS OF LEADERSHIP CHARACTERISTICS

LEADERSHIP CHARACTERISTIC RANKING	MANAGEMENT CLINICAL INTERNSHIP	
	Before n = 35 No. (%)	After n = 35 No. (%)
1 Very weak	5 (14)	0 (0)
2 Weak	10 (29)	1 (3)
3 Moderate	15 (43)	5 (14)
4 Strong	2 (6)	12 (34)
5 Very strong	3 (9)	17 (49)

Watzlaf VJM, Abdelhak M: Descriptive statistics. J Am Medical Record Assoc 1989;60(9):37–41. Reprinted with permission from American Health Information Management Association.

TABLE 9-12 FREQUENCY TABLE—DISCRETE DATA. UNIVERSITY HEALTH CENTER HOSPITAL ADMISSIONS BY RESIDENCE

	CITY n = 77 NO. (%)	SUBURBS n = 38 NO. (%)	RURAL n = 29 NO. (%)	TOTAL n = 144 NO. (%)
Hospital A	20 (26)	8 (21)	12 (41)	40 (28)
Hospital B	30 (39)	4 (11)	9 (31)	43 (30)
Hospital C	10 (13)	12 (32)	6 (21)	28 (19)
Hospital D	17 (22)	14 (37)	2 (7)	33 (23)
Totals	77 (100)	38 (100)	29 (100)	144 (100)

Watzlaf VJM, Abdelhak M: Descriptive statistics. J Am Medical Record Assoc 1989;60(9):37–41. Reprinted with permission from American Health Information Management Association.

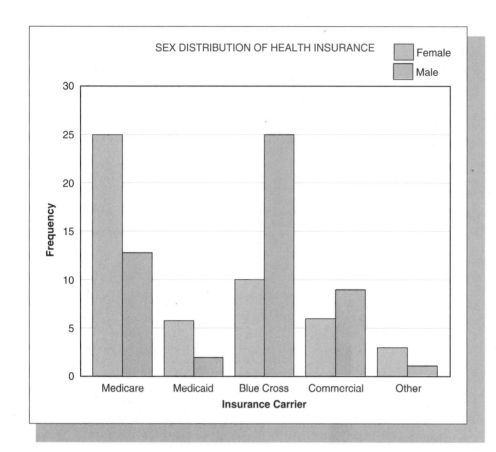

FIGURE 9–1. Bar graph. (From Watzlaf VJM, Abdelhak M: Descriptive statistics. J Am Medical Record Assoc 1989;60 [9]:37–41. Reprinted with permission from American Health Information Management Association.)

FIGURE 9–2. Bar graph and line graph. (From Infectious Disease Epidemiology Report. Pennsylvania Department of Health, Bureau of Epidemiology and Disease Prevention, 1990.)

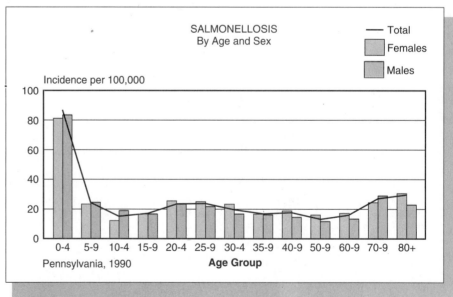

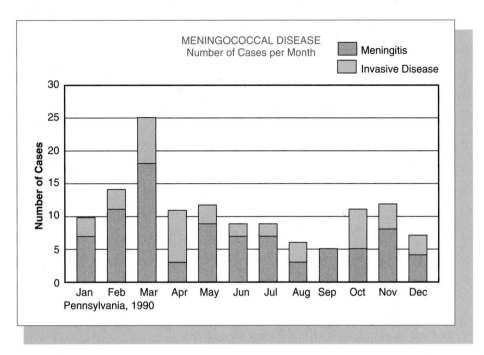

FIGURE 9–3. Stacked bar graph. (From Infectious Disease Epidemiology Report. Pennsylvania Department of Health, Bureau of Epidemiology and Disease Prevention, 1990.)

Measures of Central Tendency

The common measures of central tendency are as follows:

- Mean
- Median
- Mode

These measures are used to locate the middle or typical value in a frequency distribution. Any one of the three may be the most suitable to use, depending on a particular situation.

Mean

The **mean** is the most common measure of central tendency because it can be used for further statistics, such as the variance and standard deviation, which are discussed later. The mean is calculated by adding up the values of all the observations and dividing the total by the number of observations. The purpose of the mean is to summarize a collection of data by means of a representative value.

EXAMPLES

The lengths of stay in the hospital for eight patients in a pediatric department are 6, 4, 2, 5, 20, 25, 18, and 4 days. The mean, or average, length of stay equals the following:

$$= \frac{6 + 4 + 2 + 5 + 20 + 25 + 18 + 4}{8}$$

$$= 84/8$$

$$= 10.5 \text{ days}$$

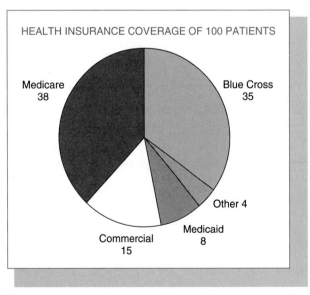

FIGURE 9–4. Pie chart (From Watzlaf VJM, Abdelhak M: Descriptive statistics. J Am Medical Record Assoc 1989;60 (9):37–41. Reprinted with permission from American Health Information Management Association.)

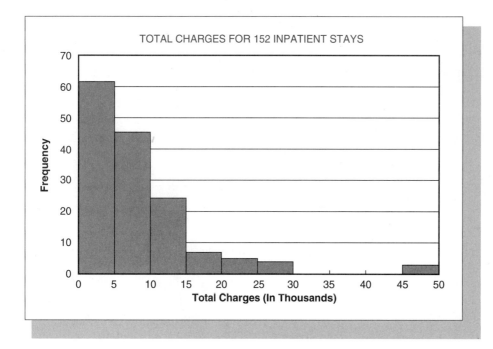

FIGURE 9–5. Histogram. (From Watzlaf VJM, Abdelhak M: Descriptive statistics. J Am Medical Record Assoc 1989;60 (9):37–41. Reprinted with permission from American Health Information Management Association.)

FIGURE 9–6. Frequency polygon/line graph. (From Watzlaf VJM, Abdelhak M: Descriptive statistics. J Am Medical Record Assoc 1989;60 (9):37–41. Reprinted with permission from American Health Information Management Association.)

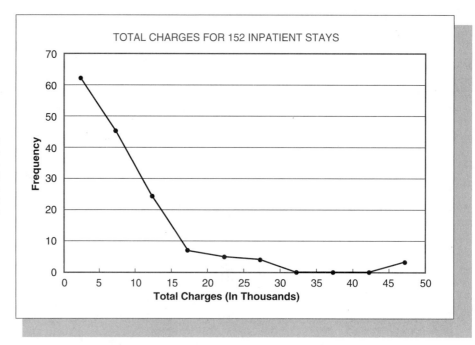

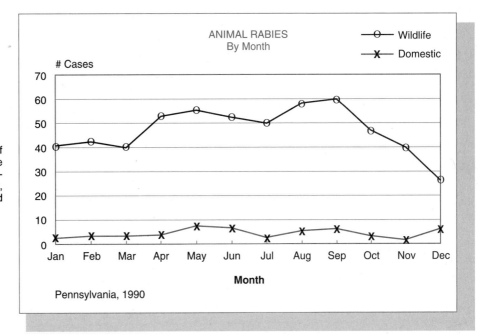

FIGURE 9–7. Frequency polygon comparing two types of data. (From Infectious Disease Epidemiology Report. Pennsylvania Department of Health, Bureau of Epidemiology and Disease Prevention, 1990.)

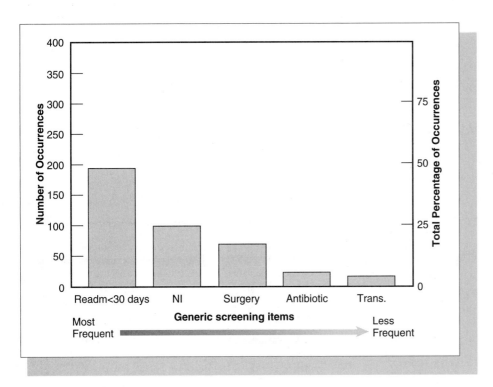

FIGURE 9–8. Pareto diagram.

Weighted Mean

If the average lengths of stay are 6, 4, and 2 days for three departments that have seen 40, 20, and 5 patients, respectively, the weighted average length of stay is as follows:

$$= \frac{(40 \times 6) + (20 \times 4) + (5 \times 2)}{40 + 20 + 5}$$

$$= 330/65$$

$$= 5.1 \text{ days}$$

Median

When the values are ranked, the **median** is the value above which there are the same number of values as below. It is the middlemost value when they are arranged in numerical order. For an odd number of observations, the median is the middle number in the ordered set of numbers; for an even number of observations, it is the mean of the middle two numbers.

The median is the most appropriate statistic to use for describing ordinal or ranked data because it allows for more meaningful descriptions of the data (i.e., the median response was between "strongly agree" and "agree").

EXAMPLE OF MEDIAN (ODD NUMBER)

Data: 1, 8, 6, 4, 2, 5, 9
Data after ordering: 1, 2, 4, 5, 6, 8, 9
Median = 5

EXAMPLE OF MEDIAN (EVEN NUMBER)

Data: 16, 4, 21, 100, 7, 1
Data after ordering: 1, 4, 7, 16, 21, 100 =
(7 + 16)/2
Median = 11.5

Mode

The **mode** is the value that occurs most frequently in a given set of values. Some distributions do not have a mode, whereas others may have two modes (bimodal). The mode is the only measure of central tendency that can be used with nominal data.

EXAMPLE

In Table 9–9, the modal health insurance is Medicare because it is the one that occurs the most.

Measures of Dispersion

Range

When summarizing continuous data in a frequency distribution, it is important to determine the amount of variability of the measurement around the mean or median. The **range** is one way to measure this because it is the difference between the highest and lowest values. Its major disadvantage is that it is concerned only with extreme values and ignores all other values. The following statistics show length of stay for patients with pneumonia.

EXAMPLE

Length of Stay: Patients with Pneumonia

COMMUNITY-ACQUIRED		NOSOCOMIAL	
Medical Record No.	Length of Stay	Medical Record No.	Length of Stay
207658	20	123579	15
214592	10	275816	22
221459	7	254137	18
158645	14	321096	10
129876	8	153992	8
Mean = 11.8		Mean = 14.6	

The range for the length of stay for patients with community-acquired pneumonia was as follows:

20 (highest value) − 7 (lowest value) = 13

The range for the length of stay for patients with nosocomial pneumonia was as follows:

22 (highest value) − 8 (lowest value) = 14

When displaying the range, it is important to show both the high and the low values so that one can see how these values are distributed around the mean.

Variance and Standard Deviation

The variance and standard deviation demonstrate how values are spread around the mean. The **standard deviation** is the most common measure of variation and is represented by the symbol s. The standard deviation (s) is the square root of the variance. The **variance**, or s^2, is computed by squaring each deviation from the mean, summing them, and then dividing their sum by one less than n, the sample size.[1]

EXAMPLE

$$s^2 = \frac{\sum_{i=1}^{n} (x_i - \bar{x})^2}{n - 1}$$

$$s = \sqrt{\frac{\sum_{i=1}^{n} (x_i - \bar{x})^2}{n - 1}}$$

where

x_i = each value in the sample
$\bar{x}$ = sample mean
n = sample size
Σ = sum of
s^2 = sample variance
s = standard deviation

For example, the variance and standard deviation of the pneumonia patient's length of stay is computed as follows:

Community-Acquired Pneumonia Variance

$$s^2 = \frac{(20 - 11.8)^2 + (10 - 11.8)^2 + (7 - 11.8)^2 + (14 - 11.8)^2 + (8 - 11.8)^2}{5 - 1}$$

$$= \frac{67.24 + 3.24 + 23.04 + 4.84 + 14.44}{4}$$

$$= \frac{112.8}{4}$$

$$= 28.2$$

Standard Deviation

$$s = \sqrt{28.2}$$

$$s = 5.3$$

Nosocomial Pneumonia Variance

$$s^2 = \frac{(15 - 14.6)^2 + (22 - 14.6)^2 + (18 - 14.6)^2 + (10 - 14.6)^2 + (8 - 14.6)^2}{5 - 1}$$

$$= \frac{0.16 + 54.76 + 11.56 + 21.16 + 43.56}{4}$$

$$= \frac{131.2}{4}$$

$$= 32.8$$

Standard Deviation

$$s = \sqrt{32.8}$$

$$s = 5.7$$

The greater the deviations of the values from the mean, the greater the variance. Therefore, compare the variance of the length of stay of the patients with community-acquired pneumonia (28.2) and the variance of the length of stay of the patients with nosocomial pneumonia (32.8). This shows that there is greater deviation from the mean of length of stay values in the nosocomial pneumonia group than in the community-acquired pneumonia group.

The standard deviation for length of stay for patients with community-acquired pneumonia was 5.3. This means that on average, observed length of stay values fall 5.3 units from the mean. The standard deviation for the nosocomial pneumonia group was 5.7, which means that on average, observed length of stay values fall 5.7 units from the mean. Therefore, there is greater variation or dispersion in the length of stay for patients with nosocomial pneumonia than in the length of stay for patients with community-acquired pneumonia.

Coefficient of Variation

When two samples or groups have very different means, the direct comparison of their standard deviations could be misleading. Therefore, when two groups have very different means, it is best to compare their standard deviations expressed as percentages of the mean. The **coefficient of variation** (CV) is used to do this.

EXAMPLE

$$CV = \frac{s}{\bar{x}} \times 100$$

Community-Acquired Pneumonia

$$CV = 5.3/11.8 \times 100$$
$$= 45 \text{ per cent}$$

Nosocomial Pneumonia

$$CV = 5.7/14.6 \times 100$$
$$= 39 \text{ per cent}$$

The CV was computed because it was important to determine whether the variation of length of stay valuesin the community-acquired pneumonia group was greater or less than the variation of length of stay values in the nosocomial pneumonia group. By using the CV, the variation can be computed exactly. The CV for the length of stay of the patients with community-acquired pneumonia was 45 per cent, and the CV for the length of stay of the patients with nosocomial pneumonia was 39 per cent. This means that the variation in the length of stay of the patients with community-acquired pneumonia was somewhat greater than that of the patients with nosocomial pneumonia.

Tests of Significance

When a researcher determines that a difference exists between two groups of people relative to a health characteristic, the researcher is interested in determining whether these differences are real or due to sampling variability. **Tests of significance** are performed to determine this. Before statistical tests of significance are determined, the alternative hypothesis and null hypothesis should be expressed. For example, there is a difference between the observed and expected number of deaths for DRG 127, Heart Failure and Shock. This is called the alternative hypothesis. Researchers also express their hypothesis as a null hypothesis. Null means none, and therefore, the null hypothesis is stated as if no differences exist.

Null hypothesis: Observed and expected numbers of deaths are the same for patients with DRG 127, Heart Failure and Shock.

If the observed difference between the actual number of deaths and the expected number of deaths for patients within DRG 127 is small, one should accept the null hypothesis because the difference may just be due to chance or sampling variability. If, however, the difference between the two groups is large, one should reject the null hypothesis because the difference is probably real and not due to chance or sampling variability.

Appropriately chosen tests of significance allow one to determine the *amount* of difference and, when that difference is large enough, to reject the null hypothesis. This statistic is called the *p* value. A *p* value of less than 0.05 is what researchers commonly use to reject the null hypothesis. For example, if the difference seen between the actual and expected number of deaths was $p = 0.001$, the null hypothesis would be rejected because 0.001 is less than 0.05. The value of 0.05 can be changed, depending on how much error the researcher is willing to tolerate. The value of $p = 0.001$ means that the differences in the actual and expected number of deaths are real and that the chances are only 1 in 1000 that the differences seen are due to sampling variability.

Two errors can be made by the researcher when using tests of significance.

Type I error: Reject the null hypothesis when it is true. alpha (α)
Type II error: Accept the null hypothesis when it is false. beta (β)

The maximum probability of making a Type I error that the researcher is able to tolerate is called alpha α and can be chosen by the researcher. A common choice for α is 0.05, but the researcher could choose a lower α of 0.01, 0.001, and so on.

The size of the Type II error is affected by α and the sample size. The larger the sample size, the smaller the sampling variability and the smaller the Type II error, or beta (β). However, the smaller the size of the Type I error, the larger the Type II error; the smaller α is, the larger β is.[6]

The type of significance tests used to determine a *P* value should be referred to a statistician because many different tests are available and tend to be chosen because of the types of variables used, distribution of sample size, and other factors specific to the research design.

To determine if differences between the observed (or actual) and expected number of deaths happen by chance, a statistical test of significance is needed. The statistic used to assess this is called the chi square (χ^2) test.

This statistic is calculated by the following formula:

$$\text{Chi Square} = \Sigma(\text{observed-expected})^2/\text{expected}$$

Referring to Table 9–5, the χ^2 for hospital #4 is as follows:

$$= (8 - 16.56)^2/16.56$$
$$= 73.2736/16.56$$
$$\chi^2 = 4.42$$

The smallest possible value for the χ^2 is 0 and the largest value can approach infinity. Tables developed by statisticians allow us to make probability statements about the χ^2 statistic. Therefore, each χ^2 statistic has a corresponding *p* value. The larger the χ^2 statistic, the smaller the corresponding *p* value. In this example, the χ^2 statistic is large (4.42) and the corresponding *p* value is less than 0.05. This means that for hospital #4, the differences between observed and expected deaths would occur by chance only 5 per cent of the time and that 95 per cent of the time the differences seen are real and not due to sampling variability. Therefore, the plus (+) sign in Table 9–5 is recorded in the statistical rating column to show that fewer deaths occurred in hospital #4 than occurred in hospitals in the comparative databases and that those differences were statistically significant. A minus (−) sign in Table 9–5 in the statistical rating column means that more deaths occurred in hospital #4 than occurred in hospitals in the comparative databases and that those differences were statistically significant. If the statistical rating column is left blank, then the differences seen were not statistically significant.

Sample Size

Because most populations under study are fairly large, researchers choose to study samples of those populations. This is appropriate as long as the **sample size** chosen is a true representative of the population under study. To obtain this, one should apply random sampling. A random sample means that

- every member of the population has the same chance of being included in the sample and
- the selection of one member has no effect on selection of another member—independent selection.[11]

Types of Random Sampling

Simple random sampling can be conducted with a table of random numbers. For example, if the population consists of 50 patient records and you would like to obtain a random sample of 20 of those, you can assign each patient a number or use an existing medical record number. Then refer to a table of random numbers, randomly pick a page to start on, and go up, down, or across, looking at the first two digits. If the first two digits are in the number assigned to the patient record, then that patient record should be included in your sample. Continue this process until your sample of 20 is met.

A stratified random sample is obtained by dividing a population into groups or strata and taking random samples from each strata. For example, to obtain a representative sample to study coding accuracy, medical records of the most common principal diagnoses would be the strata and random samples would be obtained for each common principal diagnosis.

Because both the simple and the stratified random sampling are cumbersome, researchers have chosen another sampling method called systematic sampling. With this method, a sample is obtained by randomly choosing an appropriate interval, such as every 10th record, and then selecting records at equal intervals along the list. This method takes much less time than simple or stratified random sampling and is less subject to error than the other sampling methods.

Determining Sample Size

How do you know how many records or patients or subjects to include in the sample? This question is pon-

dered by people doing continuous quality improvement studies, epidemiologic research studies, or studies of any kind in which a sample is being taken. There is no easy answer to this question. The answer depends on a few things, one of which is the amount of error that is acceptable between the population data and the sample data. The lower the amount of error that is acceptable, the larger the sample size should be.

One method used to estimate sample size includes estimating a population proportion. For example, a health care researcher wants to conduct a survey to determine the proportion of patients who believe that they received quality health care. The population for this facility includes 1000 patients who were discharged within the past year, and interviewing all of them would take an unreasonably long time. Therefore, because no prior information is available to estimate p (or the proportion of patients needed), $p = .5$. Also, the acceptable amount of error is $0.05 = B$. N is the population and n is the sample size. Therefore, the following formula can be used.

$$n = \frac{Npq}{(N-1)D + pq} \; ; \quad \text{where } D = \frac{B^2}{4} = \frac{(.05)^2}{4}$$

$$D = .000625$$

$$\text{where } q = 1 - p$$
$$= 1 - .5$$
$$q = .5$$

$$n = \frac{(1000)(0.5)(0.5)}{(999)(0.000625) + (0.5)(0.5)}$$

$$= \frac{250}{0.874375} = 285.9 \text{ or } 286$$

The total sample needed in which only 5 per cent error would be due to sampling variability is 286. Many other methods are used to estimate the appropriate sample size, depending on the sampling method chosen (simple random, stratified random, systematic). It is highly recommended that sample size selection be researched in more detail by using sampling books. *Elementary Survey Sampling* is an excellent book that clearly describes sample size and methods of selection.[12]

DESIGNING THE RESEARCH STUDY

Several steps should be taken when designing a research study that will make the entire process interesting, rewarding, and fulfilling.[13] These steps include the following:

1. Hypothesis identification
2. Review of literature
3. Draft of methodology

4. Research plan development
   - Specific aims
   - Significance and preliminary research
   - Experimental design and methods
   - Human subjects
   - Literature cited
5. Appendix

Hypothesis

A hypothesis is a tentative assertion that is assumed by the researcher but is not positively known until it is tested.

Suppose a researcher wanted to test whether the medical record would prove to be a useful collection tool for factors suspected of being associated with ovarian cancer. Previous research has found that at least 20 factors may be associated with this disease. However, few studies used the medical record alone to collect data pertaining to these factors. Ovarian cancer is a devastating disease that defies early detection. If a link could be made to one or more specific factors, then preventive measures could be taken by women with the factors to decrease the risk of developing ovarian cancer.

The hypothesis for this example is twofold:

1. The medical record is a useful tool for collecting data pertaining to factors suspected of being associated with ovarian cancer.
2. An association exists between factors suspected of being linked with ovarian cancer.

Review of Literature

Once the hypothesis is established, the second step of a sound research study design is to conduct an extensive literature review. A review must be conducted to determine what research has already been performed in this area. The best way to accomplish this task is to perform a literature search. Most libraries can conduct a literature search by entering key words and phrases into a computer that then searches through journals, books, and other publications. Depending on the type of request, a list will be printed out that includes the title, author's name, and journal title as well as an abstract, if one is available, summarizing the article. How far back in time to search must also be specified.

The key words and phrases that are used can make or break the literature search, so they should be chosen with care. If there is uncertainty about which key words to choose, the wording should be discussed with the reference librarian. For example, the key words chosen for the ovarian cancer study included *epithelial ovarian cancer, risk factors, epidemiology,* and *medical record.*

Once the literature search is concluded, it must be carefully examined and any articles of interest should be collected and reviewed. There are several reasons for conducting this review.

- To study any topic, one must develop a solid foundation in that field.
- To become an expert, one must review past literature to determine how one's hypothesis is different from previous research studies.
- To determine what it is about one's idea or hypothesis that makes it worth doing.
- To find gaps or problems with existing studies and begin thinking about how to design a study to fill those gaps.

Methodology (Draft)

At this point, the researcher should begin to think about how to design the study so that the hypothesis can be properly tested. The methodology can be the most difficult task and, therefore, should be started as soon as possible. The methodology should include a step-by-step process of what is done in the research study and why this process is necessary to properly test the hypothesis. A rough draft of the methodology should be developed to determine if the study is feasible. It also allows one to realize how much is known about the subject matter and to think about what the research involves.

Research Plan

Once a draft of the methodology is written and the feasibility of the study is confirmed, the research plan should be written. It includes the following:

- Specific aims or objectives
- Significance or preliminary research and experimental design and methods
- Human subjects
- Literature cited

Specific Aims

The specific aims should briefly describe the project's goals or objectives. The goals, objectives, aims, or purposes should be enumerated for better clarification. The list should include both short- and long-term goals. For example, the specific aims in the ovarian cancer study are as follows:

- Determine whether the medical record is a useful tool for collecting data pertaining to risk factors and other health history information. (Short-term goal)

- Narrow the number of factors suspected of being linked to ovarian cancer by providing evidence that a potential risk factor is found more in the cases (women with the disease) than in the controls (women without the disease). (Short-term goal)

- Identify groups of women who may be at high risk for developing ovarian cancer and work toward designing and implementing preventive measures to control the disease. (Long-term goal)

- Benefit future studies that examine chromosomal markers and ovarian cancer so that they begin to incorporate risk factors in the analysis of their data. (Long-term goal)

Significance and Preliminary Research

This section should detail the importance of the research project. It should state why it must be done, how it is different from previous research studies, and who the research will benefit. This section should also demonstrate the researcher's knowledge by discussing existing research that has been performed in the same area and showing the gaps in that research. Once these deficiencies are discussed in detail, this part of the plan should reveal how the current research will address those deficiencies.

The key to this section is to be succinct, clear, and organized to convey why the research is important. If the preliminary research is brief, it can be included in the significance section, particularly if it adds to the study's importance. If the preliminary research is extensive, it should be included in a separate section titled "Preliminary Studies" or "Preliminary Research."

An excerpt of the significance section follows to demonstrate how the preliminary research is used to show the importance of the proposed study.

A research study has been performed through a small grant from the School of Health Related Professions' Research and Development Fund in which risk factors for ovarian cancer cases and 40 randomly selected age-related controls were evaluated. Interpretation of the data has been limited because 30 per cent of the risk factors were not found in the medical record for the cases or controls. These results may be due to the small sample size and collection of data from only one hospital.

The proposed project will be able to effectively analyze the large number of risk factors suspected of being linked to ovarian cancer by evaluating the disease at an earlier stage and by incorporating an improved method

of epidemiologic assessment. By examining the risk factors in incident cases and age-matched controls from the medical record and telephone interview, we will be able to collect the risk factors cited immediately after diagnosis and follow-up with a telephone interview to collect any risk factors not collected from the medical record. This proposed project will enable us to remedy inadequacies with the past study and, therefore, determine a risk factor truly linked to the development of epithelial ovarian cancer. This identified risk factor will lead to the identification of women at high risk for developing ovarian cancer. Future prospective studies can be designed to follow women with the risk factor and women without it to determine if they develop ovarian cancer.

Methodology

The methodology should include a design in relation to time, place, and persons. It should consist of the following:

- *Population under study.* This section reveals which subjects will be in the study, how they will become part of the study, why these specific subjects will be part of the study, whether a subset of the population will be used and why, and how the size of the subset will be determined.

- *Time frame.* This should state exactly when the study will be conducted as well as why it is necessary to conduct the study for this specific time period.

- *Place of study.* This section should explain where the study will be conducted and if it will include one facility or multi-facilities and why.

The methodology should also include a step-by-step plan of how the study will be performed. This is called the "Procedures" and can include the following:

- *Data collection process.* This section should reveal how the data will be collected (by questionnaire, interview, abstracting techniques); what data will be categorized and why; how the data will be categorized and why; who will collect the data; whether training techniques will be needed and, if so, what the training will consist of; where the data will be stored; whether the data will include patient identifiers and why; and how the data will be accessed. A separate paragraph or statement regarding how the confidentiality of the subjects will be protected should be included.

- *Application to the institutional review board (IRB).* The methodology section should state that the study will be submitted for approval to an IRB. The IRB, or research and human rights committee, commonly is part of most health care facilities and meets at least quarterly. Some boards may meet more often, depending on the number of applications they receive. The aim of any IRB is to protect human subjects or patients from research risks and invasion of privacy. The IRB reviews all research studies that involve subjects or patients, including experiments, interviews, and questionnaires, as well as any study that collects data from a patient's medical record. The scientific merits of a proposal are considered in the context of assessing the risks and benefits of the proposed research.

- *Analysis of the data.* This section should describe how the data will be analyzed and the types of statistical tests that will be performed (e.g., frequency distribution, χ^2, confidence intervals, assessment of validity and reliability, to be addressed later in this chapter). One must be sure to describe why this analysis will be used. An excerpt from an actual methodology section is quoted below.

The hospital will contact our research team whenever an ovarian cancer patient is admitted. Our research team will match the case with the control and after discharge will abstract data from the medical record. The abstractors will be trained so that each one is certain about where to find specific information in the record when a risk factor or characteristic is not applicable, not documented, or not present in the case or control.

Once the data is collected, a telephone interview will be performed to collect any data not found in the medical record and to assess the validity of the data in the medical record. The data will be entered into a personal computer, and statistical analysis will include frequency distribution, χ^2, and odds ratios. Because the examination of risk factors from medical records may vary from one abstractor to another, various members of the research team will repeat the abstracting of another member and levels of agreement will be determined.

Human Subjects

This section is necessary only if human subjects are used in the research or if there are any risks to a human subject. The following should be included in this section:

- Demographic description of the subject population, including age, percentage of males and/or females, race
- How an informed consent will be obtained
- If necessary, how confidentiality will be safeguarded
- Potential benefits of the study to the people enrolled

Any letters validating IRB approval should be placed in this section to show that the facility in which the research will be conducted has approved the study methodology.

Literature Cited

All literature discussed or reviewed in any section of the research proposal should be numbered or footnoted in that section and listed at the end of the proposal.

Appendix

The appendix can comprise tables, figures, laboratory tests, data collection forms, and letters of support. It can include anything that is important and relative to the research study or that better clarifies a topic described in the study. Information that is not pertinent to the research project should be excluded.

RESEARCH STUDY DESIGNS

Another important step in designing a research study is the ability to choose the most appropriate study design to test your hypothesis. The HIM professional can appropriately choose the study design to use if he or she is aware of the many designs that exist. Because epidemiology relates so closely to the field of health information management, the study designs described in this chapter include epidemiologic research study designs. Epidemiology is the study of the distribution and determinants of disease and/or events in populations. It also includes using the results of the study to prevent and control public health problems. The most common types of study designs are described in detail below and summarized in Table 9–13. Examples of each design are provided, and common statistics that are generated from these studies are described.

Descriptive Study

The descriptive epidemiologic study describes the frequency and distribution of diseases in populations. It usually is the first study design chosen when little is known about the disease or health characteristics.

Cross-Sectional or Prevalence Study

The **cross-sectional or prevalence study** is one example of the descriptive study; it concurrently describes characteristics and health outcomes at one specific point or period in time. The cross-sectional or prevalence study cannot answer questions regarding cause and ef-

TABLE 9–13 TYPES OF EPIDEMIOLOGIC RESEARCH STUDY DESIGNS

STUDY DESIGN	DESCRIPTION
Descriptive studies—Cross-sectional or prevalence study	Examines the distribution of disease or health characteristics in populations at one point in time. Used to generate hypotheses.
Analytic studies Case-control or retrospective Cohort or prospective Historical-prospective	Examines a disease to determine if certain health characteristics are causing the disease.
Experimental studies Clinical trials Community trials	Modifies the health characteristics that are found to cause the disease by using health care interventions that control the disease from progressing or prevent the disease from occurring.

Prevalence rates can facilitate casefinding, assist health care administrators in planning for diversified health care facilities and special care units, aid health planners in developing appropriate health programs, and assist HIM professionals in further describing morbidity rates within the health care facility.

Prevalence rates can be categorized into two types: point prevalence rates and period prevalence rates. Point prevalence refers to evaluating a health condition at a specific point in time. Therefore, each study participant is assessed only *once* at *one point* in time, even though the actual point prevalence study may take months or years to conduct. Period prevalence refers to evaluating a health condition over a *period of time,* such as 1 year. Study participants are counted for period prevalence even if they die, migrate, or recur during the period.[6] Figure 9–9 demonstrates the difference between point and period prevalence when examining specific cases within a study.

fect or whether the health characteristic came before the disease. This study design is used to *generate* hypotheses, not to test them. For example, a health care facility may be interested in preventing community-acquired pneumonia in elderly people because it is debilitating and increases the cost and length of stay if an elderly person is hospitalized for another condition, thereby affecting both the quality and the cost of health care. The cross-sectional or prevalence study can be used to determine the prevalence of pneumonia in this region within the elderly population. To do this, the condition under study (i.e., pneumonia) needs to be defined. Specific criteria related to the type of pneumonia are needed as well as any other criteria necessary to further define the condition. Then the prevalence rate is determined. For this example, it would be as follows:

$$\text{Prevalence rate} = \frac{\text{Number of people age 65 or over with pneumonia in a specific region during 1994}}{\text{Number of people age 65 or over in a specific region during 1994}} \times (1000)$$

Once the prevalence rates are determined, they can be compared across certain groups. For example, further defined prevalence rates for pneumonia may be calculated for people under age 65 and a comparison of the two groups can be made. One cannot determine from this study design that being elderly (age 65 or over) causes an increase in pneumonia. However, one can make statements of associations; that is, older age may have an affect on the development of community-acquired pneumonia. One can then develop a hypothesis and suggest areas for further research.

ADVANTAGES AND DISADVANTAGES. Table 9–14 summarizes the advantages and disadvantages of the cross-sectional or prevalence study design. It is a useful study design when time and resources are limited. It is also appropriate to perform the cross-sectional study when little is known about the health characteristics and/or disease under study. This study can provide new or beginning information on a multitude of conditions with modest effort and time. Once this new information is analyzed, it can stimulate the researcher and enable the researcher to begin to develop hypotheses that would motivate further testing and the use of more extensive study designs. Because the cross-sectional or prevalence study may be considered a descriptive study, its intent is not to show cause and effect relations between, for example, a characteristic such as alcohol intake and a disease such as breast cancer. Analytic and experimental study designs, which are discussed later in this chapter, can assess the cause and effect relation. Unlike the analytic and experimental study designs, the cross-sectional design cannot assess the risk or likelihood of developing a disease. Other limitations of the cross-sectional design include dealing only with survivors, not being effective in studying rare conditions because a large sample is necessary to obtain cases, or missing an epidemic because it may occur and leave within a short period.[6]

By becoming familiar with the cross-sectional or prevalence study design, the HIM professional can better assess how prevalence rates are determined, determine if this study design is the most appropriate one to perform, and evaluate whether cross-sectional studies performed within the health care facility have formed appropriate conclusions (i.e., not cause and effect relations).

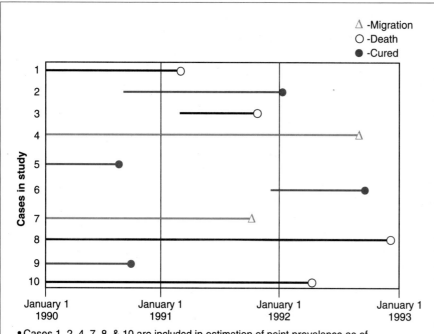

FIGURE 9–9. Chronology of cases in a community to measure prevalence.

- Cases 1, 2, 4, 7, 8, & 10 are included in estimation of point prevalence as of January 1, 1991.
- Cases 1, 2, 3, 4, 6, 7, 8, & 10 are included in estimation of period prevalence which extends from January 1, 1991–December 31, 1991.

TABLE 9–14 ADVANTAGES AND DISADVANTAGES OF CROSS-SECTIONAL OR PREVALENCE STUDY DESIGN	
ADVANTAGES	**DISADVANTAGES**
Takes less time than other studies before results are seen	Only describes what exists at the time of the prevalence study; does not answer whether the health characteristic or the disease came first
Inexpensive	Only examines survivors and those alive to be found as cases
Helpful in casefinding, program planning, planning of health care facilities or special units, and sample size determination	Not good for rare conditions or diseases
Stimulates new ideas or hypotheses	Given a health characteristic, fails to identify future likelihood of developing the disease

Analytic Study Design

Case-Control or Retrospective Study Design

In an analytic study, a disease or health condition is examined to determine possible causes. Intensive research related to the disease is necessary to determine characteristics that may cause the specific disease. These characteristics are also referred to as exposure characteristics and/or risk factors because they may increase your risk of developing the disease. The **case-control** or **retrospective study** is one type of analytic study design. It collects data on the cases (those people who have the disease that is under study) and controls (those people who are similar to the cases but do not have the disease that is under study) by looking back in time. For example, in the ovarian cancer study described earlier in this chapter, the cases included patients with epithelial ovarian cancer and the controls included patients with other diagnoses who were admitted to the same hospital during the same time period as the cases. The cases and controls also were similar in age. Specific characteristics (possible risk factors) were collected for both groups by going back and retrieving the data from medical records and through personal interviews.

When conducting a case-control or retrospective study, the following design issues must be considered:

- Randomly select cases by using incidence or prevalence rates, and obtain information on their past history of exposures. Specify criteria for the cases (i.e., epithelial ovarian cancer, ICD-9-CM code of 183.0, pathology reports, and slides indicating that the case truly is a case and does have the disease under study).

- Randomly select controls similar to the cases in characteristics such as age and sex but without the disease, and obtain a past history of their exposures. Select controls from populations such as hospitals and other health care facilities as well as residents of a community and neighbors, friends, or siblings of the cases. Cases and controls should come from similar populations to demonstrate that those who developed the disease under study are similar to other people in the community except for the disease of interest. For example, if the cases are hospital patients, controls should also be hospital patients but with a different disease or illness than the one under study.

- Determine if matching will be used. Some studies match on variables such as age and sex because these variables affect both the independent (risk factor) and the dependent variables (disease). When variables affect the dependent and independent variables, they are referred to as confounding variables. In the ovarian cancer study, cases and controls were matched on age within 5 years because age is related to several of the risk factors, such as use of birth control pills and nulliparity, and incidence of ovarian cancer.

- Design the research instrument. To collect your data, the research instrument should be developed. It can include the following:
  —Interviewer-administered questionnaire (in person or by phone)
  —Self-administered questionnaire
  —Abstract to record information from medical records
  —New forms for recording data from slides, laboratory tests, physical examinations, and so on

  List all variables you want to measure. Check and see if the instrument can collect the vari-

ables through pilot testing. Data sources should provide information of comparable detail for cases and controls. Precode the data before data collection begins by coding each variable on the data collection form with a number. When the data is entered into the computer for analysis, each variable will be recognized. Close-ended questions are preferred because they are easier to code. Improve the subject's recall with pictures and lists. An example of some sections of the research instrument used in the ovarian cancer study is presented in the Sample of Ovarian Cancer Questionnaire.

EXAMPLE

Figure 9–10 is a hypothetical example of how subjects are selected from a health care population into a case-control study. In this example, the independent variable (risk factor) is alcohol use and the dependent variable (disease) is breast cancer. The cases are those subjects with breast cancer separated into alcohol users and nonusers. The controls are those subjects with other diseases, such as heart disease, separated into alcohol users and nonusers. In most research studies, a larger number of controls than cases are chosen to better determine differences between the cases and controls.

DETERMINING THE ODDS RATIO. The **odds ratio** is an estimate of the relative risk a person has if he or she is exposed to a certain characteristic. One should only use the odds ratio with case-control studies, when the disease is rare, and when cases are true representatives of all cases and controls are true representatives of all controls.[6]

EXAMPLE

	Breast Cancer	Control	Total
Alcohol	75 (a)	100 (b)	175 (a + b)
None	25 (c)	300 (d)	325 (c + d)
	100 (a + c)	400 (b + d)	500 (a + b + c + d)

a = Subjects with the independent variable (alcohol) who developed the disease (breast cancer)
b = Subjects with the independent variable (alcohol) who did not develop the disease (breast cancer)
c = Subjects without the independent variable (alcohol) who developed the disease (breast cancer)
d = Subjects without the independent variable (alcohol) who did not develop the disease (breast cancer)

Sample of Ovarian Cancer Questionnaire (Abstracted from 119 Total Elements)

1. Do you know of any blood relatives in your family who have or have had any type of cancer?

_____ Yes   _____ No   _____ ND*

If yes, what relation?

_____ Mother	_____ Sister
_____ Father	_____ Brother
_____ Aunt	_____ Grandfather
_____ Uncle	_____ Grandmother
_____ Niece	_____ Nephew

Other: _____

_____ ND*   _____ NA*

If yes, what type:

_____ Lung	_____ Liver	_____ Lymphomas
_____ Brain	_____ Breast	_____ Colon
_____ Skin	_____ Pancreas	_____ Blood-related (leukemia)

_____ Other: _____

_____ ND*   _____ NA*

2. Do you smoke cigarettes? _____ Yes   _____ No   _____ ND*

If yes, how many cigarettes do you smoke each day?

_____ 1/2 pack or less	_____ 1 pack
_____ 1 to 2 packs	_____ More than 2 packs
_____ ND*	_____ NA*

*ND = Not documented
*NA = Not applicable

If a disease is rare, then a/(a + b) is about equal to a/b because a will be small relative to b. Also, c/(c + d) is about equal to c/d. Therefore, by assuming that a + b is about equal to b and c + d is about equal to d, the formula for the odds ratio is as follows:

$$(a/b)/(c/d) \text{ or } ad/bc$$

Therefore, in the hypothetical case shown above, ad/bc = (75)(300)/(100)(25) = 22,500/2500 = 9. This means that a person who drinks alcohol is nine times more likely to get breast cancer than a person who does not drink alcohol. Further refinement of this odds ratio could include defining alcohol levels to the actual amount a person drinks. Then 2 × 2 tables (such as the table used in the example above) could be constructed to examine levels of alcohol intake and odds ratios could be developed and compared. Other confounders for the development of breast cancer, such as age, are not addressed here. More advanced statistical analysis beyond the scope of this chapter would be necessary to examine the risk of alcohol intake and breast cancer while controlling for confounding variables.

ADVANTAGES AND DISADVANTAGES. Table 9–15 summarizes the advantages and disadvantages of the case-control study design. Like the cross-sectional or prevalence study design, it is useful when time and

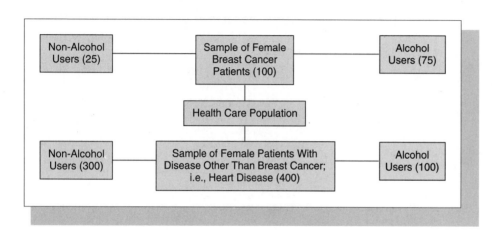

FIGURE 9–10. Example of a case-control study population.

TABLE 9-15 ADVANTAGES AND DISADVANTAGES OF THE CASE-CONTROL DESIGN

ADVANTAGES	DISADVANTAGES
Well suited for rare diseases or those with a long latency period, such as cancer and heart disease	Relies on recall or records for information of past exposures of certain factors; accuracy may be difficult to obtain
Takes less time before results are seen than the prospective or cohort study but more time than the cross-sectional or prevalence study	Validation of information collected difficult to obtain
Inexpensive	Occurrence of exposure obtained from *selected* cases and controls
Requires comparatively few subjects	Selection of an appropriate control group may be difficult
Uses existing records	Rates of disease in the exposed and unexposed subjects cannot be determined because the subjects are not being followed over time
Minimal risk to subjects	Probability of bias may be greater than the cohort study
Allows a study of multiple potential causes of disease	
Supports causal hypothesis by establishing an association but does not prove it	

resources are limited. The intent of the researcher is to establish some association between the disease and the exposure characteristic. This study design does have drawbacks because it relies on recall or past information from the subjects, making validation of that information somewhat difficult. Also, it is difficult to obtain an appropriate control group and the true relative risk cannot be determined, only estimated. However, when one wants to quickly and inexpensively determine if an association exists between a health condition and a characteristic, the case-control method is an appropriate route to take.[6]

Research using the case-control study design can be done as part of the role of the HIM professional when directing a cancer registry and when performing departmental and hospital-wide quality assessment and improvement studies. Also, performing and aiding other researchers in carrying out this study design is an important role of the HIM professional.

Prospective, Cohort, or Incidence Study Design

The **prospective study** design can do something that neither the cross-sectional nor the case-control method can do. It determines whether the characteristic or suspected risk factor truly preceded the disease or health condition. The prospective study design is the best method to determine the magnitude of risk in the population with the characteristic or suspected risk factor. A prospective study typically includes the following steps:

1. Identify subjects with the characteristic under study who are free from the disease.
2. Identify subjects without the characteristic under study who are free from the disease. These subjects are considered the comparison group.
3. Follow both groups forward in time to determine if and when they develop the disease or health condition under study.

The initial assessment to determine who should be included in the prospective study is the same as that for a cross-sectional or prevalence study because it must identify cases and noncases and determine whether they have the characteristic under study. However, once the subjects within the prospective study begin to develop the disease under study, incident cases or new cases are being collected. Those who participate in the prospective study are usually volunteers. They are examined to make sure they do not have the disease at the beginning of the study. To do this, the researcher collects data related to their occupation, medical history, and social status. Physical examinations and laboratory tests may also be needed to ensure that the subjects do not have the disease.

Some prospective or cohort studies begin in a community or an industrial setting or within a hospital. The subjects are separated into two groups based on their exposures or health characteristic and then are followed forward to determine if they develop the disease. A hypothetical example would be subjects who are asked to participate in a prospective study to determine if any time after delivery they experience postpartum depression. The hypothesis for this study is that women who deliver babies who spend some time in the neonatal intensive care unit may have a higher incidence of postpartum depression than women who deliver babies who do not spend time in the neonatal intensive care unit. Data on prenatal care, history of depression, family history of depression, and family life after delivery of the baby are collected from both groups. The women in both groups are then followed forward in time to see if postpartum depression develops.

Another common example is to compare a group of people in the community who experience certain social habits, such as exercise, with a group of sedentary people. In this example, both groups receive physical examinations and laboratory tests to be certain that they are not hypertensive. Interviews to collect data on family and personal histories are also conducted. Both groups are then followed forward in time to determine if they become hypertensive. The hypothesis for this study is that people who exercise have a decreased incidence of hypertension when compared with those who do not exercise. Data on specific types, amounts, and levels of exercise also need to be collected and analyzed.

To determine whether one group does have an increased risk of developing a disease as a result of health habits or characteristics, incidence rates must be determined. As stated previously, an incidence rate (IR) is as follows:

$$\frac{\text{Number of new cases over a time period}}{\substack{\text{Population at risk (those free of disease} \\ \text{at start of study)}}} \times 1000$$

For the examples given above, the IRs would be as follows:

$$\frac{\substack{\text{Number of new postpartum depression cases} \\ \text{during a time period in hospital}}}{\substack{\text{Women who delivered babies in} \\ \text{hospital during a given time period}}} \times 1000$$

$$\frac{\substack{\text{Number of new cases of hypertension during} \\ \text{a time period in a specific community}}}{\substack{\text{Population (both sedentary and} \\ \text{those who exercise) in the specific} \\ \text{community during a given time period}}} \times 1000$$

To determine which groups have a greater risk of developing the disease under study, the **relative risk (RR)** is determined using the following formula:

$$RR = \frac{\text{Incidence rate exposed } (IR_e)}{\text{Incidence rate unexposed } (IR_o)}$$

Using the data displayed in Table 9–16, one can calculate the RR. The IR of the group who does not exercise is 145 and the IR of the group who does exercise is 50. The RR for this study is 145/50 = 2.9.

TABLE 9–16 DETERMINING THE RELATIVE RISK: INCIDENCE RATES PER 1000 OF HYPERTENSION BY LEVELS OF EXERCISE

	POPULATION	CASES	INCIDENCE RATE
Exercise	1000	50	50
No exercise	1000	145	145
Total	2000	195	97.5

TABLE 9–17 ADVANTAGES AND DISADVANTAGES OF PROSPECTIVE, COHORT, OR INCIDENCE STUDY

ADVANTAGES	DISADVANTAGES
Describes what came first—the characteristic or the disease	Not good with rare diseases because it takes so long to follow them
Relative risk is determined, not estimated	Subjects are lost during follow-up due to death, withdrawal, migration
Analytically tests the hypothesis of cause and effect	Long time to see results
Decreases the amount of bias caused by recall or memory	Expensive
	Subjects tend to participate less because of the amount of time they must spend in the study
	Unexpected changes in environment or social habits may influence the health outcome

Therefore, the people who do not exercise are about three times more likely to develop hypertension than the people who do exercise.

Even though there are more disadvantages than advantages to using the prospective study (Table 9–17), a major benefit of this design is that it accurately determines whether the characteristic was present before the disease developed.[6] Because the IRs and RRs can be calculated, the researcher can determine the number of cases that can be prevented if a specific characteristic or exposure is controlled. This is a major advantage over the study designs discussed earlier.

Historical-Prospective Study Design

In the historical-prospective study design, past records are used to collect information regarding the characteristic or exposure under study. Then, over the next 10, 15, or 20 years, medical records, death certificates, and so on are monitored to determine the number of cases of a particular disease that have developed. The time of the actual study and the end of the follow-up period will happen sometime in the future. IRs and RRs are then calculated for the exposed and unexposed groups.

In Figure 9–11, both the obese and the nonobese cohorts were identified sometime in the past (1977 through 1985) by way of medical records and cancer registry data. The study required all subjects to be free of a breast cancer *recurrence* from 1977 to 1985. The

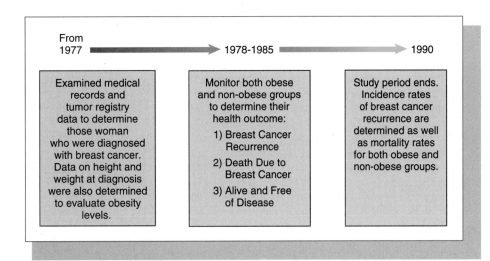

FIGURE 9–11. Historical-prospective study design.

groups were stratified based on their body mass index levels. They were followed forward in time to determine their rates of breast cancer recurrence and mortality due to the breast cancer.

ADVANTAGES AND DISADVANTAGES. The major advantages of this study design compared with the prospective study design are that less time and effort are expended and the cost is lower. All other advantages and disadvantages listed in Table 9–17 for the prospective design hold true for the historical-prospective design, except that the RR is really an estimate of risk similar to an odds ratio.

Experimental Epidemiology

Clinical and Community Trials

There are two types of studies referred to in experimental epidemiology. They are the clinical trial and the community trial.

The **clinical trial** and **community trial** are similar to the prospective study in that they comprise two groups that have different exposures and that are followed forward to determine their outcomes. It is an experiment to try a certain medication or treatment on a group and compare their outcomes with those of a control or comparison group (subjects who do not have the intervention). In the clinical or community trial, the researcher provides the "exposure" in a controlled environment by providing some intervention procedure (i.e., medicine, education, surgical procedure). The researcher decides what the intervention will be as well as which subjects will receive it and which will not.

Before beginning the trial, the researcher must obtain an informed consent from subjects and IRB approval to conduct the study and select the methods that will be used to randomize subjects into specific groups.

The researcher must also consider the following when conducting a clinical or community trial:

- How will adverse reactions and other complications be recorded and addressed?

- What criteria will be used to exclude and include subjects?

- Will the study be single blind (subject blind to which group he is in) double blind (subject and observer blind), or triple blind (subject, observer, and statistician blind)?

- Ethical considerations: If the treatment group responds favorably to treatment, should the study be stopped and the treatment offered to both groups?

The difference between a clinical trial and a community trial is that the clinical trial usually begins in a clinical setting and the intervention medication, treatment, or procedure is tested on selected subjects. In a community trial, the intervention medication, treatment, or procedure is tested on a group of subjects as a whole.[5]

Life Table Analysis

Life table analysis is most appropriate for prospective studies or experimental studies when the researcher experiences losses of subjects as a result of follow-up or the study ends before recurrence or death has occurred in some subjects. Life table analysis examines survival times of individual subjects. Survival time includes the time subjects are free of disease after diagnosis or the time to recovery or improvement after the start of a specific intervention medication, treatment, or procedure. Subjects tend to enter a study sample at different times as they enter for treatment. Each subject is followed until death, and during that time, a subject may be lost to follow-up because the researcher may not be able to locate the subject and, therefore, will not be able to determine if death has occurred. Also, some subjects may withdraw from the study because they do not want to participate in it or because it has ended. When a survival time is censored, this means that the subject is alive at the time of analysis or was alive when last seen. Survival times are flagged with a + to indicate that they are censored.[14]

Life table analysis operates on the premise called person-time denominator. This is a special denominator that must be used in calculating rates for small study groups when subjects in the study are not all observed for the entire length of the study period because of withdrawal, death, or loss to follow-up.

Assumptions for use of the life table analysis are as follows:

• The risk of the outcome event (death) should not be different if a patient enters the study during the 1st year of the study versus the 2nd or 3rd year.

• The rate of the outcome event should not be

higher at the end of 2 years of observation than at the end of 1 year.

• The rate of the outcome event is as similar among subjects lost to follow-up as among subjects who remain under observation.

One type of life table analysis is the Kaplan-Meier Product Limit Method, which is appropriate for both small and large sample sizes. The result of the Kaplan-Meier Product Limit Method is a survival curve.

The following is a hypothetical example of subjects in a clinical trial and how the Kaplan-Meier Product Limit Method is calculated.

EXAMPLES

SUBJECT NUMBER	SURVIVAL TIME (MONTHS)
1	47
2	40+
3	37
4	34
5	48+
6	41
7	41
8	45
9	23
10	43

+, censored observations, withdrawn alive or lost to follow-up.

(1)	(2)	(3)	(4)	(5)
23	1	1	9/10 = .90	.900
34	2	2	8/9 = .889	.800
37	3	3	7/8 = .875	.700
40+	4	—	—	
41	5	5	5/6 = .833	.583
41	6	6	4/5 = .80	.466
43	7	7	3/4 = .75	.350
45	8	8	2/3 = .667	.233
47	9	9	1/2 = .50	.117
48+	10	—	—	

(1) Survival time (t_i) months; (2) rank; (3) uncensored ranks (r_i); (4) proportion surviving $(n - r)/[(n - r) + 1]$; (5) cumulative proportion surviving s(t).

Column 1 lists all survival times, both censored and uncensored, in order from smallest to largest. (Uncensored observations are listed first if censored and uncensored observations have the same survival times.)

Column 2 lists the rank of each observation shown in column 1.

Column 3 lists the rank of uncensored observations only, where $t_{(r)} \geq t$.

Column 4 shows the estimated proportion of subjects in the sample who survive longer than t. To calculate the proportion of subject surviving through each time interval, n = sample size (10) and r = the

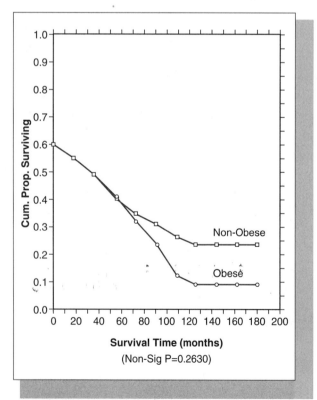

FIGURE 9–12. Kaplan-Meier estimation of survival.

uncensored rank; compute (n − r)/(n − r) + 1. Therefore, 9/10 = .90 means that 90 per cent of the subjects in the sample have survived longer than 23 months.

In *column 5*, all values in column 4 up to and including t are multiplied for each survival time. For example, 9/10 = .900; 9/10 × 8/9 = .800; 9/10 × 8/9 × 7/8 = .700, and so on.[15]

An example of the Kaplan-Meier curve for obesity and breast cancer survival is shown in Figure 9–12. This figure shows that about 80 per cent of both groups survived about 58 months, or 4.8 years. At about 110 months, or 9.2 years, about 68 per cent of the nonobese group had survived, whereas only 54 per cent of the obese group had survived.

VALIDITY AND RELIABILITY

Validity

Validity assesses relevance, completeness, accuracy, and correctness. It measures how well a data collection instrument, laboratory test, medical record abstract, or other data source measures what it should measure.

It is critical that the HIM professional be made aware of validity problems within specific types of studies. The data collection instrument and the method of data collection have a great impact on the validity of data. To determine whether the validity of a research study is upheld, specific methods should be used. One such method includes gaining confirmatory information from different sources to determine whether the information collected for the study is correct. For example, information recorded in the medical record regarding the patient's method of payment or insurance carrier can be validated by further examining financial records, physicians' office records, and pharmacy records. Brief interviews with family members can further confirm or validate the accuracy of correctness of the insurance type.

Sensitivity and Specificity

Validity also refers to correct measurement or correct labeling. Assessments of methods used to test whether or not a person has a disease are considered tests of validity regarding the correctness of measurement or labeling. One type of test to measure this is called **sensitivity and specificity.** To use sensitivity and specificity, one must know the following definitions:

True positives (TP) correctly categorize true cases as cases—valid labeling.
False negatives (FN) incorrectly label true cases as noncases—not valid.
True negatives (TN) correctly label noncases as noncases—valid.

False positives (FP) incorrectly label noncases as cases —not valid.
Sensitivity is the percentage of all true cases correctly identified—TP/TP + FN or TP/total positives (or total cases).
Specificity is the percentage of all true noncases correctly identified—TN/TN + FP or TN/total negatives (or total non-cases).[5,6]

Table 9–18 shows the accuracy of a specific blood test in detecting prostate cancer. The specificity rate of 91 per cent suggests that this blood test correctly labels noncases as noncases 91 per cent of the time and misses the noncases 9 per cent of the time. The sensitivity rate of only 83 per cent suggests that the blood test misses 17 per cent of the true cases, or those patients with prostate cancer. This blood test could pose serious health problems when true cases may be missed, and therefore, diagnosis and treatment may be delayed or missed. Each researcher must determine when the sensitivity and specificity levels are accurate enough to actually use the test.

It is difficult to assess the validity of a principal diagnosis, ICD-9-CM code, or DRG because the basis of the categorization may be subjective. However, the accuracy or validity of coding can be made once a "gold" standard is determined. The correct diagnosis, code, or DRG can be determined based on coding standards as well as agreement by expert coders. For example, the validity of coding quality can be determined by having the coding supervisor recode a random sample of records of patients with a principal diagnostic code of coronary artery disease (CAD). The coding was done by two coders— coder A and coder B. The recoding performed by the coding supervisor can be considered the "gold" standard. The validity (sensitivity and specificity) could then be recorded as shown below:

| | | CODING SUPERVISOR | | |
		True Case CAD	True Noncase No CAD	TOTAL
Coding status by coder A	CAD	9 (TP)	4 (FP)	13
	Not CAD	6 (FN)	11 (TN)	17
	Total	15	15	30
Coding status by coder B	CAD	15 (TP)	3 (FP)	27
	Not CAD	0 (FN)	12 (TN)	3
	Total	15	15	30

		CODER A	CODER B
Sensitivity =	$\frac{\text{True positives}}{\text{All true cases}}$	$\frac{9}{15}$ = 60%	$\frac{15}{15}$ = 100%
Specificity =	$\frac{\text{True negatives}}{\text{All noncases}}$	$\frac{11}{15}$ = 73.3%	$\frac{12}{15}$ = 80%

TABLE 9–18 SENSITIVITY AND SPECIFICITY. ACCURACY OF BLOOD TEST TO DETECT PROSTATE CANCER

TEST	PROSTATE CANCER	NO PROSTATE CANCER
+	TP (100)	FP (20)
−	FN (20)	TN (200)
Totals	TP + FN (120)	FP + TN (220)

Sensitivity = TP/TP + FN = 100/100 + 20 = 100/120 = 83.3%
Specificity = TN/TN + FP = 200/200 + 20 = 200/220 = 90.9%

Coder B is better than coder A in accurately coding true cases of CAD (100 per cent versus 60 per cent) and in accurately coding noncases as noncases (80 per cent versus 73 per cent).

There are specific factors that cause incorrect or inaccurate labeling. In the coding example, these factors can include inexperience and lack of knowledge regarding the disease (CAD), ICD-9-CM coding principles, and proper review and analysis of the medical record. Other factors may relate to the equipment, such as outdated coding books. Also, it is obvious that validity is influenced by the "gold" standard that is selected. When assessing results of such studies, it is important to consider the subjectivity of the standard.

Reliability

In many research studies, the data are collected by more than one research assistant. For example, in the ovarian cancer study, an abstract was used to collect the information from the medical records for both cases and controls. Because different research assistants were used to abstract the medical records to collect the data, the classification of the results might differ from one assistant to another. Reproducibility or **reliability** between more than one research assistant or observer is called interobserver reliability. However, even one individual observer's response may vary over time. Reliability within one research assistant or observer is called intraobserver reliability.

To test for the reliability of the data collected between research assistants in the ovarian cancer study, each medical record was abstracted three times to determine levels of agreement. Levels of agreement ranged from 71 to 100 per cent for all the characteristics or risk factors collected for the study. A kappa (κ) statistic was also calculated. This statistic enables the researcher to determine if the agreement levels that are seen are real or due to chance. A κ statistic can range from 0.00 to 1.00. A κ statistic of 0.60 was chosen as the standard level for this study, and therefore, anything below 0.60 was determined to not be real and due to chance or sampling variability. Therefore, the usefulness of the agreement levels for those risk factors could be limited.

Another method of testing interobserver reliability when interviewing is to use different research assistants on the first and second interviews of the same subject. One can then measure consistency of recall and variations of response to different research assistants. To measure intraobserver reliability, the same research assistant can be used at different times while measuring consistency of the subject's response.

Sometimes reliability is measured and reported in the form of a correlation coefficient (r) rather than a proportion or percentage. A correlation coefficient is a statistic that shows the strength of a relation between two variables. A correlation coefficient (r), when used to measure degrees of reliability, can range from -1 to $+1$. The closer r approaches -1 or $+1$, the stronger the reliability or the relation between two variables. The closer r approaches zero, the weaker the relation or reliability.[1] For example, if an HIM professional was interested in the correlation between the number of health care providers attending medical record documentation seminars and the number of complete medical records received in the HIM department on discharge of the patient 1 week after the seminar was conducted, a correlation coefficient can be used. A high positive score, such as 0.91, means that as the number of health care providers attending the seminar increased, the number of completed medical records at discharge increased. A high negative score, such as -0.91, means that as the number of health care providers attending the seminar increased, the number of completed medical records decreased.

BIASES

No research study is perfect. No matter how well designed a research study is, there is always some type of error or bias. Therefore, it is imperative that researchers be aware of the types of biases that can occur and the methods used to decrease the amount of bias. The following are examples of common types of error or bias.[16]

Confounding Variables

If other characteristics, such as age or sex, are known to be associated with both the independent (risk factor or characteristic) and the dependent (disease) variables, these **confounding variables** should be controlled so that they are not the reason an association is seen. Methods to control for age, for example, include matching cases and controls on age or performing age adjustment when analyzing the data.

Sampling Variability

The results of a study may be false because of improper sample size and selection, as discussed earlier in this chapter.

Ascertainment and Selection Bias

When selecting subjects, researchers are more likely to choose people who are frequently under medical care. If a disease or condition is asymptomatic or mild, it may escape routine medical attention and may have an impact on the condition under study.

In addition, volunteers and paid subjects may be very different from the general population. Volunteers may volunteer to be in a study because they are very healthy or because they have a special interest in the study.

Diagnosis Bias

Certain diseases are not easy to diagnose, and different health professionals may offer different opinions. For example, when diagnosing or determining the stage and grade of certain types of cancers, a standard review of slides by one or more pathologists who are unaware of the specimens' origin can be used.

Nonresponse Bias

Subjects who refuse to participate in a study may be different from the subjects who do participate. The solution is to collect basic demographic characteristics on participants and nonparticipants to see if the characteristics are similar. In this way, the researcher can determine if the study participants represent the general population and are not different in relation to health characteristics.

Survival Bias

Survival bias occurs with cross-sectional studies because only those who have lived long enough to be in the study are examined. The solution is to use incident or new cases to relieve this bias.

Recall Bias

Recall bias can be attributed to faulty memory or subjects who tend to remember certain types of information because of the exposure or disease. Before the study begins, list possible biases and ways to reduce them. For example, mothers of children with anomalies or complications tend to remember more about their deliveries than do mothers of healthy children. Mothers of children with anomalies are the cases, whereas controls can be mothers of children with a different type of anomaly or adverse pregnancy outcome. Mothers with healthy children could be yet another comparison group. In this way, recall bias should be reduced because cases and controls would be similar in recalling specific events relevant to their children because both groups would have children with anomalies.

Interviewer Bias

Interviewers tend to ask questions differently or may probe more if they know which subjects have the characteristic of interest. To reduce interviewer bias, the solution is to standardize the interview form and to provide intensive training for the interviewers, stressing that they must be consistent when performing the interview.

Prevarication Bias

A worker who receives disability compensation might exaggerate his or her exposure. The solution is to use several independent raters and several sources of data to validate the information collected.

USE OF COMPUTERS IN RESEARCH

Because most research studies generate large amounts of data, computers are used to sort and analyze the data. Different types of computer software can be used to do this, depending on the type of statistics that are generated. An initial database can be constructed in Lotus 1-2-3, dBase, word processing software such as WordPerfect, or statistical software such as SPSS (Statistical Process for the Social Sciences). Then further statistical analysis can be performed using SPSS or BMDP (Biomedical Data Package) to perform frequency distributions, tests of significance, and/or life table analysis.

For example, the HIM professional in conjunction with risk management personnel has been collecting data on the number of falls by both patients and employees that have occurred within the health care facility. Data collected include where and how the fall occurred; the type of injury that was sustained; the cause of the fall; and the age, sex, and race of the patients and employees who fell. The data have been coded and entered into a Lotus spreadsheet. Further analysis is necessary to determine a frequency distribution on the total number of falls and the number of falls per nursing unit. Lotus software can perform these distributions as well as generate graphics to display this data. However, using Lotus software to determine more extensive statistical analysis may not be the most efficient route to take. To determine if there is a significant association between a specific nursing unit and the number of falls, correlation coefficients and tests of significance may be necessary. These types of statistics may be more easily generated using SPSS. Further analysis to examine health outcomes 1 month, 6 months, or 1 year after the fall may include life table analysis using BMDP software.

The HIM professional should know the types of software that are available to perform certain statistical tests. Statisticians should be consulted to aid in this process as well as in the interpretation and explanation of the data. Remember that the computer software or statistical analysis performed is only as good as the data that are collected and entered into the computer. It is up to the researcher to determine whether the results make sense and, therefore, how they should be applied and interpreted.

Other types of statistical software can aid in the collection of the data for a research study by assisting in the development of the questionnaire or data collection instrument. One example of such software is EPIINFO. This software, which can be obtained for a low cost, not only aids in constructing the data collection instrument, but also includes features such as SPSS to perform basic and advanced statistical analysis of the data.

Many types of computer software and statistical analysis applications are available. It is beyond the scope of this chapter to discuss all of them. However, the HIM professional should be aware of the computer software available to assist in the database development and analysis of the data. This may be the most important step the HIM professional takes when conducting research studies in the health care environment.

Key Concepts

- Health care statistics are necessary to evaluate a specific health care system or facility and should be calculated properly and used appropriately.

- Several research study designs can be used to assess a disease occurrence or the risk of getting a disease. Knowing when to use which study design is important and should be examined carefully.

- Every research study has specific steps that should be followed, such as developing a hypothesis, specific aims, significance, methodology (sample size, how data will be collected, data sources), and analysis.

- For research statistics to be understood, clear and organized data presentations in tables, graphs, and diagrams should be used.

- Every study has within it some type of bias or error, and the researcher should be aware of these biases and discuss their impact when writing up the results.

- There are several statistical tests that should be used for certain research studies. Knowing which statistics to use and when is extremely important and has a great impact on the results.

References

1. Kuzma J: Basic statistics for the health sciences. Mountainview, CA: Mayfield Publishing Co, 1992.
2. Skurka MF: Statistics. *In* Health information management in hospitals. Chicago: American Hospital Publishing, 1994, pp 141–146.
3. Glossary of healthcare terms. Chicago: American Health Information Management Association, 1994.
4. US Bureau of Census: International population reports. *In* An aging world II. Washington, DC: U.S. Government Printing Office, 1992, pp 25, 92–93.
5. Lilienfeld A, Lilienfeld D: Foundations of epidemiology, 2nd ed. Oxford, NY: Oxford University Press, 1980.
6. Slome C, Brogan D, Eyres S, et al: Basic epidemiological methods and biostatistics: A workbook. Belmont, CA: Jones & Bartlett, 1986.
7. Watzlaf VJM, Kuller LH, Ruben FL: The use of the medical record and financial data to examine the cost of infections in the elderly. Top Health Record Management 1992; 13(1):65–76.
8. Watzlaf V, Abdelhak M: Descriptive statistics. J Am Medical Record Association 1989;60(9);37–41.
9. Logothetis N: Supporting the quality improvement process. *In* Managing for total quality—from Deming to Toguchi and SPC. Prentice Hall International (UK), Ltd, 1992, p 206.
10. Putting quality improvement into action. *In* An introduction into quality improvement in health care. Oak Terrace, IL: Joint Commission on Accreditation of Healthcare Organizations, 1991, pp 27–38.
11. Shott S: Statistics for health professionals. Philadelphia: WB Saunders Co, 1990, pp 57–67.
12. Scheaffer R, Mendenhall W, Ott L: Elementary survey sampling, 3rd ed. Boston: Duxbury Press, 1986, pp 41–77.

13. Watzlaf VJM: The development of the grant proposal. J Am Medical Record Association 1989;60(3):37–41.

14. American College of Surgeons: Module 14—Statistics Fundamental Tumor Registry Operations. Commission on Cancer, 1991, p 45.

15. Kramer S, Jarrett P: Biostatistics and epidemiology for the tumor registry professionals. Harrisburg, PA: Pennsylvania Department of Health and Pennsylvania Tumor Registrars Association, 1984, pp 83–91.

16. Schlesselman JJ: Case-control studies—design, conduct, analysis. Oxford, NY: Oxford University Press, 1982, pp 124–143.

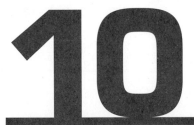

DONNA J. SLOVENSKY

KEY WORDS

Adverse patient occurrences (APO)
Aggregate data
Appointment
Audit
Benchmarking
Concurrent review
Criteria
Critical pathway
Credentialing
Discharge planning
Focused review
Incident report
Indicator
Intensity of service/severity of illness criteria
Licenture
Medical staff organization (MSO)
Monitoring and evaluation
National Practitioner Data Bank (NPDB)
Occurrence screening
Outcome measures
Outlier
Patient advocacy
Peer review
Peer review organization (PRO)
Players
Potentially compensable event (PCE)

QUALITY ASSESSMENT AND IMPROVEMENT

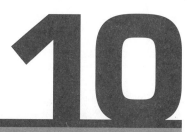

10

Privilege delineation
Process
Quality assessment
Quality assurance (QA)
Quality improvement (QI)
Quality indicator
Reappointment

Risk management
Sentinel event
Threshold
UB-92
Utilization review (UR)
Utilization management (UM)

OBJECTIVES

- Define Key Words.
- State the purpose and philosophy of quality assurance in health care.
- Outline the evolution of quality initiatives in health care.
- Identify legislative mandates and oversight agency requirements for quality review activities in health care facilities.
- Identify and describe commonly used methods for assessing and improving the quality of care and services provided in health care facilities.
- Describe the role of utilization review and management in the quality initiatives of a health care facility.
- Describe the role of risk management in the quality initiatives of a health care facility.
- Define the interaction between quality assurance activities and physician and professional staff appointment or reappointment and credentialing.
- Describe the organizational structures and communication mechanisms that are used to facilitate integration among the individual components of the quality assurance program in a health care facility.

The concept of quality as essentially symbiotic with delivery of health care is universally acknowledged. How the quality concept is measured and the specification of acceptable levels remain problematic, however. As the health care delivery system strives toward stabilization of costs and access, individuals and providers alike seek to articulate the role of clinical quality and service amenities as mediators or facilitators to achieve desired encounter outcomes. Hospitals and other service industries inevitably will compete on quality. Orme succinctly describes the goals of **quality improvement (QI)** efforts in health care as "to improve the processes of delivering care and thereby increase customer satisfaction with the quality of care (service outcomes), to improve the functional health of patients (clinical outcomes), and to reduce the costs of providing care."[1]

Purpose and Philosophy of Quality Assurance in Health Care

Japanese success in the global marketplace has brought the philosophy of QI to international attention. The initial applications in manufacturing have extended to use in service industries, including the delivery of health care. However, the familiar health care delivery issues trilogy of cost, access, and quality suggests an industry uniqueness. As Collopy notes, "the constant dilemma in the health care industry as opposed to industry in general is that of maximizing versus optimizing: clinicians must aim for the best **outcome** of care regardless of cost and health care managers at the 'macro' level are constrained, by a limitation of resources, to aim for an optimal level of care."[2] The situation is further complicated by differences in perceptions of quality: the patient may focus on delivery **processes** and amenities while physicians and other providers may be concerned primarily with technologic capabilities for clinical interventions. Players may thus rate the quality of the same episode of care differently. Goldsmith argues that "the real issue buried in the emerging quality debate is not quality per se, but value."[3] Here again, a consensual definition of "value" may not be achievable between recipients and providers. Enmeshed in this ambivalent environment, medical and administrative leaders in health care organizations strive to integrate performance measurement processes, to ensure consistent achievement of desired quality standards, and to communicate a genuine consumer orientation.

Historical Development

To comprehend the prevailing philosophy of continuous quality improvement (CQI), it is necessary to investigate the ways in which providers, purchasers, and consumers make value judgments about the quality and value of health care and how these measures have changed over time. Identifying key **players** and significant events in the evolution of the quality philosophy and techniques for assessing and ensuring quality in health care requires investigation of social and political trends as well as acknowledgment of technologic advances. For convenience, these issues are discussed from the perspective of medical education reform, hospital standardization, and health care legislation at the federal level.

Medical Education Reform

Physicians in colonial America, like other professionals and skilled craftsmen, were trained under an apprentice system.[4] This training method benefited both physicians and trainees from an economic standpoint and for a time provided an adequate geographic distribution of physicians. The number of physicians entering the market was limited only by interest, perseverance, and financial resources. However, as the nation grew and the population dispersed, a more structured approach to medical training was needed. Throughout the 1800s, medical schools teaching several medical philosophies were established by universities and commercial enterprises. These schools were unregulated and provided little scientific basis for the practice of medicine.

Although physicians were beginning to form professional societies and, thus, influence physician practice behaviors, the educational system itself did not promote standardization of medical practice or standards of professional competence.

In 1904, the Council on Medical Education (CME) of the American Medical Association (AMA) was created. Through political interactions with the state medical societies and direct contacts with the state licensing boards, the CME established a foundation for plans to establish the dominance of scientific schools. In 1905, the council surveyed all 160 medical schools in the United States and recommended closure of all schools with less than an "A" rating. Many of the 78 schools recommended for closure were homeopathic or eclectic or admitted predominantly black or female students. Lacking the legal authority or the political power to close the schools, the CME approached the Carnegie Foundation for the Advancement of Teaching and requested assistance in conducting an objective study of medical education.[4] The outcome of this collaboration was what is commonly referred to as the Flexner Report.

During 1909 and 1910, Abraham Flexner resurveyed all medical schools that had not closed since the CME inspections in 1905. His report of 148 U.S. and 7 Canadian schools provided the following information for each site visited: location, entrance requirements, number of enrolled students, number and academic rank of teaching staff, available financial resources, laboratory facilities, and clinical facilities utilized. A narrative summary of "general considerations" was given for each state.[5]

Flexner reported findings congruent with the earlier CME inspections, and this legitimation by the Carnegie Foundation provided the necessary political influence for the AMA to effect medical education reform. The medical school accreditation program established by the AMA resulted in closure of substandard schools. Standardization of curriculum requirements through accreditation provided a strong mechanism to restrict the number and increase the clinical competence of medical school graduates. *Ensuring that only competent practitioners enter the profession is a pivotal factor in improving quality throughout the delivery system.*

Hospital Standardization

The Joint Commission on Accreditation of Healthcare Organizations (JCAHO) is a not-for-profit, nongovernmental entity that offers voluntary accreditation programs for health care facilities. Since 1952, when it accepted transfer of the Hospital Standardization Program from the American College of Surgeons (ACS), the JCAHO has provided education, leadership, and objective evaluation and feedback to hospitals in the quest for health care quality.

A hospital or other health care facility requests an on-site survey by JCAHO representatives to determine compliance with standards published in the *Accreditation Manual for Hospitals (AMH)* or other standards manual appropriate to the facility type. Before the survey, the hospital performs an extensive self-analysis of compliance with the standards and prepares a written document responding to a standardized questionnaire. JCAHO staff and surveyors review this documentation before the on-site survey. During the survey, JCAHO surveyors perform the following functions:

- Review additional documentation.
- Interview selected hospital personnel and medical staff members.
- Evaluate the physical facilities.
- Collect other information necessary to assess the extent of compliance with the standards.

The surveyors look for evidence that the hospital has been in compliance with the standards for the previous 12 months. Hospital compliance with all standards that affect the accreditation decision is measured using published guidelines for determining a numerical score. Scores are aggregated into a grid and multiplied by weight factors to reflect overall performance and objectively ground the accreditation decision.

Demonstration of effective policies and procedures designed to continuously improve organizational performance is a critical factor in achieving accredited status. The JCAHO mission clearly articulates this philosophy: "The mission of the Joint Commission on Accreditation of Healthcare Organizations is to improve the quality of health care provided to the public."[6]

The original Minimum Standard adopted by the ACS Board of Regents in December 1919 was an important first step toward improving the quality of health care. *The intent of the Minimum Standard was to do for hospitals what the Flexner Report had done for medical schools— provide objective* **criteria** *for industry standardization at an acceptable level of quality.* By 1950, through the efforts of the ACS, more than one half the hospitals in the United States had demonstrated compliance with the current version of the standards.[7]

After transfer of the Hospital Standardization Program to the JCAHO, the quality focus steadily moved from standardization to **quality assessment.** Between 1952 and 1965, the standards were revised six times but continued to measure a minimum acceptable level of compliance. The publication of the 1970 *AMH* marked the transition from minimum standards to optimal achievable standards. Optimal was defined in terms of the best that could be achieved given legal, technologic, and other environmental constraints that must be accommodated.

Clinical quality assessment during this period was essentially limited to **peer review** in the form of retrospective medical "audits" conducted within the organizational units of the medical staff. Little data sharing occurred among the units, and criteria for evaluation were seldom validated outside the reviewing group. Little, if any, feedback into the physician credentialing process was evident.

Quality assessment requirements for ancillary and support service departments were initiated by the JCAHO in the late 1970s. Before incorporation of these standards in the *AMH,* quality control measures in many hospital departments were designed and implemented at the discretion of department managers. As with clinical reviews during this time, little data sharing or standardization of operational practices was achieved. The initial focus of quality reviews conducted in ancillary departments was problem identification and resolution. Department managers collected information either retrospectively or concurrently to respond to problems with employee competence or care and service delivery processes within the department's scope of operation.

The Quality of Professional Services Standard in the 1979 *AMH* signaled the beginning of requirements for using information collected during peer reviews assessing the quality of care. The guidelines specifically addressed delineation of clinical privileges for professional staff. Physician practice profiles developed through patient care quality assessments, and **utilization review** activities were incorporated into physician credentialing files, which permitted data-based decisions regarding medical staff appointment and **privilege delineation.**

In 1986, the JCAHO initiated the Agenda for Change, a 5-year plan to stimulate health care organizations to create an environment focused on continuously improving the quality of care with clinical and administrative leaders (including the governing body) committed to quality improvement. The agenda included the following goals:

- Major revision of the standards (accomplished with the 1994 *AMH*)
- Streamlining of the survey process
- Development of clinical indicators of quality

The Quality Improvement Initiative begun in 1988 clearly indicated the emerging commitment to the philosophy of continuous improvement. In January 1989, the JCAHO board of directors published the following definition of quality within the context of health care: "The degree to which patient care services increase the probability of desired patient outcomes and reduce the probability of undesired outcomes, given the current state of knowledge."[8]

The 1992 *AMH* denoted the beginning of the carefully planned transition from a quality assessment to a QI approach to health care quality, culminating in the publication of the Improving Organizational Performance chapter in the 1994 *AMH*. The preamble to this chapter declares the determination to shift "the primary focus from the performance of individuals to the performance of the organization's systems and processes."[6]

Federal Legislation

Medicare marked the entry of the federal government into the health care arena as a major purchaser of health services. The 1965 amendments to the Social Security Act provided health insurance directly to elderly people (Medicare) and through a state matching program to nonelderly medically needy people (Medicaid). These programs are administered through the Health Care Financing Administration (HCFA), a regulatory agency within the Social Security Administration. Regulations governing providers of services to Medicare beneficiaries are detailed in the *Conditions of Participation*. Revisions and addenda are published in the *Federal Register*, a Monday-through-Friday publication of the National Archives and Records Administration that reports regulations and legal notices issued by federal agencies, presidential proclamations and executive orders, and other documents as directed by law or public interest.

The original Medicare legislation incorporated two requirements for evaluating the quality and appropriateness of inpatient services.

1. Attending physicians would certify the need for continued hospitalization at 12, 18, and 30 days post admission.

2. A second physician would review a patient's health record every 14 days.

This second type of review was called utilization review (UR), a concurrent peer-monitoring process intended to ensure that inpatient services were used only as clinically indicated. For the most part, the reviews were perfunctory. Many physicians were hesitant to question clinical decisions made by other physicians practicing on the same medical staff. These review requirements were replaced through later legislation.

Legislative amendments in 1972 created professional standards review organizations (PSROs), physician-controlled non-profit entities that contracted with the HCFA to monitor inpatient services provided to Medicare recipients. These agents were authorized to deny Medicare reimbursement for inappropriate services. During the PSRO era, UR was conducted at diagnosis-specific checkpoints based on regional norms. The reviews were conducted either by PSRO personnel or by hospital employees, with review outcomes reported to the PSRO. In addition to individual patient data, hospital staff accumulated information to monitor individual physician admission and discharge patterns for comparison with statistically "expected" performance.

The Tax Equity and Fiscal Responsibility Act, passed in 1982, mandated broad-based changes in the Medicare program. The reimbursement structure was changed from a retrospectively determined cost-based payment to a prospectively established fixed price determined by the patient's final principal diagnosis. This reimbursement structure is referred to as the prospective payment system (PPS). The PSROs were replaced by **peer review organizations (PROs)** that were empowered to evaluate individual physician performance relative to quality and appropriateness of services provided and recommend punitive action to the HCFA. Recommendations for corrective action range from education to removal from the listing of approved Medicare providers and monetary fines. The PPS became operational in 1983 but allowed a 4-year phase-in for full implementation. Requirements for monitoring the quality and appropriateness of inpatient services to beneficiaries are outlined in comprehensive triennial documents, the *PRO Scope of Work*, numbered consecutively beginning in 1983. The Fourth *Scope of Work* encompasses October 1, 1993 through September 30, 1996. Organizations bid to the HCFA for 3-year contracts to operate as the PRO to fulfill mandated and elective review activities through oversight of all provider hospitals in the state or designated region. The PRO reviews individual patient cases to evaluate clinical care processes as planned and implemented by the attending physician. PRO reviews are inadequate, however, for quick feedback and response in effecting **quality assurance (QA)**. The PRO has sanction authority. Medicare reimbursement can be withheld if quality and appropriateness of care have not been demonstrated. PRO and hospital personnel work together to facilitate timely intervention in problematic cases for reimbursement.

The government assumed a stronger role in ensuring individual physician competence with the Health Care Quality Improvement Act of 1986 (Title IV of Public Law 99-660). This act established the **National Practitioner Data Bank (NPDB)**, a clearinghouse to collect and release information to eligible parties for the purpose of identifying problematic or incompetent physicians, dentists, and other health care practitioners. Under the act, a practitioner is defined as a person who is licensed, certified, or registered by the state to provide health care services. The data bank maintains the following types of adverse action data:

- Malpractice payments
- **Licensure** board actions
- Clinical privilege actions
- Society membership actions

All hospitals are required to query the data bank before granting clinical privileges to any physician and at least every 2 years thereafter. The data bank became opera-

TABLE 10–1 HEALTH CARE LEGISLATION IMPACTING QUALITY INITIATIVE	
DATE	**ACT/SYNOPSIS**
1965	PL 89-97—Medicare: Provided medical coverage for people age 65 or older, effective 7/1/66. Included provision for utilization review of inpatient services.
1972	PL 92-603—Amendments to Social Security Act: Created professional standards review organizations to monitor quality and appropriateness of inpatient services for Medicare recipients.
1975	PL 93-641—National Health Planning and Resources Development Act: Established regional planning agencies to better use health care resources. Created certificate of need program.
1980	PL 96-499—Omnibus Budget Reconciliation Act: Intended to simplify reimbursement for Medicare and Medicaid. Changed utilization review requirements.
1982	Tax Equity and Fiscal Responsibility Act: Mandated development of a prospective payment system. Created peer review organizations to determine reasonableness and medical necessity of inpatient services to Medicare recipients; authorized to approve or deny reimbursement to providers.
1983	PL 98-21—Amendments to Social Security Act: Established the prospective payment system for the Medicare program, effective 10/1/83.
1985	Consolidated Omnibus Budget Reconciliation Act: Authorized denial of Medicare payments for substandard care. Included antidumping regulations.
1986	PL 99-509—Omnibus Budget Reconciliation Act: Required peer review organizations to report information regarding substandard care to licensing and certifying agencies.
1986	PL 99-660—Health Care Quality Improvement Act: Provided immunity from liability for peer review actions in the credentialing process within specified parameters. Established the National Practitioner Data Bank.
1989	PL 101-239—Omnibus Budget Reconciliation Act: Created the Agency for Health Care Policy and Research to facilitate development of outcome measures of health care quality.
1990	PL 101-508—Omnibus Budget Reconciliation Act: Peer review organizations required to notify medical boards and licensing agencies of recommended physician sanctions.
1990	PL 101-508—Patient Self-Determination Act: Effective 12/1/91; providers must develop policies and procedures to address a patient's right to refuse treatment.

tional September 1, 1990, under a contract by the HCFA with the Unisys Corporation. Data confidentiality is maintained through a comprehensive security system to prevent unauthorized access or data manipulation by unauthorized parties.

A brief summary of health care legislation that impacts quality initiatives in health care facilities is shown in Table 10–1.

QUALITY ASSURANCE

Quality assurance refers to activities that are designed to measure the quality of a service, product, or process and encompasses taking remedial action as needed to adhere to a desired standard. In health care, the concept of QA is most often associated with the clinical components of care.

Historical Development

Although it can be said that physicians have embraced a quality philosophy since the inauguration of the Oath of Hippocrates, the historical roots of QA in medical care are frequently attributed to such early leaders as Dr. Ernest A. Codman, who promoted the concepts of "end results" at Massachusetts General Hospital in the early 1900s; Dr. George Gray Ward at New York Women's Hospital, who pioneered the medical **audit**; and Dr. Thomas Ponton, who instituted one of the first risk classification systems.

Objectives

Quality assurance presupposes that a desirable standard of quality has been defined and is measurable. Individual patient care episodes and **aggregate data** describing routine delivery of health care services are compared with the predetermined standards to identify and correct any deviation from the standard.

External Requirements

Several agents external to the health care organization delineate requirements for quality assurance activities. Some requirements are grounded in law; others are stipulated by agencies with which the hospital interacts on a voluntary basis. Because some regulatory body guidelines incorporate and surpass those of less demanding agents, only the major players are discussed here.

Medicare Conditions of Participation

The QA activities required of hospitals participating in the Medicare program are detailed in the *Conditions of Participation,* the *PRO Scope of Work,* and the *Federal Register.* Hospital personnel responsible for managing the quality program components should closely monitor directives issued by the PRO to respond to changes in regulations.

Joint Commission on Accreditation of Healthcare Organizations

As noted previously, a demonstrated commitment to a quality philosophy is pivotal to achieving facility accreditation by the JCAHO. This commitment must be evident among the hospital leadership and governance and deployed throughout the organization. Although the JCAHO does not specify a particular methodology for ensuring quality, some standards applicable to measuring and evaluating clinical care are prescriptive in orientation. These requirements are discussed under the heading "Medical Care Evaluation." As with the Medicare regulations, the standards of the JCAHO are subject to change. The JCAHO *Perspectives on Accreditation,* a bimonthly newsletter, is the official information source to monitor for standard revisions.

Internal Incentives

Purchasers and consumers of health care demand access to high-quality cost-effective care. Hospitals and other health care facilities that cannot compete on both price and quality are forced out of the market. Decreasing quality as a by-product of cost control is not an acceptable outcome. Health care providers are increasingly motivated to incorporate assurance of quality in their marketing efforts. The QI philosophy proclaims decreased costs attributed to rework as a by-product of the quest for higher quality. In a health care context, examples of rework include repeated laboratory or radiology tests or readmissions resulting from premature discharge. Organizations are reimbursed only for service that has been correctly performed. Therefore, costs associated with rework are unrecoverable.

Medical Care Evaluation

The individual programs and activities that constitute the QA initiative for a health care facility are specific to the goals and objectives established by the organization. For hospitals accredited by the JCAHO, however, certain review activities that assess both processes and outcomes are mandated. Targeted processes include those that are high volume, high risk, or problem prone. Among the

required reviews are several that are specific to the clinical activities of the medical staff. These reviews are referred to in a general sense as medical care evaluation. JCAHO standards are revised periodically to reflect advances in health care technology and health care delivery. Future trends will focus on outcomes assessment based on clinical indicators. Refer to the current standards manuals for specific requirements.

Surgical and Invasive Procedure Review

Review of surgical and invasive procedures includes evaluation of the following elements:

- Selection of the procedure
- Preparing the patient for the procedure
- Competent performance of the procedure and intraprocedure monitoring of the patient
- Postprocedure care[6]

Information available as a result of these reviews is incorporated into processes for delineation of medical staff clinical privileges.

Medication Usage Review

Medication usage evaluation is intended to investigate the following:

- Prescribing and ordering practices
- Preparation and dispensing procedures
- Drug administration
- Effects of drugs administered to patients

Sentinel events, such as significant adverse drug reactions, are subject to intensive review.[6] Information derived from these quality reviews relative to patient medication needs, effectiveness, associated risks, and cost of pharmaceuticals is used to select medications for inclusion in the hospital formulary. Individuals or committees that participate in the quality review of medications may also participate in developing organization policies and procedures for selecting, procuring, distributing, and administering medications.

Medical Record Review

Medical record review is a multidisciplinary activity performed by representatives of the medical staff, nursing staff, health information management (HIM) department, management and administrative services, and other departments or services as determined by organizational needs and objectives. Medical records are reviewed for accuracy, completeness, and timely completion on a quarterly basis. Each medical record should reflect the following:

- Diagnosis
- Diagnostic test results
- Therapy
- Condition
- In-hospital progress[6]

Blood Usage Review

Blood usage review encompasses evaluation of patients receiving either blood or blood components. Evaluation should address the following:

- Ordering practices
- Distribution
- Handling and dispensing procedures
- Administration
- Effects of blood and blood components administered to patients

Confirmed transfusion reactions are sentinel events and, therefore, subject to intensive review.[6]

Other Reviews

Under JCAHO standards, the medical staff are required to participate in other review functions, most notably the following:

- Infection control
- Internal and external disaster planning
- Hospital safety
- Utilization review

These review functions are typically addressed by multidisciplinary committees and are discussed in other sections of this chapter.

Ancillary Department Reviews

The 1994 *AMH* requires that each hospital department or service incorporate the standards for Improving Organizational Performance chapter relative to the systems and processes within its scope of operations. As with other quality reviews, departments are directed to focus on processes that are high volume, high risk, or problem prone. Within these parameters, the performance of individuals and the department as an entity is assessed from two dimensions: "doing the right thing" and "doing the right thing well."[6] In addition to the QI focus, quality control activities are required in clinical laboratory, diagnostic radiology, dietetic, nuclear medicine, and radiation oncology services.

Methodology and Models

Most quality reviews are some form or adaptation of peer review. Peer review can be defined as the evaluation of a person's professional performance by another person (or others) of equal professional standing. Time and fiscal resources typically do not permit peer review of all patient care episodes. Therefore, accountable professionals seek valid and reliable mechanisms to ensure the quality of care and services through examination of isolated events or aggregations of data. Identification of which events and what data to examine remains one of the most challenging issues in QA.

Donabedian's Model of Structure, Process, and Outcome

Avedis Donabedian's early work in the definition and assessment of health care quality resulted in one of the most widely acknowledged and conceptually sound models for assessing quality in health care. As a prelude to defining quality, Donabedian dichotomizes "care" into technical and interpersonal domains.[9] The technical domain encompasses the science and technology components of medicine ("science"); the interpersonal domain refers to social and psychological interactions between the practitioner and patient ("art"). He further acknowledges an element of care he calls "amenities," or what might be generally called satisfiers. Amenities include such features as comfortable and clean surroundings, good food, and personal convenience items. Donabedian uses these domains to conceptualize quality as a property of and judgment about some definable unit of care. *Under Donabedian's model, technical quality is quantified as the degree to which the benefits of using medical science and technology are maximized and associated risks are minimized.* The definition of health care quality published by the JCAHO in 1989 closely parallels the Donabedian definition of technical quality. Defining quality in the interpersonal domain is more nebulous because measures of values, norms, and expectations are less well defined. Most measures attempt to quantify expectations and the degree to which expectations were met. Donabedian does not attempt to quantify the amenities element of care but considers it a notable contributor to patient satisfaction with interpersonal interactions.

Expanding on the domain definition of care, Donabedian defines three approaches to assessing quality of care indirectly by using measures that examine structures, processes, and outcomes associated with the delivery of health care. Table 10–2 defines the approaches and provides examples of measures frequently used to evaluate the quality of care or services provided by individuals and organizations.

TABLE 10–2 DONABEDIAN'S MODEL OF STRUCTURE, PROCESS, AND OUTCOME

	INDIVIDUAL	DEPARTMENT	ORGANIZATION
Structure	*Professional certification *Credential review	*Staffing analysis *Equipment safety checks	*Licensure *Fire safety inspections
Process	*Peer reviews *Performance evaluations *Productivity monitors	*Review of performance indicators *Flow process analysis	*Infection surveillance *Review of utilization data
Outcome	*Practice profiles *Rework required	*Error/complication rate analysis	*Mortality rates *Quality sanctions

STRUCTURE MEASURES. *Structure measures indirectly assess care by looking at certain provider characteristics and the physical and organizational resources available to support the delivery of care.* Structure measures essentially look at the capability or potential for providing quality care. By their nature, structure measures are static: the organization or individual is evaluated at a unique point in time. The organizational structure of a facility, operational policies and procedures, technologic capabilities, compliance with safety regulations, and performance evaluation mechanisms are all examples of structure measures.

PROCESS MEASURES. *Process measures focus on the interactions between patients and providers.* Process-oriented measures examine an individual health care professional's decision-making processes as he or she directs a patient's course of treatment or, at the organization level, investigate the procedures that guide operational decisions. Examples of process measures include peer review of patient records indicating problems with patient care or documentation, compliance with **discharge planning** procedures, and patient waiting time in the emergency department before triage.

OUTCOME MEASURES. *Outcome measures look at the end results or product of the patient's encounter with the system.* One of the most commonly used outcome measures in acute health care settings is patient mortality. Although mortality is certainly an important measure, other variables may be necessary to examine the quality of care provided to patients. For instance, what if the patient's diagnosis is terminal metastatic carcinoma? Would death suggest poor quality care for such a patient? Measures such as adequate pain control and adherence to living will requirements might be more appropriate. Other examples of outcome measures that address categories of patients rather than individual patient outcomes include comparison of patient lengths of stay with regional norms, infection and complication rate review, and the number of transfers to another inpatient facility.

JCAHO Monitoring and Evaluation Model

The JCAHO promoted a **monitoring and evaluation** model to facilitate transition from a quality assessment approach to a QI orientation. The model was incorporated in the 1984 standards to establish a consistent framework for ancillary department review activities and expanded to include medical staff department activities beginning in 1990. Although the terminology changed somewhat in the 1992 *AMH*, the monitoring concept is still relevant. In keeping with the transition from quality assessment to QI, the scope has expanded to stress the responsibility of organizational leaders in the improvement process.

The goals and objectives of a monitoring and evaluation program are achieved through a 10-step process. The 10 steps and examples at hospital, departmental, and individual levels consistent with the model are shown in Table 10–3.

Quality Indicators

As implied by the general usage of the term, an indicator is an indirect measure. A **quality indicator** is an objective, quantifiable measurement that targets events or patterns of events suggestive of a problematic process or behavior. Indicators are typically classed as one of two types: sentinel events or patterns of events evident in aggregate data. A **sentinel event** is an infrequently occurring undesirable outcome of such magnitude that each occurrence warrants further investigation. Examples are obstetric mortality, transfusion reaction, and surgical misadventures that require unplanned procedures. The second type of indicator (evidenced in aggregate data) reflects outcomes that, although undesirable, are less dramatic and injurious than sentinel events and that can reasonably be expected to occur with some frequency. For example, meal trays delivered late or broken medication tablets are undesirable but can be expected to occur in the normal course of operations. Typically, these types of events are monitored until the occurrences reach a predetermined **threshold** that triggers a

TABLE 10-3 JCAHO TEN-STEP PROCESS

TEN STEPS	HEALTH INFORMATION MANAGEMENT DEPARTMENT EXAMPLE
1. Assign responsibility.	Coding supervisor is responsible for coding quality and productivity.
2. Delineate scope of care and service.	Coding personnel assign ICD-9-CM and CPT codes, enter codes and other data into a computerized database.
3. Identify important aspects of care and service.	Codes must be correctly assigned; data must be entered correctly; all activities must be completed promptly.
4. Identify indicators.	*Diagnoses and procedures are coded correctly. *All necessary codes are present. *Records are processed within 3 working days post discharge.
5. Establish thresholds for evaluation.	*Coding error rate < .05% *Data entry error rate < .03% *Records coded within 3 working days post discharge
6. Collect and organize data.	*Supervisor verifies a random sample of records processed by each coder. *Generate error reports of system edit checks. *Coders maintain checksheets to monitor record processing time.
7. Initiate evaluation.	Data are inspected to identify patterns of errors or opportunities to improve processes.
8. Take actions to improve care and services.	*Inservice training on changes in coding guidelines *Procedural changes to batch input data with minimal interruption
9. Assess the effectiveness of actions and maintain the gain.	Compare monitoring reports subsequent to actions with previous reports.
10. Communicate results to affected individuals and groups.	*Present results of quality study in weekly coding section meeting. *Document results in memorandum to HIM department director.

CPT, Current procedural terminology; ICD-9-CM, International Classification of Diseases, 9th Revision—Clinical Modification.

focused review to initiate corrective action. A focused review examines a few critical variables when a problem has been identified and is more process-directed than a random review, which typically screens for outcomes.

To achieve their potential value, indicators must be relevant, valid, and reliable. A valid indicator accurately measures the intended outcome and discriminates correctly between presence and absence of the outcome. For maximum usefulness, indicators should focus on the relation between process and outcome.[10] A reliable indicator is stable, showing consistent results over time and among different users of the indicator. The indicator must distinguish between poor-quality institutions and average- or good-quality institutions.

The logical progression in QI is to move from analysis of individual organization performance data to comparison of organization performance with data from similar organizations. When individual facilities establish unique quality indicators for internal reviews, it may be difficult to compare performance outcomes with those of other facilities.

The JCAHO Indicator Measurement System (IMS) is an interactive reference database intended to achieve the objective of external comparison.[11] Accredited hospitals collect and report objective performance data on a continuing basis. The aggregate data are adjusted for risk as necessary and analyzed on a national level. The goal is to create and maintain a national performance database to support research in health services.

The JCAHO defines an indicator as "a quantitative instrument that is used to measure the extent to which an organization or component thereof carries out the right processes, carries out those processes well, and achieves desired outcomes as a result of carrying out the right processes well."[12]

The infrastructure of the IMS is the product of multiple task forces chartered to develop sets of indicators for important health care functions.[11] Important functions are those "most affect[ing] the quality of care and services delivered in a health care organization."[12] Indicators developed by the task forces are tested in a limited number of alpha sites to evaluate face validity and feasibility of data collection. An alpha site is a facility selected to participate in the first field test under real-world conditions. The importance of establishing validity and reliability in the indicators cannot be overemphasized.

After analysis of alpha site reports, the indicators are tested in a few hundred beta sites for about 2 years. Beta testing is used to identify system weaknesses or deficiencies before full-scale implementation. Test sites investigate their ability to collect and transmit the required data with existing human and technology resources and the ease with which the indicators can be integrated into existing monitoring activities. The JCAHO also uses the beta test period to investigate the effectiveness of information technology and internal management systems that are used to analyze indicator data and provide constructive feedback to participating organizations.

Participation in the IMS is voluntary until the system has been debugged and adequately validated and until information generated through analysis of indicators is designated by the JCAHO as a component of the accrediting process. Hospitals that participated in the initial phase of the IMS began with 10 fully tested indicators in 1994 and expanded to 20 in 1995. Mandatory participation will require incorporation of all validated indicators at that time.[13] A summary listing of the indicators is shown in Table 10–4.

Hospitals may elect to either purchase vendor-developed software or develop software internally to collect IMS data for submission to the JCAHO. The JCAHO publishes functional specifications for software to support data collection and transmission and provides this information at no charge to hospitals, information system vendors, and consultants. Internal software development provides the advantage of integration with existing information systems. The JCAHO vendor product is a stand-alone personal computer application that does not integrate with other information systems. Products developed by other vendors should be carefully evaluated for integration capabilities and conformity to functional specifications.

Clinical Practice Guidelines and Critical Pathways

The 1989 Omnibus Budget Reconciliation Act created the Agency for Health Care Policy and Research (AHCPR) within the Department of Health and Human Services to foster research in clinical outcomes and effectiveness. The intended purpose of the AHCPR is "to

TABLE 10-4 JCAHO INDICATOR MONITORING SYSTEM

INDICATOR GROUP	NUMBER OF INDICATORS
I Obstetrics	10
Anesthesia	8
II Cardiovascular Care	9
Oncology care	11
Trauma care	12
III Medication use	12
Infection control	8
IV Home infusion therapy	6
V Depressive disorders	Under development

Data from Agenda for change. Chicago: Joint Commission on Accreditation of Healthcare Organizations, 1993.

TABLE 10-5 INSTITUTE OF MEDICINE CRITERIA FOR EVALUATING MONITORS

ATTRIBUTE	INTERPRETATION
Validity	When followed, a valid guideline leads to the projected health and cost outcome.
Strength of evidence	Expert judgment and other data used to develop the guideline should be documented.
Estimated outcomes	Health and cost outcomes resulting from implementation of the guideline should be projected. Patient perceptions and preferences should be considered.
Reliability and reproducibility	A guideline is reproducible if another panel of experts using the same data would produce the same guideline. A reliable guideline is interpreted and applied without variation among users.
Clinical applicability	Populations to which the guideline applies should be clearly defined.
Clinical flexibility	Clinically justifiable exceptions to the guideline should be specified.
Clarity	The guideline should be written in clear, direct language. Technical terminology should be defined.
Multidisciplinary process	Guidelines should be developed using a collaborative process involving representatives from salient interest groups.
Scheduled review	A timetable for scheduled review to assess continued accuracy and relevance should be proposed.
Documentation	The development process should be well documented, including personnel involved, data sources used, and procedures used.

Data from Institute of Medicine, Committee on Clinical Practice Guidelines. In Lohr KN, Schyve PM: Reasonable expectations: From the Institute of Medicine. QRB Qual Rev Bull 1992;18(12):393–396.

enhance the quality, appropriateness, and effectiveness of health care and to improve access to that care."[14] A major thrust of the AHCPR is to facilitate development of clinical practice guidelines, defined by the Institute of Medicine as "systematically developed statements to assist practitioner and patient decisions about appropriate health care for specific clinical circumstances."[15] Guidelines provide information about the benefits and associated risks of medical treatments drawn from current, relevant medical literature and judgments of clinical experts.

With the AHCPR as facilitator, multidisciplinary groups of experts—practitioners and consumers together—develop and test guidelines using strict methodologies to ensure clinical validity and relevance. The availability of practice guidelines is expected to standardize clinical decision-making processes and reduce variation in treatment protocols. Over time, the guidelines should contribute to improved patient outcomes.

The Institute of Medicine was charged with developing criteria for evaluating practice guidelines. It published a list of desirable attributes in 1992, which are summarized in Table 10–5.[16]

Practice guidelines under development are specific and comprehensive, clearly defining indications that a given diagnostic test or therapeutic procedure is inappropriate as well as when it is appropriate. An example of the clinical algorithm that summarizes the practice guideline for heart failure is shown in Figure 10–1. This degree of specificity is a marked distinction from earlier guidelines that focused primarily on clinical pertinence of tests and procedures within diagnostic categories. The specificity of the guidelines advances opportunities to increase communication between physicians and patients and increase patient involvement in clinical decisions.

Because practice guidelines represent "best" clinical care at a given point in time, review and revision to acknowledge advances in technology and practices are essential to continuing effectiveness. Incorporating a feedback loop between clinical outcomes and application of guidelines adds further complexity (and associated costs) to implementation.

Disseminating and implementing practice guidelines carry both clinical and financial implications for future health care delivery. Clinical validity and reliability for each guideline adopted must be established beyond question. The guidelines must be acceptable not only to providers of health care services but to recipients and payers as well. They should not be perceived solely as utilization (and thus cost) control mechanisms but as tools that enable physicians to access the wealth of clinical and technologic knowledge available to achieve the most desirable outcome from a health encounter.

Critical pathways are patient care management tools designed to achieve simultaneous goals of optimal care and appropriate resource utilization. The critical pathway is a diagnosis-specific guide to patient care delivery. Daily patient care is guided by standard physician orders for diagnostic tests, medication, and treatment. Standardizing the patient care routine allows identification and tracking of individual variations in patient response or treatment outcomes. Data sharing among facilities in a geographic region can produce critical pathways that improve community health resource utilization and ensure equivalent quality of care in all facilities.

Clinical guidelines developed under the auspices of the AHCPR are available at no charge through an online electronic service of the National Library of Medicine. This service is called HSTAT, an acronym for Health Services/Technology Assessment. Users may acquire full text, graphics, and tables in a form similar to that of the printed guidelines by using one of several electronic access methods. Access instructions can be obtained by requesting AHCPR Publication No. 94-0075, *AHCPR Fact Sheet: Using HSTAT for Online Access to AHCPR-Supported Clinical Practice Guidelines.*

Patient-Focused Care

The patient-focused care paradigm parallels some of the major concepts that underlie total quality management. Rather than the traditional inpatient care model, whereby the patient interacts with many caregivers and travels to different ancillary departments for procedures, the patient-focused approach uses a small care team. Most diagnostic procedures are performed in the patient's room or on the patient care unit. The patient is considered central to all activities, much as the customer is perceived in a total quality management organization.[17]

The patient-focused care concept is relatively new. The model emerged from practices recommended by health care consultants in the mid-1980s to improve the efficiency of inpatient care services. Although institutions may define their approach somewhat differently, the following are some common elements that are emerging.

- *Decentralized services.* Laboratory, pharmacy, radiology, and respiratory therapy services may be decentralized to the care units to reduce waiting time and provide better response to patient needs.

- *Cross-trained personnel.* Many nurses and care technicians are trained to perform tasks that might have been performed by another allied health specialist, such as phlebotomy, electrocardiogram recording, and respiratory therapy. Cross-training encourages more efficient use of technician time and decreases the number of caregivers with whom the patient interacts.

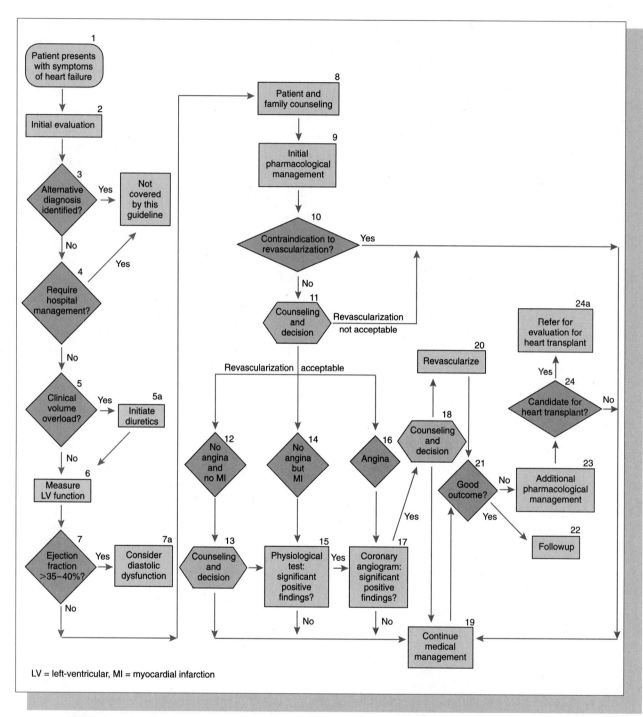

FIGURE 10–1. Algorithm for clinical practice guideline. (From Clinical practice guideline #11 heart failure: Evaluation and care of patients with left-ventricular systolic dysfunction, Uniform Hospital Discharge Data Set (UHDDS), Agency for Health Care Policy and Research. Publication No. 94-0612. June 1994.)

- *Interdisciplinary collaboration.* Care teams are taught to work together to meet patient needs. This may require crossing existing turf lines.

- *Clinical pathways.* Patient-focused care often uses critical pathways or care maps—multidisciplinary action plans—to ensure consistent practice patterns among caregivers. This approach can facilitate the effective use of resources and efficient treatment protocols.

- *Work simplification and work redesign.* Teams may diagram tasks on a flowchart to streamline patient care activities. All caregiving tasks may be performed by a smaller number of highly skilled staff or less technical tasks may be assigned to lower-skilled staff to effect cost savings.

- *Patient empowerment.* Patients are involved in their own care to increase compliance with care protocols. Increased patient involvement requires more education to support self-care.[18]

Proponents of the patient-focused care model report such outcomes as reduced length of stay, decreased staff time and associated cost savings, and improvement of patient and caregiver satisfaction with inpatient encounters.

QI Models

The QI philosophy advances the premise that the quality of a product or service can be enhanced through process or system changes that increase efficiency or effectiveness. A profusion of published literature is available that describes the problem-solving approaches championed by reigning quality gurus, promoting a plethora of tools and techniques for data collection and analysis and touting critical success factors to implementing CQI in an organization. The volume of popular or trade press reports far surpasses empirical publications. Anecdotal accounts are often difficult to assess for potential effectiveness when transferred to another organization or application. The sheer volume and diversity of information available challenge managers and workers searching for philosophical approaches and information management techniques congruous with their own QI goals.

The D*A*T model provides a conceptually simple framework to evaluate unproven processes and techniques for evidence of key interrelations and core concepts inherent in the QI philosophy.[19] The constituent elements of the model are data (D), attitudes (A), and tools (T). It is important to emphasize that merely stating the names of the model elements is insufficient for interpretation of the D*A*T acronym. The role of the asterisks (*) in denoting a multiplicative function is equally significant. The model is conceptualized as three overlapping circles arranged as shown in Figure 10–2. If the circles are visualized as different colors, the intersections of the circles would reflect the mixture of colors. If any color is absent, the center intersection is not the desired mixture of three colors. The D*A*T model is analogous in that the overlap represents the "*"—the interaction between the elements. CQI is seen as the product of the three elements such that if one element is absent (i.e., has a value of zero), CQI is also absent. This is not to imply that the individual elements are not useful in their own right. However, single elements or combinations of two elements do not produce CQI.

The model elements play unique and vital roles in achieving continual QI. Management guru Peter Drucker has said that information is data endowed with relevance and purpose. The integration of data into decision-making processes is critical to achieving QI. Attitudes are the shared beliefs, convictions, or philosophies that define the collective mind-set or expectations in an organization. The following attitudes are necessary for successful QI:

- Customer focus
- Process and systems thinking
- Data-based decision making

The tools of QI (i.e., statistical quality control, team building, decision matrices, planning diagrams) are used to achieve process improvement, facilitate databased decision making, and foster team attitudes and behaviors. As noted previously, proposed QI approaches that fail to acknowledge the importance of each element—data, attitudes, tools—and the interactions among them do not achieve the desired return. Consider this simple example. A procedure to collect and analyze patient complaint data may provide information about types and sources of complaints, but without attention to patient and worker attitudes, the improvement potential cannot be maximized.

Arguably the best-known names in quality literature are W. Edwards Deming, Joseph M. Juran, Philip B. Crosby, and Kaoru Ishikawa. These acknowledged quality gurus (and others) differ in their approaches to measuring and improving quality, but more important, they share certain similarities in their theoretical foundations. These similarities may be broadly grouped as follows:

- Leadership and vision to achieve quality objectives
- Organizational infrastructure or culture that fosters quality
- Customer focus in all aspects of operations
- Use of problem-solving methodologies
- Employee training and empowerment
- Goal of continuous improvement

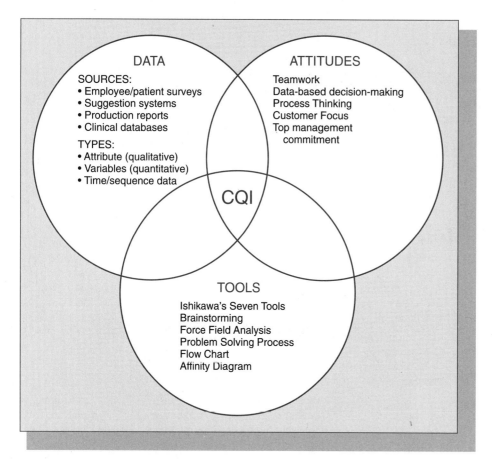

FIGURE 10–2. D*A*T model. (Adapted from Van Matre JG: The D*A*T approach to total quality management. Am Health Information Management Assoc 1992; Used with permission.)

The teachings and preferred methodologies of these men and other recognized experts are well documented in the quality literature.

Most problem-solving methodologies are essentially variations on the scientific method (i.e., controlled, systematic investigation of empirical evidence). The particular methodology chosen is not especially important. Leaders should consider the employee training necessary to ensure effective application and the adequacy of information generated from the process. Many hospitals find that the JCAHO 10-step process adequately serves their needs, but other methodologies may be preferred.

PDCA METHOD. One of the most widely used QI models is the PDCA (Plan, Do, Check, Act) method, developed in the 1920s by Walter Shewhart and popularized in Japan by Deming. The PDCA method has the benefits of being conceptually simple and easily taught and has few steps.

1. The planning phase consists of data collection and analysis to propose a solution for an identified problem.
2. The Do, or implementation, phase tests the proposed solution.

3. Checking monitors the effectiveness of the solution over a period of time.
4. The final phase, Act, formalizes the changes that have proved effective in the Do and Check stages.

The PDCA is conceived as a cyclical process, as shown in Figure 10–3. As one problem is resolved, another problem is investigated—beginning again with the planning stage and proceeding to action.

SEVEN-STEP METHOD. The seven-step method promoted by Joiner Associates, Inc., shares the benefits of the PDCA process and provides a standardized structure for documentation of QI projects.[20] The seven steps are as follows.

1. Define the project.
2. Study the current situation.
3. Analyze the potential causes.
4. Implement a solution.
5. Check the results.
6. Standardize the improvement.
7. Establish future plans.

SIX-STEP METHOD. A third basic CQI approach is presented by Re and Krousel-Wood with examples from

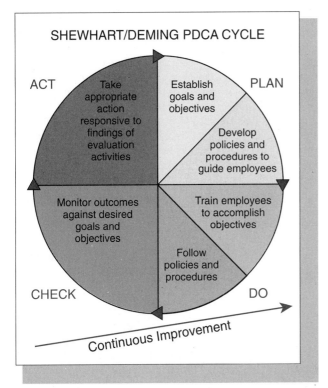

SHEWHART/DEMING PDCA CYCLE

ACT — Take appropriate action responsive to findings of evaluation activities

PLAN — Establish goals and objectives

Develop policies and procedures to guide employees

Train employees to accomplish objectives

Follow policies and procedures

Monitor outcomes against desired goals and objectives

CHECK

DO

Continuous Improvement

FIGURE 10–3. PDCA (Plan, Do, Check, Act) cycle.

a health care application.[21] This model uses the following six-step methodology.

1. Record adverse or other outcomes of interest.
2. Use statistical techniques to determine if variation is random.
3. Seek suggestions to reduce adverse outcomes.
4. Implement suggestions on a trial basis and monitor results.
5. If improvement occurs, implement suggestions and standardize.
6. Seek further suggestions for improvement.

CLINICAL AND ADMINISTRATIVE USE OF QA/QI INFORMATION

The chief executive officer, the governing body, and the officers of the medical staff share the responsibility for assuring the quality of patient care in a health care facility. This assurance can come only if the following elements are in place:

- Well-planned and well-maintained operational, clinical, and information systems
- Efficient and effective use of facility resources
- Mechanisms for objective assessment of individual and aggregate performance

- Corrective action as necessary coupled with feedback to accountable personnel

Aggregate and incident-specific QA/QI information generated through these processes is a valuable resource to medical and administrative leaders.

Information derived through performance assessment enables facility leaders to measure clinical and management outcomes and compare those outcomes with those of other facilities. **Benchmarking**, a process of comparing outcomes with those of an acknowledged superior performer, provides clear direction and objectives for performance improvement.

QA/QI information also contributes significantly to reports prepared for internal and external communications. Some information items may be collected and reported in response to direct inquiries for data. In other instances, QA/QI information may be used to adjust data to reflect case complexity, population-specific adverse risk factors, or other demographic or market characteristics. For example, an inner-city hospital that serves a primarily indigent population may experience a lower average birth weight for neonates than would be statistically expected. Including information that describes the market population served may help readers understand the data reported. *Remember relevance is a key factor in obtaining information from data.*

Personnel training and education needs may be evident from QA/QI projects. Targeting training activities to respond to identified needs offers a dual benefit; opportunities for performance improvement and monetary resources to support training are both maximized.

Patient and community education are natural outcomes of QA/QI activities. A review of clinical indicator data may identify instances in which patient noncompliance adversely affected outcomes. Perhaps patients are presenting in the emergency department with acute appendicitis, delaying their arrival until they are at risk for rupture of the appendix. The delay in seeking care may have resulted from unfamiliarity with the symptoms; from a demographic characteristic, such as lack of transportation; or from some failure of the delivery system. Each of these reasons can be addressed through community education, which can be used as a marketing tool to associate desirable behaviors and practices with facility products and services. In this example, a public service announcement describing the symptoms of appendicitis may be coupled with a hotline number in the emergency department or promotion of a hospital-based transport program.

The benefits derived from the availability of comprehensive information generated through QA/QI initiatives in a health care facility must be carefully balanced with obligations to protect the patient, the health care professional, and the organization. Assurance of confidentiality is often a key factor in gaining physician participation in the peer review process. *The confidentiality of information generated under peer review processes is statutorily recognized in every state.*[22] Because this privilege exists through state statutes, protection may differ among states. The courts tend to interpret the laws narrowly, and actions and documents not clearly defined in the state statute may not be protected. Protection under individual state statutes may be enhanced by careful attention to creating an infrastructure of policies and procedures congruent with provisions and limitations of the statute.

- Ensure that the documented purposes and structure of peer review committees conform to statutory guidelines.
- Use the formal structure outlined in medical staff bylaws, rules, and regulations rather than ad hoc or special committees for peer review activities.
- Restrict information dissemination to personnel covered by the statute.
- Provide physical security for peer review information.
- Educate all personnel and staff involved in peer review activities as to the nature and limitations of the privilege and as to policies and procedures that guide those activities in the hospital.
- Include provisions for confidentiality of all QA, peer review, and credentialing information in the medical staff bylaws.
- Channel **risk management** reports to the hospital attorney to invoke the attorney-client privilege.
- Audit policies and procedures periodically to ensure compliance with regulatory changes and protection for current practices.[22]

UTILIZATION MANAGEMENT

The goal of **utilization management (UM)** is to control inappropriate utilization of health resources. Ideally, the delivery system should be structured such that patients receive services at the least service- and resource-intensive level within the health care services continuum as appropriate to their individual health needs. The health care continuum is conceptualized as ranging from health promotion and disease prevention to hospice or terminal care. Providers of care—individual professionals and organizations—should accept patients into their segment of the continuum solely in response to medical necessity and discharge the patient as soon as maximum benefits have been achieved. In this context, "discharge" may be defined as transferring the patient into another segment of the continuum or as the patient exiting the delivery system altogether.

UM is not intended to result in lower technical or service quality. Every patient encounter is expected to be of the highest quality and to result in patient satisfaction. Health outcomes should not be diminished as a by-product of UM.

UR, the precursor to UM, has traditionally been considered a cost control mechanism that acknowledges that service intensity (considering both human and technologic resources) is positively correlated with cost. From a systems perspective, however, the higher order outcome is appropriate utilization of scarce and/or costly resources. Resource management at the micro or individual facility level is crucial to success at the macro or system level.

Historical Development

The amendments to the Social Security Act that created the Medicare program specified that provider hospitals must conduct URs for Medicare beneficiaries. Initially, these reviews were cursory examinations of the patient record by a physician (not the attending) every 14 days after admission. The reviewing physician used an informal peer review process to certify that continued inpatient care was necessary and that appropriate diagnostic and therapeutic services were being provided. If the reviewing physician determined that maximum inpatient benefit had been realized, discharge was recommended. The 14-day period before a review was initiated resulted in little effect on decreasing average lengths of stay, but the process was an important first step toward managing utilization. Physicians and other providers began learning to practice in an environment of accountability for health care costs as well as accountability for the quality of health care outcomes.

The second wave of evolution in UR came with the 1972 PSRO legislation—Public Law 92-603. This act created medical review entities that monitored quality and appropriateness of care provided to Medicare beneficiaries in inpatient facilities. Under PSROs, UR became more diagnosis-specific, with targeted lengths of stay and associated reviews based on regional norms. The PSROs were empowered to deny reimbursement for inappropriate admission and for continued hospitalization beyond the time certified as appropriate based on patient needs.

Legislation establishing the PPS restructured the PSROs as PROs and refined the focus of UR. Because hospitals are reimbursed a fixed price under PPS, regardless of a patient's length of stay, PRO review evaluates the necessity of inpatient admission and other quality initiatives with less emphasis on decreasing length of stay. A continuing objective of PRO review is identification of surgical and invasive diagnostic procedures that can be performed in outpatient settings without compromising patient safety or quality of care. Other changes in service delivery resulting from PRO reviews include restricting surgical assistants in uncomplicated cases and performing routine preprocedure diagnostic tests before admission.

The net effect of these evolutionary changes at the individual facility level has been to shift the focus from response to external mandates for UR to recognition of internal incentives for UM. Mandates still exist, but the scope of required review is insufficient to ensure the operational efficiency necessary for fiscal viability in the health care marketplace.

Objectives

Utilization management processes are intended to ensure that facilities and resources, both human and non-human, are used maximally but consistent with patient care needs. Both under-utilization (unmet patient needs) and overutilization (provision of care or services not medically necessary) are undesirable outcomes.

External Requirements

The most notable external agents that mandate UR in inpatient facilities are the federal government (for Medicare and CHAMPUS recipients) and the JCAHO. Medicare guidelines for UR are more prescriptive in orientation than JCAHO standards, which focus on the intent of UR as opposed to methodology.

Medicare Conditions of Participation

Peer review is a critical component of the reimbursement process. Individual hospitals submit claims for payment of covered services to the fiscal intermediary by way of the **UB-92**, the standardized billing form used by the HCFA to process Medicare claims, either through an electronic medium or in hard copy. The fiscal intermediary electronically transmits a duplicate of all claims submitted for a review period to the PRO. Individual claims are selected for review, using a specified sampling procedure (Table 10–6). The PRO notifies each participating hospital which discharges from its facility have been selected for review. The hospital either photocopies the designated records and mails the copies to the PRO or makes the records available to PRO personnel for on-site review. Reimbursement may be denied if a record fails review criteria. The intent of PRO review is to determine the following:

- Whether services are reasonable and medically necessary

- Whether services could effectively be furnished on an outpatient basis as opposed to inpatient admission

- Medical necessity, reasonableness, and appropriateness of inpatient services for which additional reimbursement beyond the diagnostic related group rate is sought (**outlier** cases)

- Inappropriate medical or other practices resulting in inappropriate admission or fraudulent billing for reimbursement

- Validity of diagnostic and procedural information submitted to request reimbursement

- Completeness and adequacy of care provided

- Whether the quality of services meets professionally recognized standards of care.[23]

Information derived from PRO review is available to the hospital by individual case and in aggregate reports. Annual reports aggregating data from all hospitals participating in the PRO are prepared to depict regional patterns of quality and utilization.

Joint Commission on Accreditation of Healthcare Organizations

The JCAHO defines UR as "the examination and evaluation of the appropriateness of the utilization of a hospital's resources."[6] In keeping with the systemic focus for improving individual and organizational performance, a separate UR chapter does not appear in the *AMH*. As with other performance assessment activities, UR standards have been incorporated into the Leadership, Information Management, and Improving Organizational Performance sections.

JCAHO standards are designed to evaluate how well the organization conducts UR, specifically with regard to appropriateness of inpatient admission and continuing hospitalization. Hospitals are also required to show evidence of consideration of "the appropriateness, clinical necessity, and timeliness of support services."[24] Leadership is charged with responsibility for allocation of resources necessary to ensure the effectiveness of UR activities.

Third Party Payers

Other third party payers, such as Blue Cross and Blue Shield, Travelers, and Aetna, incorporate UR requirements in their benefit plans. These requirements may include preadmission or preprocedure certification or retrospective review of patient records as a preliminary to processing claim forms for reimbursement. Some carriers require a concurring second opinion before certification for elective surgical procedures. Review mandates and procedures differ widely by payer. For this reason,

TABLE 10-6 PEER REVIEW ORGANIZATION SAMPLING PROCEDURE

REVIEW REQUIREMENT	SAMPLE
Random sample	6% beneficiary sample
Day outliers	HCFA identifies the outliers in the beneficiary sample—no specific percentage.
Cost outliers	Review when found in beneficiary sample and exceeds threshold by $3000
Readmissions	Review only when found in beneficiary sample
Transfers	Review only when found in beneficiary sample
Intervening care	Review when found in beneficiary sample to include ED, observation, outpatient continuing services, SNF, HHA, ambulatory surgery
Focused DRGs	Focused review when problem identified
Medicare code editor	Focused review when problem identified
Non-PPS hospitals	Review only when found in beneficiary specific sample
Ambulatory surgery	Review 3% facility-specific sample—procedure on ASC list (HOPD & ASC)
Requests for adjustment to higher DRG	HCFA identifies to PRO requests for higher DRG review or postpayment review
Preadmit or preprocedure	Only assistant surgeon at cataract surgery (specific codes)
Assist at cataract (preprocedure review)	Codes specified by HCFA—random sample retrospective to validate information
Freestanding cardiac catheterization facilities	No requirement
Technical denials	As necessary
Documentation review	All cases subject to review documentation to meet 42CFR 482.24(c) & 416.47(b) requirements. Documentation guidelines being developed by HCFA.
Swing bed unit waiver	Quarterly waiver determination based on denial rate
Hospital notices	All cases in which patient is liable for bill, hospital requests review, or notice issued on any "selected" cases
Beneficiary complaints	100% of beneficiary complaints re: quality in inpatient, hospital outpatient, and ASC, HHA, SNF
External referrals	100% of all referred cases
Intensified review	No specific triggers or levels; PRO identifies causes of aberrant patterns and may focus review to explore reason for unexplained aberrant patterns.
Uniform clinical data set	5% sample
Cardiovascular project	5% sample (100% review)

From Alabama Quality Assurance Foundation, Birmingham, AL.
DRG, diagnostic related group; ED, emergency department; HCFA, Health Care Financing Administration; PRO, peer review organization; SNF, skilled nursing facility; HHA, home health agency; ASC, ambulatory surgery center; HOPD, hospital outpatient department.

the admission process in most facilities includes collection of insurance information to ensure compliance with certification requirements. The actual data collection and certification procedures may be done by staff in the admitting physician's office or by hospital personnel.

Internal Incentives

Before the 1980s, hospitals had few direct incentives for UM. Cost- and charge-based reimbursement ensured patient revenue commensurate with operational expenditures. However, the rampant inflation of the late 1960s and early 1970s could not be tolerated, and cost-containment efforts at the system level eventually provided the impetus for control of resource utilization at the individual provider level. Early attempts at efficient allocation of constrained resources, such as regional health planning and certificate of need legislation, were largely unsuccessful in controlling health care costs. It was not until the monetary incentives in health care reimbursement were changed through fixed pricing, capitated prepayment, and other price controls that hospitals adopted a proactive stance toward UM.

In the health care marketplace of the 1990s and beyond, utilization controls are essential to achieving a competitive advantage. Costly technology and human resources must be used maximally to achieve acceptable per-unit prices. Efficient patient scheduling and employee staffing are important elements of an effective UM program. Increasing scrutiny by payers decrees that providers guarantee delivery of need-based services only. UM affords a degree of protection against delivery of nonreimbursed services.

Comprehensive and accurate utilization information is a critical administrative decision support tool. Executives who are negotiating preferred-provider contracts need utilization data coupled with cost reports. Planners analyze patterns and trends evident in utilization data to propose new product lines or recommend expanding or closing existing services. Utilization data that have been aggregated to reveal patterns or trends suggestive of inappropriate ordering practices for diagnostic or therapeutic procedures can be helpful to modify clinician behavior.

Program Components

Policies and procedures supporting UM programs may be uniquely designed at the facility level. Most programs, however, are similar because of the guiding influence of the JCAHO and the PRO. The primary functions in a UM program are UR and discharge planning.

Utilization Review

Effective UR requires assessment of medical necessity at a point in time when control over resource utilization can be effected. For inpatient facilities, the most critical control point is at the time of admission because an unjustified admission places the hospital at risk for absolute denial of reimbursement by third party payers for any services provided. Many insurance plans require preadmission or preprocedure certification, a form of *prospective review,* or evaluation of need before delivery of services. Admission certification by the insurance company ensures reimbursement for appropriate services provided during the course of the inpatient stay. Preadmission review consists of comparing information that describes the patient's medical condition with standard criteria that specifies clinical indications for inpatient admission. These criteria are referred to as IS/SI criteria —**intensity of service/severity of illness**—because they measure a need for health care resources that can only be provided in an inpatient facility or define a degree of acute physical impairment that requires inpatient medical intervention (Figure 10–4). Preprocedure

certification for elective surgical procedures is similar in intent and methodology to preadmission review, but criteria may be unique to individual insurance carriers. Preprocedure certification encompasses admission justification but may specify an approved length of stay or require that diagnostic testing be conducted on an outpatient basis. Hospital personnel usually must determine contract requirements for admission and procedure justification on an individual basis.

Even when not required by insurance carriers to precertify an admission, a hospital may elect to determine medical necessity for all admissions as a matter of policy. Typically, these reviews are conducted within 24 hours (or one working day) of admission and use the same procedures as preadmission certification. Admission justification conducted in this manner and evaluations to determine the necessity for continued inpatient stay are termed **concurrent reviews** because need is assessed simultaneously with provision of care and services. IS/SI criteria are appropriate for continued stay reviews because the intent is to determine the point at which the maximum benefits of inpatient care have been achieved. Discharge is indicated when information in a patient's health care record no longer conforms to the IS/SI criteria.

Medical necessity and appropriateness of care may also be investigated after the patient has been discharged through *retrospective reviews* (after services have been rendered). Retrospective review offers no opportunity to control inappropriate utilization for the patients in the sample but may provide valuable information about patterns of undesirable practices that can be used to improve future performance.

Case Management and Discharge Planning

Where UR looks at using inpatient resources maximally, case management and discharge planning functions are designed to move a patient efficiently between segments of the health care continuum. Efficient transfer between providers ensures continuity of care to the patient, permits cost control by the payer, and decreases the potential for reimbursement denial to the providers.

The incentives inherent in seeking access to care differ for patients and payers. When the patient does not bear the direct cost of care, the incentive is to seek greater access to technology and services. The payer seeks to meet the obligation to permit access to care at the lowest possible cost. Therefore, many insurance companies employ case managers, people who make decisions about the type and scope of health services a patient is entitled to access under his or her insurance coverage. The case manager certifies inpatient admission and approves transfer to other facilities or outpatient programs after discharge from a hospital. The payer goals are to ascertain medical necessity for all services

I. GENERIC

SEVERITY OF ILLNESS	NOTES/EXAMPLES

1. Oral temperature > or equal to 101°F (rectal temperature ≥ 102°F)
   a. culture/smear positive for pathogens (culture may be ordered and unreported at time of first review) or,
   b. WBC > or equal to 15,000/cu.mm.

2. Hemoglobin of < 8 grams or > 18 grams — Newly discovered

3. Hematocrit of < 25% or > 55% — Newly discovered

4. White blood count (WBC) >15,000/cu.mm. — Newly discovered

5. Serum sodium < 120 mEq/L or > 156 mEq/L

6. Serum Potassium < 3.0 mEq/L or > 6.0 mEq/L

7. Blood pH < 7.30 or > 7.50 — Newly discovered

8. PO_2 < 60 mm Hg and PCO_2 > 50 mm Hg — Newly discovered

9. Blood culture positive for pathogens

10. Sudden onset of functional impairment evidenced by one of the following:
    — Loss of sight/hearing
    — Loss of speech
    — Loss of sensation or movement of body part
    — Unconsciousness
    — Disorientation/confusion/neurobehavioral changes
    — Severe, incapacitating pain

11. Uncontrolled active bleeding at present time

12. Wound disruption (after major surgical procedure) requiring reclosure

13. History of vomiting or diarrhea and any one of the following:
    — Serum Na > 156 mEq/L
    — HCT > 55 or Hgb >16
    — Urine specific gravity > than 1.026
    — Creatinine > 2 mg% (recent onset)
    — BUN > 35 mg%

    Findings indicative of dehydration as a result of illness in any Body System and requiring in-hospital care

14. Acute onset of chest pain/pressure; dyspnea/cyanosis

15. Malignancy or recent history of surgery for malignancy — *Scheduled for IV chemotherapy or radiation*

(1)

SCREENING CRITERIA DESIGNED FOR NON-PHYSICIAN USE

FIGURE 10–4. IS/SI (intensity of service/severity of illness) criteria. (Used by permission of Alabama Quality Assurance Foundation, Birmingham, AL.)

I. GENERIC (CONTINUED)

INTENSITY OF SERVICE	NOTES/EXAMPLES
a. Special monitoring every 2 hours or more often as necessary/appropriate for patient's condition	TPR, B/P, CVP, ABGs, Pulmonary artery pressure (Swan-Ganz), arterial lines
b. Observation and monitoring of neurological status every 2 hours or more often as necessary/appropriate for patient's condition	Documented in medical record
c. Intravenous fluids (except KVO) and requiring at least 2000cc in 24 hours	
d. IV or IM medications every 12 hours or more frequently	If applicable to Severity of Illness
e. IV or IM analgesics 3 or more times daily	Pain not controlled as an outpatient
f. Respiratory assistance	Ventilator, O_2
g. Surgery performed (excluding outpatient surgery procedures list)	On admission or scheduled within 24 hours in continued stay

h. IV Chemotherapy: antineoplastic agent
1. Platinol based agent (initial or maintenance) when dosage is $\geq$ 60mg/m^2 or:
2. Methotrexate (>500mg) with Leucovorin rescue or:
3. Administered intracavitary, intrathoracic, intraarterial, intraperitoneal, or intraabdominal transfusions or:
4. Continuous or intermittent IV infusion of drugs for more than one day or:
5. Intrathecal administration for meningeal carcinoma with neurological symptoms or:
6. Intravenous antineoplastic agent with:
   a. History of previous severe adverse effect to agent or:
   b. Initial administration (not maintainence dose) for cancer or:
   c. Medical condition which prevents monitoring of patient and obtaining lab as an outpatient (bed bound)

Notes for item 4: Vinblastine Sulfate (Velban) or a combination of 2 or more agents

Notes for item 6a: Severe nausea or vomiting

i. Radiation
1. Intracavitary or interstitial therapy
2. Irradiation of weight bearing bone subject to fracture
3. Implantation of radioactive material in head, neck, or in reproductive organs
4. Isolation required due to radiation implant
5. IV pain medication necessary during radiation therapy
6. IV hydration necessary during radiation therapy

DISCHARGE INDICATORS

aa. Continued care and services could be rendered safely and effectively in an alternate setting.	
bb. Oral temperature < 101 °F for at least 24 hours without anti-pyretics.	
cc. Type and/or dosage of major drug unchanged for past 24 hours	
dd. No parenteral analgesics/narcotics for last 12 hours.	Exception: Chronic pain from terminal illness, or appropriate transfers to other facility
ee. Voiding or draining urine (at least 800cc) for last 24 hours or catheter removed and voiding sufficiently.	
ff. Passing flatus/fecal material	
gg. Diet tolerated for 24 hours without nausea or vomiting	
hh. Wound(s) healing. No evidence of infection without documented appropriate plan of outpatient treatment.	
ii. Discharged to SNF but refuses available SNF bed	
jj. Stable hemoglobin/hematocrit	

(2)

SCREENING CRITERIA DESIGNED FOR NON-PHYSICIAN USE

FIGURE 10–4 *Continued*

received and to ensure that those services are delivered in the most cost-effective setting.

Hospitals employ discharge planners to work with individual patients, their families, and their health care providers to determine the type and intensity of health care needed after discharge from the hospital. Unless postdischarge needs are identified and planned for, a patient's inpatient stay may be prolonged beyond the point of medical necessity. This places the hospital at risk for denial of reimbursement for services provided beyond the date of documented medical necessity and compromises the quality of care.

Methodology

Most hospitals use a two-stage review process with non-physician personnel conducting the initial review. Patient health records (or information submitted by the admitting physician for prospective reviews) are screened for documentation to establish compliance with predetermined criteria. If documentation is sufficient and criteria are met, admission or continued stay is deemed justifiable. If criteria are not met, the admitting physician may be asked to provide additional information or the case will be referred to a physician for peer review and discussion with the admitting physician. If documented compliance with the criteria cannot be achieved, the third party payer may withhold reimbursement for services provided.

Criteria Sources

A hospital may develop criteria for UR internally or adopt criteria from other sources, such as the IS/SI criteria used by the PRO. Whatever criteria are used, it is important that clinical validity has been determined. Criteria should be formally approved by the **medical staff organization (MSO)**.

Review Procedures

Utilization review personnel employed by the hospital conduct criterion-referenced review of clinical documentation in patient health records. Their role is to screen out cases in which documentation in the health record demonstrates compliance with accepted criteria for admission and continued inpatient stay. These acceptable cases are monitored for continued compliance, but they are not referred for physician peer review. Problematic cases, those with inadequate documentation to judge compliance or with evidence of noncompliance, are identified for administrative and clinical intervention.

When a health record lacks adequate documentation for comparison with criteria, the reviewer may contact the admitting physician to request additional information. The information needs may be met through more comprehensive admitting or progress notes, documentation of physical findings, or reports of diagnostic test results. If medical necessity is still not evident after additional information has been provided, the reviewer should refer the case for peer evaluation by a physician. Physicians who conduct peer UR may be employees of the hospital or members of the active medical staff who accept this role in the MSO peer review structure.

If, after review of the health record and discussion with the admitting physician (and sometimes examination of the patient), the UR physician cannot verify compliance with criteria, the case is deemed an inappropriate admission or continued stay. Nonjustified cases are referred for corrective action through procedurally defined channels to both the MSO and the hospital fiscal managers. For the best interests of the patient, the physician, and the hospital, adverse decisions about individual patients during the UR process must be resolved promptly.

When a physician reviewer fails to certify a patient's admission or continued stay, the hospital may notify the patient of probable noncoverage by the patient's third party payer. After receipt of the notice detailing the review process and outcome, the patient is expected to assume personal responsibility for payment of hospital charges incurred beyond the date specified in the letter. In most cases, the patient is discharged promptly. For many reasons, including the loss of community good will, the hospital prefers to avoid this type of review outcome.

Clinical and Administrative Use of UR Information

As with other medical care reviews, results of peer UR are reported through the MSO structure for evaluation of staff performance and consideration in the credentialing process. Summarized reports of all UR activity concerning the physician's patients are included in the physician's credentials file. Specific performance problems attributed to a physician may be reported to his or her MSO department chair for correction. For example, physicians who inadequately document health records may benefit from guidance by a colleague or review and discussion of UR criteria documentation requirements. Questions of clinical competence that arise from UR are properly handled through the MSO structure for self-governance. The MSO department chairs are responsible for evaluating the performance of MSO members assigned to their departments. Information generated through UR should be incorporated into the performance evaluations.

RISK MANAGEMENT

In the context of a health care facility, a risk is any event or situation that could potentially result in an injury or financial loss. An injury may be physical harm as we generally define it, but the definition used in legal terms is more encompassing. In the legal sense, harm or injury may be defined as any wrong or damage done to a person or to a person's rights or property. Although malpractice litigation often captures public visibility with large monetary awards for death or personal injury resulting from medical treatment, hospital administration and governance must be concerned with potential injury to all people who enter the hospital grounds for any reason. These potential claimants include patients, employees, visitors, contractual and business affiliates, and members of the medical staff. Risk management encompasses all policies, procedures, and practices directed at reducing risk and subsequent liability for injuries that occur in the hospital environment.

Historical Development

Structured risk management programs are essentially a response to what has been termed the medical malpractice crisis of the 1970s. Increasing numbers of claims coupled with sizable awards for damages and generous settlements pushed liability insurance premiums to unacceptably high levels. For many hospitals with unfavorable claims histories, the premiums paid for insurance coverage approached the face value of the policies purchased. Risk management programs were initiated to lower the incidence of occurrences that placed hospitals at risk for litigation and to manage effectively the aftermath of an adverse occurrence.

Few of the early risk management programs reached their potential to cultivate a safer environment and reduce the incidence of medical injuries. Program failures can in part be attributed to the lack of integration among the various activities aimed at QA. Without mechanisms to share relevant information across organizational units, problematic practices or unsafe physical facilities often were inadequately corrected because the scope of the problem was not well defined.

Objectives

Systematic risk management activities are intended to achieve the following goals:

- Minimize the potential for hospital injuries occurring
- Respond promptly and appropriately to injured parties
- Anticipate and plan for ensuing liability when injuries occur

External Requirements

Liability insurance carriers may require that hospitals engage in a structured process of risk identification and management as a condition of the policy purchased or discount premium payments if a risk management program exists. Professional liability insurance is a contractual arrangement much like any other insurance policy. Hospitals (and individual professionals) purchase protection against potential financial loss resulting from litigation through payment of premiums to an insurance company. Policy types may be broadly grouped into two categories: those that pay for *claims* made during the policy contract period and those that pay for *occurrences* during the policy contract period. The insurance carrier assumes greater risk under the occurrence format because claims may be filed after the contract has expired, with the length of time between injury and suit subject only to statutes of limitations on litigation. The policy may also be written to pay a maximum amount per year, regardless of the number of claims, or a maximum amount per claim.

The JCAHO requires that hospitals "provide a physical environment free of hazards and . . . manage staff activities to reduce the risk of human injury."[6] Responsibility for this charge is vested in the governing body, with operational responsibility delegated to a safety officer and a multidisciplinary safety committee. The standards, which appear in several sections of the manual, stipulate a risk assessment program; policies and procedures for data collection, aggregation, and reporting; and other specific organizational activities.

Internal Incentives

Claims history data and risk profiles are used to establish premium prices for liability insurance coverage. Stringent efforts by the insured to avoid or manage situations and events resulting in litigation may achieve lower premiums.

The spiraling cost of liability insurance has prompted many hospitals to self-insure for a portion or all of the coverage maintained. For example, the hospital may self-insure for the first $1 million of liability risk per year. Excess coverage that begins after the hospital has paid up to $1 million can be purchased for a much lower premium than first-dollar coverage. Under full self-insurance, the hospital assumes all costs associated with adverse judgments in the event of injury, which include the nontrivial costs of defending a claim in addition to payment of monetary awards. Attorney fees and salaries for personnel involved in the defense, loss of good will and public image, and other hidden costs should not be underestimated. These and other factors often lead to a decision to offer a financial settlement to the claimant as an alternative to defense against the suit. The value of an effective risk management program increases for hospitals that self-insure.

As social welfare agents, hospitals hold a public trust. Risk management programs acknowledge accountability to the public for a safe physical environment and adherence to accepted standards of clinical practice. Promotion of the advocacy mechanisms integral to a risk management program can be an effective public relations vehicle.

Program Components

The specific policies and procedures that constitute a risk management program at a hospital are developed in collaboration with the hospital legal counsel. Judicial interpretation of statutory law in the court system is a continually evolving process, and hospital leadership and governance are well advised to seek the advice of counsel to ensure that risk management practices adequately protect the organization. In general, the infrastructure of a risk management program is designed to do the following:

- Prevent or reduce financial loss
- Plan for and allocate funds for compensable events
- Diminish negative public image resulting from injury claims

Loss Prevention and Reduction

The best protection against injuries and ensuing financial liability is prevention. Prevention requires identifying and monitoring high-risk and problem-prone processes and physical plant locations. Historical aggregate data on injuries, identified hazards, complaints, and claims can be helpful to define risk indicators. Monitoring efforts may be directed at individual behaviors (wearing gloves to administer intravenous medications), physical safety (prominently displayed signs to indicate wet floors), personal security (functional locks on employee lockers), or some other aspect of corporate risk. Action to correct identified problems and follow-up to prevent recurrence are critical to the risk prevention process.

Loss reduction focuses on a single incident or claim and requires immediate response to any adverse occurrence. Injured people should receive prompt medical attention. Investigation of the incident should include examining the site and interviewing witnesses immedi-

ately after the occurrence to collect all pertinent facts. If the incident is considered potentially compensable, a claims representative for the liability insurance carrier should be contacted to ensure that all necessary information has been collected and appropriate responsive action taken. In many cases, prompt, sincere efforts to correct the problem can avert a claim for financial damages.

Claims Management

Claims management refers to the administrative and legal procedures initiated when adverse events are identified. For individual cases, these procedures may include the following:

- An internal audit of the hospital bill
- Examination of the health record for completeness
- Sequestration of financial and health records
- Interrogatories
- Settlement negotiations
- Preparation for trial
- Tracking of the status of claims
- Profiling of aggregate claims and losses
- Objective use of resulting information to improve individual and organization performance

Many claims by injured parties are settled without legal action. The insurance carrier or the hospital may determine that settlement is preferable to trial for several reasons, including insufficient information for adequate defense, risk of greater financial loss than the settlement amount, and adverse impact on public image. Payment is made to the claimant under the terms of the insurance contract or from reserve funds established by hospital governance.

Claims resolved through the court system often require defensive legal action over a period of several years. A finding against the hospital results in a monetary award to the claimant, usually paid out several years after the injury occurred. Substantial costs associated with the defense are incurred whether the courts find for or against the hospital. Financial planning to ensure adequate resources to meet future legal obligations requires accurate, complete information from the claims management program.

Safety and Security

All hospital personnel should assume responsibility for risk control by adhering to safety and security policies and procedures. Staff education plays an important role in maintaining a risk-free environment. The safety program should be introduced during the initial employee orientation and reinforced regularly through in-service educational programs. Training should address recognition of hazards, reporting procedures, and empowerment to correct hazardous situations that compromise safety or security. Hazard surveillance should be a routine operational procedure in all areas of the hospital with particular attention to public areas, such as waiting and vending areas, restrooms, stairs, and hallways. Areas not accessible to the public should be clearly marked and employees instructed to guide unauthorized people out of restricted areas.

Employee Programs

Employees are entitled to a safe and healthful workplace. This right is protected through the Occupational Safety and Health Act (OSHA) of 1971. The act created legally enforceable standards monitored through record keeping and reporting requirements and, in specified instances, through an on-site inspection process. Employers are required to maintain two forms that provide useful information in the risk management program. The Log and Summary of Occupational Injuries and Illnesses (OSHA Form 200) and the Supplemental Record of Occupational Injuries and Illnesses (OSHA Form 101) provide summary and detailed data, respectively, to track and analyze patterns of occurrences that involve employees.

Patient Relations

Building and maintaining a positive relationship between the hospital and the patients served is essential to an effective risk management program. Many hospitals employ a patient advocate (or patient services representative) to personalize interactions between patients and the hospital as an entity and to ensure prompt attention and response to patient complaints. A concerned person conveying the hospital's sincere desire to act responsibly after an injury or to correct a dissatisfying situation can often prevent escalation to legal proceedings.

Methodology

Occurrence screening (or generic occurrence screening) is a procedure for reviewing health records to identify documentation of any adverse clinical events for which the hospital could be held accountable if the patient chose to seek legal recourse. Adverse events that involve patients are termed **adverse patient occurrences (APOs)**. Examples of APOs might include a medication error that caused a drug reaction, performing a salpingo-oophorectomy when the patient had consented only to a hysterectomy, or failure to obtain informed consent for a procedure that resulted in sterilization. These and other events may also be referred to as **potentially compensable events (PCE)**, which means that if the hospital is found liable or agrees to a financial settlement to avoid litigation, the event will result in a financial outlay at some time in the future.

Health records can be screened for APOs as a step in the analysis procedure when processing records of discharged patients. Most hospitals have developed or adapted criteria to define what constitutes an APO and use these generic quality screens to identify cases for intervention (Figure 10–5).

Adverse clinical events identified through occurrence screening should be referred into the MSO peer review process to identify events attributable to inadequate medical care. *The validity of peer review is the true measure of the effectiveness of generic occurrence screening.*[25] Risk managers should track the number of APOs identified, the number referred for peer review, and the number attributed to medical care issues. Other useful information includes analysis of the severity of the APO, aggregations of data by the MSO department or patient care unit, and analysis of the effectiveness of response procedures. The documentation of process and behavioral changes resulting from analysis of APO data is essential to demonstration of QI.

An **incident report** is a written description of any event not consistent with routine operational procedures or patient care activities. The following are common examples of reportable occurrences:

- Needle sticks
- Patient or employee falls
- Medication errors
- Patient refusal to accept treatment

In some states, hospitals are required by law to report designated incidents to external agencies, such as the health department. More commonly, **incident reports** are prepared to assist the hospital in identifying and correcting problem-prone areas and in preparation for legal defense. Incident reports are *not* incorporated into the health record at any time. They are properly considered administrative documents prepared to facilitate intervention to minimize potential adverse effects of an undesirable event. Most hospitals use procedures to routinely submit the incident report form to the hospital legal counsel to invoke the attorney-client privilege and provide protection from discovery in the event of litigation. Incident reports should not be photocopied or prepared in duplicate. Strict adherence to procedures for preparing and routing incident reports directly to the attorney is critical to achieving protected status.

Patient advocacy is a proactive approach to ensuring patient satisfaction with the process and outcomes of care episodes. In addition to responding to individual

---

SAMPLE HOSPITAL

Unexpected Outcomes
Occurrence Screening Report

INDICATOR	PRESENT
1. Unexpected transfer to another acute facility.	
2. Unscheduled return to operating room.	
3. Unplanned organ removal/repair subsequent to or during surgery.	
4. Neurological deficit not present on admission.	
5. Patient fall resulting in injury.	
6. Nosocomial infection.	
7. Hospital-acquired decubitus.	
8. Unscheduled admission following outpatient surgery.	
9. Patient discharged against medical advice.	
10. Post-surgical death.	
11. Medication error or adverse drug reaction.	
12. Transfusion error or transfusion reaction.	
13. Return to intensive care unit within 24 hours of transfer to nursing unit.	
14. Abnormal physiological findings documented without further investigation or resolution.	
15. Complications attributed to anesthesia.	

FIGURE 10–5. Generic quality screens.

patient complaints, hospital staff monitor overall patient satisfaction with the hospital facility and staff interactions. Written questionnaires or telephone surveys are used to collect information about satisfying and dissatisfying events that happened to individual patients during their hospitalization. Complaints not identified or not resolved during hospitalization should be addressed immediately. Patterns of dissatisfying events or environmental factors evident from aggregate data should be communicated to appropriate personnel for correction.

The patient advocacy program may also encompass patient education. Information brochures, videotapes, public service broadcasts on the hospital television network, and other media facilitate communication between the patient and medical and professional staff. Better informed patients who participate in their own care are more compliant with treatment and achieve better outcomes. Patients who are informed about their treatment and prognosis and involved in decision making are more satisfied with their care providers. The American Hospital Association has published and disseminated a statement of patient rights and responsibilities. This statement is often included in patient information brochures provided at the time of hospital admission as evidence of patient advocacy.

Clinical and Administrative Use of Risk Management Information

Although quality and risk cannot and should not be considered separate issues in the administration of health care services, risk management documentation must be created and maintained in strict accordance with legal guidelines to prevent discoverability. Attorney-client privilege cannot be invoked for records maintained in the ordinary course of business or in provision of patient care.[26] Therefore, information about specific incidents or individual patients should be documented only as private communications between the risk manager or hospital leadership and the legal counsel. This communication may serve as the basis for administrative decisions or action plans to respond to an identified risk or PCE.

Aggregate data generated through facilitywide monitoring and evaluation activities, hazard surveillance, infection control, and other medical staff review activities are properly integrated into QI and peer review functions. Information is thus available to achieve the following objectives:

- Improve system processes
- Increase patient and employee satisfaction
- Improve clinical outcomes
- Decrease risk factors

CREDENTIALING

Credentialing refers to any process by which a practitioner is evaluated with the intent to effect control over his or her professional practice. More specifically within a hospital, the term refers to the policies and procedures used to determine the membership category and clinical privileges to be granted to a member of the professional staff. Clinical privileges ultimately are awarded at the discretion of the hospital governing body, although in most cases, decisions are based on the recommendations of the active medical staff through an executive committee.

Historical Development

Before 1900, physicians were autonomous craftsmen, free to choose from among multiple education or training avenues in preparation for practicing one of several medical philosophies. Clinical skills were evaluated only by patients. Physicians practiced their craft at will, limited solely by the ability to attract and maintain patients. Medical practice was typically office-based, with few hospitals in existence.

Today, physicians are products of a standardized academic curriculum, having achieved a well-defined level of clinical competence. They are permitted to offer their services to the public at the discretion of the state and may perform only those procedures allowed by hospital affiliation or within the scope of state professional practice laws.

This evolution from individual autonomy to regulated practice has been achieved through the direction and

influence of key events and players both internal and external to the medical profession. These events can be grouped into the following major areas:

- Restriction of access to the profession through control of the academic process
- Regulation of the right to practice through licensure
- Definition of a physician's scope of practice through **privilege delineation**
- Assurance of clinical competence through peer review

Objectives

The primary objective of professional staff credentialing is to ensure that staff members perform only procedures and services for which they are qualified through training and experience. Ensuring staff competence is an important factor in both QA and risk control.

External Requirements

As with other systems and processes to ensure health care quality, the JCAHO is a key player in establishing guidelines for credentialing professional staff. Other influential catalysts for credentialing mechanisms are state restrictions on professional practice and federally legislated reviews.

Joint Commission on Accreditation of Healthcare Organizations

From its inception, the JCAHO has emphasized physician credentialing as a key factor in the accreditation process. As printed in the January 1924 *Bulletin,* Standard 1 addresses the organizational structure of "physicians and surgeons *privileged* [italics added] to practice in the hospital."[7]

The Quality of Professional Services Standard in the 1979 *AMH* incorporated requirements for using information collected during peer reviews assessing quality of care in the credentialing process. The guidelines specifically addressed privilege delineation. This requirement was an important step in the evolution of physician credentialing.

The JCAHO has consistently maintained the position that privilege delineation is entirely within the purview of the individual facility and that credential reviews conducted by other facilities or agents should not be automatically accepted. As noted by JCAHO president Dennis O'Leary, the JCAHO strives to define a better approach to monitoring clinical competence of professional staff and to incorporate this information when granting clinical privileges to medical staff members. The JCAHO continues to be a driving force in maintaining an environment that stresses continuing improvement in quality, efficiency, and cost-effectiveness of health care services.

Licensure

State licensure laws played a crucial role in the restriction of physician autonomy. Early attempts at using medical licensure "to upgrade medical education, control proliferation of medical cults, and reduce competition" began in the late 1700s, but these initial nonstandard laws could not be adequately enforced.[27] During the 1800s, most medical licenses were given on receipt of the medical degree without guarantee of professional competence or were used simply as a registration mechanism by the local medical society.[4] In his now-famous report, Flexner viewed examination by licensing boards as "the lever with which the entire field may be lifted."[5] At the time of his survey, Flexner reported that no board fulfilled the conditions necessary to accomplish this objective.

Operating as agents of the state, the duty of licensure boards is to ensure that professionals are qualified to practice with reasonable skill and safety. The boards are thus empowered to award, deny, limit, suspend, or revoke a person's license and to invoke disciplinary actions specific to practice behaviors under the scope of the license granted. Graduate physicians seeking licensure in any state must pass either the sequence of examinations conducted by the National Board of Medical Examiners or the Federal Licensing Examination (FLEX) to qualify.

The National Board of Medical Examiners is a voluntary organization that assists states in developing licensing regulations. The board administers a three-part examination that may be used to qualify for state licensure. Medical schools may elect to require parts I and II as prerequisites to graduation. After graduation, a candidate must take either part III or the FLEX to qualify for licensure.

The FLEX was introduced in 1968 by the Federation of State Medical Boards and, subsequently, has been adopted by all states as a licensing examination. Nationwide adoption of the FLEX was a major step toward uniformity of state licensure requirements.[28] The Federation of State Medical Boards, established in 1912, is composed of state and territorial medical licensing boards. In addition to physician testing before licensure, the federation plays a second significant role in the credentialing process. It began collecting reports of disciplinary actions in 1915, a continuing function that has been computerized since the early 1980s. The Physician Board Action Data Bank contains reports of actions by state licensing boards and expulsions from the Medicare and Medicaid programs. This information can be accessed by individual facilities as part of their credential screening process, but there is no requirement to do so.

Health Care Quality Improvement Act and the National Practitioner Data Bank

Determination of clinical competence during the credentialing process is based on peer review of objective documentation. As corporate liability for negligent physician practice compelled hospitals to establish a more stringent credentials process, the inevitable reaction was physician litigation in response to negative decisions. Physicians whose requests for staff appointment are denied or whose clinical privileges are restricted or denied *must* have access to due process. Failure of due process to satisfy the claimant may result in litigation against the hospital and against the physicians who perform peer review for restraint of trade under the Sherman Antitrust Act or for character defamation. Denial of privileges has been upheld by the courts only in the limited context of quality of care issues.

A successful antitrust lawsuit in Oregon, *Patrick v. Burget*, subsequently upheld at the U.S. Supreme Court level, had a significant impact on physician credentialing. The court ruled that suit was permissible if denial of privileges was based solely on economic competition. Three physicians were found guilty of antitrust violations for failure to appoint a competing physician to the medical staff.

The issues emerging from the *Patrick* case had so many implications for the hospital sector that Congress passed the Health Care Quality Improvement Act (HCQIA)—Public Law 99-660—in 1986, before the Supreme Court's decision in 1988. The HCQIA denoted the initial entry of the federal government into the credentialing process, which had previously been a facility prerogative directed toward compliance with accreditation standards and accountability for provision of quality care.

The HCQIA mandated development of the National Practitioner Data Bank as a mechanism to collect physician-specific information about quality of patient care and adverse outcomes. The HCQIA legislation provided for reporting malpractice payments made (later stipulated as awards in excess of $30,000), negative actions by licensure boards or professional societies, and denial, loss, or reduction of clinical privileges for a period exceeding 30 days in any facility.[29] Noncompliance with the reporting requirements of the act carries severe penalties, including loss of immunity and suspension from the Medicare program.[30] Failure of responsible parties to report malpractice payments may result in a monetary fine of up to $10,000 per payment.[31]

The HCQIA provides protection from financial liability to health care entities, governing boards, and committees for information submitted to the data bank as a result of peer review during the credentialing process. These conditions apply when the following criteria are met.

- Action was taken in good faith and based solely on competence.
- Due process procedures were followed.
- The hospital fulfilled its reporting obligations under the act.[32]

Hospital and MSO leaders should note that the courts generally have not considered this federal privilege to extend to hospital-based peer review decisions.[22]

The data bank became operational on September 1, 1990. Since that time, hospital medical staffs considering applications for membership (either initial appointment or reappointment) or requests for clinical privileges *must* query the data bank to identify any available adverse quality of care information about the applicant. Other parties, including malpractice attorneys, *may* query the data bank under certain conditions. The confidentiality of information contained in the bank is protected and regulated by the Department of Health and Human Services through the HCFA. Individuals or organizations that violate the confidentiality regulations are subject to a $10,000 penalty.[29]

Internal Incentives

Medical staff credentialing within the hospital environment before 1965 was viewed almost entirely from the perspective of ensuring quality care. Dimond discusses several landmark legal decisions that forced hospital governing boards to consider credentialing as a protective mechanism against litigation and financial loss.[33] Perhaps the most notable case was in 1965, when *Darling v. Charleston Community Memorial Hospital* established precedent for hospital liability because of the negligent acts of members of its medical staff. This decision marked the end of the doctrine of charitable immunity for hospitals. In other cases, hospitals have been held accountable for supervising the competence of physicians and surgeons, for failure to identify incompetent physicians, and for negligence in performance of peer review activities.

Hospitals and other health care entities have a social welfare responsibility to the public they serve. A major component of this responsibility is assurance of the technical competence of those who practice their professions under the auspices of the organization. The professional staff credentialing process is an objective mechanism used by the governing body to demonstrate accountability for professional staff practice behav-

iors and associated clinical outcomes in a proactive manner.

Program Components

The credentialing process should not be viewed as static or composed of unconnected activities; however, it is important to distinguish between appointment or reappointment to the medical staff and award of clinical privileges to members of the staff. Although these two functions are conducted at fixed points in time—typically biennially—information collection to support these functions is an ongoing process.

Appointment or Reappointment

Medical staff **appointment** or **reappointment** assigns qualified applicants to an existing unit of the MSO and designates a membership category.

The MSO units may be designated in the bylaws as departments or clinical services. Some authors distinguish departments as the administrative or political unit and clinical service as the patient care unit. In the context of MSO membership, the term department is an appropriate generic term to discuss member rights and responsibilities. Department members carry out the organizational duties necessary for maintenance of the MSO structure. These duties may include committee service, peer review, recommendations to hospital leadership, and other activities that ensure accountability for department operations.

The membership category describes the degree to which members use the hospital, the length of time an appointment has been held, or some other factor specific to the hospital. Membership category titles are active, associate, courtesy, consulting, honorary, faculty, house staff, and provisional. The organizational privileges and responsibilities attached to each category title are specified in the MSO bylaws. The following are general descriptions.

Active staff members—have the full rights, privileges, and responsibilities of membership. They may include but need not be limited to voting rights, obligatory meeting attendance, and expected service on committees.

Associate status—often granted at initial appointment to permit a period of oversight by members of the active staff. Associates may be granted voting rights but face fewer expectations for committee service and other organizational duties.

Courtesy staff—hold clinical privileges but are without responsibility for organizational maintenance duties. Physicians who admit infrequently may request courtesy appointments.

Consulting staff—physicians and nonphysician professional staff who do not admit patients but who provide consulting and support services to attending physicians.

Honorary staff membership—granted to honor distinguished members of the medical community. Retired members of the active staff may hold honorary appointments to acknowledge a continuing collegial relationship with the MSO. Honorary members do not enjoy clinical privileges, voting privileges, or other membership rights or face responsibilities for organization activities.

Faculty—applicable only to teaching facilities and designates staff participating in the medical education program.

House staff—classification for interns and residents in the medical education programs of a teaching hospital. House staff practice as permitted by their medical license under the supervision of an assigned member of the faculty or active staff. Members of the house staff have no vote or membership privileges or organizational maintenance responsibilities, although some hospitals may encourage service on medical staff committees.

Applicants for initial appointment or those requesting new or extended privileges may be required to serve a period of provisional membership. The provisional period is used to permit observation and monitoring by a senior member of the staff to evaluate performance of membership duties and clinical competence. For new appointees, the duration of the provisional appointment may be specified as a period of time. For the purpose of determining clinical competence, a number of procedures or other measures may be used.

MSO applicants who accept an appointment agree to abide by the bylaws, rules, and regulations governing the MSO. A signed statement to this effect is maintained in the credentials file.

Credentials Verification

Credentials verification is primarily an administrative process to determine that an applicant has provided all required documents for review pursuant to staff appointment. Specific documentation and procedures required to apply for appointment and privileges vary among hospitals, but requirements are documented and made known to all applicants. All hospitals should require proof of the following:

- Education and training
- Liability insurance coverage
- Current licensure

- Clinical competence
- Description of health status

Privilege Delineation

Privilege delineation refers to the process of determining the specific procedures and services a physician or other professional is permitted to perform under the jurisdiction of the hospital. At the time of initial appointment and each subsequent reappointment, the applicant should formally request specific privileges. Many hospitals maintain a checklist of approved procedures. The applicant identifies those for which permission is requested. Any award of privileges should be supported with documentation of training, education, and other evidence of qualification or competence.

Failure to verify an applicant's credentials in the appointment and privileging process places the MSO and the hospital at risk of liability for injuries resulting from practitioner incompetence. The courts consistently have held hospitals accountable for the governing body's responsibility to know about the competence of people granted privileges.

Practitioner Profiles

Practitioner profiles are frequently used as a mechanism to integrate information compiled from QA/QI activities into the credentialing process. A physician's unique profile incorporates findings from all required review functions, summaries of participation in MSO committees, pertinent judgments from external review agencies such as the PRO or licensure board, and clinical activity information such as number of patients admitted. Many hospitals also include such data as the number of meetings attended and the continuing medical education credits earned at hospital-sponsored programs. Specific profile data are determined by MSO policies and procedures for credentialing (Figure 10–6).

These profiles provide a concise summary of information crucial to objective credentialing of professional staff. When properly prepared and exploited, the profiles contribute to objectivity in credentialing decisions. The inclusion of comprehensive profile documents in credentials files demonstrates the administrative mechanism used to integrate QA/QI data into the MSO appointment and privilege delineation processes.

Nonphysician Professional Staff

The nonphysician professional staff should be included in the credentialing process. These professionals are dentists, psychologists, podiatrists, and others permitted by the scope of their professional license to practice independently.

CREDENTIALS COMMITTEE REVIEW SHEET
PRACTITIONER REAPPOINTMENT PROFILE
REAPPOINTMENT PERIOD 1994–1995

1   AAEXAMPLE   DOCTOR   DPT   CATEGORY   SPECLTY

BASIC HOSPITAL STATISTICS:

DISCHARGES:	123	INPATIENT DAYS:	1234
CONSULTS:	123	OUTPATIENT ADMISSIONS:	123
INPT PROCEDURES:	123	HOSPITAL DEATHS:	123
OPT PROCEDURES:	123		

* *

THE FOLLOWING FINDINGS MUST DEMONSTRATE ACCEPTABLE PERFORMANCE FOR REAPPOINTMENT

* *

BYLAW REQUIREMENTS: 1   GS-MTG   1   DEPT-MTGS   12   CME

* * * * * * * * * * * * * * * PERFORMANCE FROM QUALITY REVIEW MONITORS * * * * * * * * * * * * * * * * *

MEDICAL RECORDS:	1	SUSPENSIONS	1	DELINQUENT
	12	RECORDS REVIEWED		
MEDICAL PEER REVIEW:	12	REVIEWED	12	JUSTIFIED
SURGICAL PEER REVIEW:	12	REVIEWED	12	JUSTIFIED
CRITICAL CARE QI:	1	REVIEWED	1	JUSTIFIED
MORTALITY REVIEW:	12	DEATHS REVIEWED	12	JUSTIFIED
BLOOD UTILIZATION:	12	REVIEWED	12	JUSTIFIED
DRUG UTILIZATION:	12	ORDERS CLARIFIED	0	LETTERS SENT
UTILIZATION REVIEW:	1	DENIALS	0	LETTERS SENT
PEER REVIEW COMMENTS:	QI COMMENTS FOR UNJUSTIFIED REVIEWS			

* *

BASED UPON REVIEW OF THIS INFORMATION, THE FOLLOWING IS RECOMMENDED:

(   ) NO   (   ) YES   ADJUSTMENTS TO CLINICAL PRIVILEGES REQUESTED
(   ) NO   (   ) YES   ADJUSTMENTS TO STAFF CATEGORY_____
(   ) YES   (   ) NO   RECOMMEND REAPPOINTMENT

_____   _____
For the Department   Credentials Committee Chairman

Hospital Statistics/Quality Review Monitor Information given is for January 1992–June 1993.
Citizenship Information and General Staff Meeting Attendance is for January 1992–October 1993.

FIGURE 10–6. Practitioner reappointment profile. (Courtesy of The Children's Hospital, Birmingham, AL.)

Methodology

In recent years, the process for credentialing physicians and other members of the professional staff has become fairly standardized among all hospitals in the United States. A flowchart of a typical application process is shown in Figure 10–7. Physician credentialing couples peer determination of clinical competence with administrative review of documents submitted for verification of education, specialty training, previous clinical experience, compliance with licensing laws, proof of insurance coverage, and other information specifically required by the hospital. As with other peer review processes, the administrative examination of documentation

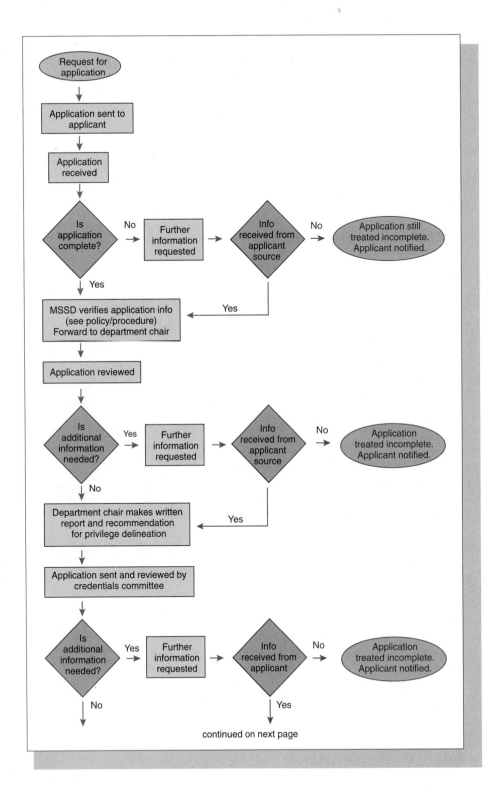

FIGURE 10–7. Application flowchart. (From Medical Staff Organization Management: Independent Study Modules, Module IV, Lesson 1. Knoxville: National Association of Medical Staff Services, 1993, pp 10–11. Used by permission.)

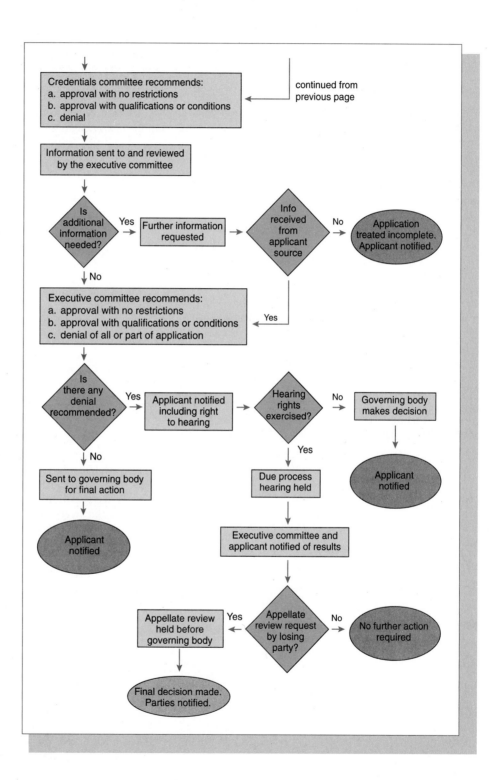

FIGURE 10–7 *Continued*

is conducted first. This procedure precludes unnecessary peer review of applicants who are ineligible for reasons other than clinical competence and ensures the presence and completeness of all necessary information to enable peer review.

Medical Staff Services Professional

The National Association of Medical Staff Services was created in 1971 and incorporated as a national nonprofit organization in 1978. The association initiated an examination-based certification program in 1981 that leads to the credential Certified Medical Staff Coordinator (CMSC) and recognizes those people who demonstrate mastery of the defined body of knowledge.[34] A minimum of 30 hours of continuing education every 3 years is required to maintain the CMSC credential. The medical staff services professional (MSSP) plays a key support role in the MSO, particularly in coordinating the administrative procedures critical to the credentialing process.

Physicians and other professionals seeking appointments to the MSO make a preliminary request for information. The MSSP responds with a cover letter and information detailing the application process. A copy of the MSO bylaws, forms used to request privileges, and authorization forms to investigate education and previous staff appointments are also included. Because of the time and costs associated with credentials verification, a preliminary screen to determine eligibility for application may be a valuable policy. All preapplication procedures must be conducted within the parameters of the Americans with Disabilities Act.

The formal application for membership and request for clinical privileges are an extensive portfolio of documents that detail an applicant's professional experience, beginning with graduation from medical school and concluding with current staff affiliation. It is important to account for all time periods.

The MSSP verifies the accuracy and completeness of each information document submitted. This is done by contacting schools, hospitals, and personal and professional associates referenced in the portfolio. Written and telephone requests for verification should be documented and all responses included in the credentials file.

The MSSP must also query the National Practitioner Data Bank and include the report in the documents available for review in the credentialing process. Hospitals are required by law to query the data bank whenever a health care practitioner applies for membership or clinical privileges and every 2 years for practitioners who hold staff appointments.[35] Queries may be submitted on a data bank form or by electronic medium. The hospital is billed for a filing fee.

Hospital-specific information requirements may include the following:

- Documentation of a physical examination
- Photocopy of the applicant's Drug Enforcement Agency certification that shows the unique registration number authorizing prescriptions of controlled substances
- Proof of a minimum specified amount of liability coverage

When all required documentation is present and has been verified for accuracy, the application portfolio should be submitted to the MSO credentials committee.

Credentials Committee

In most health care organizations, it is impractical for the entire medical staff to conduct peer review of individual applicants for staff membership. This review function (and others) is properly delegated to a committee or smaller groups of active staff members who act on behalf of the staff as a whole. The JCAHO requires a mechanism to review credentials but does not specify a committee per se. The executive committee of the medical staff is charged with making recommendations for appointment and clinical privileges to the governing body.

The credentials committee functions in an advisory capacity only and is not empowered to make appointments or grant privileges. The committee members review available information about applicants and make recommendations for staff appointment and award of clinical privileges to the governing body through the communication mechanisms designated in the medical staff bylaws, rules, and regulations. Typically, the executive committee of the medical staff serves as the formal communication link between the medical staff and the governing body regarding credentialing issues.

Clinical and Administrative Use of Credentialing Information

Accurate, comprehensive, and timely credentialing data are crucial to fulfilling the hospital's social responsibility for assurance of safe, quality health care to the population served. The profile information generated in the credentialing function is invaluable to both clinical and operational administrators. The credentials files serve as a repository for data specific to MSO criteria that are collected on individual physicians at regular intervals. In the simplest sense, the credentialing process serves as a performance appraisal of medical staff members. The individual physician data assess productivity, efficient and effective use of hospital resources, and quality of intervention outcomes. Aggregate data provide opportunities for comparisons across service units. Chiefs of medical staff units can use the data to identify continuing medical education needs and as an early-warning system of quality and risk issues. The data are also used to make such decisions as assignment of operating room time, access to diagnostic facilities, and other resource allocation issues. More productive physicians enjoy better access to constrained resources.

Hospital leaders use aggregate activity data from the profiles to support strategic plans for improving operational effectiveness or to justify expanding or decreasing product lines. Capital budget decisions are often influenced by examination of profile data. For example, purchase of an expensive laser device is not feasible if too few staff physicians have the necessary training and skill to qualify for privileges to use the device or if patient caseload is insufficient to use the equipment optimally. As with clinical administrative decisions, priority in requests for financial support for medical staff projects is often reflective of the physicians' contribution to the fiscal viability of the hospital.

MEDICAL STAFF COMMITTEES

The MSO is a self-governing entity that operates as an extension of the hospital governing body. Although the governing body retains ultimate legal and moral responsibility for the quality of professional services provided in the hospital, responsibility and accountability are operationally delegated to the MSO.

Bylaws, Rules, and Regulations

The organizational structure used to achieve this directive and to maintain the administrative functioning of the MSO is delineated in the MSO bylaws, rules, and regulations. The MSO bylaws, rules, and regulations are a collection of documents that articulate the framework within which the members of the MSO act and interact in hospital-related activities. Physicians and other professional staff members who are granted appointments must agree to abide by the bylaws, rules, and regulations as a condition of their appointment. The bylaws should be reflective of current structure and operational practices to guide behavior and to protect individual members and the MSO in legal proceedings. MSO bylaws are officially adopted by majority vote of the medical staff and formally approved by the governing board. Neither party may unilaterally amend the bylaws, and official action by both parties is required before bylaws are effective. Therefore, bylaws are of necessity global in orientation to prohibit frequent revisions. Supplemental written policies and procedures are used as guides to action in specific instances but must not be in conflict with or supersede the bylaws.

Joint Commission on Accreditation of Healthcare Organizations

The JCAHO standards do not impose a specific form of organizational structure for the MSO but do require an infrastructure supportive of self-governance, accountability to the governing body, and achievement of required functions. The standards stipulate adoption of bylaws, rules, and regulations and administrative structures within clinical departments to ensure continuing viability of the MSO. Although most standards address required functions, several standing committees of the MSO are required.

JCAHO-Required Committees

The JCAHO dictates certain standing committees to achieve compliance with required MSO functions. Committees specified in the *AMH* are described below.

EXECUTIVE COMMITTEE. The JCAHO requires an executive committee empowered to act on behalf of the MSO between formal meetings of the entire staff.[6] The executive committee is the predominant policymaking and action committee of the MSO. Typically, this committee is composed of the elected officers of the MSO and department chairpersons at a minimum. The function, size, and composition of this committee are as defined in the MSO bylaws, with two provisions dictated by the JCAHO. First, all members of the medical staff must be eligible for service, and second, a majority of committee members must be fully licensed physicians practicing on the active staff of the hospital. Additionally, the chief executive officer (or designee) attends executive committee meetings in an ex officio capacity.

The following executive committee functions are specified by the JCAHO:

- Receiving reports and taking action on recommendations from other units of the MSO
- Making recommendations to the governing body relative to MSO issues

These issues should include but are not necessarily limited to MSO structure; evaluation mechanisms and recommendations for staff membership, credentialing, and privilege delineation; QA/QI activities; and mechanisms for termination from the medical staff and fair hearing procedures.

SAFETY COMMITTEE. Members of the safety committee are appointed from the administrative, clinical, and support services by the chief executive officer or designee. The safety committee provides policy and procedural guidance to the safety officer who is responsible for operational management of the safety program. At a minimum, the safety committee meets bimonthly to review and analyze reports prepared by the safety officer.

The safety management program encompasses the following:

- Risk assessment

- Hazardous materials and waste management

- Emergency preparedness (disaster) planning

- Education of personnel to function effectively within the safety policies and procedures

- Security

- Fire safety

- Equipment

- Utilities management programs

Each of these programs is guided by written plans, policies, and procedures that delineate individual roles and responsibilities. All involved personnel are oriented to the programs and trained to assume their responsibilities. Simulations and drills are conducted at specified intervals to test the operational effectiveness of written plans and competence of personnel to fulfill their assigned duties.

INFECTION SURVEILLANCE, PREVENTION, AND CONTROL COMMITTEE. Oversight responsibility for the infection control, surveillance, and prevention processes is vested in a multidisciplinary committee. This committee, composed of representatives of the medical staff, nursing, administration, and other departments as needed, is required to meet at least quarterly. At a minimum, the following responsibilities are designated:

- Review of microbiologic reports

- Review of patient infections

- Determination of nosocomial infections

- Performance of prevalence and incidence studies

- Review of routine or special collection data appropriate to objectives[6]

The infection control function is extremely important. The scope of activities directed at infection control is organizationwide and encompasses inpatient, outpatient, service, and diagnostic areas as well as support services. Although program oversight is a committee responsibility, program management is assigned to a person or people qualified in infection surveillance, prevention, and control.

Committee Reporting Structure

The predominant requirement for committee reporting is that the executive committee of the MSO receives and acts on reports from other committees and the clinical departments and services. Committees chartered within the clinical departments and services may report to the executive committee through the appropriate department chair.

Clinical and Administrative Use of Committee Information

Information regarding the quality and appropriateness of patient care that originates from MSO committees is pivotal to the professional staff credentialing and QI processes.

Key Concepts

- The quality initiatives in health care delivery have shifted from response to external mandates to recognition of internal incentives for continuous improvement.

- Integration among the various elements of a quality program is essential to overall program effectiveness.

- Regulations and incentives guiding QA/QI activities are subject to frequent change. Program management requires dynamic leadership.

References

1. Orme CN: Customer information and the quality improvement process: Developing a customer information system. Hosp Health Serv Administration 1992;37(2):197–212.

2. Collopy BT: Do doctors need Deming? Qual Assur Health Care 1993;5(1):3–5.

3. Goldsmith J: A radical prescription for hospitals. Harvard Business Review, May-June 1989, 104–111.

4. Rosenfeld P: Protecting the public or promoting the profession: A sociological history of medical licensing law, 1990–1910. Stony Brook: State University of New York, 1984. Dissertation.

5. Flexner A: Medical education in the United States and Canada. Bethesda, MD: Science & Health Publications, 1910.

6. 1994 Accreditation manual for hospitals, Vol 1, Standards. Chicago: Joint Commission on Accreditation of Healthcare Organizations, 1993.

7. Roberts JS, Coale JG, Redman RR: A history of the Joint Commission on Accreditation of Healthcare Organizations. JAMA 1987;258(7):887–940.

8. Patient care quality defined. Joint Commission on Accreditation of Healthcare Organizations: Perspectives on Accreditation 1989;9(112):7.

9. Donabedian A: Explorations in quality assessment and monitoring. Vol 1, The definition of quality and approaches to its assessment. Ann Arbor, MI: Health Administration Press, 1980.

10. Bernstein SJ, Hilborne LH: Clinical indicators: The road to quality care? J Qual Improvement 1993;19(11):501–509.
11. Nadzam DM, Turpin R, Hanold LS, White RE: Data driven performance improvement in health care: The Joint Commission's Indicator Measurement System (IMSystem). J Qual Improvement 1993;19(11):492–500.
12. Joint Commission on Accreditation of Healthcare Organizations: Agenda for change Q & A: Indicators and the IMS. Joint Commission Perspectives 1992;12(5):9.
13. Agenda for change (information package). Chicago: Joint Commission on Accreditation of Healthcare Organizations, 1993.
14. Van Amringe M, Shannon TE: Awareness, assimilation, and adoption: The challenge of effective dissemination and the first AHCPR-sponsored guidelines. QRB Qual Rev Bull 1992;19(12):397–404.
15. Field MJ, Lohr KN (eds): Clinical practice guidelines: Directions for a new program. Washington, DC: National Academy Press, 1990.
16. Lohr KN, Schyve PM: Reasonable expectations: From the Institute of Medicine. QRB Qual Rev Bull 1992;18(12):393–396.
17. Townsend MB: Patient-focused care: Is it for your hospital? Nurs Management 1993;24(9):74–80.
18. Vogel DP: Patient-focused care. Am J Hosp Pharm 1993;50:2321–2329.
19. Van Matre JG: The D*A*T approach to total quality management. J Am Health Information Management Assoc 1992;63(11):38–44.
20. Gaudard M, Coates R, Freeman L: Accelerating improvement. Qual Progress 1991;24(10):81–88.
21. Re RN, Krousel-Wood MA: How to use continuous quality improvement theory and statistical quality control tools in a multispecialty clinic. QRB Qual Rev Bull 1991;16(11):391–397.
22. McCann RW: Protecting the confidentiality of peer review information. Am Health Information Management Assoc 1993;64(12):52–56.
23. Alabama Quality Assurance Foundation: PRO—physician—hospital outreach meeting. Information packet, 1993.
24. 1994 Accreditation manual for hospitals, Vol 2, Scoring guidelines. Chicago: Joint Commission on Accreditation of Healthcare Organizations, 1993.
25. Sanazaro PJ, Mills DH: A critique of the use of generic screening in quality assessment. JAMA 1991;265(15):1977–1981.
26. Pozgar GD: Legal aspects of health care administration. Gaithersburg, MD: Aspen, 1993.
27. Roberts JS, Coale JG, Redman RR: A history of the Joint Commission on Accreditation of Healthcare Organizations. JAMA 1987;258(7):887–940.
28. Richards RK: Continuing medical education: Perspectives, problems, prognosis. New Haven, CT: Yale University Press, 1978.
29. Galusha BL: Quality initiatives: The role of medical licensing and disciplinary boards. Qual Assur Util Rev 1988;3(3):66–70.
30. Graff D: The national practitioner data bank. Ohio Med 1990;86:703–707, 743.
31. Purtell DJ: Data bank has operational impact. Health Prog 1990;71(9):66–71.
32. Anthony MF, Crowley MA: The National Practitioner Data Bank: A catalyst for review of the credentialing process. Healthcare Executive 1991;6(2):28–29.
33. McCann RW: Federal peer review protection. Trustee 1987;40(11):24.
34. Dimond FC: The credentials process. In Orsund-Gassiot CA, Lindsey S (eds): Handbook of medical staff management. Gaithersburg, MD: Aspen, 1990, pp 105–137.
35. Independent study program, Module III, Principles of medical staff organization. Knoxville, TN: National Association of Medical Staff Services, 1993.
36. Snelson E: Quality assurance implications of federal peer review laws: The Health Care Quality Improvement Act and the National Practitioner Data Bank. J Qual Assur Util Rev 1992;7(1):2–11.

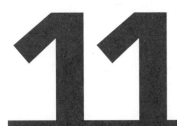

JILL CALLAHAN DENNIS

KEY WORDS

Advanced Directive	Court Order
Antitrust	Court Reporter
Arbitration	Credentialing
Assault	Defamation
Authentication	Defendant
Authorization	Delineation of Privileges
Bailiff	Deposition
Battery	Discovery
Best Evidence Rule	Due Process
Burden of Proof	Durable Power of Attorney for Health Care
Charitable Immunity	
Clerk of the Court	Emancipated Minor
Common Law	Evidence
Complaint	False Imprisonment
Confidential Communications	Fraud
Consent	Hearsay Rule
	Incident Report
Contemporaneous Documentation	Informed Consent
	Institutional Review Board (IRB)
Contract	
Corporate Negligence	Intentional Torts

HEALTH LAW CONCEPTS AND PRACTICES

11

ABBREVIATIONS

CFR—Code of Federal Regulations
FOIA—Freedom of Information Act
IRB—Institutional Review Board
MIB—Medical Information Bureau
NPDB—National Practitioner Data Bank

OBJECTIVES

- Define key words.
- Explain why health information management professionals must be knowledgeable about medicolegal
  issues.
- Distinguish between confidential and nonconfidential
  information within a health information system.
- Describe general legal principles governing access to
  confidential health information in a variety of circumstances.
- Distinguish proper or valid requests for access to
  health information from improper or invalid requests.
- Have a basic understanding of the federal and state
  court systems.
- Describe the four components of negligence.
- Distinguish properly executed consents and authorizations from incomplete or improper consents and
  authorizations.
- Identify major resources for locating information on
  laws, rules, regulations, and standards related to
  health information.

WHY ARE LEGAL ISSUES IMPORTANT TO HEALTH INFORMATION MANAGEMENT PROFESSIONALS?

At this moment, personal information about the health care or health status of millions of people is being collected, recorded, reviewed, analyzed, transmitted, used, and even misused. For every person who goes to a physician, clinic, hospital, or other treatment provider, somewhere there is a data set related to that visit or treatment. There is a record of all births, every operation, every treatment episode, every test result.

Health information management (HIM) professionals design and manage the information systems that hold these vital records. Earlier chapters discuss some of the reasons these records are kept. Scores of people and organizations want and need health information. As a result, health care providers are required by law to maintain these records. *HIM professionals must ensure that the information systems they manage, run, or design meet these obligations.* This chapter discusses some of those obligations.

Some requests for health information are legitimate. Others are not. How do HIM professionals decide which requests are valid and which are not? And for those requests that are granted, how do HIM professionals decide what can be disclosed and what can not? HIM professionals are called on to make these decisions every day. In a health care facility, the HIM professional is the resident expert on these questions. Legal counsel is not always readily available. To make wise decisions—decisions that appropriately protect the confidentiality of health information—HIM professionals must be aware of the rules, **regulations,** and laws that govern access to health information. A large part of this chapter is devoted to access issues. The rules that govern access to and disclosure of health information are fluid and often thorny. For many HIM professionals, these issues are among the most interesting they encounter in their career.

Why are legal issues so important to HIM professionals? It is because they are relied on by the following to understand these issues:

- Patients or clients whose health information
  they manage

359

- Health care organizations in which they are employed
- All users of health information

HIM professionals must take this trust seriously. By gaining a good understanding of legal issues, HIM students and professionals can be worthy of that trust.

FUNDAMENTALS OF THE LEGAL SYSTEM

In civilized societies, actions are guided by laws. These laws set forth principles and processes for our actions and for handling disputes over those actions. Laws govern both our *private* relationships (the relationships between private parties) and our *public* relationships (the relationships between private parties and the government).

Private law consists of two types of actions: tort actions and contract actions. In a tort action, one party alleges that another party's wrongful conduct has caused him or her harm. The party bringing the action to court seeks compensation for that harm. In a contract action, one party alleges that a contract exists between himself or herself and another party and that the other party has breached the contract by failing to fulfill an obligation that is part of that contract. The party bringing the contract action seeks either compensation for the breach or a court order to force the breaching party to perform that obligation.

Public law is composed of rules, regulations, and criminal law. Various governmental agencies have been charged by Congress with the responsibility of overseeing various aspects of many of our nation's most important industries, including health care. These agencies, acting under the authority of state and federal **statutes**, issue rules and regulations that touch every department of every health care organization. They cover diverse subjects, such as laboratory safety, incineration of medical waste, employment policies, confidentiality of peer review records, and mandatory reporting of medical device failures or problems. Failure to follow these rules can involve monetary penalties as well as criminal penalties. In addition to these rules and regulations, public laws include a body of criminal law—laws that bar conduct considered to be harmful to society—and set forth a system for punishing "bad acts."

Sources of Law

Laws that affect the health care system come from four main areas. They are as follows:

- Federal and state constitutions—the supreme law of the nation and state, respectively
- Federal and state statutes—laws enacted by Congress and state legislatures, respectively
- Rules and regulations of administrative agencies—acting under powers delegated to them by the legislature
- Court decisions—decisions that interpret statutes, regulations, and the Constitution and, where no such statutes or regulations are applicable, that apply **common law** (the large body of principles that have evolved from prior court decisions)

Constitutional Law

The U.S. Constitution grants certain powers to the three branches of the federal government: executive, legislative, and judicial. It also grants certain powers to the individual states. Powers granted by the Constitution may be either express or implied. Express powers are those specifically stated in the Constitution, such as the power to tax and the power to declare war. Implied powers are not specifically listed in the Constitution. They are those actions considered "necessary and proper" to permit the express powers to be accomplished.

The Constitution also limits what federal and state governments can do. For example, the first 10 amendments to the Constitution—the Bill of Rights—protects the rights of citizens to, among other things, free speech, freedom of religion, and due process before deprivation of life, liberty, or property. In a public health care facility (which is considered a governmental unit, as opposed to a private nongovernmental facility), a physician's appointment to the medical staff is considered a property right. Therefore, before that appointment could be terminated or rejected, the hospital would be obliged to provide **due process** to that physician, such as by a full hearing.

Another constitutional right important to the health care industry is the right of privacy—even though that right is not an express one. What is the right to privacy? Generally, it is considered to be a right to be left alone, to make decisions about one's own body, and to control one's own information. In the court decision of *Griswold v. Connecticut,* the U.S. Supreme Court recognized a constitutional right of privacy.[1] This right limits the government's power to regulate abortion, contraception, and other reproductive issues. The constitutional right to privacy also has been interpreted as permitting the terminally ill (or their legal guardians) to make decisions regarding the termination or withholding of medical treatment to prolong life.

Federal and State Statutes

Laws enacted by legislatures, be they Congress, state legislatures, or local city councils, are another important source of laws that affect health care facilities. One federal law that dramatically affects health care facilities as well as other business is the Americans with Disabilities Act.[2] This law not only impacts the hiring and employment practices of businesses, but also forces public facilities to remove or modify physical plant characteristics that may serve as access barriers for the disabled. The Safe Medical Devices Act is another federal statute that affects all health care facilities.[3] It requires certain incidents that involve medical devices and equipment to be reported to a national data bank.

When federal and state laws conflict, valid federal laws supersede the state laws. When state laws and local laws conflict, the valid state law controls.

Rules and Regulations of Administrative Agencies

Among the powers delegated to administrative agencies and departments of the executive branch by legislatures is the power to adopt rules and regulations to implement various laws. These rules and regulations provide guidance in how to comply with the law. Some of the most important agencies and departments that affect health care organizations are the Department of Health and Human Services and its Health Care Financing Administration, the Food and Drug Administration, the Internal Revenue Service on tax matters, the Department of Justice and the Federal Trade Commission on **antitrust** issues, and the Department of Labor and the National Labor Relations Board on labor and employment issues.

The rules and regulations of these bodies are valid only if they are within the limits of authority granted to them in their charter. Congress, in passing legislation creating these bodies, decides the broad areas in which these federal agencies may regulate, just as state legislatures do for state agencies. In promulgating their rules and regulations, federal agencies and many state agencies must follow administrative procedure acts passed by the legislature. These acts set forth the steps that administrative agencies must follow in issuing new rules and regulations and deciding disputes about those regulations. The Federal Administrative Procedure Act and most of the states' acts provide for advance notice of proposed rules and opportunity for public comment. Many federal agencies must publish both proposed and final rules in the daily *Federal Register*. An HIM professional should be familiar with the *Federal Register* and with how to scan it for notices of proposed rule-making. By doing so, a facility can have early warning of upcoming changes that may affect facility operations. By commenting on proposed rules, the facility can also influence the language of the final rule.

Court Decisions

When cases are brought before them, federal and state courts interpret statutes and regulations, decide their validity, and follow or create **common law** when no statutes or regulations apply. In deciding cases, courts generally adhere to the principle of **stare decisis** (let the decision stand). This can be described as following **precedent**. By referring to similar cases that have been decided in the past and by applying the same principles, courts generally arrive at the same ruling in the current case as in similar previous cases. Sometimes, however, even slight factual differences can result in departures from precedent. Sometimes courts decide that the precedent no longer adequately serves society's needs. One of the most important examples of this from a health care standpoint was the elimination of the doctrine of **charitable immunity,** which had until the early to mid-1960s protected nonprofit hospitals from liability for harm to patients. Courts now permit harmed patients to sue hospitals for their wrongful acts. The landmark case on this point is *Darling v. Charleston Community Memorial Hospital.*[4]

CASE STUDY

In the *Darling* case, a college football player fractured his leg during a game. He was taken to the emergency department of a community hospital, where the physician on emergency department duty was a general practitioner who had not treated a major leg fracture for several years. The physician ordered a radiograph, which revealed a fracture of the tibia and fibula. The physician reduced the fracture and applied a cast that extended from the patient's toes to just below his groin. Shortly after the cast was applied, the patient began to complain of pain, and he was admitted. The physician split the cast and visited the patient frequently while he was an inpatient. Complaints of pain continued. No specialist consultation was called.

After 2 weeks, the patient was transferred to a larger hospital and placed under the care of an orthopedic surgeon. The surgeon found much dead tissue in the fractured leg and over the next 2 months removed increasing amounts of tissue in an effort to save the leg. Finally, it became necessary to amputate the leg 8 inches below the knee.

The patient's father filed suit against the physician and the first hospital, alleging negligence. The physician settled out of court, but the hospital chose to go to court. Darling alleged that the hospital was negligent in its failure to provide enough trained nurses for bedside care of all patients at all times. In this case, Darling claimed that the nurses should have been capable of recognizing the progressive gangrene in the leg and should have called it to the attention of the medical staff and hospital administration, so that adequate consultation could have been obtained. The hospital argued that its liability as a charitable corporation—if there was liability at all—was limited to the amount of its liability insurance.

Judgment was eventually returned against the hospital in the amount of $100,000. The court decided that the doctrine of charitable immunity should no longer apply. On appeal, the Illinois Supreme Court agreed, stating: "We agree that the doctrine of charitable immunity can no longer stand. . . . [A] doctrine which limits the liability of charitable corporations to the amount of liability insurance that they see fit to carry permits them to determine whether or not they will be liable for their **torts** and the amount of liability, if any."[4]

As a result, hospitals are held liable for the negligent acts of their employees and, in some circumstances, their physicians. Health care organizations' liability is discussed in more detail later in the chapter.

Not all disputes, however, are resolved by courts. In health care, for example, sometimes health care facilities avoid the need to resort to the courts by participating in **arbitration,** in which a neutral party or panel hears both sides of a dispute and renders a decision, or by settling claims against them by negotiating a direct payment to the parties bringing the claim in exchange for the claimants dropping the claim.

THE LEGAL SYSTEM

The Court System

Federal Courts

The federal court system and many state systems have three levels of courts: trial courts, intermediate courts of appeals, and a supreme court. The federal trial courts are called U.S. District Courts. They cannot hear just any case. To be eligible to hear a case, a court must have **jurisdiction.** To be heard in a federal court, a case must involve either a federal question or diversity of jurisdiction. Federal question cases involve questions of federal law, such as possible violations of federal law or violations of a party's federal constitutional rights. Diversity cases—cases that involve citizens of different states—are heard in federal courts, but rather than use federal law, federal judges apply the laws of the applicable states in deciding these cases. In many of these diversity cases, a minimum of $10,000 must also be involved.

Appeals from federal trial courts (U.S. district courts) go to a U.S. Court of Appeals. The United States is divided into 12 circuits. These courts are typically referred to as the U.S. Court of Appeals for the First (Second, Third, Eleventh, or D.C.) Circuit.

The U.S. Supreme Court is the nation's highest court. It decides appeals from any of the U.S. Courts of Appeals. It may also hear appeals from the highest state courts if those cases involve federal laws or the U.S. Constitution. In some instances, if a U.S. Court of Ap-

peals or the highest state court refuses to hear an appeal, the case may be appealed directly to the U.S. Supreme Court. The U.S. Supreme Court need not and could not possibly hear all cases. With a few exceptions, the Supreme Court may decide not to review an appealed case. This does not mean that the Supreme Court necessarily approves of the lower court's decision; it merely means that it will not review the decision.

State and Territory Courts

In some states, trial courts are divided into special branches that hear certain types of cases. Probate court, traffic court, juvenile court, and family and divorce courts are examples. In addition to these special branches, there are trial courts with general jurisdiction—the power to hear all disputes not otherwise assigned to one of these special branches or not otherwise barred from state courts by law.

The job of the trial court is to hear the facts, review the applicable law, and decide the outcome. Sometimes there are no factual disagreements, but the parties to the lawsuit simply disagree over what the law provides. At other times, there may be no disagreement over the law, but the facts are in dispute. Often a case involves questions of law and facts.

Most states also have an intermediate appellate court that hears appeals from state trial court decisions. These appellate courts do not hold a new trial and hear new evidence; they generally limit their review to the trial court record to determine whether proper procedures were followed and whether the law was correctly interpreted.

Every state has a single high court, usually called the supreme court.* A state supreme court hears appeals from the intermediate appellate court or, if no intermediate court exists, the state trial courts. The high court often has other duties as well, such as formulating procedural rules for the lower state courts to follow.

Roles of the Key Players—Court Procedures

The **plaintiff** is the party who initiates the lawsuit. Plaintiffs initiate suits by filing a **complaint,** petition, or bill with the **clerk of the court.** This complaint is a written statement by the plaintiff that states his or her claims and commences the action. Plaintiffs sue one or more **defendants,** the party or parties from whom relief or compensation is sought. The defendant then files an

---

* In some states, the terminology is quite different. In New York, the highest court is the New York Court of Appeals, and the trial courts are called supreme courts.

answer to the complaint, which may also be called a responsive **pleading**. In this answer, the defendant denies or otherwise responds to the plaintiff's claims. If the case is not immediately settled, it proceeds into a process of **discovery**. Sometimes HIM directors are involved in the discovery phase of lawsuits by providing certain information used in the discovery devices described below.

During discovery, each party seeks to discover important information about the case through a pretrial investigation. It includes obtaining pertinent testimony (through **depositions**, sworn verbal testimony, and through **interrogatories**, sworn written answers to questions) as well as documents that may be under the control of the opposing party. For example, a patient who is suing a clinic for negligent care of an infected cut needs to obtain copies of the clinic's patient records that describe the care that was provided to the patient.

The purpose of the discovery phase is to encourage the early out-of-court resolution of cases by acquainting all parties with all pertinent facts. If the case cannot be settled out of court, it will proceed to trial. Evidence properly uncovered during the discovery phase is available in court. The judge is in charge of deciding which laws are applicable. This includes ruling on whether or not certain evidence produced in the discovery phase is admissible. The judge also keeps order and makes decisions necessary to facilitate a fair, impartial trial. If the case involves a jury, the jury's job is to determine the facts as presented in court, at least in part by deciding which witnesses and which evidence to believe, and to apply the law as instructed by the judge.

Even when a jury is present, the judge has substantial influence over the trial result. If he or she finds that insufficient evidence has been presented to establish an issue for the jury to resolve, the judge may in various circumstances refuse to send the case to the jury, dismiss the case, or direct the jury to decide the case one way or the other. In civil cases, even if the jury has already rendered a verdict, the judge may decide in favor of the other side, setting aside the jury's verdict. This is called a judgment n.o.v.—judgment non obstante verdicto (notwithstanding the verdict).

Some of the other players involved in trial proceedings are the clerk of the court, **court reporter,** and **bailiff.** The clerk of the court is the administrative manager of the court and handles the paperwork associated with lawsuits. Complaints are filed with the clerk, as are other pleadings and documents. The court reporter is responsible for creating a verbatim transcript of court proceedings. Bailiffs are courtroom personnel who are present to assist in keeping order, administering oaths, and performing other duties at the direction of the judge.

Cases That Involve Health Care Facilities and Providers

Malpractice and Negligence

One of the most frequent types of claims made against health care facilities and individual providers are claims of **negligence** or **malpractice** (professional negligence). Negligence is conduct that society considers unreasonably dangerous because "first, the [individual or party] did foresee or should have foreseen that it would subject another or others to an appreciable risk of harm, and second, the magnitude of the perceivable risk was such that the [individual or party] should have acted in a safer manner."[5]

At this point, some readers may ask, "How can hospitals be held accountable for actions when they are simply the bricks and mortar within which people work?" Two theories of negligence are used to hold hospitals and other health care organizations accountable for their conduct. Under the first theory, **respondeat superior** (meaning "let the master answer" for the actions of the servant—the doctrine of "agency"), the legal system imputes the negligent actions of the organization's employees or agents over whom it has control to the health care organization itself. Using this theory, courts hold employers responsible for those acts of their employees or agents that are performed within the scope of employment. For example, a hospital can be held responsible for the actions of its nurses while they are acting within the scope of their employment (e.g., when they are performing some aspect of their job assignment), but a hospital would not be held responsible for the actions of a nurse in its employ while she or he is grocery shopping after work.

Under a second, more current theory of **corporate negligence,** courts can hold health care organizations liable for their own independent acts of negligence. This theory holds organizations responsible for monitoring the activities of the people who function within their facilities, whether those people are employees or independent contractors, such as physicians, and for complying with appropriate industry standards, such as accreditation (Joint Commission on Accreditation of Healthcare Organizations [JCAHO]) standards, licensing regulations, and *Conditions of Participation* issued by Medicare. Health care organizations are no longer considered to be merely physicians' "workshops." They retain some responsibility for all who are authorized to function within their facilities.

The following are a few examples of the types of situations that can lead to malpractice claims against health care organizations and providers:

- Failure to properly diagnose a condition, such as cancer

- Failure to properly treat a condition—for example, not cleaning a wound before stitching it up

- Failure to monitor or supervise a patient's condition and take appropriate action; for example, in the *Darling* case described earlier in the chapter, the nurses failed to note and report the leg's worsening condition

- Failure to properly credential medical staff members (e.g., granting a physician privileges to perform some types of surgery for which he or she is unqualified)

Malpractice claims are not the only kind of claims against health care organizations and providers. The following are some of the other types of claims that HIM professionals may encounter in their professional careers.

Intentional Torts

Some of the **intentional tort** claims that may be brought against health care facilities include **assault** and **battery, false imprisonment, defamation** of character, **invasion of privacy, fraud** or misrepresentation, and intentional infliction of emotional distress.

When one thinks of assault and battery, one often thinks of a mugging or an attack of some sort. But an assault is simply a deliberate threat, coupled with the apparent ability, to do physical harm to another person without that person's consent. No contact is required. For example, if a nurse stood over a patient with a syringe, stating that he or she was going to inject that patient with a strong sedative whether or not the patient agreed to it, that would constitute an assault if the patient was aware of the threat. And if the nurse proceeded to inject the patient, that would constitute a battery. A **battery** is nonconsensual, intentional touching of another person in a socially impermissible manner. Awareness of the victim is irrelevant. An unconscious patient who has surgery performed on him without express (actual) or implied consent (such as when a patient is brought to the facility for lifesaving treatment) is the victim of a battery.

Could assault and battery ever really happen in a health care facility? In *Peete v. Blackwell,* a nurse was awarded damages after a physician with whom she was working struck her and cursed at her while ordering her to turn on some patient-suctioning equipment.[6] Even though there were no lasting injuries, the jury awarded $1 in compensation and $10,000 in punitive damages.

The laws concerning battery are one of the prime reasons behind the requirement to obtain the patient's written consent to treatment. Allegations of battery against health care facilities most often involve situations in which improper or no patient consent was obtained before a surgical procedure. Regardless of whether that procedure helps or harms the patient, unconsented-to invasions of the patient's person entitle the patient to at least nominal damages.*

False imprisonment is unlawful restraint of a person's personal liberty or the unlawful restraining or confining of a person. Physical force is not required; all that is required is a reasonable fear that force will be used to detain or intimidate the person into following orders. How could this apply to a health care facility? If a facility tried to prevent a patient's departure from the facility until the patient's bill was paid, this could qualify as false imprisonment. The use of physical restraints to keep a patient in bed for no other reason than inadequate staffing available to monitor patients could also qualify.

False imprisonment issues can be complex. For example, if an intoxicated driver involved in a motor vehicle accident is treated for minor cuts in an emergency department and now wants to be discharged to drive home but is still extremely intoxicated, must the facility release that patient or may he be restrained until he is capable of driving safely? Statutes in some states permit intoxicated or mentally ill people to be detained by a hospital if they are dangerous to themselves or others. This is one example of why it is so important for the staff in health care organizations to be familiar with state laws. In judging reasonableness of a health care provider's actions in detaining a patient, documentation in the patient record often is vital.

Defamation of character is oral (**slander**) or written (**libel**) communication to a person (other than the person defamed) that tends to damage the defamed person's reputation in the eyes of the community. To succeed in a defamation action, the defamed person must show that there was communication to a third party. Truth of the statements is a defense, as is privilege. If the defamation occurs during a **privileged communication**—such as during **confidential communications** between spouses or in a talk with a priest or minister—defamation is not found as long as those statements are made without malice (evil intent). Defamation cases in health care are unusual but they do occur, especially in the context of medical staff credentialing and granting of privileges, when the defamed party argues that the defamatory remarks were made with malice. Professionals who are called incompetent in front of others generally have a right to sue to defend their reputation. If the person making the remark cannot prove that the comment is true or that some other privilege applies, he or she may be held liable for damages. For that reason, it

---

* See, for example, *Perna v. Pirozzi,* 457 A.2d 431 (N.J. 1983), in which the supreme court of New Jersey held that a patient who consents to surgery by one surgeon but who is actually operated on by another has grounds for an action for battery!

is generally wise to refrain from making disparaging remarks about other health professionals and colleagues.

Invasion of privacy is an intentional tort with which HIM professionals must be concerned. By the very act of submitting to treatment, patients give up some privacy. However, negligent disregard for patients' privacy can and does result in actions against health care providers and organizations. Because HIM professionals and other health professionals work with sensitive information on an almost constant basis, it is easy to become callous to privacy issues. Readers who have visited friends or family members in the hospital and overheard staff members talking casually about patients and their conditions in hallways, elevators, and the cafeteria have witnessed what may have been an invasion of privacy or breach of confidentiality. Health care providers who divulge confidential information from a patient's record to an improper recipient without the patient's permission have invaded the patient's privacy and breached their duty of confidentiality. A great deal of this chapter is devoted to identifying what health information is confidential and who is a proper or an improper recipient. HIM professionals must learn these principles well and become expert in applicable state and federal laws, so that they not only avoid violating patients' privacy themselves but also can help other health professionals understand how to respect patient's privacy and confidentiality rights.

Fraud is a willful and intentional misrepresentation that could cause harm or loss to a person or his or her property. In addition to fraud associated with improper billing for procedures not performed (criminal fraud), fraud can occur in health care facilities when a physician promises a certain surgical result, even though he or she knows that the result is not so certain. For example, if a physician promises that there is no chance of a complication resulting from plastic surgery, even though such complications can occur, he or she is guilty of misrepresentation.

Intentional infliction of emotional or mental distress can also result in claims against health care facilities. In a 1975 case, a court found that a physician and hospital (through its employees) were guilty of intentional infliction of emotional distress. In this case, the mother of a premature infant (who died shortly after birth) had gone to her physician for a postpartum checkup.[7] She noticed a report in her medical record stating that the child was past 5 month's gestation and, therefore, could not be disposed of as a surgical specimen. On questioning her physician about what had happened to the body, the physician told his nurse to take the mother to the hospital. At the hospital, the mother was taken by a hospital employee to a freezer. The freezer was opened, and the mother was handed a jar containing her baby. The mother was awarded $100,000 damages, upheld on appeal. The cases are not always so dramatic. In 1985, a Georgia court found a physician guilty of intentional infliction of emotional distress for yelling at a patient and her husband.[8]

Products Liability

Products liability cases sometimes involve health care facilities. Products liability is the liability of a manufacturer, seller, or supplier of a product to a buyer or other third party for injuries sustained because of a defect in the product. The injured party may sue the seller, manufacturer, or supplier. If, for example, a hospital improperly processes or stores blood in its own blood bank, it may be liable to any patient who is harmed as a result. If the staff of a research hospital design a new type of medical equipment that is tested on patients, any harm resulting from product defects can result in product liability claims. Products liability is a complex subject beyond the scope of this chapter. It is included here simply as a reminder that there are many potential sources of liability for today's health care organizations.

Contractual Disputes

Breach of **contract** is a common claim in litigation that involves health care providers and organizations. Typically, the claims arise when one party to a contract fails to follow the terms agreed to in the contract. Interestingly, courts have been willing to enforce ethical standards prohibiting breach of confidentiality (such as the American Hospital Association's [AHA's] Patient Bill of Rights and ethical standards of the American Medical Association) as part of a contractual relationship between health care providers and their patients. Thus, an improper disclosure of health information can give rise to a breach of contract claim as well as an invasion of privacy or breach of confidentiality claim. (Invasion of privacy and breach of confidentiality claims are discussed later in this chapter.) In an important case on this subject, *Hammonds v. Aetna Casualty and Surety Co.*, the court found that a physician breached an implied condition of his patient-physician contract when he disclosed health information to a hospital's insurer without the patient's authorization.[9]

Antitrust Claims

In recent years, health care providers and organizations have been the targets of antitrust claims. Most of these claims revolve around mergers and acquisitions and alleged anticompetitive behavior in medical staff **credentialing** activities. For example, if the obstetricians on the medical staff of a local hospital seek to remove an obstetrician's staff privileges so that there will be less competition for patients, that hospital may find itself entangled in an antitrust suit. These suits usually do not directly involve the HIM department or service, but sometimes HIM professionals are involved to the extent that they support the medical staff's peer review and **credentialing** functions.

Crimes

Criminal activity can take place in any health care facility. Ask a nurse practicing in a hospital, and he or she is probably able to tell of mysterious discrepancies in narcotic counts (counts done on each unit that stores narcotics to ensure that no drugs are missing). Angel-of-death murder scenarios have been sensationalized in books and television, but they have their basis in actual events in which the weak and ill have become prey for criminal or deviant behavior by facility employees. For example, in 1989, Richard Angelo, a registered nurse in the cardiac intensive care unit at a New York hospital was found guilty of second-degree murder for injecting two patients with the drug Pavulon. He was also found guilty of manslaughter and criminally negligent homicide involving two other patients. Patient abuse and sexual improprieties are also terrible phenomena that can occur in health care facilities. In addition, falsification of business or patient records may be grounds for criminal indictment, for example, by billing Medicare for patients not seen or services not performed.

Noncompliance with Statutes, Rules, and Regulations

As mentioned earlier, health care organizations that fail to follow government-imposed mandates run the risk of a variety of potential penalties, including money penalties, removal from participation in the Medicare program, and even loss of licensure.

With this information as a backdrop, the remainder of this chapter looks at the most common legal obligations and risks that face health care facilities, health care providers, and HIM professionals in particular. First, which legal obligations and risks involve HIM professionals most directly?

LEGAL OBLIGATIONS AND RISKS OF HEALTH CARE FACILITIES AND INDIVIDUAL HEALTH CARE PROVIDERS

Duty to Maintain Health Information

One of the most fundamental duties that involve HIM professionals and their health care facility employers is the duty to maintain health information about their patients. This duty is imposed explicitly by state and federal statutes and regulations as well as accreditation standards. In some states, the hospital licensing statutes

specify not only that a medical record must be kept for every patient but also what that record must contain at a minimum. Failure to meet the requirements of these licensing statutes could subject a facility to loss of licensure as well as closure. The law and regulations setting forth the *Conditions of Participation* in federal payment programs such as Medicare also require that medical records be kept, and they outline in broad terms what those records must include.[10] Accreditation standards of the JCAHO also require accredited facilities to maintain medical records.

The duty to maintain health information is also implied in other laws. For example, vital statistics laws require the reporting of births and deaths. Under federal and state statutes, health care facilities must report to various data banks certain disease conditions and medical events, such as the treatment of gunshot wounds, suspected child abuse, elder abuse, industrial accidents, certain poisonings, abortions, cancer cases, and communicable diseases.

Mandatory reporting requirements vary from state to state. What these statute have in common is that reporting is required and the authorization of the patient is generally not needed. In fact, even if the patient expresses the wish *not* to have this information released, the health care organization must comply with the reporting requirement. This tension between the reporting statutes and confidentiality often arises with state requirements for reporting actual or suspected child abuse. Reports made in error admittedly cause much pain and embarrassment for the family involved. Many states, recognizing the natural reluctance of people to make such reports when the abuse is not proven, have exempted the party making the report from liability for erroneous reports, as long as the report is made in good faith (in other words, without malice or evil intent).

The reporting statutes attempt to encourage reporting in another important way. For example, failure to report child abuse can result in liability for injuries a child later sustains when discharged home to the suspected or actual abuser.

The problem gets even stickier when mandatory reporting statutes conflict with other laws, such as state laws that bar disclosure of mental health treatment records and federal laws that bar disclosure of substance abuse treatment. If in the course of therapy a child or an elderly person indicates that he or she has been abused, what must the therapist do? Some court decisions have permitted the protection of these confidentiality laws to be pierced but only to the extent necessary to fulfill the requirements of the reporting statute.[11] Additionally, some state confidentiality laws permit exceptions in cases of imminent harm, in which the child or abused party is in immediate danger. Other statutes, however, do not provide convenient solutions to this problem. HIM professionals who face such a situation should consult legal counsel, who may seek direction from the court in reconciling all the interests involved.

These examples illustrate why compliance with mandatory reporting statutes is not always as simple as it may seem. HIM professionals must determine their state's requirements and how those requirements may conflict with other confidentiality obligations, so that appropriate reporting procedures are in place.

Duty to Retain Health Information and Other Key Documents and to Keep Them Secure

Just as there are requirements to create patient records, there are also requirements to retain that information. Health care facilities take guidance from federal and state record retention laws and regulations and from state **statutes of limitations** in setting their own record and information retention policies. Facilities must also take into account the uses of and needs for that information, the space available for hard-copy storage, and the resources available for microfilming, creating optical disks, or for electronic storage. For example, a university-based teaching facility would probably want to retain health information longer than a small, independent rural facility because of the important role health information may play in research and teaching.

In determining a retention policy, HIM professionals must first consult all applicable statutes and regulations. Some states have specific medical record retention requirements; others regulate only parts of that information, such as radiographs. Still other states tie retention periods to their statute of limitations for contract or personal injury litigation. This can result in extremely long retention periods for the records of minor patients. For example, if the age of majority is 18 years and the statute of limitations for torts is 2 years, the minimum retention period for a neonate's record would be 18 + 2 because the statute of limitations for minors does not begin to toll until the minor reaches majority (age 18). Remember, record retention regulations are a baseline; in other words, facilities must meet these minimum retention periods but may establish longer retention schedules if desired.

It is not enough just to keep those records. HIM professionals must ensure that the records are kept in a way that minimizes the chance of their being lost, destroyed, or altered. Plaintiffs have won negligence suits against facilities that failed to safeguard their records from loss or destruction.[12] **Security of health information** has taken on new and more complex dimensions as more and more health information is stored in various electronic and other media. Medical records security used to be a simple matter of controlling access to the file area and having adequate safeguards against phys-

ical threats such as fire, flood, and severe weather. Now, with each new form of data storage and retrieval technology, HIM professionals must be alert to the new security threats that may accompany those technologies.

Health information is valuable only if it is accurate, complete, and available for use when needed. Therefore, HIM professionals must design safeguards that not only protect the information from loss or destruction and prevent the corruption of electronically stored data from power losses or surges but also protect the integrity of the information itself. In other words, the information must be protected from inappropriate alteration.

Why would anyone want to alter health information or documentation in a patient's record? In some situations, such as when a health professional is sued for malpractice, he or she may be tempted to alter the record to make the documentation appear more complete than it originally was. Some health professionals have not yet learned the importance of thorough **contemporaneous documentation** (i.e., documentation made while care is being provided, while the information is fresh in the care provider's mind), and as a result, when the time comes to defend one's actions, the record may not reflect one's care of the patient in a positive light. HIM professionals must guard against inappropriate alterations to health information by controlling access to records with extra precautions taken for those records that are involved in litigation. If presented with a request to make a change to a patient record involved in litigation, an HIM professional should refer that request to the facility's defense counsel. Rather than doing himself or herself a favor by "improving" the documentation, a health professional who makes later alterations often ends up losing the case because the plaintiff's attorney may have already gotten a copy of the original, unaltered record from the patient before filing suit. Imagine how it might appear to a jury if the plaintiff's attorney can show that the defendant altered the record once the suit was filed and that the health facility took no steps to protect the record from alteration.[13] For these reasons, it is wise to supervise all access to patient records that are involved in litigation. By doing so, the integrity of the record can be maintained while permitting appropriate access.

Falsification of records can lead to other problems as well. In some states, it is a crime if it is done for the purpose of cheating or defrauding and may lead to sanctions against health professionals' licenses.

Error Correction

Errors that are made in documenting information must be corrected as soon as they are detected, using proper error correction methods. These methods should be outlined in the facility's policy and procedure manual and taught to all people who document patient health information.

Generally, an error should be corrected by the person who made it. If the correction is a major one (e.g., erroneous laboratory results were entered on the record and resulted in a problem in the patient's care), the person making the correction should consult with the HIM manager, risk manager, and perhaps even facility legal counsel to ensure that the correction method complies with facility policy and that all appropriate steps that need to be taken are followed. Most corrections aren't that dramatic. A nurse begins to chart patient A's information on patient B's record but instantly realizes the error. Or, in the course of making up a new medication administration record, the unit clerk misspells the name of a medication, and it is quickly caught by the nurse who double-checks the record. In situations that involve paper-based health information, the person making the error should simply draw a single line through the incorrect entry, enter the correction and initial it, and note the time and date of the correction (Figure 11–1). Under no circumstances should the original entry be erased, scribbled over, or hidden because an obliteration can raise suspicion in the minds of jurors about the original entry and whether it is an attempt to cover up a major problem.

Error correction methods are different for computer-based health information systems. A system's procedures should clearly specify how errors are to be handled. Errors that are caught immediately at the time they are made can simply be changed, with no need to preserve the original entry. Errors that are caught after the point in time that someone has relied on the erroneous information pose a problem; the system must provide some way of saving the original entry and showing the new entry and the date and time it was made. Health information systems software varies, and procedures differ with each system. HIM professionals should insist that the system they use permits appropriate error correction and addendum procedures, so that the integrity of the information is preserved.

Addenda

In some circumstances, simple error correction methods are insufficient. For example, if a substantial portion of a patient's history and physical examination were left out of the original dictated report, it would be impossible to squeeze in the missing information on the original typed report. When new information is being added to a record, an addendum is used. The person making the addendum should enter a reference to the addendum near the original entry or information (e.g. "1/3/94—See addendum to H&P"—signature) and then file the addendum.

Sometimes, after they have reviewed their health in-

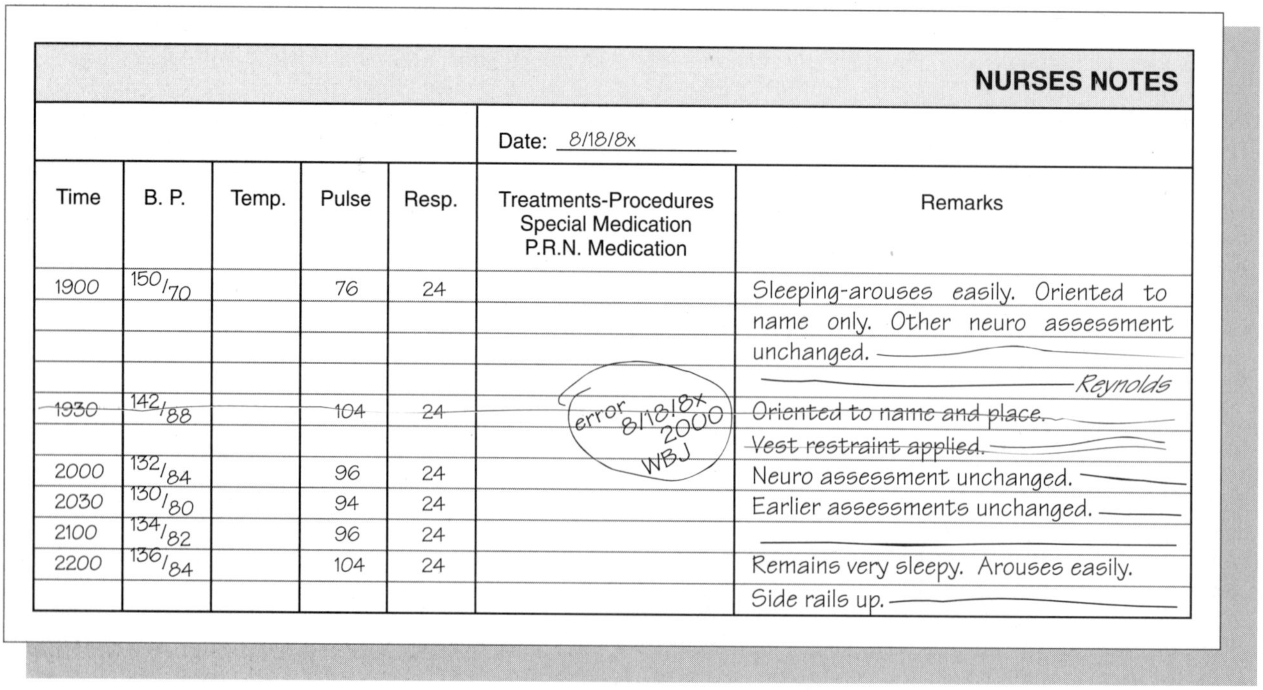

NURSES NOTES

Date: 8/18/8x

Time	B. P.	Temp.	Pulse	Resp.	Treatments-Procedures Special Medication P.R.N. Medication	Remarks
1900	150/70		76	24		Sleeping-arouses easily. Oriented to
						name only. Other neuro assessment
						unchanged.
						Reynolds
~~1930~~	~~142/88~~		~~104~~	~~24~~	error 8/18/8x 2000 WBJ	~~Oriented to name and place.~~
						~~Vest restraint applied.~~
2000	132/84		96	24		Neuro assessment unchanged.
2030	130/80		94	24		Earlier assessments unchanged.
2100	134/82		96	24		
2200	136/84		104	24		Remains very sleepy. Arouses easily.
						Side rails up.

FIGURE 11–1. Correcting errors in documentation.

formation, patients ask that their records be amended. The Privacy Act (discussed later in the chapter) permits such amendments but it applies only to health care organizations operated by the federal government, such as Department of Defense health care facilities, Veterans Administration health facilities, and Indian Health Service facilities. Requests for amendment may also arise in the context of mental health therapy, when patients have said something during therapy that they later wish they had not said. Facility policy should outline how these requests are to be handled. Unless the amendment request is pursuant to a right granted by law, such as in the Privacy Act, it should be discussed with the attending physician. If the physician believes that the request is inappropriate, he or she should discuss the matter with the patient. Otherwise, the patient's amendment should be handled as an addendum to the record without change to the original entry and identified as an additional document appended to the original patient record at the request of the patient.

Authentication and Authorship Issues

One aspect of protecting the integrity of health information that has become increasingly controversial is the issue of **authentication**. In other words, how can facilities identify the author of a particular record or computer entry into a health information system? In a paper record system, this is done through the original signature or through the use of a personal signature stamp (under the written agreement with the facility not to delegate the use of the stamp to another person). Authentication not only serves to identify the author of an entry but also indicates that the author has reviewed the entry or report for accuracy and attests to it. In computerized health information systems, authentication of documentation is often achieved through a unique identification code entered by the person making the note or report. As is true with the use of signature stamps, it is important to ensure that the identification code is not shared with others; if it is to be reliable indication of authorship, it must be used only by the person to whom it is assigned.

Validity of Health Information as Evidence

One of the reasons it is important to protect the integrity of health information is so that the information or record may be used as evidence in court proceedings. State laws governing the admissibility of health information as evidence vary.

In some states, health information can be admitted as an exception to the hearsay rule. The **hearsay rule** bars the legal admissibility of **evidence** that is not the personal knowledge of the witness. For example, a defend-

ant physician may want to use the patient record to defend a malpractice claim, but the record contains information beyond his personal knowledge—the statements of nurses, descriptions of treatments given by respiratory therapists, recording of laboratory results prepared by medical technologists, and so on. In some states, however, medical records and health information may be admitted either as a business record or as an explicit exception in the state's rules of evidence. Business records are presumed to be reliable because they are routinely prepared in the course of business and are created as business is transacted, not specially prepared months later for use in court. When submitting the record for use in court as a business record, the HIM professional must attest that the record was made in the normal course of business. If anything has happened to that record or information that departs from the normal course of business, such as an alteration of original documentation, the information no longer has that presumption of reliability and may no longer be admissible. As discussed earlier, this action can cripple a malpractice defense and destroy the information's value as evidence in other types of proceedings, such as personal injury cases.

What if a record has been microfilmed or put onto other storage media, such as an optical disk or a computer tape, and the original destroyed? Can the information still be used as evidence? Rules of evidence require that when originals are still available, they must be produced. This is called the **best evidence rule.** When it becomes necessary to prove the contents of a document, the original must be produced or its absence accounted for. The best evidence rule was adopted to prevent fraud or mistake as to the contents of a document or record. If the original has been destroyed pursuant to a facility's records retention program and only copies of that information remain, that secondary evidence (e.g., the microfilm or optical disk) will probably be admissible if the court is satisfied that the secondary record accurately reflects the original and that destruction of the original was done in good faith (e.g., as part of a facility-sponsored record retention program and not specifically to prevent the information's use in court). The testimony of the HIM professional is important in explaining the retention program and the secondary information or record system. Because of the length of time microfilming has been used, most courts admit microfilm copies without much question, but more recent technologies often must be explained by the HIM professional before the information can be used. This is one of the reasons why careful thought must go into the selection of new technology for information storage and retrieval. Obtaining the opinion of legal counsel as to the admissibility of information stored in new ways and forms is a wise step to take before adopting new technology.

Retention of Other Records and Information

Patient records and information are not the only important documents to retain. Medical staff credential files, incident reports, surgical videos that identify patients, peer review data and minutes, radiographs, surgery schedules, and emergency department logs are just a few of the items for which a retention schedule must be established. The HIM professional is often a key player in establishing this schedule. In addition to consulting applicable state and federal laws and regulations, many HIM professionals use the record retention guidelines published by the Healthcare Financial Management Association in setting facility policy.[14]

Duty to Maintain Confidentiality

Think about a past visit to a physician. What information was shared? If a patient discovered that his or her physician repeated that information to another patient, a neighbor, or the local newspaper, wouldn't that patient be angry? Today's society considers communications between patients and their health care providers to be confidential communications. For sake of discussion, this chapter defines a confidential communication as one that transmits information to a health care provider as part of the relationship between the provider and the patient under circumstances that imply that the information shall remain private. Patients rely on that promise of confidentiality in disclosing intimate details to health care providers.

Health care providers are bound by various laws and ethical standards to maintain the confidentiality of that private health information. Physicians, for example, are required by their Hippocratic Oath to maintain confidentiality— "What I may see or hear in the course of the treatment, or even outside of the treatment in regard to the life of men, which on no account one must spread abroad, I will keep to myself." The AHA's Patient Bill of Rights addresses the health facility's obligation. Number 5 of this bill of rights states in relevant part: "The patient has the right to every consideration of his privacy concerning his own medical care program." The American Health Information Management Association's (AHIMA's) own Code of Ethics sets the standard for HIM professionals to protect "the confidentiality of primary and secondary health records as mandated by law, professional standards, and the employer's policies." Although there is no comprehensive, uniform federal law that protects the confidentiality of all health care information at this time, numerous state laws address the subject, as do Medicare's *Conditions of Participation,* JCAHO standards, and a growing body of court decisions.

To fully understand the health care providers' obligation to keep patient health information confidential, those care providers need to understand what information is and is not confidential. After all, some of the information that appears in patient records is not health information. The date of a patient's admission to a general hospital is not confidential; nor is his address or date of birth. Keep in mind, however, that even though these facts may not be confidential, there may be situations in which a facility would decline to respond to requests for this information. For example, in the past, many hospitals automatically published notices of birth in the local newspaper, listing the parents' names and address and the sex or name of the child. These days, perhaps because infant abductions are on the rise, fewer hospitals do this, even with the consent of the parents.

Determining what information is confidential is not always as straightforward as it might seem. For example, for substance abuse treatment facilities, the very fact of a patient's admission for treatment is confidential, according to federal law, and may not be disclosed without patient **authorization** except under limited circumstances.[15] But generally, informational items unrelated to the treatment provided, such as the patient's name and address, name of insurer, and next of kin or other guarantor information, are not considered confidential.[16]

One practical way of separating confidential information from information that is not considered confidential is to answer the following questions:

- *Is there a patient-provider relationship?* The patient and provider must have a professional relationship. This does not imply that the patient must be paying the provider; it simply means that the relationship between them is a professional one. The patient does not have to be aware of this relationship—for example, the patient could be an infant or could be unconscious or otherwise incapacitated.

- *Was the information in question exchanged through (or in the context of) the professional relationship?* The information does not have to be related verbally but could be observed by the provider or gained through physical examination or diagnostic test or procedure.

- *Is the information needed to treat or diagnose the patient?* Data about next of kin or birthdate are not ordinarily needed to treat or diagnose.

For the information in question to be considered confidential, all three questions should be answered affirmatively.

Beyond health information, there are other documents in the health care facility that must be kept confidential if they are to adequately serve their purpose. Incident reports, in which adverse occurrences are reported and investigated, must be kept confidential to the extent permitted by state law, so that staff members will feel free to report such occurrences. Peer review records, such as committee minutes and credentialing files, also must be kept confidential to encourage candor in monitoring, managing, and improving the quality of clinical care.[17] HIM professionals are often involved in developing facility policies to protect the confidentiality of this information and in teaching staff to follow those policies.

In developing facility polices to protect the confidentiality of health information, HIM professionals must ensure that those policies adhere to federal and state laws on the subject. Many state HIM associations publish excellent legal guides to cover the basic tenets of individual states' laws. Plan to become familiar with these resources. The most important federal laws and regulations are described below.

Privacy Act of 1974

The Privacy Act was designed to give citizens some control over the information collected about them by the federal government and its agencies. It grants people the following rights:

- To find out what information about them has been collected

- To see and have a copy of that information

- To correct or amend the information

- To exercise limited control of the disclosure of that information to other parties.[18]

Health care organizations operated by the federal government (e.g., military hospitals, Veterans Administration health facilities, Indian Health Service facilities) are bound by the act's provisions. The act also applies to record systems that are operated pursuant to a contract with a federal government agency—for example, a disease registry operated under a grant from the Department of Health and Human Services.

Freedom of Information Act

The Freedom of Information Act (FOIA) became law in 1966. It requires that records pertaining to the executive branch of the federal government be available to the public except for matters that fall within nine explicitly exempted areas. Under certain circumstances, medical records may be exempt from the act's requirements. One of the nine exempt categories includes "personnel and medical files and similar files, the disclosure of which would constitute a clearly unwarranted invasion of personal privacy.[18] To meet the test of being an "unwarranted invasion of personal privacy," the following conditions must exist:

- The information must be contained in a personnel, medical, or similar file.

- Disclosure of the information must constitute an invasion of personal privacy.

- The severity of the invasion must outweigh the public's interest in disclosure.

Interpreting this three-part test has been the subject of a number of court cases.[19]

Regulations on Confidentiality of Alcohol and Drug Abuse Patient Records

These regulations, restricting disclosures of patient health information without patient authorization, apply to facilities that provide alcohol or drug abuse diagnosis, treatment, or referral for treatment—a substance abuse program in the language of the regulations. For a health care facility to be considered such a program, it must offer either an identified unit that provides alcohol or drug abuse diagnosis, treatment, or referral for treatment or medical personnel or other staff whose primary function is the provision of alcohol or drug abuse diagnosis, treatment, or referral for treatment and who are identified as such providers.[20] General hospitals and clinics are not considered to be such programs unless they have either an identified unit for this type of diagnosis or treatment or providers whose primary function is the provision of those types of services.

The regulations apply only to health information obtained by federally assisted programs, but because the definition of this is quite broad (e.g., all Medicare-certified facilities or those that receive funds from any federal department or agency, among other things), it applies to virtually all programs that meet the other requirements of the definition.

The regulations are important for several reasons. They prohibit the disclosure of substance abuse patient records unless permitted by the regulations or authorized by the patient. The regulations require specific content in an authorization to release health information. All such authorizations must include the following:

- Specific name or general designation of the program or person permitted to make the disclosure

- Name or title of the person or name of the organization to which disclosure is to be made

- Name of the patient

- Purpose of the disclosure

- How much and what kind of information is to be disclosed

- Signature of the patient and, when required for a patient who is a minor, the signature of a person authorized to give consent under §2.14 of the regulations or, when required for a patient who is incompetent or deceased, the signature of a person authorized to sign under §2.15 in lieu of the patient*

- Date on which the consent (authorization) is signed

- Statement that the consent is subject to revocation at any time, except to the extent that the program or person that is to make the disclosure has already acted in reliance on it. Acting in reliance includes the provision of treatment services in reliance on a valid consent to disclose information to a third party payer.

- Date, event, or condition on which the consent will expire if not revoked before. This date, event, or condition must ensure that the consent will last no longer than reasonably necessary to serve the purpose for which it is given.†

Interestingly, after the regulations regarding the confidentiality of alcohol and drug abuse patient records were published, many health care facilities adopted that required content as the content of their general authorization for release of health information, applying to all releases of health information, rather than use separate forms for separate purposes.

Each disclosure must be accompanied by a notice specified in the regulations. That notice is a prohibition against redisclosure. In other words, recipients of the original disclosure are put on notice that they may not redisclose the information to anyone else or use the information for anything but its intended purpose because the records are protected by federal confidentiality rules in 42 Code of Federal Regulations (CFR) Part 2. The notice states:

> This information has been disclosed to you from records whose confidentiality is protected by Federal regulations (42 C.F.R. Part 2) prohibit you from making any further disclosure of it without the specific written consent of the person to whom it pertains, or as otherwise permitted by such regulations. A general authorization for the release of medical or other information is *not* sufficient for this purpose.

There are some exceptions to the general prohibition against disclosure. In a medical emergency, for example,

the regulations do permit disclosure to medical personnel to treat a condition that "poses an immediate threat to the health of the patient."[21] Records of these disclosures must be maintained, including the following:

- Patient's name or case number

- Date and time of disclosure

- Description of circumstances that require emergency disclosure

- Description of information disclosed

- Identity of the party receiving the information

- Identity of the party disclosing the information

There are also some provisions for interagency disclosures (e.g., to the Food and Drug Administration), research, and Medicare or Medicaid audits.[22]

These regulations are lengthy and detailed. Plan to review them and become familiar with the key provisions. HIM professionals who work in health care facilities that qualify as a "program" under these regulations must become very familiar with them.

For most health care facilities, when dealing with issues other than alcohol and drug abuse program records and information, state laws are the most important determinant of the organization's policies and procedures for preserving the confidentiality of health information.

Internal and External Users of Health Information

When sorting through the maze of parties who request health information, sometimes it is useful to categorize the would-be information users as internal users or external users. Why? Because in a few but by no means all circumstances, internal users may not need patient authorization for disclosure, whereas external users almost always do. For example, employees on the facility's utilization review staff would be internal users. They would be entitled to review the records of patients on units to which they are assigned. On the other hand, an external utilization reviewer sent by a private employer to review a particular case would require patient authorization before disclosure could be made. The health care organization's in-house counsel who is coordinating the defense of a malpractice claim would be an internal user, whereas a lawyer who represents a patient, a physician, or an employee of the health care organization would be an external user and would require patient authorization.

Do not fall into the trap of thinking that just because a person works for the facility he or she has carte blanche access to all patient information. Although it is true that health care personnel involved in the treatment

---

* Whether or not a minor is empowered to sign his or her own authorizations and consents is a matter of state law and varies from state to state. Likewise, the party authorized to sign in lieu of a deceased or incapacitated patient also varies and depends on whether an executor or a guardian (respectively) has been named.

† §2.31(a) and (b) of the regulations outline the exact requirements and give sample language that meets the intent of the regulations. Most programs have adopted this sample language directly into their authorizations for release of information.

of a patient should have access to the information they need to know, it does not follow that a nurse should know the medical details involving patients for whom he or she is not caring. This can be a serious problem in health care facilities and has taken on special significance with the growing number of patients who test positive for the human immunodeficiency virus (HIV). Is there any reason for a dietary aide who delivers food trays to each nursing unit to know whether a patient on that unit is HIV positive? Certainly, one can argue that key staff involved in the patient's treatment should know. But often this knowledge goes far beyond the boundaries of those who need to know. Recognizing this problem, AHIMA has published *Guidelines for Handling Health Data on Individuals Tested or Treated for the HIV Virus.* An excerpt from these guidelines appears in Figure 11–2. The issue goes well beyond HIV status, however. HIM professionals should provide leadership and training to their coworkers on the appropriate and inappropriate uses of health information.

General Principles Regarding Access and Disclosure Policies

Health Information Ownership

As a prerequisite for discussing specific access requests, it is important to have a basic understanding of health information ownership. Who owns the record and information? It is generally accepted that the health facility owns the record itself, but the exercise of those ownership rights is subject to the patient's ownership interest in the information within that record. Health information is, after all, a legal record of what was done for the patient, proof that billable services were rendered and that standards of care were (or were not!) met. On the other hand, patients have a right to control, to the extent possible, the flow of their private health information. This is one of the reasons why every health care facility needs policies and procedures to guide employees in handling health information access and disclosure

AHIMA'S POSITION ON MANAGING HEALTH INFORMATION RELATING TO HIV INFECTION

Increasingly, health information management professionals face a dilemma: how to meet the needs for information required for patient care, providers, payers, and the community, while protecting the patient from unauthorized, inappropriate, or unnecessary intrusion into the highly personal data of his or her health record.

To protect patient privacy and the confidentiality of information relating to HIV infection, the American Health Information Management Association (AHIMA) recommends the following:

1. Screening programs should be designed to provide confidential testing of individuals and communication of their test results.

2. Specific, written, informed consent should be obtained from the individual or his/her legal representative prior to voluntary testing. [Note: State law may permit testing of a patient without consent if a healthcare worker has been exposed to the patient's blood or body fluids. In such cases, the exposure incident and the need for HIV testing should be discussed with the patient or his legal representative before the test is done.] Post-test counseling should be provided by a qualified healthcare professional.

3. Health records of patients infected with HIV should be maintained with the health records of other patients in a secure area with restricted access. Special handling procedures should be avoided, as they are more likely to call attention to the patient's HIV status than routine handling methods.

4. Each facility should implement clear policies and procedures for disclosure of health information related to HIV/AIDS and assure consistent compliance. Generally, information on HIV infection and/or AIDS is reportable to local health authorities. Depending on state law, the facility may be required to report the name of the person tested or other identifying information.

Within the facility, a patient's serologic status should be disclosed only as needed for diagnosis, management, or treatment. Others who may review patient health records for administrative purposes (such as quality improvement, billing, and risk management) must assure this information is handled in a confidential manner.

Information should be disclosed to other legitimate users (including through the billing process) only with specific written authorization of the patient or his legal representative or upon receipt of a valid subpoena. Information disclosed to authorized users should be limited strictly to that required to fulfill the purpose stated on the authorization. Authorizations for the release of "any and all information" without specifically mentioning HIV or AIDS should not be honored. Due to the sensitivity of this information, it should not be transmitted via facsimile machine or disclosed over the telephone unless urgently needed for patient care.

Redisclosure of information relating to HIV/AIDS should be prohibited, unless otherwise required by state law.

5. HIV-positive healthcare workers should be managed according to guidelines outlined by the Centers for Disease Control and Prevention and state and federal laws. The healthcare worker's privacy must be balanced against the risk of transmission to patients, employees, and others. If questions arise, the facility's legal counsel should be involved in resolving the related questions.

FIGURE 11–2. AHIMA guidelines for handling health data on people who test positive or are treated for the human immunodeficiency virus. © American Health Information Management Association. Used by permission.

requests. Those who violate the patient's right to control the flow of his or her health information may be liable to that patient.

Resources on Releasing Patient Information

In setting policies and writing procedures to guide staff in handling health information and in responding to requests for information, various resources are available. As mentioned before, many state HIM associations have published excellent legal manuals. Peers in other local facilities are usually willing to share samples. AHIMA publishes various guidelines and practice standards, updating them and addressing new issues through position statements and practice guidelines. For example, when in the late 1980s and early 1990s the use of facsimile (fax) machines to transmit health information began to emerge, AHIMA published definitive guidelines on the subject (Figure 11–3). In 1994, AHIMA published a fully updated set of guidelines on disclosure of health information. Because laws can change and case law evolves over time, it is important to use the most up-to-date sources available when establishing policies and procedures. Many health care facilities use in-house or outside legal counsel to review such policies.

Authorizations for Disclosure of Patient Information

For an authorization for disclosure of health information to be valid, it should meet the following requirements:

- Be in writing (faxes or copies may be acceptable if permitted by health care policy)
- Be addressed to the health care provider
- Specifically identify the patient (generally, full name, address, and date of birth)
- Identify the individual or entity authorized to receive the information (e.g., "Jane Doe, Esq.," or "the Law Firm of Doe and Doe")
- Identify the information that is to be released (e.g., "a copy of my entire medical record from my June 1994 hospitalization")
- Specify the reason or purpose for the disclosure (e.g., "for use in personal injury claim")
- Specify a date, event, or condition on which the authorization will expire unless revoked earlier (e.g., "this authorization is good for 90 days")
- Indicate that the authorization is subject to revocation by the patient or legal representative

(except to the extent action has already been taken on it)

- Be signed by the patient or the patient's legal representative; if other than the patient, the relationship of the party signing the form for the patient is stated (Figure 11–4)
- Be dated sometime after the patient's admission, outpatient visit, or treatment. AHIMA recommends that no more than 6 months should have elapsed between the date of the signature on the authorization and the date the form is presented. Some states may require a shorter time frame for validity of the authorization.[23]

Disclosure for Direct Patient Care

When patients come to a health care facility or provider for treatment, it is reasonable to assume that they authorize their care providers to have information about their condition and treatment. What is *not* reasonable to assume is that they are authorizing access by anyone in the facility who may be curious to know that information as well. Internal disclosures for patient care purposes should be on a need-to-know basis. This means that those who really need to know the patient's health information to diagnose or treat that patient should have access. In these circumstances, patient authorization is not required.

Sometimes requests for disclosure of health information for patient care purposes come from outside the health facility in which the information was originally collected. For example, if the patient chooses to begin seeing a new physician or is treated at another health facility, it may be important for that new health care provider to obtain a copy of the patient's past health history, a test result, or the entire record. In fact, certain regulations (such as Medicare's *Conditions of Participation*) anticipate and require the transfer of relevant patient information on direct transfer of a patient from a hospital to a nursing facility. In the situation of a direct transfer, it may be argued that the patient's authorization to release information to the receiving facility is implied in their agreement to the transfer itself, and therefore, no authorization is required. This is common practice in many areas and may be covered in written transfer agreements between health care organizations. Nevertheless, there are arguments in favor of obtaining written authorization for any disclosure under this category, which involves releasing information outside the original facility, unless there is an emergency situation in which patient authorization *cannot* be obtained (e.g., the patient is unconscious and the care providers cannot wait for the information until the patient recovers enough to authorize release).[16]

AHIMA'S POSITION ON TRANSMISSION OF HEALTH INFORMATION

The American Health Information Management Association (AHIMA) recommends facsimile transmission of health information only when the original record or mail-delivered copies will not meet the needs of immediate patient care. The sensitive information contained in health records should be transmitted via facsimile only when: (1) urgently needed for patient care or (2) required by a third-party payer for ongoing certification of payment for a hospitalized patient. The information transmitted should be limited to that necessary to meet the requestor's needs. Routine disclosure of information to insurance companies, attorneys, or other legitimate users should be made through regular mail or messenger service.

Except as required by law, a properly completed and signed authorization should be obtained prior to the release of patient information. An authorization transmitted via facsimile is acceptable. If authorization cannot be obtained in cases of explained medical emergency, information may be released for patient care without authorization from the patient or legal representative.

The cover page accompanying the transmission should include a confidentiality notice that indicates the information is confidential and limits its use. A sample statement is provided below:

CONFIDENTIALITY NOTICE

The documents accompanying this telecopy transmission contain confidential information, belonging to the sender, that is legally privileged. This information is intended only for the use of the individual or entity named above. The authorized recipient of this information is prohibited from disclosing this information to any other party and is required to destroy the information after its stated need has been fulfilled.

If you are not the intended recipient, you are hereby notified that any disclosure, copying, distribution, or action taken in reliance on the contents of these documents is strictly prohibited. If you have received this telecopy in error, please notify the sender immediately to arrange for return of these documents.

Reasonable efforts should be made to assure the facsimile transmission is sent to the appropriate destination. Destination numbers should be pre-programmed into the machine, if possible, to eliminate errors in transmission from misdialing. The sender should contact the recipient prior to transmission to assure the recipient's availability and again immediately after transmission to verify receipt of the transmitted information. (For more detailed information on patient authorizations and recommended procedures, please see AHIMA's *Guidelines for Faxing Patient Health Information*.)

Receipt of Health Information

Unless otherwise prohibited by state law, information transmitted via facsimile is acceptable for inclusion in the patient's health record. If the document is on thermal paper, a photocopy of the document should be placed in the record to avoid the fading that may occur over time with thermal paper. (The facsimile copy should be destroyed after the photocopy is made.)

If the original document was authenticated by the author prior to transmission, the facsimile copy does not need to be countersigned, unless otherwise required by state law. To verify their authenticity, physician orders should be signed by the physician prior to transmission. Unsigned orders should not be carried out until verified with the ordering physician.

Development of Policies and Procedures

Health information management professionals should take the lead in developing policies and procedures to protect patients from unauthorized, inappropriate, or unnecessary intrusion into the sensitive information in their health records. Each provider should develop and enforce its own policies and procedures for transmitting health information via facsimile that protect patient privacy and comply with legal, regulatory, and accreditation requirements.

At a minimum, these policies and procedures should:

1. assure that fax machines are located in secure areas and limit access to them;

2. identify one individual to monitor incoming documents on each machine (this person should remove incoming documents immediately, examine them to assure receipt of all pages in a legible format, seal the documents in an envelope, and send them in accordance with their instructions);

3. outline appropriate safeguards to assure that transmitted information is sent to the appropriate individual; and

4. outline the procedures to be followed in the case of a misdirected transmission.

References

Bearden, Mary M. "Fax Control: Coping with the Legal Issues," *Journal of the American Health Information Management Association 63*, No. 5 (May 1992): 58–64.

Feste, Laura. "Practice Bulletin: Guidelines for Faxing Patient Health Information," *Journal of the American Health Information Management Association 62*, No. 6 (June 1991): 29–33.

Letter No. 90-25. Bureau of Policy Development, Health Care Financing Administration, June 1990.

Tomes, Jonathan P. *Healthcare Records Manual.* Boston, Massachusetts: Warren Gorham Lamont, 1993. 62, No. 6 (June 1991): 29–33.

Letter No. 90-25. Bureau of Policy Development, Health Care Financing Administrations, June 1990.

Tomes, Jonathan P. *Healthcare Records Manual.* Boston, Massachusetts: Warren Gorham Lamont, 1993.

FIGURE 11-3. AHIMA guidelines for faxing patient health information © American Health Information Management Association. Used by permission.

SITUATION	AUTHORIZING INDIVIDUAL
The patient is:	
An adult of sound mind, (age of majority defined in state statutes)	Patient
A minor	Parent or legal guardian
Deceased	Legal representative Executor of estate
Legally judged incompetent	Legally appointed guardian
Emancipated minor	Patient
Married	
Pregnant, or treated for pregnancy	
Treated for: (varies for each state) • Venereal disease • Birth control • Drug or alcohol abuse	
Minor and his parent is also a minor	Parent

FIGURE 11–4. Form to be signed by the individual who can authorize disclosure of confidential information (the patient or the patient's legal representative).

Disclosure for Quality Monitoring or Improvement Purposes

Health information can be used to evaluate the quality of care and services provided to patients. The record provides evidence of exactly what was done, when it was done, why it was done, and how things turned out. For that reason, it is a valuable tool in quality management activities. Using the information in quality management is an impersonal use. In other words, committee members are not interested in who the patient is but in the quality of services provided. Specific patients are referred to by record or identification numbers when individual cases must be mentioned in peer review or quality management minutes and records. Members of the medical and professional staff may have access to patient health information, without patient authorization, in this context. Even so, it is unwise to hand over records to someone just because that person happens to be on a peer review committee. Do not assume that quality management is the purpose for which all requests are made. A simple inquiry as to why the record or information is needed can help to assure that the request is indeed related to the requester's quality management responsibilities.

One other caveat on this point: It is not unheard of for health professionals to use health records to gather unflattering evidence of a competitor's professional skill. Even though records may be released without patient authorization for bona fide quality management activities, these informal "research" requests may not be sanctioned, official quality management activities. HIM professionals who are approached by a physician or other health professional with a request for records pertaining to other physicians or health professionals should ask the purpose of the request. If the answer does not indicate that the activity is official quality management business, then the requester should be asked to seek the approval of an appropriate committee or department chairperson. This protects the interests of all concerned.

Disclosure for Educational Purposes

Health information is a valuable teaching tool, both for student health professionals who are involved in formal training programs and for regular staff who must continue their education. Because some student health professionals may not be employed by the facility or otherwise bound to abide by the facility policies on confidentiality, it is important to assure that any students with access to patient-identifiable health information agree to follow facility policies on confidentiality. Some facilities write such an agreement into the contract between the facility and the educational program or school; others require students to sign individual confidentiality agreements or do both.

The educational use of the record is, like quality management, an impersonal use. It matters little who the patient is; what matters is what can be learned from the case. Teaching tools, such as case summaries, test results, photographs, surgical videos, and the like, should not identify the patient. Photographs and videos should be made in such a way that the patient cannot be identified, unless authorization to do so is obtained. Valid educational uses of health information do not require patient authorization.

Again, care must be exercised in responding to these requests. Facility procedures should provide for some way to verify the validity of a student's request for information access. Sometimes this is done by having the student's preceptor or supervisor sign off on all student record requests. If no such controls are in place, students may be tempted to review health information about friends, relatives, and other people in whom they have no valid interest.

Disclosure for Research

Research, like educational purposes, usually involves an impersonal use of health information. The researchers are not interested in the identity of the patient, just that the patient falls within some predefined research population or control group. Even so, facility policies should define the circumstances under which researchers may have access to health information without patient authorization. In many facilities, researchers must have their projects approved by an **institutional review board** (IRB), an advisory board that reviews the proposed research project for its objectives and proposed methods. If the researchers will have access to patient-identifiable data, it may be important to specify expected data security provisions in a written research agreement between the facility and the researcher. For example, the facility may want to require researchers to do all data collection on site in the HIM department and not remove original records or copies of records from the health facility. The HIM professional may expect to review proposed data collection forms to ensure that patient-identifiable data are not being collected.

Research projects in which the researchers want to directly contact patients pose a special problem because the simple act of verifying whether a patient is part of a specified group may, in many circumstances, be a breach of confidentiality. For those research projects believed to have sufficient merit to warrant cooperation, some facilities agree to act as intermediaries, notifying selected patients of the planned research and giving them the opportunity to determine whether or not they want to be contacted by the researchers. Only the addresses of those patients opting to participate are provided to the researchers.

Disclosure for Administrative Purposes

Disclosure for administrative purposes refers to the many internal activities that support the day-to-day functioning of the health care facility other than direct patient care, billing, and quality management. For example, a department manager or administrator may need access to certain limited patient information if he or she is responsible for responding to a complaint about the services provided to that patient by an employee of that department. Or a security manager may need to access a patient record to review an inventory of patient valuables to determine the validity of a patient's claims of lost property. A health care organization's professional liability insurer may want to review a sample of records to evaluate documentation practices and then use its assessments in determining the organization's insurability. The health care organization's attorney, in preparation for expected litigation, may need to review the record of a patient who was involved in a serious incident. Access, based on a need to know, can often be granted to such requests without authorization, but facility policies should define the situations in which patient authorization is required. Additionally, all such requests should be funneled through the HIM department to facilitate consistency in handling them.

One of the more potentially problematic administrative uses of health information involves database marketing strategies in health care. In these marketing strategies, specific health care services are marketed to patients who are most likely to have a need for those services. For example, brochures that describe a facility's new cardiac catheterization laboratory are mailed to patients who have been treated for cardiac-related problems or who are known to be at risk for such problems. The strategies make economic sense, but unless they are handled carefully, they run the risk of breaching confidentiality by publicly identifying patients as belonging to certain disease categories.[24] HIM professionals should be involved in evaluating proposed marketing uses of patient information to guard against abuses.

Disclosure for Payment Purposes

One of the most frequent disclosures of health information involves billing insurers for services provided to patients. Through clinical codes on the bill, information about the patient's diagnoses and procedures is relayed to the insurer, who then pays for the services provided. Because the use of this information is personal—in other words, the insurance company requires information about a specific patient to pay that patient's bill—authorization of the patient or his legal representative is required.

Disclosure for payment purposes is a controversial subject because quite frequently, the patient who receives the services is not the same person who authorized disclosure as part of the application for insurance coverage. Therefore, the person whose information is being disclosed may not have given written authorization for disclosure. Many facilities try to handle this situation by making authorization for disclosure of health information part of the general consent to treatment signed by all patients on admission for treatment. HIM professionals should exercise caution in disclosing information based on a release that was signed before the information was collected. Probably the most practical way to exercise such caution is to make it clear to all patients before treatment that information will be released to their health insurer. If a patient does not want information to go to his or her health insurer for this treatment episode, he or she can make other arrangements for payment of the bill. The form suggested in the AHIMA's *Guidelines for Handling Health Data on Individuals Tested or Treated for the HIV Virus* offers the patient the option of either authorizing disclosure to the health insurer or assuming financial responsibility for the services provided (Figure 11–5).

Disclosure to Attorneys

Written authorization from the patient or the patient's legal representative or a valid subpoena is required for release of health information to an attorney, unless that attorney represents the health care provider that owns the record. In other words, the hospital's legal counsel does not require patient authorization to obtain access to a specific record, but the attorney for the respiratory therapist employed by the hospital and involved in the case does. If the records sought are from a physician's office, that physician's attorney does not require authorization, but the attorney of a codefendant hospital does require patient authorization.

HIM professionals should take care in reviewing authorizations submitted by attorneys. Some attorneys use blanket authorizations with their clients, general statements that permit just about anyone to give an attorney just about any document that relates to the client. As with all other authorizations, the content of the authorization should be reviewed to make sure it complies with the health care facility's requirements as to form and content.

Disclosure to Law Enforcement Personnel and Agencies

Occasionally, various law enforcement representatives, including the medical examiner, are interested in gaining access to health information. For example, a police officer who accompanies an unconscious injured patient to the emergency department may need access to the

---

SELECT ONE OPTION BELOW

1. _____ I authorize the forwarding of my name, address, birthdate, the name of the test(s) and charges to my insurance company.

2. _____ I consent to allow the disclosure of my name, address, birthdate, name of the test(s), and the charge to Medicaid or other medical assistance programs.

Patient's Full Name:_____ Birthdate:_____

Address: _____

City, State, Zipcode: _____

Medicaid Number: _____

3. _____ I do not give my consent to release the name of the test(s) to my insurance company, or medical assistance program. I will pay the bill myself.

Signaturer: _____

I also authorize the following persons or agencies access to my HIV antibody test results:

_____   _____ to _____
Name of Person/Agency   Date valid

_____   _____ to _____
Name of Person/Agency   Date valid

FIGURE 11–5. Patient's billing consent form for HIV testing. (Courtesy of American Medical Record Association, Chicago.)

patient's past records to contact family members. The Federal Bureau of Investigation and Internal Revenue Service investigators have also been known to request access to health information. Nonconfidential information (e.g., patient address, date of treatment) can be given to bona fide law enforcement agents who present proper identification. Confidential information should be released only with written authorization of the patient or legal guardian or in response to valid subpoenas, court orders, or mandatory reporting statutes. Involve the facility's legal counsel if health care facility policies do not address the particular situation that presents itself.

In circumstances where a suspicious death has resulted in the medical examiner or coroner being called in to conduct a postmortem examination, the medical examiner may have access to the patient's health information for use in conducting the autopsy, and no authorization for release of information is required from the next of kin or legal representative.

Disclosure to Family Members When the Patient Is a Minor

Generally, patients control access to their own health information. They may review the information themselves and choose to either share the information with family members or withhold it. However, there are some exceptions, one of which is when the patient is a minor. Before a child reaches the age of majority, his or her parents or legal guardian generally make consent and authorization decisions on behalf of the child. In some limited circumstances, there are exceptions under various state and federal laws, such as when a minor child seeks treatment without parental involvement or consent (e.g., sexually transmitted disease, alcohol or substance abuse treatment) and when the minor is emancipated. Except in those circumstances, parents or guardians have access to the health information of their child or ward, and they may sign an authorization for disclosure on behalf of their unemancipated minor or ward. In cases of divorce and separation, disclosure decisions typically are made by the parent who has legal custody of the child.

Disclosure to Family Members When the Patient Is an Emancipated Minor or an Adult

State laws permit certain minors to make their own health care decisions without parental or guardian involvement. Although the conditions vary, they generally involve minors who are married, living away from their parents and family, and who are responsible for their own support. In those circumstances, that person is considered to be an **emancipated minor** and can obtain proof of that emancipation. An emancipated minor can consent to treatment without parental involvement and may authorize disclosure of his or her health information. Because many state laws do not specifically state this, caution should be exercised in drafting facility procedures.

Disclosure to Family Members in Cases of Incapacity or Incompetency

A sad comment on the treatment of America's elderly population—especially those who are involved in residential treatment programs such as nursing facilities—is that sometimes health care providers assume that the patient is incompetent to make his or her own decisions, and so younger family members are consulted on all treatment and disclosure issues. This is a mistake. Patients typically control access to and disclosure of their personal health information. Confidential information should not indiscriminately be shared with family members without the patient's authorization. One should never assume that a patient is incompetent to make such decisions unless that patient has been legally declared incompetent. The patient should be capable of deciding what health information, if any, is to be shared with family members or others, subject to applicable laws or regulations.

Incapacity is a different issue altogether. Competent patients may otherwise be unable to make access and disclosure decisions for various reasons. They may be unconscious, under anesthesia, comatose, and so on. In cases of temporary incapacity, health care providers should use common sense, good judgment, and some restraint in sharing appropriate health information with family members who are concerned for their relative. It may be appropriate to discuss the basic facts of the patient's condition and what the immediate plan is, but it may not be appropriate to disclose each and every detail. In cases of lengthy or permanent incapacity, a legal guardian for the patient may be appointed through court proceedings. When incapacity is anticipated, a person may grant power of attorney to another person, which authorizes the designee to act on behalf of the person who is now incapacitated. The person with power of attorney or the legally appointed guardian is then responsible for making decisions regarding the disclosure of health information to others.

Patient Access to Personal Health Information

Although the health care organization or provider owns the physical record of care, state statutes grant patients varying degrees of ownership interest in the health information in their records or data sets. Patients have no constitutional right to that information.[25] Nevertheless, the generally accepted rule is that, subject to any statutory prohibition or qualification, patients have a right to review their health information. Indeed, many state laws provide for patient access to their own health information, although these laws place varying restrictions on that right.

Partly because of the variation in state requirements, health care organizations' practices with respect to granting patients access to their health information differ considerably. Even within states, some health care organizations take a consumer-oriented approach, whereas others try to discourage access requests by imposing additional hurdles for the patient to jump, such as inconvenient hours for accepting and handling such requests. Some hospitals, for example, permit patients to review their health information during their hospitalization (with the attending physician present to answer questions), whereas others require that the patient be discharged and that the record or information be completed before such access is granted. HIM professionals must ensure that their facility policies comply with state and federal laws governing patient access. Within those limitations, the facility may have some latitude in the handling of patients' requests for information.

Whatever approach is taken, the HIM professional must establish reasonable safeguards for the security and confidentiality of the information. For example, before information is handed over in response to a patient request, there should be some reliable means of identifying the requester as the patient. It is certainly reasonable to obtain the patient's request in writing by way of a signature on an authorization for release of information form. This form may also be used to document that the review or release occurred. If the original hard-copy record is being reviewed, that review should be closely supervised to guard against alterations or destruction of the record. Some facilities notify the attending physician or other health care practitioner that his or her patient has requested record access. Facilities may also choose to set certain reasonable hours for such on-site reviews. Again, any facility-imposed restrictions should not conflict with relevant laws.

Interesting questions can arise in the context of patients' requests for access to their health information. For example, what should the HIM professional do if the attending physician thinks that allowing patients to see their health information would be harmful to their recovery? Sometimes this question arises with respect to mental health therapy. Some state laws severely restrict access to mental health records. Some require attending physicians to document in the record that they believe that access to the information would harm their patients. A facility may then refuse such a request.

Other Patient-Directed Disclosures

There are many other situations in which patients authorize other parties to receive their health informa-

tion. For example, when a patient applies for life insurance, disability insurance, or admission to certain schools or programs, he or she may authorize disclosure of health information. Provided the authorization meets the facility's requirements as to form and content, these requests should be promptly honored. Although HIM professionals do not encounter these requests every day, former patients occasionally want to examine their birth records to gain information about their natural parents if they were adopted. Problems may arise because of conflicts between some state laws that grant patients access to their records and adoption laws that may require sealed records to protect the privacy of the natural parents. The sealing of adoption-related records is common. Only a few states permit the adoptee to access these records, and a few provide for the disclosure of health information to the adoptee but strict confidentiality regarding the natural parents' identities. Disclosure of health information about the parents can be important to the adoptee when health conditions that may be genetically based arise later in life. Courts are often sympathetic to these "good cause" requests to open adoption-related records, but this is a decision to be made by a court, not by an individual facility. Keep in mind that not all requests for birth records necessarily require the identity of the parents to be revealed. If the former patient is interested only in time of birth, for example, the facility may be able to honor the request without jeopardizing the privacy rights of the natural parents.

Redisclosure Issues

Once a patient authorizes the disclosure of health information to other parties, such as insurers, control of the information is out of the facility's—and often the patient's—hands. For this reason, health care organizations include a notice along with the information being disclosed that advises the party receiving the information that redisclosure of the information is prohibited. Through this notice, the third party recipient is informed of its responsibility not to further disclose the information and to protect it from unauthorized use. Many health care facilities try to discourage redisclosure by stamping a redisclosure prohibition on all information sent out of the facility to alert the recipient that redisclosure issues must be referred to the facility's HIM department.

Another interesting practice with respect to redisclosure involves the insurance industry and the Medical Information Bureau (MIB). The MIB has been described as a kind of medical "credit bureau."[26] Its data bank contains files on millions of people that are shared among hundreds of member insurance companies. The purpose of the MIB is to alert insurers to certain information about applicants for insurance—information that could be used as the basis for denying insurance. Insurers cooperatively share health information they receive through the claims payment process, pooling it in the MIB for use by all members. How can they do this? The fine print on insurance contract applications generally gives the insurer both the right to use the MIB to access health information (if any information is on file there) and to redisclose information about any health claims into the MIB. The person signing the insurance application may not have been the patient. Thus, information about any given patient may end up being redisclosed into the MIB without the patient's knowledge or permission.

Disclosure to Record-Copying Services, Microfilm Service Bureaus, and Transcription Firms

Record-copying services are being used with increasing frequency in HIM departments, and outside contractors have been used over the years to microfilm records and perform medical transcription. Many departments use record-copying services to handle routine release of information tasks. Some managers have found that these services can supply a staff person on-site in the HIM department to do the job cheaper and more efficiently than the HIM department personnel.

Whether or not these services make financial sense, their use raises some interesting disclosure issues. The function that these outside contractors perform, by its very nature, involves access to confidential health information. HIM professionals who use these services must take steps to oversee the confidentiality, security, and appropriate handling of health information. The copying, microfilming, or transcription service should also be contractually bound to handle the confidential information appropriately. In those situations where confidential health information (e.g., dictated reports or hard-copy records) must be physically removed from the facility, such as when tapes are manually delivered to an outside transcription firm or dictation is digitally transmitted over phone lines to off-site locations, the HIM professional must ensure that adequate security measures are in place to prevent theft, loss, alteration, or destruction of the information. The HIM professional must also ensure that the removal of health information from the facility under this circumstance does not violate state laws. Check state laws to determine what restrictions apply to the removal of health information from the originating facility without patient authorization.

Disclosure to the News Media

A health care organization has no legal duty to disclose health information to the news media. In past years, hospitals often released basic information about admissions and births to the news media, but many facilities have discontinued this practice. A patient's right of privacy, however, does not bar the publication of information that is of public interest. Courts hold that with regard to a public figure, the celebrity's right to privacy must be weighed against the public's right to know and the freedom of the press. Therefore, if the patient is a public figure, health care organizations usually try, when releasing information to the media, to balance the public's need to know with the patient's need for privacy. For this reason, many health care facilities have adopted policies that permit a spokesperson to merely confirm admission and classify the patient's condition (e.g., critical, poor, fair, stable, good), except under extraordinary circumstances (e.g., treatment of the president or other key public figures). Disclosure of more detailed information should be avoided to minimize the risk of liability to the organization. At the same time, even confirming a patient's admission to a program for alcohol or drug abuse treatment would violate federal law if it were done without the patient's permission.

Some segments of the media have been known to use unusual measures to try to obtain health information on celebrity patients. Staff members may even be approached with bribes. Facility policies should speak to the measures to be used in handling celebrity records. Special security procedures for preserving the confidentiality of these patients' health information may be appropriate. Some facilities use special code names on printed reports, with the code known only to the HIM director, physician, and chief executive officer, but these procedures may conflict with the laws of some states with regard to identifying the patient. Some facilities remove such records from their regular filing or computerized systems and store hard-copy reports in a locked file in the HIM department with limited access. The HIM professional should work with the organization's legal counsel or risk manager to devise an appropriate strategy for dealing with celebrity records.

Disclosure Pursuant to Legal Process

When health information needs to be used in court, the request for information comes in the form of a **subpoena duces tecum,** a **subpoena** (which may also be called a subpoena ad testificandum), a written court order, or simply a verbal order issued in court to the health care organization's attorney. A subpoena is a written order that requires someone to come before the court to testify. A subpoena duces tecum is a written order that requires someone to come before the court and to bring certain records or documents named in that order. When health information is needed in court or in pretrial discovery, such as a deposition, those orders are typically directed to the HIM department director.

State laws vary on who is empowered to issue subpoenas; judges, court clerks, and other officials may be authorized—even attorneys. The form that the subpoena must take to be valid is also a matter of state law, but generally, a subpoena must contain the following:

- A docket number

- The names of the parties (plaintiffs and defendants) involved in the case

- The name of the court or agency before which the proceeding is being held

- The details as to when and where the HIM director's appearance is being requested

- The documents that must be brought

- The signature and seal of the official issuing the subpoena

State laws vary with regard to the method by which and the time limits within which subpoenas can be properly served. Some court systems require service by sheriffs or other public officers. Other jurisdictions permit service by mail or messenger. In still other jurisdictions, service must be accomplished in person, by handing the subpoena to the HIM professional. There are also jurisdictions in which the service must be accompanied by a fee to reimburse the person subpoenaed for his or her time and expense. This nominal fee (called a witness fee) is usually set by statute or court rules. HIM professionals must become familiar with the requirements applicable to their state and federal jurisdictions to ensure that they properly respond to the subpoenas received.

Responding to any subpoena that requires the production of health information usually involves the same basic steps (Figure 11–6). These steps, especially when computerized health information is involved, vary somewhat, depending on the design of the facility's information system. Most state HIM associations' legal manuals offer good step-by-step procedures for responding to subpoenas, based on the statutes and rules of that jurisdiction. Roach, Chernoff, and Esley recommend that the procedures include the following steps at a minimum.

1. Examine the information subject to subpoena to make certain that it is complete, that signatures and initials are legible, and that each page identifies the patient and the patient's identification number. (If the information is not yet complete, try to complete it. However, one cannot ignore a subpoena because the information is not yet complete).

2. Read the information to determine whether the case forms the basis for a possible negligence action against the facility; if so, notify the appropriate administrator. (In some facilities, the HIM department performs this function in coordination with the risk management or legal department.)

3. Remove any material that may not properly be obtained in the jurisdiction by subpoena, such as notes that refer to psychiatric care, copies of information from other facilities (unless they have been properly incorporated into the patient's information), and correspondence.*

4. Number each page of the patient record, and write the total number of pages on the record folder.

5. Prepare a list of the record contents to be used as a receipt for the information if it must be left with the court or an attorney. (Most facilities use a standard form for this purpose.)

6. Whenever possible, use a photocopy of the record rather than the original in responding (in person) to legal process. (A certificate of authentication can be helpful in convincing the court to accept the photocopy as a true and exact copy of the original.)[27]

The facility's procedures should describe these steps as well as the steps to follow if a subpoena is defective in some way (e.g., issued by the wrong party, conflicts with state or federal law, asks for records not in the facility's possession). Ignoring a subpoena or court order creates trouble, possibly serious trouble. Involve the facility's legal counsel in drafting procedures for dealing with subpoenas and court orders, and do not hesitate to refer unusual problems to your facility's legal counsel. Legal counsel may decide to file a **motion to quash** the subpoena or order in which the court is asked to set aside the subpoena or order.

As mentioned earlier, court orders can be issued in writing or verbally in court to your facility's attorney. A health care organization should make every effort to comply with a court order as long as the order does not place the facility in the position of violating a statute or regulation. Again, as with the subpoena, if the court order is defective in some way (e.g., would force the facility to violate state or federal law), legal counsel must be involved immediately to work out a solution and to help the facility's leaders avoid being cited for contempt of court.

Just because health information has been subpoenaed does not mean that it will be admissible as evidence. Here again, state laws vary as to the admissibility of health information. As explained earlier, admissibility issues have become somewhat murky as new technologies for collecting, storing, and retrieving health information are put into use.

---

* For a discussion of the issues involved in relying on other health care facilities' tests and records and incorporating them into the patient's record, see King PD: Inclusion of reports from other sources in hospital records. Topics in Health Record Management 1984;5(4):81–88.

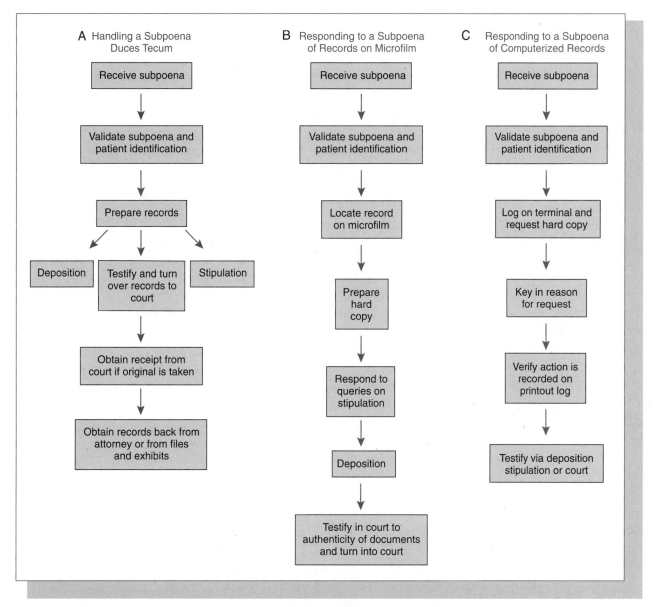

A Handling a Subpoena Duces Tecum

- Receive subpoena
- Validate subpoena and patient identification
- Prepare records
  - Deposition
  - Testify and turn over records to court
  - Stipulation
- Obtain receipt from court if original is taken
- Obtain records back from attorney or from files and exhibits

B Responding to a Subpoena of Records on Microfilm

- Receive subpoena
- Validate subpoena and patient identification
- Locate record on microfilm
- Prepare hard copy
- Respond to queries on stipulation
- Deposition
- Testify in court to authenticity of documents and turn into court

C Responding to a Subpoena of Computerized Records

- Receive subpoena
- Validate subpoena and patient identification
- Log on terminal and request hard copy
- Key in reason for request
- Verify action is recorded on printout log
- Testify via deposition stipulation or court

FIGURE 11–6. Flowcharts outlining steps in responding to subpoena duces tecum. (Adapted from Waters K, Murphy G: Medical records in health information. Germantown, MD: Aspen Systems Corp., 1979.)

HIM professionals occasionally are called on not only to produce the subpoenaed health information but to testify as well. This process typically involves being sworn in and answering questions that lay the foundation for introduction of the patient's record into evidence. HIM professionals may be asked questions about whether the record or information was prepared in the normal course of daily business or according to established policies and procedures for documentation and record-keeping. It is important for them to answer honestly and not speculate on matters that are beyond their knowledge. They should not guess at the "correct" answer to a question. When the answer to a question is not known, the proper response is simply to say, "I don't know" or "I am not qualified to answer that."

HIM Department Security Measures to Prevent Unauthorized Access

Ensuring that all formal releases of information are appropriately handled is only one aspect of protecting the confidentiality and security of health information.

Careful, thorough release-of-information policies are ineffective if internal security measures and systems are inadequate to protect health information from loss, theft, destruction, and alteration. One important aspect of protecting health information is preventing unauthorized access. In other words, how can facilities and HIM professionals keep health information out of the hands of unauthorized users?

Who might that "unauthorized user" be? It may be a curious employee or coworker who knows that his or her neighbor was recently admitted and wants to find out what is wrong with the person. It may be a private investigator who is trying to get information about someone on behalf of a client. It may be a computer hacker who breaks into the facility's health information system just for the challenge. It may even be a physician who is reviewing the records of a competitor's patients and trying to collect ammunition for a battle over delineation of privileges or medical staff membership. One of the most important responsibilities HIM professionals have is keeping confidential health information out of the hands of unauthorized users through appropriate policies and procedures, facility and space planning, information systems design and selection, staff education, and other measures.

HIM policies and procedures should specify who has access to what—ideally, as specifically as possible. In an issue of the AHIMA's confidentiality newsletter, *In Confidence,* information system security expert Dale Miller recommended that information security policies define, by specific job function, information access. "An individual should have full and timely access to the information they need to perform their current tasks, but only for the purposes of fulfilling their responsibilities."[28] When a facility employee asks to review a patient's health information, HIM professionals should not hesitate to inquire about the employee's purpose and/or need. Many times, legitimate information needs can be handled by less intrusive means than handing over a complete record. The question itself may discourage or defeat illegitimate or suspicious requests. Likewise, HIM professionals should not hesitate to verify the propriety of a request. Anyone can buy a laboratory coat and walk into a nursing station where health information is readily displayed. A person so attired may even be able to stroll unchallenged through an HIM department if staff are not adequately trained in security measures. Many health care organizations are so large that it is impossible for HIM department employees to know all the employees in other departments. Verification of employee identification is a legitimate security measure, as is checking with the employee's supervisor as to the validity of certain requests. Locked access to data processing areas is a legitimate security measure, as is locked access to record storage areas. Sometimes even these basic security measures are not observed. Part of

an HIM professional's job is to insist on adequate security measures for both manual and electronic health information systems.

Duty to Provide Care That Meets Professional Standards

In addition to a health care organization's or provider's duty to maintain the confidentiality of a patient's health information, there is a duty to provide care that meets professional standards. Simply put, health care providers must provide a reasonable quality of care to patients—care that meets professional standards. Liability can and does arise when providers fail to meet professionally accepted standards of quality, such as those issued by various medical specialty societies and other consensus groups and those dictated by statute or regulation.

Before liability can be found, the claimant or plaintiff must meet certain requirements and overcome certain obstacles. First, the complaining party must file his or her claim within the **statute of limitations.** For this chapter's purposes, what this means is that once a plaintiff knows (or reasonably should have known) that he or she has a potential claim against a health care organization or provider, he or she must file that claim within a certain period of time (e.g., within 2 years of discovering the malpractice). Otherwise, the claim will not be heard by a court. Statutes of limitations are designed to encourage the timely filing of claims, when evidence is fresh and witnesses are likely to be available. Through prompt filing of claims, the search for the truth is facilitated.

In some states, the plaintiff must also obtain a statement from a neutral health care provider (such as a physician) before filing a malpractice claim, certifying that the claim has some merit. Some states use this approach to discourage the filing of nuisance and groundless claims.

For any negligence or malpractice claim to succeed, the plaintiff must show that all of the following elements of negligence or malpractice are present.

- *Duty.* The defendant must have had some duty to the plaintiff to use care. A physician, for example, owes a duty to his or her patients to use care that meets professional standards but owes no professional duty to the letter carrier who delivers the office mail.

- *Breach.* The defendant must be shown to have breached that duty (by action or inaction). In other words, the defendant's conduct must have failed to conform to the applicable **standard of care.**

- *Proximate cause.* The breach must be the "proximate" cause of the harm that befell the plaintiff.[29]

- *Harm, or Damages.* The plaintiff must show that he or she was harmed in some way (e.g., physical pain, suffering, emotional distress, monetary losses).

How does a judge or jury decide whether a defendant acted unreasonably—breaching his or her "duty" to the plaintiff? If the claim involves simple (not professional) negligence, the judge or jury uses the **"reasonable man" standard.** In other words, the jury is told to evaluate the parties' conduct in light of jury's own general experience and background. In professional negligence (malpractice) cases, the jury has no experience and training to draw from in evaluating the parties' actions. Therefore, the standard used to judge a professional's actions is the generally accepted standard of care for that profession. For example, orthopedic surgeons' actions are judged against the current standard of care in orthopedics. Pediatricians' actions are judged against pediatric standards of care and so on. These guidelines can be established by expert testimony, professional literature, or published standards. The applicable standard of care is often determined by referring to current standards published by the relevant specialty society and the professional literature. Sometimes it is determined by referring to accreditation and licensing standards. By pointing to deficiencies in meeting those standards, plaintiffs' attorneys hope to bolster their allegations of negligence.

When a plaintiff brings a civil suit against a defendant, he or she has the **burden of proof.** In other words, unless the plaintiff can convince the judge or jury by a preponderance of evidence (making it more likely than not) that the claims against the defendant are valid, the defendant will prevail. In a malpractice case against health care providers and/or organizations, the burden of proof often shifts to the defendant under a concept called **res ipsa loquitur** ("the thing speaks for itself"). An inference of negligence or malpractice is permitted simply because an injury to the plaintiff occurred under the following circumstances:

- The event would not normally have occurred in the absence of negligence.

- The defendant had exclusive control over the instrumentality (e.g., instrument, equipment, procedures) that caused the injury.

- The plaintiff did not contribute to the injury.[30]

For example, if a patient developed postoperative abdominal adhesions after a surgical sponge was inadvertently left in his abdomen during surgery, the burden of proof would shift to the defendants (probably the surgeon and facility) for the following reasons:

- Surgical sponges are not supposed to be left in the operative site and sewn up inside a patient.

- The sponge, surgical technique, and sponge-counting procedures were within the exclusive control of the defendants.

- The patient did nothing to contribute to the injury.

All three elements must be present to successfully shift the burden of proof in a negligence or malpractice case to the defendant. Otherwise, the plaintiff retains the burden of proving the defendant's negligence by a preponderance of the evidence.

Health information is extremely important in cases that revolve around the health care provider's and organization's duty to provide care that meets professional standards. In many cases, the documentation of the care provided is the most important evidence available to the trier of fact (the jury, or the judge in cases without a jury). As health care providers soon come to realize, their documentation practices can either help them or hurt them in defending against malpractice claims. Care taken in thorough documentation can make all the difference in the outcome of malpractice litigation.

Incident, or **occurrence, reports** can be important pieces of documentation in investigating, pursuing, and defending against claims against health care organizations and providers. These reports, which should not be treated as part of the patient's health information, are factual summaries of unexpected events that have resulted (or could have resulted) in injury or harm to patients, staff, or visitors. They are used by health care organizations' risk managers and/or attorneys to investigate incidents that have the potential to become claims against the organization or individual provider and to identify areas in which improvements are needed. In many facilities, these reports serve as an important data source for the quality improvement program by identifying shortcomings and suggesting possible solutions.

State laws vary considerably with respect to protecting the incident report from discovery by plaintiffs and their attorneys. In some states, the reports are protected as part of the attorney-client privilege as long as the incident report is handled as a document prepared in anticipation of possible litigation and not used for other purposes (e.g., quality improvement). In other states, the incident report may be protected from discovery as part of the facility's peer review and quality improvement efforts. In still other states, the incident report is not protected and, therefore, users must be extremely careful about what is documented in the report. Facility legal counsel should be actively involved in defining incident report preparation and handling procedures, so that the maximum protection possible can be obtained for these reports.

Duty to Obtain Informed Consent to Treatment

One important duty to patients that HIM professionals must be aware of is the physician's duty to obtain the patient's **informed consent** to treatment. Many times, when health professionals refer to obtaining **consent**, they mean getting a permit signed by a patient. Actually, obtaining consent refers to a communication process between the health professional and the patient. Unless that communication successfully informs the patient about the anticipated treatments and meets certain basic requirements, it cannot be considered a valid consent.

For practical purposes, the duty to obtain informed consent splits into the following two parts:

- The duty to obtain a general consent for treatment (a largely administrative process that consists of obtaining the patient's signature on a form, often preprinted on the back of the facility's "face" sheet or emergency department record)

- The attending physician's or surgeon's duty to obtain a separate informed consent before the performance of surgery or other invasive procedures

Because the patient has presented himself or herself at the facility for treatment and that implies (to a certain extent) his or her consent to at least basic care, obtaining a signature on the general consent to treatment is typically a simple process. Obtaining an informed consent before the performance of surgery or other invasive procedures is often much more complex. How, for example, does the care provider know that the patient is truly making an informed decision?

For a consent obtained by a health care provider to be valid, the health care provider must meet certain requirements. These requirements may be specified in state law and commonly include the following:

- The informed consent should be obtained by the person who will carry out the procedure. In other words, the process of communicating the planned procedure or treatment and its risks, benefits, and alternatives should be handled by the person who will do or supervise the procedure. In the case of surgery, it would be the surgeon. Keep in mind that some states and case law permit the physical act of obtaining a signature on the consent form to be delegated to others, provided the process of informing the patient has already taken place.

- The patient must be capable of giving an informed consent. In other words, the patient must be legally and mentally capable of understanding what is being proposed and making a decision. If the patient has been judged legally incompetent or because of certain emergency circumstances (such as unconsciousness accompanied by a life-threatening injury) cannot give an informed consent, the guardian or next of kin (designated by state law to act in the patient's stead) must receive the information and sign the consent.

- Are minors capable of giving informed consent? In some circumstances and for some treatments they are. But how young is too young? This criterion varies from state to state. Barring any state law that prohibits this action, minors may indeed be capable of giving informed consent. Yet another aspect of this question is whether the otherwise competent patient can understand what is being said because of language barriers, hearing impairment, literacy problems, or other issues. Care providers must ensure that a patient can understand the risks, benefits, and alternatives to the proposed procedure before they obtain the patient's signature. Many facilities maintain a list of employees who can speak a foreign language. In areas where there are large populations of non–English-speaking patients, it may be important to prepare patient educational materials and consent forms in the most common non-English languages. Having access to people who are competent to use sign language is also a common need.

- The patient must be free from coercion or undue influence when giving consent. The consent of a patient who agrees to an incidental tubal ligation during gynecologic surgery because her husband threatens not to pay the hospital bill unless she does so is not considered valid.

- The consent should be granted for a specific procedure or treatment. In other words, if the physician asks for permission to do "abdominal surgery," it would be difficult to argue that the patient is giving a truly informed consent. If the diagnosis is uncertain, however, and exploratory surgery is required, the patient may indeed grant valid consent for the physician to do exploratory surgery and to proceed with more extensive surgery if, in the surgeon's opinion, it is warranted (e.g., when frozen-section laboratory results indicate cancer). The key issue is whether the patient has been adequately informed of this possibility and agrees to proceed.

- The patient must indeed be adequately informed. State laws provide some guidance on the standard to be used in judging questions as to whether the patient was given enough information. In some states, it is within the caregiver's discretion to decide whether enough information has been given. In other states, a "reasonable man" standard is used. Generally, the standards require that the patient receive information about the nature and purpose of the proposed procedure, the risks and benefits of the proposed treatment, any reasonable alternatives to this procedure, and the risks of refusing the proposed procedure or treatment.[31]

- The patient is given an opportunity to ask and receive answers to his or her questions. This is a fairly common problem faced by health care facility staff when trying to obtain the patient's signature on the consent form after the physician has discussed the procedure with the patient and left. The patient may have been reluctant to pose certain questions to the physician or may not have had time to think through all his or her questions, and the facility staff are faced with a dilemma. Does the fact that the patient still has questions mean that he or she has not been adequately informed? Facility policies should define how far staff should go, if they should be involved at all, in answering questions, or whether they should immediately contact the physician so that the patient might speak with him or her directly. Most facilities take an intermediate approach: If the question is not really related to the decision-making process (e.g., the patient wants to know about how long the procedure will take), staff may attempt to answer without questioning the validity of the consent. In cases of doubt, however, the physician should be involved. Otherwise, staff may find themselves involved in a postprocedure suit alleging a lack of informed consent.

There are a few circumstances in which informed consent is not required. In life-threatening situations where the patient is incapable of expressing consent, consent is implied by law. In addition, there are situations in which although consent is required, it need not be accompanied by the normal disclosure of risks, benefits, alternatives, and so on. For example, if there is not time to fully discuss all relevant facts because treatment must begin immediately, some care providers have been excused for giving only a brief summary of the facts as long as the patient agrees to the treatment itself. And in limited circumstances, some care providers have been excused from providing all relevant facts when the provider believes that full disclosure would be harmful. "Therapeutic privilege" could apply when a patient is clearly beyond his or her ability to cope with the details

of needed treatment, but this would have to be clearly documented to withstand court scrutiny. Patients may also waive the right to be informed. For example, if the physician attempts to inform the patient but the patient says that he or she would rather not know, just go ahead, the physician should clearly document the patient's waiver and all attempts to inform the patient. In addition, some patients may have had similar procedures or treatments before and may already be familiar with the relevant facts. Again, this situation should be documented.

Along with the right to grant consent is the right to refuse any treatment. In recent years, public attitude toward death with dignity and outcries over heroic attempts to keep patients alive at all costs (both financial and human) led to the enactment of the Patient Self-Determination Act.[32] This legislation requires health care facilities to query patients about their life support–related wishes on admission. These wishes are documented as **advance directive** to health care providers in the event they become necessary. An advance directive can be either a **living will,** a written document that allows a competent adult to indicate his or her wishes regarding life-prolonging medical treatment, or a **durable power of attorney for health care,** in which a competent adult names in writing another adult to make any medical decisions on his or her behalf in the event he or she becomes incapacitated. The documentation requirements for these advance directives vary by state. The directives, if they exist, are then maintained with the patient's health information.

Duty to Provide a Safe Environment for Patients and Visitors

A common duty of health care facilities and providers is to provide a safe environment for patients and visitors. If a patient is dropped and injured while being moved from an emergency department stretcher to an x-ray table, the facility (as employer of the people involved) is likely to be held liable for any damages. If a visitor stumbles in the facility's parking lot because the lot lights were not functioning and lawn care equipment was carelessly left in the lot's walkways by the facility's maintenance employees, the facility is liable for damages. If an infant is abducted from the neonatal nursery because the nursery was short-staffed and the babies were momentarily left unsupervised, the facility is likely to be held liable for damages.

When health care facilities open themselves up to the public and to patients for "business," they assume a duty to provide a reasonably safe environment. That is not to say that any injury is compensable. For example, if a visitor who is not watching where she is going stumbles over a clearly marked step and crashes through a plate glass window, the facility may not be responsible. Likewise, if a distraught person enters the facility's emergency department with a gun and begins firing, killing patients and employees, there might be no liability for the facility.

The key issue in determining if the facility breached its duty to provide a safe environment is whether or not the facility's actions (or lack of actions) were reasonable under the circumstances. And what is reasonable? How much is enough? That determination often is difficult to make in advance. Certainly, at a minimum, the public expects health care facilities to meet the following criteria:

- To comply with life safety and building codes as well as other recognized standards

- To provide certain training to employees

- To make sure that the equipment and materials used on patients are clean and functioning properly

Duty to Supervise the Actions of Employees and the Professional Staff

Just as health care organizations must take reasonable steps to provide a safe environment for patients and visitors, they must also supervise the actions of employees and the professional staff (including medical staff). As discussed earlier in the chapter, a health care organization can be held liable for damages when its employees fail to adequately perform their duties, under the doctrine of respondeat superior ("let the master answer").

This does not just apply to patient care duties. A health care organization can be liable for an employee's failure to perform other duties as well. For example, if an employee of a large physician group practice inappropriately releases confidential information to an unauthorized party, the group practice could be held liable in a breach of confidentiality suit filed by the patient. Employers are responsible for training their staff to properly exercise their duties. Using this example, a health care organization should certainly ensure that staff members understand proper release-of-information practices and follow them. Many facilities go even further and insist that employees with access to confidential information sign an agreement to keep that information confidential and to follow facility policies on confidentiality. Figure 11–7 is a sample nondisclosure agreement by AHIMA that is designed for use with employees, volunteers, and students in the HIM department.

EMPLOYEE/STUDENT/VOLUNTEER
Non-Disclosure Agreement

[Name of health care facility] has the legal and ethical responsibility to safeguard the privacy of all patients and protect the confidentiality of their health information. In the course of my employment/assignment at *[name of health care facility]*, I may come into possession of confidential patient information, even though I may not be directly involved in providing patient services.

I understand that such information must be maintained in the strictest confidence. I hereby agree that, unless directed by my supervisor, I will not at any time during or after my employment/assignment with *[name of health care facility]* disclose any patient information to any person whatsoever or permit any person whatsoever to examine or make copies of any patient reports or other documents prepared by me, coming into my possession, or under my control.

When patient information must be discussed with other health care practitioners in the course of my work, I will use discretion to assure that such conversations cannot be overheard by others who are not involved in the patient's care.

I understand that violation of this agreement may result in corrective action, up to and including discharge.

_____   _____
Signature of Employee/Student/Volunteer   Date

FIGURE 11–7. Sample employee/student/volunteer nondisclosure agreement. (From Brandt M: Maintenance, disclosure, and redisclosure of health information. Chicago: AHIMA, 1994. Used by permission.)

Medical Staff Credentialing Process

Under the doctrine of corporate negligence, a health care organization can also be held liable for the acts of its nonemployed staff such as the medical staff. In one of the most important cases on the doctrine of corporate negligence, *Elam v. College Park Hospital*, the court held that a hospital is liable to a patient for the negligent conduct of independent physicians and surgeons who are neither employees nor agents of the hospital.[33] A hospital owes patients a duty to ensure the competency of its medical staff and to evaluate the quality of medical care rendered on its premises. This is one of the main reasons behind medical staff credentialing programs, in which prospective members of the medical staff apply for membership and request that certain privileges to practice medicine at that facility be granted. Likewise, current members of the medical staff periodically (usually every 2 years) renew or request new or changed privileges to render certain types of care and services at the facility.

The purpose of the medical staff credentialing process

is to ensure that only qualified physicians and other credentialed health professionals practice within the facility. During the appointment and reappointment process, the applicant's background is reviewed, licenses and certifications are checked, proof of current liability insurance is verified, and practice patterns and quality review data are evaluated to determine whether the applicant should be granted the privileges he or she seeks to gain or renew. If the evaluation is done poorly, medical staff credentialing decisions can result in liability for the health care organization. In *Rule v. Lutheran Hospitals and Homes Society of America*, a hospital was liable for birth injuries that occurred during an infant's breech delivery.[34] The jury found that the hospital had failed to adequately investigate the background and qualifications of the attending physician before granting him delivery privileges. The hospital had in fact failed to check with other hospitals in which the physician had practiced. If that check had been made, the hospital would have discovered that the physician's privileges to perform breech deliveries at one of those other hospitals had been substantially curtailed. This probably would have led to similar restrictions on the physician at the defendant hospital and perhaps would have made the physician ineligible for that privilege altogether.

The actual investigative and documentation procedure that is followed in acting on initial appointment and reappointment applications is outlined in the facility's medical staff bylaws and medical staff rules and regulations. Some state statutes address credentialing requirements, and JCAHO standards impose certain criteria that should be met. The Health Care Quality Improvement Act of 1986 also imposes some credentialing-related requirements on health care organizations. These requirements are discussed in Chapter 10.

There is another body of federal and state laws that can affect the credentialing process. These laws are related to antitrust liability. Antitrust laws were developed to protect and encourage competition. Antitrust liability can arise in this context when the medical or professional staff credentialing process interferes with a physician's or health professional's ability to pursue his or her profession. This interference may be alleged to be a **restraint of trade**. This claim could arise, for example, when the only hospital for miles around enters into an exclusive employment agreement for certain specialty care consulting services and declares that any inpatients who need this specialty care may only use the employed specialist. The following laws protect against restraint of trade:

- The Sherman Act, which prohibits monopolies created by agreements among competitors[35]
- The Clayton Act, which prohibits certain arrangements that tend to lessen competition,

such as certain "tying arrangements" that deny freedom of choice in selecting services and products[36]
- The Federal Trade Commission Act, which prohibits unfair methods of competition that affect commerce

Sometimes physicians try to use these acts to support their claims that their denial of staff privileges has the effect of reducing competition. Probably the best defense to actions that arise out of the denial of staff membership to an individual is for the health care organization to show a valid basis for the denial of privileges (e.g., quality-of-care problems). The defense strategy is different when the complaint involves the denial of privileges to a whole class of plaintiffs, such as podiatrists, but that is beyond the scope of this chapter. Be aware, however, that physicians and other health professionals are increasingly sensitive to antitrust problems and that the avoidance of antitrust liability should be considered when developing credentialing-related policies and procedures.

The credentialing process has its own set of confidential information: the credentials file and the practitioner's quality profile. The credentials file is basically a dossier on each medical or professional staff member. It typically contains at least the following:

- Completed medical staff application for appointment or reappointment
- Copies of the practitioner's license, diplomas, board certifications, controlled substances permit (for prescribing certain drugs), proof of current professional liability insurance, response to the facility's query of the National Practitioner Data Bank (NPDB) (established by the Health Care Quality Improvement Act of 1986) and perhaps other organizations (e.g., the Federation of State Medical Boards and AMA Physician Masterfile), and other documents required by the bylaws (e.g., results of any proctoring or observation of the practitioner that is done during the initial "provisional" appointment to the staff)
- Completed references from various sources (e.g., program directors for residencies, department chairpersons at other facilities where the practitioner works)
- Specific listing of the privileges requested by the physician and approved by the medical staff

This background information is supplemented with a quality profile for the practitioner, which is usually kept apart from the credentials file. The profile typically contains statistical information on the volume and type of cases treated in the past by the practitioner. It also contains information on the number and type of cases that have been subjected to quality reviews and the results of those reviews. Department chairpersons and credentials committee members use this information in evaluating the practitioner's competence. This helps them to decide whether or not to grant the requested privileges. The practitioner may only treat the kinds of cases and perform the kinds of procedures for which he or she possesses clinical privileges in that facility. For this reason, credentialing and privileging decisions often involve sensitive issues and may be the subject of debate, disagreement, and even litigation (if requested privileges are denied).

Accessibility of Credentials Files and Quality Profiles

Because of their sensitive contents, the credentials file and quality profile are treated as confidential information. As a result, health care organizations need to establish clear policies on who may have access to the files and information, how the files and information are kept secure, and how long the information must be retained. HIM professionals are often involved in developing such policies.

To develop appropriate access policies that govern credentialing-related information, the HIM professional needs to understand who plays a role in the credentialing and privilege delineation process. Although the scenario may vary with individual organizations' medical staff bylaws, the following key players commonly are involved.

Applicant, or Practitioner. This refers to the person who is applying for either initial appointment or reappointment and is requesting certain clinical privileges. The practitioner has the right to review the contents of his or her own credentials file and quality profile.

Department Chairperson. This is the clinical chairperson of the medical or professional staff department to which the applicant or practitioner belongs or wants to belong. The department chairperson must meet with the applicant or practitioner, review the contents of his or her credentials file and quality profile, and make a recommendation to the credentials committee and/or medical executive committee with respect to the application or request for privileges.

Credentials Committee. Members of this medical staff committee are charged with responsibility for reviewing the contents of the credentials file and quality profile and recommending action to the medical executive committee and/or governing body. Credentials committees usually are made up of a cross section of the medical and professional staff and provide a sort of check and balance on the appointment and privilege delineation process. For example, if the department chairperson of pediatrics does not want a new pediatrician added to the staff because that would mean more competition for patients, he or she might recommend against appointment of an otherwise qualified pediatrician. A cross-sectional credentials committee would probably not have those same biases and, therefore, could help prevent claims of unfairness.

Medical Executive Committee. This committee, commonly made up of the officers of the medical staff and clinical department chairperson, often is involved in reviewing the recommendations of the individual department chairperson and credentials committee and then passing that information along to the facility's governing body with its own recommendation. Access policies should define whether executive committee members should have direct access to credential files and quality profiles in their capacity as committee members or whether their review and recommendations should be limited to the information presented by the credentials committee and department chairperson. Because the executive committee often has major responsibilities for supervising the quality of clinical practice in the facility, members often have direct access to related files and information.

Governing Body, or Board of Directors. As the group ultimately responsible for assuring the quality of services provided by the facility and its professional staff, the governing body makes the final decision on requests for appointment or reappointment and clinical privileges. This group often relies heavily on the recommendations made by the medical executive committee, department chairperson, and credentials committee but need not be bound by those recommendations. Facility access policies should define whether board members have direct access to credential files and quality profiles.

Medical Staff Coordinator. This person is responsible for collecting, organizing, filing, and controlling access to information within the credentials file and, often, the quality profile. By the very nature of his or her responsibilities, this person must have access to the files and information. Some facilities choose to separate the handling of the quality profile, delegating that responsibility to the staff who coordinate all quality management and improvement activities. In those cases, the person responsible for the credentials file might not have access to quality profile data.

To the extent that HIM professionals are involved in credentialing-related activities, they will have some access to credential and quality profile information. In some facilities, HIM professionals serve as medical staff coordinators. In other facilities, those responsibilities are separate from the HIM function, and HIM staff do not have access to this information.

Legal Risks

As mentioned earlier, the tasks of professional staff appointment, reappointment, and delineation of clinical privileges are fraught with potential problems. Physicians who are dissatisfied with the decisions made by a facility may choose to sue the facility, using a wide variety of legal theories. The elements essential to a successful defense vary with the legal theories involved, but generally, in defending these attacks, it is important to be able to show the following:

- That the facility's bylaws, rules, and regulations relating to credentialing and privilege delineation were carefully followed and that those provisions meet relevant state and federal requirements

- That the complaining party was not singled out for special treatment but was treated in the same way as other similarly situated people were treated

- That the adverse decision was clinically justified (e.g., supported by something more than just the hunches of the decision makers) and that the justification for the decision was documented within the credentials file, quality profile, or related papers

The procedures for granting medical and professional staff membership and delineating clinical privileges are closely tied to the facility's quality management and improvement activities. Health care organizations use quality management and improvement monitors and indicators not only to improve the systems that support the provision of patient care but also to gather data about the clinical performance of staff members. In this way, the governing body can fulfill its responsibilities to supervise the actions of both employees and the professional staff.

Contract Liability Issues and the HIM Department

Contracts (actual and implied) are another common source of liability for health care facilities and providers—even HIM professionals. Some courts have begun to enforce ethical and statutory obligations regarding the confidentiality of patients' health information as part of the contractual relationship between health care providers and their patients. In the *Hammonds* case cited earlier, the court found that the physician breached an implied condition of his physician-patient contract when he disclosed patient information to an insurer without the patient's authorization.[9] Thus, breach of contract is another theory under which a patient may seek relief for breach of confidentiality.

Contract liability typically arises in response to more traditional scenarios. For example, one party to a contract fails to abide by the terms of the agreement and the other party sues for damages or specific performance (basically, a court order that requires the losing party to do what it contractually agreed to do). Health care organizations enter into written contracts every day. They may contract for certain professional services, such as emergency medicine or anesthesia services. They may sign contracts for the purchase or lease of equipment or supplies. Sometimes breach of contract problems arise because a contract has been entered into without careful, advance review by legal counsel or risk manager, and as a result, the health care organization has agreed to unfavorable terms that may be difficult or impossible to meet.

How can this apply to a manager of an HIM department? Think of the potential contracts with which a typical HIM professional may be involved. There may be a contract with a transcription service. There may be a contract with a consulting company. There may be a contract with a record-copying service or a microfilming service. There may be contracts with local schools and educational programs in which liability issues regarding student-trainees are discussed. There may be managed care contracts in which the facility agrees to share certain health information with the managed care company. There may be a contract for purchase of hardware or software to support the facility's information system— the list goes on. If the HIM professional signs an agreement without benefit of legal or risk management review, he or she may be agreeing to terms that will later come back to haunt the facility.

The following are some of the typical things attorneys and risk managers look for in contracts.

- *Independent contractor clauses.* In signing a contract for professional services, the facility may want to clarify that the professional is not an employee but an independent contractor who is responsible for his or her own actions.

- *Hold harmless or indemnification clauses.* In these clauses, the health care facility generally wants the other party to accept financial and legal responsibility for its own actions and to agree to indemnify or compensate the health care facility for any claims against the facility that are the result of the other party's actions or inaction.

- *Termination or notification clauses.* Health care facilities typically want the process for terminating the contract to be clearly specified, including responsibility for advance notification of the other party of plans to terminate. The wording of such a clause is extremely important, and the health care facility will want as much latitude and flexibility as can be negotiated.

- *Confidentiality obligations.* Particularly with respect to those contractors who will have access to confidential health information, the facility and HIM professional will want to specify the contractor's obligations to safeguard the confidentiality and security of that information. The HIM professional may even want to specify the exact procedures that must be followed in handling the information.

In determining the safeguards and clauses that should be included in any contract, the HIM professional should use a variety of resources. Literature searches can locate articles specifically devoted to negotiating certain types of agreements, such as transcription contracts. The health care organization's risk manager and in-house counsel, if they exist, can also be of great assistance. Because of the expense involved in obtaining legal review of a contract, many facilities establish a policy describing the characteristics of contracts that must be reviewed by counsel versus those that can be entered into with just a departmental review or risk management review (Figure 11–8).

Legal Resources for HIM Professionals

No one expects HIM professionals to be lawyers. They are, however, expected to understand basic legal concepts, such as those described here. They are also expected to know how to find the information needed to help avoid legal problems for the HIM department, the health care organization, and, to a certain extent, the facility's professional staff. In larger facilities, HIM professionals may have access to a risk manager, in-house counsel, and outside attorneys to assist them in finding answers and developing appropriate policies, procedures, and system safeguards. In smaller facilities, there are probably fewer internal resources, and HIM professionals may need to work more closely with outside counsel.

Regardless of the setting, HIM professionals should utilize important external resources available, such as the following:

SAMPLE CORPORATE POLICY: CONTRACT REVIEW

Policy: All lease, purchase, affiliation, professional, consulting, and consignment agreements with third parties should be reduced to writing, reviewed by the risk manager (or in-house counsel), and signed by a corporate officer, or, when appropriate, by the department manager of purchasing.

Responsibility: Management committee; department managers; risk manager.

Implementation: The following is a list of types of agreements within the hospital:
- Major hospital services
- Physician services
- Professional services
- Educational affiliation agreements
- Transfer agreements
- Deeds, leases, easements, permits
- Consignments
- Equipment contracts
- Maintenance and service agreements
- Agreements with consultants
- Shared service agreements
- Provision for any other service or equipment not otherwise listed

Drafting of Contracts:
- The party contracting with the hospital may provide the contract.
- If a contract is not provided, the risk manager will assist in developing an agreement or will review a manager's draft.
- All contracts will be reviewed by the risk manager prior to signature by the appropriate vice-president or by the president.
- At least two signed originals of all agreements will be secured—one for the hospital and one for the contracted party(ies).
- The department manager/management committee member responsible for the execution of the contract may request a copy for reference to the terms of the agreement.
- File maintenance for contracts and leases is provided for in corporate policy # _____
- Requests for outside legal services should be made to the risk manager.

FIGURE 11–8. Sample contract review polcy. (From Harpster L, Veach M (eds): Risk management handbook for health care facilities. Chicago: American Hospital Publishing, 1990. Used by permission.)

- The *Journal of the American Health Information Management Association* and other professional journals and newsletters

- AHIMA's FORE (Foundation of Research and Education) Resource Center, where professional staff are available to assist in literature searches and lend library materials to members

- The state's HIM association and any legal manuals it may have compiled

- Law firms' client newsletters and client advisories. Some firms with health law departments are glad to put HIM professionals and other health care providers on their free distribution list.

- State hospital associations or other health care industry groups, which keep members up to date on medicolegal issues

- The loss control staff of any professional liability carriers that insure the health care organization

- Reference librarians at the public library or at law libraries, who can assist in locating and obtaining copies of legislation and regulations

- The *Federal Register,* a daily government publication that keeps the public apprised of proposed federal rules and regulations, so that all interested parties have an opportunity to comment and/or prepare

- HIM peers in local health care facilities, who are usually more than glad to share information

With all the information that is available, there is no excuse for ignorance. HIM professionals have important responsibilities in today's health care organizations. Patients, health care organizations, and colleagues rely on HIM professionals to protect their confidential information and to assist them in successfully navigating a maze of standards, rules, regulations, laws, and guidelines related to health information, confidentiality, and patient care issues. In so doing, HIM professionals earn their professional credentials, achieve professional success, and improve the quality of health care.

Key Concepts

- HIM professionals must make decisions every day regarding who may have access to confidential health information. These decisions must protect the patient's privacy and be based on the many state and federal laws that govern access to health information.

- There are four main sources of law: (1) federal and state constitutions, (2) federal and state statutes, (3) rules and regulations of administrative agencies, and (4) court decisions.

- The right to privacy is the right to be left alone, to make decisions about one's own body, and to control one's own information.

- The federal court system and many state systems have three levels of courts: (1) trial courts, (2) intermediate courts of appeals, and (3) a supreme court.

- One of the most fundamental duties of HIM professionals and their health care facility employers is the duty to maintain health information about their patients. This duty is imposed explicitly by state and federal statutes and regulations as well as by accreditation standards.

- It is essential that patient health information that is transmitted to health care providers remain confidential. Health care providers are bound by various laws and ethical standards to maintain this confidentiality.

- Not all information communicated to health care providers is classified as confidential information. By answering the following questions, a health care provider can determine whether or not the data item is confidential: (1) Is there a patient-provider relationship? (2) Was the information in question exchanged through or in the context of the professional relationship? (3) Is the information needed to treat or diagnose the patient?

- It is generally accepted that the health care facility owns the record or information itself but that the exercise of those ownership rights is subject to the *patient's* ownership interest in the information within that record or information.

- When health information is needed for use in court, the request for information comes in the form of a subpoena duces tecum, a subpoena (which may also be called a subpoena ad testificandum), a written court order, or simply a verbal order issued in court to the health care organization's attorney.

- Health care organizations owe patients a duty to provide care that meets professional standards. Health care providers must provide a reasonable quality of care to patients—care that meets professional standards.

- For negligence or malpractice claim to succeed, the plaintiff must show that all of the following elements of negligence or malpractice are met: duty, breach, proximate cause, and harm or damages.

- Physicians owe patients a duty to obtain the patient's informed consent to treatment. This duty is not just having a patient sign a consent form. Obtaining an "informed consent" refers to a communication process between the health professional and the patient. The patient must be informed about the anticipated treatment as well as its risks and alternatives.

- Health care organizations must take reasonable steps to supervise the actions of their employees and professional staff (including medical staff). They can be held liable for damages when their employees fail to adequately perform their duties under the doctrine of respondeat superior ("let the master answer").

References

1. *Griswold v. Connecticut,* 381 U.S. 479 (1965).
2. 42 U.S.C. §§12101-12213.
3. Sec. 51(a), (b) of the Federal Food, Drug and Cosmetic Act, as amended, 21 U.S.C. §360i.
4. *Darling v. Charleston Community Memorial Hospital,* 33 Ill. 2d 326, 211 N.E. 2d 253 (1965), *cert. denied,* 383 U.S. 946 (1966).
5. Keeton: Medical negligence—the standard of care. Specialty Law Digest: Health Care, March 1980, p 3.
6. *Peete v. Blackwell,* 504 So. 2d 22 (Ala. 1986).
7. *Johnson v. Women's Hospital,* 527 S.W. 2d 133 (Tenn. Ct. App. 1975).
8. *Greer v. Medders,* 336 S.E. 2d 329 (1985).
9. *Hammonds v. Aetna Casualty and Surety Co.,* 237 F. Suppl. 96 (N.D. Ohio 1965) and 243 F. Suppl. 793 (N.D. Ohio 1965).
10. See 42 U.S.C. §1395x(e)(2) (1974); 42 C.F.R. §482.24(c), 1994.
11. See *Minnesota v. Andring,* 342 N.W. 2d 128 (Minn. 1984).
12. See *Fox v. Cohen,* 84 Ill. App. 3d 744, 406 N.E. 2d 178 (1980).
13. See *Pisel v. Stamford Hospital,* 180 Conn. 314, 340, 430 A.2d 1, 15 (1980).
14. Healthcare records: A practical legal guide. Westchester, IL: Healthcare Financial Management Association, 1990.
15. See federal regulations governing the confidentiality of substance abuse treatment at 42 C.F.R., Chapter 1, Part 2, Section 2.13, Revised (1983).
16. See Bruce JC: Privacy and confidentiality of health care information, 2nd ed. Chicago: American Hospital Publishing, 1988, pp 24–26.
17. See McCann R: Protecting the confidentiality of peer review information. J Am Health Information Management Assoc 1993; 64(12):52.
18. 5 U.S.C. §552a(b) (1977).
19. See, for example, *Plain Dealer Publishing Co. v. U.S. Dept. of Labor,* 471 F. Supp. 1023 (D.D.C. 1979); *Florida Medical Ass'n, Inc. v. U.S. Dept. of Health, Education and Welfare,* 479 F. Supp. 1291 (M.D. Fla. 1979); and *Washington Post Co. v. U.S. Dept. of Health and Human Services,* 690 F. 2d 252 (D.D.C. 1982).
20. 42 C.F.R. Part 2, Subpart B, 2.12.
21. See §2.51 of the regulations.
22. See §2.51–2.53.
23. Brandt M: Guidelines on maintenance, disclosure, and redisclosure of health information. Chicago: American Health Information Management Association, 1994, p 7.
24. Dennis JC: Profits and patient information: Does database marketing breach confidentiality? In Confidence 1993; 1(2):4–6.
25. *Gotkin v. Miller,* 379 F. Supp. 859 (E.D.N.Y. 1974).
26. Are you "on file" in the Medical Information Bureau? In Confidence 1993; 1(1):11–12.
27. Roach WH Jr, Waller A, et al: Medical records and the law, 2nd ed. Gaithersburg, Md: Aspen Publishers, 1994, p 152.
28. Miller D: Glad you asked: Answers on information security and confidentiality. In Confidence 1993; 1(6):2.
29. See, for example, *Palsgraf v. Long Island R.R. Co.,* 248 N.Y. 339, 162 N.E. 99, *rehearing denied,* 249 N.Y. 511, 164 N.E. 564 (1928).
30. Pozgar GD: Legal aspects of health care administration, 4th ed. Gaithersburg, Md: Aspen Publishers, 1990, p 250.
31. Harpster L, Veach M (eds): Risk management handbook for health care facilities. Chicago: American Hospital Publishing, 1990, p 179.
32. Public Law 101-508, §§4206 (Medicare) and 4751 (Medicaid), 104 Stat. 1388.
33. *Elam v. College Park Hospital,* 183 Cal. Rptr. 156 (Ct. App. 1982).
34. *Rule v. Lutheran Hospitals and Home Society of America,* 835 F. 2d 1250 (8th Cir. 1987).
35. See *Patrick v. Burget,* 108 S. Ct. 1658 (1988).
36. See *Jefferson Parish Hospital District No. 2 v. Hyde,* 466 U.S. 2, 104 S. Ct. 1551 (1984).

SECTION
IV

MANAGEMENT

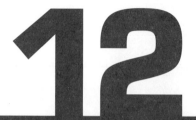

12

W. JACK DUNCAN and PETER M. GINTER

KEY WORDS

Acceptance theory of authority
Accountability
Administrative organization
Authority
Behavioral decision theory
Behaviorally anchored rating scales (BARS)
Bounded rationality
Bureaucracy
Centralization and decentralization
Closed system
Cognitive dissonance
Contingency plans
Contingency theory
Controlling
Cornerstone concepts of classical management
Critical success factors
Decision making
Delegation
Departmentalization
Effectiveness
Environmental assessment
Environmental forecasting
Environmental monitoring

Environmental scanning
Feedback controls
Formal theory of authority
Functional view of management
General managers
Goal setting
Hawthorne Studies
Human relations
Job descriptions
Leading
Management
Management by objectives
Management functions
Managers
Normative decision theory
Open systems
Organizing
Paradox of planning
Performance appraisal
Planning
Planning flexibility
Political subsystem
Power
Preventive controls
Principles of management
Process view of management

PRINCIPLES OF MANAGEMENT

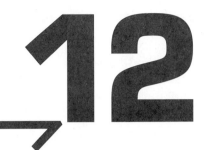

12

Progressive responsibility
Rationality
Reflective calculator
Role ambiguity
Role conflict
Satisficing behavior
Scientific management
Sequential search
Situational theory
Social subsystem

Span of control
Specialization of labor
Strategic planning
Style of leadership
Tactical planning
Task-oriented subsystem
Trait theory
Unity of command
Variance

ABBREVIATIONS

BARS—Behaviorally anchored rating scales
MBO—Management by objectives

OBJECTIVES

- Define key words.
- Define what is meant by the term "management" and discuss its key elements.
- Identify five stages (schools of management thought) through which the study and practice of management have evolved.
- Discuss the functional or process view of the manager's job.
- Identify five major functions of management.
- Discuss the relation between the major functions of management and commonly recognized principles for accomplishing these functions.
- Explain briefly additional ways of viewing the manager's job.
- Understand the strengths and weaknesses of job descriptions and the importance of job descriptions to the performance appraisal process.
- Discuss the relation among technical, interpersonal, and managerial aspects of health-related jobs.
- Apply the concept of job mix to your own professional development.

Principles of management is, to a great extent, a misnomer. Although the search for principles of management has been diligent and long-suffering, there are few, if any, true principles of management that will stand the test of scientific rigor. Herbert A. Simon, winner of the Nobel prize for economics and recognized contributor to management, stated that management principles "are little more than ambiguous and mutually contradictory proverbs."[1]

Management, after all, is an art, not a science. Looking to management for precise principles of what should be done in the numerous situations that managers face every day can lead to disappointment and frustration. Looking to management as a database of collective experience and more than a century of research and theory on how to make organizations more effective and efficient can be not only challenging but also rewarding.

Management is a mixture of experience, research, and theory. Much of the management practiced today in business, educational, governmental, and health care organizations has evolved from on-the-job training and the understudy of more experienced managers. Some is the result of serious and structured scientific investigations of organizational phenomena and of individual and group behavior in organizational settings. A portion of management knowledge is proven and can be applied with reasonable confidence. Other parts are speculative and require a degree of faith and additional trial and testing.

Collectively, management is built on organizational folklore and myth, scientific observation, and casual associations. Despite their shortcomings, today's management principles are the best available knowledge about how to improve the efficiency and effectiveness of organizations. Management knowledge is getting better, and its prescriptions with regard to improved organizational performance are becoming more precise. With these points of clarification in mind, we can proceed to examine management as a discipline and as an activity that many people—even technical specialists—will spend much of their time doing throughout their careers.

MANAGEMENT: DEFINING THE FIELD

Management is a term used to describe a variety of things in contemporary organizations. Sometimes it is used to describe a group of people who "get things done through other people," as contrasted with the people who actually do the work in hospitals, health maintenance organizations, and local health departments. Management is also used in this manner when labor-management relations are discussed. In both cases, when the term is used, we think of a group of people. At other times, the term is used to describe a field of study or an art that is practiced by the people who get things done through others. When used in this manner, we think of an academic discipline taught in a college or university, a professional skill learned from others, or a combination of both. In this chapter, the term is used to describe an activity or a series of activities, a process, that is critical to organizations in ensuring that they are doing the right things (effectiveness) and that they are doing things in the right way (efficiency).

Management, as we use the term, is the process of coordinating individual and group actions toward the accomplishment of organizational goals in a manner that is acceptable to the larger social and cultural system.

Management as a Process

Managers use a process of management that is accomplished through a series of functions that they perform. The more commonly recognized functions include the following:

- **Planning** (establishing organizational and work group goals)

- **Organizing** (structuring the tasks to accomplish goals)

- **Controlling** (ensuring performance is on target and progressing toward goal accomplishment)

- **Decision making** (generating and selecting alternative ways of accomplishing goals)

- **Leading** (motivating and inspiring behavior toward the accomplishment of organizational goals)

As might be expected, this approach to understanding management is known as the **functional** or **process view of management.** Historically, it is the most popular view and has only recently been seriously questioned as an accurate way to view the work of managers. This particular approach to management places primary attention on the **principles of management.** The reason why principles are important in the process view is obvious. If we view the manager's job as a series of functions that she or he performs, it is logical to develop a series of principles for planning, organizing, controlling, and so on. By teaching these principles to current and prospective managers, it is possible, at least

in theory, to ensure a continuing supply of effective managers. The logic is sound; the outcome is not always as expected.

Our definition of management has an additional element that cannot be overlooked. Management is an activity that takes place in a much larger social matrix. Managers are not free to plan, organize, control, make choices, and lead in ways that are not acceptable in the larger social setting. Managers are not free to abuse and discriminate against employees on the basis of their sex, religion, disability, or age because such behavior is not acceptable to the larger society. Managers cannot fix prices and illegally divide up markets because such behavior is against the law. Therefore, our definition of management needs always to keep in mind that the job of management should be accomplished in a way that is consistent with the goals and values of society.

Successful management, we have come to recognize, relies not only on the knowledge of management processes, functions, and principles, but also on the manner in which this knowledge is applied. Just as the greatest surgeon is not always the person with the most knowledge of anatomy, or the greatest courtroom lawyer is not the person with the most knowledge of jurisprudence, so it is with managers.

The best manager is not always the person with the most knowledge of management, but a person who understands people, who can adapt to changing situations, and who is of high character and has a sense of fairness. We should not, however, be misled. Surgeons do not successfully operate without an understanding of anatomy and lawyers do not win cases if they are not well versed in the law. In the same way, people who are responsible for managing others and the resources of hospitals and health centers should know the fundamentals of management. Such an understanding is our goal in this chapter.

A Brief History of Management

Action-oriented managers are not always interested in history. They have too many pressing problems to engage in the more reflective aspects of history. Although history appears to be a luxury, it can be an important tool for decision making today. At the very least, it can help us avoid repeating mistakes.[2] If the modern quality movement has taught us one thing, it is that rework is wasteful and resource-consuming. Doing things right the first time is greatly preferred. A knowledge of management history can certainly help us avoid mistakes of action and judgment.

Management, as a field of study, is only a little more than a century old. That is, even though human beings have, no doubt, managed and even planned ever since they started interacting in groups, attempts to study, teach, and develop a true field of study around management concepts have been with us for a relatively short period. Despite its relative youth, management has passed through five major stages. To see where the process or functional approach fits in this evolution, we briefly discuss the major focus of each of these stages.[3]

Scientific Management

People have been managing ever since they began living in groups. Building the pyramids required management, as did fighting wars and governing kingdoms. The rudiments of a formal management theory have been traced to the ancient Chinese, political philosophers of the early nation-states, and military leaders. It was not until the late 19th century, however, that an effort was made to systematically analyze and codify concepts of management so that they could be taught to others.

The first attempts at this type of codification took place in the United States and came to be known as **scientific management.** Scientific management was the product of the factory system and focused primarily on improving the conduct of work. Using tools like time and motion study, engineers attempted to develop the most efficient ways of doing all kinds of work. Scientific management received its name because of the commitment of most of its advocates to the application of science to the study and practice of work. This commitment is best illustrated by the determination of Frederick W. Taylor (the father of scientific management) "to prove that the best management is a true science resting on defined laws, rules, and principles."[4]

Contrary to the opinion of many, scientific management was not limited in its application to industrial or manufacturing organizations. Applications of motion study to the practice of surgery and scientific management principles to the management of city governments and universities are well documented and reached relatively high degrees of refinement. The outgrowth of scientific management, modern industrial engineering methods, is found today as frequently in hospitals as it is in manufacturing organizations.

Bureaucracy

Bureaucracy, in its contemporary usage, carries a negative connotation. This is not the case in management thought. The theory of bureaucracy finds its origin with Max Weber, a German sociologist and economist who was impressed with the organizational precision of the Catholic Church, the German army, and successful industrial firms.[5] On examination, Weber discovered that these organizations shared many things in common. Some of these characteristics accounted for their success and some accounted for their failure to realize their full potential.

In this way, bureaucracy focused on the structure of organizations, whereas scientific management had focused on the conduct and structure of work. Those organizations that functioned best appeared to possess the following characteristics:

- Specialists who were proficient at performing parts of complex tasks
- A chain of command that provided for one person having only one boss at any given time
- A system of well-communicated and well-understood procedures and rules for getting work done in organizations
- Placement and promotions based on technical competency (what you knew) rather than who you knew

The problems develop with bureaucracy not in terms of its concept or structure but in how it is administered in everyday life. When rules and procedures become ends in themselves rather than more important means to effective and efficient organizations, red tape develops. When specialists disregard the importance of the overall organization and think only of their own special units, organizations fail to realize their full potential.

Administrative Organization

In France, an important approach to management developed simultaneously with scientific management in the United States. This approach, known as **administrative organization,** was championed by Henri Fayol, an executive in the French mining industry. Fayol was the first to look seriously at the nature of management work and attempt to describe it. The process or functional school of management thought that was introduced earlier was the direct outgrowth of Fayol's thinking.[6] His ideas are the basis for much of the discussion in the remainder of this chapter.

Fayol believed that all operations in organizations could be classified as technical, commercial, financial, security-oriented, accounting, or administrative. This later category is of primary interest to us and consisted of functions like planning, organizing, commanding, controlling, and coordinating. He also believed, based on his half century of executive experience, that principles could be developed for accomplishing these administrative functions.

Human Relations

Until the mid-1920s, the preoccupation of management had been on work, organization, and, to a lesser extent, managers. In the late 1920s, the General Electric Company sponsored a large-scale research project at Western Electric's Hawthorne Works near Chicago. The

Harvard Business School was involved in this research that took almost a decade to complete. These **Hawthorne Studies,** as they became known, changed the way people thought about management and ushered in the **human relations** era of management thinking.

The focus of human relations was the worker. The job site became recognized as a social system where people came not just to earn their livings but to participate in interpersonal relations with others. According to human relations advocates, if we are to understand managing, we must understand the people being managed—how they are motivated and how they work in association with others. Human relations thought focused attention on more behaviorally oriented aspects of management, such as motivation, leadership, interpersonal and intergroup conflict, and effective communication.

Contingency Theory

Although each of the approaches mentioned to this point had its own unique focus, they shared one thing in common: All were looking for the one best way to do work and to manage. In this sense, they were all absolute in their orientation and in their quest for principles of management. However, as the Hawthorne Studies began to suggest, work is accomplished by people, and people are seldom as predictable as nonhuman resources.

Whereas clearly defined organizational structures may work well in slowly changing industries, more dynamic industries, such as health care, may be encumbered by precisely defined procedures and rules. Whereas low-skilled workers may do best when they have clearly defined tasks and deadlines, doctors, nurses, and other health professionals may function better when there is autonomy and freedom to innovate.

Contingency theory has attempted to be sensitive to the changing environment of management and look at situational factors. This approach has recognized that the great contribution of scientific management, administrative organization, bureaucracy, and human relations is to provide a knowledge base for building efficient organizations. Regrettably, efficient organizations do not always respond to changing conditions. As with IBM, General Motors, and Omega watches, organizations can become so good at making and marketing mainframe computers, powerful automobiles, and mechanical watches that they fail to see the potential of personal computers, energy-efficient cars, and quartz crystals.[7] The contribution of contingency theory has been to recognize uniqueness in situations and in people. In this sense, it represents a major departure from the primary thrust of management thought over the past century.

With this background, we begin our examination of management principles in earnest. The logical place to begin this journey is with managers.

NATURE OF MANAGERIAL WORK

It is ironic that from the time Fayol was writing at the beginning of the 20th century until almost a half century later, there were few serious attempts to understand what managers really do during a day, a typical week, or a fiscal year. Imagine studying physics without observing the behavior of physical objects or biology without analyzing the behavior of living organisms. As a result, the search for genuine management principles was greatly retarded. This changed, however, with the publication of Henry Mintzberg's *The Nature of Managerial Work.*[8] Mintzberg, reacting against Fayol's view of the manager as a **reflective calculator** who carefully planned actions, patiently structured organizations and work groups to accomplish the plans, and continuously monitored for results, proposed another view of how managers go about their tasks.[9]

Mintzberg argued that managers are far from systematic planners, organizers, and controllers. Based on his research, Mintzberg claimed that managers seldom spent more than 9 minutes on any task and that in his sample, only 10 per cent of the activities of high-level executives required more than 1 hour to complete. According to this view, the manager's job is characterized by brevity, fragmentation, and constantly moving from the demands of one moment to the demands of another.

Overview of Research

Mintzberg's writings created a great deal of interest and research on the nature of management work. One review of 30 studies concerning the activities that managers perform published between 1951 and 1982 included all levels of management and concluded that overall, the following five questions were addressed in these studies[10]:

- What do managers do?
- How do managers work?
- With whom do managers work?
- What else do managers do?
- What qualities does managerial work display?

Collectively, the attention to these five questions has provided us with a better understanding of what managers do.

Research on General Managers

Most recent research has focused on **general managers,** or those who are accountable for more than a single function, particularly chief executive officers (CEOs). In one study, 24 CEOs representing a variety of industries, including manufacturing, banking, real estate, insurance, legal services, health services, and publishing, were interviewed. The results indicated that these top-level executives dealt with three primary agendas: creating a context for change, building commitment and ownership, and balancing stability and innovation.[11] Traditional functions such as planning, organizing, and controlling were not descriptive of the work these managers performed.

Interviews with 50 CEOs of manufacturing companies regarding the degree of perceived uncertainty in six environmental sectors provided additional insights into both the sources and the domain of information search for CEOs. Again, it was found that there was little focus on traditionally defined **management functions**.[12]

Functional-Level Research on Managerial Work

Interest has also been generated in how managerial work differs for managers at different levels of the organization. One study of more than 1400 managers at various hierarchical levels found that each level valued different kinds of management tasks. First-level managers valued managing individual performance and instructing subordinates; middle managers valued planning and allocating resources to different groups, coordinating groups, and managing group performance. Top-level managers valued monitoring the external environment. Other studies envisioned lower- and middle-level managers as technically oriented people who spend most of their time on specific supervisory activities.[13]

Other functional-level research has focused on what has been called "real," "effective," and "ineffective" managers, and one study even attempted to determine whether or not CEOs were different from the senior management groups from which they emanated. Using a sample of 450 British CEOs, this study found that chief executives were not very different from other members of the top-management team with regard to domestic and educational influences. They were not, however, like the popular stereotype—atypically irreligious, highly stressed, hard-living, and capable of functioning with too little sleep.[14]

Managing in Different Industries

Because of studies like those discussed above, we are increasingly informed about management at different organizational levels. Even though many of these studies included managers from different industrial sectors, the assumed uniqueness of managing in the service sector has not been a factor that has been frequently isolated or examined. The effective management of service industries, however, is more important than ever to the economic welfare of the nation. It has been noted, for example, that almost three quarters of American workers are employed in service industries and as much as 70 per cent of our gross national product (GNP) may be accounted for by the service sector.[15]

A single area like health care illustrates the point. Whereas the GNP of the United States has increased ninefold since 1960, health care expenditures have more than doubled as a percentage of GNP. Today, health care accounts for 12 per cent of the GNP, and many believe that it will grow to 20 per cent by the year 2000. Already, according to the *Economic Report of the President* (1990), Americans spend more on health care than they spend on any other personal consumption item except housing and food. We spend, for example, almost twice as much on health care as we do on automobiles.

CASE STUDY

Mintzberg stated that if you ask managers what they do, you should expect to get a list of standard functions—planning, organizing, coordinating, and controlling—just as Fayol predicted. On the other hand, if you observe managers, according to Mintzberg, do not be surprised if "you cannot relate what they do to those four words."[16]

We decided to take him up on the challenge and enlisted 40 health care managers who agreed to participate. Twenty were top-level general managers in local health departments, hospitals, nursing facilities, and health maintenance organizations. Twenty were functional managers in the same organizations.[17] The results we obtained were interesting. Participants were personally interviewed, their telephone logs and calendars were sampled over a period of a month, and their in and out baskets were analyzed for two complete workdays.

General and functional-level managers both agreed that they spent much of their time planning and coordinating, decision making and problem solving, processing paperwork, exchanging routine information, monitoring and controlling activities, and interacting with others. General managers estimated that 80 per cent of their time was spent on these activities. About 86 per cent of the functional managers' time was consumed with these activities. Traditional managerial functions like planning, coordinating, decision making, and controlling accounted for about one third of the time of these general and functional managers.

The results of this analysis did not support the work of people like John Kotter, whose studies of general managers suggest that activities like socializing, politicking, and agenda building are tasks that successful managers do very well. Although the managers in this study might have done these things well, they estimated that less than 5 per cent of their time was consumed in this manner.[18]

These participants did confirm, however, that a sufficiently large amount of time was spent on traditional management functions to justify examining these tasks in greater detail. The ultimate goal is to use these studies as the basis for better understanding how to effectively manage organizations.

FIVE FUNCTIONS OF MANAGEMENT

Regardless of how one views the manager's job, one thing is certain. As a management career evolves, it

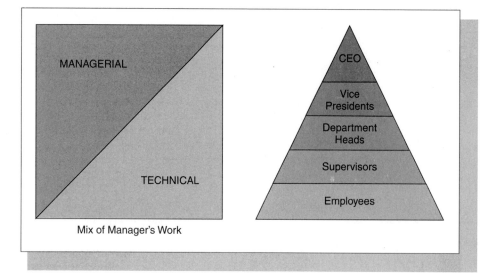

MANAGERIAL

TECHNICAL

Mix of Manager's Work

CEO

Vice
Presidents

Department
Heads

Supervisors

Employees

FIGURE 12–1. Changing mix of management work.

moves from the technical to the more conceptual or managerial (Figure 12–1). Assume, for example, that you are initially hired at University Hospital as a medical record specialist. You have no management responsibilities and your task is clearly defined as technical in nature.

After a period of time, you are promoted to supervisor of a group of three other medical record specialists. Note from Figure 12–1 that your job changes but not radically. You now perform some management functions; you set goals for the work group, coordinate activities with other work groups and among those employees who report directly to you, and are responsible for performance evaluations. Most of your time as a first-level supervisor, however, remains technical.

Next, you are promoted to a middle-level management job as assistant administrator for information services (department head). Now your job does change radically. At least one half of your time is spent **goal setting,** coordinating activities within and between groups, making management decisions about resource allocations, budgeting, and evaluating performance. Your technical responsibilities are greatly reduced. Later, your career development takes you to consecutively higher management positions as chief information officer and, eventually, CEO of the hospital. In these positions, your job is almost totally managerial. You see a computer only occasionally. Your technical skills begin to erode as you become increasingly proficient as a manager.[19]

This evolution into **progressive responsibility** has been the traditional way a management career has evolved. Although it is true that in today's organizations, with the trend toward streamlining administrative structures, reducing layers in the hierarchy, and downsizing, there are fewer management positions to aspire to, it is reasonable to view career evolution from the technical to the managerial.

Despite contemporary trends in organizational restructuring, viewing progressive responsibility in this manner is useful because it raises the important question "What are the management skills and functions that must be performed as my job becomes less technical and more conceptual in character?" Note especially the fact that the manager's job is initially one of dealing with interpersonal relations. The first-line supervisor does a little planning, organizing, and controlling, but mostly it is a job of managing interpersonal relations among employees and between employees and the supervisor. As the responsibility grows, so do the management functions.

It is important to say in the beginning that management functions are not completed in a linear or straight-line manner. Managers do not plan and then organize and then control the way our management diagrams depict the process. In fact, the process of management is quite iterative in nature; that is, all the management functions are intertwined with one another. There is a great deal of organizing, decision making, and controlling in planning, and there is planning, controlling, and decision making in the organizing function. To simplify what is a dynamic process, we resort to models that appear linear to deal with the highly complex task of management. Therefore, if there is a proper place to begin our survey of basic management functions, it is certainly with planning and goal setting.

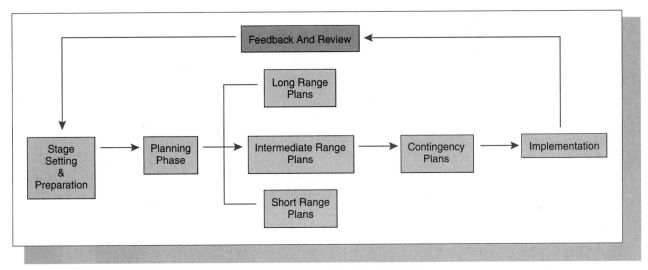

FIGURE 12–2. Overview of the planning process.

Planning and Goal Setting

Planning determines the future direction an organization will take. Planning involves setting goals and establishing priorities among all the activities that must be performed to achieve them. To fully understand the planning process, it is important to recognize that it has a number of dimensions, all of which are interrelated. We discuss a few of the more important ones. Figure 12–2 provides an overview of the planning process.

Stage Setting

The first stage of planning is stage setting or establishing the necessary conditions for successful goal setting at all organizational levels. Stage setting is basically a time of data gathering to understand the environment facing the organization and its individual parts.

For example, during the stage-setting phase, it is important to ensure that everyone has a clear understanding of the organization's mission or purpose, management's vision, and top management's strategic objectives. It is also important to carefully scan the external environment to ensure that the opportunities and threats facing the organization are clearly understood. It has been accurately stated that the keys to organizational success lie outside, not inside, the organization. The rules for success are written in the environment by customers, patients, physicians, competitors, the larger society, and so on. If we are to manage successfully, it is critically important that we understand the rules and the environmental conditions facing us.

Successful planners have to become proficient in assessing the external environment. The process of **environmental assessment** consists of the following four steps.[20]

1. **Environmental scanning.** At this point, the planner views the information received from the environment, organizes it so that it can be systematically analyzed, and identifies issues that are likely to be important for the organization and his or her area of responsibility.

2. **Environmental monitoring.** Here the database is expanded, issues and trends are confirmed or determined to be less significant, and the rate of change with regard to each important issue is determined.

3. **Environmental forecasting.** Trends are extended, relations among trends and issues are determined and specified, and projections of alternative futures are made.

4. **Environmental assessing.** This final stage involves continuously evaluating the significance of forecasted trends and the development of action plans for dealing with important external issues.

Health care reform provides an excellent example of how hospitals, health maintenance organizations, nursing facilities, and all other types of health care providers must be engaging in external environmental assessment to plan strategic directions. If you are part of the management team in a publicly supported hospital, careful attention must be given to re-evaluating your mission and generally reassessing your way of doing things.

For example, decision makers in public hospitals recognize through **environmental scanning** that health care reform is likely to involve some form of managed care that will be available to most, if not all, citizens through one of several available health maintenance organizations. Those who have been monitoring the debate relative to health care reform are probably convinced that to survive in the future portrayed by health care reform, public hospitals will have to align themselves with some type of health maintenance organization and become competitive as health providers of choice rather than merely providers of last resort. In fact, in at least one scenario of health care reform in which everyone receives a health security card and can choose a primary care provider, there may be no role for public hospitals that are not part of competitive managed care systems.[21]

How strongly public hospital planners believe in this possible course of health care reform requires a degree of forecasting to determine how likely such an alternative is relative to the other possible directions that have been discussed concerning health care reform. Finally, continuous assessing of the external environment is necessary as an aid to developing action plans for how the hospital will respond to the evolving situation in its external environment.[22]

Once the external environment is understood and the strategic issues facing the organization are identified, it is possible to move to the second stage in the planning process. This stage involves the actual development of the plan.

Goal-Setting Stage

The process of management begins with goal setting. It is difficult to imagine how one could manage without well-developed and well-understood goals. Consider, for example, the impossibility of managing your own personal affairs without clearly established goals. How could you develop your personal budget? How could you manage your time and energy effectively without an understanding of what you were trying to accomplish? How would you know when you were making progress or merely spinning your wheels if there were no goals? Good managers must be goal-setters.

There are many kinds of goals in organizations. Missions and visions are goals, but they are usually not as operational or specific as departmental or work unit goals. In this discussion, we focus on goal setting at the work unit level because this level is the place most managers need help.

Whereas higher-level goals in organizations provide general direction, work group goals should be more specific. Effective work group goals possess three important characteristics.[23] First, to be effective, work group goals should be as measurable as possible. The goals should reflect organizational priorities as well as the personal priorities of work group members. For example, a work group may set as one of its goals to reduce the amount of overtime expenditure in the data-processing department by 5 per cent by the end of the

fiscal year with no additional increase in full-time equivalent positions. This goal is specific in that it relates to overtime costs and has a time (end of fiscal year) and expenditure guideline (with no additional personnel) stated.

Second, effective work group goals should be challenging yet attainable. Nothing is less motivational than unrealistic goals. An important psychological principle states that when goals are continually unrealized, the motivation to pursue them disappears. In other words, the act of accomplishing goals provides much of the motivation for continuing to pursue even more challenging objectives. Therefore, even though goals should not be easy to achieve, they should be attainable to maintain their motivational impact.

Third, work group goals should relate to the **critical success factors** of the organization or those things that make the difference between success and failure. As an extreme example, this means that work groups should forget setting goals relating to the percentage of employees arriving late and leaving early and focus on critical things that make a difference, such as satisfaction of internal and external customers, revenue generated, and continuous quality improvement.

Plan Development Stage

Perhaps the best way to illustrate how plans are developed is to look at them in terms of the time period they are designed to cover. There are two types of **planning** in organizations: **strategic planning** and **tactical planning.** Strategic planning involves a philosophical analysis of what the organization is (its mission), what it hopes to be (its vision), and innovative ways of achieving the type of future that will ensure the organization's survival and effectiveness. This is typically the role of top management, although it is critically important to involve people at all levels in this process. The importance of strategic planning cannot be overemphasized, but this is not the major thrust of our discussion in this overview of management functions.

Tactical planning involves most middle- and first-level managers in organizations. It is the action-oriented aspect of making sure that the future visualized in the strategic plan is accomplished. Sometimes tactical plans are referred to as operational because they attempt to convert the abstract and philosophical aspects of the strategic plans into operations or actions that can be scheduled, monitored, and adjusted in light of changing conditions and priorities.

Perhaps the best way to understand tactical planning is to view it in terms of time. Managers at all levels of organizations engage in long-, intermediate-, and short-range planning. Long-range plans for most managers involve a period of 5 years or so. Plans of this nature are not precise, but at least they force some thinking about where we want to be in 5 years, how we will fit into the vision of the organization, and what human and nonhuman resources will be needed if we are to contribute as we should to our organization's effectiveness. The acquisition plans for major computer hardware systems are likely to be long term in character. Long-range planning involves being sure that we keep abreast of the developing computer and information system technology that is likely to take place over the next 5 years and being sure that we recruit and develop internally the kinds of technical expertise that can effectively use the technology.

Intermediate-term plans are for longer than 1 year but less than 5 years. Intermediate-term planning usually involves planning for major projects. The implementation of a new administrative software system requires intermediate-term planning. Large-scale software implementations cannot be accomplished in a single year. The system must be designed or adapted to our special uses, hardware alternations must be made to ensure that the system will run properly, and users must be trained to use the new system.

Project planning requires a great deal of careful scheduling to ensure that all the necessary steps in the software implementation take place in the proper sequence so that bottlenecks do not develop and costly downtime does not result in inefficiencies. Intermediate-range planning is built around the following major activities:

- Listing the activities that are necessary to accomplish a project
- Scheduling the time required to accomplish each activity listed
- Evaluating the most effective means of accomplishing each of the required activities

Short-range or budgetary planning is the third type of tactical plan. Budgetary planning encompasses 1 year or what is commonly referred to as the fiscal year. Budgetary planning is specific and attempts to specify the resources that will be available to each manager and the resources that will be required by each manager during the next year. Budgets are extremely useful planning tools because they aid managers in keeping their eyes on target and can assist in determining where resources are available and not available when various aspects of plans need to be expedited to remove project bottlenecks.

Implementation Stage

Planning is often looked on as an inefficient activity by action-oriented managers and employees. However, if done carefully and systematically, planning can reduce rework and increase the overall efficiency of organiza-tional activities. For planning to be effective, it must involve many people in the formulation and implementation processes. One of the most important aspects of the effective implementation of plans is to ensure that **planning flexibility** is built into the planning process.

Regardless of how well we scan the environment, strategically determine the mission and vision of the organization, and coordinate long-, intermediate-, and short-term plans, unanticipated events are certain to take place in the environment of health care organizations. For this reason, good plans are plans that can be easily altered and adjusted in light of changing conditions. It is usually prudent to have **contingency plans** available to allow for the most likely changes. For example, in the example presented above relating to health care reform, a good bet is that in the future, the American health care system will be organized around the concept of managed competition among a number of provider groups. This is not the only possibility. What about less likely but possible scenarios of the future? Prudent planners always allow for alternatives and contingencies.

As we would expect, the more dynamic the environment, the greater the need for contingency plans. Planners frequently talk about the **paradox of planning** that is so much a part of their job. This paradox has to do with the relation between plans and the organizational environment. In stable organizational environments, plans can be formulated that are accurate and predictive of the future. Dynamic environments cause plans to be less accurate. The paradox emerges because it is in the very environments where plans are most likely to be inaccurate (dynamic environments) that they are most needed. In stable environments, where plans can be highly accurate, they are less useful to managers.

Feedback or Review Stage

The feedback stage of planning illustrates the problem with separating the management functions. The feedback stage of planning is really control because it is always necessary to ensure that plans conform to the goals that were established early in the process. Operationally, formal programs like **management by objectives** illustrate the importance of this review process. In management by objectives and similar objectives-based management systems, the emphasis is on results and whether or not activities are proceeding according to plan. If they are, no intervention is necessary. If they are not, it is important for management to assess the reasons variances have developed and initiate corrective actions.

Corrective actions are not always directed toward inferior performance. Sometimes, to be sure, people and processes do not perform up to expectations. It is possible that the goal or standard is unrealistic, overly ambitious, or impossible because unanticipated events have taken place since the goals were established.

Principles of Effective Planning

These principles are guidelines to make planning effective and should not be thought of as principles in a scientific sense. They will serve you well in most situations.

- To plan effectively, managers should understand the environment within which their organization operates. To plan effectively in a specific department, managers must understand the mission and vision of the organization of which they are a part.

- Effective work group goals should be specific and measurable, reflect organizational priorities, and be challenging yet attainable.

- Organizational goals, regardless of the level to which they apply, should be flexible and capable of responding to changing conditions in the general environment and the health care industry.

Organizing for Action

Once goals are established and strategic and tactical plans are developed, managers must organize the resources at their disposal and direct them toward the accomplishment of organizational and work group goals.

Like planning, **organizing** is a process that consists of several distinct stages. When properly completed, organizing answers the following questions:

- What activities are necessary to accomplish the goals of the organization and the work group? Organizing requires careful thought about the individual tasks that must be accomplished if goals are to be realized.

- How can the activities listed above be logically grouped into categories consisting of similar tasks? All the things, for example, that relate to inputting information into a computer might be placed in one group of activities, whereas activities that relate to distributing the output might be placed in another group. In this manner, similar activities are arranged and classified.

- Who will be assigned the authority and responsibility for getting the different groups of activities accomplished?

To understand the management function of organizing, we examine three basic issues: the principles or concepts of organizational design, the nature of authority and responsibility, and the delegation of authority. All of these are essential aspects of the successful accomplishment of the organizing process.

Principles of Organizational Design

Three of the periods of management thought discussed at the beginning of this chapter—scientific management, administrative organization, and bureaucracy—shared certain things about their view of the proper way to organize business firms, hospitals, and other forms of organizations. They were all based on specific principles of organization that have come to be known as the **cornerstone concepts of classical organization theory.** Human relations and contingency theory differed in their approach to organization. These differences are noted in the course of discussing the cornerstone concepts.

When one looks at the organizational chart of a hospital or some other health care organization, several things become evident. Perhaps the first impression is that the organizational charts of most organizations look alike. They have several levels in the hierarchy, and the lines of communication and authority are drawn clear and seldom overlap or intersect. The jobs are specialized, and units are created that contain similar activities. All accounting activities are grouped in the accounting department, information-related activities are housed in management information systems, and so on. This similarity is not accidental. It is the result of the well-accepted principles of classical organization theory.[24]

SPECIALIZATION OF LABOR. The first principle of classical organization theory is **specialization of labor.** This principle is perhaps nowhere practiced more faithfully than in health care. The logic behind the specialization of labor is that productivity can be increased if people use their natural and acquired talents to do exclusively what they do best.

The principle of specialization of labor is one reason for the similarity in the structure of different organizations. The fact that several units are listed horizontally in the organizational chart shown in Figure 12–3 is the result of specialization. In this community hospital, there are various administrative units at the same level—marketing, accounting, admitting, and collections. These are specialized units where similar activities are grouped. There are also medical affairs and operations activities that are grouped because of their similarity. The same is true of nursing.

For example, in the finance office of a large medical practice, you find clerks who specialize in collecting accounts receivable, whereas others specialize in taking care of accounts payable. There is probably another person who specializes in keeping all the work accom-

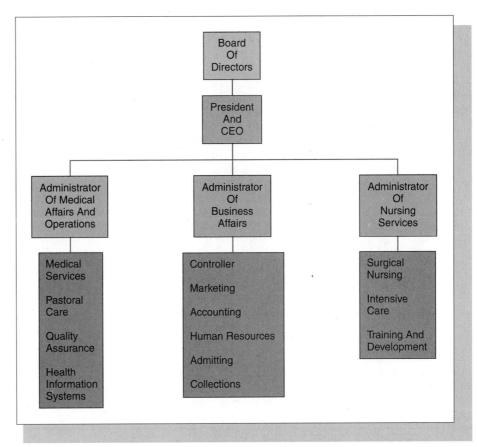

FIGURE 12–3. Functional organization of a community hospital.

plished by the clerks updated in the accounting information system to ensure that bills are collected and paid on time.

It may be that one clerk could do a little of all this work, but the specialization of labor principle argues that efficiency can be increased if a single person is responsible for all accounts receivable. This person can learn all there is to know about this area instead of being a jack-of-all-trades in three or four areas. The economic logic of specialization of labor is difficult to debate. In fact, specialists are more efficient than people who try to accomplish a number of different tasks.

Efficiency is accomplished through the specialization of labor but other things are sacrificed. The human relations school of thought, for example, taught us that the result of highly specialized work can be boredom, fatigue, and maybe even a loss of pride of workmanship. For example, the clerk who does nothing but call delinquent accounts may burn out over time. Moreover, he or she may see little effect his or her work has on the quality of patient care or the success of the hospital. The same is true of the person who inputs data into the computer system. His or her job may be such a small part of the overall work being done in the hospital that

little or no pride is taken in how the job is executed. Even if pride in the job is maintained, the routine nature of the task may cause higher error rates and reduction in quality.

UNITY OF COMMAND. The second cornerstone concept of classical organization theory is **unity of command.** The unity of command principle states that no person should have more than a single boss at any time. Figure 12–3 is effective in showing adherence to this principle. In this community hospital, it is clear who reports to whom. The nurses in charge of surgical, intensive care, and training and development report to the administrator of nursing services. The directors of pastoral care and medical information systems report to the administrator of medical affairs and operations.

The potential problems created by a violation of the unity of command principle are all too clear to many people. The secretary who works for two physicians or administrators knows the problems involved in doing the work of one before the other. The radiology technician who doubles as a patient transport attendant knows the problems when a patient has to be moved and the radiology department has need of the technician's services. These hazy lines of authority cause uncertainty, conflict, and dissatisfaction in organizations. They also place employees in the unfair position of choosing between the needs of different bosses.

This is not to say that the benefits of violating the unity of command principle never outweigh the costs. Sometimes organizational forms developed by contingency theorists violate the unity of command principle. For example, the familiar project organization may assign one person to several projects to make the most effective use of a single person. You, as a specialist in health information, might be assigned part of the time to work with a task force charged with adapting the hospital pharmacy system to the larger administrative information system. At the same time, your boss may ask you to work with the director of nursing on the development of a computerized scheduling system for nursing personnel. Technically, when you are working on any of these projects, you are responsible to the head of information systems and are also accountable to the task force director for specialized services. The possible conflicts are obvious, but the benefits from this arrangement are important enough to outweigh the problems.

For example, if health information systems did not share their expertise with pharmacy and nursing, those units might be forced to hire expensive outside consultants or a full-time information systems person who would duplicate resources already available in their department. Later, when the projects are complete, pharmacy and nursing could not justify the extra personnel and would be required to lay off someone. Project structures are useful for organizing around problems to be solved. Once the project is complete, the project can be dismantled.

SPAN OF CONTROL. The third principle of classical organization theory is **span of control,** which refers to the number of people a manager can effectively supervise. Historically, much attention has been given to this issue. In the early periods of management thought, the emphasis was on determining the optimum span of control, and some people strongly believed that managers could not effectively supervise more than 6, 8, or 10 employees. Many exceptions were found to whatever rules about optimum spans of control were developed. As a result, the emphasis changed to understanding the factors that determine spans of control in different organizations, at different organizational levels, and so on.

Perhaps few controversies in management illustrate the difference between the goals of early scientific management and administrative organization and contingency theory than this issue. Scientific management and administrative organization writers were determined to discover an absolute number of people that could be effectively supervised to aid managers in designing relations at work. Contingency theorists, however, recognized that the span of control was not so much the function of an absolute number but varied from situation to situation.

For example, one manager who is particularly well organized, has mature and motivated employees, and is responsible for a job that is geographically focused in one place may be able to effectively supervise 15 or more employees. On the other hand, a manager with jobs located in various locations, who is not personally well organized, and who is responsible for employees who are not mature or highly motivated will have to devote time to ensuring that each person is working and travel from place to place. Therefore, this manager may not be able to supervise more than five or six employees. The point is clear. Span of control is an important management concept, but there is no specific or optimum number of employees any and all managers can effectively supervise. The actual number depends on many situational variables—for example, the characteristics of the manager, the employees, and the work situation.

DEPARTMENTALIZATION. The fourth principle is **departmentalization,** which is a **cornerstone concept of classical management.** The principle relates to how managers, once the mission and goals of the organization or work groups have been established, divide or structure the work. Read over the organizational chart of a hospital or health care organization. What is the basis for the various departments? It is likely that you will find the structure divided according to a variety of criteria.[25]

In the typical acute care hospital, one finds a variety of units established on the basis of function. There are, for example, certain administrative units that are responsible for business functions, such as purchasing, accounts payable, facilities management, and data processing and management information systems. Other units are responsible for medical functions, such as surgery, medicine, and nursing. Certain ancillary functions are also performed, such as pharmacy, radiology, and nutrition services. This type of breakdown represents functional departmentalization.

Organizations can be divided in other ways. Consider the diversified health care system shown in Figure 12–4. This organization, known as Western Health System (WHS), has a number of products or services around which it is organized. One unit, Western Home Health, was organized to provide services to homebound patients and people discharged from Western Medical Center, WHS's flagship acute care hospital, who are still in need of certain services in their homes. Bailey Memorial Mental Health Clinic is an outpatient psychiatric facility devoted to assisting people with substance abuse problems and to providing care to emotionally disturbed people who are not in need of hospitalization. Western

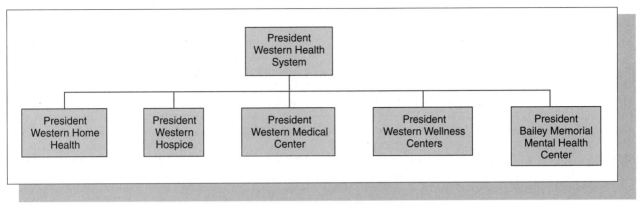

FIGURE 12–4. Structure of a complex health system.

Hospice and Western Wellness Center represent other services provided by WHS. This particular organization has chosen to departmentalize or structure itself around product units.

Another useful basis of departmentalization is geography or place. Sometimes we think of this basis of organization as useful primarily to global corporations with operations around the world. It can be equally useful to health care organizations of all kinds. The WHS's acute care hospital, for example, has six satellite ambulatory care clinics conveniently located to serve patients in different locations. In a large university hospital, the pharmacy department has satellite pharmacies in a number of places to be closer to the point of patient care.

There are two points to remember about departmentalization. The first is that there is no single basis for structure of an organization that will apply to all cases. Some organizations may be best served through a functional structure, whereas others will develop a service or product organization. Managers are free to choose the type of structure that best serves their particular needs.

The second point is that when a decision is made to functionally or geographically departmentalize at one organizational level, this does not eliminate other options at other levels. For example, WHS is organized around products and services at one level and around geography at another. The choice of structure should serve the needs of management, and managers should be free to use the type of organization that best facilitates the accomplishment of organizational and work group goals.

CENTRALIZATION AND DECENTRALIZATION. The final cornerstone concept or organizational principle of classical organization theory is **centralization and decentralization.** In the most general sense, centralization refers to the level at which decisions are made in the organization. If top-level managers make the decisions and allow few decisions to be made at lower levels, the organization is said to be centralized. If, by contrast, top management encourages decision making at lower levels—at the point of service delivery—the organization is said to be decentralized. There are some advantages of centralization of decision making. Consistency and control are encouraged. The case of software purchases is a commonly used example to illustrate the value of centralization. If each unit is allowed to purchase its own software, it is likely that little consistency will result and problems will develop. A number of word processing, spreadsheet, and database programs are used on personal computers in different departments, and when interchangeability is desired, it will not be available. Also, a centralized purchasing unit may be able to negotiate better prices with hardware and software vendors than each individual department.

On the other hand, centralized purchasing of hardware and software may force some units to use equipment and systems that are not the best for their particular applications. Decentralization makes it possible for a unit to purchase products and services that are directly applicable at the point of usage. Decentralization of decision making empowers the people who do the work to make the decisions concerning their jobs. This brings us to one final issue that is closely related to centralization and decentralization—the delegation of managerial authority.

Authority, Power, and Accountability

Authority is the manager's right to get things done. People receive these rights by the position they occupy in the organization. This association of authority with position is called the **formal theory of authority** because it views the manager's rights as always flowing from above. The CEO receives his or her rights to command from the board of directors, vice presidents receive their rights from the CEO, and so on. The president of WHS has certain rights by virtue of his or her position in the organization. **Power,** on the other hand, is a person's ability to get things done. If the president has authority but little power or ability to lead the organization, he or she will be ineffective. Power, unlike authority, is not a function of a person's position in the organization. The powerful person in the organization may be a world-renowned surgeon because of expertise. Or, it may be the president's executive assistant because this person is the gatekeeper of who sees the president. Effective managers develop abilities or power to equal the authority the organization bestows on them. This view of power is attributed to Chester Barnard and is called the **acceptance theory of authority** because it basically views authority (Barnard made no distinction between authority and power) as flowing upward from employees. In other words, the manager has authority to command because employees accept his or her right to do so.[26]

Accountability is the responsibility or liability a manager assumes for the stewardship of the authority that the organization grants to a particular position. The CEO is accountable to the board of directors for the authority he or she has been granted. The chief information officer is accountable to the CEO for the authority granted to that position. There is always accountability in proportion to one's authority.

Delegation of Authority

One of the most important determinants of a manager's effectiveness is his or her ability to delegate authority. Regardless of whether the organization is departmentalized according to services, functions, or geography, the manager always needs to be in more than one place at a time. Managers' jobs are not designed in a way that allows them to be predictably performed in an 8-hour day. Therefore, to be effective, managers must share or delegate their authority to others.[27]

Delegation accomplishes two important things in organizations:

- It allows the manager to be in more than one place at a given time.
- It allows others to make decisions, thus allowing people to develop and fine-tune decision-making skills.

That is, if authority is delegated to pharmacists in the different satellite pharmacies to make decisions within rather broad limits, the head of pharmacy can concentrate time on tasks that only he or she can do, such as interfacing with the hospital administrator and medical staff relative to departmental issues. Every organization relies on a pipeline of capable managers. How do people

learn to be managers and decision makers? They manage and make decisions. Effective delegators provide valuable training experiences for lower-level managers.[28]

The value of delegation of authority as an aid to expanding managerial capabilities and as a developer of future decision makers raises an interesting question. If delegation of authority is so essential to good management, why are most managers so unwilling to delegate? Although the question appears complicated, the answer is simple. At the personal level, some managers are threatened by delegation. Delegation reduces control and requires trust, and some managers are not comfortable with either. In times like today, when health care organizations are routinely downsizing and reducing layers in the hierarchy, it may be quite threatening to have a supply of capable decision makers below you at lower pay levels. Even well-meaning bosses might question why you, the higher-paid executive, is needed if you have direct reports from people who can make decisions almost as well as you.

Despite the risks, there is no excuse for not delegating authority. Developing and empowering employees are part of the manager's job. Admittedly, this involves some risk taking. Successful managers continuously assume such risks in the interest of the overall good of the organization.

There is a more realistic and practical reason why people resist delegating their authority. This has to do with accountability. As we noted above, anytime a person is given authority, there is a commensurate amount of accountability. What happens if your trusted employee fails to make the delegated decision? What happens if the decision is made, but the choice of action proves to be wrong, even costly to the organization? What if the pharmacist in the satellite pharmacy makes decisions that destroy relations with the nursing and medical staffs that the head of pharmacy has worked for years to build? There is a high degree of risk in delegation. There is no denying this reality. If a manager delegates authority and the results are unfavorable, the manager remains accountable for the operations under his or her area of responsibility.

Even though it is risky, managers have little choice but to assume the risks. They will not be able to perform their jobs effectively if they do not, nor will they grow professionally beyond their initial positions. The employees in their charge will not develop as they should, and overall organizational performance sooner or later will be adversely affected. Risk is part of the reality facing managers. They simply need to accept it as such and devote themselves to doing the best job they can while empowering and developing trust among employees.

In reality, a number of factors influence the extent to which authority is delegated in an organization. The following are a few of the more important.

- **Management philosophy.** Managers who are afraid to give up control, who fear for the security of their jobs, and who do not trust employees will not delegate authority.

- **Information-processing capabilities.** Limitations on information-processing capabilities can force delegation of authority. If timely information about what is happening in geographically dispersed units is not available, the managers may have little choice but to delegate. Some people have suggested that improved information-processing capabilities have enabled the effective centralization of decision making and discouraged delegation.

- **Economic conditions.** When economic conditions threaten organizational survival or the effectiveness of an individual unit, managers will be less likely to delegate authority. The emphasis will be on consistency and control to overcome the threats imposed by the external environment.

- **Necessity for innovation.** Some managers, like health services administrators, may have little choice but to delegate some of their authority. Rapidly changing environments demand innovation and change. Innovative ideas usually originate at the point of patient service. Therefore, to take advantage of all the creative ideas in an organization, delegation becomes a necessity to ensure continuous innovation.

- **Employee characteristics.** Highly professional employees demand autonomy and will insist on making decisions more than lower-skilled employees, who may be content doing what they are told to do. Professionalism usually assumes a knowledge base that can be used as the basis for decision making.

- **Organizational size.** As organizations become larger, the necessity for delegation of authority increases.

- **Importance of the decision.** More important decisions are the last to be delegated. If a decision can make or break the organization, it will be made at very high levels. Routine decisions are the most likely to be delegated.

- **Supply of potential decision makers.** In organizations fortunate enough to have a good supply of capable decision makers, authority will be delegated more willingly. In organizations where employees are reluctant to make decisions, less delegation will take place.

This discussion illustrates the way in which traditional or classical organization theory approached the issue of structuring or organizing operations. The point is that organizing, traditionally, has been viewed as consisting of several well-defined principles or concepts. Contingency theory, as noted earlier, looked at organizing in a less mechanistic way. Whereas classical theory advocated principles that applied to all situations, contingency theory, as the name suggests, was more situational. To illustrate the primary differences, we briefly survey some of the major themes of the contingency approach to organizing.

Another View of Organizing

Some regard classical organization theory as approaching the organizing problem from a **closed system** perspective. The organization was not thought of as actively interacting with its many environments. Although this is true to a great extent, it must be remembered that classical views were developed in a simpler time. Government regulations were less influential on internal operations, social values changed slower and seldom made their way rapidly into the workplace, and economic conditions seemed to remain stable for longer periods. In this more relaxed environment, decision makers could focus more on the efficiency of internal operations.

Today things are different. Organizations are generally viewed as **open systems** that actively take inputs from their environments, perform certain operations on them, and send outputs in the form of desirable goods and services back to the environments (Figure 12–5). The larger economic, social, political, and cultural environment surrounds the organization and supplies it with a basis for a philosophy of operations (i.e., a caring approach to patient care), productive inputs in the form of human (i.e., physicians, nurses, allied health personnel) and nonhuman resources (i.e., technology, physical facilities), and patients. These resources and other inputs are taken into the organizational system, and transformations are performed on them. Patients pass through the organization according to protocols and policies prescribed by the formal, **task-oriented subsystem.** Much of the quality of their care is determined not just by whether or not formal tasks are performed but how employees work as teams, the pursuit of excellence, and so on. Teamwork, excellence, and related factors cannot be mandated by the organizations but are influenced by the informal **social subsystem.** Transformations are also influenced by the **political subsystem** or how well different groups work together. Is there conflict between administration and nonmanagerial employees? Does pharmacy experience conflicts with nutrition? Is the health information management department forming coalitions with other units to lobby for a specific type of

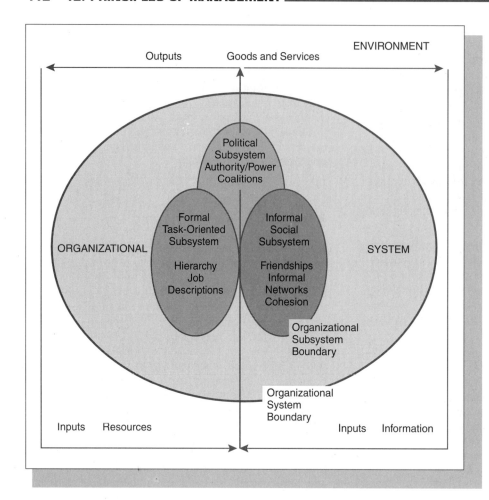

FIGURE 12–5. Organization as open system.

technology at the expense of another area in the hospital?

All these subsystems influence the quality of care that patients receive and, thus, the quality of the outputs that go back into the environment.[29] The reputation of the hospital is formed in this manner and becomes information fed back into the environment, which in turn becomes important input for the organization relative to how it is doing and how competitive it is in the marketplace.

Because of this open systems perspective, contingency theory proposes that there is no one best way to organize or manage all organizations at all times. Although this assertion may not, at first glance, appear revolutionary, it has the potential to bring into question many of the most cherished principles of classical organization theory. Is it possible that there is no limit to the span of control? Can the routine violation of unity of command improve organizational performance?

Contingency theory emphasizes the importance of organizational forces on the behavior of organizations and

managers. It focuses on the unique aspects of organizations and situations and in this way questions the universal applicability of management principles and concepts. At the same time, contingency theory recognizes the existence of a basic theory of organization and does not go so far as to propose that every situation is so unique as to make theory useless.

Principles of Effective Organizing

As with planning, there are no absolute, universally applicable principles of organizing. However, we can suggest a few guidelines for management action that are useful in practice.

- Specializing tasks is a sound organizational principle that will lead to increased efficiency if not excessively applied. In excess, specialization can overcome the positive contributions to efficiency by increasing boredom and fatigue and reducing pride in workmanship.

- Unity of command (only one boss at a time) facilitates coordination and efficiency. When violated, it may lead to certain advantages in terms of minimizing the need for redundant human resources in project management environments. There is, however, a cost associated with lack of coordination and clarity of authority relations.

- Organizations may be departmentalized according to a variety of criteria, and the bases for structuring operations may be mixed at different organizational levels.

- Decisions in organizations should be decentralized as near as possible to the point where work is performed. Where consistency is needed for managerial or legal reasons, centralization is required.

- Authority should be delegated to the extent possible to assist managers in overcoming personal limitations and to provide decision-making skills for employees who show promise as future managers.

- The application of organizational principles should consider the environment within which the organization operates and make adjustments as the realities of the situation demand.

Planning and organizing are important functions of management. Much of management theory has been devoted to an understanding of these functions. Planning provides the goals and organizing provides the structure. However, there is usually more than one way to accomplish goals. For this reason, decision making is another important management function.

Making Management Decisions

The primary function of management, according to Akio Morita of Sony Corporation, is **decision making.** Herbert Simon stated that decision making is the heart of executive activity.[30] There is certainly more to management than decision making, but there is no arguing that decision making is basically the heart of what managers do.

The management literature has focused on two things that managers need to know about decision making. The first has to do with **normative decision theory,** which attempts to assist managers by providing ways to make better decisions. If the manager has clearly defined goals such as maximizing patient satisfaction, maximizing returns to stockholders, or minimizing costs, normative decision theory can provide some tools that are useful in accomplishing these goals. In a sense, normative decision theory adapts the scientific method and

applies it to making choices that are relevant to managers.

If, for example, the manager is faced with the problem of what computer hardware to purchase, he or she should apply a systematic method to making the choice. The goal of the system should be clearly defined. Alternative systems capable of accomplishing the goal should be developed, and each should be systematically analyzed according to established criteria. Which vendors and systems can be installed in time for the planned conversion, what is the price of each competing system, and so on.

Finally, the choice should be made according to the analysis conducted. This approach or view of decision making is highly consistent with Fayol's view of management behavior because it pictures the manager as a reflective calculator who clearly defines problems, systematically generates alternative solutions, and carefully selects the best alternative in light of organizational goals. However, there is more to decision making in contemporary organizations.

The second thing that is useful for managers to know about decision making is how decisions are made. The description of this process has been the goal of **behavioral decision theory.** Whereas normative theory provides a process for making decisions, the focus of behavioral theory is on the decision maker. How does the manager go about defining the goals of the problem being addressed, how are alternatives generated and analyzed, and what is involved in the process of the final selection of the computer hardware? Both of these theories are discussed and some of their implications illustrated. This view of managerial decision making is more consistent with Mintzberg because it focuses on the manner in which decisions are made.

Normative Decision Theory

This theory of decision making is often called prescriptive because it prescribes ways of making decisions to accomplish defined goals. It is the older of the two major theories of management decision making and owes much of its origins to economic analysis.

The specific origins of normative decision theory can be traced to the operations research groups in World War II. Both the United States and Britain used concepts of mathematical decision making in areas of antisubmarine warfare and campaign planning. After the war, the potential benefits of these methods in industry were recognized and applied in selected industries, such as automobile manufacturing.

Normative decision theory makes a number of simplifying assumptions about decision makers in the interest of mathematical precision and for this reason is criticized as unrealistic in real organizational settings. Seldom is a manager in business, health care, education, or government presented with problems that allow for the direct application of mathematical decision theory. However, in a number of specialized areas, such as inventory control, process engineering, and facilities management, the techniques used by normative decision theorists have been useful.

Behavioral Decision Theory

In more recent times, close examination of the assumptions of normative theory revealed that if managers are to understand how decisions are made, alternative approaches would be needed. As a response to the unrealism of the assumptions underlying normative decision theory and the need to know more about how decisions are made as well as how they ought to be made, behavioral decision theory was developed beginning in the late 1940s.

Behavioral decision theory is most directly identified with Herbert Simon, who has been mentioned throughout this chapter. Perhaps the best way to compare normative and behavioral decision theory is to look at the assumptions they make about the decision maker (Table 12–1).

Behavioral decision theory assumes that decision makers are incapable of maximizing revenues or minimizing costs because they simply do not have the capacity to know all the alternatives and related information as normative theory assumes. In reality, the health care decision maker must consider not just the welfare of the stockholders (if the facility is privately owned) but also the needs of patients, employees, and numerous other stakeholders. Because of this, decisions are always

compromises rather than choices that maximize revenues or minimize costs.[31] The result is the selection of goals that represent compromises of the interests of several, sometimes competing value systems.

The "**satisficing**" **behavior** that results in the pursuit of satisfactory rather than maximizing goals is reinforced by the inability of decision makers to acquire perfect knowledge regarding their choices in even simple decisions. Simon argues, for example, that decision makers ultimately satisfice in their decisions because we, as human beings, do not have the "wits to maximize."[1] All decision makers operate from a base of imperfect and incomplete information. This is referred to as **bounded rationality.** There are bounds or limits to our information, and as a result, decision makers seldom, if ever, have anything near the complete knowledge of the decisional problem as visualized by normative decision theory.

Finally, whereas normative decision theory viewed decision makers as arraying a complete set of alternatives and selecting the maximizing or minimizing option, behavioral theory pictures alternative search as taking place sequentially. Because decision makers are not assumed to know all their alternatives, the process of searching for possible ways to accomplish organizational goals begins with the random selection of the first alternative and proceeds until an option is generated that satisfies the competing demands of different stakeholders. This is referred to as **sequential search.**

Unique Contribution of Health Information Systems

Perhaps the primary difference between normative and behavioral decision theory revolves around the issue of decision maker **rationality.** In management, this term is used in a very different sense than in psychology and medicine. Whereas the opposite of rationality in psychology and medicine is irrationality or abnormal behavior, the opposite term has no such connotation in management. Rationality has to do with information in management. The rational manager is the informed manager. Therefore, decision makers in normative theory were considered perfectly rational because they had complete information of the major variables in the decision-making situation. They knew the goal, the alternatives, and the outcomes associated with each alternative.

Decision makers are not thought of as rational in behavioral decision theory because they lack complete knowledge. This introduces an important role for health information systems—to increase the rationality of management through the provision of high-quality information. Managers rely on information for effective decision making. Health information systems are vital aids to both diagnostic and managerial decision making in the

TABLE 12–1 COMPARISON OF ASSUMPTIONS OF BEHAVIORAL AND NORMATIVE DECISION THEORY

ASSUMPTIONS ABOUT	BEHAVIORAL THEORY	NORMATIVE THEORY
Decision maker	Administrative person who satisfices	Economic person who maximizes
Extent of knowledge or understanding	Possesses limited knowledge of alternatives and related conditions surrounding decision	Possesses complete knowledge of available alternatives and related conditions surrounding decision
Search behavior	Sequential search beginning with random generation of alternatives	Clear ordering of preferences and available alternatives

For additional details on these processes, see Duncan WJ: Descriptive decision theory in health administration: A brief review and extension. Journal of Health and Human Resources 1980; 3(1):67–78.

sense that they provide decision makers with information on which to base well-informed decisions. This is a critical role and one that is essential to the success of organizations.

When the Decision Is Made

An important contribution of behavioral decision theory is the recognition that the consequences of decision making for the decision maker are not over when the decision is made. Have you ever made a decision, for example, perhaps to buy a car or a house and in the process obligated yourself to making payments over an extended period of time? Do you remember the feeling you had when you signed your name to the contract? Perhaps you wondered if you did the right thing. Was there a better car or more valuable house that should have been purchased? This is a natural feeling known as **cognitive dissonance.** All of us have experienced it, and it is a natural part of decision making.[32]

Because cognitive dissonance is part of decision making, it is a topic of interest to behavioral decision theory. In decision making, cognitive dissonance develops because we can usually select only one or a limited number of alternatives while rejecting all others. Only one computer system will be purchased to support the administrative operations of the health care organization. The products of other vendors will be rejected. However, we invariably select one system over another based on several of the most critical criteria. Is it compatible with our current system? Can it be delivered by a particular date?

There will, no doubt, be aspects of the systems we reject that we like or even prefer. One system may come with certain software we would like but that is not essential to our operations. Another system may be made in the United States, whereas another is made abroad. Regardless of the reason, the rejected alternatives always possess some characteristics that we like and maybe even prefer. Regardless of the alternative selected, there is always the postdecision anxiety or cognitive dissonance.

Management decision makers also experience cognitive dissonance. The more desirable the alternatives that must be rejected and the faster the decision must be made, the greater the anxiety and dissonance. Managers deal with cognitive dissonance the same way consumers deal with it. Sometimes we simply accentuate the positive of the alternative selected. In this way, we attempt to focus on the positive aspects of the system we selected while ignoring or denying the positive aspects of the systems we decided not to purchase.

In a psychological sense, managers may be said to rationalize decisions once they are made. All of us do the same thing. We rationalize the decisions made because once the choice is selected, there is little reason to continue worrying or wondering about what might have been if another alternative had been selected. The choice is made, we can learn from any mistakes made, but it is time to move on to other work and decisions. We should not, however, excessively rationalize and repeat mistakes by failing to learn from our experiences.

Essential Principles of Decision Making

Decision-making principles can be formulated as useful guides to decision makers. Although this function is, in many ways, more systematic than some of the other management functions, we should not fail to remember that the principles discussed in this chapter are guidelines to action and not absolute principles to be followed in all cases.

- Normative decision theory provides important aids for managers in selecting among alternative choices when the goals are clearly established and the bases on which choices are to be selected are clearly articulated.

- Behavioral decision theory is useful to managers for understanding how decisions are made.

- Because managers are not capable of having perfect knowledge of all aspects of the decision situation, the costs and benefits of additional information search should be part of all decision making.

Leading and Managing

The fourth management function is the subject of considerable contemporary controversy. This function has to do with influencing behavior or **leading.** In the past, leadership has been accepted by almost everyone as an essential part of management. At times, leading and managing have been used to mean the same thing. In fact, a great deal of management has dealt with different aspects of leadership.

Looking at Leadership from a Managerial Perspective

From the applied perspective of management, leadership has always been recognized as important. In fact, management has historically been interested in the following aspects of leadership:

- How do people become leaders?

- What is the best way to lead?

- What factors account for effectiveness on the part of a leader?

We will look at each of these questions and then extend the discussion of leadership beyond the customary interests of management.

The earliest concern of management regarding leadership was the question of how one becomes a leader. Although it has always been recognized that not all leaders are managers, it is hard to imagine an effective manager who does not have some qualities of leadership. For this reason, business firms, the military, and health care organizations have all been interested in how people become good leaders.

TRAIT THEORY. How a person becomes a leader was first approached, as one might expect, from a somewhat naive perspective. Early researchers looked at the physical traits of past leaders in the hope that they would find some secret to their emergence and success. This was known as **trait theory.** The research process was simple. Samples of leaders and nonleaders were compared to see if leaders possessed some traits that nonleaders did not possess. Some believed that traits like height and place or even order of birth were important to the emergence of leadership. None of these hypotheses proved to consistently predict leadership.

Some researchers expanded the naive search among physical traits to include psychological traits. Some argued that people who were successful leaders were more competitive or intelligent than others. Some were and some were not. Despite the inconsistencies, trait theory did yield some useful characteristics that at least seemed to characterize many effective leaders[33]:

- Leaders possess a strong drive for responsibility and are devoted to completing tasks that they undertake.
- Leaders are persistent in the pursuit of established goals.
- Leaders are innovative and demonstrate originality in problem solving and decision making.
- Leaders are self-confident and have a strong personal identity.
- Leaders exercise initiative and make things happen.
- Leaders are willing to accept the consequences of their actions.
- Leaders deal effectively with stress and are willing to tolerate frustrations.
- Leaders have the ability to influence the actions of others.

Although these characteristics of effective leaders all have merit and are generally legitimate, the result of both the physical and the psychological trait theories was the same. There were simply too many exceptions to all the hypotheses generated to be useful in predicting leadership ability. Despite the best efforts to identify consistent traits, the exceptions could not be denied. Most leaders were open and outgoing, but some were quiet and withdrawn. Many were tall and had a compelling physical presence; others were short of stature and unassuming. There had to be more to the issue of what makes a leader than physical and psychological traits.

SITUATIONAL THEORY. The problems of trait theory in terms of consistently predicting the emergence of leadership led to an alternative view known as **situational theory.** Situational theory was more impersonal than trait theory. Rather than focusing on the individual, this approach to leadership looked at the situation and examined the people who emerged as leaders. Some leaders, such as Winston Churchill, seemed at their best in difficult times.

At times, the victory of the situational advocates seemed assured. Careful analysis of both arguments, however, indicates that although neither of these factors—situation or traits—predicts leadership completely, both provide important insights. In fact, the best information suggests that the two views can be partially reconciled and that each can provide insights into the other. This can be done as follows:[34]

- No specific traits, physical or psychological, are essential for the emergence of leadership in all situations. The more similar the situation, the more likely will be the transfer of leadership.
- Although there are no universal leadership traits, the traits possessed by the leader must bear some reasonable relation to the situation.

The point regarding the emergence of leadership is that individual traits and situational factors interact in determining who will emerge as a leader in any particular situation. Managers can increase the likelihood that a leader will be successful in any given situation by considering the traits that are likely to be useful in accomplishing the goals of the job.

LEADERSHIP STYLE. The second leadership issue that has occupied a great deal of attention in the management literature is the appropriate **style of leadership.** Although this issue is discussed in greater detail in other chapters of this book, we briefly acknowledge the importance of the issue. Leadership style relates to how a particular person exercises influence over others. Some leaders influence others merely by their presence.

Laissez-faire. In terms of our previous discussion, some leaders can influence others without the necessity of formal authority. In a research laboratory, for example, the director may be a well-known scientist who has made many technical contributions to his or her field of expertise. Because he or she is highly respected as a scientist, people willingly follow him or her and he or she never has to use the position to require them to do their jobs. He or she simply keeps the other scientists informed about priorities and constraints and they do their jobs. This style of leadership is known as laissez-faire or free reign and is most successful in highly professionalized settings with knowledge-based workers who have a high sense of professional commitment that transcends any single organization.

Democratic Style. Another leadership style is the democratic or participative style. Leaders who display a democratic style ultimately make decisions but do so after consideration of the opinions of others. Group members are asked for opinions, and their views are seriously considered before decisions are made. Under many conditions, participative leaders achieve impressive results because involvement of the group has certain advantages, such as those listed below.[35]

- Participation helps employees understand issues and increases the likelihood that they will accept and support the decisions of the leader.

- Participation allows employees to be involved in the cooperative aspects of group decision making and gives group members a sense of belonging to something important.

- Participation allows leaders and employees to reconcile any difference they have in goals and the means to achieving the goals and thus reduces conflict.

- Participation preserves the dignity and worth of employees by acknowledging the importance of their ideas.

- Participation allows employees to understand the process through which the decisions are made, so that they are more likely to support decisions among fellow employees.

Participative leadership, however, has its down side. Participation requires time, and it can make employees question the abilities of managers. Despite the possible dangers, an offer to participate usually improves morale and the process of participation places more ideas on the table. The result often is a higher-quality decision.

Autocratic Style. Some leaders use their formal authority and behave in an autocratic manner. Autocrats usually are formal leaders who use their positions as the way to influence the behavior of others. Some people are autocratic because they feel a sense of urgency and the need to make decisions fast. Some are autocratic because they are uncertain about their abilities and see participation as a threat to their authority. In highly professional settings, autocratic leadership styles are not likely to be successful.

LEADERSHIP EFFECTIVENESS. The third major leadership concern from a management perspective is the question of leadership effectiveness. To a great extent, the interest in leadership effectiveness resulted from the concern for the appropriate style of leadership. Different advocates of various approaches to leadership have suggested that the most appropriate style of leading was autocratic, participative, or free reign. However, as we look at different organizations and different leaders, it is clear that each style is sometimes successful and sometimes not. The research of leadership effectiveness began to focus on what makes a leader effective, and some interesting findings resulted.

As with early management thought, which tended to be absolute in nature, it was found that there is no one best way to lead. Sometimes when time pressures are great and employees have little real understanding of the problem, an autocratic style of leadership may be appropriate and effective. However, when employees know a great deal about the decision under consideration, understand the goals of the organization, and want to be involved, participative leadership can be effective and appropriate. When employees know more about the nature of the work, as is often the case in highly professionalized settings, the free reign approach to leadership is the style of choice.

The point to be made is that leaders need to be less concerned about developing and perfecting a particular style and focus more on adapting their style to the demands of the situation. Leadership flexibility leads to leadership effectiveness.

An Important Leadership Controversy

One of the most recent and most important issues in leadership today is the ways in which leadership and management are different. Although good managers should be effective leaders, it is important to note that leadership and management are not the same things.

Management, as we have seen, is about planning, budgeting, organizing and staffing, and controlling and monitoring.[36] Management is concerned with ensuring that goals are clearly defined, that resources are structured in a way that helps accomplish goals, and that systems are in place to ensure that deviations from desired performance are brought back into conformance with goals. The result of effective management is order, predictability of systems, and efficiency. Management is about doing things the right way. Leadership is something different.

Leadership is about setting direction and providing a vision or hope for the future. It is about aligning groups toward the accomplishment of common goals, and it is about motivation and inspiration. The result of good leadership is change rather than order or predictability. Innovation rather than efficiency is the result of leadership.[37] This is not to suggest that management or leadership is more or less important than the other. Successful organizations require both, but both of these qualities are not always found in the same person. When organizations have management and leadership, they do the right things as well as do things right. They are efficient and they are also effective. One writer on the subject has offered the following contrast between managers and leaders[37]:

- Managers administer; leaders innovate.

- Managers are copies; leaders are originals.

- Managers focus on systems and procedures; leaders focus on people.

- Managers rely on control; leaders inspire trust.

- Managers have a short-range view; leaders have a long-range perspective.

- Managers ask how and when; leaders ask what and why.

- Managers have an eye on the bottom line; leaders have their eye on the horizon.

- Managers imitate; leaders innovate.

Principles of Leading

Leadership is a difficult job, and leading is one of the most challenging aspects of what managers do. To be effective, managers must develop leadership skills and the ability to determine what actions are likely to motivate and inspire different people in different job situations. The challenge of leadership will continue to be one of the most demanding and perplexing issues in management. Again, while not precise in a scientific sense, there are some useful guidelines managers can follow to become more effective leaders.

- There is no one best way to lead. Effective leaders are skilled at diagnosing the situation and applying the style of leadership most appropriate for the situation at hand.

- Leadership is not management and imposition of order through planning, staffing, and controlling. Instead, leadership is setting direction and providing a vision, aligning groups to pursue goals, and motivating and inspiring others.

- The identification of leadership potentials does not rest in the personality of a person but is a complex interaction of personality and situational factors.

- Effective leaders build trust and a determination to assume responsibility among those with whom they work.

Controlling: Completing the Management Loop

Controlling, like the other management functions previously discussed, is a process composed of four steps (Figure 12–6).

1. When the activity being controlled is initiated, it must be observed, monitored, and measured.

2. Because goals have been established in the planning process, they are the standard of desired performance level. These established goals are then compared with actual performance.

3. Any discrepancy between actual and desired performance is called **variance**. The type of corrective action to be initiated depends on the nature of the variance.

4. If actual performance exceeds established goals, the standard should be re-examined to ensure that it was high enough. If actual performance fails to meet the standard and if the goal is determined to be appropriate, ways must be developed to ensure that performance is improved.

The control process can be accurately viewed as an evaluation procedure whereby actual performance is measured and compared with the desired standard represented by the plan. It is also a corrective procedure because the difference between actual and desired performance provides insights into the type of action that is needed to correct the variance.

Characteristics of Effective Controls

From the perspective of health information systems, it is important to note that effective control requires accurate and timely information. Information is required at all stages of the process. However, to be effective, controls must exhibit certain characteristics.

FLEXIBILITY. For controls to be effective, they must be flexible. The overly zealous application of controls leads to excessive structure and authority on the part of the controller. It is adverse to many of the guidelines we have discussed in both planning and leadership. Consider the budgeting process of a medium-sized community hospital. The budget allows for no shifting of expenditures among the budget categories. At the end of the year, the department managers cannot take surplus funds originally budgeted for equipment and use them to cover needed travel expenses. The surplus funds must be given over to the general fund of the city and are used to cover expenditures in other government units. You know what to expect at the end of the fiscal year. Department heads go up and down the halls asking if anyone needs a new calculator, computer, or desk. Spending the funds is preferred to sending the money

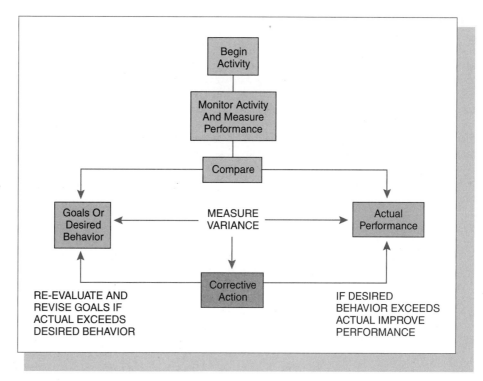

FIGURE 12–6. Control process.

back to cover the inefficiencies of others. A little flexibility in the budgeting system would probably increase the use of funds significantly.

SIMPLICITY. Controls that are simple are more effective than complex controls few can understand. Controls are of little value if they are vague or so complex that few people understand them. Many government regulations, for example, are so complex that operational managers do not understand them. Details must be interpreted by the hospital's attorney, and in the process, the real meaning of the regulation to the laboratory or maintenance is lost. When the reasons for controls and regulations are not understood or appreciated, problems also develop. Enforcement becomes more difficult.

ECONOMICAL. Controls should be economical. If controls cost more than they save, they should be questioned. For example, the maintenance warehouse at an urban hospital was experiencing a problem with employee theft. It was estimated that employees walked off with almost $23,000 worth of parts and tools each year. Because the hospital was relatively small, the loss was considered significant. The hospital administrator contracted with Health Security Engineers to provide guards and other specialized security services. The annual cost of these services was estimated to be $28,500 and would result in a savings of 90 per cent of the employee theft. This would not be an economical control.

However, we can imagine situations in which a control might be instituted even if it was not economical in the short run or for some other compelling reason. For example, if the hospital administrator above noted that employee theft was increasing every year and was likely to be even worse if something was not done, it might be appropriate to spend the extra money with Health Security Engineers to stop the escalating trend. Also, consider a slightly different problem in the pharmacy. Suppose there was a problem with the disappearance of narcotic or controlled substance drugs. The hospital administrator might be forced to spend whatever was necessary to reduce this theft. In general, however, it is not well advised to spend more on controls than you can be reasonably expected to save.

TIMELINESS. Effective controls are timely. The temperature light on your automobile is designed to be a timely control. If it does not signal you in time, you will destroy your engine. If it works properly, it will come on before damage is done. If the light comes on after the motor is too hot to run properly, it is of no value as a control.

The same is true, to a great extent, of performance evaluation systems. They function best as controls if they alert managers to problems with employee performance before serious damage is done to the organization and the employee. If the evaluation system can only identify problems that demand radical actions, the system is not an effective control.

FOCUSING ON EXCEPTIONS. Controls should focus, to the extent possible, on exceptions. Controls that unnecessarily focus on trivial aspects of operations are not useful to managers. Controls that provide managers with so much information that there is no time to review it properly are not useful. Managers can never monitor all activities under their supervision at all times. Controls are effective when they highlight exceptions or activities that are out of control. This allows managers to focus on the things that really need attention. Controls are most effective when they are flexible enough to respond to changing conditions, economical, timely, and highlight exceptional or out-of-control activities.

Types of Controls

Think about your own personal health for a moment. If you think of medical services as a type of control, there are essentially two ways medical services can help you. First, you can apply what you know about personal fitness, nutrition, and stress management and try to keep from becoming ill. You can, in other words, attempt to prevent illness. On the other hand, you can use medical services once you become ill and try to correct a health problem once it has developed. These two options are essentially the same options that organizations face relative to controls.

PREVENTIVE CONTROLS. Preventive controls attempt to keep variances from developing. They attempt to anticipate problems and avoid them. Some types of preventive controls are familiar, such as preventive maintenance. The auxiliary generators in the basements of most hospitals must be "exercised" periodically to ensure that they are properly maintained and ready for action if and when they are needed. Maintenance is performed on airplane engines at regular intervals, regardless of whether or not problems have developed.

Preventive controls are usually used in situations where the potential risk of loss is extremely high if variances develop—failure of an airliner's engine. Wellness, as a concept, represents the type of situation in which some early preventive controls can keep serious and sometimes irreversible problems from developing with your health.

Preventive controls, like preventive health, are often difficult to justify in the real world of decision makers. Sometimes maintenance expenditures are difficult to justify to the hospital administrator because it is not as easy to see how this kind of expenditure will contribute the same to the welfare and reputation of the hospital as a new surgical unit. Yet, if the facilities are not maintained, the reputation as well as the health and safety of employees and patients may be at risk. The justification of preventive expenditures is also difficult to warrant because if they are successful, they keep problems from developing. Sometimes it is impossible to convince a boss that we do not have problems specifically because we chose to invest money in preventive measures. Preventive controls are important and an integral part of all organizational control systems.

FEEDBACK CONTROLS. Feedback controls are more common than preventive controls in most organizations. Feedback controls swing into action after variances develop. They can be of two types. One type is called *non–self-correcting feedback control*. The budgeting and performance evaluation systems of most organizations are examples of this type of control (Figure 12–7).

The distinguishing characteristic of this type of control is that it highlights the variance but is incapable of initiating corrective actions. No automatic or self-correcting system is built into the control to ensure that performance problems or budget deficits are corrected. Correction requires the intervention of managers to bring things back into control. Most controls in organizations are non–self-correcting.

Another type of feedback control is *self-correcting*. Perhaps the best example of this type is the thermostat in your home or the leveling system on the elevator in your business office. Figure 12–8 shows the working of a thermostat. If we set our thermostat on 68°F., it does not mean that our office remains this temperature at all times. In fact, the temperature will seldom be 68°. This target or goal is merely an average, and if our thermostat operates with a variance of plus or minus 2°, the temperature in our office will vary from a high of 70° to

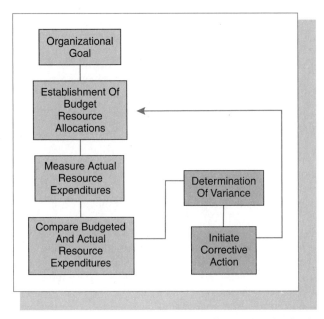

FIGURE 12–7. Budgeting as a non–self-correcting feedback control.

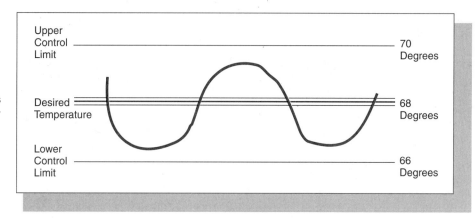

FIGURE 12–8. Thermostat as a self-correcting feedback control.

a low of 66°. The important point for our discussion is that when the temperature gets out of control, the thermostat automatically initiates actions to bring it back into control.

As noted previously, most controls in organizations require managerial intervention, which is the reason for this discussion of control as a management function. However, there are some examples of self-correcting controls. In many industrial processes, heat is a critical element to the control of quality. In steel making, for example, different types of metal are made with different levels of heat. Therefore, temperature is carefully and automatically controlled in the furnace without the intervention of management.

Control and Effectiveness

Management control is directed ultimately toward ensuring organizational effectiveness. Organizational **effectiveness,** although it has been mentioned previously and contrasted with organizational efficiency, has not been properly discussed to this point. Perhaps the reason we have hesitated to discuss effectiveness is that it is not an easy term to define. In fact, the management literature is testimony to the difficulty encountered in defining this term.

Customarily in management, an organization is considered effective if it accomplishes its goals. It may not be efficient, but the goals are realized. In this case, the role of managerial control is precisely as we discussed above—to determine variations from desired behavior and correct them or prevent them from occurring in the first place. Not everyone, however, sees effectiveness strictly in terms of goal accomplishment.

Other theories have suggested that organizations are effective when they are able to maintain internal tranquillity and minimize conflict. To others, the ability to attract the most critical human and nonhuman resources in the face of competition constitutes effectiveness. Still others believe that the ability to work effectively with the key stakeholders, such as employees, patients, physicians, and government officials, is what makes organizations effective. Regardless of the specific view of effectiveness, control plays an important role in keeping the organization focused on what it should be doing.[38]

Principles of Management Control

The theory of management control is sufficiently developed to aid us in suggesting some guidelines that will benefit management in attempting to keep planned and actual performance in line. A few of the more important guidelines are as follows:

- Organizational controls should be flexible, timely, and economical and focus on exceptions.

- When the risk of loss from variances is extremely high, preventive controls should be used.

- Self-correcting controls are rare in organizations because most variances require the conscious intervention of management to ensure that actual performance conforms to expected performance.

With this overview of management functions and selected principles, we can now move to a more in-depth look at one common management tool that is used in all types of organizations—**job descriptions.** Job descriptions are important because they constitute an important combination of planning (provide a target), organizing (assist in developing an action plan), leading (should be motivational and inspirational), and controlling (when used properly they are the standard against which performance is evaluated). In the concluding section of this chapter, we review some important aspects of job descriptions.

UNDERSTANDING JOB DESCRIPTIONS

Job descriptions are important in organizations for a number of reasons. First, they assist in offsetting uncertainty among organizational members. Without job descriptions, employees may experience both **role ambiguity** and **role conflict**. Role ambiguity occurs when people do not understand what is expected of them in their jobs. Role conflict occurs when one or more roles required by a job conflict with one another. Job descriptions can be useful in reducing ambiguity and conflict among roles.

Job descriptions also define the minimum level of expectations. This is one reason some organizations attempt to operate without job descriptions. Some people believe that job descriptions have the effect of unnecessarily "putting people in a box," so that one who wants to may say, "That is not my job" or "I do not get paid to do that" even when an important task is demanding attention. This can be an adverse result of a dysfunctional focus on job description, just as the description can define turf and cause people to be protective of their area of the organization. Despite the potential problems, job descriptions are important aids to defining performance expectations.

One of the most important functions of job descriptions is their use as a standard against which performance can be evaluated. Performance evaluation has a negative connotation to the person being evaluated and to the person doing the evaluation. This control function of managers is usually thought of as stressful and threatening. One of the reasons performance evaluations are thought of in this way is that expectations are often not clearly developed and surprises occur in the appraisal process. Job descriptions, when properly developed, can overcome some of the stress in **performance appraisal**.

Evolution of Job Descriptions

Job descriptions can be as serious and as useful as managers and organizations choose to make them. Historically, job descriptions concentrated on input factors or job specifications. Most of the space in job descriptions concentrated on specifying the job (i.e., what skills were needed to perform the required tasks) and the qualifications of the person doing the job (i.e., accounting degree, engineering degree, registered nurse). Although these aspects are important, they relate primarily to what a person brings to the job and to the minimum expectations of the organization.

In more recent times, management has insisted that job descriptions and performance evaluations be logical extensions of the organizational goal-setting process, as discussed in the beginning of the chapter. The most effective job descriptions are those that are directly anchored into the mission and goals of the hospital, nursing facility, or health maintenance organization. To accomplish this requires considerable attention.

Relating Organizational Goals to Job Descriptions

Figure 12–9 shows a sample job description for a systems programmer in technical support services in a large medical center. Note that the job description consists of several elements. The first is the job title followed by the personnel classification provided by the human resources department. This person is salaried and exempt from requirements for overtime pay and so on. The next section of the figure provides a brief description of the job.

The purpose of this mini job description within the larger description is to provide the reader with a general understanding of the nature of the job. The description makes it clear that this person is responsible for system and telecommunications software and support for all aspects of the data-processing system. A series of typical responsibilities are then provided for those who may desire some additional details. This job description also provides a statement regarding the reporting relationship of the systems programmer. In this case, the systems programmer reports directly to the associate director and systems and programming manager (one position) and has a coordinative relationship with the project manager. The coordinative relationship is important because most of the projects initiated in this department require some type of system support.

Finally, this particular job description specifies the desired qualifications of the incumbent. The appropriately qualified systems programmer should have an undergraduate degree in one of several scientific fields or accounting and 5 years of experience in specific areas. Some job descriptions indicate that relevant experience can be substituted for formal education requirements or the other combinations of experience and education that may be acceptable.

Expanding the Concept of Job Descriptions

One interesting thing that this particular organization did to relate each job to the overall success of the department was to identify critical success factors for each job and indicate the specific outcomes expected to accomplish each factor (Figure 12–10).

Note in Figure 12–10 that four critical success factors (things that absolutely must be accomplished for the department to be successful) have been identified for the department of computer and telecommunication services

Job Title:	Systems Programmer/Technical Support
Classification:	Exempt Salaried
Description of Responsibility:	Accountable for implementation, maintenance, and evaluation of systems software, telecommunications software and support, and coordination of operations. Accountable for all phases of support of data processing systems functions.

Typical Tasks:

1. Development, planning, implementing, and maintaining of network and database systems.
2. Evaluation of software and hardware changes to enhance and maintain high levels of system performance.
3. Technical assistance in areas of problem identification, debugging, and troubleshooting.
4. Technical interface among hardware and software vendors, in-house operations, and users.
5. Ensure adequate documentation and training on new system software installations.
6. Generation of new projects relating to developing technologies and work improvements.
7. Installation and maintenance of system software, utilities, language processors, access methods, and teleprocessing support.
8. Develop, monitor, maintain, and report on system performance measures.

Reporting Relationship:	Reports to Associate Administrator and Systems and Programming Manager. Coordinative relationship with Projects Manager.
Qualifications:	B. S. degree in mathematics, computer science, physical sciences, statistics, or accounting. Five years experience in technical data processing and knowledge of data management, operating system software, data communication, and networking techniques.

FIGURE 12–9. Sample job description.

within which the systems programmer/technical support job is located. These factors are as follows.

- *Project initiation and support.* For this to happen, the systems programmer was expected to provide software support on internally and externally generated projects as well as generate projects relating to new technologies and work improvement.

- *Maintenance.* The systems programmer, relative to this factor, was expected to install and maintain software, control programs, utilities, language processors, access methods, and teleprocessing support. In addition, this position must develop, monitor, maintain, and report on system performance measures.

- *Procedure development and documentation.* The systems programmer is expected to ensure documentation of all software installations and monitor the need to remedially document previous installations.

- *Technical support.* This job has a number of expected outcomes in this area, such as technical interface with vendors and users, coordination of systems planning, network and database development, planning, implementation, maintenance, and recommendations relative to hardware and software performance enhancement. The person in this position is also expected to provide technical support to programmers as well as in-house training, design systems, and write programs.

It is true that relationships such as those shown in Figure 12–10 are not parts of typical job descriptions, but they are useful to managers because they can assist in linking what is important to the overall work unit and the particular job under examination.

From Job Descriptions to Performance Evaluation

Ideally, managers are not satisfied with merely describing or specifying the job through the job description. To be of maximum value, job descriptions should be related to the critical success factors of the work unit which, in turn, should be related to the critical success factors of the organization. Specific expected outcome can then be related to the critical success factors as illustrated by the systems programmer example in Figure 12–10. The relationship, however, should not stop at expected outcomes. For job descriptions to be genuinely effective, the descriptions should have a direct link to the performance evaluation process.

EXAMPLE

In a large academic medical center, an effort was made to develop a systematic evaluation instrument for the director of internal auditing. It was determined that because the director was responsible for the overall suc-

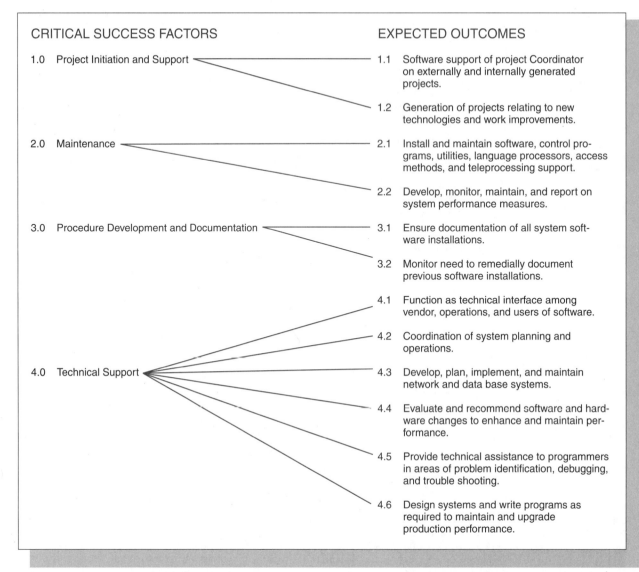

FIGURE 12–10. Systems programmer/technical support critical success factors.

cess of the internal audit function in the medical center, the first step should be specifying the mission or reason for being of the department. The mission developed by the staff in the department was carefully anchored into the mission of the medical center. The internal audit mission statement is shown below.

The Office of Internal Audit provides consultative and educational services in the identification, evaluation, and control of administrative, operational, financial, informational, compliance, and technologic risks. We provide these services to distinct administrative units for the benefit of the Audit Committee of the Board of Directors in an objective, ethical, discreet, and professional manner.

After establishing the mission of the internal audit department, the director, in consultation with the administrator in charge of the internal audit function, determined the general job description for the director of internal auditing and the critical success factors for the department. Unlike the systems programmer/technical support description, a brief statement was used for the job description of the director with most of the attention devoted to the critical success factors and outcome measures. The job description is noted below.

The director of internal auditing is responsible for the supervision of the work of internal auditors, which should be accomplished in a manner that ensures conformance with internal auditing standards, methods, and auditing programs.

The five critical success factors for the director of internal auditing job are listed below.

The following is a list of five critical success factors for the Office of Internal Audit. After each critical success factor, a brief description is provided.

Critical success factor 1. *Quality of Audits.* Preparation of audits that minimize business risks from an organizational perspective that are timely, useful to clients, consistent with internal audit procedures and standards, and responsive to changing conditions and priorities.

Critical success factor 2. *Relationship with Clients.* Reports to clients that are timely and nonthreatening analyses that are useful to them in reducing real and perceived business risks.

Critical success factor 3. *Staff Growth & Development.* Existence of a work culture in which employees contribute to the development of a mission and vision for the Office of Internal Audit that inspires high-performing teams of motivated professionals who readily accept responsibility for their own actions and the success of the office and who are constantly engaged in getting better at what they do.

Critical success factor 4. *Management of the Office.* Conduct of Office of Internal Audit operations in a manner that ensures that human and nonhuman resources are used wisely, that the most recent business practices are used, and that decisions are made in a manner that addresses the most pressing problems from an organizational perspective.

Critical success factor 5. *Leadership.* Involvement of all staff in charting the direction of the office and encouragement of everyone to grow professionally through innovative behavior while accepting their individual and collective accountability for the success of the office.

These factors are divided into two major categories: output factors and input and process factors (Figure 12–11). The output critical success factors are quality of audits and relationship with clients. These factors relate to key outputs of the department. To be successful, the quality of the audits completed by internal auditing must minimize the organization's exposure to business risks and must build confidence among the clients. The ultimate goal was that the directors of units being audited would come to look on internal auditing as a valuable source of internal consultants rather than as a unit focusing on what the unit is doing wrong.

The measures used to determine the extent of accomplishment of the output critical factors were as follows:

- Whether or not the audits met the standards expected of internal audits
- Whether or not they were conducted in a timely manner

- Usefulness as determined by the clients
- Extent to which they minimized exposure to business risks
- Nonthreatening character of the audits from the perspective of the client

The extent to which business risk exposure was minimized was further indicated by how effectively the audit plans set appropriate priorities in terms of risk exposure and the degree to which the priorities responded to changing conditions.

Three input or process critical success factors were identified for the director. They were staff growth and development, management of the office of internal auditing, and leadership. The following parameters were used to measure staff growth and development:

- Development of high-performing teams
- Extent of empowerment of employees
- Motivational level of professional employees

Some of the measures overlap, as is the case with the measures of managerial effectiveness and leadership.

The effectiveness of the management of the office was measured by the following:

- Minimization of exposure to business risks
- Efficient use of organizational resources
- Use of latest business practices

Leadership was measured by the following:

- Development of high-performing teams
- Empowerment of employees
- Development of highly motivated employees

Empowerment was further indicated by the extent to which employees were encouraged to contribute to the organization, the extent to which employees were encouraged to take responsibility, and the support employees were given in their attempts at personal and professional development.

Performance Appraisal: Closing the Loop

Performance evaluation is, in reality, an important control function in organizations. As mentioned at the beginning of the chapter, it is not accurate to think of the management process as starting with a discrete act or to think of it stopping at a specific point. Performance evaluation should take place only after there is a clear understanding of the expected goals of a job and the content of the task.

Effective performance appraisal assumes that goals have been set and communicated. If the job description

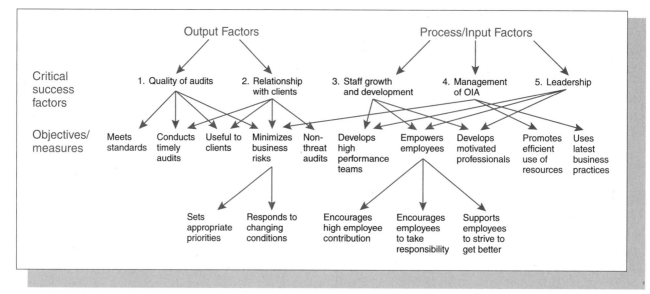

FIGURE 12–11. Office of Internal Audit. Critical success factors and objectives/measures.

is a motivational instrument, the person must understand the target and the domain of the job. If employees have participated in establishing the goals and the job content, so much the better because both will seem more relevant and personal.[39]

There are many ways to evaluate performance, and all have some advantages and disadvantages. For example, some question who should evaluate performance. Traditionally, performance appraisal has been a managerial task. Managers are responsible for assuring that the job is done, so they should be in a unique position to evaluate who is instrumental in accomplishing it. Managers, however, see the job from one perspective (above looking down). Many people believe that peers or colleagues also have important insights into who is contributing to the accomplishment of a task. For example, colleagues probably understand more than supervisors the importance of cooperation and are in a better position to say which fellow managers, nurses, or administrators cooperate in the interest of the overall organizational goals and which colleagues are primarily looking out for their own area of responsibility.

Finally, an increasing number of people have suggested that employees should have an opportunity to evaluate their supervisors. The theory is that employees have a perspective on job performance that few enjoy. By looking up in the appraisal process, employees can identify those supervisors who make their jobs easier rather than harder and those who build an effective team environment.

It is safe to say that to the extent possible and practi-

cal, a number of people should be involved in performance appraisal and evaluation. The most comprehensive evaluations are those that could consider the collective judgments of supervisors, peers, and employees. Certainly, all these perspectives can contribute to the manager's ultimate understanding of how any given employee contributes to getting the job done, the overall success of the larger organization, and the work team.

One final aspect of performance appraisal should be mentioned. This has to do with the evaluation instruments. Performance appraisals follow many models in business, education, and health care. They may range from little more than simply asking a few global questions, such as "Does the employee arrive at work on time," to more specifically designed and tested items. In a few incidents, **behaviorally anchored rating scales (BARS)** may be used where extensive research has been conducted to ensure that the appraisal takes place on the basis of behaviors that are expected in and demanded by the job. These BARS involve performance dimensions, extensive research, scale development, and, ultimately, instrument construction.

The important point is that people should be evaluated on the basis of the behaviors that are important to the successful completion of the job. This is why job goals and descriptions are critically important. It is also why we focused on the importance of developing critical success factors for each task. To illustrate, refer to Figure 12–12, a performance appraisal form developed for an internal audit. Note that each item in the form is based clearly on one or more of the critical success

OFFICE OF INTERNAL AUDIT
PERFORMANCE DEVELOPMENT AND APPRAISAL

Name: _____ **Title:** _____

1. Ensures audits are consistent with internal audit standards	Performed Below Expectation	Performed As Expected	Performed Above Expectation

Comments/Recommendations:
_____
_____
_____

2. Ensures audits are timely	Performed Below Expectation	Performed As Expected	Performed Above Expectation

Comments/Recommendations:
_____
_____
_____

3. Ensures audits are useful to clients	Performed Below Expectation	Performed As Expected	Performed Above Expectation

Comments/Recommendations:
_____
_____
_____

4. Sets appropriate audit priorities	Performed Below Expectation	Performed As Expected	Performed Above Expectation

Comments/Recommendations:
_____
_____
_____

5. Responds appropriately to changing conditions in the department and the medical center	Performed Below Expectation	Performed As Expected	Performed Above Expectation

Comments/Recommendations:
_____
_____
_____

6. Interacts with and reports to clients in a consultative manner	Performed Below Expectation	Performed As Expected	Performed Above Expectation

Comments/Recommendations:
_____
_____
_____

FIGURE 12–12. Office of Internal Audit. Performance development and appraisal.

7. Nurtures high performing teams	Performed Below Expectation	Performed As Expected	Performed Above Expectation

Comments/Recommendations:

_____

_____

_____

8. Encourages employees to take responsibility for their actions	Performed Below Expectation	Performed As Expected	Performed Above Expectation

Comments/Recommendations:

_____

_____

_____

9. Supports employees to strive to get better at what they do	Performed Below Expectation	Performed As Expected	Performed Above Expectation

Comments/Recommendations:

_____

_____

_____

10. Provides an environment that encourages motivation	Performed Below Expectation	Performed As Expected	Performed Above Expectation

Comments/Recommendations:

_____

_____

_____

11. Utilizes resources efficiently	Performed Below Expectation	Performed As Expected	Performed Above Expectation

Comments/Recommendations:

_____

_____

_____

12. Uses the appropriate business practices	Performed Below Expectation	Performed As Expected	Performed Above Expectation

Comments/Recommendations:

_____

_____

_____

OVERALL RATING	Performed Below Expectation	Performed As Expected	Performed Above Expectation

Comments/Recommendations:

_____

_____

_____

Evaluated by: _____ Title: _____

FIGURE 12–12 *Continued*

	EXPLANATION OF ITEMS	
Item Number	Explanation	Measurement
1	Generally accepted code	External review and peer review
2	(1) Audits carried out in a reasonable amount of time and (2) feedback to clients in a timely manner	Judgment and client interviews/feedback
3	Relates the audits to the needs of the client(s)	Client interviews/feedback
4	Develops an appropriate (macro) audit plan	Judgment and client interviews/feedback
5	Unplanned audits, changing needs within the audits (micro)	Employee/supervisor agreement/interaction
6	Is consultative and to the extent possible non-threatening	Client interviews/feedback
7	Emphasis is on creating teams, emphasizes working together, creates team approach	Staff interviews/feedback
8	Encourages professionalism and innovation	Staff interviews/feedback
9	Appropriately assesses staff needs, encourages continuing education, training	Staff interviews/feedback
10	Creates a participative environment where employees can be enthusiastic about their work	Staff interviews/feedback
11	Number of audits, given the staff and complexity of the audits	Employee/supervisor agreement/interaction
12	Uses contemporary management approaches, is innovative, tries new techniques	Employee/supervisor agreement/interaction

FIGURE 12–12 *Continued*

factors identified. This emphasizes the importance of evaluating people on the basis of job dimensions that are genuinely important to the success of the team and the organization. Perhaps one of the greatest failures of performance evaluation in the past is the manner in which many systems have failed to focus on job-relevant criteria. Increasingly, the importance of ensuring all performance criteria has been emphasized in the interest of fairness and for legal reasons.

Performance appraisal is usually thought of as the most objectionable part of the manager's job, yet this is a critically important control function. There may always be some disagreeable aspect of evaluating from the perspectives of the evaluated as well as the person doing the evaluation, but the importance of this activity cannot be minimized. When properly accomplished, performance appraisal can be motivational, identify early performance problems that can be corrected, and keep employees informed at all times relative to how they are performing. However, if care is not taken to ensure that clear job goals are established, that employees have

some input into establishing the criteria on which they will be evaluated, and that jobs are accurately designed and structured, performance appraisal will not accomplish its full potential.

Key Concepts

- Authority: Acceptance theory, formal theory, delegation

- Closed versus open organizational systems

- Controls in organizations
  Feedback—nonself-correcting, self-correcting
  Preventive

- Cornerstone concepts of classical management theory: Centralization versus decentralization, departmentalization, span of control, specialization or division of labor, unity of command

- Critical success factors

- Environmental assessment: Assessing, forecasting, monitoring, spanning

- Functions of management: Controlling, decision making, leading, organizing, planning

- Schools of management thought: Administrative organization, bureaucracy, contingency theory, human relations, scientific management

References

1. Simon HA: Administrative behavior, 3rd ed. New York: Free Press, 1976.

2. Neustadt RE, May ER: Thinking in time: The uses of history for decision makers. New York: Free Press, 1986, p 2.

3. For those interested in a more detailed overview, see Wren DA: The evolution of management thought, 4th ed. New York: John Wiley, 1994, and Duncan WJ: Great ideas in management: Lessons from the founders and foundations of management practice. San Francisco: Jossey-Bass Publishers, 1989.

4. Taylor FW: The principles of scientific management. New York: Harper & Bros, 1914, p 7.

5. Henderson AM, Parsons T (trans-ed): Max Weber: The theory of social and economic organization. New York: Free Press, 1947.

6. Fayol H: General and industrial management. Storrs, C., translator. London: Pitman, 1949.

7. For fascinating discussion of this affliction, see Miller D: The Icarus paradox. New York: Harper Collins, 1990, and Blasco JA, Stayer RC: Flight of the buffalo. New York: Warner Books, 1993.

8. See Mintzberg H: The nature of managerial work. New York: Harper & Row, 1973, and Mintzberg H: The manager's job: Folklore or fact? Harvard Business Review 1975;55(4):49–61.

9. Duncan WJ: When necessity becomes a virtue: The case for taking strategy seriously. Journal of General Management 1987;13(2):28–42.

10. Hales CP: What do managers do? A critical review of the evidence. J Management Studies 1986;23(1):88–115.

11. Jonas HS III, Frey RE, Srivastva S: The office of CEO: Understanding the executive experience. Academy of Management Executive 1990;4(3):36–48.

11a. Jonas HS III, Frey RE, Srivastva S: The person of the CEO: Understanding the executive experience. Academy of Management Executive 1989;3(3):205–215. See also Adams B: The limitations of muddling through: Does anyone in Washington really think anymore? Public Administration Review 1979;39(6):545–552.

12. Kraut AI, Pedigo PR, McKenna DD, Dunnette MD: The role of the manager: What's really important in different management jobs? Academy of Management Executive 1989;3(4):286–293. See also Kaluzny AD: Revitalizing decision making at the middle management level. Hospital and Health Services Administration 1989;34(1):39–51.

13. Luthans F: Successful vs. effective real managers. Academy of Management Executive 1988;2(2):127–132. See also Luthans F, Lockwood DL: Toward an observational system for measuring leader behavior in natural settings. In Hunt JG, Hosking D, Schriesheim C, Stewart R (eds): Leaders and managers: An international perspective on management behavior and leadership. New York: Pergamon Press, 1984, pp 117–141; Luthans F, Hodgetts RM, Rosenkrantz SA: Real managers. Cambridge, MA: Ballinger, 1988; Luthans F, Rosenkrantz SA, Hennessey HW: What do successful managers really do? An observational study of managerial activities. Journal of Applied Behavioral Science 1985;21(3):255–270.

14. Norburn D: The chief executive: A breed apart. Strategic Management Journal 1989;10(1):1–15.

15. Quinn JB, Doorley TL, Paquette PC: Beyond products: Service-based strategy. Harvard Business Review 1990;68(2):58–60.

16. Mintzberg H: The manager's job: Folklore or fact? Harvard Business Review 1975;55(4):49.

17. Duncan WJ, Ginter PM, Capper SA: General and functional level health care managers: Neither "manage" very much. Health Services Management Research 1994;8(2):11–27.

18. Kotter JP: The general managers. New York: Free Press, 1982.

19. Gauss JW: A decade of change: The emerging role of the CFO. Healthcare Financial Management 1991;45(5):54–62.

20. See Fahey L, Narayanan VK: Macroenvironmental analysis for strategic management. St Paul: West Publishing Co, 1986, and Duncan WJ, Ginter PM, Swayne LE: Strategic Management of Health Care Organizations. Cambridge: Blackwell, 1994.

21. Eckholm E: Introduction to the president's Health Security Act. New York: Random House, 1993, pp vii–xvi.

22. For an example of the application of this process in a health care organization, see Duncan WJ, Ginter PM, Capper SA: Keeping strategic thinking in strategic planning: Macro-environmental analysis in a state department of public health. Public Health 1992;106(3):253–269.

23. For a complete discussion of organizational goal setting, see Locke EA, Latham GP: A theory of goal setting and task performance. Englewood Cliffs, NJ: Prentice-Hall, 1990.

24. Details of the logic behind these principles are presented in Robey D: Designing organizations. 2nd ed. Homewood, IL: R. D. Irwin Publishers, 1986.

25. Hoskisson RE, Johnson RA: Corporate restructuring and strategic change: Effects on diversification strategy and R & D intensity. Strategic Management Journal 1992;13(6):625–634.

26. Barnard CI: The functions of the executive. Cambridge, MA: Harvard University Press, 1938, and Scott WG: Chester I. Barnard and the guardians of the managerial state. Lawrence, KS: University of Kansas Press, 1992.

27. Belasco JA, Stayer RC: Flight of the buffalo: Soaring to excellence, learning to let employees lead. New York: Warner Books, 1993.

28. Boje DM, Dennehy RF: Managing in the postmodern world. Dubuque, IA: Kendall/Hunt Publishers, 1993, ch 4.

29. Melum M, Sinioris MK: Total quality management: The health care pioneers. Chicago: American Hospital Publishing, 1992.

30. Morita A, with Reingold EM, Shimomura M: Made in Japan: Akio Morita and Sony. New York: Dutton Publishers, 1986, and Simon HA: The new science of management decisions. New York: Harper & Row, 1960, ch 1.

31. See Cantu C: A CEO's perspective: The role of the CFO. Financial Executive 1991;7(4):30–31, and Rapport A: CFOs and strategists: Forging a common framework. Harvard Business Review 1992;70(3):84–91.

32. Festinger L: A theory of cognitive dissonance. Stanford, CA: Stanford University Press, 1975.

33. Stogdill R: Handbook of leadership: A survey of theory and research. New York: Free Press, 1974, p 81.

34. For a classic article on this subject, see Carter L, Haythorn W, Howell M: A further investigation of the criteria of leadership. Journal of Abnormal and Social Psychology 1950;45(2):350–358.

35. Bethel SM: Making a difference: Twelve qualities that make you a leader. New York: Berkley Books, 1990.

36. Kotter JP: A force for change: How leadership differs from management. New York: Free Press, 1990.

37. Nanus B: Visionary leadership. San Francisco: Jossey-Bass Publishers, 1992. List constructed from quotation of Bennis WG: On becoming a leader. Reading, MA: Addison-Wesley, 1989, p 45.

38. For a discussion of different views of organizational effectiveness, see Cameron KS: Critical questions in assessing organizational effectiveness. Organizational Dynamics 1980;9(3):66–80.

39. Whetten DA, Cameron KS: Developing management skills: Motivating others. New York: Harper Collins, 1993, p 27.

13

WILLIAM J. RUDMAN and WESLEY M. ROHRER III

KEY WORDS

Accommodation
Achilles' heel
Action model of prob-
 lem solving
Affinity diagrams
Aggressive problem em-
 ployee
Avoidance
Belt lines
Brainstorming
Character assassination
Charismatic leadership
Collaboration
Communication
Competition
Compromise
Conflict resolution
Contingency theory
Continuous quality im-
 provement
Control chart
Correlation analysis
Courtroom
Delphi process
Effective listening
Empowerment
Feedback loop
Fishbone diagram
Fists and tears
Flowcharts
Force field analysis
Good loser
Group maintenance
Group process
Gunny sacking

Histogram
Hit n' run
Human diversity (in the
 workplace)
Kitchen sinking
Leadership
Line graph
Managerial grid
Matrix
Moping
National Labor Rela-
 tions Act
Negotiation
Nominal group process
Organizational culture
Pareto charts
Passive problem em-
 ployee
Path-goal theory
Problem solving
Processual change
Quality management
Round robin
Run chart
Silent treatment
Statistical process con-
 trol
Team building
Temper tantrums
Theory X
Theory Y
Time-out
Total quality manage-
 ment
Transactional leadership

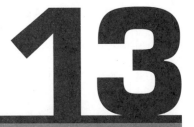

13

Transformational lead-
ership
Translational leadership

Win-win
Zero defects

OBJECTIVES

- Define key words.
- Make a convincing argument that leadership is a complex sociocultural process that is affected by leader, follower, task, and other environmental variables.
- Identify three distinct leadership models, and explain what each might contribute to enhancing leadership practices.
- Describe and apply four group problem-solving approaches (brainstorming, nominal group process, Delphi method, and the action model).
- Discuss how these decision-making processes assist the manager in dealing with ongoing and pervasive change.
- Discuss differences between transformational and processual change models.
- Explain how an effective negotiation strategy can overcome the impasse resulting from a "zero sum game" approach.
- Identify the factors that the manager should consider in determining to what extent the individual employee or work group should participate in decision making associated with a problem situation.
- Discuss the three models of communication in terms of both organizational and interpersonal communication strategies.
- Outline and apply the 10-step process to enhance organizational communications.
- Provide a rationale for top management, giving priority to diversity management, and identify the obstacles to effective implementation.
- Explain the five basic approaches to resolving conflict, and critique their usefulness in various situations.
- Detail the basic components of the formal negotiation process.
- Discuss how an effective negotiation process relates to communication and conflict resolution.
- Present an organizational (departmental) strategy for employee empowerment.
- Diagram a model of interpersonal communications, indicating the sources of potential interference and distortion.

- Briefly discuss and critique gurus of the quality management movement.
- Describe and explain the quality management pyramid.
- Outline the relations between statistical process control, employee empowerment, and continuous quality improvement.
- Briefly discuss the statistical tools of quality management.
- Discuss the impact of human diversity in affecting workplace relationships.

Successful health information managers are equally skilled in understanding and managing both technical and human factors within the work process. A productive work environment often depends on the manager's ability to manage people. How individuals interact with one another provides valuable insights on formal organizational processes as well as on informal interpersonal networks within the workplace structure. This chapter examines how human relations or interactions are established and impact work processes. Specifically, the focus is on communication patterns and conflict resolution; group dynamics and decision-making and **problem-solving** processes; leadership styles; management techniques and theory; and redefining the workplace in relation to multicultural and human diversity issues.

Underlying the discussions on interaction and the development of work relationships is a belief in the value of each person within the work process. This suggests the importance of adopting a human diversity perspective where individual differences are accounted for in management style and where individual contributions and variability are valued. Not all employees have the same goals, desires, and abilities. As health care reform shapes the way health care will be delivered in the future, it is important that managers both respect and nurture individual strengths and contributions as well as serve as visionaries in helping to redefine health information management (HIM) departments to meet future demands. This suggests a philosophy of personal empowerment based on respect and development of self-efficacy. All members of the health care team are encouraged to become part of the solution in meeting changing demands placed on health care facilities. Within work boundaries, each person should be encouraged to explore personal interests and strengths and to participate within the problem-solving and decision-making processes at the workplace.

COMMUNICATION

About 70 per cent of a manager's time is spent communicating with others. It is not surprising, therefore, that the development of communication skills is at the heart of most management philosophies.[1–12] At an organizational level, development of open communication skills is often associated with prevention of excessive internal conflict and competition, elimination of unnecessary barriers, and an increase in work productivity and worker satisfaction.[13–19] At a personal level, career advancement and work performance often depend on a person's ability to effectively communicate within formal and informal organizational structures.[1–12,14,19,20]

Communication is defined in terms of the transference of understanding between two parties (e.g., individuals or organizations).[11] Under this type of definition, communication may be verbal, nonverbal (e.g., body language), or written. Although this definition of communication may be simple, understanding the communication process can be complex and difficult. Communication models examined in this chapter focus on both interpersonal and organizational levels of communication. The most common types of communication models directly examine interpersonal communication patterns. These models are based on the direct transference of information from an initiator or source to a receiver, who immediately translates the message and provides feedback (Figures 13–1 and 13–2).[4,11,21–26] In contrast, an alternative model of communication introduced in

this chapter focuses on the simultaneous exchange of verbal and nonverbal information. This model suggests that the communication process is not one of initiators and receivers but one in which all parties involved in the communication process are viewed as initiators. This model may be expanded to patterns of organizational communication by emphasizing both written and nonverbal forms of communication.

Models of Communication

Traditional models of communication are represented in Figures 13–1 and 13–2.[4,11,20–26] The model of communication shown in Figure 13–1 is perhaps the most general and the simplest. This model consists of a message initiator, medium of transmission, message receiver, and **feedback loop**. Within this model, it is the responsibility of the initiator to ensure that coded messages use signs that are familiar to the receiver, that appropriate references are used when interpreting signs, and that the appropriate medium of transmitting messages is used. It is the responsibility of the receiver to provide adequate feedback to the initiator that understanding has occurred. Feedback is used to clarify the intended message and to facilitate future exchange. Understanding is established through a series of interactive message transmissions in which the message content is refined through the feedback process. Meaning or understanding is a negotiated process by which both parties come to a consensus of meaning.

The model of communication suggested in Figure 13–2 (based on Hay's communication model)[26] focuses more on the interpretive or interpersonal nature of communication. Understanding the communication process is based on examining the following:

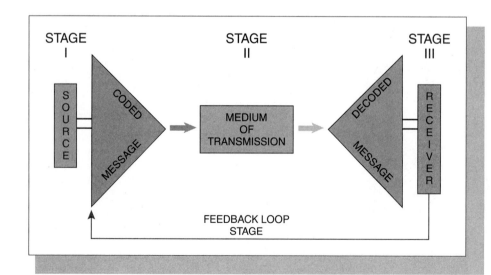

FIGURE 13–1. Informative (one-way) communication model.

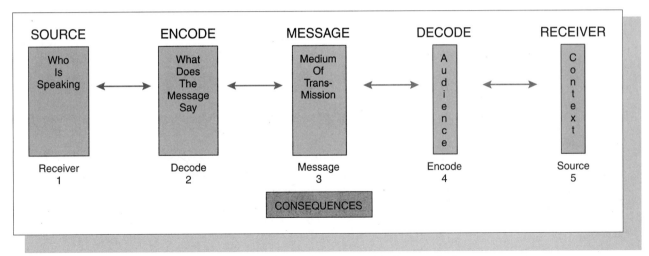

FIGURE 13–2. Interactive feedback model of communication.

- Who is speaking
- Message content
- Medium of transmission
- Context of the message
- Consequences of the interaction

Communication becomes a process of encoding and decoding in which thoughts and feelings are transformed into understanding. This requires the identification and use of appropriate words and symbols, packaging the message from the initiator in the most meaningful form, and constant feedback from the message receiver to ensure the accuracy of interpretation. Understanding occurs through a series of checks and balances of coded messages between the initiator and the receiver. Here, the filtering process of appropriate (i.e., meaningful) information selectively identifies core concepts in identifying a common ground for understanding.

The model of communication suggested in Figure 13–3 takes a more holistic view of how understanding and meaning are communicated. Whereas other models take into account nonverbal cues during interaction, this model suggests that both verbal and nonverbal cues, environmental factors, and past histories are equally important in creating understanding. It suggests that communication between two parties is always simultaneous. All parties involved in the communication interaction are initiators of understanding. For example, when one party is using words to communicate, the other party is providing simultaneous nonverbal feedback, such as shaking the head or furrowing an eyebrow. Consequently, both parties are seen as simultaneous transmitters of information or understanding. Moreover, in addition to the simultaneous exchange of information, this model suggests that each sequence of communication is discrete, bounded by environmental factors, including past interactions, time, and culture. We are linked to one another through a common language, meaningful experiences, and social structure. Both environmental factors and internal perspectives of the situation shaped by the individual's history and values define the interaction and exchange of understanding. This suggests that

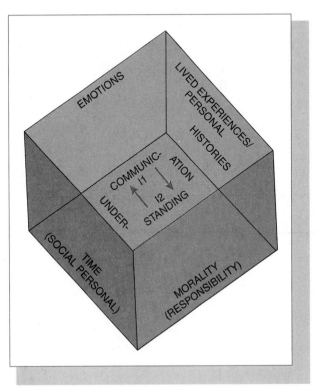

FIGURE 13–3. Interpersonal model of understanding communication.

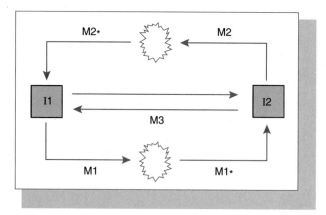

FIGURE 13-4. Interpersonal communication at an individual level.

each interaction is different, given personal and environmental factors, yet a common bond exists that allows shared meaning to be communicated.

This model also recognizes that perfect understanding is never transmitted (Figure 13-4). Understanding is never perfect because interpretation of the message varies from person to person. Figure 13-4 focuses on verbal messages (M1 and M2), the interference or barriers that occur as a result of miscommunication, and the nonverbal communication (M3) that simultaneously occurs. From this model, it becomes easier to understand why miscommunication occurs and the importance of nonverbal cues that are exchanged during face-to-face communication. Understanding or meaningful interaction occurs as a result of shared histories at both a social and a personal level.

This type of model of communication may be extrapolated to organizational networking at both a formal and an informal level (Figure 13-5). As organizational networking becomes a reality in today's health care organization, it is becoming increasingly important to understand the communication process outlined in Figure 13-5. This model suggests that written as well as verbal communication follows a similar process of interpretation and distortion. Here, transference of information is seen as a series of either interpersonal interactions or written communications in which message content is interpreted at an individual level. Even when communication is in the form of a written memo, each employee defines the message according to personal histories and past experiences. In other words, as the employee interprets the memo, understanding is based on past experiences with both the organization and the personal relationship with the individual message giver. Response to the memo, either formally or informally, is governed by perceptions related to such factors as power relationships within the organization and deliberation over the validity of the memo, which are related to expectations

about the credibility of the transmitter, expected consequences, or desired outcome. As a result of differences in perception and experience, the degree of understanding varies from employee to employee. Transference of understanding at an organizational level is related to personal relationships or shared culture. The more social and personal histories are similar, the higher the degree of understanding. Miscommunication is likely to result over differences in contextual references or meaning. To minimize miscommunication, it is important to become an active and effective listener. Following this line of reasoning, it is important that both the manager and the employee who communicate through a written format understand that written messages are interpreted in a manner similar to verbal messages. When using a written communication format, therefore, attention must be paid to detail and to structuring the message in a logical (i.e., sequential) format.

To improve communication, the following steps to **effective listening** are suggested[2,4,11,12]:

1. *Stop talking.*
2. Show you want to listen.
3. Put the talker at ease.
4. Remove distractions.
5. Empathize with the talker.
6. Be patient.
7. Hold your temper.
8. Ask questions.
9. Go easy on criticism.
10. *Stop talking.*

CONFLICT RESOLUTION

Understanding organizational communication as a series of interpersonal interactions helps to explain why miscommunication or misunderstanding exists and why conflict arises. As messages are transferred through the organizational network, each employee interprets organizational messages from a personal perspective. This interpretation, as noted earlier, is based on a unique set of personal values, histories, and experiences. Consequently, as noted earlier in this chapter, perfect communication is highly unlikely, given the uniqueness of each person. Miscommunication is a natural part of any type of social interaction. At times, however, miscommunication is deliberate and conflict unavoidable. About 75 per cent of a manager's time is spent dealing with some sort of conflict. The key to managing conflict is to create an open atmosphere of communication and trust. This is a difficult proposition at best. Consequently, how you as a manager resolve conflict among employees will, to a large extent, determine how successful you are as a manager.

In general, research suggests that **conflict resolution**

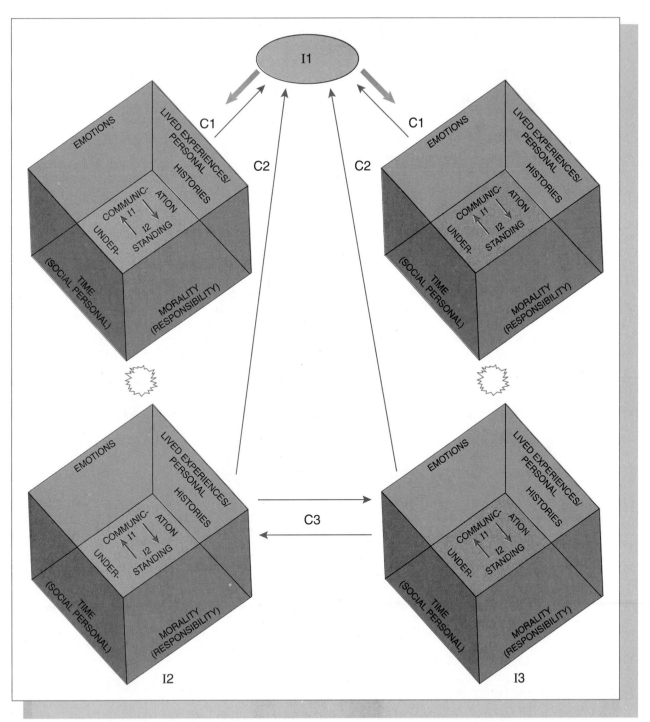

FIGURE 13–5. Expanded process of interpersonal communication at an organizational level.

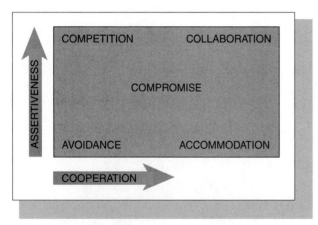

FIGURE 13–6. Conflict resolution model.

models may be based on one of five basic scenarios, ranging from assertiveness to cooperation (Figure 13–6).[26–35]

Avoidance

Perhaps the most common way of dealing with interpersonal conflict is through **avoidance.** Here, you are neither assertive nor cooperative. Instead of actively confronting the problem, you ignore it and hope it goes away. When avoidance is used to deal with problems, neither your needs nor the needs of the other party are satisfied.

In most cases when avoidance is used to deal with conflict, the conflict is not resolved. Both parties are likely to be frustrated and resentment is likely to occur. This is usually the least satisfactory way of dealing with conflict.

Accommodation

When **accommodation** is used as a way of dealing with conflict, one party is highly cooperative and responsive to the needs of others, while denying personal needs or concerns. The other party is both aggressive and highly assertive. The solution reached in dealing with the conflict is one of denial. In fact, the solution may not even address the source of the conflict.

Again, in most cases, the conflict is not resolved. The person who is accommodating is likely to become frustrated when personal needs are not met, whereas the other person may not be aware that the conflict exists. Because there is no true resolution of the conflict, the conflict is likely to occur at a later stage and time and perhaps with greater intensity, given that feelings are not dealt with.

Competition

Similar to the accommodation model of conflict resolution, when there is **competition** between parties, only one person's needs are met and the other person's needs are ignored. The solution reached is framed solely in terms of the more assertive person.

As in the case of accommodation, the conflict is not resolved. Here, the other person becomes frustrated when needs are not met. Given that the "solution" has been acted on, outward or external problems may subside through denial on the part of one or both parties. Because an acceptable solution that meets the needs of both parties was not reached and the root of the problem itself not addressed, conflict will probably arise in the future.

Compromise

When **compromise** is used as a way of resolving conflict, both parties are moderately assertive and moderately cooperative. Partial needs are being met for both parties involved in the conflict. Consequently, only a partial and unstable solution is reached in which neither side is completely satisfied.

Although a partial solution is reached, the core of the problem is *not* likely to have been adequately addressed. Both parties involved in the conflict are likely to be frustrated and to believe that they gave up more than they gained. This may lead to resentment and the likelihood of the conflict's recurrence.

Collaboration

Collaboration is the method of conflict resolution that is most likely to end in a successful resolution of the problem. Here, both parties are highly assertive, yet highly cooperative and responsive to the needs of others. Collaboration requires a great deal of patience and commitment as well as an understanding that a lasting solution requires a mutual commitment to work together. Collaborative solutions are based on active listening, honest interaction, and working within an atmosphere of open communication. Finally, what distinguishes a collaborative from a compromise solution is the belief in the need to continue to address the problem after the initial resolution.

Barriers to Resolving Interpersonal Conflict

Studies suggest that most people have a genuine desire to resolve conflict. Although there is a desire, the

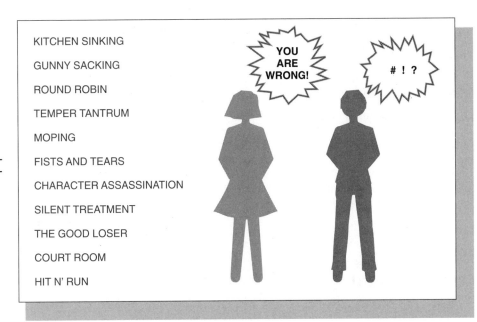

KITCHEN SINKING

GUNNY SACKING

ROUND ROBIN

TEMPER TANTRUM

MOPING

FISTS AND TEARS

CHARACTER ASSASSINATION

SILENT TREATMENT

THE GOOD LOSER

COURT ROOM

HIT N' RUN

YOU ARE WRONG!

! ?

FIGURE 13-7. Barriers to understanding interpersonal communication.

way in which a person responds to conflict may exacerbate the original condition. Research has identified 11 basic barriers that hinder resolution of conflict (Figure 13-7).[33–37]

Kitchen Sinking

"**Kitchen sinking**" refers to not sticking with the current issue. Past grievances are used to strengthen your position. The goal is to win the conflict by overwhelming the other person with evidence of past indiscretion. The most common result of this type of interaction is confusion. The issue at hand becomes secondary as the party being attacked feels the need to defend personal integrity rather than to discuss openly the current issue.

Gunny Sacking

"**Gunny sacking**" refers to hiding your true feelings concerning the conflict, usually under the guise of denying its importance. This usually results in verbal explosions in which one party overwhelms the other party. This often creates an atmosphere of mistrust and anticipation of continued conflict.

Round Robin

"**Round robin**" describes the situation in which one or both parties reassert the issue over and over, ad nauseam. The purpose is to wear down the other person and win the conflict through attrition. This usually results in an argument about who is in control rather than

a serious attempt to resolve the problem. The symptoms are discussed rather than the root causes of the problem. Both parties are likely to become upset over issues that are unrelated to the initial conflict.

Temper Tantrum

Temper tantrum may best be described as emotional blackmail of one party over the other party. Here, one party attempts to overwhelm the other party by using an emotional ultimatum. The person using the temper tantrum is assertive and cares only about personal needs. Although the person resorting to the temper tantrum usually receives immediate gratification, the conflict is far from being resolved. The other person is likely to be resentful and will be uncooperative in the future.

Moping

Moping refers to putting on your best "ain't it awful" face to win the conflict through pity. In this case, the person attempts to shift responsibility for the conflict to others and not assume any personal responsibility. This is likely to result in social isolation and feelings of rejection from others.

Fists and Tears

Although anger and pain are natural human emotions that should be expressed during conflict, when taken to extremes, these emotions can be used to intimidate others into meeting your needs (i.e., **fists**) or to induce guilt (i.e., **tears**). There is an attempt to shift responsibility to the other person for how you are feeling. This usually results in a roller coaster effect in which important issues are avoided.

Character Assassination

Character assassination occurs when one party may use a legitimate issue or conflict to attack another party personally rather than discussing the immediate problem. This type of barrier is often characterized by the use of "always" and "never" statements. Such a confrontation usually results in frustration and confusion. Seldom are important issues discussed in detail or resolved.

Silent Treatment

The **silent treatment** is often used to communicate negative emotions, such as anger, hurt, and frustration, while avoiding the risk of direct confrontation. In this approach, the silent partner attempts to gain control over a situation by inducing guilt and shifting responsibility to the other person. The party using the silent treatment often denies that a problem exists and avoids entering into a discussion in which failure is a possibility. This may result in depression and internalizing anger. Once again, the problem itself is not addressed, but issues of power and control become the focal points of the discussion.

The Good Loser

The **good loser** method of dealing with conflict is another method of shifting responsibility to the other party. You enter into discussion by stating, "It is all my fault. I take full responsibility for the situation." As a good loser, you try to win the confrontation by replacing the other person's anger and frustration with guilt. Issues related to solving the problem are ignored. The person playing this role is likely to internalize anger and become socially alienated. The ultimate rip-off for the good loser is suicide.

Courtroom

The **courtroom** style always includes a third party to validate your position and refute the other person's position. The role of the other person may take the form of written "testimony," by reference to a credible expert or through face-to-face intervention. The goal here is to win at all costs. Although the person using the courtroom technique may win the initial argument, he or she is likely to lose the other person's respect and trust. Because there is reliance on a third party to settle the dispute, people who use the courtroom technique are likely to diminish their own personal base of power.

Hit N' Run

Hit n' run uses the ambush technique of catching the person off guard as well as avoiding direct confrontation. For example, a person using the hit n' run may initially approach a problem without scheduling time to deal adequately with the possible confrontation. The goal is to avoid taking responsibility for airing grievances or considering other viewpoints on a particular issue. The other person is likely to see this as a personal attack and respond by assuming a hostile and uncompromising position.

Steps in Dealing with Interpersonal Conflict

For a collaborative solution to occur, it is important that a foundation of trust based on mutual respect and open communication be established. This requires a mutual commitment to developing and maintaining a standing protocol for dealing with future problems. In developing a protocol, the following steps may be useful.[28,29,31,32]

1. *Identifying the issue.* Communication is most effective when both parties understand the issue and agree to stick to that issue when resolving conflict. This suggests that discussions are bound both to the topic and to a specific time frame. When discussions stray from the original topic, it is likely that past problems will arise and cloud the current issue. Similarly, when time boundaries are not established, it is likely that the problem will be revisited ad nauseam without real progress in achieving an equitable solution. In both cases, the source of the conflict is not adequately addressed. It is important that time is spent clarifying the issue before solutions are offered or considered. Constant feedback is important in establishing direct and open lines of communication.

2. *Make appointment to talk.* Open and honest communication is best when both parties have adequate free time to discuss the issue. Making appointments avoids distractions, preoccupations, and obsessions. It is important to give each participant in the conflict the courtesy of knowing the issue to be discussed beforehand, so that both parties have an opportunity to prepare.

3. *Identify* **belt lines.** You need to know what issues or statements "push your buttons" and make you defensive. It is your responsibility to inform those with whom you are in conflict what your belt lines are and how you are likely to react when they are not honored. You must both agree not to hit below the belt lines without expecting retaliation. When you establish these boundaries, you should avoid personal attacks so that the real issues can be dealt with effectively.

4. *Identify the **Achilles' heel**.* An Achilles' heel is similar to a belt line but is much more sensitive. This refers to taboo issues or statements that one or both parties believe should not be discussed. Both parties must agree that these issues and statements are off limits. You must develop an understanding with the other party that if an Achilles' heel is introduced, the conversation should stop immediately and resume at a later time. By continuing the conversation, resentment is likely to build up and a meaningful solution to the conflict becomes highly unlikely. When both belt lines and Achilles' heels are broached, issues become personalized and emotional, and the source of the conflict is ignored. It is important, therefore, that when belt lines and Achilles' heels are brought into the resolution process, time-outs are called to allow both parties to cool down and reflect on the initial source of the conflict.

5. *Agree to **time-outs**.* Agree beforehand that it is acceptable for either person to ask for a time-out to reflect or respond during the resolution period. If necessary, set up a new appointment to meet at a later date. Make sure that the time-out does not last so long that the issues become blurred or forgotten.

6. *Use "I Feel" Statements.* Speak for yourself and state your position clearly. Do not make use of authorities unless necessary. Avoid bringing others into the conflict to help solve personal problems until you exhaust all possible lines of initial communication. It is important that *all* employees learn how to resolve interpersonal conflicts if a department is to run smoothly. If employees fail to take the responsibility for handling personal conflict, the manager is likely to spend an inordinate amount of time dealing with personal (non-work) issues.

7. *State your position as an opinion, not as a fact.* Try to be open and respectful to the other person's point of view. It is easier to modify an opinion than a fact. Leave room for collaboration.

8. *Negotiate solutions.* If you are truly open to alternative ways to resolve the problem and react cooperatively, you usually will find a mutually beneficial solution. If you insist on trying to win or prove your point, both parties lose.

9. *Do follow-up checks.* Regardless of the intention, resolutions to problems do not last forever. Both personal and environmental conditions change over time. It is important to establish an open line of communication to meet changing environmental conditions. Remember that for each problem, there are several equitable solutions. Do not be afraid to re-examine your position if the current solution is not working. It is important to understand that as the environment or situational context changes, adjustments must be made to the initial solutions.

10. *Seek help, if needed.* Do not be reluctant to seek help of a third party if resolutions are not forthcoming or if the conflict escalates. This often shows a sign of maturity and a willingness to seek a more lasting solution.

Dealing with a Problem Employee

As a manager, it is important that you develop a process not only to deal with conflict but also to prevent potentially destructive conflict whenever possible. Preventive steps may reduce the amount of conflict and lessen the disruptive effect if conflict occurs. Suggestions for dealing with problem employees are based on the following assumptions:

- Most people are easy to get along with (i.e., most people would rather be at peace than at war).
- People are the most valuable resource to the organization.
- Most people want to resolve conflict if they believe that the potential benefits outweigh the likely costs.

When dealing with a problem employee, there are four basic steps that may be followed.

1. Pinpoint the issue or source of conflict.
2. Examine working relationships with other employees.
3. Determine the costs of direct confrontation.
4. Search for a solution, and obtain an agreement and a commitment from this employee to work toward this solution.

Pinpointing the Conflict

The ability to clearly and accurately define boundaries of the conflict is the most difficult step in dealing with the problem employee. To clearly identify the issue requires self-examination and self-questioning as well as the ability to focus on facts rather than allowing emotion to cloud your judgment. As a manager, you must ask yourself: Is this a difficult employee? Am I the only one who is having problems with this employee? Remember, behavior tends to be repetitive. If an employee is continually having problems with other employees as well as with yourself, it is likely that this is a problem employee.

Examining Work Relationships

To determine whether this employee is indeed a problem employee, it is important to examine interactions with others. A difficult employee may not know even that a problem exists because of conflict in role expectations and failure to realize the effect on others. If possible, before confronting the problem employee, the supervisor or manager should collect information detailing both the actual behavior and the effect of that behavior on co-workers. To avoid the appearance of having the conflict resolution steps perceived as a personal attack, it is important to document disruptive behavior. Presentation of this documentation must be given with the intent of solving the problem, not as a means of discrediting the person. Documentation is extremely important if effective action is to occur.

Determining Costs of the Confrontation

With every confrontation of a problem employee, a price is paid. When confronting a problem employee, therefore, it is important to understand that this confrontation will come at some personal cost. The costs of confrontation may be addressed in terms of the following:

- Personal dissatisfaction
- Morale of others
- Disruption of the work environment

In determining the costs of confrontation, it is also important to determine the costs of nonconfrontation. Remember that avoidance of a problem never solves the problem but, in most cases, exacerbates the initial confrontation. In general, confrontation is necessary to come to an equitable solution.

Searching for a Solution

In developing a solution to your problem, it should be noted that there are two types of difficult employees: aggressive and passive. When developing your plan of action for dealing with the immediate problem, it is important that you consider which of these types of difficult employees you are facing.

When you are involved with an **aggressive problem employee,** it is important to proceed as follows:

- Choose a time that is not stressful or hurried, so that you may openly and honestly discuss issues involved in the conflict.
- Create an atmosphere of collaboration, not competition.
- Stay calm.
- Be descriptive, not judgmental.
- State openly and honestly the costs of the difficult behavior.

- Actively listen.
- Set short-term goals.
- If things do not go as planned, assess the cost of your actions, and if an important issue or principle is involved, stand your ground.
- Explain the costs of the behavior to the difficult employee.
- Be positive and constructive.

When dealing with a **passive problem employee,** a slightly different approach is suggested. Here, you should make an effort to do the following:

- Confront the employee openly in a nonthreatening way.
- Ask for the employee's help in dealing with the problem.
- Involve the difficult employee in defining the solution.
- Re-evaluate the outcome.

If the outcome of your efforts appears to be satisfactory, you have made progress toward resolving the conflict. If, on the other hand, the outcome does not appear to be satisfactory, you may need to change your strategy. If you decide to confront the difficult employee again, proceed as follows:

- Remain calm because the confrontation will probably be awkward.
- Decide beforehand which outcomes you will and will not accept.
- Be consistent and positive.

Perhaps the most important rule you should follow when dealing with a difficult employee is that there are limits or boundaries of acceptable behavior. Not all confrontations end in a solution that is perceived to be equitable for both parties. Do not be afraid to take action. Make sure that when you take action, you have carefully considered alternative actions (including no action), have appropriate documentation, and are prepared for the consequences of your action.

Coming to an equitable solution to a conflict is never an easy process. Because organizations are made up of individuals, conflict is inevitable. The better you learn to deal with conflict, the more efficient and productive you become as a manager. When developing your strategies to resolve conflict, you must remain calm, focus on the process, have patience and respect, and, most important, seek a win-win solution in which both parties emerge from conflict resolution with self-respect and an investment in collaborative problem solving.

GROUP PROCESS AND PROBLEM SOLVING

In his justification of the "learning organization," Senge argues that "team learning is vital because teams, not individuals, are the fundamental learning unit in modern organizations."[38]

In one of the most influential studies of worker behavior in industrial organizations, the Hawthorne Studies (1927–1932), the importance of **group processes** at the workplace is a central theme.[39] These studies identify and characterize the social dynamics of the informal organization with the work group as the basic unit of structure. Indeed, much of the current work on group efficacy is based on the Hawthorne Plant (General Electric) studies. The research done in conjunction with these studies demonstrates that groups often re-create a suborganization complete with its own leadership, norms, goals, and formal hierarchy distinct from the formal organizational structure. Increased productivity and improved attitudes of workers are seen to be the result of changes in the social empowerment of individuals because of group involvement. This includes the nature of supervision, management's recognition of employee needs, and development of informal employee networks. The studies conclude that the work group often serves as a social support network that buffers the worker against alienation and powerlessness within the work environment.[40]

It was not until the early 1970s, with the emergence of quality management, that interest in the role and importance of the group re-emerged. With the success of a group-based quality management philosophy in Japan, after decades of indifference, American industry began to adopt a group-based philosophy of quality control. Indeed, concepts of group process and **team building** are at the heart of most modern management philosophies.

The use of groups within any given organization depends on the source and nature of authority, the duration or time horizon, and the group's primary purpose and function. The source of the group's authority or legitimacy may be found in the formal structure and policies of the organization (e.g., a medical ethics committee, a quality management team). Alternatively, the group may be a manifestation of the informal organization (e.g., a great books club, informal grievance committee). In terms of duration or time horizon, the group may be characterized as ad hoc or temporary (short term) or permanent (long term). The actual life of most groups varies within a wide range (e.g., from 1 hour or less to a number of years). The primary purpose of formalizing the group is to define both the role and the function that the group is to perform within the organization. The purpose or mission of the group will then be a function of the following:

- The values, priorities, and norms of the leaders, members, and constituencies of the group
- Environmental forces and constraints

Team building as part of the group process is an increasingly important function in the organization. This seems to be especially true in health care organizations, given the interdisciplinary coordination of healing, restorative, rehabilitative, and preventive services to the patient. Team leadership may be provided either formally by a person serving in an official role within the organization or informally as a result of the group process. The leader is responsible for ensuring that both **group maintenance** and goal-oriented performance processes are supported by team members if the team is to remain viable and effective.

Group maintenance includes the following:

- Recruitment and replacement of team members
- Orientation and training
- Establishing goals and procedures
- Communicating performance expectations
- Monitoring and measuring performance
- Providing rewards and incentives for performance
- Conflict management
- Personal empowerment

Concurrently, the team should be engaged in appropriate goal- and role-directed behavior to further both the group's and the organization's mission. Much of this behavior can be characterized as decision-making or problem-solving activities. Without ongoing attention to group maintenance (lower-order) functions, the team becomes impaired. This will in all likelihood hinder the group's achievement of its primary (higher-order) purposes.

Various models of group formation or team-building processes have been proposed. Although approaches differ in detail, they are based on a common set of processes or phases. For example, Griffin provides a clever and mnemonically useful characterization of "forming-storming-norming-and-performing" phases of group development.[41] This approach recognizes that subsequent to bringing together the group as individuals, a turbulent phase of intragroup tensions and conflict will arise. This conflict serves as both a cathartic and a bonding mechanism for the group. The emotive phase is followed by a process of reconciliation through identifying common ground (e.g., shared values, group norms). The group reinforces performance by establishing goals, objectives, and action plans.

Incorporating the common elements of these more traditional models of group formation with various management styles, the team-building process may be characterized as follows:

- Coming to task
- Coming unglued
- Coming around (becoming restored)
- Coming home (to goal achievement)
- Becoming (empowered)

In the first phase, coming to task, individuals are identified as team participants on a voluntary or mandatory basis, selected and oriented to the problem context, and assigned areas of responsibility.

Conflict arising from both the anticipated stress and the friction of group effort as well as the force of external variables (e.g., tight deadlines) may be experienced almost immediately. The group is most vulnerable during the initial experience of conflict and, in a figurative sense, may come unglued. Individuals may retreat into isolation or even become hostile toward the group. As a result, group efforts directed toward task achievement become unfocused and inefficient or cease altogether as leaders focus on group maintenance and group survival.

Effective team leaders anticipate and nourish this conflict phase. This phase, although difficult, may be beneficial to the group by creating a sense of oneness or bonding in dealing with future tasks. The group as a whole has a greater sense of its identity, competence, power as a team and of its capacity to handle difficult situations and survive. During this process, those team members who have made the investment of active participation have grown as individuals through personal empowerment.

Having achieved this renewal of energy and commitment, the team redirects its focus on task accomplishment, problem solving, and performance. At this stage of team building, the leader should be able to allocate fewer resources to group maintenance activities than in earlier stages. The leader's role in the "coming home" phase is to reinforce the sense of mission, vision, and core values and to reward and celebrate individual and team achievements.

Empowerment is an ongoing process rather than an end state. In effective teams, empowerment is a continuous commitment to quality and excellence. The empowered team should reflect the energies and commitment of empowered individual team members and may serve as a microcosm of and catalyst for the organization.

As employees become empowered within the organization, traditional roles and job tasks are likely to expand. Empowerment suggests greater autonomy and control over work-related tasks. As a result of expanded work responsibilities, employees become increasingly involved in the decision-making process. Involvement in

decision making requires an understanding of group process and knowledge of how to develop and refine problem-solving abilities.

There are various models of decision making that group leaders may follow. The decision to use one method over another depends on the type of problem identified. In this section, we identify four models of problem solving: brainstorming, nominal group process, Delphi, and an action-oriented model of problem solving.

Brainstorming

Brainstorming is a structured but flexible process designed to maximize the generation of ideas. This model is primarily used in the exploratory phase of problem solving. It requires a leader who serves primarily as a facilitator and recorder. The following are the basic steps in the brainstorming process:

1. Identifying the problem context
2. Structuring the task in terms of process and outcome
3. Encouraging active participation of employees
4. Recording all individual responses
5. Avoiding criticism
6. Clarifying ambiguous responses
7. Inviting participants to expand the number of responses
8. Repeating the cycle[42]

Nominal Group Process

The **nominal group process** is an extension of group brainstorming to incorporate a consensus judgment about priorities or alternatives. Specifically, the nominal group is designed to make explicit the criteria the group would apply in making a decision or solving a problem.[42] The nominal group leader plays the role of facilitator-recorder. The following steps are usually associated with the nominal group process:

1. The leader-facilitator reviews the process to be followed and states the problem or issue to be addressed. (For example, the leader would ask the group to identify all the factors to consider in developing a policy for reforming the U.S. health care system.)
2. Group members are asked to work independently with each individual, creating a list of ideas and suggestions.
3. Participants then share ideas with the whole group in a round-robin style.
4. At this stage, participants are discouraged from commenting on individual suggestions.

5. The leader documents all responses (with clarification, if needed), so that all members can easily review them in the following steps.

6. Participants are encouraged to consider and discuss the meaning and implications of each response.

7. Group members prioritize the final set of responses by a rank-ordering process.

8. The leader tallies the votes and documents the rank order.

9. The participants are encouraged to discuss the results and determine whether another cycle of the process is required.

Delphi Process

The **Delphi process**, named after the Greek oracle, was developed to elicit group expertise while controlling for bias and distortion. This technique is most appropriate for forecasting future trends or events and when a range of expert opinion or the perspectives of various constituencies are desired in developing a consensus judgment. This technique allows for the expression of multiple perspectives, feedback, evaluation, refined judgments, and the emergence of expert consensus. The outcome of the Delphi process is to reduce variability of judgment. The benefits are the presumed gain in quality. The complete Delphi process is described as follows:

1. A panel of experts are identified and asked to participate.

2. Each expert is asked to make a prediction about some future end state, usually in the form of a numeric estimate.

3. The leader compiles individual responses.

4. Summary data of responses are provided to members.

5. Participants are asked (a) to justify their initial prediction in light of the group response and (b) if they want to revise their initial estimate based on the data provided from the group.

6. Responses are compiled and analyzed, and summary data are distributed.

7. The cycle is repeated until no further revisions are offered.[42]

Action Model

As noted earlier, the initiation of working groups in the decision-making process is the first step in the employee empowerment process.[1-3,5-12] Creating an atmosphere of team work and personal involvement, however, is much more involved than simply bringing employees together and providing opportunities for input. Employees must be provided appropriate training and mentorship. Moreover, an atmosphere of action must be established. The problem-solving model suggested below outlines an action-oriented approach to employee empowerment. This position suggests that although it is important to collect and carefully analyze information, it is equally important for health information professionals to act promptly and thoughtfully. Consequently, the **action model of problem solving** offered in this chapter is broken down into eight general steps. Steps 1 through 4 focus on assessing the problem and steps 5 through 8 are action-oriented.

The first step in developing a philosophy of quality management based on an evaluative scheme is to create a problem-solving culture at the workplace. Based on the problem-solving model introduced in this text, the manager can analyze the most important problem that should be addressed at an organizational, a departmental, or an interpersonal level.

1. Actively listen.

- How do you know a problem exists? (25 words)

- What are your sources of information? (List three.)

2. Define the issue.

- Briefly state your problem. (25 words)

3. Examine the evidence.

- What are the primary sources of the problem?
  People:
  Policy:
  Structure:

- In your organization, who would be the most effective person you could go to to solve this problem? (What is this person's current position?)

- To solve this problem, what would you do first? (List three steps.)

4. Analyze biases and assumptions.

- How do you benefit from this problem being solved?

- What are the consequences if this problem is *not* solved?

- What are the concrete facts? (25 words)

5. Separate emotive and cognitive reasoning.

- In what way has this problem personally affected you? (25 words)

- List three ways this problem has affected your work performance.

6. Consider alternative solutions.

-   List three alternative courses of action.
-   What do you perceive as the consequences of these actions?

7. Do not oversimplify.

-   Re-evaluate step 2. What would you add or delete?

8. Tolerate uncertainty.

-   What type of information is necessary to deal with this problem? (25 words)
-   What type of information is helpful but not necessary? (25 words)

ACT!!!
Briefly justify the course of action you would select. (50 words)
What type of follow-up would you initiate to ensure success? (50 words)

Actively Listening

Step 1 consists of active listening and asking questions. As a problem solver, it is important that you understand that problems do not occur in a vacuum. The number of viewpoints that exist on even the simplest problem is directly dependent on the number of people involved. To effectively solve a problem, consideration should be given to all viewpoints and the opportunity to participate offered to all people who have a direct stake in the conflict. You must examine the sources of the problem and the methods you might use to obtain information concerning the problem.

Defining the Issue

In step 2, the current issue must be clearly defined and separated from prior situations. This does not mean that past experiences are ignored but recognizes that old problems may cloud judgment or interfere with the current decision-making process.

Examining the Evidence and Analyzing Biases and Assumptions

Steps 3 and 4 focus on examining the evidence and understanding both personal and situational bias. You need to determine whether the source of the problem stems from the employees involved or policy of your organization, or whether it is a result of the organizational structure or culture. Next, it is important to determine who the most effective person in the organization would be to resolve this problem, and briefly outline your immediate steps in resolving the problem. When solving a problem, it is virtually impossible to eliminate bias; however, by understanding personal bias, the probability of making a more enlightened decision based on facts should increase. It is important to examine how you personally benefit from the action you take, and what are the consequences if the problem is not solved.

Separating Cognitive and Emotive Reasoning

Understanding the emotional nature of a problem is perhaps the most critical and important step in this process. Although we cannot eliminate emotions, separating emotional and rational issues is necessary. It is important to understand that emotions may play an important role in solving simple as well as complicated problems. Appropriate decisions often are made on feelings or gut reactions to problems. Understanding both the emotional and the rational elements of a situation allows for higher levels of intimacy and for a more informed and impartial decision. In separating out your emotional response, you need to assess how this problem has affected you in both your personal and your professional interactions.

Considering Alternative Solutions and Not Oversimplifying

When involved in the decision-making process, it is important to understand the complexity of the situation and that there is more than one solution that will provide equity for all parties. Respect should be given to those involved in the decision-making or problem-solving process by providing sufficient information and opportunity for involvement. Flexibility and creativity are stressed in developing appropriate solutions.

Act

Given the transitory nature of human interactions and relationships, it is impossible to collect all information of potential relevance to a particular problem even if costs were not considered. It is important to set boundaries around a problem situation and to have the confidence to act on the problem as defined. By creating an atmosphere of personal empowerment and problem solving within the decision-making process, action is likely to be prompt yet focused.

These problem-solving approaches provide structured methods for accomplishing the following goals:

-   Identifying, defining, and analyzing problems
-   Generating alternative strategies for problem resolution
-   Prioritizing problems and strategies
-   Reaching consensus on preferred actions

Of these methods, brainstorming is the one most associated with creative problem solving because it encourages uninhibited expression of ideas. Other methods discussed—nominal group, Delphi method, and the action model—all use a structured process to focus the knowledge and skills of group members upon thorough analysis of a problem situation, to consideration of alternative solutions, and then to a consensual decision about preferred action. Other problem-solving games and role-playing exercises have been developed to train people in creative thinking, but they are beyond the scope of this text.

Increasing the decision-making skills of employees and work groups should better train them for changes in the environment. Managers are better prepared to deal with change effectively if they view the change as a set of problems to be analyzed and an opportunity for creative conflict management strategies. No skills or strategies will ensure that change management is easy or certain. However, developing effective problem-solving, analytical, and conflict management tools will ensure that the manager is better prepared as a change agent or facilitator.

LEADERSHIP

The ability to develop effective leaders is crucial to the long-term viability and growth of health information management as a profession. It is becoming increasingly apparent that the management of information will be a crucial function within both the individual health care organization (i.e., hospital, rehabilitation center, home health agency, health maintenance organization) and the health care delivery system as a whole. Although the shape of health care reform will continue to be debated, one can predict that any comprehensive program that attempts universal coverage and is structured on managed care principles will depend on comprehensive, integrated health information networks. Only through closer linking of clinical, financial, human resource, and other operational performance data can we fully realize the potential of information technology available to ensure cost-effective, useful, and valid information for clinical research and management applications.

The health information manager is in a position to exercise considerable influence over the design, implementation, and management of the integrated health information networks of the future. Indeed, it may be argued that the HIM professional is crucial to this development. This suggests the need to develop the foundation skills for effective leadership in entry-level HIM education. **Leadership** clearly is a situational process with social, cultural, and political dimensions. Effective leadership behavior then is developed through application in real-world situations. Individuals grow as leaders as they interact with followers in confronting problems and opportunities in their organizational and broader environments.

The implication of this view of leadership is that potential leaders are not born with a set of necessary and sufficient traits that will ensure their acceptance as leaders and their success in exercising leadership independent of their education and other life experiences. It is evident that no educational program alone can guarantee the development of effective leadership. However, trait-based studies of leadership and subsequent studies of leadership behavior have identified a set of behaviors and characteristics that are often associated with those accepted as leaders (e.g., persuasive communicators, visionary, action-oriented). These and other behavioral patterns can be reinforced through curricular emphasis on the theory and practice of communication, decision making, conflict management, and other aspects of leadership; in-class role playing; fieldwork project assignments; and experience in leadership opportunities within the academic institution or the broader community.

Most leadership and **quality management** themes reflect either implicitly or explicitly the assumptions presented in McGregor's **Theory X** and **Theory Y** formulations.[8] Theory X, which reflects traditional management assumptions about the worker, includes the following:

- Workers are predisposed to be passive about, if not resistant to, applying their energies toward formal organizational needs and goals.

- Workers react in this way because they are inherently lazy, indifferent, self-absorbed, not very bright, resistant to change, and likely to shirk responsibility and avoid risk.

- To overcome this ongoing resistance, management must apply the carrot-and-stick method to elicit worker compliance and effort. Management must use control techniques, coercion, punishment, bribes, promises, monetary incentives, and cajoling to ensure productivity.[43]

In contrast to Theory X, Theory Y assumptions provide a more favorable picture of the worker. Theory Y assumptions include the following:

- Workers are not passive, indifferent, or resistant by nature. Rather, they are susceptible to these attitudes based on lived experiences within organizations.

- Work and the opportunity to utilize skills, knowledge, and talents are basic human needs.

- People underutilize their intellect and other capacities in the typical organization.

- Under the appropriate circumstances, which management can generally control, workers will seek out responsibility and challenging work as long as their own needs are being addressed in the process.

As noted later in this chapter, which of these sets of assumptions or combination of the two the organization or manager subscribes to influences greatly the leadership and management style that prevails in the organizational culture.

Leadership Models

Leadership has generated a vast body of research in both scholarly and popular literature. Researchers have attempted to understand the social, psychological, political, and cultural processes that affect leadership behavior, the effects of leadership on the organization, the political entity, and society as a whole, and the conditions that affect the attribution and maintenance of leadership status. Executive and organizational consultants have focused on the processes of recruiting, selecting, developing, rewarding, and retaining effective organizational leaders. Both managers in training and practicing managers may aspire to become organizational leaders, perhaps associating leadership with power and authority in the organization. Health care professionals may alternatively seek to be recognized as leaders in their disciplines or professions. The degree to which the individual HIM professional exercises effective leadership within the work unit affects the attitudes and behavior of employees. Furthermore, even if the HIM professional does not seek out a leadership role, the department's performance is directly influenced by the quality of leadership from above. Because the impact of leadership is unavoidable, professional education and development programs for the HIM professional should give priority to the nature and development of core leadership skills. Various theoretical models have been developed and tested to explain leadership and enhance our understanding of how it affects organizational performance. An overview of some of the more useful perspectives on leadership is discussed in this section.

Charismatic Leadership

The attempt to understand and model leadership as a distinct set of personal characteristics or character traits has persisted over time. The "Great Person" approach to leadership entails biographical and historical analysis of personal characteristics and environmental circumstances. From these studies, 10 qualities ranging from high energy, sense of purpose, and self-direction to intelligence were found to be necessary and sufficient for

effective leadership.[44] Although this approach has some intuitive appeal, subsequent research to specify necessary and sufficient traits for effective leadership has failed to identify reliable characterization. The primary deficiency of this approach was not, however, in the inability to provide a reliable list of traits of the effective leader but in the static and incomplete view of leadership that was offered.

Behavior Models

Leadership models that attempt to demonstrate the influence of the leader's behavior, style, or orientation on leadership effectiveness and organizational performance grew out of the Ohio State University leadership studies.[45] Models developed by this line of thought suggest that leadership styles fall along a continuum with production-centered and people-centered styles at the extremes. A two-dimensional model was developed where characteristics of the leadership behavior were identified in terms of the leader's effort to structure and control the task environment (initiating structure) and the leader's activity in developing effective interpersonal relationships (consideration).

Managerial Grid Models

One of the most popular models of leadership style is the **managerial grid**.[46] This model characterizes managerial leadership style on the dimensions of "concern for production" on the X axis and "concern for people" on the Y axis. Four anchor positions representing the extreme points are identified on the grid. This model is used as a diagnostic tool with which managers can assess their own leadership style as well as the dominant leadership style of the organization. A score representing high concern for people and high concern for productivity is defined as a team management style, whereas a low score for both people and production is regarded as a laissez-faire style of management.

Decision-Making Models

The leadership style model developed by Bonoma and Slevin differs from other models by emphasizing the decision-making role of the leader (Figure 13–8).[47] This model incorporates two dimensions based on the following two questions:

- To what extent do you obtain information input from the group (subordinates) in decision making?
- To what extent do you delegate decision authority to the group (subordinates)?

Individual managers are asked to position themselves on the matrix by responding to a set of Likert Scale

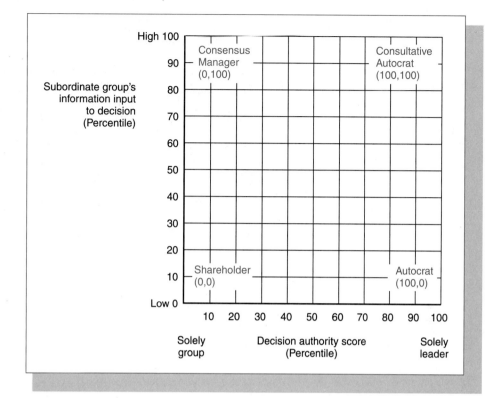

FIGURE 13–8. Bonoma-Slevin leadership model.

items. The corners of the matrix represent extreme points of management style, including Autocratic, Consultative Autocrat, Consensus Manager, and Share Holder. Although the model is primarily descriptive, it can be used to predict effectiveness of a given management style in participative management, delegation, and response to personal and organizational pressures. Bonoma and Slevin do not identify a normative style that is best for all circumstances. This position suggests that leadership flexibility in responding appropriately to the contextual situation is an ideal approach in most cases.

An alternative approach to modeling the leader is the Vroom-Yetton decision-making model of leadership.[48] This model provides decision rules for leaders to follow in the decision-making process. A set of leadership methods is arrayed, based on the degree to which the leader involves the group in the decision-making process. The leader selects an approach, using a decision-making tree based on the following attributes:

- Does the problem have quality dimensions?
- Does the leader have enough information to make an effective decision?
- Is the problem structured?
- Is acceptance of the decision by the group important for implementation of the problem resolution?
- Would the group accept the leader's decision if the leader acted alone?
- Do group members share the same organizational goals served by the decision?
- Is conflict among group members likely?[48]

By analyzing the problem in terms of these attributes, a leader can identify a feasible set of decision-making approaches.

EXAMPLE

Suppose the director of health information in an expanding health maintenance organization is required to develop a space and work-flow plan for the department for relocation to temporary offices in anticipation of newly renovated facilities. Some employees will probably gain needed space at the expense of others in response to more efficient space utilization. The steps in the Vroom-Yetton or a more simplified decision tree could be used to assist the director in determining how to make the required decisions most effectively and the extent to which the group (staff) should participate in the decision making. Addressing the questions in the Vroom-Yetton model, a reasonable set of responses would be as follows:

Does the problem have a quality dimension? Yes

Does the leader have enough information to make an effective decision? No

Is the problem structured? Yes

Is acceptance of the decision by the group important for implementation? Yes

Would the group accept the leader's decision? Yes/Maybe

Do group members share organizational goals? Yes

Is conflict among members likely? Yes

By applying the Vroom-Yetton decision tree, the feasible set of alternative actions would be identified as the following:

- The leader obtains needed input from the group and then makes a decision without further group participation. (autocratic style)

- The leader shares the problem with the group (individually or in a group meeting), obtains feedback, and then makes the decision. (consultative style)

- The leader involves the group fully in analyzing the problem, develops alternatives, and reaches a consensual decision. (consensual style)

This framework offers the leader considerable discretion in developing an appropriate decision-making strategy. According to this model, the leader would then choose among alternative decision-making approaches based on time and cost considerations. If maximizing efficiency is given priority, this supports the autocratic rather than the consensual style.

Contingency Theory

The **contingency theory** of leadership in Fiedler's model specifically recognizes the influence of situational variables on leadership effectiveness.[49] Leadership styles are characterized as "task-oriented" or "relationship-oriented." Effective leadership is a function of leader-group interpersonal relations, degree of job-task structure, and the leader's position relative to the group. Task-oriented leaders were found to be the most effective when the situation was either very favorable or unfavorable, whereas relationship-oriented leaders were more effective when the situation was more ambiguous. For example, a contingency model may focus on leadership style with reference to group characteristics. Hersey and Blanchard suggest four leadership styles on the basis of low to high values on the dimensions of "task" and "relationship" behavior.[50] The resulting styles are as follows:

- Coaching (telling)—high for both task and relationship

- Directing (selling)—high task, low relationship

- Participating—low task, high relationship

- Delegating—low for both task and relationship

The work group (followers) are characterized from low to high values on the dimensions of maturity, which include group motivation, responsibility, competence, and training. This model then associates the most appropriate leadership style with the state of the group maturity as follows:

Group Maturity	Leadership Style
Low	Directing (telling)
Low to moderate	Coaching (selling)
Moderate to high	Participating
High	Delegating

An important implication of this model is that the group leader should modify leadership style to best meet the needs of the group.

Path-Goal Models

An elaborated version of the contingency approach is the **path-goal theory**.[51] The path-goal model is based on the expectancy theory, which considers a person's motivation to perform a function.[52] This theory focuses on the following:

- The person's perception of effort needed to complete the task

- The perceived probability of the performance ending in desired rewards

- The value the person places on anticipated outcomes

The path-goal approach views the leader's role as instrumental in satisfying the needs and goals of the employee. The leader is instrumental in facilitating the employee's efforts in attaining desired results. The leader is effective in increasing employee motivation and satisfaction to the extent that the leader provides an increased awareness of valued rewards and outcomes; clarifies paths between effort, performance, and rewards; and eliminates obstacles along the path.

Based on the path-goal model, the following leadership styles have been identified:

- Directive

- Supportive

- Achievement

- Participative[51]

These four styles complete the model by recognizing the influence of intervening factors identified as subordinate characteristics (e.g., locus of control) and environmental factors (e.g., nature of the task). These variables are seen as affecting the relation between a given leadership style and employee satisfaction.

Transformational Leadership

Current leadership theories, both scholarly and popular, have drawn heavily from the literature in corporate culture, quality management, and organizational excellence. Indeed, **transformational leadership** theory with its roots in corporate culture and organizational excellence perspectives as well as a renewed interest in the charismatic aspect of leadership has become the prevailing paradigm of the current trend in leadership modeling. The transformational leader is perceived as both a manipulator and an architect of organizational culture.[53,54] The leadership role is one of facilitating the organization's ongoing process of accommodating to and catalyzing environmental change. The effective leader articulates a vision of the organization's future and models the values, priorities, and behaviors consistent with achieving that future. The transformational leader transmits a vision of the future of the re-created organization, infuses meaning into organizational processes, interprets and attempts to anticipate environmental change, and continually invigorates organizational culture.

This is in contrast with the conception of **transactional leadership.** The transactional leader's role involves an ongoing process of exchanges with subordinates to reward and reinforce appropriate behavior supporting organizational objectives.[55] The transformational leader goes beyond reinforcement of the status quo to sustain acceptable levels of performance under given constraints of the moment. Rather, the transforming leader acts as a catalyst to empower followers to envision goals that transcend short-term predictable objectives and to focus on continuous growth and personal development.[56] The transactional leader facilitates, whereas the transformational leader empowers.

Rohrer proposes the concept of **translational leadership** to complement the transactional and transformational roles.[31] In this translational role, the leader communicates and interprets the vision of the transformational leader into policies, procedures, and plans to be implemented at the transactional level. Although most managerial positions should have the opportunity to engage in each of these types of behaviors, the middle manager is seen as having a special responsibility for the translational role. Certainly the quality management movement (as discussed later in this chapter) entails the kind of visionary, catalyzing leadership associated with performance exceeding expectation and empowered followers.

What Do We Really Know About Leadership?

Few issues have received the attention that the study of leadership has received. Although an attempt has

---

The Three T's of Leadership

Transformational (T1)
- Has a charismatic identification
- Creates vision and meaning
- Challenges the culture (norms and values)
- Articulates broad mission and goals

Translational (T2)
- Translates broad mission and goals into operating policies, procedures, and standards
- Provides feedback to upper management about employee performance and productivity, client satisfaction, employee concerns, and resource needs

Transactional (T3)
- Involves day-to-day exchange between manager and employee
- Clarifies performance expectations and job requirements
- Monitors performance and provides coaching and resources
- Provides rewards for effective performance and sanctions for ineffective performance

---

been made to understand "the leader," a great deal of uncertainty surrounds both definitions and role expectations of leaders. The following statements, although not inclusive or definitive, are intended to provide a brief overview of what we know about leadership.

- Leadership is essentially a relational process that involves social, political, and cultural aspects of behavior rather than being a reliable set of personal characteristics.

- Effective leaders present a charismatic aspect in their behavior (i.e., they attract followers and stimulate emotive responses of attachment, affection, loyalty, and commitment).

- Leadership is arguably the single most important factor that influences organizational effectiveness. The effects of the leader's actions are mediated by the interaction of situational variables, including the task, the core technologies, and the characteristics of the followers.

- Effective leaders understand their organizational culture and fit within an ever-changing and increasingly complex set of environments.

- The effective leader has a vision of the future, a passion about organizational excellence that can be communicated, and a capacity to convert followers with a transformed vision of the organization and of their role in re-creating the organization.

- To survive well, the transformational leader must be responsive, tuned in, and adaptable and become accustomed to confronting turbulence and conflict. The leader must be able to create opportunity out of chaos.

- Quality management is essentially a leadership commitment made throughout the organization to encourage ongoing empowerment of individuals and teams and to demand an escalation in performance expectations.

- Whatever leadership is exactly, we are convinced that we will continue to need more of it if we are to survive and thrive in the face of an increasingly uncertain future.[57]

In no environment is this more relevant than in health care in the 1990s and beyond.

QUALITY MANAGEMENT: QUALITY, EXCELLENCE, COMMITMENT

Quality management as a management philosophy has become a mainstay of most health care organizations. Philosophically, quality management has fostered a cultural revolution of leadership style focused on a commitment to excellence and service. Quality management may be defined as a cultural commitment to quality performance through the empowerment of all workers in a process of continuous improvement through use of innovative scientific methods. This suggests an integrated, organizationwide system that ensures standards of conformance in both process and outcome that is communicated to all employees and that anticipates meaningful participation of all employees. Innovation, empowerment, education, excellence, and quality are the bedrock principles of quality management. A **total quality management** approach suggests a transformational leadership style that emphasizes ongoing employee development and participation. Every employee is perceived as being a service provider. Integrated team building that uses various strengths of employees within the organization is stressed. Rigid task performance and satisfaction is *not* acceptable. Rather, emphasis is placed on futuristic planning and implementation of innovative technologies for continuous improvement.

Theoretical Foundations of Quality Management

Several quality management philosophies exist, but in general, the foundations of quality management can be traced to the writings of Deming, Juran, and Crosby.[1-3,5-12] Although the work of all three authors falls under the generic label of quality management, there are important differences that need to be discussed. Indeed, at certain points, beliefs concerning management among these three theorists are diametrically opposed.

Deming and Quality Management: 14 Points to Total Quality

Deming, in his classic *Out of the Crises,* is seen as the original quality management advocate.[3,5,9] For decades after his original works, Deming's philosophies were not endorsed or accepted by mainstream American management theorists or practitioners. Deming's initial success in promoting his management style came from the Japanese adoption of his ideology after World War II. American interest in Deming did not occur until the early 1970s. Deming, more than any other quality management philosopher, takes a more humanistic approach to management.[3,5,9] Deming bases his theory of management on a belief that employees want to come to work, perform with maximum effort, and recognize personal excellence, and they are committed to the best interests of the organization as long as these interests are in agreement with personal needs and priorities, which is consistent with the basic tenets of Theory Y.

Deming is process- rather than outcome-oriented in his management philosophy. Given the process orientation, Deming strongly disagrees with the use of formal individual evaluations or goal setting. Assuming that workers are committed both to excellence and to working at maximum capability and that management is leading in the desired direction, worker evaluation becomes superfluous. Deming suggests that problems of the organization are more likely to be a result of inefficient management rather than lack of worker commitment. Indeed, Deming suggests that about 85 per cent of the problems with quality experienced within organizations lies with management and 15 per cent with workers. Within Deming's conception of management there are no merit raises, formal evaluations, or individual "stars." Differentiation at the individual level leads to conflict, dissatisfaction, and lower rates of productivity.[3,5,9]

Deming's view is that economic stability of the organization depends on developing an atmosphere of constant change and innovation. Economic stability is ensured through a belief in the constancy of innovative change. A reactive strategy of knee-jerk response to adversity without a guiding vision or strategy will lead to economic decline and threaten the survival of the organization. Top management must take initiatives to ensure an open atmosphere of creativity, innovation, and creative risk taking, even if negative consequences result in the short term. This philosophy implies a belief in developing continuous educational programs for all employees. In this way, management is able to make use of all the skills and expertise of the empowered workforce.[3,5,9]

Juran's Quality Trilogy

Juran's major contribution to the quality management field centers around the quality trilogy of quality planning, quality control, and quality improvement and the redesign and emphasis on control charts as a primary method of evaluating performance (i.e., the belief in the need to initiate continuing **statistical process control**).[5,7,8] Juran's emphasis on planning, control, and improvement suggests that both process and outcome measures must be continually monitored. Unlike Deming, Juran believes strongly in the continuous use of performance appraisals to evaluate work productivity. When performance falls short of goal expectations, corrective action should be initiated. Corrective action, according to Juran, may be in the form of either incentives or coercive action to ensure excellence and quality performance. This approach suggests that Theory X assumptions have a role in Juran's quality management perspective. Merit pay and individual monitoring are part of Juran's quality management program.

To implement organizationwide evaluative standards of performance and evaluation criteria, Juran suggests the use of control charts based on the reduction of both error rate and variation over time. According to Juran, after quality standards have been established, it is necessary to continually monitor performance to detect nonconformance and initiate change to reduce both error and variation. Perhaps the most intriguing feature of Juran's modified control chart is the extreme fluctuation that occurs during change periods. Juran seems to recognize that as change is introduced and the status quo is disrupted, work performance becomes erratic during the adjustment period. After workers become acclimated to the change, performance should improve in terms of a reduction in the number of errors and the degree to which performance fluctuates.[5,7,8]

Crosby: Quality Equals Zero Defects

Crosby is much more rigid in his definition of quality performance and excellence than either Deming or Juran.[1,5] For Crosby, the definition of quality is complete conformance to standards. The performance standard is defined as zero defects. As Crosby notes, accepting even a 99.9 per cent efficiency level would be unacceptable. This is especially true in health care, where errors are likely to lead to irreversible consequences (e.g., death). Prevention or the elimination of error is of paramount importance to Crosby.

In contrast to Deming, Crosby is a strong advocate of goal setting, merit pay, recognition of "champions" or "stars," and exhortation of employees through slogans and competitions. Quality is implemented through development of educational programs, mass media and human relation promotionals, and management's total and visible commitment to quality. Although Deming and Juran both advocate team building and group process, Crosby strongly focuses on the value of team decision making as the primary method of worker empowerment.[1]

Tools of Quality Management

As quality management practices have evolved, greater emphasis has been placed on developing evaluation procedures. Indeed, quantitative documentation has become the cornerstone in the application of most quality management theories.[1,3,5–7,58–60] Evaluation measures have generally fallen under the framework or heading of statistical process control.[5,58] Under this scheme, both process and outcome measures are considered. Statistical process control techniques, as defined in most quality management theories, are used for the following purposes:

- To generate ideas
- To organize information
- To analyze, evaluate, and present data

Although the list of statistical process control techniques is limitless, it can be reduced into 10 general techniques that overlap and that best summarize the list of potential evaluation techniques. Idea-generating techniques generally fall under processes related to brainstorming or affinity diagrams. Data organization methods are usually related to the matrix, fishbone, or force field analyses. Data evaluation and presentation methods are usually related to histograms, run charts, pareto charts, control charts, or correlational analysis.

Idea-Generating Techniques

BRAINSTORMING. Most quality management theories begin evaluation processes by discussing the value of brainstorming. Brainstorming, as mentioned earlier, requires a team of 6 to 10 persons who are brought together to generate ideas about a relevant issue. Brainstorming is a process by which an issue is defined, a time limit for discussion is set, and ideas are recorded for all team members to discuss. All ideas should be expressed vocally, and criticism should be limited. The goal is *not* to come up with a final solution but to examine various options. Brainstorming has become an integral part of quality management because of an emphasis on worker empowerment and the need to solicit various opinions from all levels of workers within an organization.

AFFINITY DIAGRAMS. Affinity diagrams may be used to bridge the gap between idea generation and data

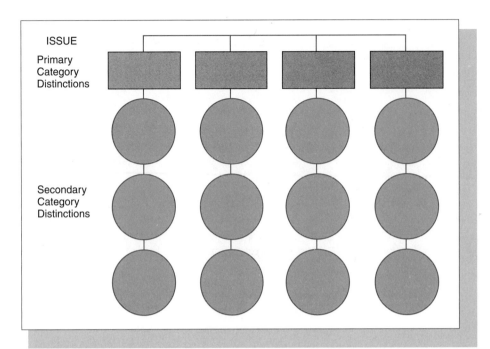

FIGURE 13–9. Affinity diagram.

organization. After the initial brainstorming session, affinity diagrams are often used to organize and prioritize information into clusters or categories (Figure 13–9). Affinity diagrams are particularly useful when dealing with large amounts of complicated information. This technique reduces what may be considered an unmanageable amount of information into smaller sets of homogeneous groups. In addition to organizing information, affinity diagrams may be effectively used in generating new ideas and in solution planning. By organizing data into homogeneous groups, teams may begin to prioritize action according to importance, need, or resources of a particular issue to an organization. As in the case of brainstorming, time limits should be set to facilitate action and keep the amount of new information generated to a manageable amount.

Data Organization

FLOWCHARTS. Flowcharts are graphic representations of a specific sequencing of steps in a decision-making process. A flowchart is a pictorial representation of the decision-making process that consists of a series of symbols connected together to represent an expected or logical sequencing and networking of ideas (Figure 13–10). Flowchart analysis begins by deciding on the starting and ending points. Ideas generated by brainstorming are time ordered in a causal manner. Activities should be arranged around decision-making points in the time sequence. Options for potential outcomes should be mapped at all decision points. This should include necessary impacts and outcomes. Flowchart analysis should help answer questions related to resource management (both material and personnel), necessary process and outcome factors, and potential paths (e.g., networks) involved in the decision-making process. The ultimate goal of flowchart analysis is to accurately portray real-life situations in an ordered and understandable format.

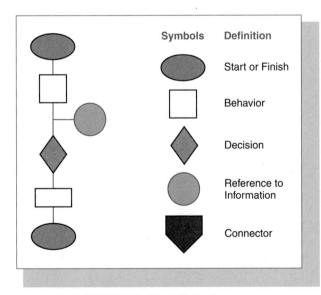

FIGURE 13–10. Affinity diagram.

MATRIX. The **matrix** is a multidimensional tool that may be used to organize, categorize, and reduce information into a more usable form. Both qualitative and quantitative data may be used in the matrix. As an organization and reduction tool, the matrix may be used in the decision-making process by weighting information or in the evaluation of performance over an extended period. In addition to focusing on internal processes, the matrix may be used to examine influences of external factors (e.g., economic conditions). To use the matrix, first the information that is to be collected must be identified. Then, after the information is collected, relevant categories that may be maintained over time are developed. The matrix is used in conjunction with both qualitative and quantitative methods to store data and to retrieve data for performance evaluation or in various aspects of the decision-making process. The matrix allows for a quick reference to information over time by synthesizing and integrating ideas into manageable forms.

FISHBONE. The **fishbone diagram** is used to place factors that are expected to affect a problem, condition, or project in causal order. This diagram is useful in graphically representing a time-ordered process in relation to outcome variables. Used in conjunction with brainstorming and affinity diagrams, the fishbone diagram allows for an integration of probable causes toward a clearly defined outcome measure in the decision-making process. When using a fishbone diagram, first, outcome variables are placed on the right side of the paper at the end of the causal line (Figure 13–11). Second, major causes are directly linked to the causal line in an ordered sequence. Finally, minor causes are linked to

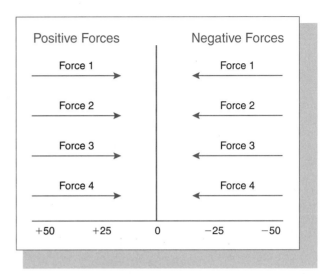

FIGURE 13–12. Force field analysis.

each of the major causes along the time line. This allows the manager to visually connect related processes to specific outcomes.

FORCE FIELD ANALYSIS. Force field analysis is similar to fishbone analysis in connecting process to outcome variables. In addition to identifying the causal order, force field analysis estimates the relative effect of each process variable on the outcome variable. In force field analysis, the outcome variable is placed in the center of the paper (Figure 13–12). Process variables can then be identified by both causal ordering, if desired, and expected strength of effect, either positive or negative, on the outcome variable. Expected positive effects and negative effects are identified by being placed on either side of the outcome variable. By identifying positive and negative effects as well as estimating the relative effect of each variable, both factors that facilitate and factors that impede change are pictorially identified. Force field analysis is particularly useful in developing strategic plans when resource allocation must be prioritized.

Data Analysis and Presentation

HISTOGRAMS. Histograms are graphic representations of frequency distributions. They are useful in helping to clearly identify whether or not the variation that exists in the frequency distribution is normal or skewed, suggesting areas of further attention (Figure 13–13). When using a histogram, first a vertical and a horizontal axis are created. Values are placed on the vertical axis and classes are placed on the horizontal axis. Second, the range of scores on relevant data points to be marked on the vertical and horizontal axes must be determined. If

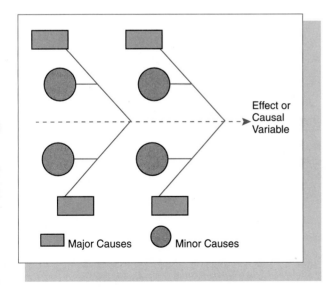

FIGURE 13–11. Fishbone analysis.

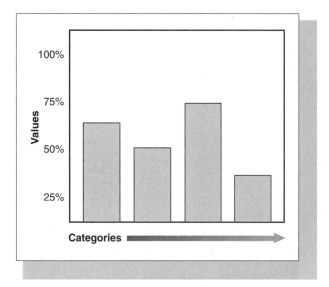

FIGURE 13–13. Histogram.

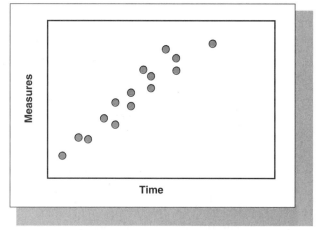

FIGURE 13–14. Scatter diagram.

using ratio-level data, it must be decided first whether grouped data are representative and then which categories are most representative of the data. All processes have variation; a histogram can quickly identify both the level and the type of the variation.

RUN CHART AND LINE GRAPH. Run charts and line graphs provide the health information professional with a simple yet highly graphic visual method of monitoring trends over time. A run chart is an excellent method of establishing performance trends and standards of evaluation over a lengthy period. When using a run chart, the time period for which data are to be collected and analyzed (e.g., ongoing or time-bounded) must be decided. Second, a graph is drawn with a vertical and a horizontal axis. Here, the horizontal axis indicates increments of time, and the vertical axis indicates increments of measurement. Finally, data points are plotted and the results for trends in the data are evaluated (for an example see Figure 13–14).

PARETO CHARTS. Pareto charts are similar in form to bar charts and histograms. The primary difference when using a pareto chart is that occurrences are categorized from most frequent and most important to least frequent and least important. When using a pareto chart, first the types of causes and conditions to be studied are selected. Second, the standard for comparison (i.e., frequency, cost, or amount) is determined. Third, the vertical axis is drawn and labeled with standards used for comparisons and the horizontal axis is drawn and labeled with categories. Finally, bars are drawn that represent the frequency of each factor according to a predetermined rank ordering (Figure 13–15). Pareto charts

are often used in conjunction with brainstorming as a visual aid to demonstrate where attention to specific problems should be focused.

CONTROL CHARTS. For most quality management practices, **control charts** have been adopted as the primary tool for performance evaluation. Control charts provide an effective, visual way of statistically detecting significant variation from expected norms (Figure 13–16). There are two basic types of control charts that may be used, depending on the distributional form of responses. In industry, the most commonly used control chart is based on a normal distribution and makes use of standard deviations to determine confidence intervals and statistical significance. In health care settings, given the greater need for accuracy as a result of the consequences for error, control charts based on a Poisson distribution are more appropriate than the normal distribution for many types of incidence data. To use a control chart, first a mean score for the data under analysis must be calculated. Second, it must be determined whether the confidence intervals are based on a normal or a Poisson distribution. At this point, the acceptance level of statistical significance (i.e., .01 or .05) must be decided. Third, data are plotted on a graph of horizontal axis for time and vertical axis for performance standards. Finally, significant differences or deviations from the expected mean score are noted. Control charts are a quick and efficient way of determining statistically significant deviations in performance.

CORRELATION ANALYSIS. Correlation analysis allows the HIM professional to determine the strength, direction, and statistical significance of a relation between one or more performance variables or standards (Figure 13–17). Correlation analysis provides information concerning the importance of various factors on perform-

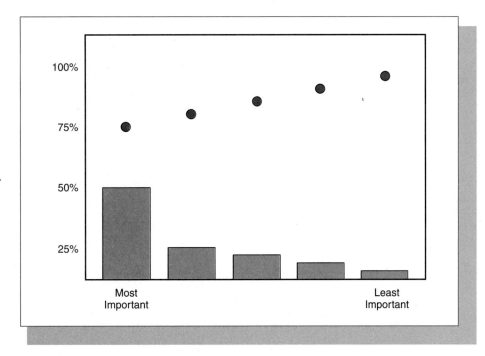

FIGURE 13–15. Pareto chart.

ance evaluation that can be used in conjunction with brainstorming, affinity diagrams, and other methods. Correlation coefficients provide an exact interpretation of the relation noted on the run chart. In correlation analysis, scores range from −1.0, signifying a perfect negative relation, to 0.0, signifying no relation, to 1.0, signifying a perfect positive relation. To use correlation analysis, first a variable believed to be related is selected. Second, the acceptance level of significance (.05 or .01) is determined. Finally, the relation is analyzed to determine significance (usually a t-test at .05 or .01), direction (positive or negative), and strength of association. Correlation analysis provides easily interpretable num-

bers and a straightforward method of examining how various performance measures are related.

Introducing Change into the Work Environment

A changing sociopolitical environment and the introduction of new technologies and quality management efforts toward streamlining health care reform

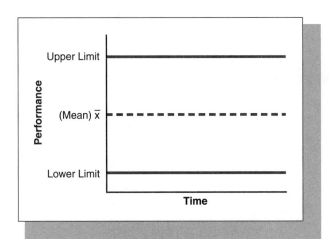

FIGURE 13–16. Control chart.

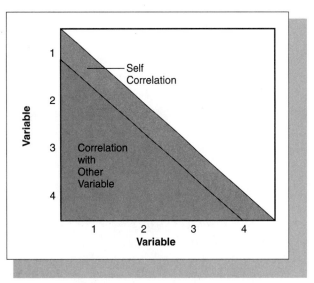

FIGURE 13–17. Correlation measure.

have resulted in a rapid re-engineering within HIM departments.[61-63] The use of computer-based patient records (CPRs), smart cards, voice recognition, and electronic interchange as well as changes in reimbursement procedures, funding, and patient advocacy have forced HIM professionals to redefine work processes.[61-63] Given this rapid change, it is important that HIM departments develop work environments in which change becomes an acceptable and a desirable part of the workplace culture.

Prior research has clearly documented high levels of employee resistance to and fear of change. For most employees, change is perceived as being very personal.[2,4,64] Fear of change is most often a result of uncertainty of the unknown, personal insecurity of new work environments or responsibilities, self-interest, or disruption of the status quo.[2,64-66] Employees generally believe that hidden agendas accompany organizational change. It is commonly thought that change will result in increased workload responsibilities, time commitments, and management expectations or that it will affect advancement and disrupt formal and informal networks of communication.[2,4,64-66]

In response to employee fears concerning change, management is most likely to deal with a proposed change from a structural or an organizational perspective. Management response usually takes the form of depersonalizing change, demystifying the **processual**

nature of the **change,** and opening up formal communication channels.[64,67-69] Management fails to understand that to successfully implement change, a more personalized approach should be implemented. Indeed, the way in which people process change messages should in turn determine the way in which change messages are positioned to better ensure success. Moreover, recent studies suggest that all employees are willing to accept change when it is presented in a format consistent with past experiences.[65,66] Studies conducted with health care professionals indicate that the way in which change is perceived (based on past change experiences) can be divided into five categories (Figure 13–18).[65,66] Each category suggests differences in the way past experiences with change influence how employees process new change messages. Moreover, these data provide insights for improving how management might personalize change messages to gain support from employees.

In Figure 13–18, Level 1 employees (represented by a triangle) have little cognitive experience with change. They have followed a structured sequence of advancement, lived in the same area, and developed long-term friendships in the community. These people are resistant to change, fearing a disruption of the status quo. Change messages should be simple, visual, nonthreatening, and incremental. They should focus on opportunities for personal growth.

Level 2 employees (represented by a triangle turning

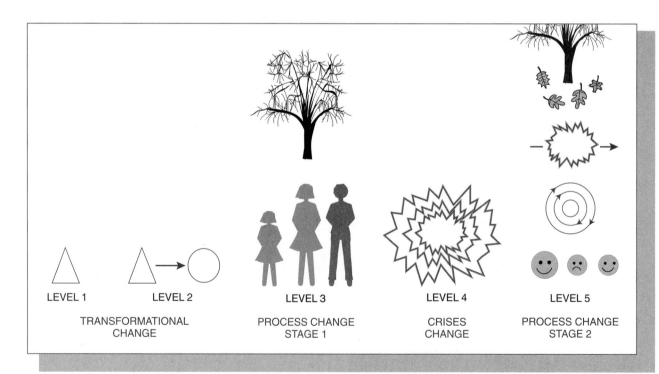

LEVEL 1	LEVEL 2	LEVEL 3	LEVEL 4	LEVEL 5
TRANSFORMATIONAL CHANGE		PROCESS CHANGE STAGE 1	CRISES CHANGE	PROCESS CHANGE STAGE 2

FIGURE 13–18. Categories of perceived self-actualized change: processing change message.

into a circle) are likely to have had minimal but positive change experiences. Focus is on outcomes rather than on the process associated with change initiatives. Change is viewed as inevitable and transformational, not incremental or processual. There is a belief that change will result in disruption and restructuring of work and social roles. Change messages should again be visual but contain a substantive message structure that focuses on the content of the change. Change should be positioned as a natural part of life and work experiences. Opportunities for personal and professional growth should be emphasized.

Level 3 employees (represented by either a tree or stick figures) perceive change as a natural and ongoing process. Although experienced with change, these people are not likely to have experienced a change crisis. Here, the distinction between a tree and a stick figure represents the type of support networks that is needed to help the employee when change occurs. For example, those who draw flowers or trees are likely to rely on structure or traditions, whereas those who draw stick figures are likely to rely on significant others for support. For Level 3 employees, the content of the message is more important than the presentation format. These people should have sufficient information to assess both the quality and the effect that the proposed or implemented change will have on personal and professional goals. Change messages should reflect the type of support needed to accept change. If the employee relies on structure, change initiatives should focus directly on organizational benefits and indirectly on benefits enjoyed by the employee. If reliance is on other people, creating change support groups to help orient the employee to accept change would be the preferred strategy.

Employees in Level 4 (represented by an uncontrollable explosion) are undergoing a crisis of change. The drawing suggests that these people are experiencing a change crisis perceived to be uncontrollable (e.g., death of a loved one, divorce, loss of a job). Because the outcome of the change is unknown, personal and professional stability are threatened. Message development must reflect a sensitivity to the disruption the employee is facing by focusing on whatever stability might be associated with the proposed change. Messages should be highly visual and incremental, yet provide a rationale that focuses on the positive aspects of change in stabilizing life activities.

Level 5 employees (represented by leaves falling from a tree, arrows through an explosion, concentric circles, or detailed faces) are likely to have experienced a major change crisis or a sequential series of minor change crises. Employees within this category, if they believe in the proposed change, think that, regardless of the magnitude of change, they can adapt and contribute to the success of the change initiative. In determining whether an employee's perception of change belongs in category

3 or 5, focus should be directed toward both the detailed nature of the drawing and the processual growth or decay, as suggested in the drawing (e.g., changes in the face, leaves on the tree). Although employees in category 5 may draw support from either structure or significant others, they are more self-motivated and self-reliant in acceptance and promotion of change. Those respondents who draw an arrow through an explosion or concentric circles are likely to rely on personal strengths to deal with change. An arrow through an explosion represents a person who perceives change as a series of minor crises, whereas the concentric circles represent a person who perceives change as more natural and processual.

Employees in Level 5 are likely to be change agents. Consequently, messages should include information that contains the rationale for the proposed change, practical application, immediate impact, future implications, and an invitation to become part of the proposed change. Employees in this category need to be involved in the development and implementation to buy into the proposed change. Message content should focus heavily on personal and professional growth as well as an invitation to participate in the change.

Prior studies suggest that, depending on both the value and personal belief system of the employee and how the message is positioned, all employees are amenable to accepting change.[65,66] As a manager or director of an HIM department, you probably have either recently implemented or are in the process of implementing a CPR system. The implementation of such a system should increase both the efficiency and the effectiveness of HIM departments. As the CPR is introduced into HIM departments, managers will have to deal with employee fears and concerns about the new technology. Using the paradigm suggested in this chapter, the manager may take a different approach with employees, depending on past experiences with change. This does not suggest that the manager must have employees make drawings and then analyze them. It simply means that the manager develops some working knowledge of the diversity in experiences of those directly supervised and then acts according to that knowledge. For employees at Levels 1 and 2, before the actual implementation, it might be helpful to place displays of the CPR in appropriate areas. Here, messages would be highly visual and focus on the increased freedom gained by having a CPR. The manager might, on a personal level, reassure the employee that this change will not transform the environment but will add to the credibility of the profession and allow more time for personal development, if desired. For Level 3 employees, in addition to the posters, the manager might offer more detailed information on the value and process of implementation. Here, personal reassurances on how the CPR will add to personal growth and advancement possibilities will help in acceptance of a new technology. In this situation, messages must be more direct and content-oriented. For Level 4 employees, the manager must take a more personalized and interactive approach. (Note: In all likelihood, no more than one or two employees will be at this stage.) The manager must spend time reassuring these employees that this new technology will not disrupt regular work routines. Moreover, follow-up sessions must be initiated to ensure that the Level 4 employees are coping with the change. Finally, Level 5 employees, in addition to being exposed to the orientation suggested above, must be brought directly into the implementation process. Their advice on how best to implement, train for, and use the CPR must be solicited. A manager may use a Level 5 employee, for example, to run a support group for Level 3 employees or to conduct training and in-service seminars to gain support for the change.

It is important that change messages be personalized. This will, for most employees, increase the likelihood of acceptance of the intended change. Managers should take time to better understand the way employees process change messages. The way most employees perceive change is heavily dependent on past life experiences. This suggests that managers need to better understand employees and to discuss the proposed changes on a personal level.

NEGOTIATION

Negotiation is a complex social exchange process that is pervasive in our society, both within and outside of health care organizations. It occurs both as a formally structured process with clearly established mechanisms, roles, norms, and rules (e.g., contract negotiations) and as informal bargaining between people (e.g., employee bargaining about vacation time). The negotiation may involve two parties, each forwarding individual interests; two parties, one forwarding individual interests and the other forwarding organizational interests; or two or more parties, each representing the interests of different constituencies. Negotiations may be established ad hoc to deal with a specific, unique situation or may be structured as an ongoing or recurring process.

Whatever its specific application, the negotiation process has some common elements, including the following:

- Structure

- Initial positions

- Unresolved conflict

- Communication (transaction)

- Realigned positions

The structure of the negotiation may be formalized and predictable by regulation or agreement of the parties or established by practice, or it may be informal, idiosyncratic, and unpredictable. The process may be time-bound (e.g., to meet contract expiration deadlines) or indefinite (e.g., commitment to diminish personal conflicts at the workplace).

Each party brings an initial position to the negotiation process whether or not it is articulated explicitly. This position might be perceived as the desired end state of the negotiation and/or as the party's "bottom line"—the unreducible set of expectations or value commitments that the party regards as beyond compromise. The strength of commitments and emotional intensity associated with these positions influence the nature, duration, and perceived success of the negotiations.

pa.Given that the negotiation process is essentially one of conflict resolution, it follows that unresolved conflict lies at the foundation of all negotiations. Each party attempts to advance, if not fully achieve, a bargaining position. The basic assumption underlying the decision to enter negotiations by at least one of the parties is that the position of the other cannot be achieved without cost to or compromise of a personal position. Given that both parties share this perception, the process is likely to be conflictual because each party will act to protect personal turf and to prevent the other from gaining at the expense of each party's perceived best interests. The negotiation process provides a mechanism for keeping conflict within acceptable boundaries, so that a mutually agreeable settlement may be achieved at a reasonable cost to both parties.

Communication is fundamental to effective negotiation. Failed negotiations often can be the result of dysfunctional and ineffective communication. A model of the communication process and obstacles to effective communication have already been presented. Given that negotiations are founded in conflict, there is considerable potential for interference, noise, and distortion. The use of negotiation strategies that entail deception, withholding of information useful to the other party, and masking one's actual final position or willingness to compromise further complicates the communication dynamics.

A completed negotiation—not necessarily one that is perceived as successful by either party—inevitably entails some revision or realignment of the initial position of one or both parties. Inability or unwillingness by at least one party to move from the initial bargaining position results in a blocked negotiation, perhaps terminating any further communication or prompting an escalation of conflict. The use of mediation and conciliation interventions in stalled contract negotiations represents an effort to avoid this worst-case scenario. The negotiated agreement may be achieved by one or both parties sacrificing or modifying an initial position. For each party to experience increased satisfaction with the negotiated outcome, that party must perceive a tangible gain from the process. This is often expressed in terms of the extent of attainment of the initial position, but it could be associated with the achievement of the settlement itself, regardless of the actual gains and losses relative to the initial position. For example, a dispute between family members about a "do-not-resuscitate" option for an elderly parent will permit only one of two alternative actions: do or do not resuscitate. One party may yield an initial position to preserve family harmony and take satisfaction in facilitating an agreement even at the sacrifice of the initial position.

Negotiations in actual experience can be difficult and personally demanding experiences even when outcomes are perceived as successful by both parties. Otherwise self-confident and proactive people are likely to avoid negotiation or approach it with anxiety and trepidation. Why is the process perceived to be such a high risk, even a treacherous endeavor? Can the process itself be changed so as to be less threatening to the participants? By what criteria should we evaluate the effectiveness of a negotiation? How do we maximize the likelihood of perceived success?

Most problems associated with real-world negotiation as experienced are based on the underlying logic of the zero-sum game. This simple economic model structures any transaction between two actors as a game of resource exchange in which one party can gain only at the expense of another because the total resources in the game are fixed. For example, consider the following situation:

1. Mr. Jones has 5 value units and Ms. Stone has 3 value units.

2. A total of 8 value units are available.

3. Neither Mr. Jones nor Ms. Stone can gain resources without the other suffering a corresponding loss of resources.

4. For example, for Ms. Stone to obtain the level of resources that Mr. Jones controls, she can gain 2 units $(+2)$ only if Mr. Jones gives up 2 units (-2).

5. The net result of this transaction, $(+2)(-2) = 0$, is zero. Consequently, this transaction and any other equitable transaction in this system is zero sum.

6. To obtain equal distribution of wealth (value units) and, consequently, a power equilibrium, the more powerful person must willingly sacrifice this resource advantage to the benefit of the other. Mr. Jones gives up 1 unit and Ms. Stone gains 1 unit $(-1)(+1) = 0$. Applying a strictly economic logic, this transaction is irrational from the perspective of Mr. Jones, and it would be irrational for Ms. Stone not to accept this exchange.

7. The system as a whole is indifferent to the reallocation because the level of total resources remains constant.

As long as negotiation is perceived to be a zero-sum game, the process is inherently conflictual and encourages passive-submissive, aggressive-dominant, or withdrawal behavior by the parties involved. This is counterproductive behavior relative to the primary goal of the negotiation process of achieving a long-term equilibrium.

This analysis suggests that reducing the negative attitudes of potential participants and enhancing the likelihood of a mutually successful negotiation require the replacement of a zero-sum logic with one that permits resource expansion. In the zero-sum game, one participant can win only if the other loses a given transaction; therefore, a win-lose outcome is assured. What is desired is a situation in which both parties are able to achieve gains in the negotiation process. The outcome should be one perceived by both parties as **win-win.** Both parties achieve net gains (real or perceived) and experience satisfaction with the negotiation process and the final agreement.

Fisher and Ury developed a practical model for enhancing outcomes of negotiation processes to enable the parties to reach an agreement without either party sacrificing real interests.[70] The method they propose requires the following elements:

- Dealing with personal concerns separate from problem analysis

- Focusing on the real interests of the parties rather than the declared or unstated positions

- Developing alternative strategies that result in mutual gains

- Identifying and applying mutually acceptable and objective criteria in evaluating alternative problem resolutions and the terms of negotiated agreement

Separating people issues from problem attributes allows for balanced attention to both personal needs and sensitivities and the substantive issues to be negotiated. Also, it should minimize the interference of affective and emotional responses rooted in personal conflict.

Focusing on interests rather than intransigent positions should encourage mutual problem analysis and shared perspectives. This approach leads participants to identify and articulate their genuine interests, values, and priorities. The assumption is that both common ground for agreement and significant obstacles are better understood through both parties engaging in this mutual exploration.

Effective negotiation entails an unfreezing of assumptions and opinions as a foundation for creative thinking and idea generation. Each party should be encouraged to participate fully in exploring problem resolution options that benefit both parties. If both parties pursue a strategy of mutual gain (i.e., win-win or collaboration), then neither is forced to accept a settlement of disadvantage, which places one party in a losing position. However, this strategy of mutual gain may not result in the maximum gain possible for either party. This choice is somewhat analogous to a "minimal regret" strategy in which the rational decision maker selects a course of action that minimizes the maximum loss among an array of alternatives.[42]

Specifying and applying objective, mutually determined criteria independent of initial positions in establishing a negotiated agreement are the final prerequisites for effective negotiations. This element is important for its role in facilitating the unfreezing of positions, reinforcing efforts at mutual inquiry and understanding, and establishing the negotiated agreement on the satisfaction of the real interests of both parties. The resulting agreement is likely to yield greater overall satisfaction and prove more durable than an agreement based on compromised positions and short-term trade-offs.

Negotiations in Labor Relations

Negotiation of the written agreement (i.e., the contract) between representatives of union and management has been the keystone of the labor relations system in the United States.[71,72] This literature suggests the various perspectives that might be applied to characterize negotiations in stating that "collective bargaining has been described as a poker game that combines deception, bluff, and luck; as an exercise in power politics; as a debating society marked by both rhetoric and name calling; and as a rational process" (footnote 71, p. 437).

The negotiation process clearly serves to reduce and manage conflict to facilitate the achievement of a written agreement that is acceptable to both parties. Alternatively, the negotiation process can be viewed as an important mechanism for labor management communications. The system of collective bargaining structures and channels what could become a fragmented, inefficient, and even chaotic process. Given that traditional labor management relations have been founded on conflict and hostility, the need for an effective communication process is clear. Certainly, the negotiation process can be seen as an exercise in power politics in which each side attempts to increase its relative power at the expense of the other, independent of concerns about the details of the written agreement. Finally, negotiation may be regarded as an art or technology.[73]

Beyond its functions of conflict management and communications, the contract negotiations process serves a symbolic function. The process assumes ritualistic characteristics with its predictable plot line, posturing with initial show of force, progression toward a climactic conclusion, delaying tactics, threats and bluffing, and dramatic last-hour concessions. While serving the explicit purpose of reaching an agreement, the process also allows the parties to re-enact symbolically the historical, economic, political, and sociocultural tensions and conflict between the laboring class and the owners of capital. This periodic playing out of the struggle between labor and management can be seen as contributing to conflict reduction over the long term.

In the typical contract negotiation process, representatives of both the organized employees (union) and management come to the table to bargain collectively over the terms of a written agreement (i.e., the contract). The agreement may address any items related to "wages, hours, and terms and conditions of employment" as mandated by the **National Labor Relations Act** and applicable to state laws governing collective bargaining. Both sides are represented by teams that advocate the collective interests of the parties. Typically, the union presents a list of demands that constitute its initial bargaining position. The list contains items that are intended as bargaining chips to be offered in exchange for more highly valued gains later in the negotiation process as well as items that are perceived (at least initially) as non-negotiable.

Management evaluates the union demands in terms of projected costs, perceived impact on employees not included in the bargaining unit, related human resource management policies, and preservation of management rights. It presents a written response stating its position on each of the demands. During a series of scheduled bargaining sessions, the area for common ground is explored as the less difficult issues are resolved first. At the same time, both parties indicate which issues have highest priority, those considered to be "sacred" and not subject to trading off or compromise. Considerable posturing and bluffing may characterize this phase as each party attempts to maximize its own bargaining position and identify points of vulnerability of the other side. Growing tensions and unresolved conflict may result in aggressive behavior, acting out emotional responses, breakdown in communications, and temporary withdrawal from the bargaining table.

If negotiations involving a health care organization reach an impasse on mandatory bargaining issues, under the 1974 Health Care Amendments to the National Labor Relations Act, parties must notify the Federal Mediation and Conciliation Service to initiate the mediation process to resolve the issue at impasse. A board of inquiry, appointed to serve as fact finder and mediator, presents a written report and set of recommendations for resolving the impasse. Although nonbinding, these recommendations typically carry considerable weight in the reaching of a final agreement between the parties. In some situations, a process of interest arbitration has been established within prevailing written agreements that requires an impartial external party to make a legally binding decision about unresolved issues to effect the final agreement. Under other circumstances, the union may call for a strike or other form of work action to dramatize its position on unresolved issues.

In the best case, the parties with or without formal mediation come to final agreement on all issues. Each party signs a written agreement that the union officials present to members in the bargaining unit for final ratification. On ratification, the written agreement becomes the basis for ongoing communication, conflict resolution, and problem solving for both parties during the life of the contract, typically 3 years in health care. The grievance procedures and rights arbitration process that are almost universally included in the written agreement provide mechanisms for ongoing administration of the contract, the resolution of conflicts in application of the contract, and the identification of areas for clarification or revision of contractual terms during subsequent negotiations. This becomes the basis for productive employer-employee relations and for the resolution of conflict.

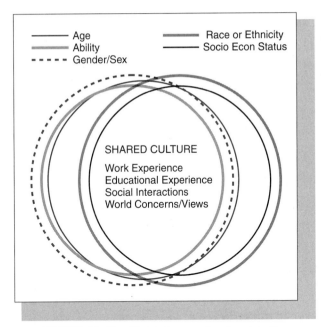

FIGURE 13–19. Model of occupational community.

HUMAN DIVERSITY AND MULTICULTURAL SENSITIVITY

As the workplace becomes increasingly segmented along both demographic and sociocultural dimensions, it is important for HIM professionals to develop a greater understanding and sensitivity to **human diversity** and multicultural issues. To be more effective, it is becoming increasingly important that managers actively facilitate an environment sensitive to individual differences and respectful of employee interests and abilities. By doing so, communication should improve, conflict decrease, and employee satisfaction and productivity increase.[74–82]

Although creating an ideology of personal employee empowerment and sensitivity may seem simple, in point of fact, this is a difficult task for any manager. Current political issues (e.g., political correctness toward Afro-Americans and women entering mainstream professional careers) may have raised the consciousness of a few, but in practice, little has changed. Indeed, concerns over the lack of sensitivity to individual differences are clearly reflected in trends to initiate human diversity and multicultural issues into management-training curricula.

As noted earlier in the quality management section of this chapter, the quality management philosophies being adopted by most health care organizations seem to argue for a standardization of organizational performance policies and practices and in viewing all employees as having the same levels of commitment, dedication, and ability.[1–3,5–12] Indeed, both traditional and quality management philosophies have focused on the importance of **organizational culture** in developing the employee's world view, ideology, and definition of self (Figure 13–19).[83–85] Behavioral and ideologic standards associated with organizational culture are perceived to be at the

center of how an employee defines personal attributes and determines specific responses to various social situations (i.e., defining the situational context). Individual differences are believed to be subsumed by organizational culture and values. Organizational and job identification become the primary sources of personal identification. For example, this perspective suggests that personal identification of the HIM professional would be as follows: first, as an HIM professional (i.e., the profession); second, as a specialist, manager, or director of an HIM department (i.e., position within the organization); and third, with the organization (e.g., hospital, health maintenance organization, university). Gender, age, marital status and children, and socioeconomic status demarcations are relegated to being peripheral identification markers. Consequently, the way you act, your values, and your personal associations become intimately tied to both professional and organizational values.

As noted earlier in this chapter, several quality management principles are based on the notion of the organization's being the primary determinant in defining self. Quality management principles are focused away from meeting individual needs and toward meeting organizational needs. This requires the acceptance of standardized organizational principles and beliefs about appropriate behavior. **Continuous quality improvement,** commitment and dedication to increasing productivity, and striving for zero defects are a few of the quality management buzz words that are based on theories of organizational culture.

In contrast to the organizational model, a management philosophy based on human diversity or multicul-

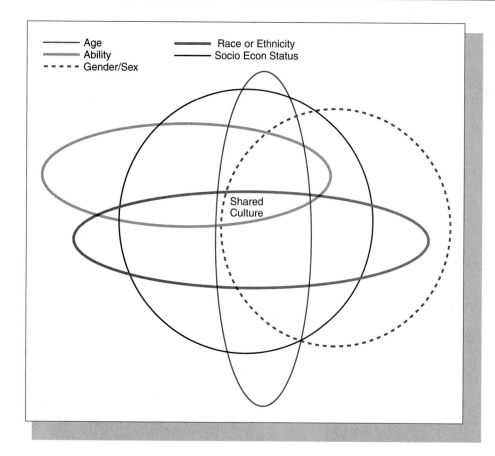

Age
Ability
Gender/Sex
Race or Ethnicity
Socio Econ Status

Shared Culture

FIGURE 13–20. Model of management sensitivity.

tural sensitivity emphasizes the value of individual attributes and contributions.[74–82,85] There is a recognition that each person has a unique past, characteristics, responsibilities away from the workplace, and personal strengths, weaknesses, and abilities. This position recognizes the importance of professional and organizational affiliations; however, employees are seen as much more than simply actors within the organizational culture. Age, marital status, children, community ties and responsibilities, ethnicity or race, socioeconomic status, and ability all play an important part in how a person comes to a definition and understanding of self (Figure 13–20).

Past histories and relationships play an important role in how each person perceives the world and selectively processes messages. As a result of these differences, each employee has the ability to play a dynamic role in shaping work relations. The way communication networks are created and maintained, how excellence and commitment are culturally operationalized and accepted, and how performance standards are administered are based on the dynamic integration of each employee into the work environment. To disregard past histories or sociocultural influences in all likelihood results in restricting or hindering the HIM manager's ability to ef-

fectively manage. For example, managing change is a primary responsibility for most HIM managers. The way in which change messages should be positioned is based on the ability of the manager to personalize messages in the most appropriate manner. This suggests that the manager should be sensitive to employee needs, understanding of employee abilities, and respectful of employee differences.

Earlier in this chapter, it was noted that the success of an HIM manager often depends on his or her ability to manage people. To effectively manage employees, it is important that HIM managers earn and maintain respect from employees. To earn and maintain respect from employees, HIM managers must, first, demonstrate respect for employee differences and, second, encourage employee involvement within the organizational structure at a personal level. Understanding that your employees are the organization's most valued resources implies that you as a manager must take the initiative to act in developing the personal strengths of each employee. Consequently, two of the most important keys to becoming a successful quality manager are developing high levels of sensitivity to employee differences and similarities and taking proactive action that will integrate all employees into a cohesive unit.

INTEGRATING QUALITY AND EXCELLENCE INTO DAILY ROUTINES

As an HIM manager, it is easy to get caught up in total quality management exhortations of commitment and dedication, quality, and excellence. Cost containment, downsizing, striving for **zero defects,** and an ever-increasing emphasis on improving productivity have become a reality within most health care organizations. Although it is important for HIM managers and professionals to strive toward excellence in their work, it is equally important that an atmosphere of civility and equity be established. An effective management style should be focused on creating a work environment of integrity and honesty, open communication, respect, and compassion. To be effective as an HIM manager, you need to be responsive to organizational demands as well as employee needs. More often than not, this requires you as a health care manager or HIM professional to walk a fine line where you must judge between equally compelling demands. Striking a balance where organizational and employee needs converge may be one of the most taxing yet important tasks of the manager.

For the HIM manager to be responsive to employee needs and to be increasingly productive in terms of organizational expectations, high levels of trust between management and employees must be established and maintained. For trust to be developed and maintained, a work environment of open communication, honesty and integrity, and respect for employee differences should be created. The first step in creating an atmosphere of trust is to ensure that open communication exists between management and employees (see Achieving Excellence). It is important that the manager clearly communicates work expectations and priorities. Employee input into the decision-making process should be encouraged when appropriate. The staff should feel comfortable in approaching the HIM manager with any type of work-related issue. Second, as an HIM manager, you must establish a pattern of honesty and integrity in your dealings with employees[10] (see Creating Integrity). As a manager, you must honestly care about your employees as people by demonstrating a belief in basic human values. There should be a high degree of consistency in work-related decisions regarding employee behavior. The HIM manager should demonstrate the ability to deal equitably and in a timely manner with all employees. Honest mistakes, especially those based on creative risk taking, should never be punished. The third step in establishing a work environment of trust centers around respect of each employee[10] (see Achieving Success in Management). Effective management begins and ends with respect and concern for the needs of employees. Your employees are the most valuable resources of your organization. It is necessary that each employee feel important and that he or she is making an integral

Achieving Excellence

- Communicate to employees what is expected of them on the job day to day.
- Operationalize work priorities to avoid confusion and plan for progress.
- Manage by walking around to better understand the needs of employees.
- Maintain a professional atmosphere in which employees are respected for their individuality.
- Understand that change is an integral part of the process of excellence.
- Never discourage innovation or creativity.
- Initiate unbiased evaluation standards.
- Concentrate on asking questions and listening rather than on telling.
- Appreciate and reward success. This will, in all likelihood, create repetition of the behavior.
- There are no stupid or silly questions that are beneath your full and immediate response.
- Immediate response to any situation is necessary.
- Open communication channels to allow employee input and participation in work-related decision making.
- Never close yourself off to employees.

contribution to the success of both the department and the organization. This suggests that the HIM manager should respect and value the contributions of all employees. Not all employees will have the same commitment, time, or ability to contribute equally in meeting organizational demands. The ability of the manager to understand differences and then help develop strengths often results in higher levels of productivity and job satisfaction. Employees should be rewarded for contributions and encouraged to be involved at personal levels of comfort. Creating a two-tier culture in which a few

Creating Integrity

- Honestly care about your employees as people, not just their work performance.
- Orient management goals to create an open atmosphere of trust.
- Never punish honest mistakes or failures or place responsibility for failure on the employees (scapegoating).
- Establish an atmosphere of customer service and follow-up.
- Show a belief in basic human values of human dignity, human fallibility, and human needs.
- Tell subordinates when they do not meet standards, and show them how to improve performance.
- You must build trust and win the participation of all workers.

Achieving Success in Management

- *Respect*. Good management begins and ends with respect and concern for the needs of employees and self.

- *Stimulate*. Every person in your organization can and will make a contribution if given the opportunity. No bad questions or answers. Your job is to stimulate interest and development.

- *Serve*. You are there to serve your employees. A good manager will facilitate personal growth and development among employees.

- *Prepare*. Prepare for tasks each day. Employees know if you are not prepared. It is a sign you do not care.

- *Pay Attention*. Every person in your organization is an individual. Each person has a different history and life agenda. You must be cognizant of individual differences.

- *Use Common sense*. Do the right thing.

- *Be Flexible*. There are no hard and fast rules in management that cover all situations. You must be flexible.

are valued and rewarded while others are perceived as second-class citizens of the organization will, in most cases, lead to conflict and lower levels of overall productivity among employees.

The human diversity management style offered in this chapter does *not* mean that all employees will be rewarded equally, or that employees will *not* be held accountable or responsible for assigned responsibilities and performance effectiveness, or that employees are *not* expected to strive toward excellence. The type of management or leadership style based on personal empowerment, as suggested in this chapter, is based on a philosophy of employee responsibility and the need for health care professionals to strive for continuous quality and excellence in providing health care services. It is the manager's responsibility to motivate and facilitate employee involvement and growth within the organization. This perspective suggests that the most effective way of ensuring productivity is to create an atmosphere of collegiality and cooperation. The goal is to create a collaborative culture in which all employees are placed in a win-win situation. This is likely to be accomplished by developing a leadership style that is respectful of employee differences and nurturing of employee strengths and abilities.

Unlike the more technical areas of health information management (e.g., coding, medical terminology), when dealing with employees in social settings, there are no formulas that provide answers for all management situations. There is no laundry list describing set patterns of behavior that will explain all the dynamic combinations of interactions between workers in an HIM department. At times, you will make mistakes in judgment. At other times, you will exceed expectations. There is no cook book solution that can tell you how to interact with others or how to manage. The essence of succeeding in both areas is to develop your own knowledge base, skills, and insight in human relations, so that over the long term, you will "do the right thing."

References

1. Crosby PB: Quality is free: The art of making quality certain. New York: McGraw-Hill, 1979.
2. Bassett LC, Metzger N: Achieving excellence: A prescription for health care managers. Rockville, MD: Aspen Publishers, 1986.
3. Deming WE: Out of the crises. Cambridge, MA: MIT Center of Advanced Engineering Study, 1986.
4. Haimann T: Supervisory management for health care organizations. St. Louis: Catholic Health Association of the United States, 1989.
5. Logothetis N: Managing total quality: From Deming to Tagguchi and SPC. Englewood Cliffs, NJ: Prentice-Hall, 1992.
6. Juran JM: Quality planning and analysis. New York: McGraw-Hill, 1980.
7. Juran JM: Juran on planning for quality. New York: The Free Press, 1988.
8. Robbins SP: Organizational Theory: Structure, Design and Application. Englewood Cliffs, NJ: Prentice-Hall, 1988.
9. Deming WE: Quality, productivity and competitive position. Cambridge, MA: MIT Center of Advanced Engineering Study, 1982.
10. Rudman WJ, Mazzoni J: Myth of the empowering manager: Communicating a vision. Topics in Health Information Management 1992;13(2):29–35.
11. Peters T, Waterman RH: In search of excellence. New York: Alfred A. Knopf, 1984.
12. Peters T, Austin N: A passion for excellence. New York: Alfred A. Knopf, 1986.
13. Lewis PV: Organizational communication: The essence of effective management. Columbus, OH: Grid Publishing, 1980.
14. Baird JE, Diebolt JC: Role congruence, communication, supervisor-subordinate relations, and employee satisfaction in organizational hierarchies. Western Speech Communication 1976;40(4):260–269.
15. Disalva V, Laesen D, Seiler W: Common skills needed by persons in business organizations. Communication Education 1976;25:273–275.
16. Downs CW, Hazen MD: A factor analysis study of communication satisfaction. Journal of Business Communication 1977;14(3):63–73.
17. Golden S, Boissoneu R: Health care supervisors identify communication barriers in their supervisor subordinate relationships. Health Care Supervisor 1987;6(1):26–36.
18. Roberts DF: The nature of human communication effects. *In* Schamm W, Roberts DF (eds): Process and effects of mass communication, Rev ed. Urbana: University of Illinois Press, 1971.
19. Umiker W: Powerful communication skills: The key to prevention and resolution of personnel problems. Health Care Supervisor 1986;4(3):30–34.
20. Carnevale AP, Gainer LJ, Meltzer AS: Workplace basics—the essential skills employers want. San Francisco: Jossey-Bass, 1990.
21. Westly BH, Maclean MS: A conceptual model for communication research. Journalism Quarterly 1957;34:31–38.
22. Fisher D: Communication in organizations. St. Paul: West Publishing, 1981.
23. Goldhaber GM, Porter DJ, Yates MP, Lesniak R: Organiza-

tional communication. Human Communication Research 1978;5(1):76–96.

24. Berlo DK: The process of communication. New York: Holt, Rinehart & Winston, 1960.

25. Rogers EM, Kincaid DL: Communication networks. New York: The Free Press, 1981.

26. Huffman EK: Medical record management. 9th ed. Berwyn, FL: Physicians Record Company, 1990.

27. Thomas KW: Conflict and conflict management. In Duncan MD (ed): Handbook of Industrial and Organizational Psychology. Chicago: Rand McNally, 1976, p 889.

28. Lyles RI, Joiner C: Supervision in health care organizations. New York: John Wiley & Sons, 1986.

29. Kramer M, Schmalenberg C: Conflict: The cutting edge of growth. Journal of Nursing Administration 1976;VI(8):19–25.

30. Robbins SP: Management: Concepts and practices. Englewood Cliffs, NJ: Prentice-Hall, 1984.

31. Robbins SP: Managing organizational conflict: A non-traditional approach. Englewood Cliffs, NJ: Prentice-Hall, 1974.

32. McConnell CR: The effective health care supervision. 3rd ed. Gaithersburg, MD: Aspen Publishers, 1993.

33. Robbins SP: Organization theory: Structure, design and application. 3rd ed. Englewood Cliffs, NJ: Prentice-Hall, 1989.

34. Banker LL, Whalers KJ, Watson KW, Kibler RJ: Groups in process: An introduction to small group communication. 4th ed. Englewood Cliffs, NJ: Prentice-Hall, 1991.

35. Vecchio RP: Organizational behavior. Chicago: Dryden Press, 1988.

36. Bach GR, Wyden P: The intimate energy. New York: William Morrow & Co, 1969.

37. Tompkins PK: Communicator as action: An intro to rhetoric and communication. Belmont, CA: Wadsworth Publishing Co, 1982.

38. Senge P: The learning organization. New York: Doubleday/Currency, 1992, p 10.

39. Homan G: Fatigue of workers: Its relation to industrial production. New York: Reinhold Publishing Corp, 1941.

40. Mayo E: The human problems of an industrial civilization. New York: Macmillan, 1933.

41. Griffin R: Management. Boston: Houghton Mifflin, 1984.

42. Huber G: Managerial decision making. Glenview, IL: Scott, Foresman & Co, 1980.

43. Bennis W, Schein E (eds): Leadership and motivation: Essays of Douglas McGregor. Cambridge, MA: MIT Press, 1966.

44. Tead O: The art of leadership. New York: Whittlesey House, 1935.

45. Hemphill J: Situational factors in leadership. Columbus, OH: Ohio State University, Bureau of Educational Research, 1949.

46. Blake R, Mouton J: The managerial grid. Houston: Gulf Publishing Co, 1964.

47. Slevin D: The whole manager. New York: AMACOM, 1989.

48. Vroom V, Jago A: The new leadership: Managing participation in organizations. Englewood Cliffs, NJ: Prentice-Hall, 1988.

49. Fiedler F, Chermers M: Leadership and effective management. Glenview, IL: Scott, Foresman & Co, 1974.

50. Hersey P, Blanchard K: Management of organizational behavior: Utilizing human resources. Englewood Cliffs, NJ: Prentice-Hall, 1982.

51. House R, Mitchell T: Path-goal theory of leadership. Journal of Contemporary Business 1974;3(4):81–97.

52. Lawler E: Job design and employee motivation. Personnel Psychology 1969;22:426–435.

53. Bass B: Leadership and performance beyond expectations. New York: The Free Press, 1985.

54. Avolio B, Bass B: Transformational leadership, charisma, and beyond. In Hunt J, Baliga B, Dachler H, Schriesheim C (eds): Emerging leadership vistas. Lexington, MA: Lexington Books, 1988, pp 29–49.

55. Hollander E: Processes of leadership emergence. Journal of Contemporary Business 1974;3(4):19–33.

56. Burns J: Leadership. New York: Harper & Row, 1978.

57. Rohrer W: The three T's of leadership: Leadership theory evisited. Topics in Health Records Management 1989;9(3):14–25.

58. Omachonu U, Ross J: Principles of total quality. DelRay Beach, FL: St. Cucie Press, 1994.

59. Joint Commission on Accreditation of Healthcare Organizations: A pocket guide to quality improvement tools. Oak Brook Terrace, IL: 1992.

60. Joint Commission on Accreditation of Healthcare Organizations: The measurement mandate. Oak Brook Terrace, IL: 1993.

61. Abdelhak MA, Anania-Firouzan P: Hospital information systems applications and potential: A literature review revisited. Topics in Health Information Management 1995;13(4):1–14.

62. Lytle SJ, Lytle BV: Getting back to healthcare: The new automation strategy. Journal of the American Health Information Management Association 1992;63(10):66–71.

63. Billings M: Be a re-engineer. For the Record, January 25, 1993, 5, 28.

64. Wilson A: A strategy of change. London: Routledge, 1992.

65. Rudman WJ: Implementing change in the work redesign process. Topics in Health Information Management 1994;14(4):59–67.

66. Rudman WJ, Lippiny A: Evaluating and inventing change in health care procedures, association of management. Association of Management International Conference 1993;5(9):13–19.

67. Plant R: Managing change and making it stick. London: Fontaner, 1987.

68. Morgan G: Riding the waves of change. London: Sage, 1989.

69. Dunphy DC, Stace DA: Transformational and coercive strategies for planned organizational change. Organizational Studies 1988;9(3):317–334.

70. Fisher R, Ury W: Getting to yes: Negotiating agreement without giving in. New York: Penguin Books, 1984.

71. Metzger N, Malvey D: Negotiating and administering the labor relations contract. In Fottler M, Hernandez SR, Joiner C (eds): Strategic management of human resources in health services organizations. New York: Wiley Medical, 1994, pp 438–479.

72. Fossum J: Labor relations: Development, structure, process. Homewood, IL: BPI/IRWIN, 1989, p 247.

73. Asante MK: Afrocentricity. Trenton, NY: Africa World Press, 1988.

74. Gould SJ: The mismeasurement of man. New York: WW Norton, 1981.

75. Grossman HW, Grossman S: Gender issues in education. Boston: Allyn & Bacon, 1994.

76. Hale J, Benson J: Black children: Their roots, cults, and learning styles. Baltimore: The Johns Hopkins University Press, 1988.

77. Heath SB: Wars with words. New York: Cambridge University Press, 1983.

78. Kent G: Department of Education: Sexism: What no one even said, but everyone told you. Frant Pert, Dept. of Education, 1986.

79. Kenben L: Women of the republic: Intellect and ideology in revolutionary America. New York: WW Norton, 1980.

80. Cochman T: Black and white styles in conflict. Chicago: University of Chicago Press, 1981.

81. Nieto S: Affirming diversity: Political context of multicultural education. White Plains, NY: Longman, 1992.

82. Banks J: Introduction to multicultural education. Boston: Allyn & Bacon, 1994.

83. Schein EH: Organizational culture and human performance. San Francisco: Jossey-Bass, 1986.

84. Van Mannen J, Barley SR: Occupational communities: Culture and control in organizations. Research in Organizational Behavior 1984;6:287–365.

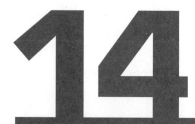

RITA A. SCICHILONE and CAROL J. BARR

HUMAN RESOURCES MANAGEMENT

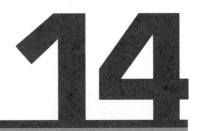

14

Employee handbooks
Employment "at will"
Equal Opportunity Employment
Ergonomics
Factor comparison
Flextime
Grievance procedure
Halo effect
Human resource audit
Human resource planning
Job analysis
Job description
Job enrichment
Job evaluation
Job grading
Job performance standards
Job ranking
Job sharing
Layoffs
Office landscaping
Open office design plan
Performance appraisal

Placement
Point system
Preventive discipline
Proactive human resource management
Progressive discipline
Promotion
Protected group
Proximity chart
Rating scale
Reasonable accommodation
Recruitment
Relative humidity
Replacement charts
Selection process
Seniority
Sexual harassment
Staffing table
Task (accent) lighting
Task-ambient lighting
Training
Trip frequency chart
Undue hardship
Workstation

ABBREVIATIONS

ADA—Americans with Disabilities Act
ADEA—Age Discrimination in Employment Act
BLS—Bureau of Labor Statistics
CTD—Cumulative trauma disorders
db—decibels
EAP—Employee Assistance Program
EEOC—Equal Employment Opportunity Commission
EPA—Environmental Protection Agency
FLSA—Fair Labor Standards Act
FMLA—Family Medical Leave Act
FTE—Full-time equivalent
HVAC—Heating, ventilation, and air conditioning
NIOSH—National Institute for Occupational Safety and Health
NLRA—National Labor Relations Act
NLRB—National Labor Relations Board
OFCCP—Office of Federal Contract Compliance Program
OSHA—Occupational Safety and Health Administration/Act
RSI—Repetitive Stress/Strain Injury
VDT—Video display terminal

OBJECTIVES

- Define key words.
- List and explain the human resource management responsibilities of all managers.
- Discuss the external and internal environmental challenges that face a health information services department manager into the 21st century.
- Apply the legislative and regulatory agency requirements for managing employees in a health care organization.
- Describe the societal, organizational, functional, and personal objectives and activities of human resources management in health care organizations.
- Understand the systems model of human resource management as it applies to health information services.
- Develop methods of recruiting, selection, retaining, and terminating employees that staff a health information services department.
- Describe various performance evaluation and compensation management programs used in health care organizations.
- Implement effective strategies for building a health information management team.
- Describe orientation and training needs for health information services departments.
- Define and explain career planning programs for health information management personnel.
- Outline the considerations that must be examined in designing work space for health information services.
- Apply the employee's individual needs to the design of work space.
- Describe the components of a work station.

CHALLENGES OF HUMAN RESOURCES MANAGEMENT IN HEALTH INFORMATION SERVICES DEPARTMENT INTO THE 21ST CENTURY

Managing health information in the 21st century will place special demands on health information management (HIM) professionals to recruit and manage the human resources required to achieve the goals of health care organizations. It is predicted that the health care labor force of the future will demand multiskilled

469

workers who have the flexibility of working in various provider settings within new integrated health care systems. Health information managers and specialists will be required to staff health care delivery systems that emphasize preventive and longitudinal care, which may not be restricted to one provider or level of care. As organizational changes mandated by health reform converge during the next century, health information managers must be prepared to respond to the accompanying restructuring of the workforce that will follow.

This chapter explores the requirements of human resource management, with a special focus toward managing health information services in a dynamic environment. Scattered throughout the chapter are some examples drawn from actual human resource management situations that HIM professionals have experienced. The questions included with the examples are intended to be rhetorical, to encourage creative thinking and problem solving by the reader. In most of these situations, as in the reality of the workplace, there is no one right answer. A manager of people must learn to evaluate and react to situations based on limited information. The reader is encouraged to use these scenarios to consider possible options in human resource management and examine the resulting consequences of taking action.

One of the most important roles that the HIM professional can assume in human resource management is strategic planning. This is a **proactive human resource management** activity rather than reactive in managing the workflow in health information services. This type of planning anticipates and prepares for future staffing needs. The greater the number of workers employed by the service and the greater the degree of complexity in the interrelationships between jobs that exists in the organization, the more important systematic **human resource planning** becomes in providing health information services.

Planning improves utilization of resources by providing a planned method of matching personnel with organizational or departmental goals and objectives. A human resource plan can achieve economies in hiring new workers because similar positions can be recruited at the same time, saving multiple expenses, and be oriented and trained as a group rather than individually.

As health information services become more distributive, with organizationwide accountability rather than departmentalized functions, astute planning becomes an essential role for the HIM executive.

A major advantage of human resource planning for the HIM professional is the readily available reference document that shows the departmental resource considerations impacted by expansion or downsizing of department operations. This allows the health information manager to respond to a number of "what if" questions for the organization. For example, if a digitized patient

record is to be implemented within the year, record filing positions will no longer be needed. If a plan is prepared 6 months to 1 year in advance, these employees can be retrained or transferred to another division so that terminations and **layoffs** are prevented. On the other hand, more data imaging and analysis staff will be required, so **recruitment** or **training** can be initiated early on to meet this need. Planning assures that both external environmental challenges and internal challenges can be confidently met by the HIM professional.

EXAMPLE

Memorial Hospital has decided to provide medical language specialists to process medical dictation for a large group practice that adjoins the building. The human resources plan will analyze how many specialists will be needed and then recruit, train, and orient them at the same time. It is believed that this will be more cost-effective than training each specialist individually. The plan could also lay the groundwork for hospital employees to be trained as backup staff. Because this work is likely to ebb and flow, contingency plans for contracted transcription support should also be made. Because this plan exists, the health information manager can be confident when she guarantees reliable and uninterrupted services for these physicians.

What other applications are there in health information management for human resource planning?

External Challenges

The structure and function of health care organizations and providers are constantly changing to adapt to the external environment. The organization is often powerless to control these outside forces, so it must create the appropriate human resource management processes that allow challenges to be met in the most cost-effective ways. Some challenges evolve slowly, such as the impact of women joining the workforce over the past 20 years. As women began working outside the home in increasing numbers, a need was created for different types of benefit programs and work schedules.

Other challenges occur suddenly, as when new laws or court rulings are passed and must be immediately followed. For example, in 1990, the Americans with Disabilities Act (ADA) created regulations that affected human resource management in every health care organization. Also in 1993, the Family Medical Leave Act (FMLA) was signed into law, which forced many employers to examine and revise policies and procedures concerning time off and job security when a family illness occurs.

Today's organizational environmental challenges may be as close as the neighborhood where the building is located or as far reaching as the global community. There are a number of environmental factors that impact health care organizations that merit further discussion as they relate to human resource management and information management.

Health care reform measures taken to reduce costs and improve the efficiency and access to health care systems are one example. Any deep budgetary cuts in Medicare and Medicaid reimbursement by the government will force many organizations to trim staffing and look for ways to decrease health care resources and functions provided per visit. Unless increased access to care and its associated reimbursement will improve health care revenues and profit margins, health care reform legislation measures will probably reduce the number of new jobs and opportunities for growth within the health care sector.

Managed-care programs and health networks will redefine the organizational structure and business processes of delivering health services. Recommendations proposed by some reform plans will change the way business is conducted and information is managed between providers and payers. This opens up a whole new industry centered around electronically based clinical information collection and transfer, perhaps using patient-carried cards or accessing clinical data repositories by way of fiberoptic networks. A number of similar external challenges will continue to be significant factors in how health care providers manage information services and the human resources required to provide them.

Technology

Technology continues to be the most significant change agent that will impact human resources in the HIM profession. Repetitive, clerical, and filing functions performed by people in the past are being replaced by computerization. Because this evolving technology facilitates easier and more meaningful methods of collecting and displaying data for analysis, new jobs are being created for HIM professionals to use information from these newly developed management tools.

New medical equipment and techniques are changing the way medicine is practiced. This affects the types and methods of data collection that are required. Health care providers are seeking new ways to keep clinicians free to provide care to patients instead of spending a disproportionate amount of time documenting past events. Event-capturing information systems, such as videotape, can provide more accurate and timely information capture with less effort by clinicians and provide a higher value back to the patient than after-the-fact, text-based documentation methods. This type of information management can change the job titles, **job descriptions**, and the duties of health information services departments.

Digitized documentation can be transmitted over fiberoptic networks, which may cause facilities to manage incoming and outgoing data from other organizations as well as internally generated information. Human resource managers must accommodate continually changing approaches to information capture, transfer, and retrieval.

EXAMPLE

The health information manager at the University Medical Center is a key department head position. A new telemedicine program has been developed so that rural hospitals can use university specialists as consultants without the patient being transferred. The system transmits digital signals over a fiberoptic network, using special equipment. The "record" that results from this interchange is videotape that is captured during the interchange between the consultant and the referring physician. The chief executive officer has asked the health information manager to decide how many additional full-time equivalents (FTE) are needed to manage these records.

How will this new technology affect current record-processing staffing patterns?

What types of information are needed to decide if the human resources in the health information department will be affected?

Economy

Economic challenges always have an impact on human resources because the economy determines the number of staff as well as the compensation packages the organization can afford. Economic cycles in the local, national, and even the global economy always affect management of human resources.

It is critical for managers to try to anticipate economic climates. Organizations that monitor economic trends can avoid sudden crises in the human resources function by anticipating and planning shifts in the economy. If the economy is in a recession because of local unemployment or natural disaster situations, open positions should not be filled until the economy stabilizes. Instead, contracted services or temporary help can be used until the organization is sure that jobs are secure. This minimizes the human suffering of layoffs and reduction of hours for regular staff.

Sometimes, for economic reasons, downsizing of the workforce must occur. Termination for this purpose is termed layoff, involuntary separation, or required staffing adjustment. Layoffs, or "staffing adjustments," can take several forms. Reduction in worked hours, changing a full-time position to a shared position, and loss of positions by attrition are all methods of cost reduction that minimize the human suffering experienced by laid-off workers. Severance pay and outplacement assistance may be offered to assist the employee in the transition to another job or a period of unemployment. Respect for the employee's feelings and preservation of the worker's dignity are of utmost importance.

In a prosperous economy, the focus may be on recruitment of new workers to fuel organizational expansion. Health economic cycles may demand examination of staffing and compensation programs to remain competitive as workers become more mobile and turnover increases. Sometimes this is referred to as "right sizing."

EXAMPLE

> The manager of health information at a 50-bed rural hospital has a variety of duties, including human resource management. Because of Medicare and Medicaid budget cuts, the hospital lost more than $1 million last year. The hospital administrator announced at a department meeting one day and told each department head that they must reduce staffing by 25 per cent. There are four full-time employees. Two are single parents who have no other source of income. One is married to a successful lawyer and works "just to stay busy." The other employee is a recent graduate of the Accredited Record Technician (ART) program who has introduced some innovative and money-saving ideas into the department.
>
> What options are available to this manager to comply with the request that would result in a minimum of adverse reactions?

One of the most ominous challenges in the external environment for the 21st century is the introduction of strong competition and managed-care plans into the health care services industry. This makes health care organizations more cost-conscious, profit-driven, and business-oriented than ever. The effect on human resource management and staffing is the assurance of efficient health care delivery without a decline in the quality of services. Right sizing is a necessary function in human resource management just to survive.

Cultural Changes in the Workforce

MULTICULTURAL WORKFORCE. A number of cultural changes evolving in the United States present challenges in human resource management. The population continues to become more diversified in all areas of the country as minority groups increase in the workforce. The U.S. Department of Labor Statistics predicts an influx of Asians, Hispanics, blacks, and women into the workforce, followed by an exodus of white men (see Workforce 2005). Current workers scheduled to retire are likely to be men and almost one half will be white. The Bureau of the Census predicts that by the year 2000, whites will represent only 72 per cent of the population, down from 80 per cent in 1993.

Workforce 2005

Who's entering the workforce?
Hispanics: a 75% increase
Asians and others: a 74% increase
Blacks: a 32% increase
Women: a 26% increase

Who's leaving the workforce?
White, non-Hispanic males: 82% of those leaving

Source: Kutscher, Ronald E. "New BLS projections: findings and implications." *Monthly Labor Review,* Nov. 1991, Vol. 114, Number 11

WOMEN IN THE WORKFORCE. Over the past two decades, there has been a rapid increase in the participation of women in the workforce. This trend has increased the labor pool for the traditionally female health services jobs of nurses, housekeepers, food service workers, and clerical staff.

The increase of women in the workforce and the subsequent increase of working parents have affected benefits and work schedules. **Cafeteria benefit plans,** in which employees can choose from an array of benefits to fit their needs or lifestyle, are common. For example, working parents may choose a discount on child care, whereas a childless worker may choose dental insurance. Paternity leaves for both mother and father and personal days for sick children are additional examples of ways employers have responded to this cultural trend.

Job sharing and **flextime** are used to accommodate individuals' needs. Job sharing occurs when a full-time position is shared by two or more persons. This has advantages for both the employer and the employee. The employer has built-in coverage for vacations or illness. If additional work hours are needed, two persons are able and available to perform the job without overtime pay. Advantages for the employee are that schedules may be arranged to accommodate child care or other lifestyle situations.

Flextime allows employees to control their work schedule within parameters established by management. The employer usually has some type of core structure, such as days or hours, that the employee must work to provide needed services. The start and stop times can be flexible around these core hours. Other employers allow flexible scheduling but require the employee to schedule themselves in advance (i.e., 2 weeks to 1 month ahead). The use of flextime often depends on the tasks performed and how they affect department operations. If a certain amount of work must be performed in a given time period, the start and stop times and day of the week worked may be unimportant and the employee may be allowed to work at will, provided the required number of hours or tasks are completed.

Work Ethics Over the Generations

1930–1940	In the depression era, people feared their bosses as they worked to survive. Human resource management consisted of the boss's threat "Work, or else you'll lose your job." Workers from this era seldom spoke up about problems on the job. They were grateful to have the job and still feared the manager.
1940–1950	In the decade after World War II, the economy was booming. Workers from this period were motivated by higher salaries. Communication skills became recognized as important for leadership of employees rather than fear.
1950–1970	In this time period, personnel management became a profession in its own right. Participative management began to allow workers some input into how things were done, and the importance of the psychological rewards of work was stressed.
1970–1990	From 1970 through the end of the 1980s, human resource management programs experienced the **"job enrichment"** years. Employees began to relate job content to personal preferences so that work could be meaningful to them. Management by objective methods placed strong emphasis on individual potential and creating short- and long-term goals to achieve it. Personal sacrifices were common to achieve promotions and climb career ladders. This was the period of the women's movement, and the stereotype of the superwoman who could "do it all" was created. Yuppies and dinks were born (young, upwardly mobile professionals and dual-income no kids couples) and were written and spoken about as part of the workplace culture.
1990s	During the 1990s, some human resource professionals believe that the culture is moving from this job enrichment era to a culture with a 1990s lifestyle enrichment emphasis. This suggests that the workforce of tomorrow will value their leisure time more than they do their jobs. This baby-buster generation is the newest generation in the workplace and the smallest in the United States. They grew up with the information and communication revolution as a result of satellite television and personal computers. They are more educated than any other generation, and because they are so well informed, they take a global view of events. These workers are goal-oriented but want to actively participate in work procedures and management. They value their not-at-work time more than previous generations and are willing to trade job enrichment for lifestyle enrichment.

Another cultural trend plays itself out in many of the interpersonal relationships that are found in health care organizations. As the roles of men and women in our society become less defined, some groups need to learn to work effectively together. For example, perceptions of the nurse-physician relationship are changing. In the past, nearly all physicians were men and nurses were women. Now increasing numbers of physicians are women and male nurses are more common.

In health information services, most positions have been traditionally held by women in the past three decades. As these male/female roles continue to dilute in our culture, it is expected that more diversity in the staff of the health information services department also will occur.

AGE. Various sources cite three generation groups present in the workplace today. People who were raised in the depression era, born in the 1930s and 1940s, who are approaching retirement; the baby boomer (now middle-aged) generation; and the newly christened baby busters, born after 1963, each approach their work life with a slightly different philosophy. The members of each group have their own outlook and similar opinions about what they expect from their jobs and their managers (see Work Ethics Over the Generations).

Regulatory Requirements for Human Resource Management

An array of regulatory requirements mandated by the government through state and federal legislation affect human resource management in health care organizations (Table 14–1). These laws affect personnel management through the recruitment and hiring process to the safety of the workplace.

EXAMPLE

Health information services had been 100 per cent female for as long as the current department director can remember. Then last summer, two young male college students applied for health record analyst positions on the evening shift. Because they met the job qualifications and were eager to work, they were hired. At the last manager's meeting, the evening supervisor expressed a concern about the behavior of these employees. Because they are avid sports fans, they often bring in a portable television set and watch sporting events as they work. Female employees have always been permitted to play a radio on the evening shift, provided they used earphones.

What two cultural factors may be at work here? How can this problem be handled with a minimum of conflict and work disruption?

TABLE 14–1 FEDERAL REGULATIONS AND AGENCIES THAT AFFECT HUMAN RESOURCES

LEGISLATION OR AGENCY	EFFECTIVE DATE	PEOPLE AFFECTED AND KEY POINTS
Joint Commission on Accreditation of Healthcare Organizations	Ongoing	Voluntary accreditation Leadership and organizational performance
Occupational Safety and Health Act	1970	Safe and healthy environment for all workers
Fair Labor Standards Act	1938; amended 1963	Sets minimum wage, overtime pay, equal pay, child labor, and record-keeping requirements for employers; 1963 Equal Pay Amendment forbids sex discrimination in pay practices.
National Labor Relations Act (Wagner Act)	1935	Gives employees the right to collective actions and outlaws unfair labor
Labor Management Relations Act (Taft-Hartley Act)	1947	Outlaws unfair labor practices by unions
Labor Management Reporting and Disclosure Act	1959	Forces unions to properly represent their members' interest
Civil Rights and Affirmative Action	1964	Prohibits discrimination on the basis of race, color, religion, sex, or national origin
Vietnam Era Veterans' Readjustment Assistance Act	1974	Affirmative efforts to provide employment for qualified disabled veterans and veterans of the Vietnam era
Age Discrimination in Employment Act	1967	Protects employees between the ages of 40 and 70
Americans with Disabilities Act	1992	Outlaws discrimination against disabled people and assures reasonable accommodation for them in the workplace
Family Medical Leave Act	1993	Grants unpaid leave and provides job security to employees who must take time off for medical reasons for themselves or family members

JOINT COMMISSION ON ACCREDITATION OF HEALTHCARE ORGANIZATIONS. Many organizations also submit themselves to voluntary accreditation by agencies such as the Joint Commission for the Accreditation of Healthcare Organizations (JCAHO). The JCAHO publishes standards to measure the effectiveness of leadership, human resource management, and organizational performance in health care organizations. The 1994 *Accreditation Manual for Hospitals* contains standards that assess the human resources management service functions of planning, directing, implementing, coordinating, and improving services. These organizational performance standards address such issues as doing the right things and doing the right things well in collective employee performance.[1]

SAFETY THROUGH THE OCCUPATIONAL HEALTH AND SAFETY ACT. The Occupational Health and Safety Act (OSHA) was passed in 1970. In passing OSHA, Congress declared that the intent was "to assure so far as possible every working man and woman in the nation

safe and healthful working conditions and to preserve our human resources."

OSHA covers all workers except those who are self-employed or protected under other federal agencies and those who work on family-owned and -operated farms. It has jurisdiction over every chemical substance, piece of equipment, and work environment that possesses even a potential threat to worker health and safety. The extremely detailed OSHA standards are administered by the Occupational Safety and Health Administration. This agency issues work and safety standards and inspections on a routine and surprise basis.

Health care organizations are not exempted from OSHA's oversight. They are required to communicate to employees information on the known risks associated with any hazardous materials encountered on the job. All hazardous materials must be labeled as such. A written orientation and training program must be developed and used to educate all employees.

Examples of hazards that may impact health information management are the safety of electronic equipment operation and exposure to hazardous materials, such as alkaline batteries. Protection from exposure to communicable disease may also be required by OSHA for employees who have patient contact.

Record-keeping requirements are extensive but constitute the only effective method of tracking, identifying, and correcting safety and health hazards. Detailed reports must be filed for all occupation-related injuries, illnesses, and deaths.

Through OSHA, the U.S. government has tried to provide physical security by imposing a duty on employers to provide a safe and healthy workplace. Severe penalties are imposed on organizations that violate this law because violations could lead to serious injuries or industrial diseases.

COMPENSATION

Fair Labor Standards Act. The Fair Labor Standards Act (FLSA) of 1938 affects compensation management in the United States. It sets minimum wage, overtime pay, equal pay, child labor, and record-keeping requirements for employers. For every "covered" job, overtime pay at one-and-a-half times the employee's regular rate of pay must be paid for every hour past 40 worked in a week. Several categories of workers—executive, administrative, and professional—are exempt from this act and hence exempt from the overtime provisions.

Equal Pay Act. In 1963, Fair Labor Standards Act was amended by the Equal Pay Act. This was passed to eliminate sex-based discrimination in pay practices. It requires employers to pay men and women equal wages when the jobs that they perform are equal in skill, effort, and responsibility and are performed under equal working conditions. Exceptions are allowed for valid merit or seniority award systems or when personal productivity determines compensation, such as in sales commissions.

LABOR UNION LEGISLATION

National Labor Relations Act. This legislation, also known as the Wagner Act, became law in 1935. It was passed during the depression years in an attempt to minimize disruption of interstate commerce by labor strikes. This law gives employees the right to collective action free of employer interference or repercussion. It gives employees the right to form labor unions and bargain with organizational management about wages, hours, and working conditions.

It also prohibits the following unfair labor practices:

- To interfere, restrain, or coerce employees who desire to act collectively or refrain from such activities

- To dominate or interfere with the formation or administration of any labor organization by contributing money or other support to it

- To discriminate against anyone in hiring, stability of employment, or any other condition of employment because of their union activity or lack of involvement

- To discharge, discipline, or otherwise discriminate against employees who have exercised their rights under this act

- To refuse to bargain in good faith with employee representatives

To make the National Labor Relations Act (NLRA) work, the National Labor Relations Board (NLRB) was created to enforce it. The role of the NLRB is to protect workers from management. The NLRB conducts the secret-ballot elections that determine whether or not a union will be organized and adjudicates any unfair labor practices by the employer.

Labor Management Relations Act. After World War II, in 1947, the Labor Management Relations Act was passed by Congress. Also known as the Taft-Hartley Act, it amended the earlier National Labor Relations Act by adding unfair labor practices by unions. This act made it illegal for unions to engage in the following conduct:

- To restrain or coerce employees or employers in the exercise of their legal rights

- To force an employer to discriminate against an employee because of the employee's membership or nonmembership in the union

- To refuse to bargain with an employer in good faith

- To engage in strikes or threats to force members of management to join a union (usually to collect large initiation fees) or to force an employer to do business with another employer

- To require an employer to bargain with a union other than the one employees have selected

- To demand excessive or discriminatory initiation fees

- To picket an employer to force it to recognize the union as the employees' representative without requesting a government election within a reasonable time period

Labor Management Reporting and Disclosure Act. This act was passed in 1959 when it became apparent that some union leaders were not properly representing their members' interests. The major provisions of this act are listed in the Components of Labor Management Reporting and Disclosure Act chart.

Components of Labor Management Reporting and Disclosure Act

Major Provision	Effect
Title I	Created a bill of rights for union members in working with their union. It assured members equal rights, freedom of speech and assembly, the right to sue the union, and other safeguards.
Title II	Imposed detailed reporting requirements on those who are responsible for union funds.
Title III	Established safeguards to ensure that the rights of members to elect leaders will not be lost when a national union takes over a local union and creates a trusteeship.
Title IV	Requires that fair elections for union officers be held periodically.
Title V	Sets forth the fiduciary responsibility of union officers and prohibitions against certain people from holding union office (primarily convicted felons).
Title VI	Grants the secretary of labor the right to conduct investigations into possible abuses under this act.
Title VII	Includes a series of miscellaneous provisions that limit strikes, picketing, and boycotts.

Managing Human Resources in a Unionized Organization. The primary objective of labor unions is to present a unified and organized front to the management for improvement in wages, benefits, and/or working conditions. Unions exist to perform the following functions:

- Protect jobs
- Secure preferred hours of work
- Defend workers' rights
- Negotiate for the best benefits possible for their members

Unions often have some political and societal objectives as well. These objectives are accomplished through support of political candidates and lobbying for legislation on issues pertinent to the union.

The role of any manager faced with union organization is to provide complete, unbiased information to counteract the union drive. The most important factor is the management's attitude toward unionization. Data can be collected and displayed about union dues, strike records, salaries of officers, and any other relevant facts that the management would like employees to know about the union. These data must be limited to facts, and management must be careful not to express its opinions about unions (see Do's and Don'ts for Managers and Supervisors During a Union Organizing Campaign).

Do's and Don'ts for Managers and Supervisors During a Union Organizing Campaign

Do
- Tell employees that the organization does not believe that they need union representation and that you would like them to vote no.
- Answer employees' questions about organizational policies and discuss the union campaign issues.
- Tell employees that if they join the union, they will be expected to pay union dues and fees.
- Assure employees that union or no union, management is going to continue to try to make the organization a good place to work.
- Explain to employees that the organization will recognize the union and bargain in good faith if the majority of the employees really want it, but that any improvements in wages and benefits are negotiable and not automatic, as the union might want them to believe.
- Administer appropriate disciplinary action or terminate any employee who threatens or coerces other employees, whether for or against the union.
- Request outside union officials to leave facility property if they try to solicit employees there. Escort them off the property or, if appropriate, call the police to have them removed.

Don't
SPIT
S—Spy on employees or conduct surveillance of any kind to determine the level of union sentiment.
P—Promise anything. You should not do anything to suggest that you are soliciting grievances.
I—Interrogate anyone. Asking questions about union sympathies or union activity is an unfair labor practice under the law.
T—Threaten, coerce, or intimidate any employee because of their union activity.

Data from Werther, William B., Jr., and Keith Davis. Human resources and personnel management. 3rd ed. New York: McGraw-Hill, 1989, pp 500–519.

EXAMPLE

> The HIM employees of Holy Hospital belong to a union. Cindy Black, a union member, wants to leave work early to attend her son's Little League baseball game. Cindy offers to work through her lunch hour so that she will put in a full 8 hours of work.
>
> If she is allowed to do this, what problems may result?

Civil Rights Legislation

CIVIL RIGHTS ACT OF 1964. The Civil Rights Act, passed in 1964, prohibits discrimination in employment based on race, color, religion, sex, or national origin. **Equal opportunity employment** constraints emerged during the 1960s and 1970s from federal acts, state and local legislation, and executive orders of the president of the United States. The intent of these laws was to provide equal opportunities in employment to these protected groups.

Affirmative action programs are written, systematic human resource planning tools that outline goals in hiring, training, promoting, and compensation of minority groups that are protected by equal employment laws. Employers may discriminate among workers on the basis of effort, performance, or any other pertinent work-related criteria. The law allows employers to reward excellence in employees and penalize employees for unacceptable performance. The laws require, however, that both these actions be related to work-related criteria, not sex, race, religion, or other prohibited factors.

Disparate treatment occurs when members of a **protected group**, such as women or minorities, receive unequal treatment. If a health care provider regularly hired female applicants as file clerks and did not allow them to apply for higher-paid positions, such as hospital orderlies, the result would be disparate treatment.

Disparate impact occurs when employment practices have a different impact on one or more of the protected groups. Requiring a high school diploma, for instance, for all jobs in an HIM department may have a discriminatory effect on minority workers, who, by history, have a greater percentage of high school dropouts in their population. Any standard applied should be shown to be necessary for performance of the job and not result in screening out any protected classes.

REHABILITATION ACT OF 1973. This is a series of laws designed to assist the handicapped. Section 501 applies only to the federal government and requires affirmative action to employ qualified people. Section 502 provides that handicapped people have free access

EXAMPLE

> A large urban hospital has an affirmative action program because it is a major government contractor ($20 million a year was received from government research contracts and Medicare payments). Under this program, the hospital agreed to promote two women into supervisory positions for each man. This practice was to continue until 45 per cent of all the supervisors were women.
>
> Health Information Services had the first open position that qualified for this program—that of clinical data supervisor. The director was one of the few female department heads in the hospital. The department employs 3 men out of 75 employees. The assistant director who manages this area maintains that a male employee, John Jones, is the most qualified for the position. He has spent 2 years in medical school, is a graduate of a health information management program, and holds Registered Record Administrator (RRA) and Certified Coding Specialist (CCS) credentials. John has worked as a health data analyst in this hospital for 1 year.
>
> Another employee, Kate Kessling, has also applied for the position. Kate has more experience and **seniority** in the department than John but does not have the same educational background or credentials. Kate has worked as a health data analyst at this hospital for 10 years.
>
> The human resource specialist recommends that Kate be given the job in compliance with the affirmative action program. What should the director of Health Information Services do? Who should be promoted and why?
>
> How will the choice be justified to the human resource specialist?

to federal and federally financed buildings constructed after 1968. Section 503 of this law mandates that employers with federal contracts in excess of $2500 must avoid employment discrimination against handicapped people and take affirmative action to employ and advance such people. Section 504 of the act outlaws discrimination by recipients of federal financial assistance against qualified handicapped people. Because Medicare Part A and Medicare are considered to be federal financial assistance, most hospitals are covered by this act.[2]

EXECUTIVE ORDERS ON AFFIRMATIVE ACTION. Executive order number 11141 issued in 1964 bans federal contractor discrimination against employees or applicants because of their age "except upon the basis of a bona fide occupational qualification, retirement plan, or statutory requirement."[2]

Executive order number 11246 and its establishment of the Office of Federal Contract Compliance Program (OFCCP) prohibit job discrimination based on race, color, religion, sex, or national origin by contractors and their subcontractors doing business with the federal government and require that they take certain affirmative action. A federal contractor's noncompliance with these obligations can result in the government's withdrawal or termination of the contract and/or a refusal to enter into any future dealings with the employer. The OFCCP could also sue the contractor to require compliance. In such an action, the OFCCP can seek appropriate relief on behalf of women and minorities, including back pay.[2]

VIETNAM VETERANS. The Vietnam Era Veteran's Readjustment Assistance Act of 1974 requires federal contractors with contracts for $10,000 or more to engage in affirmative efforts to provide employment for qualified disabled veterans and for veterans of the Vietnam era.

AGE DISCRIMINATION. The Age Discrimination in Employment Act (ADEA) protects employees and applicants between 40 and 70 years of age from age discrimination. This act applies to private employers who employee 20 or more workers during at least 20 weeks in the current or prior year. State and local government employers also are covered by this law. Although the term "employer" does not include the federal government, the act contains special provisions that are applicable to federal employees. The Equal Employment Opportunity Commission (EEOC) administers this law.

If the employer is covered, then all its employees are protected by the ADEA with the following major exceptions:

- Employees are not covered if they are 65 years of age but less than 70, have been employed for at least 2 years preceding retirement in a bona fide executive or high policy-making position, and have an immediate and vested retirement benefit of at least $27,000.

- Elected state and local government officials and members of their staff are excluded from the act's protection.[2]

AMERICANS WITH DISABILITIES ACT. Title I of the ADA makes it illegal for organizations with 15 or more employees to discriminate against an otherwise qualified person with disabilities if that person can perform the significant job duties with or without **reasonable accommodation.** Recruitment, hiring, **promotion,** compensation, termination, leaves, layoffs, job assignments, and benefits are all covered under this act.

The definition of disability is broad, stating that a disabled person is one who has a physical or mental impairment that substantially limits one or more of his or her major life activities, has a record of substantially limiting impairment, or is regarded as having a substantially limiting impairment.

Although the ADA was the most sweeping civil rights legislation since Title VII of the Civil Rights Act of 1964, this act was not intended to be an affirmative action initiative for the disabled. The employee must be qualified by meeting all the job requisites. The act requires that qualified employees with disabilities receive reasonable accommodation in the workplace to perform the essential job functions without causing **undue hardship** to the employer. If a job description has marginal functions included, the disabled person cannot be excluded because of inability to perform them if they could easily be assigned to someone else.

Some examples of reasonable accommodation are the following:

- Modifying existing facilities to be readily accessible to and usable by a person with a disability

- Restructuring a job to allow the disabled person to do it

- Modifying work schedules

- Acquiring or modifying equipment

- Providing qualified readers or interpreters

- Appropriately modifying examinations, training, or other programs

- Reassigning a current employee to a vacant position

What constitutes undue hardship? Any action that would require significant difficulty or expense when considered in light of the nature and cost of the accommodation in relation to the size, resources, nature, and structures of the employer's operation is viewed as undue hardship.

The health information manager can comply with this law by doing the following:

- Determine and *document* the essential functions of each job.

- Review job applications for unlawful questions or statements regarding people with disabilities.

- Inform and train anyone doing employment interviews about the ADA regulations.

- Pre-employment physical examinations must be done as a condition of employment. If a disability is found in the physical examination and the hiring supervisor rescinds a job offer, it must be proved to be for job-related reasons.

- Post the ADA poster provided by the EEOC in an accessible format to applicants, employees, and members of labor organizations.

FAMILY MEDICAL LEAVE ACT. Passed in 1993, the FMLA grants unpaid leave and job security to people who must take time off for medical reasons or to care for ill family members. The U.S. Department of Labor's

Employment Standards Administration, Wage and Hour Division, administers and enforces the FMLA for all private, state, and some federal employees.

To be eligible, an employee must work for a covered employer for a minimum of 1250 hours over a period of 12 months and at a location where at least 50 employees are employed by the employer within 75 miles.

Leave entitlement is ensured by the act for any of the following reasons:

- For the birth or placement of a child for adoption or foster care

- To care for an immediate family member (spouse, child, or parent) with a serious health condition

- To take medical leave when the employee is unable to work because of a serious health condition

On return from FMLA leave, employees must be restored to their original jobs or equivalent jobs with equivalent pay, benefits, and other employment terms and conditions. Advance notice of leave of at least 30 days is required from the employee for "foreseeable" circumstances. An employer may require medical certification to support all medical leave requests, including second or third opinions and a fitness-for-duty report to return to work.[3]

SEXUAL HARASSMENT. **Sexual harassment** can produce a number of negative effects in the workplace: decreased productivity, high turnover and absenteeism, low morale, higher recruitment and training costs, and potential legal liabilities. Sexual harassment may take two forms: quid pro quo, which are sexual favors for a benefit, or interference with work performance by creating an intimidating, a hostile, or an offensive work environment.

Both men and women may be victims of sexual harassment at work, and the victim may not be of the opposite sex of the harasser. The victim is not always the person to whom unwelcome sexual advances are directed. The manager should be aware that it is not required that a formal complaint be filed for the employer to be held liable.

To prevent problems with sexual harassment in the workplace, specific policies should be developed against such harassment and be widely communicated. All supervisory personnel should be trained concerning these policies and be aware of the resulting penalties for infraction. All complaints of sexual harassment should be fully investigated. The employer's liability is judged by whether the management knew or should have known about the harassment and what action, if any, was taken to stop it.

Every complaint should be treated seriously. Managers should conduct themselves in a manner that conveys that all parties involved have rights. Facts should be gathered before any judgment is made. Complete documentation at each step of the process is important. It should describe who was involved as well as the form of the harassment and when, why, where, and how it occurred.

Internal Issues

Organizational Culture

Every organization has its own unique culture. This culture is the product of its people, its mission, and its successes and failures. The challenge for supervisors is to be proactive to this culture. In every organization, there are a few core values or beliefs that shape its culture. In some health care organizations, it is service to patients; in others, service to physicians; and in others, revenue enhancement and cost containment at all costs. Conflicts arise when person's or group's desires are not consistent with the culture and values of the organization.

Information Systems

Information systems continue to improve in efficiency and ease of use. For efficient management of human resources functions, appropriate utilization of information systems is necessary. Because managing people requires large amounts of detailed information, an adequate information system should be developed to facilitate decision making and accomplish more work with less effort. It is now possible to computerize much of the paperwork required for human resource management. This results in improved services to employees, better planning tools for the manager, and improved information capture for the administration or owners of the organization.

Managers and supervisors have an important, continuing responsibility in maintaining complete and accurate information concerning their human resources. Basic data should be maintained on each employee. Although the Fair Labor Standards Act does not dictate the manner in which records are kept, it requires that accurate records be maintained and include the following:

- Employee's name (the same as is used for social security) and any identifying symbol or number used in lieu of the employee's name on any time, work, or payroll sheet

- Employee's home address, including zip code, as well as date of birth if under 19 and occupation

- Time of day and day of week when the employee's workweek begins

- Regular hourly rate of pay, basis on which wages are paid, and the amount and nature of each payment excluded from the regular rate (e.g., bonuses)

- Hours worked each workday and total hours worked each workweek

- Total daily or weekly straight-time earnings

- Total weekly premium pay for overtime

- Total additions to or deductions from wages paid each pay period

- Total wages paid each pay period

- Date of payment and the pay period it covers

- Copy of the agreement or understanding if the 8-and-80 option is in effect; if the agreement is not in writing, a memorandum summarizing its terms and showing the date it was entered into and the period for which it remains in effect.[2] The 8-and-80 rule is available to hospitals and other facilities primarily engaged in caring for the sick. It requires that overtime be paid for the greater of the number of hours of work in excess of 80 hours in a biweekly pay period of 14 calendar days (rather than in excess of 40 hours per week) or the number of work hours in excess of 8 in a day.

Beyond the data above, additional information is needed on each employee. Hire dates and anniversary dates of promotions are needed for **performance appraisal** administration. The pay rate and range or job grade must be recorded. Copies of performance appraisals and disciplinary action should be kept. Documentation of orientation and training programs in which the employee has participated is important. These records are essential to provide a defense of compensation or performance appraisal decisions and to show compliance with wage and hour laws.

OBJECTIVES AND ACTIVITIES OF HUMAN RESOURCE MANAGEMENT IN HEALTH CARE ORGANIZATIONS

Human resource activities in the HIM department mirror the activities found in many non–health care businesses (Figure 14–1). Certain key objectives and activities are required to provide and maintain an adequate workforce that accomplishes the work to meet the needs of the consumers of health information services.

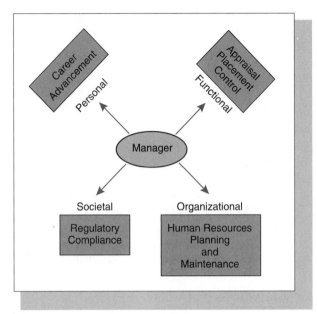

FIGURE 14–1. Activities and objectives of human resources management.

Societal Objectives—Regulatory Compliance

The primary mission of health care organizations is meeting the health needs of society. Being a labor-intensive industry, the human resources of the health care organization are needed to achieve this mission. Society's needs are often expressed through statutes and regulations. Compliance with these laws, such as the *Conditions of Participation* for Medicare and Medicaid, is an example of activities that fulfill this societal objective of meeting the public's health needs.

Other societal objectives fulfilled by health care organizations involve the rights of employees for a safe and fair work environment. The human resource activities that involve the policies and procedures that assure compliance with equal rights legislation, regulatory mandates, and union-management relations fulfill this societal objective.

Organizational Objectives

Human resource management is also used to assist an organization in fulfilling its mission and meeting its goals. Human resources planning, selection processes, training and development programs, performance appraisal systems, and employee controls are the human resource activities carried out to meet the organizational objectives.

Functional Objectives

The functional objective of human resource management is simply to maintain the level of services that are appropriate to the organization's needs. A human resources department exists only to serve the rest of the organization.

Human resource activities that meet the functional objectives include position appraisal and **placement** assistance as well as selected management control activities.

Personal Objectives

The human resource function also has the objective of assisting employees in meeting their individual goals, at least to the extent that these goals remain consistent with the goals of the organization. It is important for employee's personal objectives to be met if they are to be retained and motivated in today's dynamic health care environment.

If personal needs are not met, employee performance and satisfaction decline and turnover rates increase. These developments result in increased cost to the company both in direct costs (recruitment, selection, and training) and in lost productivity. The indirect cost of high turnover rates may be public relations problems.

The personal goals and objectives of employees are met through training and development programs, career ladders, and placement assistance as well as through compensation administration.

Individual personal assistance objectives may be met through an **employee assistance program** (EAP). EAPs are organized departments or divisions of the human resources department staffed by professionals such as social workers and counselors. They may also be independent organizations that a health care organization contracts with for services. The purpose of these programs is to help employees who may have personal or family problems that interfere with job performance. Some common employee problems are substance abuse, financial problems, family conflicts, coping with stress, and both physical and mental health problems.

Employees may seek out this confidential service on their own or be referred by a supervisor. The goal of an EAP is to help employees help themselves. In addition to the personal rewards gained from this help, these programs make good economic sense for the organization because the cost of excessive absenteeism, reduced productivity, and turnover can be substantial. An EAP referral may save an employee who would otherwise leave the organization and/or it might eliminate or minimize barriers to optimal performance of the employee.

A SYSTEMS MODEL OF HUMAN RESOURCE MANAGEMENT FOR HEALTH INFORMATION SERVICES

Definition of a System

A systems approach to human resources management is useful in health information services departments because it enables recognition of complex interrelationships of the individual parts to the whole service (Figure 14–2). In the systems view, it is less likely that the balance and interdependency of these subsystems will be overlooked. When a systems model is used, the manager can clearly see the internal and external boundaries of the system and the relations of the subsystems to the boundaries.

As information technology advances and changes, an HIM department may be termed more appropriately a "service" because much of the work done is performed throughout the facility rather than within the confines of a single department. This makes a systems view especially useful in understanding where health information services fit within the organization. This systems approach also aids in understanding where organizational control ends and the external environment begins. This is always a key issue in the management of human resources. Whenever activities are interrelated, a system exists.

Applications to Human Resource Management

The subsystems of the human resources functions are as follows:

- Recruitment, selection, and training
- Employee and labor relations
- Compensation, benefits, and security provisions
- Performance appraisal and employee development
- Response to environmental challenges

All these subsystems relate to and affect one another. The health information manager must remain aware of the interdependency to minimize conflicts and problems that may occur when the system gets out of balance. An applied systems view describes human resource management as transforming the inputs (employee skills and abilities) and processing them into outputs (desired results or outcomes).

Applying a systems view to health information management assists in defining the variables that affect production within the department (Figure 14–3). Processing of the information for a discharged hospital inpatient

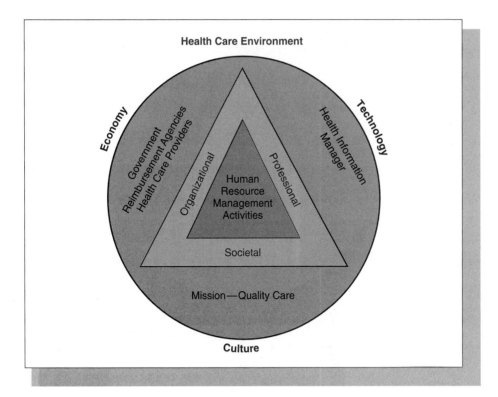

Health Care Environment

Economy

Technology

Government
Reimbursement Agencies
Health Care Providers

Health Information
Manager

Organizational

Professional

Human
Resource
Management
Activities

Societal

Mission—Quality Care

Culture

FIGURE 14–2. Systems model diagram.

is a good example of the interdependency required using the systems model. After the patient is discharged, the data must be gathered, scanned, or otherwise abstracted and collated in a prescribed order or format. The next step is analysis for missing elements followed by routing to the clinical coding staff to assign diagnosis and procedure codes for billing and indexing. Next, the records are forwarded to the physician for completion, if necessary. When complete, the records are committed to a storage medium. Unless the organization is small, one person cannot perform all these functions. Several employees with different skill levels are needed to perform the various functions in the required sequence at appropriate times. If the information is not collected and available in one place, it cannot be coded or analyzed, and if data elements are missing, the record cannot be committed to permanent storage.

Human resource activities function the same way. Performance appraisal must take place before decisions can be made concerning compensation adjustments. Orientation and training cannot occur until the recruiting and selection process is completed. Environmental challenges from legislation, the current economy, and employee lifestyle and cultural influences continually affect the other subsystems that make up the whole.

A systems model is used to suggest options for the manager to pursue in the following example.

EXAMPLE

Delta Diggins has just been promoted to manager of health information services at Happy Trails Health Center. A team of physicians, administrators, and department heads has decided to convert to a patient-centered environment. Health information currently is digitally stored on optical disk by scanning paper documents. The patient-centered care project calls for a completely computerized patient record, with information coming from various sources throughout the organization. Health information services will manage the central data repository. Delta is excited about this innovative approach but is concerned about how to communicate the changes to staff and how the new system will affect the department's operations.

How can a systems view of human resource management assist Delta in this situation?

A systems model facilitates a comprehensive and integrated approach for human resource management. To provide highly skilled and challenged workers, it is critical for the health information manager to match the right employees with the positions that best fit their abilities and desired skill levels. It is also the manager's responsibility to maintain staff competence and motivation through continuing education and staff development. In addition, it is important to facilitate career ladders and/or professional growth pathways. These programs should be implemented and coordinated whenever possible to

Resources × Processing = Product

Employee Skills and Abilities × Organization Structure × Organizational Procedure × Teamwork

Equals

Productive, Successful Outcomes

Health Information Services:

| Access and Retrieval Systems Data Collection and Analysis Confidentiality and Data Security Reimbursement and Optimization | × | Effective Human Resources Management in Health Information Services | = | Efficient and Effective Utilization of Health Information Throughout the Organization and Community |

FIGURE 14–3. Application of the systems model to productivity.

promote qualified and motivated HIM workers who will competently serve health care organizations for years to come. Using a systems model will help to accomplish this goal.

HUMAN RESOURCE PLANNING

The management of staffing always requires timely and thorough planning. Both short-term plans and long-term strategies are important. Careful human resource planning to maintain the desired level of service is essential and helpful in times of reduced resources or inadequate skilled labor supplies. As budgets tighten to meet shortfalls in reimbursement, departments may be asked to do more work with less help.

Plans are needed to assure that a supply of trained workers is available when needed. Cross-training technical staff by a regular rotation of job duties accomplishes more than one objective. It assures a ready substitute for absent employees or open positions. It also alleviates some of the boredom that causes turnover in highly repetitive positions.

A strategic plan for coding staffing may include teaching a coding class regularly, so that a constant supply of trained coders is available. Planning for peak workloads in transcription by contracting with an outside service on an as-needed basis can be a lifesaver in the event of an unexpected loss of a skilled transcriptionist or a sudden increase in the workload.

With these plans, staffing adjustments can be managed with a minimum of lost productivity and compromise of essential services.

EXAMPLE

Generating the physician profiles for reappointment to the medical staff is a demanding responsibility of the HIM Department at Memorial Hospital. It involves pulling together activity statistics and performance data on 450 physicians each year. Virginia Smith has done this job for 2 years and has developed an efficient and organized system for producing accurate reports. The hospital will be credentialing about 30 per cent more physicians next year because the hospital has formed alliances with several large group practices.

Lana Lockhart is the administrative director of Medical Staff Affairs. She is responsible for all medical staff credentialing functions. Late one afternoon, she is notified that Virginia has just been seriously injured in an auto accident. Lana's assistant tells her that Virginia is the only one who knows how to do the profiles. There are written procedures, but they are not clear enough for the other staff to follow. The reports must be completed next week to go out to the medical staff departments. Lana's assistant is in a panic over what to do about this situation.

What should have been done to prevent this crisis or at least minimize its adverse effect on the operations of the organization? How will Lana cope with the current situation?

Tools for Human Resource Planning

Some tools are useful in writing a human resource plan.

Date Compiled: _____

Possible HIS Position Vacancies	Name of Employee	Attributes
Manager, Health Information Services	M. Jones	A, 1
C. Smith, Incumbent	B. Benson	B, 2
	J. White	B, 1
Assistant Manager, HIS	J. White	A, 1
M. Jones, Incumbent	B. Benson	B, 2
Supervisor, Clinical Data	F. Brown	A, 1
J. White, Incumbent	J. Jones	B, 2
Supervisor, Medical Language Division	S. Green	A, 1
B. Benson, Incumbent	C. Black	B, 1

Key to Attributes:
A = Ready for Promotion
B = Needs More Experience Before Promoting
C = Not Suitable for Promotion At Present

1 = Performance Appraisal Rating Excellent
2 = Performance Appraisal Rating Acceptable
3 = Performance Appraisal Rating Unacceptable

FIGURE 14–4. Replacement chart.

Job Title	1	2	3	4	5	6	7	8	9	10	11	12	Total FTE's
HI Analysts			2						1		1		4
Data Entry Specialists		3			1					2			6
Optical Imaging Specialists								1					1
Release of Information Coordinators					1				1				2
Director of HIS													
												Total	13

FIGURE 14–5. Staffing table. Anticipated openings for this budget year by month of the year.

Replacement Charts. These charts are a visual representation of who will replace who in the event of a vacancy. The development of this chart is based on information collected during a human resource audit. In Figure 14–4, the replacement chart shows that if there is a vacancy at the manager level (M. Jones leaves), J. White is more likely to be promoted than B. Benson. If J. White moves to manager, then B. Benson moves up to assistant manager and F. Brown or S. Green could be moved into the second slot for consideration for the next vacancy.

Staffing Table. A staffing table is also a graphic representation of job titles and potential slots with anticipated position openings (Figure 14–5). Because of increased computerization, it is projected that data entry clerks will be hired in February, May, and October. A total of six FTEs will be needed in the current calendar or budget year.

Human Resource Audits. An audit is conducted to assess which openings can be filled with internal candidates (people already employed). An audit puts all the important information about the skills and abilities of the workforce together in one document to make recruiting, training, and career planning activities more coordinated and effective.

Skill Inventories. These inventories are conducted for nonmanagerial employees, and management inventories are conducted for supervisory staff. Demographic information, such as job title, job experience, and length of service with the organization, is required. Critical factors to include in an inventory are the employees' present performance level and their potential for promotion. This tool allows for detailed information concerning employees' specific skills.

Job Analysis and Design

Every manager in an HIM department is required to know how to perform **job analysis** and job design of all the positions in his or her area of accountability. The importance of well-designed jobs is best illustrated in the example below.

EXAMPLE

A hospital information system was introduced in the mid-1990s in this 180-bed long-term care facility. When a new manager was recruited, she discovered that none of the procedures or job functions had been restructured to maximize use of this technology. Statistics were still gathered manually, and tabulation was still accomplished by the use of an adding machine using information from daily employee logs. The computer had an adequate statistical reporting feature, but the jobs in the department had to be reorganized before any benefits of this automation could be appreciated by the organization. Once the jobs were regrouped and procedures and responsibilities outlined, statistical reporting took 2 hours compared with 4 working days each month.

Other job functions were restructured as well, and within 2 years, the department was doing twice as much work without additional staff. Job restructuring also has some additional yet not so tangible benefits.

What are some of these intangible yet desirable effects?

Improvements in worker productivity, quality, and cost usually begin with an analysis of job functions and responsibilities. The manager must have a clear understanding of each job and how it relates to other jobs within the system. Knowledge about these jobs and their requirements is collected through a process called job analysis. This process analyzes key components and requirements of each position, not the person in the position. The following tools can be used to perform job analysis:

- Job analysis forms, such as shown in Figure 14–6
- Questionnaire for written completion or interview
- Checklists
- Review of employee logs or diaries

Direct observation by the manager is another option, but it is time-consuming, costly, and more likely to be biased than the other methods.

Managers perform job analysis for the following reasons:

- Evaluate the affect of external challenges on a specific job.
- Force elimination of outdated and/or unnecessary job requirements that may cause discrimination in employment practices.
- Discover job elements that affect the quality of work life.
- Plan for future departmental needs.
- Match applicants with job openings.
- Determine training needs.
- Develop untapped potential in a position. For example, a review of the position of insurance clerk at a neighborhood health clinic reveals that basic knowledge of ICD-9-CM coding is

---

Position Title: Health Information Secretary

Department: Health Information Services

Supervisor: Manager, Health Information Services

Current Supervisor's Name: Kathy Castlerock

General Job Objectives:
- Acts as department receptionist and first telephone contact.
- Processes daily work schedules.
- Coordinates completion and filing of birth certificates with the Bureau of Vital Statistics.
- Demonstrates effective relationships with co-workers, patients, public, physicians, administration, and outside agencies.

Essential Job Duties:
(List all tasks required to perform the routine functions required for the position.)
Example:
- Completes birth certificates or fetal death certificates as required.
- Greets visitors to the department
- Routes incoming phone calls and takes messages when intended party is unavailable.

Meets Standards of Performance By: (Example)
(For Greeting Visitors) Receiving no complaints in the performance period concerning discourteous service.

Exceeds Standards of Performance By: (Example)
(For Greeting Visitors) Receiving compliments by visitors, coworkers, or physicians on helpfulness and courteous service.

FIGURE 14–6. Sample job analysis form.

---

required. There is often a backlog in coding of outpatient service records. By identifying this untapped resource, the insurance clerk can be trained to help with backlog coding. This accomplishes two objectives: It helps the facility provide better service while enhancing the job of insurance clerk.

- Place employees in positions that use their skills effectively.

- Assess employee compensation so that salaries are fair and based on the work and the skills needed.

- Form a foundation for the creation of productivity standards.

Job Descriptions

A job description is a written document that explains the qualifications, duties, working conditions, and all other significant aspects of a job. Within an organization, all job descriptions follow the same format. Form and content of job descriptions between health care organizations vary. Job descriptions can be simple, one-page documents or complex and detailed reports. All job descriptions should contain, at a minimum, the key elements (see Job Description Requirements).

Some job descriptions also include **job performance standards** and are used as the primary criteria for performance evaluation.

EXAMPLE

Joan Hellman, the clinical data supervisor at St. Elsewhere, a Community Mental Health Center, noticed that within the job description for health information services there was a requirement that clinical coding specialists must keyboard at 45 words per minute. It came to her attention that an experienced specialist from a competitor applied for an open position but failed to pass the initial screening conducted by the human resources department.

Joan discovered that in the past, the specialists in this position were required to type diagnoses and procedures on the face sheet of the record, and this was an important skill. At the present time, coders only input the five-digit codes into the system, using a computer keyboard. The codes are transmitted through an encoding software package on the center's information system, which generates a completed face sheet. Employees never use a typewriter.

What process should Joan have explored before the clinical coding specialist position was recruited? What methods can be used to conduct this process?

Job Description Requirements	
Element Required	**Purpose**
Date	Date it was written and revised
Author	This is included so that questions can be directed to the appropriate person.
Department or Division	Location of the primary workplace
Job grade or job level	Ranks the job's importance for compensation purposes
Supervisor or reports to	Outlines organizational or departmental structure
Job status	Exempt or nonexempt from overtime
Job summary	Concise description of what this job does
Essential job duties	Major tasks and responsibilities of this position
Job specifications	Qualifications in terms of education, experience, and skills needed to perform the essential job duties
Working conditions	Physical demands and working environment. If there are any unusual demands of the job or strenuous physical demands, they should be mentioned here.

Employee Handbooks

Employee handbooks provide a written reference manual for human resource management. The following guidelines pertain to their content and use.

- Employee handbooks must conform to written policies used in the organization.

- Handbooks must be continually updated to reflect changes in policy and procedures.

- Handbooks must be issued to all employees.

- Employees should sign a statement stipulating that they have received a handbook, that they will review its contents within a definite time period, and that it is their responsibility to inquire of the manager or supervisor if they have questions. This signed statement must be maintained by the employer.

- The receipt should not have the employees acknowledge that they have read and understood the handbook; because they sign the receipt at the time they are given a copy, this type of statement, although common, is a factual impossibility.[2]

Once job analysis, job descriptions, and employee work rules are in place, either by policy and procedure manuals or by employee handbooks, the next step is to find the right person to place in that position.

RECRUITMENT

Recruitment is the process or set of activities performed to find and influence talented people to come to work in an organization.

Steps in the Recruitment Process

The steps involved in recruitment are performed whether the recruiter is a professional or works for the organization.

1. The job opening is identified through review of the human resource plan or by a request by a manager.

2. The recruiter learns what each job requires by looking at the job analysis information, the job description, and any additional job specifications documentation. This review enables the recruiter to match the right job with the right person. It is important to make sure that the job description and specifications are up to date and that no significant changes are planned for the position. If new duties are going to be added or old ones taken away, the job description should be revised before the position is recruited.

3. Once the significant characteristics needed to perform the job are identified, various channels are used to seek out and entice people to apply.

Sources of Applicants

Entry-level positions are usually filled by newspaper or trade journal ads or by walk-in applicants. Sometimes health care organizations use professional recruiters for

EXAMPLE

> Helpful Hospital uses professional recruiters after professional positions have gone unfilled by way of traditional methods for 3 months. The manager of health information services is anxious to get a clinical information coordinator position filled as soon as possible to begin work on some big projects. Six weeks after the recruiter has been engaged, she still does not have a single applicant.
>   What is the next step? What questions should the recruiter be asked? What action can be taken?

EXAMPLE

> Memorial Hospital had a difficult time finding competent entry-level clerical staff on the evening and night shifts in health information services. The assistant director previously was an instructor in health information management at the community college. She suggested that they try recruiting HIM students for their open positions.
>   What are the pros and cons of this plan from the view of department manager?

managerial and skilled technical positions. If a professional recruiter is used, the manager should watch for recruiter biases that limit the applicant pool. Recruiters may be biased toward one gender or age-group or toward graduates of certain programs or with certain degrees. Professional recruiters also charge a fee for their services. An agency's policies and contracts should be carefully reviewed to understand the obligations. State employment agencies may be used without fees.

Recruitment avenues readily available to health care organizations large enough to be recognized as a potential employer are walk-in and write-in candidates. Targeted advertising is the most common channel of recruitment. Local newspapers, professional journals, and trade magazines are the most likely places to advertise. Some organizations post or publish new positions on bulletin boards or in-house newsletters.

Educational institutions are an excellent source of recruitment for HIM workers. Medical assistant, medical transcription, medical secretary, nursing, and business programs are sources of potential employees as are institutions that prepare HIM professionals. Students in these professions can become motivated, knowledgeable, part-time and temporary workers.

Constraints

Constraints arise from the organizational and compensation policies, environmental conditions, job requirements, costs, and affirmative action programs.

Organizational constraints can include a promotion-from-within policy that mandates that already-on-board employees (who are qualified) be hired before outside job applicants. Another example is the policy to give preference to veterans for Veterans Administration positions.

Compensation policies may constrain recruiting. For example, if the pay range for coders is more than $2 an hour less than the market rate, the number of applicants may be limited and not as qualified as if the pay range were at the market rate. If the pay rate cannot be

improved because of organizational constraints, the job can be made attractive in other ways, such as flextime scheduling or a 36-hour workweek being counted as full time for benefits.

Some organizations may have employment status policies that can be a constraint for effective recruitment. For example, an organizational policy against hiring part-time workers (or the opposite—hiring only part-time workers) limits the applicant pool. The health information manager may use the advantages of job sharing described earlier as reasons to request a variance on policy.

SELECTION

Once an adequate pool of applicants has been recruited, then the **selection process** begins. The selection process is also a series of steps that results in the hiring of an employee to fill the open position. The number of available and qualified applicants for the position is an important consideration. For example, if there is a shortage of medical transcriptionists in the region and 10 persons apply, it is likely that selection of a qualified candidate can occur. On the other hand, if it is known that the local college is graduating 25 HIM professionals each year and only one person applies for the position, recruiting methods should be reviewed to see that the advertising was appropriate and actually reached the target market.

Another consideration is the accuracy of the personal résumé. Many employers find exaggerations or outright lies on written résumés. Credentials of potential applicants should be verified with the organization that issued them. In the case of credentialed HIM professionals, the validity of the credential should be confirmed with the American Health Information Management Association.

In each health care organization, some general steps are followed in the employee selection process. Depending on the circumstances, some steps can be combined and/or adjusted to fit the needs of the situation.

Steps in the Employee Selection Process

1. *Preliminary Reception.* The screening process often begins here as the employer forms an opinion and may assign a rating based on a preliminary or courtesy interview.

2. *Testing.* Performance tests assess the applicant's ability to do the required work. Coding tests, mathematics tests, keyboarding and transcription tests, and medical terminology tests are examples found to be useful in HIM departments.

All tests must be reviewed and validated so that they are not or will not be perceived as discriminatory. Discrimination against an applicant based on an invalid test is illegal, even if it is unintentional. The tests must be useful and valid indicators of future job performance and must be given to all applicants for a position. For example, a math proficiency test is not appropriate when the position does not require statistical computations or accounting functions.

Aptitude and psychological tests are not considered performance tests. Aptitude tests determine the probability of a person's success in some activity in which he or she is not yet trained. Psychological tests measure anything from personality preferences to behavior patterns. Both aptitude tests and psychological tests should only be given with careful consideration and consultation with a human resources professional.

3. *Screening Interview.* This interview, conducted by the hiring supervisor, evaluates the applicant's acceptability for the position. Most managers or supervisors have more confidence in the personal interview as a screening technique than any other step in the selection process. As a mechanism of two-way communication, not only does the employer have an opportunity to evaluate the applicant but the applicant has a chance to evaluate the employer and the job.

4. *Reference and Background Checks.* The main objective of this step is to verify the accuracy of the work history and to avoid the hiring of an employee with known performance problems. In HIM positions, protection of confidential information is critical, so that anyone with a known history of indiscretion is not hired. The extent of this process depends on the job duties the applicant will be responsible for performing.

5. *Medical Evaluation.* The medical evaluation certifies that the applicant is physically fit for the intended position. This step is critical in health care organizations where the employee may have contact with patients. An estimated 70 to 80 per cent of employers now require drug screening tests before an applicant may be considered for employment.

6. *Supervisory Interview.* This interview is usually conducted by the person to whom the applicant would report. In some cases, both the department head and the supervisor interview the applicant. For some positions, such as quality improvement specialist or tumor registrar, an administrator or a physician may want to participate. One person should be designated as the final hiring authority, and it is critical that the immediate supervisor have significant input, if not complete authority. This manager has a vested interest in the applicant and is the person most likely to evaluate a good job fit.

The job description and specifications should be reviewed with the applicant during the interview and a copy given to the applicant for consideration. Technical questions about the job may be asked at this point, and the applicant should view the actual work environment. This helps applicants decide if the environment is a good choice for them.

7. *Realistic Job Preview.* This step enables the applicant to better understand the actual job and job setting before the final hiring decision is made. The intent of this extra step, which many managers omit, is to identify job expectations and dispel any misconceptions that the applicant may have about the position. By this honest exposure to the actual work environment, it is hoped that job dissatisfaction and early turnover would be minimized.

These steps can be streamlined if necessary by combining 1, 2, and 3 into one unit. In some cases, the reference check has limited value but should only be skipped if the manager or another reliable source has personal knowledge of the applicant's background and work history. Steps 6 and 7 can be combined into one integrated session. Most employers provide a probationary period that can substitute as the realistic job preview. At the end of a designated period, generally 3 to 6 months, either the employer or the employee may end the relationship without adverse effects to either party.

RETENTION

Retention of staff is one of management's most important responsibilities. Employee turnover is costly to the organization. Not only are there significant costs in the recruitment and selection process but there are also costs in establishing new employee records, orienting and training the new hire, and losing productivity when positions are vacant.

Orientation

Human resource management involves more than finding and hiring people for positions within the organization. Once the employee reports for the first day of work, many additional activities must be performed.

A good orientation program gets the employee off to the right start. The premise that if employees are properly selected, orientation programs are not needed is false. When one moves to a new neighborhood, starts classes in a new school, or joins any type of group as a new member, one has a feeling of discomfort or at least unfamiliarity for a while. The process of becoming a productive and satisfied employee is critical to the organization as well as to the employee, and it must begin the very first day with orientation and instruction. The instruction should include areas that most people consider common sense. Orientation programs are discussed in greater detail later in this chapter.

EXAMPLE

Anna Smith, a bright young girl, was hired as temporary help to abstract health records for a special project. The release of information supervisor showed Anna where to find the information, how to operate the equipment, and where to put the abstracts when she finished. What she neglected to mention was that the records were in a specific, indexed order and that they should stay that way through the abstracting process. Two hundred fifty records were already re-indexed with information out of order within them before this error was discovered.

What are some things the supervisor could have done to prevent this from happening? Should Anna be reprimanded?

Communication

Open, honest two-way communication between managers and employees is the best defense against employee dissatisfaction. A proactive approach to identifying and solving problem areas before they disrupt department operations is a desirable objective.

Regular department meetings with agendas that include an open forum can keep small problems from becoming crises. Regular one-on-one touch-base meetings between supervisor and employee also go a long way toward making an employee think that he or she is making an appreciated contribution to the work of the department.

Performance Feedback

Providing regular feedback on performance to employees is one of the most important management roles in encouraging and retaining employees. Employees need to know the areas in which they need improvement, guidance, and instruction. Otherwise, they believe that their work is satisfactory.

EXAMPLE

Jeri Jones stops by Rosemary Stone's office early one Monday morning. She is obviously nervous about speaking to Rosemary, the department director. Jeri works Sunday through Thursdays as a tumor registrar. Recently, she joined a new church. She loves her job, has an excellent work record, and doesn't want to jeopardize her position. After some encouragement from co-workers, she asks why her position must work every Sunday. After a review of her duties and a documentation review of the position, it becomes apparent that the work no longer needs to be performed on Sundays. At the time the position was created, no computer-equipped desk was available Friday and Saturday, so the Sunday-through-Thursday schedule was created. Tumor registry no longer shares desks or computer terminals with other positions.

What might be some other valid reasons for job-specific scheduling?

Does Rosemary have the right to make Jeri continue the Sunday schedule? What should Rosemary do?

TERMINATION

In today's environment, it is rare that people stay in the same position until they retire. More likely, the employee will be promoted (given a better job with more responsibility), will be transferred to another department, or will leave the organization. Other possibilities are **demotions** and terminations. Some employees just do not work out. Because of a poor attitude, refusal to cooperate with organizational philosophy, or personality conflict, the employee causes more problems than he or she makes up for in productivity.

Most organizations have termination-for-cause events that require immediate dismissal. Those situations are usually clearly defined and, although unpleasant, not usually as troublesome for the manager as subtler difficulties. The following are examples of for-cause behavior:

- Prolonged absence from work without notification

- Coming to work under the influence of drugs or alcohol

- Being caught in the act of stealing materials from the employer

Before taking steps to terminate a problem employee, managers should review the following considerations to protect themselves and their organization against wrongful discharge allegations and further conflict:

- Were any promises made to the employee when hired or at any time during employment that were not fulfilled?

- Is there a good cause for the termination, or a pattern of behavior that when considered collectively could be considered good cause?
- Has this employee filed any claim, charge, or complaint with any government agency or engaged in any "protected" activity (as in a union)?
- Is the decision to terminate fair, deliberate, and reasonable? Do other people in the organization support the decision? Is there complete documentation of the events leading to the decision to take action?
- Is this employee in a particularly vulnerable position at the time of termination?

For additional safeguards concerning disciplinary action, please refer to Figure 14–7.

Wrongful Discharge

Negotiated resolutions are recommended if an employee is likely to take court action to pursue a wrongful discharge. Severance pay, outplacement assistance, and transfer to another, more suitable position are some suggestions that may be mutually acceptable. The health information manager must be aware of the legal consequences and the legal constraints placed on employers to protect employees from wrongful discharge.

Historically, employers and employees have operated under the doctrine of **employment "at will."** Under this doctrine, an employment contract without a specified term could be terminated by either party, with or without cause. Recently, this doctrine has been eroded in the courts. The claims are generally based on the following.

Tort Law. The termination is based on a premise that violates public policy. For example, an employee is discharged for filing a workers' compensation claim or for threatening to report abuse of hospital patients to state authorities.

Implied Contract. Courts in many states have recognized claims based on statements made in employee manuals and handbooks or oral statements made by managers.[3] The managers' statements or the handbooks *implied* that an employee would be retained for a certain length of time or as long as the employee met outlined standards.

Implied Covenant of Good Faith and Fair Dealing. This would apply to employees discharged for reasons other than just cause. The covenant is most often recognized on the basis of long service, personnel policies, and oral representations. Relatively few states recognize such an implied covenant in the employment context.[4]

Prior to taking disciplinary action, a manager may complete this checklist. If one or more "no's" are checked, it is a good idea to discuss the action with the Director of Human Resources or someone from Administration to assure the disciplinary action planned is appropriate under the circumstances.

Yes No

1. Has the work rule or the policy that was violated been published or otherwise clearly communicated to this employee?
2. Did this employee ever receive a written copy of this rule or policy?
3. Is the rule posted on bulletin boards or similar areas?
4. Is the infraction reasonably related to the orderly, efficient, and safe operation of the unit, department, or organization?
5. If others have similar infractions, did they receive the same disciplinary action as is being contemplated for this employee?
6. Are there factual records available on all employees covering violation of the rule or policy in question?
7. Does this employee have the worst record of all employees on violation of this rule or policy?
8. Have there been any previous warnings for violation of this rule or policy given to this employee?
9. Does the documentation surrounding the infractions include dates, times, places, witnesses, and pertinent facts on all past violations?
10. Is there a factual written record showing the steps taken by the manager to correct the improper conduct of all employees?
11. Is the degree of discipline to be imposed related to the seriousness of the offense, the degree of fault, and any mitigating factors?
12. Has this employee had an opportunity to tell his or her side of the story?

FIGURE 14–7. Disciplinary checklist.

Layoffs

Involuntary separation occurs when the employer terminates the employment relationship for whatever reason, sometimes as a result of low patient counts or economic conditions. As previously discussed, layoffs should be avoided when possible if the same effect can be achieved by reduction in hours, early retirement, or job sharing.

Involuntary separation usually has no benefits. Voluntary separation for a troublesome employee may be negotiated for a solution that saves face for the employee and benefits the organization.

Retirement

Retirement is another type of separation, which the manager can sometimes minimize by offering the worker part-time work. This serves as a means of assisting people to move into more leisure time while retaining access to their considerable knowledge and skills and the stability of tenure that they have to offer the organization.

EXAMPLE

> Molly Madsen, the director of the HIM department, came to work early on Saturday morning only to find a weekend transcriptionist, Ima Nocount, slumped over her keyboard. In a Thermos at her **workstation** the remnants of an alcoholic drink were evident. When her production from the Friday night shift was reviewed, the printout consisted of "I hate that *&#!@#$ Molly Madsen" and various other strings of unflattering text about various employees of the facility.
>
> How should Molly handle this situation? Suppose Ima hadn't been caught with any liquor and her production, although consistently below standard for speed, is fairly accurate for content and spelling. How does that change the situation?

Employee **counseling, discipline,** and communication are strategies for preventing employee turnover and the need for termination or supervisor-requested transfers. Anything managers can do to prevent terminations of any type benefits the organization. Unless for personal reasons, workers do not resign if they enjoy a satisfying work environment, a challenging job, communication with their supervisors, and personal opportunities for growth.

All organizations have policies and procedures that serve as guides to employee behavior. These policies and procedures should be documented in organizational and departmental employee manuals. Within these personnel policies should be an outline of the disciplinary process and the **grievance procedure.** The competent health information manager communicates these policies and procedures to staff as they are hired and reinforces pertinent policies and procedures as critical incidents occur. When employees fail to follow these work rules or do not meet the standards outlined for their positions, it is

the manager's responsibility to assist and motivate them back into compliance.

COUNSELING

Employee counseling is the process of modifying the behavior of the employee according to the objectives of the manager. These objectives should be in accordance with the recognized standards of performance and be consistent with the goals and mission of the organization. When the employee is out of compliance, the right type of coaching, education, or counseling must be undertaken to correct the problem as soon as possible. Communication should be timely, tactful, and truthful. Criticism should be constructive, not accusing, and directed at the employee's behavior. Follow-up meetings should be scheduled at the close of counseling sessions to assess progress toward the goals or problem resolution.

EXAMPLE

> Tanya Tuckerman, an information system analyst, works closely with the physicians in data management and distribution. She has an excellent work record and meets all the productivity standards specified in her job description. She works the 3-to-11 P.M. shift. Tanya's supervisor, Ronda Hammond, sees her report to work every afternoon at 3, but because Ronda often leaves by 5 P.M., she doesn't interact with Tanya a great deal.
>
> Ronda has noticed that sometimes Tanya's dress is inappropriate business attire, but she is not in literal violation of the departmental dress code. The evening supervisor reports that a member of the house staff (resident physician) called her and said that Tanya had made overfriendly and inappropriate comments to him. The supervisor admitted that this is not the first time that physicians have complained about Tanya. The evening supervisor has tried to speak with Tanya about more professional dress and attitude while at work. The physician involved wants this to be taken care of or he will go "straight to the top" and have Tanya fired.
>
> What should Ronda Hammond, the department director, do about this situation?

Typically, three types of counseling may occur in the workplace: directive counseling, nondirective counseling, and participative counseling. Directive counseling is the process of listening to an employee's problems, making a joint decision about what should be done about them, and then telling and motivating the employee to follow through and take action. In a nutshell, it is an advice-giving function. In nondirective counseling, the process focuses more on the employee's working through the problems by explanation, analysis, and problem-solving exercises. It emphasizes changing the person's perception of the problem or his or her reaction to it rather than dealing only with the problem itself. Participative counseling is conducted by professional counselors only, such as might be found in a formal employee assistance program. This makes it the most expensive type of counseling to be undertaken. It is a middle ground between directive and nondirective counseling because it establishes a cooperative exchange of ideas to help solve an employee's problems. The functions of reassurance, communication, emotional release, and clarified thinking are all used in participative counseling.

DISCIPLINE

Preventive Discipline

Preventive discipline encourages compliance with standards or rules so that infractions are avoided. Self-discipline is expected of all employees after being informed about the rules and the expected standards of performance.

Corrective Discipline

Corrective discipline is an action that follows an infraction of the rules or failure to meet the standards of performance. Typically, the disciplinary action is a penalty of some kind that discourages repeat offenses and serves to discourage other employees from the same behavior.

Progressive Discipline

Progressive discipline is a system that has stronger penalties for each successive repeated offense. Its purpose is to give the employee several opportunities to correct the offensive behavior before more serious action is taken. The last (fatal) step in progressive discipline is termination. In many situations, progressive discipline works fine, the problems are corrected, and termination is avoided. When the infraction is something like tardiness or absenteeism, employees correct themselves when they become aware of the seriousness of the warnings and the potential for losing their jobs. In other situations, progressive discipline may not be as effective.

Progressive discipline programs begin with a verbal warning from the supervisor to the employee. The warning includes a description of the problem, what is needed to correct it, and the time frame within which it should be corrected. A summary of this conversation should be documented in the manager's records but not in the employee's personnel file.

If the behavior is not corrected in the expected time frame, the next step is a written warning. The written warning does become part of the permanent personnel file. This documentation should clearly and concisely describe what the problem is, the date of the verbal warning, and the employee's behavior since that date. Any documented evidence that substantiates the inappropriate behavior should be attached. After written warning (depending on organization policy) may come suspension without pay or involuntary termination.

Progressive discipline works well with rule infractions but is not as effective in skill deficiency or quality of work performance problems. In fact, it may produce an attitude problem that was not an issue at the outset. In-service education and/or counseling may be more effective in these situations.

When a progressive discipline program is not applied tactfully, does not use constructive correction methods, and just makes threats of taking the next step, it will not be effective. In most cases, when action is threatened, the manager has no choice but to follow through so that order is maintained. This system is something like the parent-child relationship. If the parent says that certain behaviors will result in specific consequences and does not follow through when they occur, the rules are not taken seriously.

GRIEVANCE PROCEDURES

Employees should have the same communication and problem resolution avenues as managers. This is done by the use of complaint or grievance procedures and effective communication channels. Depending on the complexity of the organization, this may be a simple meeting between a manager and an employee or a formal, documented process that transcends departmental lines.

Employee complaint procedures are established because no matter how clear or well defined an organization thinks that its policies and procedures might be, they are misunderstood or miscommunicated at times. Questions and problems often arise that require a systematic investigation and mutual resolution for a satisfying work environment.

Any complaints or disagreements that arise over work-related issues should be dealt with promptly. Ideally, employees who think that they have been unfairly treated should be able to discuss their concerns with their supervisors. However, sometimes misunderstandings, emotions, and personality conflicts make the issues difficult to resolve on a one-to-one basis. When this occurs, a grievance procedure assures that the employee has a fair hearing, that the issue will be thoroughly and equitably investigated, and that all questions will be answered to the satisfaction of both parties.

The most common form of a grievance procedure provides an employee with the opportunity to present her or his case to increasingly higher levels of management. The immediate supervisor is the first level, and then, depending on the depth of the organization, the case may proceed through managers, directors, vice president, president, and, ultimately, the governing board. The emphasis is placed on resolution of the issues at the lowest possible level, so that the time and energy of people beyond the supervisor and employee are not expended to solve an issue that could be worked out within this relationship.

Goals of Grievance Procedures

Grievance procedures should share the following goals:

- To make sure all employees are treated with consideration and fairness
- To enable the organization to handle employee problems and complaints quickly to the satisfaction of both parties
- To enable employees to obtain answers to their questions about their jobs, management practices and policies, and other subjects of concern or importance that are not addressed by the supervisor

Essential Points

When writing a grievance procedure, the following essential points should be covered:

- Clearly state the goal of the process.
- List which items may be grieved. This includes examples of appropriate issues and instances in which the grievance procedure *may not* be used, such as dismissals for cause due to evident drug use, theft, or breach of confidentiality.
- Specify who is to hear the grievances and the time frames for each step.
- Delineate the step-by-step procedure for the process.
- Describe mediation and arbitration proceedings, if applicable.
- Establish time limits for grievance handling to facilitate prompt action, investigation, and resolution.
- Outline responsibilities of the management at each step concerning documentation, notification, and action.

Union—Nonunion

In a unionized organization, the handling of employee grievances is regulated by the union contract. Even if the employee works for a nonunion employer, some aspects of the grievance procedures are regulated by the National Labor Relations Act, which was discussed earlier. The presentation of a grievance by an employee or a group of employees is a protected activity under this act. This means that the employer cannot discriminate against an employee because he or she has registered a grievance. For example, it is illegal to fire or in any other way penalize someone for filing a grievance. If the employer would take such an action, the employee has the right to file a complaint with the NLRB.

Sample Health Information Management Complaint Procedure

GOAL. This procedure was established to create an avenue for problem resolution so that questions or conflicts could be investigated and resolved quickly, thoroughly, and within the appropriate organizational structure.

VALID COMPLAINTS

- Questions about or concerns with policies and procedures
- Disagreement with performance appraisal
- Concerns about the physical work environment
- Questions about or concerns with compensation and benefits management

INVALID COMPLAINTS. Appeal of termination for cause as specified in the policies and procedures is an invalid complaint.

PROCEDURE

1. Complaints should be presented orally to the immediate supervisor.
2. The employee may present the complaint personally or organize a group to present the complaint.
3. The supervisor will hear the complaint and make every effort to resolve the problem at this step. The supervisor shall write out the complaint, whether it is resolved or not, sign it, and then ask the employee or the employee group representative to also sign, so that the complaint is documented and clearly defined.

If the complaint cannot or will not be resolved by the supervisor immediately, the supervisor will outline the plan to accomplish resolution and document the estimated time frame for this to occur on the same document. If the problem can be resolved right away, the solution is documented. This report will be filed in a special file labeled "Complaints."

4. If the outlined plan or the resolution proposed by the supervisor is unsatisfactory to the employee or group, a copy of this report is sent to the division chief with the "Request for Review" box checked.

5. The division chief will conduct a review and respond to the employee or employee group representative within 3 working days with a plan for problem resolution.

6. If, after this step, the employee or group still believes that the problem is not resolved, the last step is to present the issue to the Personnel Action Committee for consideration. This committee will convene in special session within 10 working days. The decision of this interdisciplinary committee will be binding, and no other appeals will be heard. Members of this ad hoc committee will be the division chief, the supervisor involved, three members of the division at large not involved in the issue, and two human resource management specialists.

EXAMPLE

Gertrude Grump, a record retrieval specialist, is scheduled to work every Saturday. She was hired part-time to cover Saturdays when the full-time staff are off. She believes that it is unfair that the full-time record retrieval specialist should have every weekend off. When she brought up this concern to the supervisor, the supervisor explained that her position was designed to be a regular Saturday employee and that there are no plans to change scheduling.

Gertrude appears in the department director's office with a grievance form that has been filled out. What will the department director need to do now?

PERFORMANCE APPRAISAL SYSTEMS

Performance appraisals are used to evaluate how well an employee does her or his job. When correctly administered, they benefit the employee, the manager, and the organization. The main purpose of performance appraisal is to assess performance and provide guidance on how the employee can improve by suggesting behavior changes or additional skill development. It provides a framework for setting individual goals that fit into the departmental and organizational strategic plan.

Formal evaluation of employee performance provides valuable information for management. Increases in compensation and promotions are often linked to performance appraisal results. Managers use the results of this assessment to monitor patterns or trends that reflect success or failure in recruitment, selection, or training programs.

A performance appraisal system should produce an accurate picture of the employee's job performance. To do this, job performance standards must be created, agreed upon, and accepted by both managers and employees. The performance appraisal system must then use these standards as the basis for the evaluation.

Some performance standards are common to every job within an organization, such as attendance, but no two positions are likely to have the same criteria for evaluation. The essential job duties and standards are identified during job analysis, and many organizations place them within the job description as well.

Types of Performance Appraisal Systems

Rating Scales

Various methods are used to rate performance. A **rating scale** is probably the oldest and most widely used method (Figure 14–8). A continuous scale range of unsatisfactory through average to outstanding, perhaps using a numeric scale, is a common method. Other systems use a discrete system in which the manager assigns "Does Not Meet Standards," "Meets Standards," "Exceeds Standards," or something similar. To be useful, the ratings must be easy to understand, be a reliable indicator of performance, and be based on the critical behaviors that determine job performance.

The manager must take action for any unsatisfactory or "not-meeting-standards" employee. This usually takes the form of a written action plan to improve performance with a designated target date for improvement and the consequences for continued poor performance. A sample of such a plan is shown in Figure 14–9.

EXAMPLE

Karen Kline is the director of Health Information Services at Mercy Memorial. The corporation that Mercy is affiliated with has a rating scale type of performance appraisal system, and its use is mandated for all departments. Employees are rated in four areas—dependability, adaptability, quality of work, and quantity of work—using a scale of 1 to 5. Karen's managers have expressed dissatisfaction with this system because of numerous complaints by employees about perceived unfairness in its administration. They think that the system is too subjective and generic and does not always apply to their jobs. In addition, the managers think that this system does not allow for encouragement of continuous improvement in performance.

What are the possible options for Karen as the department director in this situation?

Employee Name:		Department:			
Supervisor:		Date:			
Position:					
Employee Attributes	Excellent (5)	Good (4)	Acceptable (3)	Fair (2)	Poor (1)
Dependability					
Initiative					
Productivity					
Quality					
Total By Categories					

Overall Score (Sum of Categories):

Comments:

FIGURE 14–8. Sample performance evaluation system—rating scale.

Checklists

Checklists may be used to select statements or words that most clearly describe an employee's performance (Figure 14–10). They may contain weights so that the more critical job duties have greater impact.

A forced-choice method requires the supervisor to choose the statement in each pair of statements that is most descriptive of the employee being evaluated. Often both statements in the pair are positive or negative. The following are examples of paired statements:

Fast learner	Hard worker
Work is accurate and thorough	Employee sets a good example for peers
Absent often	Usually tardy

Forced-choice methods are usually standardized, so that there may be few job-specific criteria used in evaluation. Another disadvantage is the perception of an employee when one statement is chosen over another. For example, an employee may think that he is both a hard worker and a fast learner.

Critical Incident Method

The **critical incident method** of employee performance evaluation requires the rater to document either extremely good or bad behavior related to job performance. The statements gathered are termed "critical incidents." Although this is a helpful method for providing job-specific feedback, it is dependent on the rater faithfully and honestly recording *every* critical incident.

Behaviorally anchored rating scales is a variation of the critical incident method. It identifies and evaluates relevant job-related behaviors. Specific named behaviors are used to give the rater reference points in evaluating the employee. These reference points may be called significant job duties, key result areas, or job performance benchmarks (Figure 14–11).

There are also systems that evaluate employees by comparison with coworkers. These methods include the ranking method, forced distribution method, point allocation method, and paired comparisons. Each one has advantages and disadvantages that must be considered before a choice is made as to which will work best.

For professional development and growth, the following goals will be established to improve personal productivity and enhance contributions to department objectives and the hospital mission.

Within each goal, selected objectives are outlined to serve as benchmarks and measure progress towards that goal.

**Area of Accountability—Clinical
Data Coordination**

I. Reduce unbilled accounts due to coding to 0 days with minimum oversight.

   A. Report status every Monday to department head using the Health Information Services weekly statistics form.

   B. Outline reasons for variance from the standard.

   C. Perform timely follow-up to assure that all records are released for billing within the time parameters established.

II. Improve productivity in coding and abstracting. Industry standards for coding Medicare inpatients are 15 to 20 minutes per record. Emergency room and Outpatient services 2.5 minutes per record and Ambulatory Surgery 10 minutes per record.

   A. Document obstacles that prohibit this level of performance at this hospital.

   B. Increase coding expertise through continuing education from a variety of resources.

   C. Code all patient types to enhance skills.

III. Use Continuous Quality Improvement (CQI) principles to improve work efficiency in your responsibility area.

   A. Organize work area to exhibit neatness and efficiency.

   B. Prioritize daily work to optimize adherence to department CQI standards. Report when not attainable to reasons beyond your control.

FIGURE 14–9. Sample performance development goal plan.

Administration of Employee Performance Appraisal Systems

Administration of performance appraisal systems can be the most rewarding or the most difficult job that a manager undertakes. A good system facilitates a better outcome, but a good manager can even make a poor evaluation system work effectively. The manager must combine as many objective measurements as possible with a subjective assessment of the employee's performance.

Methods to Assist the Manager

There are several effective tools that can assist the manager with administering performance appraisal. Employee self-appraisal is useful when the goal of the evaluation process is self-development. In many cases, employees are more critical of themselves than is the manager. The most important dimension to the self-appraisal method is the buy-in and commitment of the employee to improvement because goals and objectives are jointly developed.

Management by objective is used with self-appraisal so that the manager and the employee establish joint goals. The idea is that if manager and employee agree on goals, behaviors will be adjusted to assure that they are met. To be effective, management by objective requires regular and timely feedback about progress.

Rater Biases That Affect Appraisal

The main problem with subjective assessments is the potential for rater bias. A supervisor may fail to remain emotionally detached during the evaluation. The most common rater biases include the **halo effect** (strong personal like or dislike), the error of central tendency (inclination to make everyone average), and the leniency or strictness tendency (inclination to be too lenient or too strict in general).

The following are other biases that may affect performance appraisals:

- *Cultural bias.* A manager may be biased for or against a given cultural background because of his or her own life experiences with others from that culture.

- *Personal prejudice.* Personal like or dislike of a person because of sex, religion, or past experiences should not affect performance evaluation. Assessments should be strictly criteria-based on key result areas determined before the review period begins and communicated to the employee in language that she or he can understand.

- *Recency effects.* An employee's behavior in the most recent period, whether it be weeks or months, should not color an annual performance evaluation. The whole performance period should be reviewed and assessed. This requires systematic review and documentation as events occur.

COMPENSATION MANAGEMENT

Definition

Performance evaluation and compensation management are often linked together so that employees who perform well are rewarded with increased compensation.

Weights	Performance Appraisal Criteria	Check
	Employee Name _____ Department _____ Position _____ Date _____ Supervisor _____	
6.5	Employee is accountable to essential job duties.	
4.0	Employee keeps work area well organized.	
3.9	Employee works cooperatively with others as a team.	
4.3	Employee considers consequences before taking action.	
0.2	Employee adheres to dress code.	
etc.		
Total 100		
	Total of All Weights Checked	

FIGURE 14–10. Sample weighted performance checklist.

Employee: Kay Smith   Department: Health Information Services
Supervisor: Marion White   Date: Jan 15, 1996
Rating Period: Oct 1 through Dec 31, 1995   Position: Clinical Coding Specialist

Accuracy of Coding

Date	Positive Employee Behaviors Noted	Date	Negative Employee Behaviors Noted
9/15/95	Monitoring and Evaluation shows 98%	11/13/95	M & E of inpatient coding revealed
	accuracy on outpatient coding		error rate of 7%
10/13/95	M & E shows 97% accuracy	12/15/95	M & E of inpatient coding still
			shows error rate of 7%
			Corrective Action Plan given.

Accuracy of Abstracting

Date	Positive Employee Behaviors Noted	Date	Negative Employee Behaviors Noted
10/5/95	No errors found on 50 records	12/31/95	None recorded to date
11/17-95	No errors found on 100 records		

FIGURE 14–11. Behaviorally anchored rating performance appraisal system.

Compensation management is defined as a system to develop a comprehensive, systematic salary-and-benefit program. Compensation includes not only wages and salaries but also benefits such as health insurance and, in some cases, profit-sharing and incentive rewards. When compensation is not competitive, employees are likely to become dissatisfied and leave. Recruitment of replacement workers of the same quality is difficult.

By fairly rewarding desired results and commitment to the organization, the organization is more likely to obtain behaviors that are consistent with managerial strategies. Human resources planning, recruiting, selection, placement, **career planning,** employee development, and performance appraisals all contribute to this effort as well, but compensation management programs have the advantage of being modified quickly and tied to changing objectives of the organization.

Objectives of Compensation Management

The following common objectives are pursued through effective compensation management:

- Attract desirable, qualified applicants.
- Retain current competent staff.
- Assure quality results in services provided.
- Reward desirable work behaviors.
- Control costs and facilitate budgeting by managing resources appropriately.
- Comply with laws and regulations for wage and salary administration.
- Improve efficiency by using a system that is easy to understand.

Job Evaluation

Job evaluation is an important component of a compensation management program. It is a systematic procedure used to determine the relative worth of the position to the organization. To be effective, the job evaluation process is based on the job description. Because job evaluation requires special knowledge and training, it is usually performed by human resource professionals.

Understanding the process used by the organization to determine the worth of a job to the organization—in reality its pay grade—is important for the HIM manager. The manager wants to be sure that the wages set for the health information services positions are equitable within the organization and competitive within the community. If the health information services personnel

are paid less than organization staff in similar positions or in different organizations, the health information services department will become a training ground for other departments and organizations.

EXAMPLE

The health information services department has some of the lowest salary ranges in the hospital. Jane Jurgens, the department director, is concerned with increasing dissatisfaction from the data management staff, who stated that they must have highly technical skills and work under stress and still do not make as much as the medical secretaries in other areas of the hospital. When Jane visits with the human resource specialist about this problem, she confirms that the secretarial positions earn a full $1.72 an hour more than the data management staff positions. She advises Jane to examine the job descriptions and compare them with those of the medical secretary positions.

What factors should Jane consider as she performs this job analysis?

Job ranking, job grading or classification, **factor comparison,** and the **point system** are some methods used to evaluate jobs. Figure 14–12 compares these methods along two matrixes: whether they compare the whole job or divide the job into factors and whether jobs are compared against one another or against a standard.

The simplest method, but also the least precise, is the ranking method. Jobs are ranked by comparing them with other positions within the organization. A file clerk in the health information services department may be ranked near the bottom (10), whereas the diagnosis related group (DRG) coordinator is closer to the top (2). This ranking is due to the magnitude of responsibility of the DRG coordinator position and its impact on revenue generation. The ranking method is best used in organizations with a small number of positions.

Job grading is more sophisticated than ranking but is really not any more precise. This process classifies each job to a grade that it most closely resembles. A common example of this method is civil service classification. It is not precise because the job is grouped with jobs that it is most similar to on an overall basis. The health information manager should be knowledgeable about the descriptions of the job grades and which grades would be appropriate for HIM positions.

The factor comparison method requires comparison of elements of the job, not the entire job. Factors are used that are common to all positions, such as responsibility, required skills, mental effort, physical effort, and working conditions.

To discern the effect of using the factor comparison method on the HIM positions, one needs to understand

	COMPARES EACH JOB AS A WHOLE	COMPARES EACH JOB ONE ELEMENT AT A TIME
Measures job against job	Ranking methods	Factor comparison methods
Measures job against predetermined scale	Classification or grade methods	Point methods

FIGURE 14–12. Job evaluation systems chart.

how the method works. The steps of this process are as follows:

1. Establish the factors on which the jobs will be compared (e.g., responsibility, working conditions).
2. Determine the key jobs. Key jobs are those that are commonly found within the organization and that are common in the employer's labor market. The current wage rate for the key jobs is not controversial.
3. Rank the key jobs according to the factors, one factor at a time for the key jobs.
4. Establish the average salary for each key job and apportion the money to each factor according to how the job was ranked on the factor—the higher ranking, the greater the proportion of wage to the factor.
5. Place key jobs on a factor comparison chart.
6. Evaluate other jobs using the key jobs as benchmarks.

As with the factor comparison method, a point system compares elements of job, but it compares the factors to a descriptive standard rather than to other key jobs. The descriptive standard is a definition of each factor and the levels within the factor. For example, if education was one of the factors, degrees within this factor would be as follows:

- Master's degree or beyond
- Bachelor's degree
- Associate degree or specialized training beyond high school
- High school diploma or equivalent

Points are assigned to each degree within the factor. Job grades are determined by the total number of points in a range. Therefore, to apply this method, the health

information manager needs to be knowledgeable of the factors used, the degrees within the factors, the points assigned to each degree, and the point ranges for the job grades. This information is usually not available to anyone outside the human resources department. But the health information manager could determine a job's worth by comparing various jobs and analyzing their job grades.

Many variations of these methods are used. Large organizations modify these standard approaches to meet their specific needs. The Hay Plan method is marketed by a large consulting firm and is popular in health care organizations. This is a proprietary method and relies on a committee evaluation of critical job factors to determine each job's relative worth.

Why Job Evaluations Are Used

Regardless of the method used, all job evaluation approaches seek to determine a position's relative worth to provide internal equity within an organization and competitive position in the community.

No matter which method is chosen to evaluate the job and establish the pay rate, the manager should review and request adjustment for any assignments that do not appear reasonable and fair. For example, health record analysts review the patient record after discharge and identify missing documents or data. The supervisor of the health record analysts discovered that workers doing the same type of job in the outpatient surgery center were ranked two job grades above the health record analysts. Investigation revealed that the inpatient health record analyst position had been ranked lower because of the lack of emphasis in the job description of the medical terminology skills, data entry experience, and interaction with the medical staff. After the job descriptions were revised, the job was re-evaluated and the health record analysts were awarded a well-deserved pay increase.

Salary Surveys

Some organizations use data from wage and salary surveys to determine the market value of a given position. These surveys are often done by professional associations, such as state hospital associations. In using this information to determine wages, management decides where it wants its organization to be within the market (i.e., at the top, near the middle, on the low side). One problem with reliance on wage and salary surveys for compensation is comparability. A position that one facility considers a health record technician can vary significantly from the same position at another facility. Surveys often unknowingly lump unlike jobs together and may skew the data high or low. Also, if the sample is small, as in a survey of a small state for the position of manager of Health Information Services, a disproportionate number of experienced or, at the other extreme, entry-level personnel would skew the results.

To maintain an effective compensation management program, large organizations group jobs into classifications or grades for pay rates. Even a medium-sized organization with 2000 employees and 325 separately identifiable jobs would have a complex task to administer compensation. The existence of different pay ranges for all 325 jobs would probably be meaningless because many jobs would differ by only a few cents. Instead, rate ranges are assigned to each job classification or grade. Employees are placed within ranges according to related job experience and longevity with the organization.

Managers should be aware of the challenges that affect compensation administration. Prevailing market forces cause some jobs to be paid at a higher rate. For example, if there is a shortage of qualified clinical coders, the prevailing wage for clinical coders may be much higher than their relative worth in the organization. Computer programmers enjoyed this phenomenon during the 1980s before supply caught up with the demand.

When union is involved, even for a portion of the workforce, union contracts may drive wages past the relative worth of the jobs. This is particularly true if the union controls most or all of a particular skill area.

TRAINING AND DEVELOPMENT

Training and development of an HIM team is a worthwhile goal of any manager of health information services. A sound training program assures employee involvement, growth, and competency through the changing needs of the future environment. Although training and development programs are costly, failure to provide them can also be expensive. For example, if the coding staff has not kept abreast of coding and DRG changes, a hospital could have huge revenue losses as a result of inappropriate DRG assignment or returned claims because of outdated code use. Failure to keep abreast of changing regulatory and accreditation requirements may place an organization in danger of unfavorable accreditation decisions or sanctions.

Starting a Training Program

Needs Assessment

A needs assessment is the first step a manager should take in structuring the training program. This diagnostic process identifies weak areas or changing work requirements and then determines what is needed to correct the deficiencies.

Potential training needs can be identified in the following ways:

* Review professional journals to identify changing requirements in the collection, analysis, and dissemination of health information.

* Question employees about their need for new skills or knowledge.

* Retrieve and analyze key indicators from internal and external sources such as quality assessments, management feedback, grievance reports, claims denial reports, and productivity monitor systems.

Assess Impact on Staff

Once the needs are identified, the next step is to assess the impact on the current staff.

* Will the training be welcomed and appreciated, or resented?

* Will the training program have the desired outcome?

* Which employees will receive the training?

* How will taking time out for training affect department operations?

Training and development programs are especially helpful to prevent obsolescence and career plateaus. Obsolescence occurs when employees no longer have the skills required to perform successfully in a changing workplace—for example, medical transcriptionists who cannot operate word processors and record retrieval specialists who do not understand how to use the computer to look up patients' numbers in the master patient index.

Career plateaus are points in employees' work lives when their performance is good enough to keep them from being fired or demoted to a lesser position but their skills are not adequate to earn them a promotion. Employees should be steered away from getting stuck on a plateau by being encouraged to participate in appropriate training and development programs. Key signs of career plateaus are reluctance or refusal to adapt to new technology and insistence that "the old way was better." These employees may lose interest in volunteering for professional growth activities and may require assertive direction or a mandate to attend training sessions.

Training Programs

Orientation

Formal orientation programs may be provided for all new employees within a health care organization by the human resources department. This orientation *never* substitutes for the job-specific departmental orientation and the personal interchange between the new employee, the supervisor, and the peer group.

Orientation programs are a key ingredient of employee satisfaction in an organization. Even experienced, superbly qualified new hires can benefit from an effective orientation. The central objectives of orientation are to reduce a new employee's anxieties about how she or he will fit in and to make sure that she or he knows the ropes of the new position at the outset. The program helps the employee learn about the social, technical, and cultural aspects of the workplace, as discussed previously.

One of the major benefits to the employer from a formal orientation program is the consistency of advice given, compared with the information that may be distributed by the employee's coworkers or peer group. The best orientation includes participation by all three groups.

1. The employee should attend the formal orientation, which includes personnel policies and organizational information.
2. There should be a work site orientation by the supervisor as to what the job entails and how the job fits into the department and organization.
3. The most meaningful orientation session will probably be a show-and-tell by the appropriate peer group. This portion trains the new employee by example and fills in the details missed by the first two types of orientation. Here the employee finds out who to ask and where to go for additional information.

BENEFITS OF ORIENTATION. The benefits to the organization of orientation by the peer group include the facilitation of employee acceptance into the social structure of the organization. By being introduced to key people, the new hires become comfortable within the workplace much sooner than they would on their own.

Staff Development

After orientation, managers must be alert to any training that employees need to stay current and productive. During the first departmental orientation session, the manager should review the job description in detail and outline the expectations for performance on every significant job duty listed. The staff will never hit the target if the manager has not pointed out the direction in which they are to aim and what it takes to score a bull's-eye. Many employees quit a job because they become frustrated with a manager who reprimands them for deficiencies in performance that they did not clearly understand. The supervisor must never assume that employees instinctively know anything. Job responsibilities, procedures, productivity standards, and expectations must be explicit and sometimes repeated several times.

Educational programs may be obtained outside the facility or consist of presentations by coworkers or other health care professionals from within the organization. The type and extent of the programs depend on the type of staff development needed and the budget available to fund it.

Career Planning

Career planning enables employees to be promoted from one level of job to another within an organization. It also provides an incentive for longevity in the workplace and keeps the staff interested, challenged, and continuously improving their skills. It also has the organizational advantage of assuring a continuous supply of qualified workers to accomplish the objectives of the organization.

For example, Sally is a health information specialist whose main responsibility is inserting late reports in discharge records. As a result of this job, Sally knows the document filing system well and is familiar with the various parts of the record and the sequence required by various users. She could be easily trained to assist with release of information requests several times a week. The release of information coordinator position has a higher pay rate and requires more skills than Sally's position. When Sally has had time to learn the extra skills, she will be an excellent choice for promotion to release of information coordinator.

The health information manager can assist in career planning within the organization as well as within the profession. Executives from the organization can be asked to give presentations on opportunities for advancement within the organization or affiliated institutions. **Career counseling** may be offered formally by the human resources department through an employee assistance program or casually by mentoring of staff.

Written materials on professional advancement with additional education should be made available. Another means of promoting career planning is to post job descriptions within the department, so that requirements for higher positions are known. Trainee positions can be created for people who want to advance but lack the job experience to apply for a particular position.

EFFECTIVE TIME MANAGEMENT STRATEGIES

A busy manager needs to set priorities to remain productive and energized for the various demands that arise in the course of a day's work. Here are some effective time management strategies.

- A personal calendar system helps keep track of accountabilities and schedules. A number of excellent products are available, and creative managers have also devised their own.

- Know yourself. Identify strengths and acknowledge shortcomings. Put strengths into action, and set personal goals to improve areas of weakness that you can live with. Allocate time for personal needs as well as professional demands or burnout will occur.

- Surround yourself with supportive people who know how to get things done. Learn from them and also use employees as a resource for time-saving ideas.

- Adopt the attitude that "there's got to be a better way to do my job that takes less time," and always be looking for even small things that will work toward this goal.

- Keep staff in the know, so that they can be proactive within the department. This saves time and frustration by avoiding "fires" that only a department head or manager can extinguish.

- Be sensitive to customers' needs. Time spent building relationships and developing alliances is time well invested. Make customers priority one every day by being accessible. Customers include staff, physicians, management peers, and the administration. Treat everyone with respect and dignity, and spend time talking with them, soliciting opinions, and listening with an open mind.

- Spending time keeping people informed regarding the status and direction of the health information services for the facility is the best possible time management strategy.

ATTRIBUTES OF AN EFFECTIVE HEALTH INFORMATION MANAGER

- Effective health information managers start a project with their time, not the task at hand. They regularly record and analyze their use of time for optimal productivity.

- Competent health information managers focus on results, not work, and start with what they can do, not with limitations and constraints.

- Perceptive health information managers recognize that no one functions alone in a health care organization. Support from administration, peers, and subordinates should be cultivated to facilitate greater accomplishments and multiply efforts.

- Smart health information managers concentrate efforts on areas in which outstanding performance will yield big returns. Rather than simply doing things right, they seek to do the right things as well to save time and materials.

- Excellent health information managers are decisive. They identify the strategic and generic elements in situations and avoid solving the same problem or making the same errors twice.

DESIGN AND MANAGEMENT OF SPACE IN HEALTH INFORMATION SERVICES

Most of this chapter is concerned with the methods and mechanisms that are used in managing the human resources of an HIM department. The environment in which these human resources function is extremely important to the success of the human resources management function. This section focuses on the arrangement of the physical components of furniture, equipment, and lighting with the goal of providing maximum effectiveness and coordinating these physical components into an efficient and comfortable work area.

Work Space Design

Health information managers need to pay attention to the design of the work space. Health information processing requires the use of both paper and computers.

How do both the old and the new fit into an environment that is comfortable to work in without creating the stress of physical problems such as **carpal tunnel syndrome**? New pieces of equipment are introduced and must be integrated into already crowded offices. Not only is the space at work changing to accommodate new technology, but the new technology is changing the location of the workplace. The number of employees working at home is increasing.

Considerations in Designing Work Space

When designing the work space, the following aspects should be considered.

Work Flow

Considering the purpose of the organization, the primary objective in work space design is efficient and effective work flow. Is the work moving to the next person with a minimum of backtracking and bottlenecks? Work flow is a greater concern in an environment where paper is used than in a totally computer-based system.

Traffic Patterns

Along with work flow, the traffic patterns of employees and visitors to the area are important considerations. To determine these patterns, the location of entrances to the area, the employees who work together, and the employees who frequently receive visitors or leave the area frequently need to be identified. A **trip frequency chart** shows which employees frequently interact with one another (Figure 14–13). The various employees and locations are listed in the horizontal and vertical axes. The number indicates how many times one employee visits the work space of another employee. Low numbers indicate which employees do not interact frequently and, therefore, do not need to be close to one another, whereas high numbers indicate a need for closeness.

Work groups and/or teams are commonly found in today's workplace. Space design must facilitate the work of these teams, not prohibit it. The supervisor or team leaders also need to be located in proximity to their staff to provide more effective supervision and facilitate communication.

The work space allotted to a particular departmental function or work group should conform to the number of employees performing that function. Equipment, references, and other materials needed to perform the job

TO / FROM	Director	Secretary	Health Information Analyst	Release of Information Specialist	Clinical Coder	Optical Image Specialist
Director		14	5	3	7	8
Secretary	30		4	9	2	10
Health Information Analyst	8	3		4	12	20
Release of Information Specialist	16	9	5		5	14
Clinical Coder	12	4	10	6		9
Optical Image Specialist	25	19	9	11	7	

FIGURE 14–13. Trip frequency chart.

can then be located in one central area so that they are easily accessible to all employees performing similar tasks.

Functions Performed in the Work Space

When designing the work space, an obvious consideration is the type of function performed in the space. Some specific functions beyond the data entry–clerical type functions must be considered. The reception area has a public relations aspect. Because visitors see this area first, it should be neat, well organized, and functional. It should be located so that visitors do not interrupt the work flow. Serving as a buffer zone between the outside and the place of work, the reception area provides privacy for the staff. This area should be monitored constantly to assist and screen visitors, letting only those people enter who have legitimate business.

Another special purpose area is a conference room. This area is needed for meetings that are too large to take place in a private office, that might disturb others in the office, or that need special equipment (e.g., an overhead projector). This area can also be used for training.

In the overall design of a department, it is often desirable to place certain areas next to each other and other areas far away from each other. A restaurant designer would not place the patron waiting area near the garbage dump. This would be undesirable. A **proximity chart** shows the need to place some areas close to or far from each other (Figure 14–14). It can also show why the proximity is important.

Need for Confidentiality of Work Performed

If the work being performed is of a confidential nature, access to the work area may need to be controlled. If the confidential information is audible—for example, physicians dictating reports for the patient record or employee conferences—then the space design must provide for this speech privacy. If the work is performed on a computer, the use of screens or panels around work areas may be advisable to prevent others from reading information displayed on the computer screen. The location of a fax machine also has security concerns. In a health care organization, confidential information is often transmitted by way of fax machine. Fax machines should be located in areas that are secure from access by unauthorized employees.

Shift Workers—Sharing Work Space

Sometimes it is necessary to divide a particular job function into shifts. This is true if space is restricted or if equipment to perform the job is costly and limited in supply. Shift work may mean that employees must share their work space. Under these circumstances, each employee should have some private space in the work area that is his or her own for displaying photos and for storage of personal items. Employees sharing work space need to respect one another's privacy. Adjustability of chairs and other work equipment is important so that the needs of all may be met.

Flexibility for Future Needs

Work space design should be as flexible as possible to accommodate the future needs of the organization. These needs might include downsizing, expansion, or further computerization. The use of partitions instead of solid-wall offices is recommended for organizations that anticipate change, either in size or in the work functions being performed. Workstations whose components may be added or subtracted as necessary (i.e., modular furniture) increase the capability of organizations to implement change without loss of efficiency.

Expanding technology demands increase the need for power capabilities of the work space. Regular electrical power and "clean" power for computers and telecommunications systems are located beneath access floors so that necessary power is available at any given location. This system allows for flush-to-floor outlets and flexible placement of furniture and equipment.

Employees' Personal Needs

The work environment is composed of people gathered together to perform work that will accomplish the objectives of an organization. These people have physical, social, and psychological needs that must be met as well as the need to collect a paycheck. Today's workforce wants a comfortable, safe, user-friendly environment.

In 1978 and again in 1980, a Steelcase National Study of Office Environments was performed.[5] The second study showed that office workers saw a strong connection between their overall satisfaction with their work environment and their level of job performance. Management and workers alike believed that there were fewer errors and higher concentration on work when comfort was improved.

PHYSICAL NEEDS

Ergonomics. Ergonomics is the science concerned with the relationship of people to their work environment. Its purpose is to determine how the physical environment affects workers' morale and performance. The goal of ergonomic design is to integrate the needs of the organization with the needs of the worker in a healthy, productive environment.

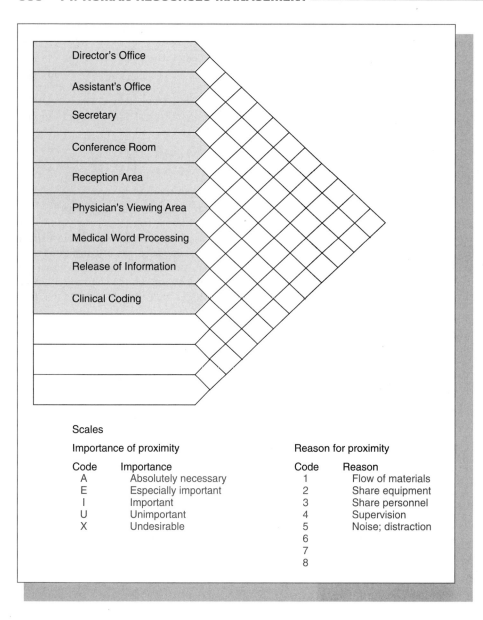

Director's Office
Assistant's Office
Secretary
Conference Room
Reception Area
Physician's Viewing Area
Medical Word Processing
Release of Information
Clinical Coding

Scales

Importance of proximity

Code	Importance
A	Absolutely necessary
E	Especially important
I	Important
U	Unimportant
X	Undesirable

Reason for proximity

Code	Reason
1	Flow of materials
2	Share equipment
3	Share personnel
4	Supervision
5	Noise; distraction
6	
7	
8	

FIGURE 14–14. Proximity chart.

The following aspects of ergonomics are important for design of the work space:

- Design and adjustability of the furniture to the individual employee

- Design of the work processes to include breaks and changes in jobs with a high degree of repetition

- Arrangement of the workstation components so that all the employees' tools and equipment are within easy reach

Physical Size and Structure. Because employees vary in physical characteristics such as height, weight, and length of torso and extremities, workstation components should be as flexible and adjustable as possible. Chairs should be adjustable as to seat height, the angle of backrests and armrests, and back tilt. Work surfaces should have the capability of being raised or lowered according to the height and needs of the user. Computer monitors should swivel, and their height should be adjustable. The position and height of the computer keyboard are especially important. Ongoing training programs for the ergonomic use of chairs, computers, and their peripherals (printers, keyboards, monitor supports, computer and printer stands, and printer enclosures) should be conducted routinely in the office.

Age. Older people may require special consideration

in the workplace. Because visual and hearing problems are more prevalent with increasing age, lighting needs to be adequate for the task being performed and background noise should be considered. Older employees also like a warmer temperature.

Medical Conditions. In addition to the special considerations of age, workplace requirements for physical handicaps or other medical conditions of the worker must be addressed. Adjustments to the work space to accommodate special equipment or handicaps without causing the employer undue hardships is required by the ADA.

Shared or Multifunction Workstations. Workstation furniture or components must accommodate a number of functional tasks. Many workstations used by general or technical employees are shared, either on the same shift or between shifts. This means that it is even more important to purchase furniture with as many adjustable features as possible.

Ergonomics looks not only at the construction and adjustability of furniture and equipment but also into design of the work processes. Repetitive tasks require frequent changes in position. Employees can develop muscle strain and aching if seated in one position for too long. From an ergonomic standpoint, taking frequent breaks and varying the type of work performed are essential. Medical transcriptionists commonly sit at word processing stations for many hours without changing position or routine. Breaks do not always have to be rest breaks. Interspersing different functions into the transcriptionist's day can alleviate the strain and muscle fatigue that comes from sitting for long hours in the same position. Transcriptionists should break their routine occasionally by answering telephones or filing transcribed reports. This procedure helps to reduce boredom as well as fatigue. Changing the routine may not work well if an incentive or other type of productivity program is in place.

INJURY PREVENTION. Musculoskeletal injury may occur during the performance of repetitive tasks, particularly if physical capabilities are exceeded. Injury risk can be reduced by proper design in physical support, equipment, and the work process. Effects of poor ergonomic design include muscle pain and strain, pinched nerves, headaches, dizziness, eyestrain, neck strain, carpal tunnel syndrome, backache, and fatigue. Sometimes these injuries are called cumulative trauma disorders (CTD) and repetitive strain (or stress) injuries (RSI). They were formerly associated with manual labor; today, they are commonplace in the office setting.

SAFETY NEEDS. A safe work environment is important to management as well as to office workers. It reduces the number of work-related accidents that are costly to the organization in terms of lost work time and workers' compensation claims.

Management is responsible for providing a safe work environment for employees. These responsibilities include the following:

- Maintaining a favorable climate for safety
- Assuring that the equipment and furniture are in the best working condition
- Being a good example
- Teaching principles of safety (see Basic Safety Principles)
- Stressing an orderly work environment
- Stopping unsafe acts

SOCIAL NEEDS. The atmosphere in the office affects employees' happiness and feelings of well-being. A positive environment can motivate employees to improve productivity. When work occurs in an enjoyable place,

---

Basic Safety Principles

- Cords for telephones or electrical equipment should be out of sight, if possible. Furniture often has cable channels to accommodate the multitudes of cords required in today's workplace. Cords should never be draped across aisles or walkways. Whenever unplugging an electrical appliance, one should always pull on the plug, not the cord. Yanking on the cord breaks insulation or loosens terminals.

- File and desk drawers should not be left open for people to trip over or walk into. They should not be used as a step stool because they will not hold a person's weight.

- Office tools such as scissors, staples, razor blades, and pencils should be used only for their intended purpose. Pencils are not to be used as hole punchers. Letter openers are not to be used for prying open stuck drawers.

- Paper cuts are an annoying type of injury that can be avoided by proper handling: using rubber fingerguards, picking up individual sheets of paper at the corner instead of the side, and encouraging the use of hand lotion for dry skin, which is more susceptible to paper cuts.

- Drawer files can tip over if more than one drawer at a time is opened or if heavy objects are placed in top drawers or far in the front of a drawer.

- Stepladders should be fully open and locked before use. Move the ladder to the desired location instead of reaching from the ladder. Do not use boxes, chairs on rollers, or tables in place of ladders.

- Open-shelf files should be bolted to a wall or to the back of another file. Trying to remove records from files that are too tightly packed causes the files to sway or topple if they are not bolted to some other support.

employees work harder with fewer sick days than when each day begins with dread.

Employees, especially those who are engaged in similar activities, like to work in proximity with one another. They can easily ask questions or otherwise confer on the work at hand. Workstations in clusters are effective in encouraging the team approach.

PERSONAL SPACE. Personal space is the private area that surrounds an employee and is felt to belong to her or him. Personal space requirements vary between cultures, with those from Middle Eastern countries typically requiring less than Americans.

Territoriality is another concept that should be considered in office space planning. Territoriality refers to the physical area under the control of the employee or that which is specifically for his or her use. It may be the employee's workstation or it may refer to a private office.

Employees take pride in their physical surroundings. The workstation becomes a reflection of employees' personalities. They like the freedom to decorate or personalize it to suit themselves.

Reflection of Status in the Organization (Is the Corner Office Dead?)

The status of an employee within an organization, especially the managerial staff, used to be reflected by whether or not the employee had a private office, the size of that office, and whether or not the office had windows. The large corner office in a building or suite was seen as the most desirable space in terms of status within the organization.

Private offices are not as common or as widely used as they were in past years. The trend is toward a more open type of **office landscaping.** The private office still denotes prestige, however, and most executives prefer to have some degree of privacy in their work setting. The work may be of a personal or confidential nature that requires a location in which business matters cannot be overheard by other employees. The work may also require a high degree of concentration. Such a case would require locating the workstation in an area free from distractions and interruptions.

The disadvantages of private offices are interferences with heat and air-conditioning systems, a decrease in supervisory effectiveness, and increased construction costs.

Managers can enjoy almost as much privacy with an open plan as with a private office by using high divider panels to surround the office furnishings. Panels with doors are available in a wide variety of fabrics and materials, including glass.

Evaluation of individual needs is necessary to decide whether a private office is needed. Combining the con-

ventional office plan with private offices with the open plan maintains the status and privacy needs of the executive. Such a combination is referred to as the **American plan of office design.**

Legal Requirements and Recommendations

Many of the laws and regulations previously discussed in this chapter affect the design of work space. OSHA requires that employers furnish a workplace that is free from hazards that are likely to cause serious harm or death. OSHA has safety requirements for equipment, noise level standards, and lighting requirements for computer users. For workers who keyboard for a "cumulative total of four or more hours, inclusive of breaks, during a twelve-hour period,"[6] OSHA requires adjustable hardware and chairs as well as antiglare screens for computer monitors. Armrests, wristrests, and foot supports must also be provided at the request of the employee.

Most workers prefer challenging and varied work. Providing variety in tasks reduces the risk of repetitive stress injuries at the same time it improves morale. Minibreaks, which may only consist of a stand-up stretch, are recommended throughout the day. OSHA concludes that frequent short breaks increase productivity and comfort, especially for computer users.

The National Institute for Occupational Safety and Health (NIOSH) sets standards in office design, construction, and use of equipment, especially in the use of computers. The results of a 1980 NIOSH study showed that computer users experience various types of health complaints. Among them are optical problems, gastrointestinal upsets, emotional problems (thought to be brought on by stress), painful or stiff muscles and joints, and loss of strength in arms, hands, wrists, and fingers. After the study, NIOSH stressed ergonomic solutions to these problems. In other words, they recommended that managers provide employees with furniture and equipment that can be adjusted to the physical traits of each individual worker to eliminate strain. NIOSH sets standards for lighting as well.

The Vocational Rehabilitation Act of 1972 requires that federal buildings as well as buildings that were built with more than $2500 in federal funds be accessible to handicapped people. These requirements include wide aisle space for wheelchairs, 28-inch height for desks, 32-inch-wide doors, ramp entrances to buildings, and appropriate (time-delayed) entry doors.

The ADA provides that if a facility is a "public accommodation," it must take "barrier removal" steps. Public accommodations include many types of service establishments, such as professional offices of health care providers, pharmacies, insurance offices, banks, and hospitals. Barriers that affect work space design can be modified in the following ways:

- Installing ramps where steps are located
- Repositioning shelves
- Installing flashing alarm lights
- Widening doors
- Installing offset hinges to widen doorways
- Installing accessible door hardware
- Removing high-pile, low-density carpeting[7]

Environmental Considerations

The results of the Steelcase Study II on office comfort showed that the ability to control temperature is important to office employees. Workers who participated in the study stated that if they could change physical conditions in their offices, they would most often make improvements in the heat and air-conditioning, regulate temperature, reduce noise, obtain more space and privacy, and acquire more comfortable chairs.

Given a choice between getting a raise with no improvements in the office environment and getting a smaller increase with improvements, more than one half of the employees in the Steelcase Study selected the larger raise. A substantial number, however, stated that they would select a smaller raise if they could control heat and air-conditioning (30 per cent) and general office comfort (27 per cent), had a chair with back support (26 per cent), had a private office with a door (21 per cent), and had a quieter place in which to work (20 per cent). It is interesting to note that heat and air-conditioning ranked highest as the item employees most wanted to control; it ranked 11th as the item that executives believed that their company would consider a motivator or reward for high employee performance. Employers greatly underestimated the need of employees to control their own environment.

AIR QUALITY. Heating, ventilating, and air-conditioning (HVAC) systems are an integral part of office design. Heating and air-conditioning systems are easier to operate in the **open office design plan** of most modern offices than in the traditional or closed plan.

Good air quality improves productivity. Air pollution (stale, dusty air), on the other hand, produces undesirable effects, such as headache and fatigue. Air circulation is important in the work environment. Fifteen cubic meters of fresh (outside) air per hour per person is desirable in a nonsmoking environment. Air-conditioning not only cools the air but also removes undesirable pollutants such as smoke, asbestos, soot, dust, and chemicals. Clean air is important for equipment operation as well as for its effects on employees. Mechanical air filters are helpful, as are frequent cleaning, sweeping, and vacuuming.

OSHA has set indoor air quality standards and can take action against employers who fail to comply. The Environmental Protection Agency (EPA) lists indoor air pollution as one of its top five environmental issues, causing a wide range of problems such as bronchitis, asthma, emphysema, cancer, and heart disease. The EPA states that a common problem in businesses is that the HVAC system operates only on weekdays and not when the building is unoccupied. It suggests starting the system several hours before workers arrive and continuing it for several hours after they leave for maximum effectiveness. The EPA also promotes restricted areas for smokers. The agency recommends regular inspections of the building and the HVAC system. Data on symptoms suffered by building occupants and likely contamination sources should be collected and analyzed periodically.

TEMPERATURE. Temperature is the hotness or coolness of the air. A comfortable office temperature is about 70° Fahrenheit or lower, with older employees requiring a slightly warmer environment. Thermostats are often set at 65° during the heating season to conserve energy. Human bodies in large numbers generate heat, especially when they are performing physical tasks such as walking and typing. A computer also generates heat equal to one person.

HUMIDITY. The percentage of moisture in the air is called **relative humidity.** The most comfortable standard for office workers is 30 to 60 per cent with a temperature ranging between 65 and 70°. Automated equipment requires a relative humidity range between 20 and 80 per cent. Too much humidity causes short-circuiting in equipment and too little humidity produces static electricity.

LIGHTING. Proper lighting is more important today than ever before with so many people using computers. Lighting affects not only productivity but employee health as well.

In planning a good lighting system, the following factors should be considered:

- Flexibility and adjustability
- Ease of installation
- Low energy use
- Low initial cost
- Efficiency of the system
- Safety
- Effect on employees (comfort level)
- Integration of sunlight into lighting systems

Amount and Type of Light. The amount and type of light should be evenly diffused over the work area.

Moving from areas of greater light intensity to areas of lesser intensity causes eyestrain, fatigue, and headache because of pupil expansion and contraction.

The amount and type of light used depend on the color scheme in the office decor, the type of work being performed, and the age of the worker. Less light is needed in areas that are decorated with light colors because light colors reflect light, whereas darker colors absorb light.

High levels of illuminance are needed for many tasks that involve paper documents, whereas lower levels are needed in computer-user environments, reception areas, storerooms, and stairways. In areas where work is both paper-based and done on computers, appropriate lighting is difficult to achieve because of the different lighting needs.

Also, older workers require more light for performing the same tasks as younger workers. After age 50, light requirements may be 50 per cent higher and after age 60, 100 per cent higher than for younger workers.

Light Source Design. Light sources are designed as direct lighting, indirect or reflective lighting, or combinations of the two (Figure 14–15). Direct lighting reflects directly on the work surface. Semidirect lighting reflects some light off the ceiling but most shines directly on the work surface. Indirect lighting reflects all light off the ceiling. Lights may be suspended from the ceiling, recessed in the ceiling and enclosed, placed in troughs near the top of the wall, suspended from partitions, or attached directly to modular furniture.

Task Lighting. The number one priority for lighting is to achieve the best task visibility possible. A second priority should be to create the most comfortable visual environment possible. **Task lighting,** also referred to as accent lighting, often involves building the light fixtures into the furniture or workstations to illuminate specific work areas. Task lighting is especially important in an open office design.

Sometimes variable-intensity task lighting is used in work areas. Variable-intensity lighting achieves adjustability by using a plastic cylinder with a network of dark lines enclosing a fluorescent lamp. By turning the cylinder, employees can adjust the illumination to suit themselves or the tasks.

Ambient Lighting. Indirect lighting fixtures provide **ambient lighting.** Light is directed upward so that it is reflected off the ceiling onto the work area. It provides light for a large area, but the light is insufficient to work by. Ambient lighting is often combined with task lighting to provide a lighting system that is flexible, lower in energy costs, and easier to install than direct overhead lighting. **Task-ambient lighting** can be used with reduced overhead lighting, or it can supply light by means of fixtures that emit light both upward and downward. It is an attractive and economical means of providing adequate light for an open office design.

Lighting and Computers. The lighting at computer workstations should be lower than for areas in which concentrated work on paper documents is performed. Glare on the monitor from lights and windows can be avoided by using antiglare filters, with proper placement, and with the capability of adjusting the computer screen. Computers should be placed at right angles to outside windows. The user should not directly face the window when working at the computer. Window coverings such as louvered blinds can be used to adjust the amount and glare from sunlight.

SOUND AND ACOUSTICS. Sound control is important for a healthy and productive work environment. Without a sound control program, employees experience physiologic and psychological problems such as increased blood pressure, accelerated heart rate, increased muscle tension, mental stress, and irritability.

Sound is measured in decibels (db). One decibel equals the smallest degree of difference or change in loudness that is detectable by the human ear. Maximum sound levels for various types of office environments are as follows:

- General offices—60 db
- Private offices—40 db
- Data centers (with computers, printers, copiers, telephones, and other equipment)—70 db

The sound control system has two main goals: speech privacy and controlling noise generated inside and outside the work area.

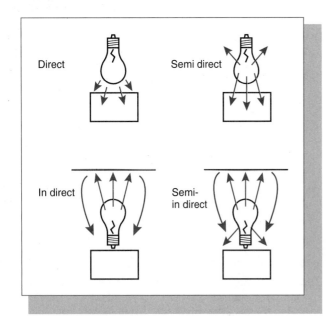

FIGURE 14–15. Light source design.

Levels of Speech Privacy. Various levels of speech privacy can be attained through the use of construction materials, acoustic decorations, and sound-masking devices. Levels of speech privacy are as follows:

- *Absolute*—nothing can be heard, not even mumbling. It is the most difficult and expensive level to achieve.

- *Confidential*—cannot understand what is said but mumbling can be heard

- *Normal*—sound of incoming conversation is loud enough to distract people from their work; a fair amount of conversation could be heard if one concentrated on listening; recommended where the confidential level is not needed

- *None*—most common level; incoming speech is distracting and easy to understand

Guidelines for Controlling Sound. Controlling sound can be done by confining the source of the noise within a separate room, muffling the sound source with acoustic materials, or submerging it into the background hum of a white noise system. The following are some additional guidelines for controlling sound that should be considered in work space design:

- Use barriers to block sound.

- Locate desks so that employees do not face traffic.

- Use sound-absorbent materials.

- Position overhead lights so that sound reflection is minimized.

- Angle windows outward, if possible.

- Use acoustical covers on printers and other equipment to reduce noise levels.

- Use felt or rubber cushions under equipment.

- Carpet the work area where equipment is being used.

Pleasant background noise such as music is often used in the workplace. Music has a calming effect, reduces fatigue, and lessens monotony. Music appropriate for the office environment and the type of work being performed should be selected.

An effective sound control system results in increased efficiency, decreased errors, a higher level of concentration, increased physical comfort, and elimination of distractions.

The Workstation

A **workstation** is a collection of desks or work surfaces, equipment, storage facilities, and chairs shaped by technology, the task to be performed, and various human needs. It is a tool used to accomplish an objective of the task at hand.

Components

The basic units are desktops or work surfaces, pedestals that contain various-sized drawers, end supports, shelves, filing units, and housing for electronic equipment. Many components are interchangeable or modular, and different configurations can be achieved with the same components. Because of this, standardized workstation components should be used throughout the organization.

DESK OR WORK SURFACE. The office desk serves as a work space, storage space, filing area, and place where office and communications equipment sits. Efficiently organized, the desk can enhance productivity. Made-to-order drawer arrangements facilitate storage and make supplies accessible.

The height of the work surface should be adjustable, if possible, to accommodate the height of the user and the task to be performed. Work surface height should be about 28 inches for tasks other than keyboarding. Keyboard or typing tasks require a lower work surface than other tasks. Keyboards should be at least 2 to 3 inches lower than the regular work surface so that the users' arms do not have to be raised to type. Keyboards may be attached under the desk in a pull-out arrangement, or a special lower work surface may be built into the workstation to accommodate the keyboard.

The size of the desk often depends on employees' organizational levels and the tasks assigned. Unless the employee is a full-time computer operator, the desktop should not be crowded with equipment. Managers who do many types of desk work need a larger work area.

Guidelines for Work Surface or Desktop Arrangements. The positioning of key workstation components is extremely important in an organization concerned with efficiency and ergonomics. Employees should be able to reach all work surfaces and equipment with a minimum of movement. Frequent stretching to reach key workstation components causes fatigue as well as other musculoskeletal problems relating to the arms, neck, and back.

The positioning of the components on the work surface depends on the frequency, sequence, and duration of the task. The more frequent and longer-duration tasks are done in the primary zone; the materials that are used to support the more frequent tasks are stored in the secondary zone.

Writing, keying, and reading use the primary zone, or front area of the work space. This is the area of the work surface that is within bent arm's reach. Computers may be located in the primary space in the workstation for full-time computer operators and in the secondary space for managers and others who operate computers only part of the time.

Supporting materials and equipment only occasionally used or waiting to be used are placed in the secondary area, or the area of extended arm's reach.

Space that does not fall into the primary or secondary zone categories should be used for storage.

THE CHAIR. The office chair is probably the single most important component of the workstation because of its ergonomic impact. To be effective, chairs must provide employees with the proper back and leg support. Because of varied body size and structures, chairs must be adjustable. Proper chair adjustments lessen fatigue and muscle strain, and the employee can work for longer periods without breaks or changing tasks, thereby increasing productivity.

Chairs should have the following adjustments:

- Seat pan tilts forward and backward
- Pneumatic height adjustment
- Independent back adjustment
- Individualized lumbar support both in height and firmness

COMPUTER AND PERIPHERALS. As with the chair, flexibility and adjustability are prime factors in computer monitor selection and placement. Monitors should swivel and tilt and, if possible, be adjustable in height. The monitor should be positioned at the user's eye level and close enough to the employee to prevent eyestrain and fatigue. It should be provided with hanging components to accommodate task lights and hold copy.

Printers should be located so that the user does not have to get up from his or her chair to retrieve printed pages.

The design of the keyboard should allow the hand to be in a neutral position while keying. A neutral position is similar to a handshake position. Traditional keyboard design forces the palm downward and the wrist outward, called an ulnar deviation. New designs for keyboards attempt to alleviate these problems.

PARTITIONS. Partitions surrounding the workstation are usually less than ceiling height and designed to house shelves or closed-in storage space, bulletin boards, and other components that may be useful to the employee. Such panels or partitions provide privacy and diminish distractions from the surroundings.

SHELVING, FILING, AND STORAGE SPACE. The efficiently designed workstation contains filing and storage space located convenient to the seated worker. Lateral files and portable file units are newer options available that replace the traditional filing cabinets. Electronic movable files and circular files may be used in conjunction with the workstation. Shelves may be located above

the workstation within easy reach of the worker, and drawers for supplies can be attached to the work surface for easy accessibility.

TELEPHONE. The telephone and any accessory equipment should be positioned so that it is convenient to the user but does not interfere with the primary work space. Telephone cords should be long enough to permit the employee to reach the phone from any position in the workstation. Cordless telephones and headsets are useful for various applications.

Key Concepts

Managing human resources in a health information services department through the next century will be an exciting challenge. New technologies for information processing, a national agenda of health care reform, and a continuing quest for quality improvement in delivery systems will provide numerous opportunities for health information management professionals.

This chapter has provided only an overview of the dynamic and complex field of human resource management. A command of the following key concepts is essential for the health information manager meeting the challenge of managing human resources into the twenty-first century:

1. Maintaining an awareness and working knowledge of the changing external environment concerning health care organizations and systems that will affect human resource functions.

2. Ensuring organizational compliance to increasing regulatory control of the employer-employee relationship by keeping abreast of current employment laws and guidelines.

3. Managing human resources in accordance with organizational culture and ethnic diversity in the workplace.

4. Creating operational plans to carry out the objectives and activities for human resources used in health information services.

5. Using a systems model to examine and explore useful alternatives and solve problems in human resource management.

6. Employing a variety of methods and tools for planning and controlling human resource functions.

7. Developing effective recruitment, selection, compensation, and evaluation programs and methods to be used in health information services departments.

8. Providing key management strategies for performance appraisal, discipline, and motivation of individuals and groups of employees.

9. Orienting, training, and developing health information services employees for career growth and skill acquisition.

10. Providing leadership in a health care facility by directing human resources to accomplish the mission of the organization.

11. Designing a work place that integrates the needs of the organization with the needs of the employees in a healthy and productive environment.

References

1. 1994 Accreditation Manual for Hospitals. Oakbrook Terrace, IL: Joint Commission on Accreditation of Healthcare Organizations, 1993.

2. Henry KH: The health care supervisor's legal guide. Rockville, MD, Aspen, 1984.

3. U.S. Printing Office, 1993, pp 353–844.

4. Ulterino ED, Robfogel SS: Discipline and discharge: Avoiding legal pitfall. *In* Metzger N (ed): Handbook of health care human resources management. Rockville, MD: Aspen, 1990. pp 465–478.

5. Minor RS, Fetridge C (eds): The Dartnell office administration handbook. Chicago: Dartnell Press, 1984, pp 710–712.

6. Schneider MF: Why ergonomics can no longer be ignored. *In* Galitz WO (ed): The office environment: Automation's impact on tomorrow's environment. Willow Grove, PA: Administrative Management Society Foundation, 1984, chap 3; Makowe J: Office hazards. Washington, DC: Tilden Press, 1981, chap 4.

7. American jurisprudence, 2nd ed. New York: Lawyers Cooperative Publishing Co, 1992.

15

ROSE T. DUNN

KEY WORDS

Accounting rate of return
Accounts receivable
Accounts receivable turnover ratio
Accrual basis accounting
Action steps
Activity ratio
Assets
Balance sheet
Budgets
Business plan
Capital budget
Capital expenditure
Capital expenditure committee
Capitation
Capitalization ratio
Cash
Cash basis accounting
Cash budget
Certificate of Need
Charge master (charge description master)
Chart of Accounts
Compounding effect
Controlling
Current ratio
Days of revenue in patient accounts receivable ratio

Depreciation
Discounting
Double-distribution method
Environmental assessment
Equity
Financial accountant
Financial accounting
Financial analysis
Flexible budget
Fund balance
Goal
Liability
Liquidity ratios
Long-term debt/total assets ratio
Managerial accountant
Managerial finance officer
Master budget
Master charge list
Matching principle
Medicare
Mission
Net
Net operating revenue
Net present value
Objectives
Operating budget
Operating margin ratio
Opportunity costs

FINANCIAL MANAGEMENT 15

ABBREVIATIONS

AHA—American Hospital Association
CDM—Charge description master
CFO—Chief financial officer
CHAMPUS—Civilian Health and Medicine Program of
  the Uniformed Services
DRG—Diagnosis related group
HCFA—Health Care Finance Administration
HFMA—Healthcare Financial Management Association
HMO—Health maintenance organization
PPS—Prospective payment system
RBRVS—Resource-based relative value scale
SWOT—Strengths, weaknesses, opportunities, threats

OBJECTIVES

- Define key words.
- List different reimbursement methodologies.
- Decipher the differences between financial accountants, managerial accountants, and managerial finance officers.
- Use fiscal terms with understanding.
- Calculate key financial ratios.
- Understand the difference between cash and revenue.
- Cite the role of the health information professional in the budgeting process.
- State the key phases in strategic planning and how strategic planning drives financial management activities.
- Prepare a business plan.
- List the budget types.
- Perform capital evaluation methods.
- Describe various cost allocation methods.

HISTORICAL PERSPECTIVE

Financial management has become increasingly complex over the past 20 years. Concurrently, the roles held by the health information management (HIM) professional and health information services have become pivotal positions in the fiscal success of any health care organization. The dependence on the health (medical) record's content to define accurately and completely the services provided and conditions treated for reimbursement purposes contributed to this escalation in status. Skilled HIM professionals have the expertise to cull the health record for pertinent data and information to maximize reimbursement without compromising the integrity of data quality.

During this dynamically changing period, the financial aspects of health care organizations have become much more important for good management decisions. All managers involved in health care organizations must be aware of the impact of regulatory changes on the financial environment. Health care managers must know how to adjust their operations to respond to the dynamics of the economy. The government and other regulatory agencies focused attention on the financial aspects of health care during a time when health care expenditures were increasing at double-digit inflationary rates, resulting in more regulation and closer scrutiny of fiscal activities by external agencies (Figure 15–1).

Health Care Expenditures

In the 1930s, the customary method of paying for health care was direct, out-of-pocket remuneration. Some payments were monetary, others were in goods. When hospitals started being used more often than physician offices or house calls, both hospitals and industry explored ways to insure for the cost of health care. This exploration resulted in the establishment of insuring agents that served as the forerunner for what became Blue Cross and led into multiple private insurance companies, both nonprofit and for-profit. These companies provided a new service to the public—coverage for health care expense.

As more people paid health care insurance premiums, they began exercising their "right" to make use of services paid for by their premiums. The increasing use of

515

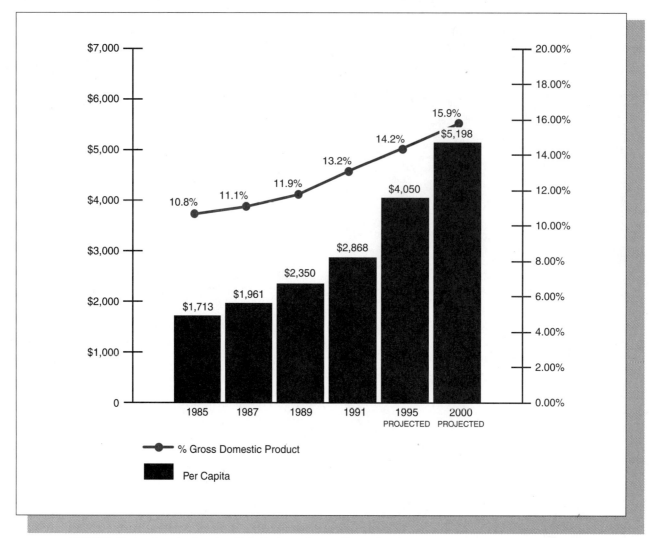

FIGURE 15–1. Growth of national health expenditures. (From The Universal Healthcare Almanac, Silver & Cherner, Ltd.)

health care services contributed to rising premiums and greater than anticipated demands on health care providers and organizations. The demand was but one factor leading to building more hospitals and more people seeking training in health care as physicians. Insurance provided an avenue that not only insured the individual but also assured the hospital that it could receive payment for the care provided. Such assurances were atypical before the 1930s and provided the insureds no incentive to limit or judiciously seek health care services. Access to full or nearly full payments for services did not encourage hospitals to limit the realm of services provided or control duplication of services within the same community.

By the mid-1960s, social reform required the establishment of a government-subsidized health care pro-

gram. This program became known as **Medicare**. The Medicare program further encouraged hospitals to provide services without regard to cost because most costs were reimbursed under the Medicare reimbursement program. Over the past 30 years, the government's perspective has become one that embodies the philosophy that all citizens have a right to health care. This trend began with the passage of Titles 18 and 19 to the Social Security Act in 1965.

As health care expenditures continued to increase from year to year, the federal government found it necessary to impose controls on its insurance costs. It was not until the 1980s that the reimbursement formula was modified to restrict reimbursement and control the government's expenditures for health care. In 1982, the Health Care Finance Administration (HCFA) implemented the Tax Equity and Fiscal Responsibility Act. The law mandated a prospective payment system (PPS). The PPS became effective in 1983. This program attempted to balance the payments made for the same services rendered by different providers and pay the providers based on the diagnosis at a fixed rate. Diagnosis related groups (DRGs) were established in the United States and case mix groups in Canada.

Reimbursement modifications occurred in the private insurance industry as well. Some contracts established between insurance companies and hospitals paid the hospital a specific rate for care provided to its subscribers (covered insureds). Different reimbursement methodologies now exist, including prenegotiated amounts, reimbursement based on a discount off of billed charges, **per diem** payments, reimbursement based on audited costs, and payment for services at billed or full charges. Billed- or full-charge reimbursement seldom occurs. Some insurance organizations provide payments directly to the subscribers, who then must pay the hospital.

The sequence of events that have occurred over the past 30 years has created the third party payer concept. A **third party payer** (the insurance company) pays for services received by others (the insureds) obtained from yet another party (the provider) who the payer may not have selected to provide the services.

Reimbursement modifications have extended beyond hospital providers to home health agencies (converted from **whole service** cost-based to discipline cost-based), skilled nursing facilities (resource utilization groups), outpatient departments (studying the idea of ambulatory visit groups or ambulatory patient groups), ambulatory surgery centers, and rehabilitation facilities (proposed function-related groups). The philosophical change in reimbursement to control costs impacted physicians as well. The Resource-Based Relative Value Scale (RBRVS) was implemented in 1992. The intent of the RBRVS was to ensure equity in payment between physician and other individual practitioner providers and between physician specialties. In effect, payments were based on CPT-4 codes, regardless of the provider's specialty providing the service. Under the RBRVS, a physical therapist is paid the same amount as an orthopedic surgeon (in the same geographic location) when heated massage is provided.

Other attempts at controlling costs included reducing the options available to a person to obtain health care services. In the 1980s, the growth of managed care programs (i.e., health maintenance organizations [HMOs], preferred provider organizations [PPOs], and prepaid group practice plans) was significant. Growth continued through the 1990s. Some communities had as much as 60 per cent of its insured population enrolled in a managed care program. The programs require the insured person to comply with some rules of access,

obtain approval for routine care, seek services from a preselected set of providers, and fulfill other utilization requirements. Substantial financial disincentives are imposed on those who choose to receive services outside the predefined network of providers or without obtaining the necessary approvals.

The bottom line is that health care costs increased uncontrollably when health care was paid for "in full." Controls using a variety of methods, fee structures, prospective rates, access mandates, and so on have regulated costs to some degree. Provider dropout through hospital closure and state-mandated authorization processes such as **Certificate of Need** programs to set up new services or purchase expensive equipment has reduced some duplication of services. These activities have reduced the amount of payment a health care organization or provider receives for services rendered. It is essential for management to provide services **efficiently and effectively** at a cost lower than or equal to the payment that will be received. The health information manager's role now includes more than effective and efficient management practices. This chapter discusses how the health information manager contributes to an organization's fiscal viability through productive and proficient data collection and information processing for reimbursement, patient care, and research. It primarily addresses reimbursement information and the HIM professional's role.

HEALTH INFORMATION TERMINOLOGY

When the HIM professional interacts with the accounting staff of her organization, she is probably conversing with those professionals involved with **financial accounting**. These people are responsible for recording and reporting the financial transactions of the organization. Transactions include such things as issuing a payment to a publisher for the coding staff's coding books. The payment is recorded as an expense to the HIM department and classified by the type of expense—for example, books and subscriptions. Besides recording the expense, these professionals also must reduce the cash balance to allow for the payment to be issued to the publisher. The people employed in the financial accounting section of fiscal services capture the data necessary to build the foundation for reports used in understanding the financial management of the organization. This chapter describes the duties of the **financial accountant, managerial accountant,** and **managerial finance officer** (Table 15–1).

The transaction processing can be accomplished in one of two manners: **cash basis accounting** or **accrual basis accounting**. In a cash basis environment, each transaction is recorded when cash is exchanged, similar

TABLE 15-1 FINANCIAL MANAGEMENT DUTIES

FINANCIAL ACCOUNTING	MANAGERIAL ACCOUNTING	MANAGERIAL FINANCE
Record financial transactions (payments, orders, expenses, revenues, accruals, etc.)	Prepare reports such as budgets, cost reports, productivity and volume schedules, etc. Set rates or charges. Monitor variances.	Financing and funding activities. Planning for future expenditures. Investment decisions and planning.
When: Past and current activities	When: Current and future activities	When: Future activities
Titles: Staff accountant, accountant, bookkeeper	Titles: Cost accountant, budget coordinator	Titles: Chief financial officer, treasurer

to one's personal finances. Revenues are recognized when money is received for services provided, and expenses are recognized when money is paid out for the resources used to provide those services. The cash basis accounting method may have worked in years past but not today because services rendered today are seldom paid for today. Instead, health care providers must wait 30 or more days to receive payment from a third party, typically an insurance company.

Just as there are principles for filing and classification, accounting has principles as well. These principles are known as generally accepted accounting principles (GAAP). The **matching principle** is one. This principle states that revenues should be matched with the expenses incurred to produce the revenue. To do so, the accrual basis of accounting must be used. The accrual method records the revenues expected as "revenues," although the "cash" has not yet been received. The revenues are matched as closely with the expenses as possible. For example, if an operation occurred today, the expenses associated with performing the operations are operating room staff, anesthesia, medications, disposable medical-surgical supplies, and so on. The charges associated with each of these items are recorded as revenue, and the actual cost or expense of these items is recorded as expenses of the operation.

Profit represents the amount of money (cash) actually received from the payer (patient or insurance company) less the actual cost to do the service, assuming that the cost is less than the cash received.

Each transaction must be recorded during the financial accounting process. Transactions are assigned to

RKK Memorial Hospital- Income Statements for years ending December 31 (Revenues and Expenses)	(thousands of dollars)	
	1995	**1994**
Net patient services revenue	110,500	98,500
Other operating revenue	7,300	8,800
Total operating revenue	117,800	107,300
Operating Expenses		
Nursing services	54,300	50,200
Dietary services	5,200	4,640
General services	12,680	11,450
Administrative services	11,290	10,360
Employee health and welfare	9,560	9,240
Provision for uncollectibles	4,220	3,980
Provision for malpractice	1,450	1,220
Depreciation	4,200	4,050
Interest expense	1,890	2,300
Total operating expense	104,790	97,480
Income from operations	13,010	9,860
Contributions and grants	3,290	890
Investment income	540	345
Nonoperating gain or loss	3,830	1,235
Excess of revenues over expenses	16,840	11,095

FIGURE 15-2. Balance sheet.

RKK Memorial Hospital Balance Sheets for years ending December 31 (thousands of dollars)		
	1995	**1994**
Cash and securities	7,250	5,850
Accounts receivable (estimated net)	22,760	20,850
Inventories	4,780	3,440
Total current assets	34,790	30,140
Gross plant and equipment	152,420	145,780
Accumulated depreciation	26,930	21,550
Net plant and equipment	179,350	167,330
Total assets	214,140	197,470
Accounts payable	5,680	5,250
Accrued expenses	5,790	5,420
Notes payable	945	2,870
Current portion of long term debt	2,670	2,200
Total current liabilities	15,085	15,740
Long-term debt	29,420	30,800
Capital lease obligations	1,720	2,140
Total long term liabilities	31,140	32,940
Fund balance	167,915	148,790
Total liabilities and funds	214,140	197,470

FIGURE 15–3. Financial statement.

designated accounts. Several health care associations, such as the American Hospital Association (AHA) have developed a standard **Chart of Accounts**, although there may be slight variations from one health care organization to another. Typically, the largest expense items are in the lower-number account categories, whereas the expense categories that have limited expenses appear in the higher-number account groups. Labor expenses may be classified to the 100 series, and dues expenses may be classified to the 900 series. A chart similar to the standard chart of accounts for expenses exists for revenues.

Financial accounting using the accrual basis requires the accountant to comply with the double-entry method of transaction recording. This means that when revenues and expenses are matched and recorded, another set (double) of entries must occur simultaneously. These entries typically record an amount equivalent to the revenue in a category called **accounts receivable**, while the expense amounts reduce categories of assets, such as medical-surgical supply inventory and pharmaceutical inventory, or increase liability categories, such as wages payable.

The statement of revenues and expenses and **balance sheet** result from the double-entry activities. The statement of revenues and expenses are where the revenues and expenses are reported (Figure 15–2). The balance

sheet displays the organization's **assets, liabilities,** and **fund balance** or **equity** at a fixed point in time, e.g., December 31 of a given year (Figure 15–3). Assets are cash or cash-like items or other items that can be converted to cash. Furniture is an asset because it can be sold for cash. Liabilities are those bills the organization owes. They may be wages accruing between paydays, mortgage payments due to the bank, and so on. The fund balance category is the residual category that collects the profits and losses that result from the differences between revenues and expenses. The statement of cash flow provides additional information about the source and use of funds (Figure 15–4).

USING THE REPORTS TO PROVIDE MANAGEMENT INFORMATION

The value of the recording efforts of the accounting staff is the reports created from their activities. The reports allow management to compare the success of providing services cost-effectively. **Financial analysis** or **ratio analysis** is the management process of formulating judgments and decisions from the relation between the numbers represented on two reports: the statement of revenues and expenses and the balance sheet.

A ratio expresses the relation between two numbers,

RKK Memorial Hospital Statement of Cash Flow for 1995 (thousands of dollars)

Cash Flow from Operations

Total operating revenue	117,800
Total cash operating expenses	(100,590)
Change in acounts receivable	(1,910)
Change in inventories	(1,340)
Change in accounts payable	(430)
Change in accruals	370
Net Cash Flow from Operations	13,900

Cash Flow for Investing Activities

Investment in plant and equipment	(6,640)

Cash Flow from Financing Activities

Repayment of long term debt	(1,380)
Repayment of notes payable	(1,925)
Capital lease principal repayment	(420)
Change in current portion of long-term debt	470
Net cash flow from financing	3,255

Nonoperating Cash Flow

Contributions and grants	3,290
Investment income	540
Nonoperating cash flow	3,830
Net increase (decrease) in cash	7,835
Beginning cash and securities	5,430
Ending cash and securities	14,285

FIGURE 15–4. Statement of cash flow.

such as one asset category, cash, to all assets. Professional associations such as the Healthcare Financial Management Association, the Medical Group Management Association, and the AHA, and health care systems collect data from their member organizations and members and publish average ratios. Sometimes the data are reported by region, facility size, and facility type. The publication of average ratios permits organizations to compare their individual ratios with the average to determine how well they compare with others.

When doing ratio analysis, it is important to be consistent in defining the ratio components. When HIM professionals calculate the average length of stay of adult patients, they must be careful not to include infant discharges or infant days. This means that the definition for adult length of stay demands that the composition of the denominator and numerator be consistently determined. Additionally, one should not assume that published average ratios are developed in the same way by all who submitted data to the collecting organization.

RATIO CATEGORIES

There are four commonly recognized ratio categories. They are as follows:

- Liquidity
- Turnover
- Performance
- Capitalization

Liquidity and capitalization ratios focus on balance sheet numbers (assets, liabilities, and equity/fund balance accounts). They measure the ability of the health care organization to meet its short- and long-term obligations. Performance ratios use data from the statement of revenues and expenses. Ratios in this category evaluate the effectiveness of resource use to deliver services and products. Turnover or activity ratios use data from the balance sheet and the statement of revenues and expenses. These ratios measure the organization's ability to generate net operating revenue in relation to its various assets.

Liquidity Ratio

One of the most common **liquidity ratios** is the **current ratio.** This ratio compares current assets with current liabilities. Both categories appear on the balance sheet. What the current ratio tells a manager is whether there are sufficient cash and cash-like assets to cover the immediate liabilities (bills) that will come due in the short term (1 year).

Example

> The Citywide Surgi-Center has cash, marketable securities, and accounts receivable of $300,000. Citywide has payroll liabilities, payables due to their suppliers, and the mortgage on the surgery equipment and building due this year in the amount of $150,000.
>
> Current Assets = $300,000
> Current Liabilities = $150,000
> Current Ratio = 2/1 or 2.0
>
> The ratio says that Citywide can meet its current obligations twice. It has twice as much cash and other liquid assets as it needs to meet its bills.

Turnover Ratio or Activity Ratio

One ratio that is affected by the activities of the health information services department is the **days of revenue in patient accounts receivables ratio.**

This **turnover ratio,** or **activity ratio,** divides patient accounts receivables by the average daily patient revenues. Patient revenues are found on the statement of revenues and expenses and patient account receivables are found on the balance sheet because accounts receivable are considered an asset to an organization. Accounts receivables eventually are paid and converted to cash. Patient revenues can be expressed as either net or gross. Gross patient revenues, sometimes referred to as patient services revenues, refer to the value of services provided at full-billed charges. Net patient revenues, sometimes referred to as net patient services revenues, refer to the amount the health care provider expects to receive as payment for the services. Therefore, net revenue is gross revenue less any contractual discounts or adjustments agreed to between the insurance company and the provider or the difference between full charges and fixed fees established by the government (e.g., DRG) or insurer. The 1990 American Institute of Certified Public Accountants' audit and accounting guide,

Audits of Providers of Health Care Services, requires that reports prepared for public use reflect net patient revenues, not gross patient revenues.

When using net patient revenues in the **accounts receivable turnover ratio** (AR days ratio), one must be certain to use net accounts receivables. For consistency purposes, if gross patient revenues is used, then the divisor must be gross accounts receivables.

Days of revenue in patient accounts receivable	=	Patient accounts receivable / Average daily patient service revenue *or*
Net days of revenue in patient accounts receivable	=	Net patient accounts receivable / Average daily net patient service revenue
Average daily patient service revenue	=	Patient service revenue for the period / Days in the period *or*
Average net daily patient service revenue	=	Net patient service revenue for the period / Days in the period

The days of revenue in the patient accounts receivable ratio provide a measure of the average time that receivables are outstanding or the period that a health care organization extends credit to its debtors. High values for this ratio imply longer collection periods and may signal the need for the health care organization to seek cash or financial resources from other sources to pay its ongoing day-to-day expenses until the receivables are collected.

Example

> Compare Citywide Surgi-Center's days of revenue in patient accounts receivables (also known as AR days) with the hypothetical average published by U.S. Surgi-Centers.
>
> | | May | June | July | August | Sept | U.S. Surgi-Center Average |
> |---|---|---|---|---|---|---|
> | AR days | 37.6 | 37.9 | 38.4 | 39.1 | 39.7 | 21.3–75.0 |
>
> Citywide is collecting their receivables effectively, yet the collection period is increasing, so management should assess whether staff are becoming lax.

Performance Ratio

The **performance ratio** evaluates the use of resources to achieve a goal. A common performance ratio is the

operating margin ratio. This ratio displays the relation between the net revenues received and the expenses required to supply the revenues. If Citywide had net operating revenue this month of $100,000 and expenses of $96,000, the revenues in excess of expenses would be $4,000 ($100,000 − $96,000). This amount would be compared with an amount known as net operating revenue.

Net operating revenue is the amount of revenues *expected* to be received or total charges less those deductions expected by third party payers resulting in revenues **net** of deductions or net operating revenue. Citywide's operating margin ratio would be 4 per cent.

Capitalization Ratio

There are several **capitalization ratios.** One that may be experienced by anyone who works in an organization that has a building project anticipated is the **long-term debt/total assets ratio.** This ratio compares the amount of long-term debt the organization has (bills that will come due in a period more than 1 year from now [e.g., mortgages]) with the amount of assets (things the organization can convert to cash [e.g., furniture, land, inventories, marketable securities]) it has to pay those debts. The banks will consider the organization's ability to pay back the estimated additional debt it will incur.

PARTICIPATING IN THE MANAGEMENT OF REVENUE

Because services rendered generate revenues, it is imperative that services be priced (charged for) effectively and consistent with the cost to provide the service. This requires regular analysis of expenses associated with services or product costing. HIM professionals have access to all data associated with various procedures to resolve conditions and the resources used to treat a condition medically because they have access to the health record. The HIM professional can be key to collecting and classifying tests and procedures performed for the various conditions treated.

HIM professionals can assess the various expenses (costs) associated with a service. Charges must be assigned so that costs are covered for the various supplies and services used. Each health care organization has a **master charge list,** sometimes called the **charge master** or **charge description master.** This list reflects the charge for each item that may be used in the treatment of a patient and the charge for most services—that is, respiratory therapy treatments, physical therapy services, laboratory tests, and so on. The charge description master is usually automated and linked with the billing system. In some organizations, it is also linked with the clinical data system maintained by HIM services and can be used to perform fiscal-clinical analyses.

Associated with each service is a charge and either a CPT-4 code or an HCPCS code from the HCFA's Common Procedural Coding System. CPT-4 codes are updated annually by the American Medical Association. HCPCS codes are updated periodically by the HCFA. The HIM professional's knowledge of classification systems can be beneficial in ensuring that the master list is up to date at all times.

Insurers pay for services in one of the following ways:

- Full charges
- Discounted arrangement
- Per diem arrangements
- Per case or according to a fee schedule
- Capitation arrangement

Routinely analyzing paid claims to determine how much was paid by the insurer for a service, test, procedure, and so on and comparing the payments with the master list charges are important. If the insurer pays full charges, no variances are noted, but for other arrangements, the payments may be less than or more than the amount charged by the health care provider.

DRGs are an example of a **per case** or fixed payment system. Care provided for a given condition classified into a DRG may cost more than the approved payment for the given DRG. If payment rates are less than the amount charged, a revenue deduction or adjustment will occur. If adjustments are significant, expenses may not be fully covered. If expenses are not covered, management must consider alternatives to providing the care, such as modifying the supplies and services included in the treatment of a condition. Coding professionals who recognize the effectiveness of different tests in treating a condition can identify the more effective tests for utilization management professionals and physicians to consider in establishing treatment guidelines for other physicians to follow.

If payment rates are higher than the amount charged by the health care provider, the provider should assess its charges. Typically, health insurance companies set their rates based on community averages. If the amount paid by the insurance company is higher than the provider's charges, then the provider's charges are lower than the community average. Insurers also pay based on a practice of paying the lower of the insurance company's fee schedule or the provider's charges. Whenever charges are paid, the same analysis of the provider's charges should occur. This type of periodic review of payments to charges helps the provider maximize reimbursement for the organization.

In some areas of the country (West Coast, Arizona, Minnesota) where managed care is a dominant method of insurance, another payment arrangement known as **capitation** may apply. Capitation payments are used in health maintenance organizations (HMOs). Insureds enroll with an HMO. For each month an insured remains with the HMO, the HMO's providers are paid a fixed amount (capitated amount), usually at the beginning of the month. The providers (physicians, therapists, and sometimes facilities such as hospitals and ambulatory surgery centers) are required to provide any care needed by the insureds during this period, regardless of whether or not the capitation amount is sufficient to cover the cost to do so.

REVENUE VERSUS CASH

We have studied several issues that refer to **revenue** and **cash.** For most health care organizations or providers, cash often results from the collection of payments for services rendered. Revenues result from performing the services. Revenues are the charges for the services provided. Typically, services are not paid for at the time they are received. Health care entities must set up procedures to reduce the time between when a service is recorded as revenue (on or about the date it was provided) and the time the revenue is converted to cash (the date it is paid for). This timing factor forces management to create the **cash budget.** The cash budget is an estimate of future cash receipts and disbursements.

The cash budget is equally as important in an HMO. As noted earlier, these organizations receive their cash before services are rendered. They must carefully spread the use of the cash throughout the month or period to ensure that enough cash is available to cover the expenses that they estimate will occur.

The HIM Professional's Role in the Cash Budget

The cash budget predicts for management when cash will be received and when cash will be disbursed. If we consider the operating room example discussed earlier, the wages of the employees probably will be paid before the insurance company pays for the patient's claim. All medical-surgical supplies used during the operation probably were obtained before the operation and held in the medical-surgical supply inventory. These items were paid for before the surgery was performed. In this scenario, cash for the supplies was disbursed before the surgery, cash for staff wages was disbursed after the surgery, and cash was not received for the surgery until about 30 days after the surgery.

The HIM manager holds one key to expediting the time lapse between the recording of revenue and the receipt of cash. This key is in the coding and classification function. Because codes are required for proper billing and complete, accurate codes are required for maximum reimbursement, the health information manager must ensure that the coding and classification staff are up to date in their work and in the application of coding rules and principles and professional review organization (PRO) and HCFA regulations and that they have current coding references and guides. Further, the health information manager must implement procedures and practices to monitor workflow to ensure the timeliness of workflow through the coding and classification section of the department and identify causes for delay.

The following causes can delay the processing of patient records, delaying in turn the coding function and thus the billing of patient services.

- *Untimely receipt at discharge.* Patient records should be received promptly at patient discharge from an inpatient facility or discharge from care during an outpatient procedure or outpatient encounter. Some organizations have found that by leaving the record with the provider for a limited period of time (e.g., physicians, nurses, therapeutic testing area), the record is more complete on receipt by the HIM department than it would be if it were removed or received immediately after the treatment. If this advantage exists, the health information manager must monitor the value of the delay and weigh the value of having more complete information from which to code and classify conditions against the delay in days that result and the delay in processing the claim.

- *Physician noncompliance.* Some records cannot be adequately coded without additional input from the physician or other providers. This problem may occur when a discharge summary (clinical résumé), operative report, or, possibly, a pathology report is needed. To avoid delays because of these situations it is imperative that the HIM department develop a positive rapport with all physician and provider areas. In these cases, a member of the HIM department calls the provider or his assistant and explains the reason for urgency in completing the record. Some organizations have special incentives and disincentives to expedite record completion, such as gifts or suspension programs, respectively, but these procedures are time-dependent and several days can pass before the provider is even aware of a record needing completion. The best alternative is to identify techniques that ensure that the record is complete at the time the service is rendered.

- *Lost records.* Occasionally a record is misplaced during the encounter or treatment period. This occurrence can be a medicolegal concern, but more likely it will turn up eventually and was probably placed in a drawer in error or dispatched to a treatment area that held the record to complete its documentation. The manager's role is to monitor record movement and to ensure that there are adequate and timely alerts to identify missing records promptly so that staff can be assigned to begin tracking the record's last appearance.

- *Inadequate coding staff or scheduling.* If this is the cause for delayed coding and claims processing, the HIM manager's responsibility is to work with the health care organization's administration and human resources department to rectify the shortcomings. The manager also should quantify the cost of delayed claims processing; that is, if the claims are delayed by 5 days, this will result in delay of payment by 5 days. Based on the organization's current rate of interest on its funds, how much has been lost in interest earning by not having the payments in the bank for 5 days? The latter analysis may require the health information manager to work with the accounting, finance, or patient accounts staff to calculate the cost.

- Untimely transcription of key reports. Coding professionals often require the pathology report, discharge summary, operative report, and/or radiology reports to code conditions accurately. If delays exist in the transcription of these reports, coding may be adversely affected. HIM department directors must monitor routinely the transcription timeliness and have controls in place to ensure that reports are typed promptly. Such controls may be the use of part-time or on-call transcriptionists when backlogs accrue or the use of a transcription service.

Cash flow is the lifeblood of any organization. Enhancing cash flow is the responsibility of management staff, especially those who contribute to the final preparation of the claim. The HIM health department is key to this process.

As mentioned earlier, the cash budget is one of several budgets prepared for the management of an organization. It is equally important in a fee-for-service environment as in a capitated environment. In a capitated environment, however, the emphasis on maximizing cash flow for the HIM professional may differ from the role in a fee-for-service environment.

In a capitated environment, the HIM professional should concentrate on activities that identify clinical practice patterns that result in the most cost-effective outcomes. For example, based on analysis of a sample of records, the HIM professional may find that the number of visits required when a certain drug is administered for a condition is less than when another drug is used to treat the condition. This finding may reduce resources used to see a patient more times under a capitated payment. In a fee-for-service environment, the HIM professional may do the same study, but the key is to determine if the costs incurred to treat using either drug are covered by the fee that is charged.

In either case, the HIM professional should also concentrate on simplifying all record documentation processes for providers. By doing so, the providers are able to use their time effectively to treat more patients rather than spending time documenting. The HIM professional should also be involved in data collection areas to ensure that data are collected accurately and retained for future retrieval. For example, a registration system that does not retain demographic information from a prior encounter and requires data re-entry is inefficient.

Other budgets used by management include the **statistics budget,** operating budget, and **capital budget.** These budgets are discussed more fully later. All budgets are an outcome of the strategic planning activities of an organization.

STRATEGIC PLANNING

Kevin McArdle, a strategic planning consultant from Saint Louis Park, Minnesota, uses analogies to describe the strategic planning process.[1] During his work with the American Health Information Management Association (AHIMA), he portrayed the strategic planning process as a bicycle. The board of trustees or board of directors has the responsibility for steering the bicycle. Management and staff are charged with the duty of turning the wheels of the bike to get the organization to the location (goals) desired.

Strategic planning requires a methodical approach. Several phases are traditionally involved. All staff have a role in the process, but the most important role is providing input for the organization's management to consider. Input often is not limited to the thoughts each employee may have about how to improve the organization's services and image in the community; sometimes it also entails how the employee perceives the institution or provider as a consumer of the services offered by the institution or the provider. McArdle has created a strategic planning process and has established a language pertaining to strategy planning (Figure 15–5 and The Language of Strategy).

McArdle's model of strategic planning requires the senior-most management staff (administration, board of trustees or directors, medical staff leaders) to determine where the organization should be in the future **(vision).**

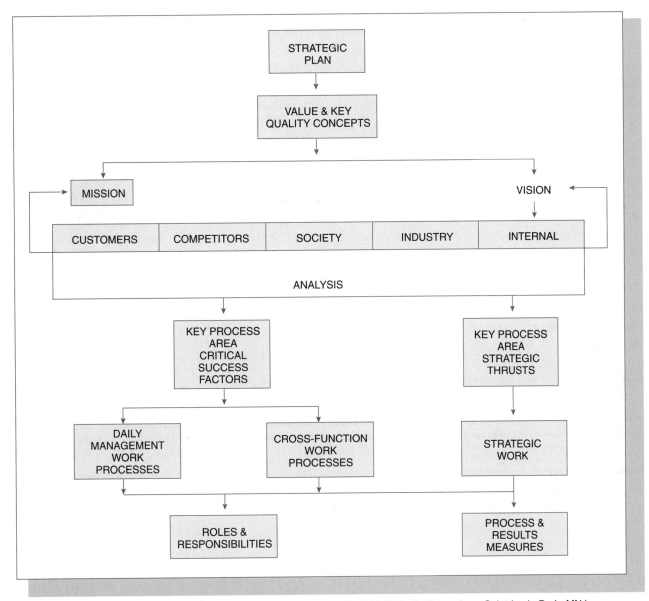

FIGURE 15–5. Strategic planning model. (Courtesy of McArdle K: McArdle Enterprises, Saint Louis Park, MN.)

Comparing the vision with today's business (**mission**) demands a thorough analysis of the business's customers and competitors, society, industry, and internal customers and services. This analysis is similar in scope to the **environmental assessment** described later in this chapter.

The analysis process identifies weaknesses and strengths that must be fine-tuned. These weaknesses and strengths are those areas that are critical to the organization's achievement of its vision and success of key process areas.

Phase 1—Environmental Assessment

Unlike some industries, health care operates in a dynamically changing environment that often depends on the dominance of the political party controlling the United States government at any given time. Except for children's hospitals and pediatricians, most hospitals and providers care for elderly or Medicare-covered patients. This population typically represents more than one half the total patient population served. This phenomenon is

The Language of Strategy

The strategic planning process requires flexibility and involvement. A strategic plan must be relevant to the environment in which it operates and to the people who implement it. Having a strategic plan is not enough to drive an organization toward its vision. A strategic plan must also be carefully executed and deployed throughout the organization.

Strategic Plan—A strategic plan provides an organization with working definitions, descriptions, and details of who it is, what it does, and what it will do in both the short and long-term future.

Vision—The vision represents the dream that the organization hopes to accomplish—"Where do we want to be in the future?"

Mission—The mission represents the mandate that the organization perceives it has from its customers and community—"What business are we in today?"

Guiding Beliefs—The guiding beliefs represent the values and guiding principles that should drive behaviors and decision making within the organization—"What do we believe in?"

Purpose—The purpose of an organization is a somewhat permanent statement to communicate the nature of the organization in terms of corporate purpose. It often is a combination of vision, mission, and guiding beliefs.

Environmental Analysis—An environmental analysis is a collection of data and information that describes the current state of an organization and its business environment. It often is formatted using a SWOT analysis—Strengths, Weaknesses, Opportunities, and Threats.

Key Strategic Initiatives—The key strategic initiatives describe the major or critical initiatives necessary to manifest the organization's vision and future perfect scenario by defining what would have to be done differently in the distant or long-term future. Key strategic initiatives are more strategic and long term in nature.

Key Process Areas—The key process areas describe the critical processes in which an organization must excel in order to be successful. These are processes where effective performance is critical to the achievement of the organization's mission and satisfaction of its customers. Key process areas are more tactical and near term in nature. Key process areas are also known as Key Result Areas.

Strategic and Tactical Process Assignments—The strategic and tactical process assignments describe the specific strategic (long term) and tactical (near term) activities that must be accomplished to drive the organization forward. They are typically defined in terms of goals and objectives.

Goal—A goal is a destination to which the organization commits itself. Goals tend to be general, unqualified statements that describe the outcome or attribute the organization seeks to achieve.

Objective—An objective is an established milestone that once achieved, demonstrates progress towards a goal.

Process Results and Measures—Process results and measures are key indicators that show how well the key process areas are progressing and improving as well as how well customers' needs and expectations are being met.

McArdle K. McArdle Enterprises, Saint Louis Park, MN, 1993.

expected because people are living longer and with age typically comes illness.

The changing environment requires health care management to plan and anticipate future events that will impact their ability to survive and deliver services effectively and efficiently. The reimbursement practices of insurance companies, including Medicare and state-funded aid programs, are emphasizing more fixed payments or case-based payments, similar to those of the DRGs. Health care providers are being required to provide services for a fixed fee rather than being paid at their billed charges.

The environmental assessment phase requires management to consider both the internal and the external environment separately and how they affect each other.

The external environment is composed of those factors outside the control of management. It may include such things as the following:

- Regulation
- Labor availability
- Economic conditions
- Environmental issues

For example, if Citywide Surgi-Center decided to build another center and purchased a site in another part of the community only to find that the land contained dioxin residue, this environmental condition is outside its control but impacts its plans and availability of resources. Some inner-city health care organizations have difficulty recruiting staff because the staff believe that the location is not as convenient or safe as organizations in the suburbs. This perception affects labor availability.

A comprehensive environmental assessment begins at the broadest scope—international—and narrows the assessment through a series of steps until it reaches the local evaluation. If strategic planning is done at the departmental level by the HIM department management, the external environment may address the organization of which the department is a part or other departments that impact the HIM department.

Some organizations subscribe to a planning analysis

approach known as SWOT. This approach defines the organization's as well as its competitors' strengths, weaknesses, opportunities, and threats. For example, the discovery of dioxin on Citywide's recently purchased and proposed new site is a threat to Citywide because it has consumed some of its limited resources, cash, to purchase property that could be considered valueless and inappropriate for further development. All the work to identify the site has triggered the awareness of a need for a facility in this location to Citywide's competitors. The competitors now have the advantage of knowing that before they purchase property in this locale, they should have the property tested for hazardous chemical deposits.

Regulatory changes stimulated by the Reagan administration in 1980 demonstrate how government can impact the health care environment dramatically. The issue of competition in the health care industry became a major concern, and cost reimbursement was abolished with the implementation of a PPS in 1983. These changes proceeded rapidly, and health care providers who had not planned adequately failed. Closure of hospitals became a newsworthy occurrence with increasing frequency.

The internal environment is composed of such items as resource availability, patient volume, condition of equipment and building, new technology demands, and staffing, including practitioners with privileges to use the facility. The internal environment items are assessed at the same time as the organizational structure, the composition of the board of directors or trustees, the mission of the organization, and the resources available to support the organization. The SWOT approach can be used to direct management's efforts in its planning activities.

Once the internal and external environments are evaluated, there are several areas that require management's attention for its long-term survival. These areas can be considered key program or key process areas. The plan covers a period longer than 1 year. In the United States, health care organizations typically prepare 3- to 5-year strategic plans. The actual planning to support the key process areas is programming. During the programming process, management translates its predictions of what the future holds into steps to achieve a viable program that responds to the future's demands and organization's mission. Programming efforts require all management to review and reflect on the meaning of the mission to decide if it continues to describe the purpose of the organization. However, missions do not change often.

Mission

The mission is a statement of the organization's purpose in broad terms. It defines the geographic environment and population that the organization serves—for example, "The Mission of Citywide Surgi-Centers, Inc. is to provide convenient, state-of-the-art, surgical services for all residents of the City of Citywide and its surrounding neighborhoods."

Goals

To implement the mission, administration defines **goals** to support the mission. A goal is a statement of what the organization wants to do. One of Citywide's goals may be to increase the number of nontraditional surgeries performed at the center by supporting research into safe surgery techniques. The goals established by senior administration serve as the direction management needs to figure out the organization's intent.

Objectives

Once the intent is known, management can formulate **objectives.** Objectives are more specific statements that define the expectations or outcomes given the goal direction. Citywide's objective may be to begin performing normal vaginal deliveries on an outpatient basis by the second quarter of next year. Objectives provide clear guidelines for junior management and supervisors to define the **action steps** to achieve the objective. The action steps define the date when certain activities will be completed, how much labor or funding will be required, how resources will be used, and the expected outcomes or results. During action step formulation, budgets are developed.

THE BUSINESS PLAN

As planning becomes more refined in health care organizations, planning activities often are delegated to department management. Some organizations require their managers to prepare business plans. A **business plan** is a formal written document that evolves from the input of others, listing objectives that support the organizational goals. The plan includes the following:

- Specific actions steps
- Quantifying resource requirements and cashflow benefits
- Prediction of expected outcomes
- Programmatic outline that may span a fiscal year or a longer time frame

All budgets and business plans rely on data. Collected data must be in a format that conveys information to the manager. The following are some common data sources for the HIM department:

- Monthly discharge, surgeries, and visit statistics by payer type—Medicare, public aid, commercial, managed care
- Monthly discharge, surgery, and visit statistics by service type—Medical, surgical, obstetrical, and so on
- Length of stay by clinical service and payer type
- Incomplete medical records, per week or month, per physician, per clinical service, and so on
- Requests for records from insurers, patients, other health care providers
- Average pages per record, number of pages generated by automated sources, number of pages handwritten
- Lines, minutes, or words of dictation per month, per physician, per report type
- Records requested and pulled
- Discharges by DRG
- Cases by physician (encounters, discharges, surgeries)

Many of these are volume statistics. The HIM professional also must maintain data on the department's activities that affect the fiscal viability of the organization, such as the following:

- Days from discharge or encounter to code
- Days from code to entry into billing system
- Balances unbilled
- Timeliness in transcribing dictated reports for referring or primary care physicians

Although the first grouping of data sources may have been self-explanatory, the second grouping may require some discussion.

Days from Discharge to Code

This refers to the average number of days it takes for the coding staff to code discharged patient records. Zimmerman and Associates, an accounts receivable consulting firm, recommends that this period be less than 7 days. To do this requires the following:

- That transcription activities be timely to ensure that reports are typed and filed in the records for the coding staff
- That loose materials, especially pathology and cardiology reports, are filed on receipt
- That records be assembled promptly

- That physician relations are positive so that the coding staff can confer freely with the physicians if additional information on any phase of the case is needed

Any of these activities can extend the days from discharge to code.

Days from Code to Entry in the Billing System

This period refers to the time it takes for the codes and other abstracted information to be entered into the organization's billing or abstracting system. Health care organizations often rely on automated methods to receive data from other departments to complete the billing claim for insurance companies. A centralized information system ties information gained at the time of registration with the services and supplies received throughout the episode of care. The final component is recording the conditions treated that correspond with the services and supplies issued. This is the coding function of HIM personnel. Once all necessary coding operations are completed, the patient accounts or business office personnel can proceed with their billing activities.

Any delay in entering required data into the centralized information system results in billing delays. Delays can occur as a result of staffing shortages. The health information manager must be attentive not only to the time lapse between discharge and coding but also to the time lapse between coding and data entry. There is no benefit to having all records coded in a timely manner if the data are not entered into the abstracting or billing system until several days later. Data entry should occur the same day or the day after coding.

Balance Unbilled

This category of records includes all records whose codes have not yet been entered into the billing system *and* been released for billing. Data and documentation in the record may be insufficient to allow accurate coding. Additionally, some payers require physician involvement before permitting the provider to bill for the services. Civilian Health and Medical Program of the Uniformed Services (CHAMPUS), and some state and public aid agencies require physicians to complete a statement attesting to the accuracy of the listing of diagnoses and procedures prepared by coding personnel before billing for the services rendered. This is the attestation process. All HIM activities could be complete but the physician may have not yet completed the attestation form. This one step can delay billing. Systems must be put into place to expedite record completion.

Some health care facilities use medical staff rule and regulation sanctions to force the physician to complete records and the attestation form within a given time frame. This can result in adversarial relationships between the medical staff and the HIM department. Others use giveaways to entice the physician to complete required documentation, such as lunches and gifts.

To expedite the process, some HIM departments do some of their coding duties during the episode of care (hospitalization). This practice of concurrent coding allows the HIM staff to interact with the physicians and nurses on the patient care unit. This interaction can improve the turnaround time of the variables we have been discussing.

Timely and accurate recording of sufficient data by providers is a requirement for participation in the health care process. Physicians and other health care practitioners need to know what is required and expected of them. An educational, business-like approach is most successful in addressing documentation requirements and expectations. The HIM specialist, in addition to providing information and education to physicians and other practitioners, brings creativity and knowledge to the documentation process. More options are constantly being presented to facilitate the recording, authentication, and transfer of patient data. HIM specialists can evaluate and apply new methods and technology to achieve effective documentation of care. Quality documentation supports the direct care process and many administrative processes, including payments for services.

Trends

To complete the business plan data gathering, the statistics gathered should be compared with those of prior periods to identify trends that imply a change in operations or staffing is required. If the statistics showed that the number of minutes of dictation was increasing by 10 per cent per month, it could be anticipated that additional transcriptionists would be required or external assistance would be needed to transcribe the dictation.

Staffing Information

Staffing information is a necessary component of business planning. Staffing information maintained by the HIM manager should include the following:

- Current organizational chart by function and by name
- Productivity standards
- Skills assessment inventory for each staff member
- Training obtained or needed
- Average time off by categories of staff (nonproductive time)

Maintaining this data allows management to know which staff members are prepared to assume new duties, what training must be planned or budgeted for to allow other staff members to take over activities, and the true productive time of staff members. **Productive time** is the time a worker is present and working. A full-time position is typically 2080 hours annually (40 hours per week × 52 weeks). Yet a full-time position does not equate to 2080 productive hours. Some hours will be nonworked because of vacation, holidays, sick time, and so on. Productive hours are further reduced by training and meeting hours. Monitoring time off allows management to know the true productive hours available to meet work load demands.

Other Items Considered Before Preparing the Business Plan

Two assessments may be completed before proceeding with a business plan: automation assessment and program assessment. These assessments are similar to doing an internal environment assessment of the HIM department. When the assessments are completed, the health information manager will know whether the tools are available to achieve the outcomes necessary. If administration has determined that no additional staff can be added this year, then a manager's dependence on automation may increase. Automation may be less expensive to add than staff and increase productivity as well. The assessment of programs requires the staff to consider seriously the adequacy of each service it offers and decide if the services meet the users' or customers' needs.

The Four M's

All managers have the responsibility to manage the four M's:

- Manpower
- Machinery
- Materials
- Money

When preparing the business plan and, ultimately, the budget, all proposed expenditures must balance the M's; that is, an increase in one should attempt to offset the cost of another. If we request a computer to help us do our work, we should be able to do the work with fewer persons. This is a trade-off between machinery and manpower. Sometimes, however, machinery is needed to offset the need for more manpower to meet volume increases.

The organization's goals include increasing cash flow. Your proposal is to establish a courier service to deliver incomplete records to physicians' offices to decrease the number of incomplete records.

Objective
To decrease the number of incomplete records by 25%.

When do you plan to do it?
By second quarter of next year

What will be achieved?
• Reduction in accounts receivable days by 2 or $140,000 by delivering records to physicians' offices. This will reduce the time for the physician because he/she does not have to come to the HIM department to do his/her records.

• Reduction in physician complaints or increase in compliments.

• Avoidance of purchase of additional file shelving units to store incomplete records.

What is needed to achieve the objective?

Resources: Capital: Small Car*: $10,000

              Operating Expenses:

                          Labor: .5 FTE $ 7,200

                          Auto Costs: 4,000

Collaboration Required: Security, Personnel and Purchasing Departments

*Car to be used by courier. Courier must be licensed driver.

How does the hospital benefit from this objective?
Cashflow impact: The reduction in incomplete records will result in 2 fewer days in accounts receivable or the equivalent of $140,000. Invested annually at 10%, the $140,000 will yield at least $14,000 interest income.

FIGURE 15–6. Questions to be asked when preparing a business plan.

Developing the Business Plan

Now that we have gathered and assessed the data, we have identified the needs we want to address. The first step is to figure out if the needs we identified are consistent with the organization's mission and goals. If the organization establishes a goal to increase services to the elderly and you think that this is the year you should propose establishing a child day-care center for the community, your proposal probably will be rejected.

If your proposal is consistent with the organization's mission and goals, then you must decide what you want to do and how you want to do it. Several questions can be answered during the process (Figure 15–6).

Each objective is developed accordingly, and action steps must be prepared in detail to ensure that the objective is attained. Costs to do each step of the planned objective must be determined and associated with the timing of the steps. If the car for our objective is to be purchased in March, the funding should be budgeted in March. Gasoline and other automobile costs will be incurred throughout the year, probably at the same rate each month. Therefore, the $4000 in automobile costs should be spread evenly throughout the year and so forth. Once the costs are identified, the budget can be prepared.

BUDGETS

Budgets are numerical documents that translate the goals, objectives, and action steps into forecasts of volume and monetary resources needed. The managerial accounting process includes the activities of planning and preparing budgets consistent with the strategic plan. Just as we have an accounting component responsible for recording transactions as they occur (financial accounting), there are other people who work with administration and management to assign the anticipated fiscal resources of the organization. These people may work in the budget or controller's office. Their primary responsibilities include helping management to prepare budgets, conduct cost-finding studies (to be discussed later in this chapter), set rates, and determine productivity. The reports they produce include the budget, the budget variance reports, cost reports, and third party reimbursement reports. The types of budgets that result from the planning process include the statistics budget, the operating budgets, and the **master budget.**

Statistics Budget

The first of several budgets developed from the planning process is the statistics budget. Future volumes are often predicted from historical data. The HIM department is the primary source of historical data, such as discharges by clinical service, payer type, DRG, and physician; operations by type and surgeon; length of stay by DRG, diagnosis, clinical service, and physician; number and type of ambulatory visits; number and type of home health visits; number and type of ambulatory surgery cases; number and type of emergency department visits; and many other volume indicators. Unless significant changes have occurred in the regulatory, and external and internal environments, relying on historical data to predict the future is appropriate. But history should not be the only source of volume predictions.

Key medical and other clinical staff members should be interviewed for their prediction of future demands for services. The medical staff is a valuable source of information and may be aware of plans for service changes and expansions of competing organizations. They also have access to literature that describes technologic advances in patient care. Such advances could drastically reduce volumes experienced in the past. In the 1970s, it was not uncommon for patients who had cataract extractions to be hospitalized for 3 or more days. Today this procedure is a common outpatient procedure.

The statistical analysts in the HIM department also can predict declining volumes by comparing data from month to month and identifying trends in utilization of the facility by different physicians or by the community. Sometimes physician utilization declines as a physician ages and cuts back his or her practice or when a physician finds a facility that is more convenient to his or her office.

When new services are contemplated, the staff involved in providing the service should be involved in predicting the utilization of the services or the volumes anticipated. Staff optimism should be tempered by management querying staff and the anticipated users of the service. Sometimes administration uses marketing research firms to predict volumes based on the demographics of the community. If a hospital is anticipating opening a long-term care facility or skilled nursing facility, an analysis of the age demographics of the community should be done to ascertain the number of elderly

people residing in the community today and the number expected to be residing in the community in the next 5 to 10 years. Further, an assessment of the competition would be completed.

Operating Budgets

Once patient, physician, and procedure volumes are determined, managers can begin building their operating budgets. These budgets predict the labor, supply, and other expenses required to support the work volume predicted.

Example

If Citywide implements an outpatient normal vaginal delivery service with a volume of 2800 vaginal deliveries annually, what does Citywide's HIM department need to do to support this new service? The supervisor may predict the following:

- An average of 10 deliveries will occur per working day.
- The department will be responsible for gathering prenatal information by telephone because a vaginal delivery is usually not precisely scheduled weeks in advance.
- A coder will need to be trained to code obstetric services.
- Additional file folders will be needed if the facility uses paper records—one each for baby and mother (2800 × 2 = 5600).
- A staff member will need to be hired and trained to prepare birth certificates, and the department will need to obtain a personal computer to run the birth certificate software.
- The birth certificate software should interface with the registration function to permit download of pertinent parental information and upload of the infant's name to the registration system. Ideally, the software should also interface with the state vital statistics system for direct reporting. The state is the official repository for birth certificate data.

The supervisor must now assign costs to each of these items and budget them in the correct categories: labor, file supplies, training and education, hardware, and software. All items except hardware will traditionally appear in the expense portion of the operating budget.

The departments that provide direct patient care prepare an expense portion for their operating budgets, but additionally, these areas must prepare the revenue portion of their operating budgets. The patient care departments assign estimated charges to the services they will be delivering based on the statistics budget.

Master Budget

After all departments develop their operating budgets, the same categories of expenses (e.g., labor, supplies, training and education) and revenues (patient care, nonpatient care [e.g., cafeteria]) are consolidated into one **master budget** with each of the operating account's combined balances.

Who Participates in Budget Development?

Many people participate in the budgeting process. Facilities find it advantageous to include supervisory and front-line staff members in the development of budgets because they are closer to the consumption of resources. This is known as the participatory approach to budgeting. But management is ultimately responsible for the budget and its compliance with organizational objectives, goals, and mission. Because the budget is a prediction of expenses, revenues, services, and volumes to come sometime in the future, it cannot be exact but should be used as a guide to measuring and improving management's predictive capability.

Budget Periods and Types

The budget period may differ from organization to organization. Budgets may be prepared for 1 year or several years. Typically, budgets are prepared for 12 months. Some organizations use a **rolling budget method.** This method requires management to prepare a budget for a period of time and add to the end of that period another month when a month is consumed. For example, a budget may be prepared for 6 months (January through June), and when the first of the 6 months (January) ends, the manager would prepare the budget for the new 6th month (July).

Another type of budget is the **flexible budget.** This budget is predicted on volume. All supplies, labor, and other variable expenses are budgeted in proportion to the anticipated volume. If the volume anticipated is not reached, then labor and other expenses are expected to decrease accordingly and vice versa if the volume exceeds expectations.

Zero-Based Budgeting

Because many facilities are experiencing reduced reimbursement for their services, modified approaches to budgeting are being considered. One such approach is the **zero-based budget.** In the zero-based budgeting approach, management must complete the program assessment addressed earlier and define consequences if programs are terminated or reduced. William Cleverley, in his 1992 text *Essentials of Health Care Finance,* defined the seven steps of zero-based budgeting.[2]

1. Define the outputs or services provided by the program or department (statistical reports, coding, quality assurance study preparations, responses to requests for information, transcription, filing, and so on).
2. Determine the costs of these services or outputs.
3. Identify options for reducing the cost through changes in outputs or services (modify current procedure, eliminate an activity).
4. Identify options for producing the services and outputs more efficiently (use of a contracted service, voice recognition, optical imaging, and so on).
5. Determine the cost savings associated with options identified in steps 3 and 4.
6. Assess the risks, both qualitative and quantitative, associated with the identified options of steps 3 and 4.
7. Select and implement those options with an acceptable cost-risk relation.

FISCAL PERIODS

Budgets often correspond with fiscal periods. Organizations can choose a calendar year—that is, it begins January 1 and ends December 31—or a fiscal year—that is, it begins during another time of the year, such as July 1 through June 30. Fiscal periods are selected by organizations because they more consistently conform to activity cycles of the organization. A teaching institution may choose the fiscal period of July 1 through June 30 because students finish one level of training in June and are ready to start the next level beginning in July.

CAPITAL REQUEST PROCESS

The computer that Citywide's patient record supervisor needed would be categorized as capital. Each facility defines its capitalization value. For the sake of this example, any expenditure in excess of $500 for equipment or furniture is considered a **capital expenditure.** The computer will cost $2500. Capital items usually have a high initial cost and a "life" or more than 1 year. The personal computer is expected to be used for more than 5 years (the computer's life).

Some facilities establish a **capital expenditure committee** to evaluate all capital requests, so that cash resources are used to purchase those high-cost items that

Example

Assessing a Record Storage Section

We will assess the record storage section of our department.

1. *Define the outputs or services provided by the program or department.*
   Record filing
   Record retrieval
   Loose material filing
   File purging

2. *Determine the costs of these services or outputs.*
   Record filing

2 Employees:	$24,000
Supplies:	$3,600

   Record retrieval

2 Employees:	$25,200
Outguides:	$4,325
Printer:	$1,200
Other Supplies:	$3,700

   Loose material filing

1.5 Employees:	$18,000
Supplies:	$3,600

   File purging

2 Part-timers:	$12,000
Purge boxes:	$5,000
Purge logs:	$200
Other supplies:	$1,800

3. Identify options for reducing the cost through changes in outputs or services.
   Record filing
   Option 1: File at night when less congestion in files—savings: none.
   Record retrieval
   Option 1: Permit all requesters to pull their own records; assume only one half will be willing to do so—savings: $12,500.
   Loose material filing
   Option 1: Stop fastening in loose material; drop file loose materials only—savings: .25 employee ($4,000).
   Option 2: File pathology reports and dictated reports only; drop sort remainder in boxes with first letter of patient's last name—savings: 1 employee ($12,000); costs—boxes ($260).
   File purging
   Option 1: Do not do annually; do only when out of space—savings every other year: $12,000; costs—1 additional part-timer: $6,000; supply costs will not change but will occur in the year purging occurs.

4. Identify options for producing the services and outputs more efficiently.
   Record filing
   Option 1: Implement optical storage at cost of $250,000—savings: eliminate filing staff; costs: New equipment ($250,000), scanner/proofer staff ($30,000).
   Record retrieval
   Option 1: Implement optical storage at cost of $250,000 to permit all requesters to access records automatically—savings: eliminate retrieval staff; costs: included above in record filing.
   Loose material filing
   Option 1: Implement optical storage at cost of $250,000 to permit scanning of loose materials—savings; eliminate loose materials filing staff; cost: add 1.5 scanner/proofers to store and index materials ($22,500).
   File purging
   Option 1: Allow the microfilming company to do this at a cost of $2.50 per box.

5. *Determine the cost savings associated with options identified in steps 3 and 4. See savings and costs above.*

6. *Assess the risks, both qualitative and quantitative, associated with the identified options of steps 3 and 4.*
   Record filing
   —Filing at night. No risks; will result in improvement of activity
   —Optical imaging. Risks: customer buy-in, timeliness of implementation, potential duplication of records at user sites, misindexed records, staffing requirements
   Record retrieval
   —Permit requesters to pull their own. Risks: customer dissatisfaction, misfiles, nonuse of outguides
   —Permit requesters to retrieve directly from optical station. Risks: customer training and dissatisfaction, customer printing and making duplicate records, system malfunction and downtime
   Loose material filing
   —Drop filing. Risks: if staff does not fasten loose materials in record when record is taken from file, loose materials may be lost.
   —File only dictated and pathology reports. Risks: customer dissatisfaction resulting from lack of all data; must search through boxes if requester specifically requests a loose sheet that is "boxed"
   —Optical imaging: Risks: may not be able to keep up with volume of loose materials, misindexing, staffing estimates
   File purging
   —Do every other year. Risk: files become tight
   —Allow microfilmer to do. Risks: may purge records incorrectly

7. *Select and implement those options with an acceptable cost-risk relation.* (This step would occur in concert with a conversation with one's supervisor. Once determined, the options accepted become the budgeted activities for the department or section. All costs associated with the activities approved are budgeted. All costs associated with the activities not approved are eliminated.)

will yield the most benefit to the organization. Once the final list is approved, then proposed acquisition dates are assigned. The proposed acquisition date does not guarantee a manager that he or she will be able to purchase the item on that date. The chief financial officer or controller must assess the condition of the cash budget to determine if sufficient cash will be available to meet not only the upcoming expenses to support the upcoming service levels but also the one-time expense associated with the piece of capital.

The health information manager is obligated to contribute to conserving the facility's cash and adjusting the department's operations to meet the actual levels of service. For example, if Citywide's plans do not develop as expected and only 1400 deliveries are predicted by year end, then the number of folders ordered may be excessive but may not be returnable. Yet the coder hired to do the obstetric coding may be able to prepare the birth certificates, thus reducing the need for a birth certificate coordinator. If volume is such that the birth certificates can be typed, then a personal computer and the software may not be needed.

Because capital requests are typically considered by a committee, it is important for department managers to know how to prepare a well-developed and justified request for the equipment needed for their departments. To do so requires an analysis of the opportunity cost of funds.

CAPITAL INVESTMENT DECISIONS

In most organizations, there is a formalized process for obtaining approval of a capital expenditure. The process usually is initiated by a department manager preparing a written request on a capital expenditure approval form (Figure 15–7).

Some forms are elaborate, requiring the manager to calculate various financial analyses. Others are more verbiage-oriented, requiring the manager to define the need, alternatives considered, volume of business related to the item being requested, analysis of various vendors or suppliers considered or bids obtained to determine the item's cost, and an economic feasibility study.

The capital expenditure committee considers all requests received. A capital investment should be evaluated by the following:

- From the perspective of its contribution to the mission and from a financial perspective relative to the cost of the capital acquisition

- Revenues it may generate for the organization

- Period of time the acquisition will contribute to the organization (economic life)

- Cost to the organization to borrow the funds or loss of interest on the funds

- Regulatory hurdles, such as requirements to obtain approval from planning or rate-setting agencies, and any reimbursement opportunities through Medicare or taxation

Any organization has limited funds to invest in new capital. Each decision to use funds for one acquisition means that another must be forgone. Financial managers describe this process as weighing opportunity costs. **Opportunity costs** are benefits that would be received from the next best alternative use of the investment funds. Some providers use as a measure of opportunity cost the interest rate received on invested funds.[3] Cleverley defines opportunity costs as "values foregone by using a resource in a particular way instead of in its next best alternative way."[2]

Who Has Organizationwide Responsibility for Capital Decisions?

You may ask who has the overall responsibility for capital decisions. This responsibility is another component of the fiscal services area. The overall capital planning function is part of the managerial finance role. Some institutions assign this duty to a chief financial officer (CFO); others, a treasurer. The role of the managerial finance officer is one of planning for the future. We have discussed the role of the financial accountant. It is one of recording what has happened today or in the past, such as paying staff for work performed. We have also discussed the role of the managerial accountant during the budget review. This person helps record what is happening currently or previously (variance analyses) against what was anticipated and what is still anticipated to happen (the budget).

The managerial finance officer, CFO, or treasurer works with financial organizations (banks, investors, and so on) to obtain funding and financing for an organization's plans. If an organization wants to build a new building, financing support is required. This person also may make investment decisions to maximize the income on idle money the organization may have at any given time. The thrust is to ensure that the organization is effective in delivering the services suggested by the mission statement while doing so efficiently, so that funds are not being spent on inappropriate items. The following reports result from these activities:

- Balance sheet

- Statement of changes in financial position

- Investment reports

- Financing reports

Description _____ Budget Year _____
                                        Budget Cost $ _____
Manufacturer _____ Unity Cost _____
                                        Quantity _____
Model # _____ Total _____
                                        Freight _____
Vendor _____ Installation _____
                                        Quorum Discount _____
Materials Manager Signature _____ TOTAL COST $ _____

1. Type of expenditure: Replacement _____ New _____

2. Briefly define function of capital expenditure _____
_____
_____

3. Estimate # of procedures to be done _____ **4.** Average Charge per procedure _____

5. Will the number of FTE's increase or decrease _____ **6.** By how many _____

7. Briefly describe why item is needed _____
_____
_____
_____
_____

8. Financial Analysis   Annual   **REQUESTED BY:**

  a. Gross revenue $ _____
  b. Less: Salaries   _____   Department Director   Date
  c.   Supplies   _____
  d.   Depreciation   _____
  e.   Professional Fees   _____
  f.   Other (itemize) _____   _____   **APPROVED BY:**
  g.   _____   _____
  h.   _____   _____
  i.   (Total sum b-h)   _____   Dept. Asst. Administrator   Date
  j. Gross profit (a-i)   _____
  k. Less: Contractual adjustments   _____
  l.   Bad debts   _____   Maintenance Director   Date
  m. Policy discounts   _____
  n.   Total (sum k-m)   _____
  o. Gross margin (j-n) $ _____   Asst. Admin.– Finance   Date
  p. Asset cost   _____
  q. Return of individual asset O/P   _____ %
  r. Payback—years (P/O)   _____   Administrator   Date

FIGURE 15–7. Capital expenditure justification form. (From Huron Regional Medical Center)

Illustration continued on following page

Capital Expenditure Request Instructions

Description	Please list the exact item you are requesting.
Manufacturer	If known, please list the manufacturer of the product you are requesting.
Model #	This is important to ensure you are ordering the item you really want.
Vendor	If known, please list who the vendor is from which this item can be ordered.
Budget Year	This should always be our fiscal year that ends on June 30 each year. e.g., October 4, 1993 is budget year 1994.
Budget Cost	This is the amount you list on your Capital Equipment Budget. If the item wasn't budgeted please insert "NONE."
Quantity	How many do you want to order?
Total	Multiply the number in Unit Cost by the number in Quantity.
Freight	Please include this total if known. You may ask the Materials Manager for this total. If the Unit cost included freight, insert "NONE".
Installation	Please have our Maintenance Department give you a figure to include here.
Quorum Discount	This must always be completed. If there is no discount, please insert "NONE".
Total Cost	This is the total you receive when adding together the freight and installation with the Cost.

The financial analysis, section 8, must be completed prior to approval by the Assistant Administrator–Finance and Administrator. Should you need any help in completing this section, please contact the Controller or the Assistant Administrator–Finance.

FIGURE 15–7 *Continued*

TIME VALUE OF MONEY

No discussion of capital expenditures would be complete without including the concept of the **time value of money.** This concept includes several premises. The first is that a person who invests his money should be entitled to a return or interest. The return is based on at least two conditions: the length of time the money is invested and the degree of risk associated with the investment. If the investment carries great risk, the rate of return should be higher and vice versa.

The time value of money says to the layperson that it is more beneficial to receive a dollar today than to receive it 1 year from now. The reason is that a dollar received today can be invested and gain interest for 1 year longer than a dollar received 1 year from now. That is, a dollar received today and placed in a savings account at 5 per cent interest accrues a minimum of $.05 in interest. At the end of the year, the savings account closes at $1.05. If the dollar is not received until the end of the year, there would be $1.00, not $1.05.

Compounding

The value of the investment is determined by the length of time the investment is in place because of the **compounding effect.** In the example previously discussed, we started with $1, but at the end of the year, we had $1.05, simply by selecting a safe bank in which to deposit this dollar. If that dollar was left in the bank for 3 years at the 5 per cent interest rate, we do not end up with $1.15, but rather $1.16. An extra $.01 is earned because of the compounding effect. By the 4th year $.22 is gained. Although the gain may not seem significant in this example, consider the effect if $10,000 is invested. Compounding can mean significant gains for the investor.

Discounting

The concept of **discounting** is the opposite of compounding. The question we ask ourselves when we are considering discounting is, How much must one invest today at a compound interest rate of x to receive a given amount at the end of N years? What we know is how much we want to have at the end of the period—say, our retirement age. What we do not know is the *present value* of the money we need to invest today at today's interest rate to accumulate the sum we want by retirement age.

For example, if you were to retire next year and today's interest rate is 5 per cent and you want $105,000 next year, what is the present value we would need to invest today? ($100,000)

When the capital expenditure committee evaluates capital requests, they are evaluating the opportunities available to the organization. Should the organization leave its funds in the bank at a certain interest rate, or should it invest in a new program that predicts it may yield yet another level of revenue and do so for several years? Decisions like these are confronted by managers every day. The managers must weigh the risk associated with the new program against the considerably lower risk of leaving the money in the bank. Unfortunately it's not this simple because each year many capital requests are submitted and each must be compared with one another.

Helping the capital expenditure committee is the fiscal management staff. Financial managers assess or weigh the value of an investment in equipment or other capital request against the interest that would be received on the funds if left in the bank by using one or more of the following capital evaluation methods.

- **Accounting rate of return**
- **Payback method**
- **Net present value**

Net Present Value

In its simplest format, a new piece of equipment or new program will have cash outflows and cash inflows. For example, St. Elsewhere Medical Center has two capital requests. One is from the HIM department for a new dictation system. The other is from the business office for a new charge auditing program.

We know that both will require some cash outflows. The dictation system vendor will expect to be paid a certain sum at the time of installation. The charge auditing program will require additional staff and training costs before it is fully productive. Both proposals will have cash inflows. The HIM manager predicts that she will be able to eliminate the contract typing service expense and do all work inhouse, thus eliminating payments to the outside contract service. The business office manager says he will find items that have been used in the patient care process and not been charged. Once found, his staff can add these charges to the bill and obtain third party reimbursement for them.

Both proposals have an expected life of 5 years. That is, the equipment will operate optimally for 5 years before the technology will be outdated. Each will be depreciated over 5 years as well. Straight-line **depreciation** is calculated by dividing the capital cost by the years of life (in this example, the life is 5 years). The resulting amount is considered the annual depreciation expense.

The charge audit program includes a training program

for those departments that provide services. The program proposes that it will use a continuous quality improvement approach to identify where charges are lost and assist these areas in reducing errors. Over a period of 5 years, all departments will have improved their charge-entering procedures to ensure that no charges will be overlooked or lost.

The proposals will subtract cash outflows from cash inflows to result in a new cash inflow or outflow at the end of each year for the full 5 years. Depreciation expense is considered an outflow. The proposed annual nets for each project must be evaluated against the rate of interest the moneys would have earned if left in the bank. Because the net amounts are the remaining amounts received at the end of each year, we must use a discounting factor to determine the present value of each net amount.

To find this factor, use a table that can be found in most finance textbooks. Table 15–2 represents a portion of such a table.

Example

You want to bring the copy service in-house. Because you know the volumes intimately, you can accurately forecast the service's growth. Your current contracted copy service pays your organization a retrieval fee, but your staff does all the logging, pulls all the records, and answers all the calls about the records requested. Based on the volumes you have experienced in the past and anticipate in the future, you can estimate the revenues from the copies and the related expenses. The revenues less the expenses are the net cash flows.

1. Prepare your proforma (expected revenues and expenses) to provide this service internally.

2. Meet with your CFO and ask him what interest rate he expects on his investments or what return he expects from new programs. Review the table in a finance book labeled "Present Value of One Dollar Due at the End of N Years" and the interest column that corresponds to the CFO's expectations. He expects 13 per cent.

From this example, one can see that even though the program is projected to generate $38,000 in net cash flows, the real value of those flows in today's dollars is $23,587.13. In other terms, if we had $23,587.13 today and invested it at 13 per cent interest, at the end of 5 years it would yield $30,000. If we need $25,000 in capital to start this program, the investment ($25,000) would not be recovered in the 5 years and may be turned down. If we need only $19,000, perhaps to buy a personal computer and a big copy machine to support the logging effort, then the project may be approved because the investment is less than the net present value of the cash flows ($23,587).

Comparing Competing Projects

	Medical Records	Patient Accounts
The project	Dictation system	Auditing program
Net cash flows	$25,000/year	$15,000/year
Project life	5 years	5 years
Initial capital	$75,000	$60,000
Annual depreciation	$15,000	$12,000
Return required	10%	10%
Net present value (NPV)	$94,775	$56,865
NPV − initial capital	$19,775	($3,135)

Decision: The medical record project meets the criteria to have a 10 per cent return and exceed the initial capital outlay.

Accounting Rate of Return

This evaluation method uses averages. The annual net inflows or outflows are averaged over the project's life for each project. The asset value or investment value is averaged over the life of the project as well. The asset value is depreciated on a straight-line basis for the life of the program.

TABLE 15–2 INTERNALIZING THE COPY SERVICE PROPOSAL

YEAR	NET CASH FLOWS	PRESENT VALUE 13%	VALUE OF CASH FLOWS TODAY
1	$1,000	.88496	$ 885.00
2	3,000	.78318	2,349.54
3	7,000	.69305	4,851.35
4	12,000	.61332	7,359.84
5	15,000	.54276	8,141.40
TOTAL	$38,000		$23,587.13

Example

If we use our same copy service example's facts, we can use the following *accounting rate of return* formula:

$$\frac{\text{Average Net Income}}{\text{Initial investment}} = \frac{\$38,000/5}{\$19,000}$$

(the total cash flows/5 years)

(the initial capital investment)

Accounting rate of return: 40 per cent
   Before proceeding further, we need to revisit our CFO and determine if an accounting rate of return of 40 per cent is acceptable.

Comparing Competing Projects

	Medical Records	Patient Accounts
Net cash flows	$25,000/year	$15,000/year
Depreciation	− 15,000/year	− 12,000/year
Average net income	$10,000	$ 3,000
Average investment	$75,000	$60,000
Accounting rate of return	13%	5%

Decision: The medical records project has a higher accounting rate of return.

Payback Method

The payback method is probably the simplest of all methods. The payback period determines the number of years it will take for the cash inflows from each project to payback the initial investment (cash outflow).

Example

Internalizing the Copy Service Proposals

Year	Net Cash Flows	Initial Investment	Remaining
0		$19,000	
1	$ 1,000	− 1,000	$18,000
2	$ 3,000	− 3,000	15,000
3	$ 7,000	− 7,000	8,000
4	$12,000	− 12,000	
5	$15,000		
Total	$38,000		

We can see that by year 4, our initial investment will be paid back. To calculate the portion of year 4 that it consumes, we divide the remaining amount ($8,000) by the net cash flow ($12,000). Therefore, this investment will be paid back in 3.67 years.

Comparing Competing Projects

The medical record project's initial investment is $75,000. Annual cash flows of $25,000 will result in a payback period of 3 years ($75,000/$25,000).
   The patient accounts project's initial investment is $60,000. Annual cash flows of $15,000 will result in a payback period of 4 years ($60,000/$15,000).

Arguments: Pro and Con

Each of the evaluation methods has advantages and disadvantages. No one method is more effective than the other and occasionally financial managers use more than one method to weigh the opportunities. The payback method is the simplest to use. No special tables are required, but it ignores the basic concept of money management—the time value of money.

The accounting rate of return is simple to use. No special tables are required, but it ignores the time value of money and does not take into consideration when inflows are received. The same average could result if the heavier inflows are received later in the project's life or earlier. If the time value of money was considered, a money manager would want to receive the larger inflows earlier rather than later.

The net present value approach requires calculations of the discounted amounts or the use of special discounting tables. It assumes, however, that net inflows are reinvested at the same rate as the cost of capital or the interest rate the investment would have received had the money been left in the bank. It also requires the evaluators to assume a rate of return.

COST OF ALLOCATIONS

To determine the approximate costs to provide services, an organization must develop and maintain a cost allocation system. The cost management system allocates direct and indirect costs. Costs are classified by department or responsibility center. Non–revenue-generating departments are considered indirect cost departments, whereas revenue-generating departments are considered direct cost departments. Cost allocation allocates the costs of indirect, non-revenue departments to direct, revenue-generating departments.

Why Does Allocation Occur?

Some payers reimburse on the basis of the full costs of direct departments and permit the allocation of indirect departments to the direct departments only to the extent that the indirect departments contribute to the direct departments' provision of care or generation of revenue.

Many indirect departments support the provision of care through the assistance provided to the direct departments. For example, telecommunications is an indirect department. If no one answers the organization's phone during an emergency, services are not provided. The HIM department supports the efforts of the nursing service, the therapy departments, and the ancillaries by serving as the central controller of all records and reports. The HIM department is considered a non–patient revenue generating department. The total costs of the department are, therefore, considered indirect and must be allocated to the patient revenue–generating departments of nursing, therapy, and laboratory, and so on.

The HIM department does have revenue-generating opportunities. Some departments charge for copies of medical records provided to insurance companies and lawyers. Other departments provide transcription services for their physicians and charge accordingly. These services are revenue-generating; however, they are not directly related to the primary mission of the organization—patient care.

Allocation Methods

Step-Down Method

The **step-down method** is a common method that is supported by Medicare in its cost-reporting requirements. In this method, the indirect department that receives the least amount of service from other indirect departments and provides the most service to other departments has its costs allocated first.

The chaplain service is an indirect department that may offer less service to other departments than the HIM department offers to direct departments. Both provide services to nursing, but seldom does the chaplain provide services to the therapy departments or the laboratory. So the HIM department costs would be allocated before those of the chaplain service.

The allocation is made based on ratio of services provided to each department or some other allocation, such as square footage, employees, or worked hours.

EXAMPLE OF COST ALLOCATIONS

Housekeeping serves more indirect departments than laundry/linen or medical records. Housekeeping's services are used 20 per cent of the time by laundry/linen, 5 per cent of the time by medical records and radiology, and 70 per cent by nursing. Laundry/linen's services are used 3 per cent by medical records, 5 per cent by radiology, and 92 per cent by nursing. The allocation results in all the costs ($147,760) of the indirect departments to the direct departments of nursing and radiology.

The step-down approach is most common in health care institutions. The steps in the allocation table's appearance show how the approach was named.

Double-Distribution Method

The **double-distribution method** is similar to the step-down method. This method assumes that the allocation of costs cannot be linear and that some indirect departments need to be allocated to less commonly dispersed departments before the costs of these departments are fully allocated. In the example discussed earlier, housekeeping was fully allocated to the remaining departments of laundry/linen, medical records, radiology, and nursing. Then laundry/linen's costs were fully allocated. In the double-distribution method, we would

	DEPARTMENT TOTAL COSTS	HOUSEKEEPING	LAUNDRY/LINEN	MED RECORDS	TOTAL
Housekeeping	$ 30,000	$ 30,000			
Laundry/Linen	15,000	6,000(.20)	$21,000*		
Medical Records	100,000	1,500(.05)	630(.03)	$102,130	
Radiology	135,000	1,500(.05)	1,050(.05)	10,213(.10)	$147,760
Nursing	270,000	21,000(.70)	19,320(.92)	91,917(.90)	402,240
Total	$550,000	$30,000	$21,000	$102,130	$550,000

* The laundry/linen department costs were $15,000 plus the allocated housekeeping costs were an additional $6,000.

now have the opportunity to distribute some of laundry/linen's costs back to housekeeping. In the step-down method, that option is not available.

Simultaneous-Equations Method

The **simultaneous-equations method** (also known as the algebraic or multiple apportionment method) permits multiple allocations to occur through sophisticated mathematical software and the use of simultaneous mathematical equations. This method may require 10 to 12 different distributions of costs.

Why Is Cost Allocation Methodology Important for the HIM Professional?

Some forward-thinking facilities provide comprehensive budgeting reports to their department managers. The managers see not only the direct costs incurred by the department—that is, the supplies they order and pay for, the labor they paid for, and so on—but also the allocations of costs from other departments. The HIM department may find it unusual to see costs for the laundry department allocated to the HIM department. If the HIM department uses no laundry services, then the allocation should be removed and reallocated to the departments that use this service. The health information manager must fully investigate the services of laundry before removing the allocation because the laundry department may assist housekeeping in removing stains that may appear on the carpet in the HIM department.

Further, the HIM department should assess whether costs are being properly allocated to its user departments. This may require HIM department management to monitor for several months the user demand, perhaps by counting the number of records, reports, or statistics requested and then determining what percentage of all requests should be allocated to each user department. For example, the HIM director may decide that the simplest method to allocate the HIM department costs is by record requests (Figure 15–8).

RECORDS REQUESTED FOR FIRST NINE MONTHS OF YEAR

Requestor	Number Requested	% of All
Administration	5	.004
Fiscal Services	210	.16
Quality Management	400	.30
Risk Management	17	.01
Nursing Service	323	.24
Respiratory Therapy	105	.08
Physical Therapy	90	.07
Anesthesiology	47	.04
Surgery	143	.11
Medicine	180	.13
Social Work	12	.01
Total	1340	1.01 (due to rounding)

FIGURE 15–8. Example of record request.

Given this information, the HIM professional can now approach the cost accountant and review current allocations to the new data, and she may make adjustments as indicated based on the factual data provided.

Some facilities allocate costs in a less scientific manner for simplicity purposes. Some methods include allocating costs of other departments to user departments based on the total square feet occupied by all user departments. In our example, if the HIM department represented 5 per cent of the total square feet served by housekeeping, then 5 per cent of housekeeping's costs would be allocated to medical records. Clearly, one could argue that the HIM department area requires less cleaning than perhaps the operating room, but the allocation method is simple to apply and keep up to date.

OTHER PHASES OF FINANCIAL MANAGEMENT

Implementing

Throughout this chapter, we have alluded to the actual implementation precautions and things that managers must take care to do and to avoid. The implementation process is probably the most rewarding activity of management, because it confirms whether your ideas were correct, your plans were accurate, and your achievements are worth reaching. It requires support from your entire staff as well as from management above your level.

Controlling

The activity of **controlling** is one of several management duties. In this chapter, it refers to the activities that management must pursue when what was planned does not occur—financially.

HOW DOES MANAGEMENT CONTROL THE FINANCIAL ASPECTS OF ITS DEPARTMENTS?

One tool that most organizations have is a **variance report.** This document reflects the budget that was prepared and approved and shows the actual results on at least a monthly basis. If the business plan proposal for a courier service to reduce incomplete records is approved, the effectiveness in reducing the receivables, reducing the incomplete records, and using our half-employee and car at the limited amounts projected will

be monitored. Should more labor hours be needed or higher than expected car expenses be incurred, this information will show on the variance report. The impact on accounts receivable and incomplete records will *not* show here.

The reduction in accounts receivable is monitored by the business office or patient accounts and probably the CFO. The actual results of the accounts receivable appears on the balance sheet. The incomplete record count is a regular management report prepared by the director of the HIM department.

NEW TRENDS

With reimbursement pressures certain to increase, even in an economy operating under ideal conditions and in an environment of total health care reform, the need to closely monitor all activities to ensure that services are delivered as cost-effectively as possible will be management's greatest challenge.

Seeking Alternatives

No manager can identify *all* alternatives to doing a task. Just as the composition of the business plan requires the involvement of all staff, during times of economic downturns and lower volumes, all staff need to be involved to find other methods to achieve the same outcome. Management should meet with staff in teams if the staff size is large or as a whole if the staff size is small at regular intervals to brainstorm alternatives to performing tasks. Ideally, this process should occur before the budgeting process so that management can fully investigate the options that surface and prepare any justification materials at budget time. This participative management approach is becoming more common in health care with the increased awareness of continuous quality improvement processes in a total quality management environment.

Increasing Communication Among Departments

In the past, departments within an organization had little interaction. With the advent of DRGs, a cooperative relationship has evolved between the HIM department and patient accounts. The need to keep each other informed of account receivable status requires that each area's manager and staff work closely and respect the other's constraints. Each area has expertise that should be shared with the other.

The HIM department has learned to work with sometimes demanding medical staff members. Patient accounts has extensive experience working with patients and insurance companies to collect balances due on the accounts. Sharing techniques with each other on how best to get results from people will benefit both departments.

Both departments receive newsletters, regulatory notices, and other information sources that can be shared with each other to allow both departments to be more knowledgeable.

Each area works with medical terminology. The staff in patient accounts often is trained from within. HIM professionals can teach medical terminology to the patient accounts staff and educate them in medicolegal aspects, such as patient confidentiality and proper release rules.

The HIM department also can support increased reimbursement by ensuring that the organization's CDM (master listing of services) is kept up to date with current CPT-4 codes.

Role of the HIM Professional in Financial Management

The need for HIM professionals to be more adept in fiscal activities is apparent. This chapter cannot review all aspects of financial management. To be truly successful, HIM professionals of tomorrow must be able to communicate as easily with the CFO as they are able to deal with the medical staff. If the HIM professional is to gain this level of expertise, additional training must be sought beyond the contents of this chapter.

References

1. McArtle K: Personal communication, 1994.
2. Cleverley WO. Essentials of health care finance, 3rd ed. Gaithersburg, MD: Aspen Publishers, 1992, p 299.
3. Neumann BR, Suver JD, Zelman WN. Financial management—concepts and applications for health care providers, 2nd ed. Baltimore: National Health Publishing, 1988.

16

KAREN YOUMANS

KEY WORDS

Benchmarking
Critical path
Decision grid
  (or matrix)
Decision table
Decision tree
Flowchart
Flow process chart
Gantt chart
Informal organization
  (unwritten organiza-
  tion)
Methods improvement

Movement diagram
  (layout flowchart)
Operation flowchart
Organization chart
PERT network
Productive unit of work
Productivity
Productivity standards
  (work standards)
Project management
Re-engineering
System

METHODS FOR ANALYZING AND IMPROVING SYSTEMS

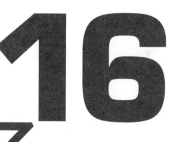

16

Systems analysis and
design
Systems flowchart
Work breakdown struc-
tures

Work distribution chart
Work sampling
Work simplification

OBJECTIVES

- Define key words.
- Describe various methods of organizing work.
- Define productivity, productivity standards, and a productive unit of work.
- Describe the various methods of measuring output to establish productivity standards.
- Apply the work simplification process to improve a system.
- Explain the concepts applied to the systems model.
- Utilize the systems analysis and design process to analyze and improve a system.
- Differentiate between the formal and the informal organization.
- Examine the characteristics of projects and project management.
- Utilize the project management process to achieve an organizational goal.
- Define re-engineering.

INTRODUCTION

Health information is not limited to one department or even to one organization. It is developed, disseminated, and used throughout the organizations and communities. The effective use of health information depends on the systems that can create, analyze, disseminate, and utilize it. To be effective, the systems must effectively use the resources of people, processes, and equipment.

An important skill for the health information manager is to be able to analyze the processes that create and handle health information to be sure that they are functioning in the most efficient and effective manner. These processes could involve paper, computer systems, or both.

This chapter describes the tools that can help to analyze and improve the methods used in health information systems. The discussion begins at the micro level of individual jobs and procedures and moves through a mid level looking at systems analysis and design and organizational concepts to a larger macro or organizationwide level with the concepts of project management and re-engineering.

INDIVIDUAL WORK PROCESSES (MICRO LEVEL)

Organizing Work

The method of organizing, or allocating, the work among the employees depends somewhat on the type of organization and the nature of the work to be accomplished. Work division can be accomplished by any of the following methods:

- *Function*—Similar tasks are performed by one unit within a department or an organization.
- *Project*—A work unit performs all steps for a particular project (an example is a task force).
- *Product*—In a manufacturing company, one unit performs all the work to produce a single product.

Sections on Organizing Work, Work Distribution Chart, and Productivity were contributed by Carol J. Barr.

Serial Work Division

Employee	Poly Ester	Justin Case	Cindy Rella
Processes	Tasks 1 & 2 on all records	Tasks 3 & 4 on all records	Tasks 5 & 6 on all records
Sequence	Before tasks 3, 4, 5, & 6	After tasks 1 & 2 and before tasks 5 & 6	After tasks 1, 2, 3, & 4

Parallel Work Division

Employee	Poly Ester	Justin Case	Cindy Rella
Processes	Tasks 1, 2, 3, & 4 on 1/3 of the records	Tasks 1, 2, 3, & 4 on 1/3 of the records	Tasks 1, 2, 3, & 4 on 1/3 of the records
Sequence	First to work on this group of records	First to work on this group of records	First to work on this group of records

Unit Assembly Work Division

Employee	Poly Ester	Justin Case	Cindy Rella
Processes	Tasks 1 & 2 on all records	Tasks 3 & 4 on all records	Tasks 5 & 6 on all records
Sequence	First to work on record, or after tasks 3 & 4, or after tasks 5 & 6, or after tasks 3, 4, 5, & 6.	First to work on record, or after tasks 1 & 2, or after tasks 5 & 6, or after tasks 1, 2, 5, & 6.	First to work on record, or after tasks 1 & 2, or after tasks 3 & 4, or after tasks 1, 2, 3, & 4.

FIGURE 16–1. Methods of organizing work.

Territory—Sales forces are divided in this manner, with each representative responsible for a certain geographic area. Another example may be the organization of the hospital nursing service by patient care units.

- *Customer*—This concept can be applied in a health information management (HIM) department when teams are organized to work on patient records of particular doctors.

- *Process*—Similar work processes or procedures are grouped together and performed by a particular unit or group of employees.

Work processing can be further subdivided to the individual employee level. This subdivision can be classified into serial, parallel, and unit assembly (Figure 16–1).

Serial Work Division

The serial work division is one of consecutive handling of tasks. A series of small tasks are grouped together. Each task in the series is performed by a specialist in that type of work. The work passes from one employee to another until all tasks have been performed and the work is complete. An example of the serial arrangement is an assembly line in a factory where each step in the process is performed by a different person.

Parallel Work Division

Parallel work division demonstrates a concurrent method of handling work. One person performs a series of tasks. The tasks may be, but are not necessarily, related. Several employees may be performing the series of tasks at the same time. An example of this method in an HIM department is where four persons are employed to assemble and analyze patient records. Each employee assembles and analyzes records.

Unit Assembly Work Division

In unit assembly work division, each employee specializes in a particular task, as in serial work division, but the sequence of tasks on each unit is not identical. For example, in Figure 16–1, Poly Ester specializes in tasks 1 and 2. She may perform these tasks before anyone else works on a particular item, after tasks 3 and 4 are done, after tasks 5 and 6 are complete, or even after all steps—3, 4, 5, and 6—are done. A great deal of coordination is necessary in the unit assembly method because the amount of time needed to perform individual tasks differs. The advantages and disadvan-

TABLE 16–1 ADVANTAGES AND DISADVANTAGES OF WORK DIVISION METHODS		
SERIAL	**PARALLEL**	**UNIT ASSEMBLY**
Advantages		
• Employees are skilled in their own tasks. • Causes of delays are easily identified. • If one step in the process requires a specialized skill or use of specialized equipment, fewer skilled staff and/or equipment are needed.	• Because employees know all functions, absences and volume fluctuations are managed. • Work is more interesting to the staff because they see it through to completion and it encompasses a wider variety of functions.	• Saves time; employees can work on the item without waiting for others to finish their task. • Employees are skilled at their own tasks.
Disadvantages		
• Employee absences can cause backlogs. • Slow employees can delay the final product. • Work can become boring because employees' work has limited variety and scope. • The work items are handled numerous times because each step is performed by different employees. This may increase the total processing time for all steps.	• If one or more of the steps require specialized skills or equipment, more skilled staff and/or equipment are needed, making the process more expensive. • Recruiting and training of staff to complete multiple functions may be difficult.	• Work can become boring because employees' work has limited variety and scope. • Difficult to use unless work can be easily divided into tasks that do not depend on the results of other tasks. • Coordination of work flow and scheduling of completion of individual items would be difficult.

tages of the three methods of organizing work are delineated in Table 16–1.

Work Distribution Chart

The **work distribution chart** is a useful tool that provides data to analyze the processes performed by a work group and the individual employee within the work group (Figure 16–2). Examination of the data assists in identifying problems but not solutions. The work distribution chart is a matrix that displays the tasks being performed in a work group, the employees who perform them, and the amount of time spent on each task by each employee and the work unit as a whole.

Analysis of the work distribution chart can answer the following questions.

	CLERICAL SUPERVISOR	TIME (HOURS)	INPATIENT ASSEMBLY & ANALYSIS	TIME (HOURS)	INPATIENT ASSEMBLY & ANALYSIS	TIME (HOURS)	OUTPATIENT ASSEMBLY & ANALYSIS	TIME (HOURS)	OUTPATIENT ASSEMBLY & ANALYSIS	TIME (HOURS)	TOTAL TIME
Supervise	Supervision Duties	4									4
Clerical	Birth/Death Certificate	$3\frac{1}{4}$	Assembly & Analysis	$3\frac{1}{4}$ 4	Assembly & Analysis	$2\frac{1}{2}$ 4	Assembly & Analysis Correct med rec numbers	$2\frac{1}{2}$ 4 $\frac{3}{4}$	Assembly & Analysis Correct med rec numbers	$2\frac{1}{2}$ 4 $\frac{3}{4}$	$3\frac{1}{4}$ $10\frac{3}{4}$ 16 $1\frac{1}{2}$ $\frac{3}{4}$
	Statistics	$\frac{3}{4}$									
Filing			Loose Sheets	$\frac{3}{4}$	Loose Sheets	$1\frac{1}{2}$	Loose Sheets	$\frac{3}{4}$	Loose Sheets	$\frac{3}{4}$	$3\frac{3}{4}$
Reception											
Total		8		8		8		8		8	40

FIGURE 16–2. Work distribution chart.

What tasks are employees performing? Are these tasks important to achieving organizational goals? Question the total time of the group on a particular activity and then that of individual employees. Are the activities that take the most time really the most important ones? Is a lot of time spent redoing work that had errors? Handling complaints?

How are tasks distributed among employees of the work group? Does each employee do a little bit of one task? Does any one employee do the bulk of one task while the others are not using their time effectively?

Are employees' qualifications being utilized? Are highly skilled, highly paid employees using those qualifications? For example, are medical transcriptionists filing the reports that they type? On the other hand, are employees doing tasks that they are not qualified to do—for example, a person with only knowledge of medical terminology assigns codes to Medicare patients' diagnoses and procedures?

How are individual jobs constructed? Are employees performing too many unrelated tasks, or are they doing one thing all day long? Performing too many unrelated tasks wastes effort and is costly. Changing from one task to another decreases productivity because of the time spent setting up and ending each task. The monotony of performing one or a few tasks for most of the work time causes boredom and, possibly, dissatisfaction with the job.

Analysis of the work distribution chart may also aid the manager in choosing one of the aforementioned types of work division (serial, parallel, or unit assembly). By including the number of units produced in the work distribution chart, managers can use the chart to establish **productivity standards** in an organization.

Preparation of the work distribution chart requires the following steps.

1. *Each employee prepares a task list.* Over a 1-week period, each employee lists the tasks he or she performs and the amount of time spent on each. The task statements should be brief and specific and include no more than 15 statements. The duties should be listed in order of importance. Every minute need not be accounted for. Hours should be entered to the nearest 15 minutes, and breaks and other nonproductive time should be included in a miscellaneous category.

To gain cooperation from the employees, the supervisor should explain the purpose of gathering this data. The purpose is not punitive but to analyze how time is spent in the work group to improve the jobs.

2. *Supervisor prepares a list of the major activities of the work group.* This is a list of general categories into which all activities of the employees can be classified. As a rule, no more than 10 activities should be listed. They should be listed in order of importance with the most important listed first.

3. *Supervisor combines the employee task list and the activity list into the work distribution chart.* The work distribution chart is complete when

- the major activities are listed in the left-hand column;
- the employees are listed across the top of the chart;
- the tasks performed by each employee and the amount of time required for performance of each task are listed in the column under the employee's name; and
- the total time spent on each major activity by all employees is recorded in the right-hand column.

Productivity

Productivity is the process of converting an organization's resources (labor, capital, materials, and technology) into products and services that meet the organization's goals. A productive organization is one that produces quality products and/or services with the least expenditure of resources.

Productivity is often expressed as a ratio of:

$$\frac{\text{OUTPUT (Services or products)}}{\text{INPUT (Resources consumed)}}$$

Some related definitions are important to the understanding of productivity. A **productive unit of work** is an item produced that meets established levels of quality. The quality level is an important aspect of this definition. When a product does not meet the quality level, it often has to be redone. Therefore, if products that do not meet the quality level are counted as output, the number of products would be inflated because of having to count the rework as well as the original work as outputs. Examples of outputs in an HIM department are coded patient data, completed response to a request for information, and a transcribed report.

Productivity Standards

Productivity (also known as performance or work) standards are the tools that are used to specify the expected performance and to measure actual performance. Productivity standards have many uses in managing an HIM department. They can assist in determining the number of personnel, equipment, and supplies needed to accomplish the projected workload; in scheduling completion and distribution of tasks; in evaluating proposed changes in processes or systems to see if a savings in personnel time would occur; in setting goals for a work group or individual employee; and in evaluating performance of a work group or individual employee. Productivity standards can also be used to determine the actual cost of producing a given product or service.

SETTING PRODUCTIVITY STANDARDS

Measuring Input. To set productivity standards, certain determinations must be made. First, the methods of quantifying inputs must be determined. This is usually in terms of employee time expressed in paid staff hours worked. Second, the unit of work for measuring output must be established. For given processes, this can take various forms. For example, for the coding function, should the number of codes be counted or the number of records? Should the output be classified by level of difficulty (e.g., outpatient versus inpatient, Medicare versus non-Medicare)?

Measuring Output

ACTUAL PERFORMANCE. Various methods are used to measure output. They range from using past performance data to using time studies and work sampling. Using data from actual performance is the most common method of measuring output. It is the easiest, quickest, and least expensive. Data can be collected by the organization's own staff. Specialists are not needed. Methods used to collect this information include employee-reported logs in the form of time ladders or diaries. Equipment can also be used to count items of work; for example, dictation equipment can record the number of minutes transcribed or characters entered.

WORK SAMPLING. **Work sampling** is another method of collecting actual performance data. This method is based on the statistical laws of probability. The research concepts of population, random selection, and sample must be comprehended to understand the work sampling methodology.

Population: All items or members of the group to be studied

Sample: The group of items chosen to represent the whole population. The size of the sample is important because it must be large enough to represent all members of the group but small enough to be manageable and cost-effective

Random Selection: The method of choosing the sample that gives each item in the population an equal chance of being chosen

In work sampling, the supervisor observes employees at times randomly selected and records the task the employee is doing at the time of the observation. The observations are tallied to determine the percentage of all work time (the population) spent on each task. Combining these percentages with the number of items produced determines the productivity standards for these tasks.

Using actual performance data has several problems. These productivity standards are based on existing procedures, employee performance, and qualifications—all of which might not be the most effective for this process. Therefore, expected results would be based on poor performance and ineffective processes.

BENCHMARKING. **Benchmarking,** another method of setting standards, is the comparison of one organization's performance with that of another organization that is known to be excellent in that area. Benchmarking is beneficial because it is more than comparing productivity. It involves discovering how the benchmark organization achieves its goals and incorporating these methods into your organization. The aim of benchmarking is the improvement of the organization's processes.

SYNTHESIS. Synthesis methods using stopwatch studies are the most expensive techniques for setting productivity standards. Stopwatch studies require a skilled analyst to observe the employee performing the task and to record stop and start times for each portion of the task. The selection of the employee to be observed is an important element of this technique. The employee should be one who performs the task at an average speed, not the fastest or the slowest. This method also is the poorest in human relations. Having every move one makes be watched can be quite unsettling and put one on edge.

Whichever method is used to collect data and set productivity standards, the concept of quality cannot be overlooked. Techniques for assuring the expected quality level of the output must be built into the methods for measuring the quantity.

Efficiency is as important in setting work standards as it is elsewhere in the organization. If it becomes too expensive to set standards and measure work, the goal of productivity monitoring is defeated.

Productivity standards must be understandable, realistic, reliable, and attainable under normal working conditions. Clear communications between employers and employees is important for the program to be a success. An effective productivity management program is based on accurate, reliable standards that have earned credibility with the employee.

INCREASING PRODUCTIVITY. Productivity can be increased by the following methods:

- Increasing output while holding input constant
- Decreasing input (resources) while maintaining the same level of output
- Increasing output while decreasing resources

- Increasing resources and output but with a proportionately greater increase in output
- Decreasing output and resources with a proportionately greater decrease in resources

Research findings on productivity improvement show the following[1]:

- Productivity goes up when it is measured.
- Productivity improves as it becomes a primary goal of management.
- Productivity increases as managers and staff are held accountable for its measurement and evaluation.
- Productivity increases as its benefits are shared with those employees responsible for the increase.
- Productivity increases as employees are rewarded for extra output.
- Productivity increases as the resources allocated are in direct proportion to the productivity improvement potential.

IMPLEMENTING A PRODUCTIVITY PROGRAM. To be useful, an organization needs a focused approach to improving productivity. A productivity improvement program needs well-defined goals. To be effective, as many employees as possible should be involved in the development of the program. Organizational goals should be integrated with employee goals. All employees should be part of the program and be accountable for productivity improvement in their own work areas. Employees should share in the benefits of improved productivity and should be rewarded and reinforced for their contributions. Implementing a productivity improvement program is a six-step process.

1. Identify an area in the organization for improvement.
2. Establish a unit of measurement (productivity ratio) and measure current performance in that area.
3. Develop a *measurable* productivity objective.
4. Identify a strategy for meeting the objective.
5. Establish time frames and identify checkpoints.
6. Analyze results and provide feedback.

An example of a productivity improvement program in an HIM department is shown in Figure 16–3.

Work Simplification or Methods Improvement

An organizational goal is to provide the best service or make the best product with the least expenditure of resources while maintaining a healthy and contented workforce. The effectiveness of the individual employee depends on the effectiveness of the processes used. **Work simplification**, sometimes called **methods improvement**, is an organized approach to determine how to accomplish a task with less effort in less time or at a lower cost while maintaining or improving the quality of the outcome. It uses commonsense concepts to eliminate waste of time, energy, material, equipment, and space when performing work processes. Sometimes work simplification is misunderstood to mean work speed up. When work simplification tools are correctly used, the rate of production is enhanced by performing only the essential steps in the best way possible at a standard pace.

The fundamental objectives of work simplification are as follows:

- Simplify
- Eliminate

Productivity improvement area:	Coding
Productivity Ratio:	Number of records coded per man hour
Current Level of Productivity:	6 correctly coded patient records per man hour
Productivity Objective:	10 correctly coded patient records per man hour
Improvement Strategy:	Weekly educational programs on coding. Each coder will attend a coding seminar each year.
Time Frame:	Six months
Checkpoints:	Monthly
Evaluation and Feedback:	Measure productivity, if level meets goal, praise and congratulate. Establish incentive pay program.

FIGURE 16–3. Productivity improvement program for coding.

- Combine
- Improve

The simplest means of performing the work is usually the easiest and most practical.

Questioning is fundamental to improving work processes. The first question that must be asked is, "Does this process assist in achieving the organization's goals?" When the answer is no, the process should be eliminated. Remember to question the statement "That's the way it has always been done." The questions of who, what, when, where, and how must be answered.

The philosophy of work simplification is that there is always a better way to perform each and every task. The statement that the process has always been done this way is a red flag that the process could use change and that the employee does not understand why the procedures are done in this way. The goal of a work simplification program is to increase efficiency through the elimination of unnecessary work and through the optimal structure of necessary work.

The human being who performs these tasks must be given significant attention when dissecting individual jobs. Employees need to be involved in the process because they are the experts in their own processes. If they are involved in the change, they are more likely to accept the change. However, care must be taken so that the content of the job does not become oversimplified and boring.

The steps in the work simplification methodology are similar to those in the scientific method.

1. Identify a problem area or select a work process or function to improve.
2. Gather data on the problem.
3. Organize and analyze the data gathered on the problem.
4. Formulate alternative solutions or improvements.
5. Select the improved method.
6. Implement the improved method and evaluate the effectiveness of the improvement.

Identifying a Problem Area or Selecting a Work Process or Function to Improve

The identification of a problem is not an easy task. A competent manager must be able to differentiate between a symptom and its cause or problem. What appears to be the problem may only be a symptom. This step is essential because if the symptom's cause is not correctly identified, the problem will not be solved and the symptom may only be temporarily eliminated.

In health care, distinguishing between symptoms and diagnoses (problems) is a familiar process. The patient presents to the emergency department with the symptom of abdominal pain. On testing and evaluation, the patient is diagnosed with acute appendicitis. Once the cause of the abdominal pain is identified, treatment can be initiated to remedy the symptom.

Using the same approach of symptom versus diagnosis, common work symptoms can be examined to find the diagnosis or problem. For example, the symptom of poor productivity may be traced back to the problem of inefficient work flow. High employee turnover may be a symptom of low morale caused by poor workload distribution.

The following list of symptoms indicate a potential problem and should be investigated:

- Duplication of work processes
- Overlapping of responsibilities
- Frequent backtracking
- Inconsistencies
- Frequent delays and interruptions
- Poor workload distribution
- Inaccuracies and errors
- Lack of controls
- Lack of instructions or procedures
- Low employee morale
- High absenteeism
- Complaints from customers and employees
- Waste of materials, effort, personnel, time, and space
- Obvious fatigue
- Poor safety record
- Excessive time required to carry out an activity in comparison with results achieved

Managers need to be sensitive to cues from their employees and their surroundings. When managers are not responsive to these cues, a potential problem may develop into a crisis situation. Once a sign is recognized as a potential problem, the manager must proceed to investigate and move to resolution of the problem. Nothing is more discouraging to employees than to raise a concern and have no response from management. After a while, employees will complain among themselves and fail to make management aware of problem areas.

Another approach to selecting an area of work to be simplified is to review areas with high labor requirements and a large number of diverse work activities as well as those in which excessive time is needed to perform the work, the costs are high, or the end product is inadequate.

Gathering Data About the Problem

Data collection methods vary with the type of problem and work performed. Data-gathering methods include the collection of blank forms used in the process, completed forms, organizational charts, job descriptions, procedures, interviews with employees, and observation. Additional facts may be obtained from supervisory staff.

The key to gathering data is to ask the right questions to find out how the work is being performed. The following are key questions to ask:

- Why is this process performed? How does it move the organization toward achievement of its goals?
- Who does the work? What are their qualifications for performing these processes?
- What work is currently being done?
- When (in what sequence) is the work being performed?
- Where is the work being performed?
- How is the work being done? Why is it being done this way? Is there a better way to achieve the same result?
- At what rate does the work flow to the employee? Is the rate consistent?

A flow process chart can be used to analyze procedures and determine opportunities for improvement through eliminating, combining, or resequencing any part of the process.

FLOW PROCESS CHART. A **flow process chart** is a tool used to collect information on the steps of a work process and to analyze and improve the process. It is especially helpful in analyzing manual operations.

The symbols used to represent each step in the process are shown in Figure 16–4. The symbols that represent each step are connected with a line to facilitate analysis.

A flow process chart briefly describes each step in the process, identifies the distance that objects are moved, and shows the amount of time consumed by each delay. The following are typical problems that can be identified by using a flow process chart:

- Duplication of effort
- Too much travel time from one workstation to another
- Delays in transferring work

Each step in the process should be subjected to the following questions:

- Is that particular step necessary or of value?
- Can the step be eliminated?
- Can the step be streamlined or combined with another step?
- Is the step properly sequenced within the process?

Figure 16–5 shows a completed flow process chart for the release-of-information function.

FLOWCHARTS. Additional types of **flowcharts** are used to verify and obtain information about how a procedure is being performed. Flowcharts are essentially road maps that show the logical steps and sequence

SYMBOL	PROCESS	END RESULT	EXAMPLE
○	Operation Make-ready	Get-ready to do	Sorting
●	Operation Do	Produces or accomplishes	Coding, data entry
⇨	Transportation	Moves	Walking
▽	Storage	Keeps	Object placed in permanent storage
□	Inspection	Verifies	Proofreading
D	Delay	Interfaces	Object is in temporary storage or waiting

FIGURE 16–4. Flow process chart symbols.

	Present	Proposed	Difference
○ No. of Operations	8	7	1
⇨ No. of Transportations	4	1	3
☐ No. of Inspections	3	2	1
◻ No. of Delays	1	1	0
▽ No. of Storages	1	1	0
Distance Traveled	65	20	45
Minutes Delayed	60	30	30

Job _Processing a request for copies of medical records_

Charted by _S. Smith_

Department _HIM_

Date _4/4/95_

Present Method	Operation	Transportation	Inspection	Delay	Storage	Distance in Feet	Time in Minutes	Proposed Method	Operation	Transportation	Inspection	Delay	Storage	Distance in Feet	Time in Minutes
written request opened by receptionist	●	⇨	☐	◻	▽			written request opened by ROI	●	⇨	☐	◻	▽		
request forms alphabetized	●	⇨	☐	◻	▽			ROI clerk checks for completeness	○	⇨	☒	◻	▽		
receptionist transports to release of info	○	⇨	☐	◻	▽	15 Ft		ROI alphabetizes request forms	●	⇨	☐	◻	▽		
ROI clerk checks for completeness	○	⇨	☒	◻	▽			ROI reviews chart locator system	●	⇨	☐	◻	▽		
ROI clerk makes outguides for charts	●	⇨	☐	◻	▽			ROI prints list for clerk	●	⇨	☐	◻	▽		
ROI waits for clerk to pull charts	○	⇨	☐	◼	▽		60 MIN	ROI waits for clerk to pull charts	○	⇨	☐	◼	▽		30 MIN
clerk pulls charts	●	⇨	☐	◻	▽			clerk pulls charts	●	⇨	☐	◻	▽		
charts transported to ROI	○	⇨	☐	◻	▽	20 Ft		charts transported to ROI	○	⇨	☐	◻	▽	20 Ft	
ROI reviews medical record	○	⇨	☒	◻	▽			ROI reviews charts	○	⇨	☒	◻	▽		
ROI tags pages to copy	●	⇨	☐	◻	▽			ROI copies charts	●	⇨	☐	◻	▽		
ROI copies charts	●	⇨	☐	◻	▽			chart to file	○	⇨	☐	◻	▼		
chart and copies transported to supervisor	○	⇨	☐	◻	▽	15 Ft		copies mailed	●	⇨	☐	◻	▽		
supervisor inspects request and copies	○	⇨	☒	◻	▽				○	⇨	☐	◻	▽		
chart and copies transported back to ROI	○	⇨	☐	◻	▽	15 Ft			○	⇨	☐	◻	▽		
ROI documents copies sent	●	⇨	☐	◻	▽				○	⇨	☐	◻	▽		
chart to file	○	⇨	☐	◻	▼				○	⇨	☐	◻	▽		
copies mailed	●	⇨	☐	◻	▽				○	⇨	☐	◻	▽		

FIGURE 16–5. Flow process chart for release of information (ROI).

involved in a procedure. Flowcharts are used to depict all levels of operations from whole systems that involve many departments and people, as in a systems flowchart, to the work of one person or procedure, as in an operations or procedure flowchart. The **systems flowchart** depicts the flow of data through all or part of the system, the various operations that take place within the system, and the files that are used to produce various reports or documents. Figure 16–6 shows an example of a systems flowchart for the master patient index.

Flowchart Symbols and Guidelines. The standard symbols shown in Figure 16–7 are used to construct flowcharts. When unique symbols are used, their meaning should be identified in a key or legend on the flowchart (see Guidelines for Constructing a Flow Chart).

Operation or Procedure Flowchart. The **operation flowchart** is a graphic representation of the logical sequence of activities in a procedure. In addition, it points out the decision points encountered in carrying out that function. The operation flowchart should specify how a function is performed, not the methods used. This type of flowchart is a superb communication tool between employees and management (Figure 16–8).

Movement Diagrams. The **movement diagram,**

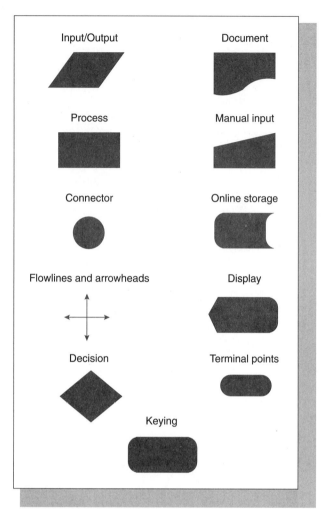

FIGURE 16–7. Common flowchart symbols.

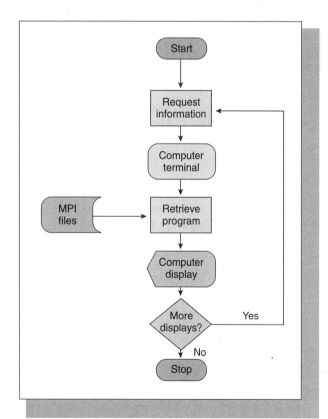

FIGURE 16–6. Systems flowchart for master patient index.

Guidelines for Constructing a Flowchart

• Title the chart with the name of the procedure or system, the name of the department and organization, and the date.

• Describe each step of the process, using concise, brief phrases (e.g., file record, transcribe discharge summary). If possible, write the step description inside the symbol for the step.

• Write decision steps in a question form that can be answered with a yes or no (e.g., Is record complete?). Decision steps are usually followed by two steps: one leading from the yes response and one leading from the no response.

• Draw the flowchart from top to bottom and from the left-hand side to the right-hand side of the page. Use on-page connectors to show flow without drawing lines over the diagram. Use off-page connectors to show the links to subsequent pages. Note the start and end of an activity.

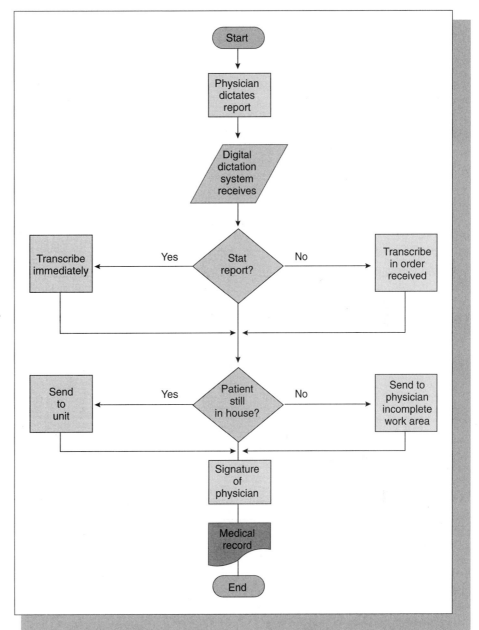

FIGURE 16–8. Operation flowchart for transcription.

sometimes called a **layout flowchart,** represents graphically the physical environment in which the processes are performed. The purpose of a movement diagram is to depict the flow of work activities through the desks and equipment. A movement diagram can show movement of paper or employee. This type of chart can be beneficial in indentifying the problem of backtracking or bottlenecks in procedures. With a graphic display of the physical layout, a more efficient route for accomplishment of the task can be achieved.

Movement diagrams or layout flowcharts are espe-

cially useful in the analysis of manual systems (Figure 16–9).

Organizing and Analyzing Data Gathered on the Problem

The third step of the process entails organizing and analyzing the facts or data obtained from step two. As with all steps in work simplification, the employees who perform the work need to be included in this process.

Data can be organized in many ways. One is by

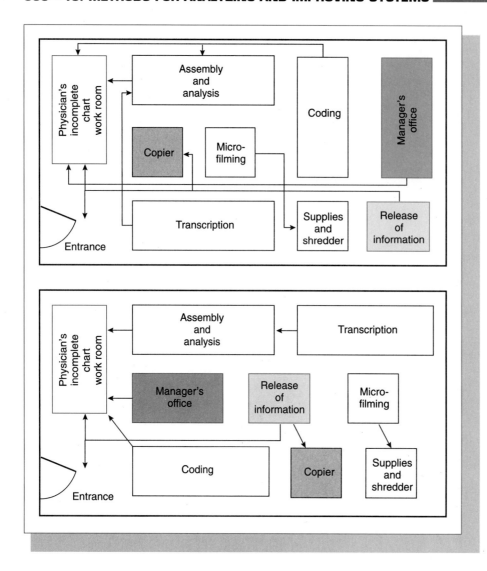

FIGURE 16–9. Movement diagram or layout flowchart. *Top,* Shows an inefficiently arranged section of an HIM department. The release-of-information employees are not located near the photocopier, and the manager and coding staff are far removed from physician access. *Bottom,* Improved physical layout, making movement and work flow more efficient.

chronologic sequence of the work under study. Another is by problems or source of problems, such as the department or function in which they originate.

Formulating Alternative Solutions and Improvements

Using the fundamental belief of methods improvement that there is always a better way as well as the information gathered, questioned, organized, and analyzed from the prior steps, several alternatives should come to mind. Employees who are close to the situation might not see the value of making changes, but their input must be acquired. Journal articles and conferences with colleagues within and outside the organization may stimulate some new and different thinking.

Selecting the Improved Method

To identify the best alternative for rectifying the problem, several decision-making tools are available.

DECISION GRID OR MATRIX. The **decision grid** or **matrix** (Figure 16–10) is the most basic of the decision support tools. The alternatives are compared with one another by various criteria. The alternatives are listed down the left side. The elements or criteria are listed across the top. Examples of frequently considered criteria in selecting alternatives are cost, feasibility, desirability, acceptance, effect on productivity, and effect on quality.

This grid may be used to arrive at a decision concerning any type of problem once the alternatives are defined and the criteria selected. Another option is to

Alternative	Cost	Feasibility	Desirability & Acceptance	Decision
1 Hire new coding supervisor	$28,000 position	Requires recruitment; few qualified applicants; usually new grad	Coding staff will resist new graduate	3rd priority
2 Promote lead coder to coding supervisor	$8,000 raise ($28,000) $20,000 savings	Places heavy burden on work load	Coding staff may resist	2nd priority
3 Promote operations supervisor to Assist. Director supervising both operations and coding	$12,000 raise ($28,000) $16,000 savings	Excellent; supervisor has previous coding experience	Poses minor acceptance problem with coders; very desirable to operations supervisor	1st priority

FIGURE 16–10. Decision matrix or grid showing the elements considered by the director of the HIM department in the hiring decision for a coding supervisor.

weigh the criteria. The element of cost may be weighted three times any other element. This would mean that cost is the first priority in this decision-making process. The grid's primary advantage is that all relevant information can be displayed and viewed at the same time. This is useful when a committee or group is attempting to arrive at consensus.

DECISION TABLE. A **decision table** is an analytical tool that provides a means of communication of the logical sequence of a particular operation. This type of decision support tool can be used in situations where the logic and sequential flow of data cannot be clearly shown on a flowchart. The decision table was originally designed to explain the logic found in computerizing a manual process.

A basic decision table is divided into four segments:

- **Conditions segment.** These are usually questions that form the conditions that may exist in a system. Condition statements or questions are assigned row numbers and entered in the left-hand column. A heavy line separates the condition statements or questions from the action statements.

- **Condition-entry segment.** This is the set of rules that provide yes or no answers to the questions in the conditions segment. The rules should be numbered. The rule numbers are then assigned horizontally across the top of the form. The condition entries are entered opposite the applicable condition questions.

- **Action segment.** This lists the action to be taken for fulfilling each condition. Action statements are assigned row numbers and are entered below the condition statements below the heavy line.

- **Action-entry segment.** This section uses an X to indicate the suitable action concluded from the answers entered in the condition-entry segment.

A decision table may be simple and characterize only a few conditions. It can, however, be complex and contain dozens of conditions and actions. Examples of the usage of decision tables in the HIM department may involve a complex process within the department or may assist in employee decisions (Figure 16–11).

DECISION TREE. Decisions are often linked to other decisions. In effect, sometimes one decision necessitates future decisions. A **decision tree** is used to chart alternative courses of action for solving a problem. It also depicts some of the probable consequences or risks resulting from each course of action. Decision trees are a valuable tool for evaluating decisions that are linked together over time with assorted potential outcomes. As an example, the transcription supervisor experiences an unanticipated heavy load of dictation. She has insufficient staff to handle the workload. The obvious alternatives to this situation include (a) hire more transcriptionists, (b) pay overtime to current transcriptionists, (c) contract work out to a transcription service, or (d) hire temporary help (Figure 16–12).

In using this decision tool, the decision centers on the objective of making the wisest expenditure of money. This decision tool is effective when probabilities can be determined for the various outcomes. In this example, it would be helpful for the transcription supervisor to determine the probability of an increased demand for transcription services or the probability of the continuation of the heavy load of dictation. After evaluation of additional services rendered and reflection of previous year figures, the supervisor may estimate that there will

Employee Raises	Rule 1	Rule 2	Rule 3	Rule 4
Employed less than 1 year	Y	N	N	N
Employed 1–3 yrs	—	Y	N	N
Employed 3–5 yrs	—	—	Y	N
Employed 5 or more years	—	—	—	Y
No Raise	X			
3% Raise		X		
5% Raise			X	
7% Raise				X

Conditions / Actions — Condition Entry / Action Entry

FIGURE 16–11. Decision table used to determine employee raises.

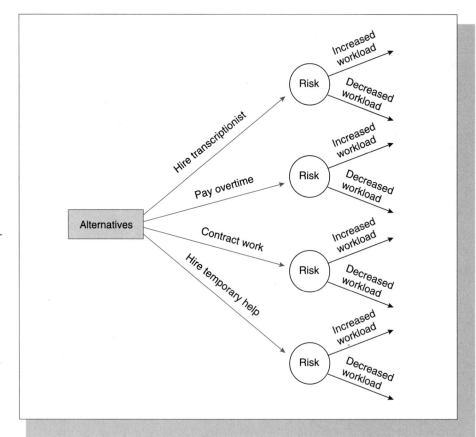

FIGURE 16–12. Decision tree.

Guidelines for Work Simplification

- Encourage employee participation in planning for work simplification. Promote employee knowledge of work simplification objectives, process, and results. In-service training may be necessary.

- The series of work activities needs to be simple and productive. Each adopted activity must be justified for its necessity. All unnecessary activities must be eliminated. Those activities that contribute directly to the goal should be maximized.

- Whenever reasonable, combine work activities. Duplication of effort is frequently found when you begin to evaluate a procedure. In various activities, certain data are copied over and over again. If feasible, these writing activities should be combined into a single method or operation.

- As much as possible, reduce the distances traveled. Sometimes the movements of people and papers are costly and may be wasteful. Closely examine such movements and attempt to reduce them to the shortest distance possible. However, when movement is essential, it is typically a more efficient process to move the paper than to move the person.

- Strive to arrange activities to provide for a smooth work flow. When more than one clerical step is included in the process or activity, a pattern of steady, constant flow of work is ordinarily desirable. The employee may feel overwhelmed by workloads that are too heavy. On the other hand, the employee may get frustrated and bored if workloads that are too light appear frequently. Hesitations and delays in the flow of work should be minimized.

be a 70 per cent probability that the workload will increase next year and a 30 per cent probability that the workload will decrease. Monetary values will have to come into play in evaluating the risks compared with the alternatives.

Implementing the Improved Method and Evaluating the Effectiveness of the Improvement

Provided that the employees have participated in the entire process, this step should be easy and simple to apply. The improved method should result in a more simplified, better, faster, more convenient, and less costly method of performing the task. The purpose of the work simplification and the reasons for its importance should be made clear to each and every employee affected by it.

To assure success with the improved process, document the new procedures and review them with all employees involved. People, by nature, tend to resist change. However, if employees realize that this change is part of their own efforts, resistance should be minimal. Sometimes it is helpful to demonstrate work simplification examples from other departments. If the

employees can see results in reducing waste and accomplishing the work effectively, they will work together with you to meet the challenge that work simplification offers (see Guidelines for Work Simplification).

SYSTEMS AND ORGANIZATIONAL LEVEL (MID LEVEL)

Systems Analysis and Design

Systems analysis and design is a methodology used to evaluate and study all types of systems. This process is usually used at an organizational level involving several departments and functions. The main benefit to using this process is that it is a defined and accepted methodology for gathering and "analyzing a great quantity of data in a logical, documented format."[2] Like work simplification, it follows the scientific method of problem solving, using tools of description, investigation, research, creativity, and judgment. The analysis portion involves examining the way things currently are done and defining the users' requirements for the system. The design segment determines the best way to meet the users' specified requirements for the system.

The systems analysis and design process can be used for various types of systems, ranging from paper and pencil systems to paperless computer-based systems. Its use with computer information systems is detailed in Chapter 18. The process can be lengthy and time-consuming and requires a dedication of staff and financial resources. It is usually used when an existing system no longer meets the organization's needs or new needs are identified.

The health information manager can be involved in this process in a variety of ways, including as a user of a system, defining its requirements with a systems analyst or even assuming the systems analyst role.

The use of the systems analysis and design methodology does not guarantee success. The choice of solutions (designs) is still a human one and fraught with possibilities of human bias and error.

Systems Model Concept

The process of systems analysis and design is based on the systems model concept. A **system** is an assemblage of things that form a connected whole; a complex but ordered whole; a plan or scheme; method. A system refers to various elements that are interrelated according to a plan for achieving a well-defined goal. In an organization, the elements are employees or human resources, equipment and supplies, and raw material. These elements are linked together by processes or procedures to achieve the organization's goals or desired outcomes (Figure 16–13).

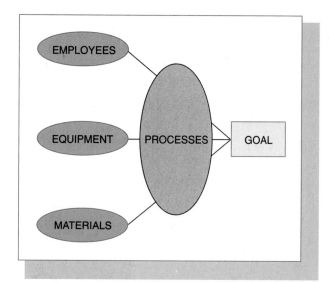

FIGURE 16–13. Diagram of a system.

HIERARCHICAL STRUCTURE. Systems model also recognizes the hierarchical structure of systems. Large systems are composed of subsystems, which in turn are composed of subsystems. For example, the human body is a system composed of subsystems of the digestive, respiratory, and cardiovascular systems. The digestive system is composed of the stomach system, the small intestine system, the large intestine system, and so on.

UNITY OF PURPOSE AND BOUNDARY CONCEPTS. Embedded in the systems model concept are the principles of unity of purpose and boundary or integrity of the system. These concepts are important for effective application of the systems analysis and design process. A system has unity of purpose when the system and its subsystems all focus on achieving a single purpose. The boundary concept refers to separating the system from other systems. It identifies what is included and what is excluded in the system being studied. The boundaries define the scope of the study as well as possible limits of the system. For example, the process under study may involve several departments, but the study may be limited to the part of the process that occurs only within one department. Determination of the system's boundaries is often an administrative or management decision.

Input–Output Cycle

Systems are composed of input, processing, output, feedback, and control.

INPUT. The flow of work through a system begins with some type of input. Examples of input include labor, energy, money, and attitudes. In a health infor-

mation system, the types of input are commonly data, information, and/or materials. Examples of materials include the mail, demographic data on the health care facility's patients, and telephone calls received by the receptionist. Incorporated into this input are employees' skills and knowledge and the equipment and supplies needed to perform the task.

PROCESSING. The processing element transforms the input into a desired output. Sometimes this phase is called the transformation process. The following are traditional processing activities:

- Classifying
- Storing
- Sorting
- Filing
- Calculating
- Retrieving data and information

Processing refers to the procedures and methods involved in the system. Procedures are established series of work steps used to accomplish a goal and commonly include the efforts of several people. Procedures handle recurring transactions consistently and uniformly. In viewing procedures microscopically, we see that they consist of a progression of methods. Procedures consist of related methods that are essential to complete various work processes. Methods apply to the tasks of an individual employee and may represent a manual, mechanical, or automated way of performing a procedure. An example of a method is to alphabetize the names of the physicians on the medical staff by their last names.

OUTPUT. The ultimate goal of a system is output. Output is a result of transforming input into a desired form. For example, the transcriptionist transforms the physician's dictation into a typed report. Other output examples are release-of-information correspondence, coded diagnoses and procedures, and productivity reports. Output is usually in paper or computer screen format and is needed as the input for another process or system.

FEEDBACK. Feedback is crucial for success of the entire system. It compares the output with expected standards of performance. In other words, feedback contrasts what was produced to what should have been produced. An example of feedback would be the physician's evaluation of the typed report or the quality improvement plan. If the feedback shows that the quality standards were not met, a modification is sent back to the input phase for improvement of the system.

Feedback can also occur concurrently with the input-processing-output cycle. The input and processing are evaluated and improved before the preparation of the output.

CONTROLS AND CONSTRAINTS. Systems do not operate in a vacuum and are controlled and constrained by internal and external factors. These factors dictate what can and cannot be done in every phase of the system. An internal dimension of controlling encompasses the organizational policies, procedures, and standards that impact the system. An example of an internal control for a health information process is the policies and procedures that govern the release of health information. This policy stipulates the type of information that may or may not be released without the patient's written authorization. Additional internal controls may be those required for profit as a profit margin or for quality of service and those required by the customer.

The external controls include the local, state, and federal rules and regulations as well as social, economical, and ethical values. External controls that affect the HIM department are the federal regulations on the confidentiality of drug and alcohol patient records, the information management standards of the Joint Commission on Accreditation of Healthcare Organizations, and the diagnostic related group (DRG) weights published in the *Federal Register*.

Goals of Systems Analysis and Design Process

The goal of the systems analysis and design process is to produce a well-designed system that can be described as follows:

- Effective. The system accomplishes its purpose and achieves its established goals.
- Efficient. The system accomplishes its purpose while remaining cost-effective.
- Dependable. The system meets established time frames.
- Flexible. The system can accommodate unusual circumstances.
- Adaptable. The system can absorb changes, if necessary.
- Systematic and logical.
- Functional. The system serves its intended purpose.
- Simple.
- Resourceful. The system is useful within the organization.
- Accepted. The system is accepted by those who work with it.

Components of Systems Analysis and Design

The major components of systems design are as follows:

- Determination of the need and objectives of the system
- Systems analysis
- Design of the system
- Evaluation of the proposed system
- Implementation of system

DETERMINING THE NEED FOR THE SYSTEM. Before beginning the analysis process, the users must determine the need for the system. The needs are often determined by management and are in the form of objectives. They should provide answers to the following questions:

- What information is needed?
- Who needs the information?
- When do they need it?
- In what format do they need it?

SYSTEMS ANALYSIS. The analysis of the system has three components: Accumulation of facts, organization of facts, and evaluation of facts.

Accumulating the Facts. The gathering of data is possible by envisioning the course that a piece of paper follows in a process and then tracking each step in that particular process. The tracking can begin at any point and work backward or forward from there. Sources that may be used in the accumulation or gathering of facts include the following:

- Organization charts
- Procedure manuals
- Job descriptions
- Flowcharts
- Financial data

Investigation methods include group discussions and interviews with managers and operations employees as well as questionnaires to all affected personnel and users of the system. Before the investigation is begun, the existing manuals and charts should be reviewed. The interview should focus on obtaining facts pertinent to the system analysis. At this point in the process, solutions should not be suggested. Strategic questions should be devised to verify facts from previous sources.

Organizing the Facts. The facts obtained in the previous step must be organized or classified in some way. Conventional methods to organize facts are by the following categories:

- Interrelated objectives
- Organizational structure
- Input and output
- Processing modes
- Major complaints or problems disclosed

Organizing facts by organizational structure can be advantageous because it shows who has authority to decide and the flow of data among organizational units. Organizing facts by major complaints or problems is also beneficial because only valid problems and significant complaints should be included. The organization of facts is helpful to proceed with their evaluation. The means of organization should also show meaningful relationships.

Evaluating the Facts. As much as possible, the facts should be ranked, rated, measured, weighed, and evaluated. The assignment of quantitative values to facts should be accomplished in as many areas as possible. In reality, some evaluation may be subjective and based on opinion. Information tends to include some nonquantifiable components. Again, try to adhere to the facts, not to feelings or beliefs. At this point in the process, possible solutions to the problems may be examined.

Designing the System

After the facts have been gathered, organized, evaluated, and analyzed, a design of a new system or a proposed revision to an existing system is explored. People must be committed to this process. The design of a system should be a team effort that includes management, operations personnel, and users of the system. Many times, numerous systems could fit the requirements. However, they can differ in many aspects, especially cost.

The following factors should be considered when designing the new system:

- Effects on employees (retraining, layoffs, transfers, schedules)
- Profits and costs (salaries, space, materials and supplies)
- Customer service

System design should not be performed in a rush. Various possibilities must be considered with their strengths and weaknesses. The term "trade-off" is routinely used in this part of the process. In other words, sometimes one need must be sacrificed for another.

Evaluating the Proposed System

In this step of systems design, the proposed system should be evaluated to determine whether it is satisfac-

tory. A review of the overall arrangement and a specific check of the design's critical areas are crucial. The proposed system must meet the needs of the employees and managers as well as the organizational needs.

Implementing the System

The last step in systems design is the implementation phase. This phase may be time-consuming. To implement a new system smoothly, it is imperative that the employees have a stake in the new system. Again, the employees and management should have been actively involved in the entire system design process. The new system may be implemented on a trial basis by a few employees. Employee acceptance should be taken into consideration. Some retraining may need to take place at this time. Modifications to the new system may occur during this trial period. If the new system involves a large operation, parallel operations may be conducted. This procedure allows the old system to continue to function while the new system "bugs" have been worked through and removed or modified. After the trial period, the old system can be phased out.

Effective Organizations

To be effective and efficient, processes and systems must occur within an effective organization. Organizational structures include both formal and informal.

Formal Organizational Infrastructure

The formal organizational infrastructure is designed to plan work, assign responsibility, supervise work, and measure results. The formal relationships between various people and the organizational structure are identified on an **organization chart.** This chart clearly identifies hierarchical relationships, the lines of authority, responsibilities, and span of control. In an organization chart, the primary functions of the organization and the subfunctions within each primary function are identified. It should also aid in the identification of any areas of overlap in responsibility. The major disadvantage of the formal organization chart is its inability to show the informal interaction between employees as they carry out their everyday activities.

Informal Organization

The **informal** or **unwritten organization** refers to the many interpersonal relationships that occur in an organization and do not appear on the formal organization chart. A typical informal organization is composed of two or more persons who develop mutually satisfying interactions pertaining to personal and/or job-related matters. An informal organization develops over time.

POSITIVE ASPECTS OF INFORMAL ORGANIZATION. The most positive aspect of an informal organization is its blend with the formal organization to produce an operable system for the accomplishment of the work. If management can motivate the informal leaders to accept a new procedure, these leaders may be able to convince others to accept it. The informal organization provides the necessary social values and stability to work groups.

A well-known benefit of informal organization is that it provides an additional channel of communication. It is capable of efficiently sending and receiving communications. This informal channel is called the "grapevine." The grapevine can be described as the informal oral communication network that aids employees in learning more about what is happening in the organization and how it might affect them. Many times it is more effective than the formal line of communication in distributing information, obtaining feedback, solving problems, and revising procedures.

In addition, informal group discussions should be linked to the team concept used in total quality management, which is discussed at length in Chapter 13.

NEGATIVE ASPECTS OF INFORMAL ORGANIZATION. Information organizations can also be a hindrance to management. In some organizations, the disadvantages far outweigh the benefits. A common example of abuse of the informal organization is where the employees find opportunities to work together even when no such work assignments have been made.

When an informal group loses confidence in a manager, they may combine forces to make life miserable for the manager. On occasion, informal groups may develop cross purposes with the goals and objectives of the formal organization.

Potentially negative impacts or conflicts resulting from informal organization must be weighed against its constructive and practical function in nurturing creativity and innovation. A relatively conflict-free organization tends to be rigid, static, and inflexible.

ACCEPTANCE AND BALANCE. Managers must accept three additional facts about the formal and informal organizations.

1. Informal organization is inevitable. Management creates the formal organization and can alter it as it so desires. The informal organization is not created by management. As long as organizations are composed of people, informal organizations will exist.

2. Small groups are the central component of the informal organization. Group membership in the informal organization strongly influences the overall behavior and performance of its members. Many sociologists agree that the group, not the individual, is the basic component of the human organization.[3]

3. Informal organization will always coexist within the formal structure. This is a fact of organizational life. The formal and informal organizations must be balanced to achieve optimum performance and attain organizational objectives. Management trying to suppress the informal organization creates a destructive situation that results in reduced effectiveness. On the other hand, if the formal organization is too weak to accomplish its objectives, the informal organization can grow in strength, resulting in abuse of power, insubordination, and disloyalty.

The ideal situation is where the formal organization is strong enough to achieve its objectives and at the same time permit a well-developed informal organization to maintain group cohesiveness and teamwork. The informal relationships that exist in an organization deserve the attention from employees and managers concerned with the organization's effectiveness.

ORGANIZATIONWIDE LEVEL

Project Management

Project management as defined by some experts is management plus planning.[4] It uses the basic management principles of planning, organizing, directing, and controlling (with an emphasis on planning) to bring a project to a successful conclusion. Because projects are unique and demand that people do things differently from before, the team is following an unknown path and must plan ahead.

Project management techniques are used by many and varied professions—engineers, construction contractors, and military and government agencies. Today's health care managers also find project management techniques helpful in confronting the conflicting responsibilities of completing ongoing and routine work while exploring and implementing new health care delivery models and technologies with less resources, greater time constraints, and continuous communication links across organizational units.

Characteristics of a Project

To understand the concepts of project management, the characteristics of a project must be defined.

Unique. This process has never been done before. It is a one-time event or one-of-a-kind activity. It will never be repeated in precisely the same way again. There is no practice or rehearsal. Experience can be gained from previous projects. However, this particular combination of time, place, people, and project is unique.

Product or result. The outcome of the project is a single, definable product, such as build that bridge, launch that rocket, or construct that hospital. Projects are goal-oriented and work through the process to achieve that goal. The product is different for each project.

Finite. The project is usually on a fixed time scale with a start and finish date. It can be viewed as a temporary activity. The project is undertaken to accomplish a goal within a set period of time. Once the goal is achieved, the project ceases to exist.

Complex, numerous, and sequenced activities. Projects involve a variety of complex and sequenced activities used to achieve the goal or objective.

Team. Projects are completed by a team of people from diverse professions and organizational units. Projects may be task interdependent and use advanced technology. However, projects are human endeavors and cannot be performed by technology alone.

Cross-functional. Many times projects cross several functional areas in an organization, involving multiple skills and talents from many people. The actual work may be performed by many functional areas. Because of this, the project does not neatly fit into the organizational structure.

Limited resources. Projects usually have a set limit of resources and budget. The end result is specified in terms of cost, schedule, and performance requirements.

Change. Projects have the characteristic of being somewhat unfamiliar. Projects may comprise innovative technology and possess pivotal elements of uncertainty and risk. However, the essence of project management is to create change. When the project is completed, the world (i.e., organization, department) is a little different.

Characteristics of Project Management

The following are some characteristics of project management.[5]

- A single person, the project manager, administers the project and operates independent of the normal organization chart or the chain of command. The project manager has the authority to plan, direct, organize, and control the entire project from start to finish.

- Decision making, accountability, results, and rewards are shared among the members of the project team.

- Although the project activities are temporary, the functional areas performing the work are usually a permanent part of the organization. After the completion of the project, the individual workers are returned to their original assignments or reassigned to a new project.

- The project focuses on delivering an end product or end result at a certain time, with certain resource allotments, and to the satisfaction of performance or technical requirements.

- Project management can set into motion other support functions, including personnel evaluation, accounting, and information systems.

Project Planning

Planning is essentially thinking ahead. In project management, planning involves two phases: defining the project and planning the project.

DEFINING THE PROJECT. Defining the project is often called project overview. Four areas are detailed in the definition phase.

1. The *problem statement* answers the following questions:

What is the problem?
What is the opportunity?
What is to be done?
Who is responsible for the project?
When must it be completed?

2. The *goal statement* is the final outcome of the project. It serves as a point of focus and reference that keeps all activities on track. A goal statement tells precisely what the outcome will be and when it will be done. It needs to be action-oriented, short, simple, and straightforward. An example of a project goal is to implement a computer-based patient record by the year 2000.

3. *Objectives.* To achieve the stated goal, several steps have to take place. These steps represent milestones in the project and are considered objectives. They define major components that must be accomplished to achieve the overall goal. Objectives are more precise and measurable than the goal statement. A project objective for the goal of implementation of a computer-based patient record is the on-line connection between the hospital computer system and the medical staff offices within 6 months.

4. *Resources.* Resources include people (human resources), materials, space, and money that are needed to achieve the goal.

PLAN. A project is initiated with the preparation of a written plan. The purpose of the plan is to direct and guide the project manager and the project team members through the project. Basically, planning is thinking ahead, communicating the plan, and using the plan as a yardstick to measure the progress toward achievement of the goal. The five areas detailed in the planning phase are as follows:

1. *Project activities.* Every objective of the project should encompass separate activities. These activities define the work to be accomplished to attain the objective. **Work breakdown structures** is a method often used in projects. It divides the project into major objectives, partitions each objective into activities, further divides the activities into subactivities, and creates work packages that must be done to complete the project.

2. *Time and cost.* The amount of time and cost for completion of each activity are estimated. Variations in time may be due to the skill level of the people performing the activity, material availability, technology or machine variations, and unexpected events, such as illness and employee turnover. Estimates in time may contain the most optimistic completion time, the most pessimistic completion time, and the most likely completion time. Cost estimates are typically categorized into labor, materials, other direct (i.e., telephone, postage) costs, and indirect costs or overhead.

3. *Activity sequence.* Once the activities have been identified along with their time and cost estimates, they need to be sequenced. Some activities are dependent on another; that is, one activity cannot be started until another is completed. They must be done sequentially. Other activities may be done simultaneously.

4. *Critical activities.* Management tools such as the **Gantt chart** and **PERT network** can be used to determine the sequence and the amount of time needed to complete the project. The sequence of activities that makes up the longest path to complete the project is called the **critical path.** When activities are completed on schedule, the whole project will be completed on time. However, sometimes activities take longer than anticipated or materials cannot be obtained, and then the project completion time is extended.

5. *Project proposal.* The purpose of a project proposal is to provide a complete description of the project activities, time lines, and resource requirements. It is a statement of the general approach being taken and the results expected. It is a decision-making tool, a key to management control, a training aid for new project team members, and a reporting document. The project proposal portrays the transition from project management planning to project management implementation.

PROJECT IMPLEMENTATION. Once the project has been approved, the work begins. The implementation process contains three phases: organize, control, and termination.

Organize. Organizing includes the assembly of the required resources (materials, manpower, and money) to accomplish the work defined in the plan. Organizing also includes the development of the structure needed to administer the plan. The following three areas are detailed in the organization phase.

1. *Project manager.* The most important element of project management is the project manager. This person has the responsibility to integrate work efforts and plays a major role in planning and executing a project. The project manager is accountable for the project and dedicated to achieving its goals. The criteria for selection of a project manager vary according to organizations. The usual characteristics include the following:

- Background and experience
- Leadership
- Strategic expertise
- Technical expertise
- Interpersonal skills
- Managerial capability

Selecting the most qualified project manager can be the key to the project's success or failure.

2. *Project team.* Project management entails bringing individuals and groups together to form a single, cohesive team working toward a common goal. Project work is teamwork accomplished by a group of people. Once the project manager is selected, he or she can assist in the selection of the project team members.

The size and composition of the project team depends on the resources allocated to the project. The following characteristics are desirable in a member of a project team:

- Commitment to the project goal
- Communication skills
- Flexibility
- Technical competence
- Task orientation
- Ability to be a team player
- Experience with project management tools
- Dependability, history of meeting deadlines

3. *Work activities.* Now that the planning and organizing have been done, work on the project gets started. The project manager assigns responsibilities for completing activities to members of the project team. As discussed previously, activities can be subdivided into subactivities and work packages. A work package as one continuous activity is assigned to a project team member

who has the authority, expertise, and access to the appropriate resources necessary to complete the assignment.

A work package has beginning and ending tasks with a definitive description of each task. The project manager schedules the start dates of each work package. Because many activities are interrelated, work packages must be clearly documented so that their completion can be tracked.

Control. Controlling is the monitoring and maintenance of the structure of the project. Part of control is the reporting at specified points throughout the project. The reports should indicate potential problems. The following two areas are detailed in the control phase:

1. *Effective project leadership.* The project manager and the project team must work together to reach the project goal. Group cohesiveness, open communication, team development, and empowerment of members are top priorities for the project manager. The following are some guidelines for effective project leadership:

- Do not overdirect.
- Recognize individual differences.
- Allow individual team members the freedom to guide their own work.
- Become a resource person instead of a controller.
- Become a facilitator instead of a boss.
- Become a buffer between team members and outside problems.
- Insist on feedback.
- Do not over-observe.
- Appreciate each project team member for his or her unique characteristics and contributions.
- Develop conflict resolution strategies.
- Improve communication techniques.
- Maintain group cohesion.
- Facilitate effective meetings.

2. *Control tools.* Controls focus on performance levels, cost, and time schedules. Controls also track progress, detect variance from the plan, and allow the project manager to take corrective action.

The project manager reports the status of every activity in the project at least monthly. This report summarizes the progress for that month and for the length of the entire project. The project manager should also report the variances from the plan. These variances may be related to budget, labor, time, or materials. Positive variance examples are being ahead of schedule or under budget. Negative variances may include an extended time schedule or a greater budgetary item than anticipated. Negative cost variances may not be under the project manager's control, such as unexpected equipment failure or increased cost of supplies.

When each milestone of the project is completed, the project manager should review the project. Despite all the extensive planning, things will not automatically happen according to the plan. To get back on schedule, the project manager may have to reallocate resources, consider alternatives, and re-evaluate activities. This is where good project managers prove their worth by getting the project back on schedule.

Termination. There are three types of project termination.

1. *Termination by extinction.* The project work as scheduled is either successfully or unsuccessfully done and the decision to terminate is agreed upon.

2. *Termination by inclusion.* The successful project is institutionalized or transformed into the organization as a unit.

3. *Termination by integration.* A common way of closing successful projects occurs when equipment, material, and personnel are distributed back into the organization.

TERMINATION PROCESS. The four phases in the termination process are as follows.

1. *Approval.* Obtain the client's or administration's approval of the project. The termination or close down of the project depends on their satisfaction and the quality of service the project provided.

2. *Logistics.* Assign a termination manager and team to assist in the termination phase, conduct a termination meeting, prepare personnel reports, and terminate work orders and contracts.

3. *Document.* Document the entire project. Document the completion and performance of all team members as well as the performance of vendors, consultants, and contractors.

4. *Final report and audit.* The final project report is a history of the project. Items included in the final project report are the overall success and performance of the project, techniques used, strengths and weaknesses, organization, and recommendations from the project manager and project team. An audit of the project should be conducted after implementation. The essential questions that need to be asked in evaluating the success of the project are the following:

- Was the goal achieved?
- Was the work done on time? Within budget? Within specifications?
- Was the client or administration satisfied with the results?

PROJECT TOOLS. Project tools may be used in the planning or controlling phase of project management. The two most common tools are the PERT network and the Gantt chart.

PERT Network. PERT is the acronym for program evaluation review technique. It is a scheduling device that was originally developed early in the space age as a tool for missile development programs. It is a system of diagramming the steps or component parts of a complex project. The various components and the estimated completion time for each component must be identified. Lines illustrate the sequential flow of activities as well as the components that are dependent on one another and must be performed sequentially and those that are not dependent and can be performed concurrently. The estimated completion time is shown for each activity.

Included in the preparation of a PERT network is the determination of a critical path. The critical path is the longest route and estimated completion time in the PERT network for a given project. This route would consist of the components or activities that must be completed, the order in which they must be completed, and the time frame in which they must be completed for the project to be accomplished (Figure 16–14).

EXAMPLE

The transcription supervisor of an HIM department in XYZ Hospital is responsible for supervising the installation of a new dictation system. The supervisor reports to the director of HIM the length of time needed to complete the project. The following must be accomplished to complete the project.

START: Administration approved the purchase of a new dictation system.

Step A: Hospital electricians need to rewire the transcription area to accommodate the new dictation system. They estimate that this will take 10 days.

Step B: The equipment vendor installs the equipment into the prewired area. This step will take 3 days.

Step C: The transcriptionists are trained on the new dictation system once it is installed at the hospital. The training will take 2 days.

Step D: The equipment vendor orders the system from Atlanta. They estimate that the equipment will take 15 days to arrive.

Step E: The transcription supervisor is taken to the equipment vendor's office to be trained on the new equipment for a 1-day session. One day of travel time will need to be allowed.

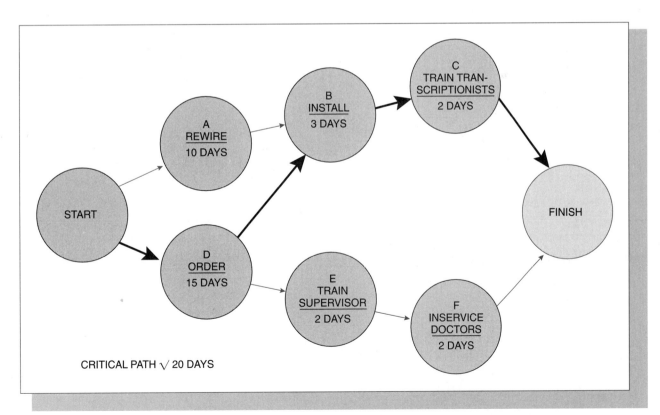

CRITICAL PATH √ 20 DAYS

FIGURE 16–14. PERT network. The black arrows indicate the critical path and determine the amount of time needed to complete the project (20 days).

Step F: The vendor presents the system to the hospital physicians. This includes a slide presentation and a mock dictation station. The presentation will be given at various times over a 2-day period.
FINISH: The new dictation system is ready to go.

As shown in Figure 16–14, some activities may occur at the same time. Other activities must wait for an activity to be completed before they can begin.

Gantt Chart. Named after the famous management consultant, Henry Gantt, a Gantt chart is a common project scheduling tool. Gantt charts are appropriate for complex projects with multiple steps. The chart consists of a horizontal scale divided into time units (days, weeks, months) and a vertical scale depicting project work elements (tasks, activities, work packages). The length of the horizontal bar corresponds with the expected length of time to complete the activity. As time progresses, the bar is filled in with symbols that relate to projected completion, actual progress, and actual completion (Figure 16–15).

The Gantt chart can also be used for manpower planning, resource allocation, and budgeting and is often used to track the progress of computer-based projects. It provides an excellent view of project status. It is a useful tool for monitoring progress. As with the PERT network, the Gantt chart plays an important role in the planning and controlling of projects.

Re-engineering

Re-engineering (also known as business process re-engineering) has been used in the business world and is now finding its way into health care. Business process re-engineering, endorsed by *Harvard Business Review*, is a

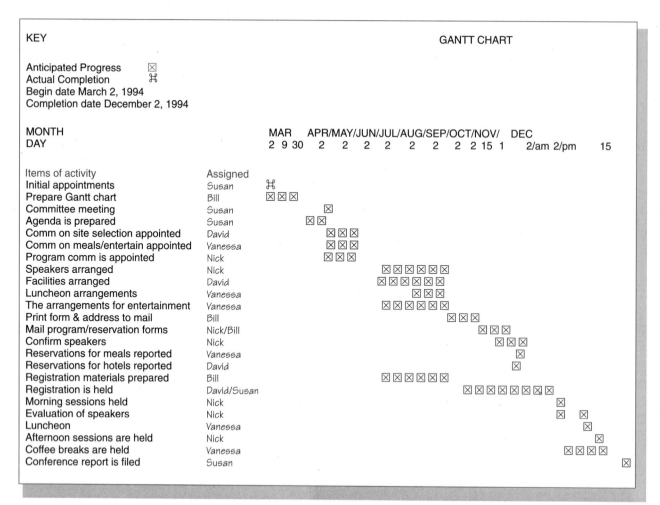

FIGURE 16–15. Gantt chart showing scheduling of a professional conference.

theory in which the way business is done is radically re-evaluated to achieve dramatic performance improvement. It encourages streamlining functions to reduce time, cost, and effort while enhancing the quality of service. In health care, this means meeting the challenges of becoming efficient and productive while providing quality care. This concept is new and different in health care possibly because the terms "radical" and "health care" usually do not go hand in hand.

Re-engineering means challenging every aspect of the way of doing business to substantially improve performance. Re-engineering the process means "starting with a blank sheet of paper," starting all over, starting from scratch, and challenging the status quo with the goal of vast improvements.[6] It explores new ways of doing the work as well as questions why processes are done at all. Each process performed should contribute to achieving the organization's goals. The processes that do contribute are called value-added activities.

Once a process is determined to be necessary, each step of the process is questioned. Does the step add value? Can it be simplified? Would resequencing the steps smooth the work flow? When practical, can the steps be automated?

Objectives

The main objectives of re-engineering are as follows:

- Reduce cost.
- Increase revenue.
- Improve quality.
- Reduce risk.

Re-engineering is a complete rethinking and transformation of key processes. Using the re-engineering approach, a key hospital process of admitting an inpatient could be transformed or virtually eliminated perhaps by using an interactive computer process from the patient's home.

Re-engineering emphasizes streamlining of cross-functional processes to achieve organizational objectives. Patient-focused care is an example of a cross-functional process in a health care environment. The nursing units are transformed into self-contained mini hospitals in which the delivery of care is closer to the patient. The unit might contain a mini laboratory, a mini radiology department, and a mini pharmacy. A health care team is selected by the patient's diagnosis, procedure, or severity of illness. That health care team delivers all the care to the patient. The actual number of health care workers the patient has contact with is less than in the traditional health care delivery models. Business process re-engineering entails the assimilation of several interrelated changes, including policies and procedures, organization and staff, facilities, and technology.

Relationship to Quality Improvement

Because re-engineering advocates radical change that might be too risky for health care organizations, the more cautious and acceptable approach of quality improvement is often used in conjunction with re-engineering. Sometimes total quality management is used in conjunction with re-engineering to restructure a process to create the most efficient operation model for delivering an outcome. Total quality management starts with minor successes and builds.

Applications to Health Information Management

Health information management professionals need to become involved in the organizationwide re-engineering process. They need to look at processes and procedures in a whole new light. Looking forward to the computer-based patient record, HIM professionals need to view how it will radically change the delivery of patient care and management of information. To gain its full potential, HIM professionals have to be willing to let go of old ways and change things dramatically.[7] The same forms as used in paper records cannot simply be computerized and expected to meet the information needs of the future. Given the HIM role in the health care field and the dramatic changes in health care delivery systems, HIM professionals need an understanding of and commitment to the re-engineering process.[8]

Key Concepts

- Work division can be accomplished by function, project, product, territory, customer, or process. The three methods of dividing work are serial, parallel, and unit assembly.

- The work distribution chart can be used to answer the following questions:
  —What tasks are employees performing? Are these tasks important to achieving organizational goals?
  —How are tasks distributed among employees of the work group?
  —How are employees' qualifications being utilized?
  —How are individual jobs constructed?

- Productivity standards are used to accomplish the following:
  —Determine the number of personnel, pieces of equipment, and amount of supplies needed to handle the projected workload.

—Schedule completion and distribution of tasks.

—Evaluate proposed changes in processes or systems to see if a savings in personnel time would occur.

—Set goals for a work group or individual employee.

—Determine actual cost of producing a given product or service.

- The fundamental objectives of work simplification are to simplify, to eliminate, to combine, and/or to improve the work processes. The simplest means of performing work is usually the easiest and most practical. The philosophy behind work simplification is that there is always a better way to perform each and every task.

- The steps in the work simplification process are as follows:

  —Identify a problem area or select a work process or function to improve.

  —Gather data about a problem.

  —Organize and analyze the data gathered on the problem.

  —Formulate alternative solutions or improvements.

  —Select the improved method.

  —Implement the improved method and evaluate the effectiveness of the improvement.

- Systems are hierarchically structured in that a system is composed of subsystems. Subsystems can be further broken down.

- Identifying the boundaries of the system—what is included and what is excluded—identifies the scope of the study.

- Systems design consists of five major components:
  1. Determination of the need for and objectives of the system
  2. Systems analysis
  3. Design of the system
  4. Evaluation of the proposed system
  5. Implementation of the proposed system

- In systems analysis, the sequence of steps is the accumulation of facts, the organization of facts, and the evaluation of facts.

- The formal organizational infrastructure is designed to plan work, assign responsibility, supervise work, and measure results.

- Facts about the informal organization are as follows:

  —Informal organizations are inevitable as long as there are people in the organization.

  —Small groups are the central component of the informal organization. Group membership in the informal organization strongly influences the overall behavior and performance of its members.

- —The informal organization will always coexist within the formal structure.

  —Informal relationships deserve attention from employees and managers concerned with the organization's effectiveness.

- Project management focuses on completion of a project with the following attributes:

  —Unique; never having been done in precisely the same way before

  —Focused on producing a single definable product

  —Has defined deadlines

  —Involves a variety of complex and sequenced activities

  —Completed by a team of people with diverse qualifications and skills

  —Does not fit neatly into the formal organizational structure

  —Has a set amount of financial resources

  —Creates change

- The major objectives of re-engineering are to reduce cost, increase revenue, improve quality, and reduce risk.

References

1. Management for productivity. Presented by John Sheridan Associates, Inc., Southeastern Medical Record Conference, Miami, May 13, 1981.
2. Waters K, Murphy GF: Systems analysis and computer applications. *In* Health Information Management and Systems Analysis. Rockville, MD: Aspen Systems Corp, 1983, p 118.
3. Longest B Jr: Management Practices for the Health Professional, 3rd ed. Reston, VA: Reston Publishing Co, 1984, p 122.
4. Reiss G: Project Management Demystified. London: E & FN SPON, 1992, p 16.
5. Cleland D, Kin W: Systems Analysis and Project Management. New York: McGraw-Hill, 1983, pp 191–192.
6. Hammer M, Champy J: Re-engineering the Corporation: A Manifest for Business Revolution. New York: Harper Business, 1993.
7. Brandt M: Re-engineering—starting with a clean slate. J Am Health Information Management Assoc, May 1994, p 62.
8. Fox L: Organizational change: Re-engineering the work flow. J Am Health Information Management Assoc, April 1994, p 35.

Bibliography

Brodnik M (ed). Reengineering in health information management. Top Health Information Management 1994; 14 (3).

Kallaus N, Keeling BL. Administrative Office Management. 10th ed. Cincinnati: South-Western Publishing Co, 1991.

Kish J Jr. Office Management Problem Solver. Radnor, PA: Chilton Book Co, 1983.

Littlefield CL, Rachel F, Caruth D. Office and Administrative Management. 3rd ed. Englewood Cliffs, NJ: Prentice-Hall, 1970.

Minor R, Fetridge C (eds). Office Administration Handbook. 6th ed. Chicago: Dartnell Corp, 1984.

Nicholas JM. Managing Business and Engineering Projects. Englewood Cliffs, NJ: Prentice-Hall, 1990.

Quible Z. Administrative Office Management: An Introduction. 5th ed. Englewood Cliffs, NJ: Prentice-Hall, 1992.

Stallard J, Terry G. Office Systems Management. 9th ed. Homewood, IL: Richard D. Irwin, Inc., 1984.

Weiss J, Wysocki R. 5-Phase Project Management. Reading, MA: Addison-Wesley Publishing Co, 1992.

Wulf P. Performance Improvement: A Case Study. Presented by Patrick Wulf from Ernst & Young, FHIMA mid-year symposium, Orlando, FL, February 4, 1994.

SECTION
V

INFORMATION SYSTEMS

17

GRETCHEN F. MURPHY

KEY WORDS

Application software
Architecture
Audit trail
Bedside workstation
Biomedical device
Clinical data repository
Clinical information system
Community health information network
Computer-based patient record
Confidentiality
Cooperative processing
Data
Data dictionary
Data security
Database
Database management system
Decision support system
Document imaging
Electronic mail
Encoders
Executive information system

Expert system
File server
Hardware
Health care data networks
Health care information
Information warehouse
Intelligence factor
Internet
Knowledge base
Local area network
Mainframe
Medical decision support systems
Medical informatics
Medical information system
Microcomputer
Minicomputer
Multimedia processing
Niche vendor
Open systems
Operating system
Order communications
Order entry
Pen-based device

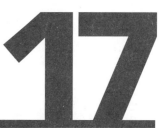

Picture archiving and communication system
Point of care system
Privacy
Re-engineering
Results reporting
Software
Sponsors
Standard query language

Telemedicine
Terminal
Text processing
Turnaround document
Voice recognition
Users
Wide area network
Workstation

TMR—The Medical Record
WAN—Wide area network

ABBREVIATIONS

AAMRS—Automated Ambulatory Medical Record System
ALGOL—Algorithmic Language
ANSI—American National Standards Institute
ASTM—American Society for Testing and Materials
BASIC—Beginners All-purpose Symbolic Instruction Code
CHINS—Community health information network system
COBOL—Common Business-Oriented Language
COSTAR—Computer Stored Ambulatory Record System
CPHA—Commission on Professional Hospital Activities
CPR—Computer-based patient record
CPRI—Computer-based Patient Record Institute
DBMS—Database management system
DRG—Diagnostic related group
DSS—Decision support system
EIS—Executive information system
GUI—Graphical user interface
HIS—Hospital information system
HISPP—Health Care Informatics Standards Planning Panel
HL-7—Health level 7
IEC—International Electrotechnical Commission
IEEE—Institute of Electrical and Electronic Engineers
IOM—Institute of Medicine
ISO—International Standards Organization
LAN—Local area network
LISP—List processing
MS/DOS—(Microsoft) Disk Operating System
MUMPS—Massachusetts General Hospital Utility Multiprogramming System
PACS—Picture archiving and communication system
PC—Personal computer
PC/DOS—(IBM) Disk Operating System
PL/1—Programming Language One
RMRS—Regenstrief Medical Records System

OBJECTIVES

- Define key words.
- Define and describe the overall scope of health information systems in the health care industry.
- Describe the current drivers that impact health information systems developments.
- Explain the fundamental purposes of health information systems.
- Illustrate emerging reliance of health care providers as primary users of health information systems data.
- Differentiate between individual and aggregate uses of health information systems data.
- Review the historical development of health information systems as forerunner to computer-based patient record (CPR) systems.
- Explain how hospital systems fit in health information systems development and related computer-based patient record efforts.
- Describe landmark efforts in computer-based patient record developments.
- Explain functional requirements and expectations for computer-based patient records.
- Discuss data and information concepts for health information systems and computer-based patient records.
- Build a case for computer-based patient records as central components in integrated and networked systems.
- Redefine and forecast a growing role of computer-based patient records in health care and review the progress in their development.
- Review basic information technology concepts and terms.
- Describe technical building blocks and illustrate information system components.
- Characterize health information systems applications for administrative and clinical needs.
- Outline and discuss key issues involved in developing health information systems for now and the future.
- Develop an understanding of transition management in planning and implementing new technology.
- Identify resources and strategies needed by health information management professionals to lead and participate in CPR projects.

HEALTH INFORMATION SYSTEMS' ROLE, PURPOSE AND USE

The ideal scenario of a patient experience is one in which, as the patient arrives at the physician's office, hospital, or another health care setting, he or she is quickly identified as someone who has been seen before. The patient's previous laboratory tests and imaging results are viewed at a computer workstation. These test results, combined with other historical and care data already collected into the computer system, are reviewed in minutes. If necessary, data are transferred through a network to a specialist for immediate feedback. The referring physician and the specialist view the information simultaneously while conferring by phone. New treatment is documented and automatically added to a central repository, from which the patient as well as other care providers can retrieve information in the future. Special reminders and flags that alert the physicians about special conditions that need to be investigated, such as drug/drug contraindications and new reports on patient allergies, are automatically presented when the patient's care information is retrieved. Even reminders for annual immunizations and screening procedures are generated with automatic notification to the patient. As well, claims for services are automatically processed through computerized systems and forwarded electronically for billing and reimbursement. Scenarios such as this are becoming more accepted, addressing patient and provider expectations regarding health information systems (HISs).

In the midst of the 1990s, the health care industry has committed to very focused goals. We need more information in health care than ever before. We need to achieve better health care quality outcomes and cost efficiencies in providing health services. We need to extend access to larger patient populations and health care information to more users. To meet these goals, we are applying new technology in information systems and communications to multiple business processes within the industry. Computer-based patient record systems have emerged as a unifying principle of the health care industry information structure and many health care information systems today. The overall purpose of this chapter is to demonstrate this principle through examining the current health information systems environment, the technology used within it, and key applications and challenges associated with it. Health information professionals need to develop a greater appreciation of the role and potential of the computer-based patient record (CPR) and information systems in their expertise.

The term *health information management system* serves as an alias for many specifically defined information systems. These include hospital information systems, clinical information systems, decision support systems, medical information systems, management information systems, community health information systems, and others. Lindberg, a pioneer in medical information systems, defines a medical information system as "the set of formal arrangements by which the facts concerning the health or health care of individual patients are stored and processed in computers."[1] Blum describes a clinical information system as one that is dedicated to collecting, storing, manipulating, and making available clinical information important to the delivery of patient care.[2] Clinical information systems focus on clinical information that may be limited to a single area, or a more comprehensive treatment of clinical information appropriate for a computer-based patient record. At the beginning of this decade, challenges of increasing information demands, an expanded patient record definition, more sophisticated functionality, and a set of strategic recommendations for the health care industry were clearly identified.

This chapter begins with a general discussion to paint a current overall picture of health information systems and describe some of their features; this is followed by a review of their historical evolution, demonstrating the emergence of the computer-based patient record in its current role. The history and the basic building blocks of computer technology are described. Current issues and applications are examined. Finally, the role of managing transition and change is explored. As health information professionals, our understanding of the environment is essential in planning for the future.

An Agenda for the 21st Century

In the 1993 report "Toward a National Health Information Infrastructure" the Work Group on Computerization of Patient Records published a vision statement that focused on harnessing the capabilities of computers to improve the quality and efficiency of patient care.[3]

> This work group believes that we must harness the capabilities of computers to improve the quality and efficiency of patient care. More complete and accurate patient information will become available across time and place (with appropriate safeguards for patient privacy). Caregivers and patients will have access to practice guidelines, prompts, reminders, and other decision support tools to enhance diagnosis and treatment and to evaluate the likely outcomes of alternative treatment options. Patients and purchasers will be able to obtain information on the cost and quality of health plans and providers. Researchers, regulators, and evaluators will have access to data support decisions about health care delivery and financing. Costs will be reduced by eliminating redundant functions and streamlining inefficient processes.

To achieve this vision, we need a health information infrastructure consisting of several components. At the cheart of the infrastructure are CPR systems—maintained by providers to capture, store, retrieve, transmit, and manipulate patient-specific health care–related data, including clinical, administrative, and payment data. Using standard definitions, codes, and formats that enable data to be universally recognized and processed, CPR systems would be linked (with appropriate mechanisms to control access) through high-speed communication highways capable of transmitting multimedia data (including voice, image, and text) electronically.

Support for better patient care decision-making and analysis of patient outcomes would be available through reference data bases and computerized knowledge based systems which use decision logic and practice guidelines to help caregivers make decisions about diagnoses and treatment options and evaluate outcomes of health interventions.[3]

This vision statement describes the multiple resources that must come together to accomplish that goal. In fact, the adoption of this vision was an evolutionary process and still drives strategic planning today.

Recent major strides have been made toward better managing of essential information. One such stride is automating the exchange of clinical and financial data needed by health care providers and those charged with managing the health services delivery process.[4] Another major stride is the belief of systems designers and providers alike that information linkages in health information systems must be viewed from multiple perspectives and gathered along a longitudinal continuum. In the 1990s, the concept of longitudinal data has expanded to include networked systems that extend beyond individual institutions into community, state, and national data systems. The steady expansion of information processing has reinforced the need for new partnerships as well. The recognition that teamwork is an underlying principle paramount to achieving quality and cost goals in health care systems of all kinds is another major stride. Finally, it is evident that we have advanced efforts to accomplish the vision toward a national health information infrastructure.

The emerging CPR, which allows for automatic transmission of information required for case and utilization management, claims processing, and other core activities, is advancing rapidly. **Health care data networks** are meeting the challenge of widespread access. Networks provide access to an individual's **health care information** to care providers and payers, as well as aggregate data to administrators, employers, policy makers, and other support organizations through centralized and distributed data bases.[4] Through them, the patient can rely on access to health services supported by more coordinated information allowing greater efficiency and better quality.

Purposes of Health Information Systems

More than any other industry, health care is extraordinarily information intensive and demands systematic information tools for effective management. Health information systems are designed to provide **individual** and **aggregate** health care data to health care delivery environments. Systematic collection, organization, and retrieval of information are fundamental to providing health care services. The complexity and features of information systems are determined by the individual information needs of the **users** and **sponsors** of these systems. Users are the health care team, clerical and technical personnel, analysts, and managers that rely on these systems to perform their job. Sponsors are those that authorize, endorse, and fund the information system.

Blum noted in 1984 that information systems are accepted as an integral part of the modern health care facility and provide three overlapping classes of services:

- cost reduction
- operational scope
- patient care

For example, a hospital information system can reduce the clerical burden on nursing personnel, allowing fewer nurses to provide a comparable level of care with more patient-centered activities. The data-dependent tasks are minimized. Operational scope replaces manual processes—such as patient appointment scheduling—with automated ones. Accuracy, improved coordination of services, and speed can be demonstrated as benefits when the appointment-scheduling process is automated. Clinical laboratory processes are another example in which operational tasks can become far more efficient with computer systems. A third class of services described by Blum is direct patient care, which can be enhanced through automating patient record information as well as applying reminders and alerts that offer consistent surveillance and timely intervention opportunities.[5]

In 1991, Malec categorized health care information systems to help conceptualize their functions within organizations in a hierarchical manner. Figure 17–1 depicts a pyramid structure to illustrate the manner in which information systems are developed within organizations.

The pyramid base includes transaction-oriented systems, or transaction processing systems, that automate basic operations. Examples of these are foundation systems such as patient registration and patient accounting. Departmental applications used in pharmacies and laboratories fit in this category as well. With these applica-

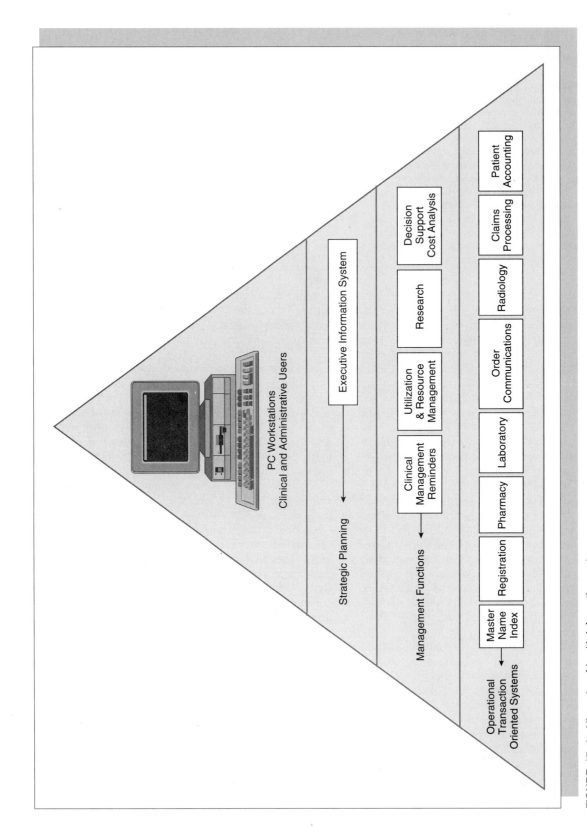

FIGURE 17–1 Hierarchy of health information systems.

tions the daily business activities in the organizations are carried out. Many of the benefits noted in Blum's earlier observations can be realized in these applications. The second layer includes management applications. Diagnostic Related Groups (DRGs) management systems, product line analysis applications, utilization management systems, and the like are used by managers for resource management within organizations. The top layer of the pyramid focuses on strategic functions. Here, **decision support systems** and **executive information systems** are examples. A decision support system is one in which data are combined with analysis tools, allowing the user to understand current activities and perform "what if" questions that enable future optional scenarios to be posed. These systems may be broad based and equipped to answer overall program questions concerned with financial viability of a proposed course of action. They may also be applied to clinical programs and utilization questions. An executive information system typically draws a limited amount of data from contributing systems and offers similar analysis for strategic questions only. The focus is on high-level summary data.[6] By means of the viewing of information systems benefits, broad purposes and potential for organizations can be identified.

Understanding a variety of perspectives helps us understand features and benefits of information systems and their evolution. The first perspective described by Blum focuses on specific benefits in service improvements. The second perspective proposed by Malec focuses on how systems are coming together to provide key functions for organizations. Levels of applications must come together so that foundation systems accomplish daily tasks but also provide data for additional uses. Applications are implemented in layers to add management functions needed to meet primary service goals. Data must be exchanged among users more efficiently and accessed in a more timely manner for day-to-day functions, and assembled for administrative tasks as well. Consider the range and scope of health information systems suggested in our discussion thus far. Together they are connected to achieve an initial set of purposes, i.e., to:

- Support direct patient care delivery events

- Ensure coordination of care processes through coordinated scheduling activities

- Manage financial processes of the organization

- Provide data that managers use for resource planning and management

- Provide data to manage patient care populations as components of preventive care medicine

- Generate data to maintain specific information registries

- Support outcomes research

- Offer tools for use in strategic and tactical planning

Health Information Systems Data Users' Individual and Aggregate Needs

Users can be classified according to their need for data. Individual data are patient care and provider performance data or aggregate data viewed from an institutional perspective for research purposes and to better understand the overall performance of the institution, as well as community data drawn from multiple settings for local and state health care analysis and planning. From a national perspective, data users require cost and outcomes research data for planning and administering broad-based initiatives. Uses of individual data are illustrated by the caregivers on the health care team and by health care managers. Uses of aggregate data begin with care delivery planning and extend to institutional, community, and national levels.

Changes in the Role of Physicians

The physician provider today is either actively using or planning to use a PC workstation to access, collect, and share information. Technology already connects individual office practice systems with local hospital information systems for the mutual benefit of the patient, the physician, and the health care organization. Today, many physicians access patient records through workstations using a point and click device and little typing.[6] Touch screens and graphic displays enhance use and contribute to more efficient business functions within their practice.

Preadmission administrative tasks expedite patient admission to the hospital. Viewing ancillary test results and transmitting changes in physician orders are effective ways to streamline care processes. In addition, tools such as **electronic mail** allow easy connection to colleagues and facilitate collaboration among providers. Electronic mail is a communication system in which computers are connected through networks. The system may be a local one or extend to the national or international community. Because information is already vast and continues to grow, the careful management of this information as a strategic and tactical resource remains a challenge. Organizations today are seeking to provide physicians with access to information when, where, and in the form needed in the most efficient manner possible. This means offering technology support in user-friendly ways so that solutions are practical and mutually beneficial. In working with physicians as computer system users, organizations have learned that facilitating ease of use, limiting the training component required to learn system functions, and avoiding incremental time commitments have encouraged these partnerships with busy practitioners.[6]

The access needs have become extensive, and the complexity and coordination required to meet them are increasing. Because physicians today require information technology to successfully deliver care, the answer to their needs will eventually be the computer-based patient record. Not only will patient information be stored in electronic form, but the physician will be able to bring a new **intelligence factor** through access and employment of external resources for research, quality monitoring, and diagnostic aids. Physicians will require access to external **expert systems** in the midst of patient care delivery through automation. This means that the health information system they use will need to network to such reference sources as the National Library of Medicine and electronic mail to conduct the information flow. By the early 1990s, many health care organizations were connected to results of external research through their libraries. Clinical support tools such as clinical guidelines and expert systems were readily accessible. Workstations were deployed in local physician offices as well as in hospital work areas to access these external data bases. Consider the following prediction published in 1991:

> With national networks for data sharing, the physician wishing to search Medline during a patient encounter and online chart review will be able to request rapid direct connection to the National Library of Medicine (NLM). With adequate system integration, the physician will make such connections through simple point and click features on the screen—no worrying about the phone number for the network or how to log onto the NLM system. All that should be totally invisible to the user.[6]

The Nurse User and Documenter of Individual Patient Data

Nurses require unique capability in information systems. The nursing department consumes 40 plus per cent of hospital budgets and utilizes a major component of an organization's payroll. It comes as no surprise that productivity demands have yielded a number of applications for nurses. Patient acuity systems have been in place for 20 years. These systems provide a rating or assessment of the patient's level of acuity and condition severity. They help allocate hours and skills needed to meet patient care demands. Staffing and utilization reports help hospitals plan for future needs. Nurse scheduling systems are dovetailed with acuity systems to bet-

ter manage overall nursing resources. From the vantage point of direct patient care services, nurses are primary customers of physician orders, pharmacy, laboratories, radiology, physical therapy, central supply, operating rooms, and more. Hospital information systems typically automate the processes associated with the nurses' uses of these resources.[6] Yet these systems do not directly support nursing care delivery. That is better supported through point-of-care **bedside workstations** that streamline patient care documentation and feed directly into patient record systems.[6]

Special Care Team Users Bridge Institutional Data

Special care providers such as physical therapists, occupational therapists, speech therapists, and the like require health care information in both private practice and through facility-wide information systems. Just as physicians use the computer to link office to hospital, so do other team members in even more diverse settings. Home health care today uses health information management systems that connect the field staff including nurses, therapists, social workers, and others through lap-top personal computers and hand-held devices. They use these devices to retrieve and collect information in the field and update to an agency information system for tracking, managing care plans, and scheduling patient services. In hospital environments, these providers access hospital information systems for relevant information on their patients and participate in data capture for such applications.[7] Long-term care facilities have implemented information systems that generate care plans and worksheets for rehabilitation and daily activities. Care plans and computer-generated worksheets are tools used by physical and occupational therapists to facilitate documentation.

Individual Patient Data in Utilization Management

Utilization managers are professionals charged with monitoring and overseeing individual patient cases to ensure that they are managed utilizing the appropriate services and resources. These managers, as well as quality planning personnel, require health information systems that enable them to view data for individual case tracking. They also need to see data in the aggregate to analyze and coordinate ongoing management and future activities. Utilization managers understand how patients use health services, and they rely on the information to promote effective utilization strategies. Information systems can offer reports that are used to educate care provider staff in their utilization practices and to illustrate trending data for the organization. Utilization management is a vital pulse point in health services today. Efforts of the federal government have extended over three decades to address optimal utilization. The advent of DRGs was an attempt to bring a rational analysis to understanding the resources required to deliver health care services in hospitals. The goal was to determine appropriate utilization of services according to similar clinical conditions (adjusted for similarities and differences in various parts of the country) so that a more equitable distribution of resources could be established. The work with DRGs brings focus to information systems and their use of data beyond that of patient care use. What became evident in utilization management was that information systems and the right data contained in them were essential to overall survival of health care organizations in an increasingly competitive environment.

The Move Beyond Individual Patient Data to Prospective Management of Patient Populations

Providers, focusing on outcomes, expect information systems to allow them to view individual patient information for care purposes and to incorporate clinical reminders or messages that help them maintain a given plan of care for that patient. They also need to review their patient population according to specific types of problems and services to maintain an effective assessment of the overall services they are providing. Health care organizations review patient population categories to compare and contrast their own performance with guidelines and standards. In an outpatient setting, assessment data are typically drawn from a computerized outpatient data system that collects encounter information on problems, diagnoses, and procedures. In hospitals, it is drawn from the discharge analysis data initiated from the point of admission, often through admission-discharge-transfer applications, and completed following discharge analysis data collection performed in the health information department.

Immunization tracking and cancer screening are examples of information systems that are used to manage populations of patients for purposes of prospective planning. As the national health care industry steps up to the need to manage chronic health care problems over time and to improve the health of the patient through increasing the focus on prevention, the associated need for data systems will grow. The development of immunization tracking applications that monitor immunization status and notify physicians and patients that immunizations are due has improved the rates of immunization. Vaccination rates increased when reminders were provided to these patients and their physicians. The computer system was used to alert physicians of the immunizations, and provide physicians with information about the immunization status as a management tool. This example illustrates how attention paid to prospective clinical management yields benefits in patient care.[8]

Health Information Systems Aggregate Data Use in Cost Containment

Health information systems have demonstrated significant impact on cost containment. As noted in the mid 1980s by Blum and others, reduced labor occurs in manual communication of information from one department to another when communications technology is used. Streamlined documentation procedures in bedside terminals for nurses contained costs. Improved claims processing applications also reduced costs. Costs were also reduced in test ordering when physicians accessed an online patient record system prior to test ordering to verify availability of already-captured test results. Additionally, pharmacy costs were lowered when cost data alerts were provided through an online ordering system. In one significant study published in 1993, physician inpatient order writing on microcomputer workstations that were linked to an electronic medical record system demonstrated a 12.7 per cent reduction in admission charges. The organization projected that this would amount to savings of more than $3 million in charges annually for the hospital's medicine service. In addition, cost savings were also noted in the following:

- Patient length of stay was 10.5 per cent shorter.
- Physicians ordered fewer tests.
- Medication costs were lower.
- Costs of all types of patient charges were reduced.

One limiting factor was that the system required more physician time than did the paper charts. For many institutions, the physician time component remains a barrier to physician ordering success. The conclusion was that more study was required to increase the gains from this process and determine additional alternatives that contribute to efficiency.[9]

What is known is that streamlining processes through applications such as automated registration and appointment scheduling, test and medication ordering, and test results reporting can improve overall efficiencies in health care organizations. Savings include eliminating data collection and data entry redundancies. More efficient use of personnel time occurs when communications automatically notify and trigger departmental systems. Better organization and presentation of data itself contributes to the evidence mounting in favor of investing in HISs. Providers and managers have realized significant benefits from information systems, but they are not the only users to realize such potential. Computer systems are used to track patient satisfaction with overall health care services and provide health care organizations with strategic information needed to better plan and manage the care delivery process. Customer satisfaction data are a well-recognized commodity. Finally, advocates of integrated hospital systems have cited advantages that include the use of a central database shared among applications, elimination of data redundancy, and reduced costs when application code is shared by user groups.[10]

Health Care Outcomes Data Within Organizations and Beyond

The health care delivery system is considered a business enterprise. Thus it undergoes the same kind of business assessments necessary to maintain an effective business in operation. Products of health care services should be measured for quality and efficiency just as in any business activity. The cost of health care has become so vast and unmanageable over the past few decades that patients, providers, and payers are more and more focusing on the outcome of the services provided. All are asking key questions: Is the patient's health improved? How much are patients themselves participating in their own health care? Are quality measures in place, and what do they tell us? Do we employ effective and least costly interventions during care planning and delivery of care? Are we moving to identify ways to accomplish prospective care management of populations so that we are one step ahead of problems?

Not only are aggregate treatment and health services data used to assess outcome status but also patient perspectives are now incorporated into outcomes evaluation. Research has shown that patients appreciate the opportunity to provide information that will facilitate collaborative decision making with their providers. As members of their own health care team, some patients are asked to submit self-reported functional health status questionnaires. Facilities are tracking patient satisfaction surveys, and providers are more aggressive in thoroughly explaining patient care options so that the best decisions for each patient can be made. In 1994, Casper and Brennan stated that ". . . Patients hold unique insights into their preferences and desires for health care and clinical outcomes.[11] There is growing cognizance of the lack of the patient input in the existing record. Further, the emergence of health outcomes research in the last decade has resulted in a growing body of evidence supporting the importance of incorporating patient preferences in health care decision making and in the assessment of the quality of health care."[12] We can see that objective clinical measurement data combined with patient-generated data provide improved outcomes.

Community Health Information Networks

Along with administrative uses and screening and tracking applications that meet key users' needs, individual organizations are now accountable to payers, researchers, planners, and other data users outside the enterprise. A **community health information network** (CHIN) is designed to meet the need for health data beyond the individual organization through a community-wide focus. They are proposed to meet the community need for shared data. The American Hospital Association defines a CHIN as "an integrated collection of computer and telecommunications capabilities that facilitate communications of patient, clinical, and payment information among multiple providers, payers, employees, and related health care entities within a community."[13] The purposes of typical questions are to:

- Improve efficiency of the health care claims process and financial settlement transactions
- Provide a valuable data system to improve access to data for community users
- Supply information on the cost, appropriateness, and effectiveness of health care providers
- Provide health services purchasers with the data needed for benefit plan and workplace health analysis
- Offer the community the capability to perform special wellness/health studies
- Provide researchers and physicians with the capacity for medical effectiveness studies

To accomplish these objectives, the CHINs would link providers, purchasers, payers, and patients to an integrated system that would maintain eligibility, utilization review, and encounter and claims processing data. It could perform standard billing and related business functions as well. Further, it could acquire and maintain basic demographic, financial, employment, insurance, and encounter data using standardized data collection procedures already in place; and position itself to incorporate additional standardized processing when it is developed. Two major deliverables could be an extensive data repository made up of interrelated databases that would serve all users via patient profiles drawn from the data collected from the participating organizations, and an improved capacity to process, consolidate, and route encounter and claims transactions more efficiently as well as assist in the processing of remittances. Thus, both clinical quality and cost management could be addressed.[13,14]

In practice, CHINs are selecting a variety of approaches to accomplish their goals. Some concentrate on administrative and/or financial data only. Others are collecting clinical data. The next few years will afford the opportunity to observe and learn from CHINs for planned community data uses.

Health Care Delivery Management and National Policy

Health care delivery management extends across multiple care settings and over time. From the management of acute care focused, short-term illnesses in the 1950s and 60s, the United States' requirements have shifted to long-term management of chronic illness and an emphasis on prospective management of "preventable" health problems. As noted in the 1993 report on Computerization of Patient Records, the "cost and quality of health care are currently of major concern to the American public. . . . Ways to improve the value of care— what quality can be purchased for what cost—are at the forefront of today's health reform agenda."[15] Here, indeed, is where we saw the major shift and emphasis on adopting automation and finding ways to share it. It is clear that the information intensity of health care delivery is the major driver of improved information processing technology.

One cited example of the use of technology to accomplish these national goals is **telemedicine.** Identified as an excellent resource to expand services to rural areas and positively affect the health outcomes of patients, this concept was proposed to link providers to effect widespread access to health resources. Along these lines, personal health information systems were proposed to provide the means for individuals to be able to access health information resources 24 hours a day using telephones and home computers. Basic health practices and first aid guidelines for family and household use and consulting nurses were suggested as universal resources. Advice from such resources could result in reduction of unnecessary health care services. Population data structures and system coordination would enable secondary users to research large populations for purposes of more effective overall health strategies and improvements. This research could occur without access to personal identifiers, yet be focused enough to benefit specific diagnostic populations as well as occupational and geographic ones.[16]

The Health Security Act proposed a new framework for the health care system. The proposed legislation included the establishment of a national data and information framework, nationwide electronic networks for health data exchange, and strong privacy, confidentiality, and security protection. The implications for health care information systems are significant. Information systems must meet organizational needs as well as specific external needs, primarily the elements of a national information infrastructure—the foundation piece. One set of issues and recommendations submitted to the White House and National Academy of Science task forces on the national health information infrastructure included discussion of value added specifically through information systems. Administrative information systems were challenged to save significantly through unified claims processing and electronic data interchange. In general, information systems were identified as key to access, store, and transmit information to support access and use of patient records anywhere in the United States. One study estimated that $15 billion a year could be saved through the use of such systems.

Summarizing Common Purposes

As these individual information system needs are acknowledged and developed, common components can be identified that cross sponsor and organization boundaries. In fact, we can say that successful HISs today are those that must meet a common set of operational objectives, i.e., to:

- Deliver data for the more efficient operation of daily business activities
- Demonstrate cost effectiveness
- Provide extensive patient data to a growing number of authorized users
- Contain easy tools for management analysis
- Offer streamlined data capture—capture once
- Make summary and aggregate data readily available
- Minimize duplicate data
- Minimize immediate data transfers
- Localize processing
- Standardize communications
- Establish an architectural custodian responsible for the technical specification of the data for institutional data dictionaries
- Define/deliver data as an organizational resource through a data repository
- Improve managerial effectiveness
- Enable linkages within and beyond organizations to community, regional, and national data systems

- Contribute to executive information system functions
- Maintain effective data security measures[6]

Organizations that deliver health care need to provide internal and external data on the outcome and efficacy of their services. This requires detailed, timely clinical and financial data. Organizations will need to identify and monitor optimal medical care decisions. This means that clinical guidelines and their effective applications will need to be incorporated into the care processes in efficient ways. The care delivery processes will need to be re-engineered and streamlined. Enhancement of interorganizational data sharing and coordination in order to meet the demands of longitudinal patient data become paramount. Comprehensive long-range planning efforts that develop organizational philosophies and strategies for advanced health information management systems and their implementation are integral to the health care industry. The tools must be available to accomplish the work. It is acknowledged that today's health care facilities need to share integrated patient information within their own environments as well as across service providers. They need to capture and compute the accurate costs of clinical care, track clinical outcome data in relation to services provided, and ensure longitudinal collection and storage of patient information with universal access in whatever environment that care is rendered.[17]

COMPUTERS IN HEALTH CARE— PAST AND PRESENT

Early Efforts, 1960s–1980s

Computers were introduced into the health care arena through punch card data processing. Early work in epidemiologic and public health applications that performed statistical analysis on the incidence, distribution, and causes of diseases in society provided the early experience with computers.[18] Applications grew into information systems in which specific problems of medicine were addressed. While some of the early activities were focused on decision making for physicians, many developers worked on building total information systems for hospitals. Also, during the 1960s and 1970s, significant work was undertaken by Octo Barnett at Massachusetts General Hospital in the ambulatory care environment with the development of COSTAR (computer-stored ambulatory record system). Another historic effort of note was work in information systems done by Morris Collen at Kaiser-Permanente in Oakland, California.[18] The first patient care system that claimed to

automate the patient record was initially marketed as the IBM Medical Information Systems Program in the late 1960s and sold until 1972. While a number of other companies were involved in patient care information systems during this period, only the system devised by Lockheed Aircraft—now the Technicon Data System (TDS)—is still in existence. In fact, the TDS today has been installed in about 120 hospitals and remains one of the successful experiences well worth study.[19]

During the 1970s, HISs were developed in several ways. Many hospitals approached information systems development through departmental systems and began with financial information systems. Others adopted a goal of a single integrated or monolithic system that was designed to use one large database that shared its resources among departments. In contrast, others acquired versions of hospital information systems through departmental applications such as a clinical laboratory system to which custom features were later added. While the intention was to create common data through a single shared database, this proved difficult to achieve.[19] In large part, database structures and the tools needed to use them effectively were still immature during the 1970s. During this period, hospital databases were derived largely from discharge analysis of medical records. Many hospitals participated through contracts with external computer service organizations by submitting discharge abstracts to the service computer companies for processing and receiving printouts of hospital statistics. The most extensive program was maintained by the Commission on Professional Hospital Activities (CPHA). Its program brought health information professionals into the computer age as they worked with computerized data in new ways. Expectations were expanded as CPHA and others introduced more computing power and offered better ways to retrieve data and provide comparative reports.

As the minicomputer became more established in the 1970s, more and more separate departments were able to acquire departmental systems that met their specific needs. Vendors began to offer packages of functions for hospital departments such as laboratory, radiology, pharmacy, and accounting. In addition, software tools emerged that reduced the mystery associated with computers, and medical practitioners became more interested in leading and participating in computing activities. Minicomputers provided as much and more computing power than the huge mainframe computers. With expanded sophistication of computer system users, the emergence of system development teams became more evident.

By the late 1970s, microcomputers and the PC rolled into place. This major technologic development gave rise to additional empowerment and expectations by health care practitioners. In effect, technologic advances produced computers of reliability, small size, and small cost. Hardware reliability and availability became highly affordable. Computer and business communities recognized that the greatest cost involved in information systems development was in the software. Thus, software engineering emerged as a field dedicated to management of the software development process.[17] The three major activities that characterize the 1970s were significantly improved reliability of hardware and software, reduction in cost, and significant investment in research and development. All this laid a strong foundation for the work to come.

Evolution of Hospital Information Systems: 1980s to mid 1990s

In the 1980s, communication technology grew to provide foundation applications in health care organizations. Demographic and associated information was already available on patients who registered into clinics or were admitted into hospitals, and data were automatically sent to hospital departments that needed to commence service. Thus admission notices were communicated to dietary, housekeeping, laboratory, radiology, and other ancillary services electronically. In turn, order communications enabled physician orders to be sent from a nursing station directly to an ancillary area. In addition, significant gains were made in building computer networks that linked a variety of diverse applications together.[18,19]

In 1980, Ball and Jacobs described HISs at three levels. A Level I HIS included admission-discharge-transfer application with bed and census reporting, order entry communications, and charge capture and inquiry functions for billing purposes. A Level II HIS focused on systems that included part or most of the patient record. This provided fundamentally clinical databases and improved collection and use of clinical data within these systems. The Technicon System at El Camino, Mountain View, CA, is an example of a Level II HIS system. Level III was used to describe an HIS in which data were linked to knowledge bases that provided diagnostic support and actual intervention for patient care activities. In these systems, special alerts were made available that responded to specific data content and messages and notified providers through the system.[20]

By the end of the decade, a HIS was defined as an institutional information system that links basic business process functions (registration, admission, discharge, and transfer [R-ADT]) to **order communications** and **results reporting** functions to discharge abstracting and patient accounting processes. In the 1990s, hospital information systems are required to operate on many functional levels. For instance, they typically embrace and connect multiple functional areas through the information systems. This may occur through integrating information as well as connecting departmental systems through network communications. A comprehensive HIS contains six components:

- Core applications such as patient scheduling, admission, discharge, and transfer (R-ADT) provide the central notification to the hospital of patient admission.

- Business and financial systems such as patient accounting, billing, and payroll provide data processing for the business activities of the organization.

- Communications and networking applications transmit messages among departments such as nursing and ancillary areas. Communications are used to notify these departments of patient admission and provide for tracking orders and responses to them.

- Departmental systems such as pharmacy, radiology, and laboratory are designed to manage the business functions of those departments and connect data to institutional data bases.

- Documentation systems are used to collect, store, and retrieve patient data. Applications in this category range from point-of-care bedside terminals for nursing documentation to transcription modules that capture and store clinical reports.

- Reminder and advice functions assist physicians in planning patient care activities. Such reminders can include messages to alert for significant test results, utilization criteria, and drug/drug interaction data. This component includes the monitoring of compliance to clinical pathways. We will see how this component has emerged as a fundamental tenet of envisioned computer-based patient record systems.[18]

In reality, hospital information systems can be viewed along a continuum from the first three major components to acquisition of all six. Figure 17–2 depicts a schematic representation of the major applications in a hospital information system and illustrates the six components. Note that information needed for admission is captured at preadmission and may be entered into the master patient index, where it is maintained as a permanent name index for all patients. Applications are shown as connected through communications. Data are viewed as the common resource. Data are also aggregated and used in high-level planning and evalua-

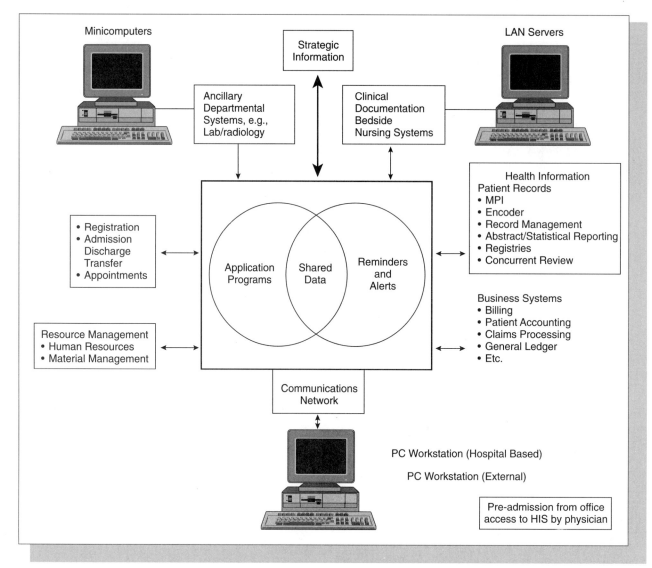

FIGURE 17–2. Hospital information system schematic.

tion efforts. The organization relies on the HIS for daily processing activities and for follow-up analysis work.[6]

Recent Trends in Hospital Information Systems

By 1993, Bleich and Slack characterized hospital information systems as primarily communications foundations that supported a database management system. In HISs, hundreds or thousands of terminals throughout the hospital continually collect data in one form and display or print them in another.[21] As the HIS has evolved, so has its breadth and depth. It has become more and more common to see key functions automated at the department level. Some hospitals acquired computer systems incrementally, driven by their individual priorities. Others developed and followed some form of master plan established to acquire the computing resources necessary to meet their needs. Along with this growth, hospitals also adopted a specific overall strategy. In hospitals, a decision was made to build toward an interfaced system or an integrated one. Table 17–1 shows how these two systems differ. They not only represent different technologic approaches but they also represent different operational strategies. The role and decision-making activities of departmental managers would reflect these differences.[21]

TABLE 17-1 INTERFACED INFORMATION SYSTEMS VERSUS INTEGRATED INFORMATION SYSTEMS	
INTERFACED INFORMATION SYSTEMS	**INTEGRATED INFORMATION SYSTEMS**
Interfaced computer systems require programming to communicate with one another. Basically, single department systems are designed to meet the needs of that department. They are characterized as systems in which each department is responsible for maintaining its own data base. Personnel of each department are the only ones authorized to change data. Data needed by another department must be sent from one computer to another. Often this necessitates maintaining duplicate data. The programming required to connect these systems can be expensive. Recent developments in communications standards to link independent computer systems have gone a long way to reduce the complexity and cost of these interfaces.	These are systems in which all the departments share a common database. All data elements are maintained in a single data dictionary, and users must follow specific rules for updating and editing.
The advantage of this approach is that it is department centered. Each department has more power over system decisions and can select the "best of breed" for its area. For this approach to be effective, standard communications protocols such as one designed as a communication standard must be used to connect one system to another.	The advantage in this approach is that once a data item is updated or modified in any way, all users are immediately notified of the change. So in cases where the data may be stored more than once for ease of use, the automatic synchronization and update of the data element offers consistency and reliability. The major trend for all organizations' systems is to combine networking, database management, data standards, and new analysis and design methods. Integration builds common data and access to them in a way that minimizes department boundaries and supports data as an organizational resource.

Health Professionals Adopt New Agendas

Also in the decade of the 1980s, health professionals from diverse backgrounds came together to work on medical computing in a variety of ways. Physicians, engineers, administrators, nurses, software developers, and others adopted new roles. They sought to define and describe their unique information needs. By the mid 1980s, the overall domain of **medical informatics** had emerged and became a recognized, yet still evolving, field. The variety of clinical computing endeavors had coalesced into a more commonly understood domain with a corresponding need to define and describe them with an information handling perspective. Medical informatics became more clearly defined, and health care professionals became more team oriented as their involvement in systems development expanded. In 1990, Greenes and Shortliffe defined medical informatics as "the field that concerns itself with the cognitive, information processing, and communication tools of medical practice, education, and research including the information science and the technology to support these tasks."[22] The unique challenges involved in medical computing depended on the evolution of informatics as a focus of study for a variety of health care professionals. Health information professionals initiated alliances with the American Medical Informatics Association and others during the late 1980s to participate in and lead aspects of patient data computing that advanced the effectiveness of health information management. These activities included work on research, standards, systems, and policy issues.

Automated Health Record Systems— Historical Landmarks

Significant pioneering work has been accomplished over the past three decades in medical record systems. Three notable medical record systems are the Computer Stored Ambulatory Record System (COSTAR), the Regenstrief Medical Record System (RMRS), and The Medical Record (TMR). COSTAR was originally developed in 1968 for implementation at the Harvard Community Health Plan. One of the earliest systems designed at the outset to replace the paper record, this system is one of the most widely used automated medical record applications and became a milestone in the development of automated ambulatory medical record systems (AAMRS). It initially included six modules:

- Security and integrity
- Patient registration
- Appointment scheduling
- Medical record
- Billing and accounting
- Medical Query Language

Its scope provided comprehensive information relationships and tied the flow of data through the modules.

The system supports codified clinical information through its own **data dictionary** in seven major divisions. Established and maintained by technical developers, the data dictionary contains definitions for all the entities, attributes, and relationships of the user view of the data and denotes the physical system in which the data resides. COSTAR established data dictionaries in physical findings, diagnoses, laboratory tests, medications, nonmedical therapies, procedures, and personal patient history.

When patients make appointments in COSTAR, the appointment scheduling module serves as a trigger to generate a printout encounter form for a patient visit. As patients are seen for care, providers collect new data on computer-generated encounter forms that contain preselected clinical data and are precoded for consistent data capture and data entry ease. All patient encounters, including ambulatory, home, hospital, and telephone, are captured either via encounter forms or through dictation. The COSTAR system has been implemented in multiple sites, including county-wide public health programs, hospital and physician office settings, and others. The breadth of linked functions in COSTAR served as a model for subsequent system developers.[23]

The RMRS was implemented in 1972. Originally designed to create a "summary" computer-based patient record, the RMRS contained records for approximately 1 million registered patients in 1995. Modules include patient appointments, laboratory test processing and results reporting, inpatient drug orders, and outpatient prescriptions. It is part of a larger health information system that also supports hospital information components. Computer-generated encounter forms are used to collect information that is later entered by data entry specialists. The encounter form includes a master problem list and medications and serves as a **turnaround document** for clinicians. A turnaround document developed for the RMRS system is usually a one- to three-page summary computer generated for a patient visit. It includes a format that is completed during the visit or encounter to record the events and is subsequently "turned around" and returned for follow-up computer data entry. An order communications module was developed in RMRS, and, by 1991, physicians in the general medicine clinic of the Regenstrief System in Indiana were entering orders directly through PC workstations. In addition to laboratory and pharmacy data, clinic subsystems and tapes from the affiliated Wishard Hospital (a participating Regenstrief System hospital) case abstracting service provide for comprehensive data collection in this landmark system. In it radiologic procedures, electrocardiograms and echocardiograms, occult blood studies, spirometries, bone marrow diagnoses, vital signs, and weights are stored. Text reports for x-ray, surgical pathology, hospital admission histories, and discharge summaries are also stored in the computer in a separate file. RMRS has demonstrated that a system designed to automate the medical record can evolve naturally into an organizational, administrative, and clinical information system and that clinical point-of-care data are the data foundation. The RMRS system has contributed significantly to outcomes research and, through the use of clinical reminders to trigger analysis and planning for the providers, has demonstrated that significant cost benefits are obtainable through the automation of medical record content linked with appropriate information systems applications.[23]

The TMR System is a comprehensive medical information system that was developed at Duke University Medical Center. TMR sought to eliminate the paper record in an outpatient setting. It has evolved over 25 years and currently supports both outpatient and inpatient settings. It is known for developments in the database and data dictionaries. In TMR, the data include:

- Problems and diagnoses
- Subjective and objective findings
- Orders
- Therapies
- Encounter data
- Accounting data
- Links to an appointment scheduling module

These data can be entered interactively by authorized health care team members. **Audit trails** are maintained for security purposes. An audit trail can record the access and/or action that occurs in a computer record by logging the user identification and the file identification, recording date and time of access, and the action done. Patient monitoring, laboratory, and other ancillary system data are entered directly into TMR from host systems. Of particular note are TMR retrieval capabilities that facilitate multiple views of the data. Providers can view data from problem, time, task, and encounter perspectives. The system supports research and medical effectiveness studies.[23]

Computerized Patient Records in the Inpatient Setting

The HELP system, a comprehensive hospital information system that combines clinically based modules with a financial data base, integrates information from admitting, radiology, pharmacy, pathology, radiology, nursing, respiratory therapy, and clinical laboratories and creates a computer-based patient record for all patients. HELP was designed to meet the following objectives[24]:

- Support an ever-expanding medical database with automated tools for acquisition, storage, and review that was planned to replace the paper record.
- Implement a system to process medical information that would facilitate interventions and links to protocols so that physicians would be able to modify care plans on the basis of an interactive computer system environment.

- Accommodate research subsystems to facilitate clinical research including cost and quality components.

HELP combines communications and clinical alert features through time- and data-driven rules. For example, if a particular data or data value arises, rules are invoked that communicate interactively with the physicians responsible for care. In one study, the HELP system demonstrated the use of these features to alert physicians to monitor and better manage infection control for hospitalized patients. It provided intervention messages directly through the system to a terminal that resulted in modified behavior for individual patient care. In turn, these experiences were used collectively to strengthen hospital policies and procedures for infection control.[25] HELP also demonstrated the benefits in applying quality-based guidelines and criteria directly to individual patient information. Latter-Day Saints Hospital, Salt Lake City, establishes a set of physician-approved criteria for ordering blood transfusions. The criteria, linked to supportive data in the integrated data base, are then used to "qualify" each order for a blood transfusion. These orders were entered directly into the system by physicians and nurses. Orders are then "qualified" as appropriate or referred to the staff member responsible for review. The Quality Assessment staff member further researches the order against details of the case and institutional criteria and approves or denies the request. HELP remains an excellent example of a constantly evolving computer-based patient record system that embodies the principles of quality clinical alerts and reminders in the active care process.[26]

THE PRESENT GOAL—THE COMPUTER-BASED PATIENT RECORD (CPR)

The patient record is the principal repository for information concerning a patient's health care, uniquely representing patients and serving as a dynamic resource for the health care industry. When viewed over time, it paints a longitudinal picture of health problems and services. Remarkably, it has changed very little over the past 50 years. As of the mid 1990s, it is still primarily paper based.

The emphasis today is, and into the next century will remain, on the computerization of the patient record in order to serve multiple demands and to expand and multiply value to patients and health care providers. Data have been abstracted from the patient record into computer systems since the 1950s. Today, our understanding of patient data origins has led us to establish a system that will automatically collect and assemble patient data ranging from information provided by patients

themselves to information generated from biomedical devices such as electrocardiograms and other data sources internal and external to the institution into a longitudinal repository with access to clinical intelligence. We have a clear goal and are striving to meet it. While the evolution of computer-based patient record systems continues and has demonstrated effective progress through the landmark systems already described, the real impetus began with the Institute of Medicine (IOM) study conducted from 1989 to 1991. (This originally was named the Committee on Improving the Medical Record in Response to Increasing Functional Requirements and Technological Advances.) The committee's charge was to[27]:

- Examine the current state of medical record systems, including their availability, use, strengths, and weaknesses
- Identify impediments to the development and use of improved record systems
- Identify ways, including developments now in progress, to overcome impediments and improve medical record systems
- Develop a research agenda to advance medical record systems
- Develop a plan, design, and/or other provisions for improved medical record systems, including a means for updating these systems and the research agenda as appropriate
- Recommend policies and other strategies to achieve these improvements

One phase of the initial work was the establishment of key definitions. These definitions are used today as work continues to develop and implement the CPR.

Patient record—The repository of information about a single patient. This information is generated by health care professionals as a direct result of interaction with a patient or with individuals who have personal knowledge of the patient (or with both). Traditionally, patient records have been paper and have been used to store patient care data.

Primary patient record—This is used by health care professionals as they provide patient care services to review patient data or document their own observations, actions, or instructions.

Secondary patient record—This is derived from the primary record and contains selected data elements to aid nonclinical individuals (i.e., persons not involved in direct patient care) in supporting, evaluating, or advancing patient care. Patient care support refers to administration, regulation, and payment functions. Patient care evaluation refers to quality assurance, utilization review, risk management, and medical or legal audits. Patient care advancement refers to research. These records are often combined to form what the committee terms a secondary database (e.g., an insurance claims database).

Computer-based patient record—An electronic patient record that resides in a system specifically designed to support users by providing accessibility to complete and accurate data, alerts, reminders, clinical decision support systems, links to medical knowledge, and other aids.

Patient record system—The set of components that form the mechanism by which patient records are created, used, stored, and retrieved. A patient record system is usually located within a health care provider setting. It includes people, data, rules and procedures, processing and storage devices (e.g., paper and pen, hardware and software), and communications and support function.[29]

The committee noted that patient record systems could be part of hospital information systems, medical information systems, or a type of clinical information system.

CPR to Meet Challenges of Increased Demands

The increased demands on the patient record act as drivers for change. Physicians and other clinicians need the patient record for clinical data collection, problem definition, systematic clinical planning and follow-up, and population-based management.[28] Patients require records to obtain their clinical history for caregivers and information for claims processing, for participation in their own care evaluation, delivery, and planning activities, and for decision making. They may also require patient record data for genetic tracking, legal needs, and other business activities.[29] The question is, Can the record meet these needs in its current mode? The answer can be seen in a review of its weaknesses.

Drawbacks of Using Paper Records

The paper record suffers from basic limitations inherent in its nature. As a physical entity, it must be located in a single location for a single use at any given time. This restricts the record to one user at a time. By its very nature, the paper record cannot meet the needs of the complex care environments that exist in health care; its use is becoming unrealistic in the face of pressures to control operational costs.

The record's ability to serve as the communicator from one provider to another and to maintain continuity of care is limited. Providers must rely on the documentation by other practitioners. The style and completeness of that documentation varies from one setting to another. In fact, there is no method to identify where

information is lacking due to incomplete data or incomplete documentation of the data—a support mechanism that could be used when computer applications incorporate "required" data fields to strengthen data capture. Consider that the record may not even contain data from companion care events. For example, data contained in the personal logs of the practitioners are not included. There is no mechanism to contain documents or images produced by external resources such as radiologists, special study programs, and education. Part of the reason for this is that the record cannot contain unlimited information in such varied formats and still remain effective for daily use. This is changing with technology that will offer multimedia and faster electronic transmission of data. We know that there may be extensive additional information on patients that must be accessed and incorporated in the patient's record from external sources.[29]

The current record suffers from weaknesses in understandability, legibility, chronology, and data organization. We cannot rearrange data on paper to display it in alternative formats that might help view data relationships in new ways. We are limited to the fundamental chronologic flow of information as it is collected. Investigators must page through thick documents and try to connect related information from many and often diverse locations.

The content of the record is the evidence needed to determine the effectiveness of care and, collectively, it provides the foundation for clinical planning. We must have data in aggregate form to understand these areas. Health services research currently requires data to effectively evaluate cost and quality. Dependence on the paper record with manual retrieval methods adds cost and complexity to overall data aggregation and analysis activities. While the primary activity of the patient record is to support patient care, alternative uses can interfere with its availability for the care process. Patients and providers need the patient record to function beyond a basic data repository. Today we need the repository characteristic of the record to combine with intelligent commentary to give evidence that the data were applied against clinical guidelines and protocols.

Finally, it is clear that we have shifted to a new paradigm over the past 10 years. The patient record itself must be newly defined both in content and in functionality. Health care organizations are in the midst of determining the new definition and health information professionals are assuming a leadership role in this activity.

Defining a New Model

There is a new model of a patient record. The definition proposed by the IOM study offered a start in 1991.

For many organizations, the expansion of the definition will continue to be controlled by external accrediting organizations or by statute. Perhaps we need to view the patient record as the entity that collects, records, and manages health care information in a way that supports multifaceted health care experiences. Note the definition of **health care information** itself. In legislation passed in Washington state early in the decade, it was defined as "all information, oral or recorded in any form, related to any care, service, or procedure to diagnose, treat, or maintain the physical or mental condition of an individually identified patient. It is obtained in the course of a patient's health care from a health care provider, from the patient, from a member of the patient's family or an individual with whom the patient has a close personal relationship, or from the patient's legal representative."[30]

This definition opened up the content sources beyond the traditional patient record by including all forms of information as well as the longitudinal component of the information. It offers a broader view of content and replaced the term *record* with *information*. Today, the patient record contains not only data from the care givers but also from the patients themselves in self-reported tools such as functional health status surveys. We have also seen that data may come directly from biomedical devices and are transformed into information for clinical use. The period of transition we are in is not likely to change in the next decade. Defining and redefining work will continue as new and more complex data collection and generating devices emerge.

More Sophisticated Functionality Through a CPR Model

Shortliffe et al. noted that computer-based patient record systems must fulfill the following from a content perspective. They must provide clinicians with a readily accessible, intelligible assembly of clinical data that characterizes the condition, prior management, and current treatment plan of a patient. Furthermore, there must be reliance that data from multiple sources are included. CPRs must provide a clearly defined and well-organized database to permit epidemiologic assessment of patient outcomes and patterns of practice so that management strategies could be viewed within specific clinical contexts. From an applied intelligence perspective, new functionality must allow the record to access current research and practice guidelines as well as include interactive decision support tools that are based on information derived from analyzed population data, thereby building on best demonstrated practices.

When viewed as an operational entity for health care organizations, the CPR systems must have a positive impact on workflow operations. Decrease in administrative record keeping and form submission responsibilities that burden health care providers was targeted early in this decade as a significant cost saver. Improved claims processing has helped. However, other administrative processing can also be improved. Referrals, occupational injury reporting, and other functions will benefit from similar streamlining efforts.[29]

Another commentator, H. D. Covvey, cites the functionality of the CPR in some detail as well.[28] The record content will include uniform core data elements (minimum data standard) and standardized coding (standard nomenclature and standard classification systems). Based on a common data dictionary (data standard), the CPR will include information on all phases and aspects of care as well as have the capability to include all essential data types.

The record format will display a front page problem list and similar data contained on paper record face sheets. Users will be able to flip through content to review carefully. Searches will be possible by problem, within a time period, and according to other constraints; the record will be internally structured for audit and quality assurance. Basically, the CPR will be structured to address needs of all stakeholders and will be integrated among disciplines and sites to meet data exchange standards.

From a system performance perspective, rapid retrieval and user-intuitive 24-hour access will be essential so that users will be able to use the CPR with little or no instruction. The access will be accomplished via standard networks and workstations and available at convenient places of care and work. Easy data input will be available and multimedia support required. Interfaces with high-performance networks will be expected.

Linkage to other information systems will enable easy transferability of information and access to scientific literature and other information resources such as hospital information systems, research databases, and community data systems. Covey notes that appropriate registries and databases will also be linked along with family members' records: Providers will be able to use E-mail to communicate with other providers for referrals and consultations.

Intelligence will be available in the form of medical decision support and clinical guidelines. These investigation and monitoring tools will be available to support clinicians in managing individual and groups of patients and will operate on personal computers as well as on larger applications. Guidelines can provide the basis for clinical reminders and custom "alarm" systems. For instance, a patient who is receiving IV medications for a cardiac condition may be monitored for low blood pressure. In certain kinds of heart failure, some patients maintain a lower blood pressure by medical protocol. A low blood pressure reading may signal an "alarm" at a point different from that for another patient who has a different kind of medical condition.

Report capabilities will offer summary views. They will include derived documents (e.g., workers compensation, insurance) and easily customized user interfaces. Standard reports (e.g., discharge summary) will be system generated. Ad hoc reports and trend reports and graphics will allow diverse views. Abstraction through selected data sets per time and data orientation will be possible. Chemotherapy-response data may be recorded in tandem with key vital signs. Trend data displays and graphics may need to be tailored in individual cases.

The CPR will be structured for easy access for patients and advocates. Safeguards regarding confidentiality, reliability, security, and recoverability will be in place with appropriate management structures. Finally, training and implementation will rely on innovation, such as intuitive user interfaces, so that minimal training is required for use. CPR systems will be planned with as graduated an implementation schedule as is possible.[28]

CPR Building Blocks—Data and Technology

The nature of data and health information applications are the building blocks that come together in a health information system. **Data** elements themselves can be viewed as the raw material of information systems. Users require data that are transformed into information and then into knowledge. Blum characterized data as the uninterpreted data elements that are given to the problem solver. This includes something as elementary as a patient name as well as numeric data such as age or a pulse rate. A test result, a diagnostic code, and height and weight are other examples.[18]

On the other hand, information refers to a collection of data that contains meaning as when data are processed, that results in a display or report containing information. In this context, data and information can be stored in a permanent, accessible database. The computer-based patient record, stored on line, would include data and information resulting from the analysis and processing of other data. For example, results reported from laboratory tests and presented through a computer workstation flowsheet provide time-oriented information to the provider of care.

Knowledge is defined as the "formalization of the relationships among elements of information and data." That is, that new data or information can be inferred from the data and information already present.[28] The example of the flowsheet might move from test results (data) to a diabetic care management flowsheet (information) to the awareness that a patient's condition has undergone a change (knowledge). Perhaps the most easily understood description of knowledge in this context is the use of rules that are applied to the data and information that enable providers to apply medical judgment to the care processes. How does this affect health information systems and, in particular, computer-based patient record systems?

Covvey notes that the "contents" of computer-based patient records and health information systems can be expressed as data types or as data elements. Some of the significant complexity of the record is due to the multimedia data type characteristic. This characteristic has only been addressable through multimedia information systems in the first half of this decade. Table 17–2 lists the variety of data types required in patient record systems.[28] Data types should be present in ways that provide information when comparisons, trends, and confirmation of differential diagnostic investigation are sought by clinical providers. If we understand the role of data types more clearly, we can better comprehend the complexity of the challenges that must be faced. Significant thought must come into transforming data into information for the purposes of medical knowledge. The ability to collect, organize, analyze, and retrieve data via computers in a meaningful way extends and expands the discriminating capacity and problem-solving abilities of providers. Data, information, and knowledge are essential building blocks for health information systems.

Coded Data Versus Text Processing

Patient data are expressed in coded form and natural language or text. Coded data are exemplified by the use of standard coding systems such as the ICD9-CM and CPT systems. There are multiple coding systems in place that bring standard expression to clinical data. Coded data have the advantage of consistency of expression for

TABLE 17–2 DATA TYPES REQUIRED FOR CPRs	
DATA TYPE	**EXAMPLES**
Text	Hospital discharge summary; history and physical; narrative operative report
Numbers	ICD9 codes
	CPT codes
	Blood pressure value recording 140/86
Voice	Stored dictation accessed by phone or PC; voice recognition of radiology dictation results
Image	Radiology film, document image
Video	Echocardiogram
Drawings	Drawing of a burn distribution on a body surface
Signal	Electroencephalogram or electrocardiogram tracings

diagnoses, procedures, laboratory tests, drugs, and so on. Yet, due to strengths and weaknesses in these systems, none completely addresses the clarity and precision required to capture and represent clinical facts. The National Library of Medicine project to establish the Unified Medical Language System is an ambitious attempt to bring together diverse coding schemes with general medical terms to create a vast thesaurus that will link together related terms for the benefit of diverse users. This work includes, for example, initial COSTAR terms for problem statements. Even though these were developed for a specific application, the content has provided a starting point for CPR designers to develop problem list directories that can link to associated codes such as the ICD9-CM when appropriate and can be compared with data from other institutions for analysis and research.

Many health information system developers bring significant energy to work on coding systems as they currently are used for claims processing and billing as well as epidemiologic and outcomes research efforts. Thus efforts are focused on improving the current coding schemes and seeking or developing an ideal replacement. Advocates believe that strong coding schemes are essential components in health information systems and that the fastest way to establish and secure consistent data from health care organizations is through standard coding systems. There continues to be national and international interest in identifying an "ideal" coding system that will secure accurate, efficient data capture from the care delivery experience and that accurately represents the clinical concepts. These tools address part of the problem but do not fully support current models of thinking used by physicians and other health care team members in the care delivery process.

The majority of the patient record in most institutions still consists of unstructured text. This is the most natural medium of expression and, to date, best details the thinking and conclusions of those planning and delivering care. In fact, the majority of the content of paper records is free text. Because of this reality, the value of technology for natural language processing is well recognized. "Medicine needs a system based on an architecture that could capture medical data in natural language form, structure it in alternative ways and retrieve it through queries that allow users to retrieve and display information in multiple forms including conversion into standard codes as well as natural language expressions. **Text processing** may be defined as the computer processing of natural language."[31] This is a far more sophisticated endeavor than the notion of searching text by key words, a process well known in library research today. It requires a comprehensiveness and completeness of content such that a given domain of medicine will be adequately represented. Therefore, natural language processing for cardiology, for instance, would need to include all the terms and expressions used by cardiologists in their models of thinking. Symptoms, related medical terms, and specific cardiology expressions (including semantic linkages and relationships) would all be required elements.

One example of a current approach to this problem includes semantic systems that focus on semantic information to process the natural language text. Pattern matching is used to match like or similar patterns and convert them into standard encoded forms. Pattern matching is very useful in some areas of medical terminology when content is highly structured. Anatomic pathology would be an example. For patient record hospital discharge summaries, however, this approach is not effective.[29]

Script-based systems, an alternative approach, have made a significant contribution to this work as well. Script-based systems combine keywords and scripts. Scripts may be a predesigned expression that represents information about consequences of care processes. Scanning for keywords invokes a particular script. The script itself then serves as a building block for the remainder of the text-processing event. It may act as a template that specifies necessary components and the properties required. When the entity in the text is found, the template is completed. Medical transcriptionists apply a similar concept when they develop and maintain stored phrases that can be invoked to quickly assemble reports such as history and physical examinations. This allows single key words to be indexed to longer medical expressions. Thus physician dictation, for instance, would be significantly streamlined when such tools are in place. As we consider the role of natural language processing in medicine, the emphasis is placed on how natural language is used by clinicians and others to communicate between and among clinical data, knowledge bases, expert systems, and others. Friedman and Johnson point out that this occurs in three ways: as input submitted by a user to a system that will be new information stored in the data base; as query expressions used to seek information from the system; and information retrieved that may be converted into natural language for the user.[31]

We can look to additional work in this area to advance the automation of clinical data while preserving the natural thinking patterns and communication models employed by clinicians. In 1994, Sager et al noted[31]:

> In the evolution of computerized patient record systems, the controversy between free text and preset categories for recording patient data has not been resolved. The need for standards pushes toward preset categories and controlled vocabularies, while the need for expressive power, so as not to distort the patient data, speaks

for allowing some amount of free-text reporting. A compromise that is not compromising is calling.

Strategic Recommendations

With these features clearly laid out, how then will we move the United States healthcare industry in this direction? The IOM tackled that question and identified strategic recommendations. These were broad-based initiatives combined with practical strategies. The IOM study resulted in strategic recommendations designed to promote and facilitate the rapid development of computer-based patient records (see Institute of Medicine's Strategic Recommendations).

Institute of Medicine's Strategic Recommendations

• Health care professionals and organizations should adopt the computer-based patient record (CPR) as the standard for medical and all other records related to patient care.

• To accomplish the first Recommendation, the public and private sectors should join in establishing a computer-based patient record Institute (CPRI) to promote and facilitate development, implementation, and dissemination of the CPR.

• Both the public and private sectors should expand support for the CPR and CPR system implementation through research, development, and demonstration projects. Specifically, the committee recommends that Congress authorize and appropriate funds to implement the research and development agenda outlined herein. The committee further recommends that private foundations and vendors fund programs that support and facilitate this research and development agenda.

• The CPRI should promulgate uniform national standards for data and security to facilitate implementation of the CPR and its secondary databases.

• The CPRI should review federal and state laws and regulations for the purpose of proposing and promulgating model legislation and regulations to facilitate the implementation and dissemination of the CPR and its secondary databases and to streamline the CPR and CPR systems.

• The costs of CPR systems should be shared by those who benefit from the value of the the CPR. Specifically, the full costs of implementing and operating CPRs and CPR systems should be factored into reimbursement levels or payment schedules of both public and private sector third-party payers. In addition, users of secondary databases should support the costs of creating such databases.

• Health care professional schools and organizations should enhance educational programs for students and practitioners in the use of computer, CPRs, and CPR systems for patient care, education, and research.

Progress Toward a CPR

Progress has occurred. The institute recommended by the IOM study was established in 1991 and has steadily grown in its mission. A national will has been embraced by providers and those who deliver care. Significant investments are in place. Major vendors today are marketing CPR software. Others are serving as **niche vendors** who develop and market one or two applications only. In an effort to meet limited needs, vendors then form partnerships to integrate and build comprehensive systems. The consistency of purpose has aligned planning and development efforts on multiple fronts. The progress made by the Computer-based Patient Record Institute to date:

• Demonstrated leadership and initiative in its growth and sponsorship of landmark efforts since its inception in 1991.

• Formed alliances with federal and state agencies and consortiums with companion sponsors.

• Supported and engaged in work in standards development needed to advance the pace of development of automated systems that can conform to common content and information exchange conventions.

• Fostered education and research through publication of a compendium on cost-benefit experiences of computer-based patient record initiatives.

• Underscored the professional leadership of the American Health Information Management Association in a leadership role.

• Endorsed and employed work groups focused on key development areas such as work on confidentiality and privacy matters and others that needed legislative efforts supporting demonstrations of CPR systems.

Envisioned by the IOM as a necessary sponsor and driver needed to achieve computer-based patient records, the CPRI has been a leader in this work. It has been an appropriate partner to the health care industry efforts to work toward the same goal, and it has not worked alone. The parallel work has moved ahead as well.

New Ideas in Development

Progress under way at institutional levels incorporates many of the recommendations of the IOM study. Let's consider them briefly.

Some organizations have selected one vendor's integrated product; some have elected to combine multiple vendors. Others have adopted preliminary strategies for increasing automation for their organizations in a stepwise manner, moving toward integration at some point in the future. In these cases, it is thought that there is time to take some key steps and still wait to adopt a single-focus direction. The benefit of working with one vendor offers speed of implementation and tight integration of applications. A number of vendors are offering CPR software and have included multimedia functionality in their products. For many hospitals and other health care organizations, this is the best approach. They rely on a vendor's history and experience and support the necessary interfaces to existing applications already in place in their organizations. Further, many of these vendors have brought in experienced health information professionals in positions ranging from design consultants to vice presidents. This has strengthened their products from the patient record management perspective. Health information professionals have made significant gains in leading efforts to transform the paper record into electronic formats in many of these cases. Some have chosen to market on-line transcription as an opening step to beginning work on the CPR. This, in concert with increased availability of PC workstations linked to hospital data systems, has offered practitioners access to increased data and the experience of retrieving it in automated form. There have, of course, been management issues around volumes and organization of data in these efforts. The support from current word processing tools that offer powerful formatting and other text handling tools has made these efforts worthwhile.

The limitation is that there are, as yet, no vendors who can deliver all of the components in consistent strength needed to produce the CPR as we envision it today. One current approach combines the data from existing older systems and new applications that may exist within a single institution—data transferred from diverse applications (perhaps running on different computer platforms)—to a combined resource and reorganized into a **clinical data repository.** The benefit of developing a data repository offers organizations the ability to establish the data base and use standard data base management systems to create the ability to retrieve information in a tailored fashion. Healthcare organizations establish **information warehouses** that receive clinical data from the transactions systems such as a pharmacy system or a radiology system and combine them with other organizational data. Data can be reconciled and made available through a variety of current tools such as:

- report writers
- statistical packages
- graphics tools

It can also be presented in a series of clinical views or profiles designed to deliver the CPR content to users. Golob characterizes the purposes of a clinical data repository as follows[32]:

- Provides easy access to patient information for providers and demonstrates time saved over the paper record use
- Expedites results reporting through customizable displays
- Provides quick and easy access to longitudinal patient data
- Supports a common user interface for accessing patient information—usually via a workstation
- Provides information in a comprehensive, integrated manner rather than by departmental orientation
- Provides an easy vehicle for applying population management for the prospective clinical planning needed today
- Supports monitoring and analysis of patient care outcomes

State and other data systems that require data from hospitals and/or participating organizations are examples of data repositories. In fact, the advances made in community-based health information systems have relied on the principles and benefits seen in the repository approach. Its ability to provide utilization and resource analysis information across institutional settings is a key value for participating providers. Even organizations taking a slower approach to acquiring a CPR within their institutional setting may already be involved in community-based health information through their participation in state data systems.

Finally, progress in education for the CPR and, in the larger context, medical informatics has occurred. Health educators are teaching students about the CPR and the potential for the integration of computer technology within their respective disciplines. Computer technology is used in computer-assisted instruction and is available in settings where students complete practicums.

INFORMATION TECHNOLOGY FOR HEALTH CARE

In order to deliver cost-effective health information management systems and CPRs, we must rely on information technology—hardware, software, and telecommunications to collect, store, manage, and transmit health information. The following briefly reviews key concepts in these areas and illustrates their role in health care information systems. Consideration of how information technology has evolved will help in understanding how we have moved to the current expectations in information systems.

Hardware

Hardware is the physical equipment that makes up computers and computer systems. This includes the electric, electronic, mechanical, and other equipment. The computer requires a central processing unit with

TABLE 17-3 DATA INPUT AND OUTPUT OPTIONS

KEYBOARDS AND TERMINALS (CATHODE RAY TUBE OR VIDEO DISPLAY MONITOR)

Link monitor screen to the computer and use for data entry and retrieval. Terminals may use a keyboard, a point and click device, or touch screen in which finger touch selection guides the user through the process.

PC WORKSTATIONS

PCs used for "one-stop" access and retrieval. They perform the same functions as the keyboards and terminals and contain programs that can manipulate the information locally. PC workstations often contain standard software tools such as word processing, spreadsheets, databases, and electronic mail applications.

HAND-HELD COMPUTERS (ALSO CALLED PERSONAL DATA ASSISTANTS, PDA)

Devices available for point of service input; travels with caregiver; can be wireless. These are also known as pocket devices.

MINIATURIZED CRTs

Very small terminals (less than 3 inches across) that can be mounted and made available for users at eye level, freeing user from moving to check data.

SCANNERS AND WANDS

Used for quick reading of bar codes or other scannable input documents such as service billing sheet data or patient self-recorded history questionnaires. Some scanners enable the computer to read a printed or handwritten page. See optical scanning.

SENSORS

Devices used to sense and record changes in temperature, weight, and others. Monitoring equipment uses sensors to collect, display, and record data.

VOICE RECOGNITION

Computer capability to understand human speech. This allows practitioners to talk directly to devices and record findings. Emergency and radiology departments have applied this technology.

VOICE RESPONSE

Units that use prerecorded messages or speech synthesizers and are capable of communicating directly to users.

PRINTERS

Used to print reports and copies of screen displays. Printers are valued according to speed, print quality, noise, reliability, and size.

MICROFILM/MICROFICHE (COMPUTER OUTPUT MICROFILM)

Produced by computers for such uses as master patient indexes, these retrieve data through special readers. They are a less costly alternative to maintaining data on-line.

DISK DRIVE/DISKETTE

Part of the computer that reads software and data files into memory. As an output device, it writes information from the computer to the disk, thereby allowing backup of the completed work.

OPTICAL DISK

A disk that is written and read by light. CDs, CD-ROMs, and video disks are recorded at the point of manufacture and cannot be erased. WORMs (write once read many) are optical disks recorded in user locations that cannot be erased.

capacity to hold data being processed as well as the equipment needed to carry out the data processing functions. Peripheral equipment including magnetic disk and tape drives, data input devices such as terminals and PCs, and output devices such as printers and plotters are also hardware. Computers come in mainframe, mini, and micro sizes. **Mainframe** machines are used for major applications, to maintain large databases, and for high-volume work. **Minicomputers** are often used in departmental systems such as laboratory or radiology systems. And **microcomputers** are used in individual applications such as a single-user donor registry and as workstations for larger systems. Most managers use microcomputers on a daily basis.

Input, Output, and Storage Devices

Data can be collected automatically from other computer systems or it can be entered through a manned data entry process. Biomedical devices such as automated electrocardiogram systems and patient monitoring systems convert data from one form to another and transmit it to a database. Terminals, PCs, optical scanning devices, and pen-based devices are operated by users to capture and enter data into computer systems. Computers can receive input directly from remote computers through communications networks. Collen noted that, "With respect to medical information systems, the most important innovation in the 1980s was probably the improved connections among machines into more general, local, national and worldwide high-speed networks. Using network technology, hospitals could unite all the different computers throughout their various departments, even though the computers were located in geographically dispersed locations."[33] Table 17–3 defines and describes input and output devices.

Terminals and Workstations

The most common method of data retrieval is the terminal and/or a workstation. **Terminals** are connected to information systems and are used to enter and retrieve information. A hospital information system has terminals located at nursing units for data entry such as ordering patient services as well as to retrieve information such as laboratory test results. While terminals are still common to health information systems of all kinds, in recent years this has given way to the PC as a more sophisticated and powerful input device. The need now is to provide such devices that are connected to one or more computer applications to serve as fundamental **workstations** for users. As currently defined, a workstation is a PC that is connected to an information system.

It is used to connect directly with the database in the system and to access and receive information from the system directly. When the information is passed to the workstation, it can be further processed at the PC level. In addition, being PCs, such workstations do house software applications as well. Electronic tools currently available such as local word processing software, spreadsheets, and database tools can be coupled with information provided through the health information system connection. The user may manipulate data on the workstation and send it through electronic mail to another user in the system. In addition, computer users may access external resources through communications equipment such as the Internet and others that offer up-to-the-minute references and clinical support tools. The Internet is a telecommunications international computer network that serves as a gateway to a multitude of users. The workstation is planned as the ubiquitous doorway for all users; and is a key concept in the computer-based patient record. Objectives of a professional workstation are listed below.[29]

Workstation Objectives

- Increase user productivity.
- Reduce data entry time and eliminate redundant data entry.
- Standardize the provider/system interface by allowing command and response specifications of a hospital information system to be user-modifiable.
- Complete the bulk of the patient care documentation during the patient encounter through on-line, point of service data capture—bedside and examination room.
- Improve quality of care through clinical guidelines availability.
- Provide intervention messages for exceptional patient conditions through innovative displays.
- Facilitate the management of free text data.
- Allow for new voice input/output, handwriting recognition, and imaging technology to be incorporated into the workstation.
- Facilitate the collection of administrative, financial, and clinical data for outcomes, research, organizational assessment, and resource management studies.
- Increase accessibility to medical information through the use of clinical decision support tools and the provision of easy-to-use links to existing medical reference data bases (MEDLINE).
- Provide easy access to output processes that integrate various result data to display medical information.
- Lessen the risk of data loss and mitigate the effects of a system failure through the local collection and storage of patient data (that can be stored for transmission to the HIS after recovery).[36]

Most health care practitioners today are already influenced by the power and communications options available through computer workstations. The home computer industry has done much to educate the consumer about software and the communications capability of computers. Managers work with electronic mail within and beyond their organizations. In small group practice settings, PCs are used to maintain the patient record with retrieval readily available for transcribed notes as well as data sent through communications links from hospitals and special care centers that are linked to these settings. Indeed, the computer is becoming as common as the telephone in business environments.

Pen-Based Devices

Pen-based and hand-held computers offer a very specialized approach to the workstation. These are devices that can be carried in the pocket. They have built-in communications and organizer software. The goal is to ultimately replace beepers, mobile phones, personal organizers, fax machines, and laptop computers. In the health care industry, one example of **pen-based devices** is use in home health organizations in which visiting nurses use the pen-based device to record the visit encounter data. In another case, a pen-based device is used to document IV therapy data in hospitalized patients. In both examples, the devices are used for daily tasks and are plugged into a "dock" or receiving component that transfers the data into a larger computer system. As of early 1994, these devices were still clearly developmental. They are limited by size and display capability and by the lack of full recognition of handwriting. In a report published in August, 1993, the technology was estimated to be able to read the user's handwritten characters about 95 per cent of the time. As an example, on average, one of every two telephone numbers written on a PDA screen is misinterpreted by the software.[34] So while additional technologic details need to be refined, these devices do offer promise for busy practitioners once these matters are resolved. They may, indeed, become an effective working tool for capturing patient information.

Document Imaging Devices

One approach to developing a computer-based patient record is to use **document imaging** as a way to capture and store text-based information. Some hospitals have already initiated this process as a strategic step in moving toward a fully computerized patient record. In these departments, patient record forms are scanned via document imaging as soon as they are sent to the department. Once the record is scanned, all functions needed to process it, such as quality review, coding, data abstraction, and others, can be done through a workstation that provides the capability to retrieve the scanned items. This offers fast processing capability and retrieval available through workstations around the hospital with extensive access for users. As a data input approach, document imaging builds an effective bridge between the paper record system and computer-based patient record through familiarizing providers with the general technology and the capability to retrieve needed information in multiple locations. Through workstations around a hospital, physicians may access records of previous hospitalizations directly through a PC. With the technology for **multimedia** coming into its own, many health care organizations are combining the use of optical storage systems with digital health information systems to offer initial multimedia features of an increasingly electronic patient record. Multimedia processing incorporates data, voice, and video to communicate through a PC workstation.

Voice Recognition

Voice recognition is considered by many to be the major breakthrough needed to fully automate the patient record. This is because it offers the most efficient means for practitioners to incorporate data capture into their normal routines. When the health care team works with many patients throughout the day, the methods used to capture the necessary clinical and service information must be easy to use. How do busy practitioners incorporate working with a computer workstation into daily activities in ways that conserve time? For many, the possibility of voice recognition offers the greatest promise. This technology has grown phenomenally over the past 10 years. Effective uses were noted in emergency departments and radiology and surgical pathology applications in the late 1980s; however, speed was generally slow and the vocabulary was limited. These systems require a voice recognition board in the computer and associated software.

Compatibility with existing software, expansion of vocabulary, techniques for establishing computer recognition of the user's voice, and cost are still issues that need work. However, there are reports of successes that are worth noting. In one example, an automated speech recognition application was used to explore the use and benefits of such a system for nursing documentation in a hospital. The system allowed nurses to create patient documentation by speaking directly to a PC. There was little or no use of a keyboard. Linked directly to a hospital information system, this application provided immediate retrieval as well as a hard copy. This hospital acquired three voice systems which contained 10,000-word, speaker-independent vocabularies. Speaker-independent refers to words that the system recognizes regardless of who speaks. Nurses in two target areas, emergency and surgery, were selected as domain experts and worked with the developers to set up a nursing documentation care plan. The user spoke a few "trigger" words into the system to call up much longer phrases that were entered into the text. For instance, a trigger word allowed the nurse to express complex observations on several key words or phrases, thereby saving significant nursing documentation time and still capturing patient data effectively. In this case, "just 12 words trigger the system to create a 44-word passage that completely, accurately, and, in accordance with standardized guidelines, describes the nursing assessment for a particular patient."[35] Once continuous voice and extensive vocabularies become available, data capture and retrieval will grow quickly and this technology will offer rapid developments in CPR systems.

Software—Operating Systems and Programming Languages for Applications

Software is the set of instructions and documentation required to operate computers and their applications. Software includes programs that are sets of instructions that direct actual computer operating functions, called the computer **operating system**, and sets of instructions used to direct specific types of business processes, known as **application software.** Software written to process medication orders is an application software. These are combined to direct the overall functions of a given information system. The operating system directs the internal functions of the computer. It serves as the bridge to application programs. Without an operating system, each programmer would have to program all the detail involved with receiving data, displaying graphics on a screen, how data would be sent to printers, and so forth. Operating systems contain all of the standard routine directions that handle such tasks. Creating a common platform for all the software that is used, operating systems act as system managers that direct the execution of programs, allocate time to multiple users, and operate the input/output devices as well as the communication lines. Operating systems are provided by the hardware manufacturer. While operating systems have developed in the complexity required for large computers, they have become simpler for microcomputers. An example of an operating system worth noting is UNIX. Capable of supporting a number of powerful utility programs and time-sharing and multiuser access, UNIX was designed to run on more than one kind of computer, thereby making it more universal for more users preparing for the interchangeability of computing resources.[33]

Programming languages refer to the variety of sets of instructions developed to operate applications and to generate instructions themselves. Software has developed significantly over the past 30 years and the evolution of new generations of programming languages has enhanced the use and rapid development of computing power. Generally speaking, all instructions to computers are ultimately expressed in their native codes. Known as machine language, this most basic level of programming refers to the system of codes by which the instructions are represented internally in the computer. To illustrate: A programmer writing in a computer's low-level machine language uses machine instructions to address memory cells for storing data, accumulators to add and subtract numbers, and registers to store operands and results. Some codes represent instructions for the central processor, some codes move the data from the accumulator into the main memory, some codes represent data or information about data, and some codes point to locations (addresses) in memory.[33]

The second-generation programming languages built on machine codes by the invention of a symbolic notation called assembly language. Assembly language used key words to invoke sets of machine instructions. Terms such as "Add" or "Load" represented specific sets of machine instructions. These low-level languages used such terms known as "mnemonic" codes to program more efficiently. The assemblers were used to translate program instructions directly into machine code. Even in the 1990s programs needing extreme efficiency are still written in assembly language because this language gives the most efficient control over the program's operations within the computer.

Programming languages evolved along with computers. More powerful programming languages applied the notion of using predetermined, available sets or sequences of machine level instructions to simplify programming tasks. The goal was and is to develop and use programming languages that simulate natural language as much as possible.

Third-generation programming languages extended the efficiency of the programmers by offering the capability to write programs in languages that were shorter, quicker to write, and had fewer errors. They combined more and more of the machine level instructions to accomplish their tasks. This generation of language also introduced a new capability. Some could run on different machines. Examples of third-generation programming languages include Fortran (Formula Translator), APL (A Programming Language), COBOL (Common Business-Oriented Language), and BASIC (Beginners All-purpose Symbolic Instruction Code). An excellent tool for learning, BASIC generated error messages as students entered their program line by line into the computer. Students could respond and make corrections easily. ALGOL (Algorithmic Language), PL/1 (Programming Language One), PASCAL, C, and ADA were additional languages considered third generation.

One programming language, MUMPS (Massachusetts General Hospital Utility Multi-Programming System), was established for specific use in health care applications. Collen notes that MUMPS was probably the most commonly used programming language in the United States for clinical applications during the 1970s and 1980s. The COSTAR system was written in MUMPS. In recent years, DXplain was developed in MUMPS. DXplain is a diagnostic decision support system in use today. DXplain can be purchased to run on local PCs and is in use in individual practices as well as in more sophisticated health information systems. As of the late 1980s, both the Department of Defense and the Veterans Administration had installed nationwide medical information systems using MUMPS.[33]

Fourth-generation languages emerged with even greater efficiencies by enabling programmers to use instructions at a higher level. They worked with program generators—sets of instructions that could be invoked as components when needed. This allowed them to focus more on the logic of the program and less on the instructions to the computer. They were designed for powerful manipulation and used program-generation techniques. LISP (List Processing) language, for example, was used to manipulate various lists such as a group or sequence of elements, numbers, words, diseases, symptoms, and so forth. This level of programming languages supported work in artificial intelligence and medical applications.

Communications

Communications technology has revolutionized both performance and expectations for data access, transmission, and use. As the backbone of health information systems, it was targeted in 1993 as a significant element of health care reform. Health care organizations are currently linked in alliances of all kinds. Health maintenance organizations (HMOs) and primary care networks (PCNs) are two examples. It addition, we have seen how the evolution of health care extends from ambulatory and hospital care to home health, occupational health, hospice, and rehabilitation facilities. Information systems are passing data to coordinate patient care, to more efficiently process claims, to facilitate collaborative planning and research, and to control costs. Consumers are expecting their clinical information to be transferred among providers to maintain the flow of health services. Most health information professionals are using communications technology to accomplish daily tasks, both within and beyond their immediate organizational boundaries.

Communications technology is used within individual organizations to connect the terminals, workstations, printers, and storage equipment to the computer. Information systems that operate with a mainframe computer utilize communications technology to network all the terminals located at nursing stations and ancillary areas. Communications technology has evolved from the basic terminal to computer connection to local and wide area networks and the client server technology. A **local area network** (LAN) connects multiple devices together via communications and is located within a small geographic area. An example of a LAN is a medical computing system at a primary care clinic in which seven PCs are connected to a server. The physicians and nurses all access the server for patient files as needed. The basic job of a local area network is to physically link a few to several hundred PCs together and often to a mainframe or minicomputer. The mainframe or minicomputer—and even some microcomputers—provide the location for all or some of the data needed by the PC users. Other data and programs needed for processing them may be located on each PC locally. Communications technology consists of a variety of materials such as twisted-wire cables, fiberoptics, phone lines, and even infrared light and radio signals.

Typically, a message is sent from one PC to another. This may be a query for data, a response to a request, or an instruction to run a program that may be stored on the network. The action may require data stored locally in the PC or data maintained on the **file server.** A file server is a specialized PC, or larger host computer, that is used only to provide a common place to store all the data that the PC users may need. The configuration of the LAN enables the users to retrieve and use the data as rapidly as possible. The network must receive requests from individual PCs, handle simultaneous requests, and send messages to the appropriate requester. In effect, it must manage traffic. LAN topologies refer to the physical configurations of the networks.

Wide area networks (WANs) are used for extensive, geographically larger environments. They are often used for computer systems connecting separate institutions. They are also used for computer systems in large single institutions. An extensive WAN was installed at the Columbia-Presbyterian Medical Center. Beginning in the late 1980s and supported by a federal grant program, this institution has installed an extensive network that encompassed 18 buildings at seven geographically separate sites. Based on the goal of a workstation for "one-stop shopping," this institution has combined clinical and research computing facilities with library and PC utilities such as word processing and electronic mail. Columbia-Presbyterian Medical Center has demonstrated the value of implementing this technology as an overall technical strategy in building a comprehensive information system.[36]

Client Server Technology

Client server computing is the splitting of an application into tasks that are performed on separate computers, one of which is a programmable workstation. Put another way, client server computing is a form of **cooperative processing**. Figure 17–3 illustrates the five types of this technology: distributed presentation, remote presentation, distributed logic, remote data management, and distributed database.[37]

Cooperative processing distributes the processing tasks to different systems for optimal responsiveness. By separating shared data, for instance from the application program, it can provide more efficient computer functions. It seeks to achieve the best performance for low-volume and high-volume processing, optimal network

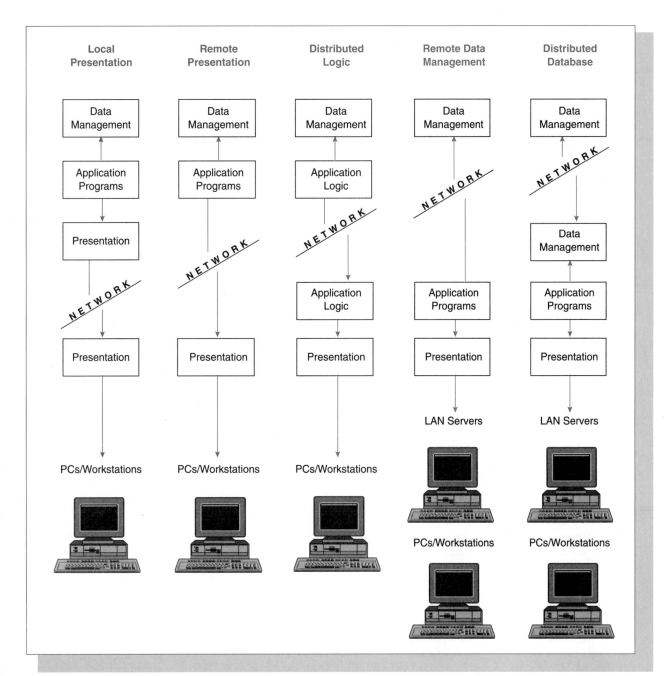

FIGURE 17–3. Client server configurations.

traffic, and realistic security and control. The benefits are improved user experiences because the workstation capability improves through custom presentations and reduction of the traffic on the system network. In cooperative processing, the host computer typically works with a microcomputer. The host computer may perform the tasks associated with maintaining the application database and the microcomputer controls the presentation of the data and the user's interaction with the data.

An example of client server technology occurs when clinical data from transaction systems such as laboratory and pharmacy systems are sent to a workstation. Programs housed in the workstation then direct the format of display and data. For instance, customer-designed flowsheet data display formats may differ from one medical discipline to another at the workstation level yet the information may be retrieved from the same source (server) because the client workstation uses local application logic to retrieve that presentation. Client server technology employs networks for data transmission. The technology must combine and connect technical functions at three levels: the host server (often mainframe systems), the network functions, and the intelligent workstation capability. Simply expressed, large computer applications are in the process of employing networks and their associated operating systems to distribute and extend computing operations to workstation customers who are operating diverse machines. In a large customer environment, for instance, the organization may employ this approach to connect to both PC/DOS and MacIntosh machines. Implications for this technology are many. For those involved in developing CPR systems, integrity of data is a major concern. There must be adequate data management tools to ensure the integrity of updates so that every user is assured of having reliable, timely data. This technologic approach gained significant ground in the 1990s.

Databases

A **database** is a collection of stored data—typically organized into fields, records, and files—and an associated description. A **database management system** (DBMS) is an integrated set of programs that manages access to the database.[18] Databases have evolved with emerging technology and advances in software tools. They are used to store the data required by the application programs to accomplish the system objectives. The goal of data structures within a database is to be able to represent the basic meaning of data in a medium that allows powerful retrieval and manipulation for users. Major database designs are:

- hierarchical
- relational
- object-oriented

Database Alternatives

HIERARCHICAL DATABASE. This is a tree-like network in which nodes are connected by links such that all links reference from child to parent. The way this kind of database operates can be illustrated in the manner it is searched. A user questions (queries) the database and the search seeks the answer from parent to child. The nodes that meet the conditions of the question are identified by searching downward through the tree. Retrieving involves gathering the root record and following pointers to the record in the next lower levels, which, in turn, contain pointers to the level below them. Each datum has only one parent. In cases in which a particular datum may need to be represented in more than one part of the database and related to more than one parent, the data may be managed through pointers that refer to the multiple locations of the data item. Hierarchical databases can be very effective when the questions are predetermined and pointers can be used to effect shortcuts. Flexible methods are required to update the database. It is not flexible for those questions that were not yet determined at the time the database was designed. The tree structure is an effective database structure only as long as the levels of the hierarchy are limited. The problems with this structure arise when the data are needed for more than one purpose. Then multiple hierarchies have to be superimposed on a single data structure, or the data have to be copied.

NETWORK DATABASE. This is a variation of the hierarchical database in which pointers are used extensively to provide greater flexibility to the hierarchical model.

THE RELATIONAL DATABASE. The most widely used database model, this design utilizes a straightforward and easily understood concept. A relational database is made up of tables. Each table names a relation and consists, in turn, of rows and columns. A relation scheme can be defined as a set of attribute names for the relation. Retrieval uses relational algebra to manipulate relations. In a relational database, relationships between files are created by comparing data, such as medical numbers and names. A relational system can take any two or more files and generate a new file from those that meet the matching criteria. Key fields are used as indexes to speed the process. Relational database vendors have optimized their systems for speed, and, for most applications, they are sufficient. This database structure has gained popularity for use on personal computers. It is easily understood and lends itself well to medical applications such as registries that are used in health information management departments. These systems provide convenient direct retrieval and limited update, but processing for deep data analysis is not supported. Relational technology handles less complex transactions such as registering a patient and is organized so that data are independent of the programs that manipulate them. It does not handle arrays and repeating groups efficiently and does not easily accommodate data types such as unstructured text, video, and voice. The relational database was a natural for the application of **standard query language** (SQL). Now an ANSI standard, this tool includes database query techniques as well as features for defining the structure of the data, modification, and specifying security constraints within the database.

OBJECT-ORIENTED DATABASE. This is the most recently developed and newest philosophy for information storage. The object-oriented model is broader than the relational model and can be applied to a wide range of contexts outside database management. The object-oriented approach is designed for more complex transactions, such as those required to manipulate the patient record. It handles arrays more efficiently than relational technology. Object-oriented databases contain characteristics to control, manage, and query the database.

Data Structure

The data structure specified for the CPR is an integrated, distributed database. Foundation to the CPR will be a standard dictionary of data items that will be used in constructing the database. The database requirements for an optimal CPR have been outlined:

- Must accommodate reading of transaction level detail—such as that found in a hospital order entry module—if the CPR is to be created as a byproduct of the care processes as well as accommodate operational and clinical research and serve as the sole legal record

- Must have the capability to record original data, changes, and/or updates to those data and maintain access to prior versions

- Must maintain a record of who performed them and when the changes occurred

- The level of detail must accommodate statutory requirements such as those required in prescription detail

- There must be a single integrated source of data about the patient

- Users must be able to trust the completeness of the data

- Standardized methods for updating patient data must be in place

While the physical design of the database can and likely will be spread across multiple databases, the logical access and retrieval for users should look and feel like a single database. There will also be a need to access and retrieve patient information according to selected data views that represent specialty care, longitudinal high-level summaries, and other elements. Distributing the processing among different applications and computers is also necessary to permit use of different types of processing resources in multiple institutions and sharing common data with local additions. Integrated access of remote information/knowledge databases to automatically invoke intelligence and incorporate expert knowledge, alert and reminder features, and tools will bring the "intelligence" to the CPR. It will be crucial to establish standards for transmission and coordination and management of new information within the databases to provide a virtual patient record with currency and accuracy.[29]

Architecture

Architecture is defined as the composite of specific components and the way in which they interact to form a computer system.[38] Architecture provides a metaphoric way to describe business environments as well as tangible hardware and software configurations. It depicts the relationships and the general functions of a computer system's equipment and how it fits together to constitute the system. Architecture refers to the ways specific hardware and communications equipment are technically organized and connected within organizations to operate the ongoing information systems that support the business functions. Overall, the technical architecture is used as the storage, road map, and transmission base for data to be processed. On the other hand, data architecture tends to the collection, management, and storage of the data for organizations.

Consider another example using database architecture and the associated hardware. We can describe a database architecture as having three layers:

- First, a user interface interacts directly with a user to accept information about specific criteria to search for information about the topics considered.

- Second, an analysis module, the "thinking" part of the system, makes decisions about the patterns that should be sought and submits queries and statistical questions to the search engine.

- Third, the search engine executes the queries and statistical questions against the database.

These queries may be SQL statements to be handled as standard routines by the database architecture. The hardware configuration may be a client server arrangement in which the client is a workstation manned by a nurse or analyst user and the server is where the database resides. The architecture consists of all components of the system. We typically view architecture in graphic displays or drawings that show a top-down picture of the various components of the system (Figure 17–4).

Open Systems

Open systems architecture refers to the use of computers based on industry-standard hardware and software components. Unix and the PC/DOS and MS/DOS operating systems are examples. Standards typically define the interfaces between system hardware, operating

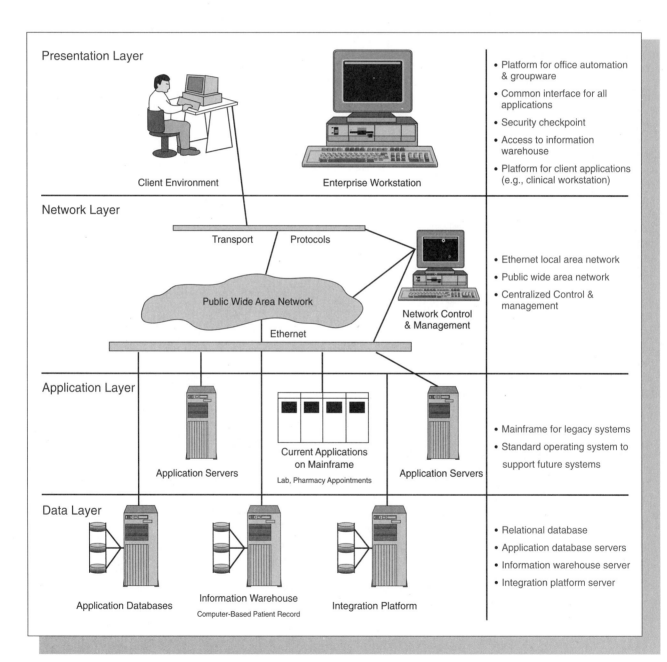

FIGURE 17–4. Future architecture technology.

systems, and databases, and even the look and feel of user interfaces. The theory is that when open systems are used, users can select from multiple vendor products, thereby increasing their flexibility. The goal is to move to a computing environment that supports a variety of applications. Organizations are working to bring together existing systems with new applications. Information systems departments are working with new software that transforms data from older "legacy" systems and places it into a repository. Open systems is playing a major role in shaping the computer industry in the 1990s.

HEALTH INFORMATION SYSTEM APPLICATIONS

Throughout this chapter, illustrations have been provided to express the common goals, features, and problems of health information systems. In this section, several examples of administrative and clinical applications that are typical components of health information systems are reviewed. Health care organizations today are heavily involved in acquiring or developing these applications and bringing them together to work in a formally integrated information system or in a well-coordinated set of information systems.

Administrative Applications

Administrative applications include those applications that operate the daily business functions in the organizations. These typically include registration-admission, discharge, transfer applications (R-ADT), the business functions carried out in health information management departments, material management, claims processing, financial systems, and decision support systems. The clinical systems include those associated with ordering, receiving, monitoring, and documenting patient care.

The R-ADT system is an example of a foundation administrative system. A basic module contained in hospital information systems, this application collects the initial set of data that is used to establish a "record" of the new admission in all affected hospital departments and to "append" follow-up data and functions after discharge. As an application customer, a health information services (HIS) department links to the R-ADT application in order to accomplish the following functions:

- Create and update the institutional master patient index
- Generate census displays and associated reports as needed throughout the institution

- Initiate utilization protocols where appropriate
- Initiate patient record retrieval through automated record tracking modules
- Notify transcription and provide identification data for early reports
- Pass data to outpatient scheduling systems to facilitate clinic appointments
- Notify and send preliminary data to local applications such as cancer and implant registries
- Connect, where established, with physician office systems through telecommunications to notify and provide data directly to involved physicians

At the point of discharge, it generates similar notification to the necessary departments. This would include discharge and transfer notification to ancillary and service areas so that the information on that case can be closed and notifications initiated for new activities such as room set-up and materials ordering that begin when one patient leaves the institution. In HIS departments, the data collection work continues directly with record completion modules, transcription, and discharge abstracting functions directly from the patient record. The same notice generated from R-ADT can activate record tracking modules and quality monitors for follow-up action, and the discharge abstract function builds on the initial database. In many health care organizations, hospital discharge data are collected into a database that also includes outpatient data and may include additional service information if the organization extends to alliances with physician office practices as well.

Encoders are another example of an administrative application found in HIS departments that automate the coding function. Providing automatic code assignment when the diagnosis is entered, these systems have brought consistency, speed, improved accuracy, and expert system tools to the coding function. Coding functions require the combined skill level of trained practitioners and the automation supplied through encoders. Linked to DRG management systems, encoders illustrate how technology has affected business processes in health care organizations.

Decision Support Systems

Decision support systems are information systems designed to support planning functions of an organization. They range from simple analysis of cost per patient for specific departments or clinics to high-level strategic analysis, marketing, and policy development. They draw from multiple databases to analyze the day-to-day business activities of the organization.

EXAMPLE

In constructing a decision support system for a health maintenance organization that includes a hospital, ambulatory long-term care, and home health agency, the planners collected data from on-line transaction systems, including the HIS, the outpatient pharmacy system, the radiology information system, and the long-term care system. Data from these systems were reorganized into both detailed and summary form data sets. It was then combined with cost data to support analysis. Figure 17–5 illustrates how this activity was carried out. In this model, analysis can be performed from both clinical and administrative perspectives.

Benefits of Using Decision Support Systems

What are the benefits of such systems and how do they contribute to the ongoing technology impact on health care professionals?

- Improved productivity for both management and health care professionals

- Improved profitability for organizations

- Improved access to specified population data such as a medicare population or diabetes patient population

- Competitive advantages in the market place

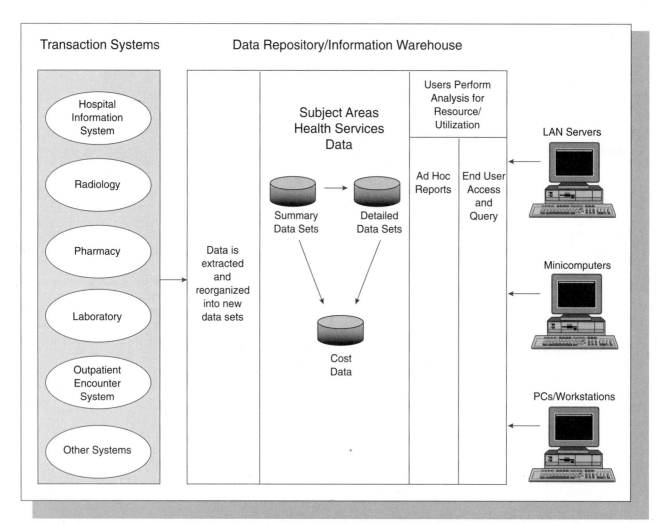

FIGURE 17–5. Feeding data for decision support. The data repository is part of an information warehouse. This approach increases the value of existing data stores and empowers end-users to meet simple reporting needs through local workstations.

- Improved access provided health care professionals by means of workstation tools to access data and query information of direct interest to them. Such capabilities provide added value to physicians interested in viewing data about their patient populations in comparisons and trends

- Improved strategic planning to health care organizations, with tailoring of such plans to their service area and beyond

In the new world of health care alliances and organizational consortiums that have emerged in this decade, the demand for more sophisticated access and critical analysis of health care data continues to increase. Appropriate cost for reliable quality of care remains a driver in health care today.[6]

Executive Information Systems

Executive information systems (EIS) are a subset of decision support systems.[6] An EIS is a system that extracts data from institutional databases, which are then analyzed, reorganized, and reformatted for presentation in graphic color-oriented forms. Designed so that top executives can view a "snapshsot" of summary and trend data, these systems focus on financial "readings" that allow both summary and trend data views and the options of drilling down to detail. Executives use a mouse or touch screen tools to query the data and can produce hardcopy reports as needed. These systems are designed to work on intelligent workstations and are available as timeshare options that allow comparison of an individual hospital performance with others in a peer group. Executives access external data as well as internal through EIS systems. Examples of these would be community data systems that contained data supplied by local or state hospitals, external demographic databases that supply population trends by age and sex, and statistical analysis packages designed to calculate potential service demand.

Clinical Systems

There are some key clinical systems that serve as fundamental components of a complete CPR system. They are components of current health information management systems or are systems that will combine with such systems to create a new model. They serve as transaction systems that perform routine daily operations and may provide patient data directly to a CPR system. In other cases, they are new systems that are being connected to developing CPR systems through telecommunications. An understanding of the basic functionality of these systems will enhance our understanding of fun-

damental data ebb and flow throughout a given institution and over time among many institutions and care events. Extensive discussion of these applications is beyond the scope of this chapter. However, in the next section four of them and their impact on health information management are discussed.

Order Entry

Order entry systems are designed to organize and communicate order processing functions in health care environments. Originally driven by and connected to charge capture, they have evolved significantly and currently include order management functions that have already proven beneficial in health care. In an HIS, **order entry** refers to an online entry of orders for drugs, laboratory tests, and procedures, usually performed by nurses or physicians.[18]

In an HIS, orders are initiated at the nursing unit (usually by physicians) for diagnostic tests, supplies, treatments, and general care direction.

EXAMPLE

An order for a diagnostic radiology examination or an echocardiogram is entered through an order entry system in a hospital. The order is transmitted through communications directly to the departments responsible for carrying out the order. Data noting date, time, conditions, and required functions are included. The receiving department may transfer the order into a departmental system that receives all orders, prioritizes them according to institutional criteria, and places them in a queue for processing. They may emerge on a worksheet for the radiology department personnel to follow as they set up and execute a day's schedule. Once the work is completed, the results of the test may be recorded locally, then transmitted back to the ordering source so that hospital personnel can view the status of the order and either see a result directly or follow up if appropriate. The results may be a message that an examination is complete and will be available at a specified time or the examination results may be displayed directly on a terminal or workstation. At the same time, the necessary charges are captured simultaneously for services provided to the patient. Now the basic function of order entry can be extended to include order management features in the following example.

EXAMPLE

An order placed for blood work is received by the laboratory system and compared with data housed within a patient record system. The comparison identifies that the same blood analysis was completed recently. The system invokes a standard message to the ordering location; the physician may reconsider the need for the order. This example is drawn from known experiences with enhanced order entry systems. In fact, the current focus on such systems is to build them so that such interventions are standard options.

Sittig and Stead discussed a current view of order entry capability and expectations in 1994. They characterized the approaches to order entry in two ways. First, order entry was developed as a component of HISs that were intended for physician use. Second, order entry was established in ways that combined inpatient and outpatient data and incorporated interventions designed to influence the ordering physician at the point of ordering itself. In the first, the direct ordering function was carried out to plan and execute services for hospital inpatients. There is evidence that this approach was successful in some cases. In the Technicon Data System, 78 per cent of the physicians participated in ordering or reviewing results through the system. In the second expectation, benefits have been shown as well. Notably, the study at the Regenstrief Institute demonstrated cost savings when physicians used an order entry system that incorporated online access to a computerized medical record and to intervention messages about cost and utilization.[39]

Benefits anticipated from physician order entry both in outpatient and inpatient environments are expected to include process improvement, cost improvements, clinical decision support, and optimization of physician time in many ways:

- Elimination of lost orders
- Elimination of ambiguities caused by illegible handwriting
- Automatic start/stop orders
- Reduction of order processing
- Maintenance of cost targets for tests and drugs
- Access to online pharmacy and test resources

Physician and other staff time can be saved because of availability of ordering capability in multiple locations and reduction of telephone calls currently needed to clarify orders and directions. In order for this important system to realize its benefits, work needs to be done in the area of policy development, behavioral change, and technical components.[39]

Results Reporting

Results reporting applications are systems designed to retrieve diagnostic test and treatment results from feeder systems such as laboratory, radiology, and other departmental settings and present them directly on inquiry by the care provider. Results reporting particularly features laboratory results in flowsheets and graphics displays. Such systems may operate in tandem with an order entry system. They can also present transcribed reports and images such as those scanned from external sources. They may be a module with an HIS that displays results for selected areas on a local terminal. Increasingly, they may be designed to retrieve designated results through a data repository using SQL or some other query tool. The ideal sought in results reporting systems is the capability to custom display data so that they meet the information needs of individual providers. Thus, results reporting displays for diabetic patients may look different from those needed for chronic congestive heart failure patients.

Although it is most associated with laboratory test results, results reporting has expanded to include a broader range of retrieval options. Online access to image and voice will be combined in these systems so that more and more complete diagnostic and assessment results will be delivered as components of CPR evolving systems. It is also worth noting that the results reporting modules offer the best marketing for developing CPR systems. Physicians, nurses, and other care providers must see results that are timely, information-rich, and dependable if they are to develop an allegiance to computer-based data in general. When incremental strategies are considered for automation that build on current systems, the results reporting area should have a priority.

Medical Decision Support Systems

Medical decision support systems can be characterized as systems that provide diagnostic investigation tools, clinical guideline advice, and expert system resources to clinicians. An **expert system** is a program that symbolically encodes concepts derived from experts in a field and uses that knowledge to provide the kind of problem analysis and advice that the expert might provide. Expert systems provide the capability to perform tasks that would be carried out by an expert in the field. A **knowledge base** is a collection of stored facts, heuristics, and models that can be used for problem solving.[18] These systems have been successfully implemented in a number of locations. One example is the software developed to help users move through specific steps designed to identify a specific diagnosis. Software packages that accomplish this can be purchased for use on PCs as well as incorporated into larger systems. Another example of this kind of resource is a pharmacy information support application, which maintains information on drugs, their uses, and potential contraindications for clinicians to reference. In yet another example, software may scan patient data collected and/or maintained in a database, apply analysis criteria to them, and deliver a message to the clinician. An example of a medical decision support program that combines decision support criteria and patient information would be one that reviews computer-stored patient information for timeliness of monitoring blood tests when seizure medication is re-ordered. Identified as resources to strengthen the diagnostic investigation, evaluation, and treatment processes, these programs are seen as powerful tools for clinicians. At the same time, challenges arise in updating and maintaining these systems for dynamic use, for research is ongoing and system updating is a demanding task.

Medical decision support functions have been applied to assist in data collection, assess the quality of medical reports, and extract relevant clinical data from natural language reports in the HELP information system.[40] They are used to help in data collection by using interactive processes that lead the data collector into responding to the desired questions. These programs provide support by strengthening the information gathering function and ensuring that consistent and more complete information is collected. This has been done with patient history taking with considerable success. Another example of a knowledge system is when specific criteria are established to monitor the completeness of transcribed reports. When the criteria indicate that information is missing following a scan and search process, notification can be provided to the clinician—a direct assessment of the quality or thoroughness of the transcribed report. This approach was applied to analyzing and improving the expertise applied in reading x-rays by tying the patient diagnosis with the radiology findings. A third way to use medical decision support logic is to use it to search and analyze natural language text by seeking matched terms that the language processor knows go together. It enables the program to match like concepts to confirm diagnostic results indicated in the narrative text. These illustrate innovative ways and program logic that can be applied to computerized patient information to strengthen the completeness, accuracy, and prognostic validity of the data. They demonstrate the potential for innovation and critical support functions required in a computer-based patient record.[40]

Problems with Medical Decision Support Systems

While the medical community acknowledges the potential of computer programs that are capable of bringing expert knowledge to their fingertips, a few obstacles have been noted. In recent surveys reported in the *Journal of Family Practice,* reactions expressed a variety of perspectives. All physicians saw the computer as a potential physical entity and barrier that could result in the loss of rapport with patients. Many believed that computers represented a loss of clinical control, particularly as decision support ranging from clinical to cost interventions became more prevalent. The anticipated changes in the practice environment were viewed as weighing down providers and contributing to an inertia in the face of change. Also, many approved and welcomed programs that increased their access to expert knowledge, but rejected the insertion of interactive decision support tools that gave directions on how to treat individual patients. Many indicated that decision making tasks were too complex for the computer to be a significant tool in completing them—often because patients presented with multiple and chronic problems.

A question of legal liability arose. Will such decision aids become part of a legal argument on the appropriateness of an individual physician's decisions in planning and overseeing an individual patient's care? Finally, many expressed the opinion that such tools had the most potential for new physicians who were prepared for a different care environment that was expected to include more innovation.[41]

Because these systems are expected to extend the patient record from a repository to a dynamic and interactive information processor, it is important to anticipate and plan for their use. For many health information professionals, pilots and demonstrations of these tools will be part of a planned CPR development and implementation strategy. The operational access and uses of patient records are in the midst of change. As workstations and facility/office practice networks continue to grow, leadership and problem solving will be required to validate general development strategies as well as transform environments for implementation.

Point of Care Systems

A **point of care system** is a system by which data are captured at the place where the service of care is provided. One of the most common examples is a bedside terminal system designed for patient data capture at the bedside. These systems can be viewed as those that are located where the patient is receiving care, such as the bedside, and those that are carried around by the caregivers, such as hand-held devices. In bedside terminal applications, nurses capture information about the patient directly—often through elaborate templates that use scripts and icon displays designed to eliminate key strokes. These systems are intended to speed up nursing data capture and ensure consistent and legible documentation. Care plans, medication administration templates, and others offer improved access and reduced dependence on paper.

The concept of point of care systems also incorporates data read from bedside monitoring devices from which information is transmitted into the computer directly. As these become more capable of providing the appropriate data, their incorporation into HISs will become more valuable. We know that reduced data entry, retrieval, and physical movement have demonstrated cost savings. It is likely that HISs will incorporate modules for point of care within their functionality.

One consideration of such systems is that all of them must be incorporated into the changing character of the paper record. Because computerized data are retrieved for inclusion in paper records, the printouts and summaries will likely increase paper volume. Planning and legislation are needed to redefine the paper record as a paper/computer-stored record in a way that allows such data to remain in electronic form. Such legislation will also need to redefine the means by which radiology results are incorporated into a patient record. Digital images and radiology reports will be incorporated into the CPR as multimedia capability allows, along with inclusion of radiology through connected picture archiving systems. A **picture archiving and communication system** (PACS) is an integrated computer system that acquires, stores, retrieves, and displays digital images.[18]

Biomedical Devices

Along with improved data collection and retrieval opportunities, bioengineering advances began to provide data automatically through **biomedical devices** used to monitor signals directly from the body. Data from patient monitoring devices were transferred directly to computers without human intervention. In fact, in some advanced systems, data from monitoring devices provided triggered "alerts" within an HIS so that the clinicians could take note of new facts and adjust therapies accordingly. Measurements at critical points provide comparisons so that the informational component can be seen as a pattern. The pattern of physiologic measurement illustrated by monitoring can be factored into the overall diagnostic strategies and long-range care management.

Clinicians need to know the change factor from one monitoring data set to another. Because much of these data come in the form of tracings and plots, transforming the items into information within computer systems is increasingly important. Growing sophistication of these devices and the information they yield can be automatically incorporated into health information systems. This offers greater consistency and accuracy of patient care data that will strengthen clinical predictability in investigation and care management.

As we note that **multimedia processing** will be the foundation of HISs being developed now, we can already see that practitioners must be able to view data from biomedical devices along with image, sound, and digital perspectives. The challenge will be to extract and manipulate information that draws from a variety of data sources to meet a specific need of the user. Biomedical engineering as a primary source of ongoing new technology will expand its influence on the collection, transformation, and retrieval of information as elements of HISs.

One example of a combined biomedical and text application is a surgical intensive care unit clinical information system that pulls the data together and makes them available for minute-to-minute care management. Because all the objective data are captured, the system can provide special messages to alert the clinical staff when a change occurs in the patient's condition. It also provides the data so that trend and multiple factors can be analyzed in a coordinated manner. In this example taken from the Cedars-Sinai Hospital, the alerting systems have been shown to dramatically reduce the time between the occurrence of a critical event and the time the response to it is initiated, thus improving the quality of care.[42]

HEALTH INFORMATION SYSTEMS AND CPRS—SELECTED ISSUES AND BARRIERS

In order to achieve the benefits sought in the HISs and associated CPRs discussed in this chapter, the health care industry must address a number of issues and barriers, including:

- Cost
- Technologic advances
- Customer expectations
- Legislation
- Organizational restructuring
- New partnerships and education

They incorporate sociologic, technical, and management responses to innovation and change within organizations and communities. From a slower, predictable environment, we have all moved to a fast-paced, unpredictable one. There is more need for flexibility and change management than ever before in our history. Among the areas for health information professionals to address are confidentiality and security of patient information, standards for vocabulary, content, and data exchange, and appropriate strategies for managing the transition from paper-based to computer-based patient records.

Confidentiality and Security

Confidentiality and security have been continuous topics of discussion and the subject of state and national legislation during this decade. What needs to be done? Who needs to do it? And how should it be accomplished?

In 1993, the Office of Technology Assessment noted that "computerization of health care information, while offering new opportunities to improve and streamline the health care delivery system, also presents new challenges to individual privacy interests in personal health care data. Technical capabilities to secure and maintain confidentiality in data must work in tandem with legislation to preserve those privacy interests while making appropriate information available for approved uses."[43] This opening to their report clearly states the need. Patients have a right to the confidential safeguard of their personal health information. Professional, regulatory, and organizational foundations for maintaining patient confidentiality and data security must be reinforced. Authorized disclosure must be adapted to fit into a current and more complete understanding of the scope of health care information. Institutional approaches to systems development and implementation will need to include appropriate strategies to maintain customer and staff awareness of privacy requirements. Certainly, regulatory and accrediting organizations address this concern. Standards in confidentiality and data security have been developed over the course of this decade. The ASTM Standard Guide for Confidentiality notes that "The goal is to computerize patient records within the next 10 years. To achieve this goal, CPR systems will need to protect the confidentiality of patient data, provide appropriate access, and use recognized data security measures."[44]

Health information management professionals are called to build on key concepts. **Privacy** is the right of individuals to control disclosure of their personal information. **Confidentiality** is an ethical concept. It is the ethical as well as a legal concept endorsed by health professionals to meet the expectation of patients that their information, when provided to an authorized user, will not be redisclosed. **Data security** refers to the technical and procedural methods by which access to confidential information is controlled and managed. Incorporating these concepts into policies for health information systems and the computer-based patient record brings new challenges. By the early 1990s proposed federal legislation had called for enforcement of laws and regulations regarding confidentiality and penalties for misuse. It also specified that systems must be able to identify where, when, and by whom data was originated; to trace all data origin and access activities. In addition, it proposed that patients be able to access and audit their data.[45] The underlying principle was based on the users' legitimate needs. Providers were to restrict access to specific elements of patient health information according to the requesting individuals' need to know information to perform their job.

The health care industry was asked to accept a clear definition of the ownership of health care data, and spell out distinctions between privacy and confidentiality. Organizations were charged with accountability for maintaining privacy through information systems in a concrete manner. These were based on a long-standing acknowledgement that patients must be assured that the information they shared with their health care practitioner would remain confidential. The American Medical Association has stated: "Without such assurance, the patient may withhold critical information which could affect the quality of care provided, the relationship with the provider, and the reliability of the information maintained."[45]

Who will accomplish the tasks needed to address these issues? Professional and organizational leadership is required, of course. Consider it within institutions. On the operations side, health information professionals are typically responsible for overseeing confidentiality matters and updating organizational policies and procedures established in manual record systems. As well, they are asked to adapt the pertinent policies and procedures to accommodate the increased automation of patient information in departmental and institution-based computer systems.[29] On the technical side, comprehensive security tools have been developed by system designers and are seen as functional system requirements. Software techniques are available to ensure that patient data remain confidential and protected from unauthorized or inadvertent disclosure, modification, or destruction. The current attention focused on these technical protections reflects the reality that computer-based patient records will expand accessibility to multiple users. Providers and other patient data users will be able to access records from multiple locations with relative ease; and we are called on to "balance patients' rights to privacy with the benefits of carefully monitored use for research, planning, and other publicly beneficial functions."[46]

How will this be accomplished? What are some of the specific organizational and systems implications? To effectively manage the confidentiality and data security needs in HISs, we need to establish:

- Institutional oversight groups to recommend policies, approve procedures, and recommend appropriate access and management strategies

- Operational policies and procedures including confidentiality statements signed by all staff

- Thorough education programs for all health facility staff on confidentiality and data security responsibility and accountability

- Individual user ID for all staff keyed to their "need to know" to perform their job functions

- Individual passwords, key cards, biometric or

other means for precise registering of system access

- Monitoring/audit capability for access tracking and follow-up

- Management reports on access and potential confidentiality breaches for line managers to use in supervising staff

- Human resources policies to manage the consequences when staff breach confidentiality

Managers are aware of the balance required to meet improved information processing, transmitting, and storage of patient data while ensuring that appropriate confidentiality protections are in place. Teamwork and collaborative efforts will be needed just as they are in other aspects of systems development. Representing patient interests through strong security programs increases confidence in the technology and reinforces appropriate behavior for providers in all settings.

Health Care Information Processing Standards

The role of standards in the HIS environment is paramount. In 1993, a Government Accounting Office (GAO) report noted that the federal government "often lacks the information needed to evaluate the effectiveness and benefits of the health care it is paying for. The automated medical record is key to this information. However, after over a decade of effort, the comprehensive set of standards needed to make an automated medical record system a reality still does not exist . . . . Without the leadership to set priorities, marshal resources, coordinate activities, and facilitate consensus-building, standards development efforts have yielded meager results."[46] Standards are agreed-on conventions for using terms, code schemes, and processes that are required to significantly advance HIS developments and, in particular, the CPR. They are used to establish information system requirements and processes and designate technical specifications as well. In healthcare, we have worked with standards for patient record content and organization beginning in 1918 with the American College of Surgeons and continuing over the years with the Joint Commission. Coding systems are standards. Computer systems that use common data definitions recognized throughout a particular industry are using standards. To meet the goals of consistent and reliable access to longitudinal health care information on patients, we must address standards development in crucial areas. We must agree on:

- A vocabulary so that the meaning of terms can be trusted and that information can be compared among institutions

- Conventions to be used to transmit data from one computer system to another

- Communications protocols if an electronic super highway is to be achieved for the health care industry

- Basic criteria for managing confidentiality and security within the information infrastructure if the American public is to accept the technology benefits inherent in patient data automation

Work on developing standards for these areas has been under way for over 10 years in the voluntary standard setting arena. Thoughtful planners, clinicians, and systems developers have recognized that agreements in standards would be essential to successfully advance interconnected systems. While individual system developers could develop and market individual systems that would meet the needs of a single organization, it became increasingly clear that compelling forces such as health care reform, market advantage, and cost containment would demand that standards development be accelerated. In 1991, the GAO issued a report on computerizing the patient record that emphasized the crucial role that standards play in meeting long-term goals for CPRs. In addition, standards development became a national focus from a national policy perspective and from that of participating standards organizations. The American Health Information Management Association (AHIMA) accelerated its efforts and participation in the work. Coordination of government, industry, and professional organizations combined to establish a cohesive oversight of standards efforts in the United States, and a national planning panel was formed to provide oversight to the standards development process that is still in place today.

American National Standards Institute

The American National Standards Institute (ANSI) is a nonprofit, privately funded membership organization that coordinates the development of United States voluntary national standards. Founded as an umbrella organization to coordinate the activities of the voluntary standards system and eliminate conflict and duplication, it represents the United States as the member body to the international standards bodies such as the International Standards Organization (ISO) and the International Electrotechnical Commission (IEC).[47] In 1991, they were asked to address the area of health care information processing standards by forming a new panel named the Health Care Informatics Standards Planning Panel with the following identified scope:

- Health care models and electronic health care records

- The interchange of health care data, images, sounds, and signals within and between organizations/practices

- Health care codes and terminology

- The communication with diagnostic instruments and health care devices

- The representation and communication of health care protocols, knowledge, and statistical databases

- Privacy, confidentiality, and security of medical information

- Additional areas of concern or interest with regard to health care information

Formed to promote coordination of the efforts of various standards groups and to be the one format channel for United States standards work in other countries, the panel does not develop standards. In their charter statement, its members specify that the planning panel would "coordinate the work of the standards groups for health care data interchange and health care informatics and other relevant standards groups toward achieving the evolution of a unified set of nonredundant, nonconflicting standards that are compatible with ISO and non-ISO communications environments."[48] Membership is open and professional associations, vendor organizations, and the standards organizations are all represented (see Health Care Information Processing Standards Activities).

The ongoing significance in standards development and refinement cannot be overstated. The very core problems with common data terminology, transfer methods, and images will require ongoing support as we advance in systems and in CPR developments. When fully applied, standards will provide interchangeability and true open systems. From a quality and cost perspective, the health care industry relies on progress in these areas. The agreements and coordination among the standards organizations illustrate the collaboration required to deliver health care services effectively in this country.[49]

Managing the Transition—Challenge to Health Information Professionals

The 20 years spanning 1990 to 2010 mark the active development and deployment of computer-based patient records as the unifying principle within HISs. The tasks before health information professionals will focus on multiple parallel efforts. Staging the technology development and deployment is only one facet of this long-range goal. There are a number of coordinated milestones that must be acknowledged and appropriate management direction adopted. Let us consider a set of

essential activities that must occur. We need to lead and facilitate these activities so that moving ahead to technology improvements becomes feasible—particularly in the direction of the CPR. We need to:

1. Educate health care organizations, practitioners, and consumers to prepare them for the changes. The technology today invites those in health care organizations to communicate with their peers, their practitioners, and their patients in new and innovative ways. Educating users to rely on computers to supply their data needs will be a continuing agenda for professional organizations and institutions. In 1993, some initial estimates for the costs of implementing the CPR were 54 million dollars.[50] Table 17–4 illustrates a national view of these projections. The consumer will also need education as we get more efficient with delivering and coordinating consumers' care information through computers. As providers can rely on up-to-the-minute data and research to communicate with patients, we will foster a different kind of patient—one who can function as a stronger member of the health care team.

2. Recognize that the technology itself must be in place. Electronic data systems and information highways continue to be dependent on fundamental and affordable technology. Foundation systems are needed to provide daily transaction processing for all health services. For many organizations, this will take up the better part of this decade. Managers will be expected to use computers in their own daily activities, including budgeting, data analysis, and writing and communication. Active participation in planning and implementation of technology within organizations will strengthen managers' skills and better prepare them to understand technologic needs.

3. Address the crucial acceptance factors. Ease of use is one we have discussed in terms of the user interface with workstations. Another issue is the necessary preparation to adequately manage the confidentiality and access concerns of patients and those associated with the user communities. It is very likely that we will need participation in public forums on this topic.

4. Model demonstrated quality and cost incentives to encourage individual organizations to adopt aggressive programs. To do this, a sound business cost/benefit rationale is required. Closer scrutiny will be directed to systems development projects to be sure that clear cost containment targets are included in the planning, and the opportunity for "nice-to-have computer systems" will give way to "cost-justified computer systems." Managers will apply cost/benefit tools in their forecasting with greater discipline than ever before.

5. Upgrade organizational policies and procedures that redefine the patient record, moving from a paper record to a combination of paper and information from data systems. This can be the lead at national levels as

Health Care Information Processing Standards Activities

American Health Information Management Association

AHIMA participates in ASTM, HL7, ANSI HISPP, X12, ACR/NEMA, IEEE/MEDIX, and CEN standards activities. Areas of special interest are the computerization of health information, the computer-based patient record, and the confidentiality/security of patient information. AHIMA provides formal representation to these organizations through alliance agreements.

Accredited Standards Committee X3

ASC X3 prepares "generic" standards in such areas as file formats and communications protocols for use by application specific groups, for example, Identification Cards—Financial Transaction Cards, Identification Cards—Magnetic Stripe, Identification Cards—Location of Embossed Characters on ID Cards. Network Database Language standards plus projects in data communications and Open Systems Interconnection (OSI). X3 develops generic standards for information technology, is administered by the Computer and Business Equipment Manufacturer's Association, and is accredited to submit its documents to ANSI for approval as American National Standards.

Accredited Standards Committee X12 (ASC X12)

ASC-X12's standards should be used for billing and remittance transactions between a care site and a third party payer. These standards for billing and information have been adopted by Health Care Financing Administration (HCFA). X12 develops standards for electronic data interchange and is administered by the Data Interchange Standards Association. X12, which is composed almost entirely of insurance companies, does not develop standards for communication of clinical data. Those standards should be handled by the standards groups with existing experience and expertise (such as HL7 and ASTM).

ASTM Committee E31 on Computerized Systems

ASTM develops and publishes standards on a wide variety of topics in health care informatics. It has been in existence since 1898. It has multiple areas of work under way within its E31 Committee on Computerized Systems. Examples of publications available include E1238—Standard Specification for Transferring Clinical Observations Between Independent Systems; E1239—Standard Guide for Description of Reservation/Registration-Admission, Discharge, Transfer (R-ADT) Systems for Automated Patient Care Information Systems; E1466—Specification for the Use of Bar Codes in Clinical Laboratory Specimen Management; and E1384—Standard Guide for Description for Content and Structure of a computer-based patient record. ASTM also has work under way in standards for health data cards, data authentication and medical transcription, and in constructing protocols for advice rules to be used in medical decision support applications.

Medical Record Content and Structure Standards (E1384)

The ASTM Committee E31 on Computerized Systems has been working on standards for the content and structure of medical records for more than 10 years. They have published a consensus standard on some aspects of the problem. This standard is E1384 Standard Guide for Description for Content and Structure of a computer-based patient record. It is currently housed in Subcommittee E31.19 on Vocabulary for CPR Content and Structure. Selected work is also being developed within Subcommittee E31.12 on Computer-based Patient Records. ASTM represents the only standards-setting group that has focused on this issue. With input from CPRI, it continues to have the formal standards responsibility for developing these content and structure standards.

Health Level 7 (HL-7)

This organization has had significant impact on systems developers, filling a need for application standards to allow internal computer systems to interface at some level. Examples of standards available are: Application Protocol for Electronic Exchange in Healthcare Environments, Version 2.1, HL7's Implementation Support Guide. HL7 is used for within-institution transmission of orders; clinical observations and clinical data, including test results; admission, transfer, and discharge records; and charge and billing information. As of 1994, HL7 was being used in more than 150 United States health care institutions including most leading university hospitals and had been adopted by Australia and New Zealand as their national standard. HL7 is also supported by most of the health care system vendors. It will not serve every communication need in a health care institution, and continued development is needed to obtain a message standard that will track and control all of the processes within a hospital or health care institution. However, HL7 will serve the immediate need.

Institute for Electrical and Electronic Engineers (IEEE) P1073 Medical Information Bus (MIB)

This organization has a long track record in standards development. Examples of IEEE work are: Standard for Medical Device Communications—Medical Device Data Language, Medical Device Communications—Physical Layer Interface—Cable Connected. This organization continues to be a primary contributor in health care information systems developments.

Medical Data Interchange (MEDIX)

Examples of the work of this organization are: Standard for Health Care Data Interchange—Overview and Framework, Recommendations for Health Care Data Interchange—User Needs.

Health Care Information Processing Standards Activities *Continued*

American College of Radiology-National Electrical Manufacturers Association (ACR-NEMA) Imaging Standards
ACR-NEMA should be used for the transmission of images in all contexts and for message transmissions with Picture Archiving Systems (PACs) serving departments such as radiology. ACR-NEMA is supported by most radiology PAC system vendors and has been incorporated into the Japanese Image Store and Carry (ISAC) optical disk system as well as Kodak's PhotoCD.

Computer-Based Patient Record Institute
This organization was formed in response to the Institute of Medicine study on the Patient Record recommendations. The mission is to initiate and coordinate urgently needed activities to facilitate and promote the routine use of computer-based patient records through health care.

American Dental Association
The ADA sponsors an Accredited Standards Committee (ASC) MD156 for Dental Materials, Instruments, and Equipment. This committee has added a task group on dental informatics. The data content has been coordinated to conform to the vocabulary work under way in ASTM E31.19.

well as within individual institutions. Milestones and "report cards" that report on quality indicators for organizations incorporate required data components for information systems. This helps clarify and encourage appropriate and measurable clinical data capture that is foundational to a CPR.

6. Coordinate programs that stage the development within institutional information systems master plans. This endorses the concept of a unifying principle. We have discussed the natural evolution of systems as they are mapped out in hierarchic views. This and other institutional strategies will serve as the basis for the

TABLE 17-4 PROPOSED CPR STRATEGIES AS OF 1993

CPR STRATEGIES	LEAD ORGANIZATION	TIME FRAME
Improve knowledge about state of the art		
Conduct provider surveys	Computer-Based Patient Record Institute (CPRI)	1993–94
Develop reference model for evaluating costs and benefits of CPR systems	Department of Health & Human Services (HHS)	1993–96
Analyze information needs and uses in a variety of provider settings	CPRI	1993–96
Evaluate issues related to organizational professional and personal change	CPRI	1993–96
Develop national standards		
Fund HISPP standards planning and coordination	HHS	Ongoing
Develop, test, and promote use of a patient data set for emergency purposes	Health Care Informatics Standards Planning Panel (HISPP)	1993–96
Compare and contrast coding schemes and develop needed coding schemes	HISPP	1993–96
Develop uniform provider, payer, and patient identifiers	HISPP	1993–94
Foster development of standards certification process	CPRI	1993–94
Establish national legal standards for protecting the confidentiality of patient information	Congress/President	1993–94
Evaluate existing data sets	HHS	1993–96
Enact legislation requiring federal agencies to demonstrate the usefulness and cost effectiveness of any mandated data set	Congress/President	1993–95
Develop linkages between existing and future computer-based information systems		
Encourage development of community health information networks	HHS/CPRI	1993–96
Collaborate with other industries and government to create the health care component of the National Information Infrastructure	CPRI	1993–ongoing

incremental steps that automate more and more clinical data. Some of these go hand in hand to cover the most return on investment and, at the same time, extend value added to multiple customers. So systems will become more affordable, dependable, and useful to more customers. A new clinical laboratory system that is added to a large organization's integrated clinical systems development plan may drive the results reporting for clinicians, send data to a clinical repository in which a growing computer-based patient record is maintained, and offer a new service that generates mailed test result reports to patients.

7. Endorse and support revised legal frameworks so that federal and state data systems that offer community-based experiences with components of computer-based patient records can be established. State laws are in the process of being realigned with federal requirements in these areas. New definitions of the patient record, accepted changes in storage requirements, and automated authentication techniques will all be needed to advance the work.

8. Design tactical implementation protocols for adoption by and among health care organizations so that high-yield components of the computer-based patient record can be introduced, evaluated, and rapidly deployed. This strategy focuses on the experience that bringing technology to the eager customers first—particularly clinicians—accelerates technology diffusion. Happy customers will market the technology most effectively. At this point in health information systems development, there are many demonstrations that illustrate this experience. If we provide new data or data in new and more effective formats, then clinical customers will be more willing to modify their data collection behaviors to contribute the value added.

9. Monitor corresponding work on intelligent databases that contribute current clinical guidelines and protocols and find ways to introduce them into the organization. Not only are they needed for reasonable support to medical providers, but they are clearly designed for inclusion into the computer-based patient record systems. In the simplest form, guidelines can be stored electronically and look-up features can be provided. In the more sophisticated approaches, organizations may tailor guidelines for internal use. Experiments that connect individual patient data to guidelines to offer feedback before, during, and after the care delivery process will best illustrate the requirements expected of the computer-based patient record systems.

10. Study the known barriers already published to develop action plans to overcome them—learn from others' mistakes. We need to survey the deployment tactics and identify the success benchmarks. Sharing experiences with other organizations will help develop a collective wisdom as we move to such a new environment. One example of this is the fact that many health professionals have not learned to type. This means that introducing computer systems—even point-of-care systems—to personnel who do not possess simple keyboarding skills will require expensive pretraining on the technology itself before a specific application can be taught. There is also time needed to adjust from character-based terminal screens to the newer graphical user interfaces (GUIs). It must be clear that newer user interface styles are going to be more effective. In some cases, such as a high-volume prescription data entry function, icons and a windows user interface style may not be the most efficient for the organization, but evidence to date indicates that the GUI benefits have led to easier and more intuitive learning for information system users.

11. Lead and participate in re-engineering needed to prepare the operational environment for the changes. One of the driving forces of this decade is re-engineering. We have learned that simply installing computer systems on existing business processes fails to realize the benefits. Business processes, the way we move patients through from appointment, check-in, care, and follow-up, must be re-examined. Along with other business processes, this work flow requires careful review to see if there are more efficient ways to accomplish it. The notion of continuously improving our business processes to be sure that the best methods are in place fits in with the total quality management philosophy and practices that have been used with positive results since the late 1980s. We can expect to re-engineer the way patients are seen and treated for long-term services and to update the processes used to move around the information and use it more effectively. Re-engineering is the fundamental rethinking and radical redesign of business processes to achieve dramatic improvements in performance such as cost, quality, service, and speed.[51] Considering that providers are expected to incorporate new technology in direct care practices, examining how data capture and retrieval can occur most efficiently will lead to new paradigms.

12. Incorporate a thorough knowledge of the impact of change on individuals in the work force and plan the changes from a top-down approach. We know that technology affects organizational culture including structure and design. It changes workflows and brings in new job designs and responsibilities. Staff will require new skills and knowledge to perform their work. Worker motivation and incentives will call for new communications and operations policies and procedures to build the kind of strong teamwork required to absorb change. Human resources will be strategic partners for all managers in the long-term change agent tasks, and new skills will be required for managers as well as workers.[52]

CPR Working Assumptions—Planning for 2000

Among the scenarios in place today, one model of CPR development is designated as part of an integrated clinical information systems master plan that defines systems in multiple developmental levels. The CPR component can be viewed from a content definition perspective associated with database planning and development, while its functional implementation may be associated with a clinical workstation within a facility-wide information system. As the critical mass of patient data maintained in systems grows more complete and devices become more available, the paper record will be needed and used less. Over time, the increased computer-stored documentation will be functionally used as the primary record. Printouts may be needed for legal purposes, but probably not for long. Progress will be made incrementally through specific projects such as order entry and results reporting and stored dictation made available through workstations for clinicians' viewing. Yet an overall strategy is required to ensure that the CPR is fully defined and can be articulated as an organizational goal. Then specific projects can be laid out as building blocks.

How do we formalize a CPR project and communicate the basis for it? For health information managers, formal liaisons are in place with institutional medical record committees, quality improvement committees, and others. One way to exercise leadership and lead others in this direction is to incorporate future thinking into current status reports. An illustration of this is a forecasting component in an annual report or as a contribution to institutional strategic planning work. We know that we will work in a transitional environment. What is it? Can we describe it? Are there working assumptions that will help describe a broad framework? Generally, in health information management, we already know and are planning for some basic assumptions (see Predictions for CPR Development).

Table 17–5 illustrates proposed standard CPR system requirements that summarize the expectations laid out in this chapter beginning with the IOM study at the beginning of the decade. Current estimates indicate that national standards will specify minimum content, data exchange, and privacy requirements. The comprehensive nature of the requirements posed in Table 17–5 are complex and meeting them remains a challenge for health information professionals and others.

Predictions for CPR Development

- The computer-based patient record (CPR) will be defined as a record of specific clinical and clinically related data and financial and assessment data that originate and are collected from multiple information systems, housed in an institutional or community information warehouse, and accessed through workstations.

- The CPR will expand and reorganize patient data currently maintained in paper records and function as an integrated system that links patient clinical data with "intelligence" features such as guidelines and alerts. The paper record is defined as the legal documentation of patient care for the organization. Current national leadership views a computer-based record as both the documentation of patient care and the documentation of providers' access and use of tools such as clinical guidelines and reminders.

- CPR development will conform to generally accepted national standards.

- Initially, the CPR may be defined as an automated record that resides in multiple institutional information systems and is a supplement to the legal medical record. Although data will reside in multiple care sites, they will be accessible for view as a whole and available when needed in paper form.

- When operational, the CPR will result in significant organizational quality and cost benefits.

- Confidentiality and data security provisions will be required by CPR customers and state and national legislation. In order for the CPR to be accepted legally, policies and procedures will need to be developed that define how data are entered, validated, updated, accessed, and protected from improper alteration.

- The functional usage of the CPR will be developed through flexible, customizable workstations that will serve as the gateway to clinical information systems.

- CPR implementation will be staged. Phase I version of a CPR may be implementation of a data set drawn from an established institutional, regional, or national data dictionary that meets mandated reporting requirements. Subsequent versions will be coordinated with institutional and community-based needs that specify additional content areas defined by combined external and internal priorities.

- Operational planning and re-engineering required to support a CPR implementation will be a major organizational initiative.

- Regardless of the planned approach, physicians will need the capability to select portions of a logical CPR from a menu to assemble either a screen summary or a paper summary for care purposes.

Selecting an Approach to CPR Development

Drawing from the assumptions noted here, appropriate goals and objectives can be formulated for health information professionals to follow. These, in turn, could support an approach to CPR development within an institutional setting. Following are goals and objectives for a model institutional CPR development project.

TABLE 17-5 USER REQUIREMENTS FOR COMPUTER-BASED PATIENT RECORDS

RECORD CONTENT

Uniform core data elements
Standardized coding systems and formats
Common data dictionary based on standard vocabulary
Information on outcomes of care and functional status
Images, tracings, video, and voice

RECORD FORMAT

"Front page" problem list
Ability to flip through the record via efficient scan and search functions
Integrated among disciplines and sites of care
Longitudinal—building toward lifetime records

SYSTEM PERFORMANCE

24-hour access
Rapid retrieval
Available at convenient places
Easy data input

LINKAGES

Linkages with other information systems (e.g., radiology, pharmacy)
Transferability of information among specialties and sites
Linkages with relevant scientific literature
Linkages with other institutional databases and registries
Linkages with records of family members
Electronic transfer of billing information

INTELLIGENCE

Medical and administrative decision support
Clinical reminders
Intervention "alarm" systems capable of being customized
Clinical guidelines–based care plans for individual and population management

REPORTING CAPABILITIES

Easily customized clinical output (summaries and other user selections)
Standard clinical reports
Customized and ad hoc reports (e.g., specific evaluation queries)
Trend reports and graphics
Derived documents (mandatory reporting, special registries, insurance)

CONTROL AND ACCESS

Easy access for patients and their advocates
Safeguards against violation of confidentiality
System tools for auditing and monitoring access activity
Strong legal and institutional data security provisions including consequences

TRAINING AND IMPLEMENTATION

Minimal training required for system use
Graduated implementation possible

GOALS

- Develop a CPR of clinical data from inpatient and all outpatient environments as a fundamental tool for patient care and as an organizational data resource. This will be completed as a component of an organizational data repository.

- Adopt a CPR model consistent with national standards that incorporates clinical "intelligence" features.

OBJECTIVES

- Identify major internal and external stakeholders to determine customer requirements for the CPR.

- Document required content and describe uses and users.

- Define a staged CPR content and clinically related information and associated attributes for the organization.

- Plan and develop an organizational CPR data model based on a warehouse repository to include broad needs of direct patient care, clinical management, outcomes measurement, research, administrative, and financial components.

- Initially assess and then monitor external forces that affect data attributes, to include regulatory and legal bodies that are mandating the data content of records.

- Establish strategic connection with relevant community, state, and national data systems and business partners as a basis for networking with real and potential contract institutions to determine mutual data needs.

- Analyze, plan, and stage implementation of computer-based "practically paperless" patient record over time in conjunction with operations and medical staff partners.

Ways of Developing a CPR Project

DEFINING CONTENT. One way to begin work on these CPR goals and objectives is to focus on defining the content. A basic strategy is to identify the content through a series of data sets in order to organize the data into defined groups that represent customers, including analyzing current patient record and associated data sources documentation practices, researching external customer needs that may affect the planned content through legislation or accreditation requirements, and determining internal customer needs by defining and documenting a series of specific customer data sets associated with internal and external priorities. Existing sources and already determined data sets could be used when feasible such as:

- Uniform hospital discharge data set
- Basic ambulatory medical care data set
- Minimum uniform data set for home care
- Minimum hospice data set
- Minimum data set for long-term care
- Health record core data set
- Occupational health data set
- Emergency medical information data set
- Minimum nursing data set
- Health care financing agency minimum data requirements
- National Committee on Quality Assurance patient record data set
- Institutional clinical data sets (e.g., diabetes, heart care, back pain)
- Community or Institutional Registry data sets (cancer, trauma, donor)

Accrediting and regulatory content requirements are examples of external priorities. A heart care service's designated data set is an example of an institutional data set that might be defined as an organizational priority. In other cases, clinical measurement objectives may set the priorities for internal data sets or national legislation may mandate required data content to build toward a CPR in hospitals. Data sets can be implemented stepwise through planned applications according to a clinical systems master plan. The acquisition and documentation of a series of data sets provide a long-term foundation approach to defining the content. Of course, common data used in the developing applications will serve as the foundation and will gradually build a longitudinal data resource.

SELECTED PROTOTYPES. Another approach directed to a short-term version of a CPR could be accomplished through selected prototypes. Offering model data sets to providers through workstations would provide modeling experiences. For instance, a designated hospital discharge/transfer data set designed for transferring patients to home health for follow-up would offer a slice of information for a trial. This may be presented through inquiry screens on a clinical workstation installed in physicians' offices. It could also be used for direct transfer to a home health agency as a remote display or printout. A next phase might expand the data to include the most recent results reporting data from the hospital ancillary departments, an obvious support for improving

the level of coordination across care sites. The developing CPR must be able to meet the current usage requirements of the paper record as well as facilitate a growing acceptance of computer stored data and provide value added re-engineering required to support a CPR implementation for organizations and the health care industry. Managing change efficiently will remain a priority.

Key Concepts

Why is the current focus on health information systems so strong? Will it affect the way work is accomplished?

- Quality and cost objectives drive information systems development and the rate of growth of health information systems is increasing.

- Users represent multiple professions and rely on health care data and health information systems as a fundamental resource to meet their individual and collective business needs.

- User interaction with computers is changing as users' data needs demand more sophisticated tools for access and manipulation.

- More thought and planning is required to develop coordinated approaches that support new models of health information systems within the industry.

What lessons have we learned from the past?

- History has provided key concepts for data collection and information flow. Benefits of technology have been clearly demonstrated, and today major health information system components are geared to be used through tools largely targeted for widespread use.

Is the current CPR goal well accepted and understood?

- Establishing strong CPRs is the current national goal. When CPR systems are established, improved functionality will allow improved information access from diverse locations and reliable health information on patients will be made available.

- Health professionals will employ data and technology in their work including immediate access to current research and recommended clinical guidelines. These are expected to play a strong role in improving the health of the public. Work in developing community health information systems illustrates widespread endorsement as well.

- It is important to track progress toward the national goal and benefit from collective experiences.

What specialized knowledge will be required?

- Health information professionals will need to be well grounded in basic technology and understand alternative approaches and pathways used to launch CPRs.

- Input/output choices will be key and database systems will be required to put CPRs together. Understanding architecture and related processes will be essential for leaders in CPR innovation.

- An understanding of how applications come together to combine data and streamline processing is crucial. Organizations will be continually learning and modifying information and data strategies to meet market, quality, and cost goals.

What are the key components of managing the transition?

- Knowing issues and barriers serves as foundation for institutional education and development programs.

- The most successful efforts include understanding, leading, and participating in re-engineering work in organizations and within organizational alliances.

- Best demonstrated practices throughout the industry provide guideposts and assurances for institutional transitions.

- Studying the impact of change on individuals and employing quality improvement tools as a basic strategy is essential.

Think about how far we have come today. Hospitals, Health Maintenance Organizations, and home health and hospice facilities use workstations to connect not only physicians but other care providers to the necessary data, allowing them to plan, analyze, record, and retrieve patient and facility-wide and management data. The health information management systems in place and in development today are geared for this world.

References

1. Dick RS, Steen EB (eds): Computer-Based Patient Record—An Essential Technology for Health Care. Institute of Medicine Report, Washington, D.C.: National Academy Press, 1991, p. 12.
2. Blum B: Clinical Information Systems. New York: Springer-Verlag, 1986, p. 35.
3. Toward a National Health Information Infrastructure: Report of the Work Group on Computerization of Patient Records to the Secretary of the U.S. Department of Health and Human Services, Washington, D.C.: U.S. Government Printing Office, 1993, p. 5.
4. Broccolo BM, Fulton DK, Waller AA: The electronic future of health information: strategies for coping with a brave new world. J Am Health Information Management Assoc 1993;64:64.
5. Blum B (ed): Information Systems for Patient Care. New York: Springer-Verlag, 1984, p. 1.
6. Ball MJ, Douglas JV, Desky RIO, Albright JW (eds): Healthcare Information Management Systems. New York: Springer-Verlag, 1991, p. 224.
7. Klein E: Automating home care, technology's impact on home healthcare providers. Health Care Informatics 1993;10(8):22.
8. Barton MB, Schoenbaum SC: Improving influenza vaccination performance in an HMO setting: The use of computer generated reminders and peer comparison feedback. Am J Public Health 1990;80:534.
9. Tierney WM, Miller ME, Overhage JM, McDonald CJ: Physician inpatient order writing on microcomputer workstations. Effects on resource utilization. JAMA 1993;269(3):379.
10. Gross MS, Hoehn BJ, Rooks CS: Clinical information systems: Why now? Topics in Health Information Management 1993(1);14:1.
11. Casper GR, Brennan PF: Improving the Quality of Patient Care: The Role of Patient Preferences in the Clinical Record. Proceedings of the Symposium on Computer Applications in Medical Care, AMIA Conference, New York: McGraw-Hill, 1994, p. 8.
12. Casper GR, Brennan PF: Improving the Quality of Patient Care: The Role of Patient Preferences in the Clinical Record. Proceedings of the Symposium on Computer Applications in Medical Care, AMIA Conference, New York: McGraw-Hill, 1994, p. 9.
13. Frawley K: Achieving the CPR while keeping an ancient oath. Health Care Informatics 1995;12(4):28–30.
14. Rubin, RD: Washington State CHIMS Status Report, CPRI Compendium, p. 4.
15. Toward a National Health Information Infrastructure: Report of the Work Group on Computerization of Patient Records to the Secretary of the U.S. Department of Health and Human Services, Washington, DC: U.S. Government Printing Office, 1993, p. 1.
16. Dowling AF: Information Management Implications of Federal Health Care Reform. J Healthcare Information and Management Systems Society 1994;8(1):21.
17. Gross MS, Hoehn BJ, Rooks CS: Clinical Information Systems: Why Now? Topics in Health Information Management 1993;14(1):1.
18. Shortliffe EH, Perreault LE: Medical Informatics Computer Applications in Health Care. New York: Addison Wesley, 1990, p. 21.
19. Dornfest S: History and Impediments to Progress in the Development and Implementation of the Computerized Patient Record. Proceedings from the Health Information Management Systems Society, American Hospital Association, 1993, p. 84.
20. Ball MJ, Jacobs S: Hospital Information Systems as We Enter the Decade of the 80s. Proceedings, IEEE Fourth Annual Symposium on Computer Applications in Medical Care, Institute of Electrical and Electronic Engineers, New York, 1980, . 183.
21. Bleich HL, Slack WV: Designing a Hospital Information System: A Comparison of Interfaced and Integrated Systems. Yearbook of Medical Informatics, 1993, p. 153.
22. Greenes RA, Shortliffe EH: Medical informatics—An emerging academic discipline and institutional priority. JAMA 1990; 263(3):1114.
23. Kunitz and Associates, Inc.: Interim Report on Data Sources for

Ambulatory Care Effectiveness Research—Descriptions of Selected Automated Ambulatory Medical Records Systems. February 5, 1992, p. 11.

24. Pryor TA: The HELP medical record system. MD Computing 1988;5(5):48.

25. Burke JP, Classen DC, Pestotnik SL, et al: The HELP system and its application to infection control. J Hospital Infection 18(Suppl A):424, 1991.

26. Gardner RM, Golubjatnikov OK, Laub RM, et al: Computer-critiqued blood ordering using the HELP system. Comput Biomed Res 1990;23:514.

27. Dick RS, Steen EB (eds): Institute of Medicine Report, The Computer-Based Patient Records—An Essential Technology for Health Care, Washington, D.C., National Academy Press, 1991, p. 10.

28. Covvey HD: The digital hostage taker's syndrome: reflections on the computer-based patient record. Managed Care Quarterly 1993;1(3):60.

29. Ball MJ, Collen MF (eds): Aspects of the Computer-Based Patient Record. New York: Springer-Verlag, 1992, p. 12.

30. Uniform Health Care Information Act of Washington State, Revised Code of Washington (RCW) 42.17.205, 1991, p. 3.

31. Sager N, Lyman M, Bucknall C, et al: Natural language processing and the representation for clinical data. J American Medical Informatics Assoc 1994;1(2):142.

32. Golob R: Securing a bridge to the CPR: Clinical data repositories. Healthcare Informatics 1994;11(2):50.

33. Collen MF: The origins of informatics. J American Medical Informatics Assoc 1994;1(2):92.

34. Kelly R, Caldwell B: PDAs: Do you need them? A special report. Information Week, August 2, 1993, p. 21.

35. Trofino J: Voice recognition technology applied to nursing documentation. Healthcare Information and Management Systems Society 1993;7(4):42.

36. Clayton PD, Pulver GE, Hill CL: Physician use of computers: Is age or value the predominant factor? Patient Centered Computing (Proceedings). Seventeenth Annual Symposium on Computer Applications in Medical Care, American Medical Informatics Association. New York: McGraw-Hill, 1994, p. 301.

37. Tunick D: Client server computing strategies for the 1990s. Part I. Industry Services: Inside Gartner Group This Week Newsletter, July 28, 1993, p. 2.

38. Webster's New World Dictionary of Computer Terms. New York: Prentice-Hall, 1988, p. 12.

39. Sittig D, Stead W: Computer-based physician order entry: The state of the art. JAMA 1994;1(2):108.

40. Haug RJ: Uses of Diagnostic Expert Systems in Clinical Care. Proceedings of the Symposium on Computer Applications in Medical Care, American Medical Informatics Association, 1994, p. 379.

41. Taylor TR: The computer and clinical decision-support systems in primary care. J Fam Pract 1990;30(2):138.

42. Shabot MM: Integrating information systems for enhanced efficacy and outcomes management. J Healthcare Information and Management Systems Society 1993;7(4):27.

43. US Congress Office of Technology Assessment. Protecting Privacy in Computerized Medical Information. OTA-TCT-576. Washington, DC.: U.S. Government Printing Office, September, 1993, p. 1.

44. ASTM Draft Standard Guide for Confidentiality, Privacy, Access for Computer Based Patient Records and Data Derived from Computer Based Patient Records, Version 6 draft. Philadelphia: American Society for Testing and Materials, 1993, p. 3.

45. Toward a National Health Information Infrastructure. Report of the Work Group on Computerization of Patient Records to the Secretary of the U.S. Department of Health and Human Services, 1993, Appendix D, p. 2.

46. Automated Medical Rrecords, Leadership Needed to Expedite Standards Development, GAO Report, 1993, p. 1.

47. American National Standards Fact Sheet, Health Care Informatics Standards Planning Panel. New York: American National Standards Institute, Memorandum 88, 1994, p. 1.

48. American National Standards Health Care Informatics Standards Planning Panel Charter Statement. New York: American National Standards Institute, Memorandum 4, 1992, p. 1–2.

49. Status Report of Health Care Informatics Standards, Health Care Informatics Standards Planning Panel. New York: American National Standards Institute, Memorandum 114, 1994, p. 2.

50. Toward a National Health Information Infrastructure. Report of the Work Group on Computerization of Patient Records to the Secretary of the U.S. Department of Health and Human Services, 1993, p. 19.

51. Melrose JP: The three Rs for CPR implementation: Regulations, reengineering and rightsizing. Health Care Informatics, October 1993;10(10):58.

52. Kissler GK: Managing the Process of Change. Proceedings of the Health Information Systems Society, American Hospital Association, 1993;3:55.

18

MERIDA L. JOHNS

INFORMATION SYSTEMS LIFE CYCLE

18

OBJECTIVES

- Define key words.
- Discuss similarities and unique characteristics among the various life cycles, including the general systems life cycle, information systems life cycle, and information systems development life cycle.
- Understand the impact on organizational resources of the juxtaposition of various information systems at different information system life cycle stages.
- Discuss the life cycle stages in Nolan's six-stage theory of information system development.
- Identify the three stages of the information systems development life cycle and the components of each.
- Apply techniques and tools, including hierarchy charts, data flow diagrams, data dictionaries, and entity-relationship diagrams to perform information systems analysis and design.
- Understand and apply investigative strategy techniques for gathering information for system design and development.
- Evaluate information system interfaces from satisfying and efficiency perspectives.
- Describe the various techniques that are used to evaluate information systems, including benefits realization, break-even analysis, payback period, and discounted payback period.
- Describe the activities that take place during system implementation.
- Describe the purpose and content of a request for proposal.
- Describe the usual process that is followed in purchasing a vendor system.

INTRODUCTION

The manager of the clinical laboratory wants to replace the department's outdated information system to better manage information relating to collecting specimens, tracking completion of laboratory tests, and reporting clinical test results. The radiology department director wants to install an information system that will help manage patient flow, track the completion of radiology tests, store transcribed radiology reports, and automatically retrieve patient demographic data from the hospital information system. The vice president for hospital human resources wants to purchase an automated system that will help manage information related to employee demographics, employment status, employee benefits, and salary administration. The director of health information management (HIM) plans to request the purchase of an automated system that will track the status and location of clinic and inpatient medical records. The goal of all these managers is to use automation as an adjunct in helping them better manage information. Most of these systems will cost several thousands of dollars; the clinical laboratory and radiology systems may even cost millions of dollars. Considering the investment to be made, how can these managers be reasonably confident that the systems selected will meet the needs of their organizations and their various departments? One strategy to help ensure that appropriate systems are selected is to follow a structured approach for analyzing user needs, identifying functional requirements that meet the user needs, selecting a system that has the required functionality, and implementing the system in an organized, well thought out manner.

Part of the health information manager's responsibility is to help analyze, design, and implement automated systems for patient-related and clinical data management on a departmental and an enterprisewide basis. This chapter outlines a structured approach for accomplishing these tasks and provides tools to assist the health information manager to be successful in this process.

System Analysis, Design, and Implementation

Faced with the challenge of analysis, design, and implementation of an automated system, the health information manager's primary goal is to provide a system that meets user and/or department needs and that also supports the strategic objectives of the enterprise. To assist in accomplishing this goal, the development process for an information system usually consists of four principal phases:

- Analysis phase
- Design phase
- Implementation phase
- Evaluation phase

Taken as a whole, these phases make up what is typically called the **system development life cycle.**

Analysis Phase

To provide an information system that meets user requirements, the health information manager must identify how an automated system can support the performance of user tasks. An understanding of the environment in which user tasks are performed is an essential part of the analysis phase if needs are to be adequately identified. The analysis phase lays the foundation and provides the map for **system design** and implementation. Several tools and approaches are available to help in the analysis process. Some of these are structured. Among structured development tools are graphic flowcharts, decomposition charts, matrix tables, and data flow diagrams.

A less structured approach to identify user needs is the development of prototype systems. In this approach, a model or "draft" system is quickly developed. This is called the prototype system. The prototype system is presented to the user and refined after initial use. Before the final product is achieved using this method, there may be several iterations of the prototype. The more structured process, however, is still the methodology of choice in most instances.

Design Phase

System design encompasses activities related to specifying the details of a new system. Typically, this includes making decisions about the logical and physical design of the system. Through the use of structured design tools such as **computer-aided software engineering** (CASE) programs, a systems blueprint is developed. This blueprint is analogous to an architect's blueprint and provides the basis for the physical system design. The physical design stage converts the system blueprint into specific detail so that computer code can be developed. In a health care setting, the traditional description of system design applies when the automated system is developed by a staff within the organization. However, in today's environment, health care organizations fre-

quently purchase already-designed systems from outside vendors. In these cases, the meaning of system design takes on a different perspective. It usually refers to the assessment of various characteristics of the design of the system rather than the development of the system itself.

Implementation Phase

System implementation involves making the system operational in the organization. Implementation characteristically covers a wide range of tasks including the following:

- System testing
- User training
- Site preparation
- Managing organization change and system impact

To achieve the primary goal of meeting user needs, the system must function efficiently and effectively. To minimize potential system defects and operational flaws, test data are constructed and entered into the system. The results of system testing are used to correct operational weaknesses and to make programming changes.

User training is an essential component for successful system implementation. If users are not proficient in system use, then the effectiveness of the system is reduced. The element of user training is not always sufficiently emphasized, and plans for user training are often ill-conceived and incomplete. Consideration needs to be given to how to organize the training effort, identifying and selecting the most appropriate training strategies for the task and users and developing the training materials and/or systems.

Evaluation Phase

The evaluation phase is important in any system development effort. Frequently, systems are developed and implemented but never evaluated to determine if the original goals for implementation are met. Lack of evaluation can contribute to a lack of realization of potential system benefits. Therefore, to achieve maximum benefits realization, all systems should be evaluated against predeveloped criteria and needs requirements.

Role of the HIM Professional

Within a health care enterprise, the health information manager should be an advocate for use of appropriate strategies and tools that will help ensure the development or selection of information systems that meet organizational needs. The health information manager usually chairs or serves on several information-related organization and department committees, including the following:

- Committees charged with enterprisewide information management
- Information security
- Strategic planning for information technology
- Departmental information technology

As an advocate for effective system development or selection, the health information manager should assume a prominent role in the system development life cycle. Tasks assumed may vary from individual to individual, depending on specific job functions. For example, the director of an HIM department may assume overall responsibility for the analysis, design, and implementation of a departmental health record tracking system. On the other hand, an HIM professional who has oversight for enterprisewide clinical information systems may have responsibility for assisting clinical areas in carrying out the processes of the system development life cycle. The HIM manager may assume a more technical role and be responsible for direction and day-to-day operations of individual phases of the system development life cycle for a specific project. It is not unusual to see HIM managers leading project development teams for a variety of clinical and patient-related information systems.

SYSTEM LIFE CYCLES

To fully appreciate the development of a system and its place within the organization, a knowledge of the life cycle of systems is necessary. Like human beings, all systems go through a life cycle. Systems originate, develop, and, finally, decline. Several models have been developed that illustrate the concept of a system life cycle. In this section, four perspectives of system life cycles are discussed.

- General system life cycle
- Information system life cycle
- Discontinuity of information system life cycle
- Organization-wide information system life cycle

General System Life Cycle

Information systems are similar to biological, social, and political systems. All systems go through a system life cycle. All systems have a birth or development period, a period of growth and maturity, and a period of decline or deterioration.[1] The following example demonstrates the four phases of the **general system life cycle.**

EXAMPLE

Birth and Development

Ten years ago, the health records department of a community hospital implemented a system to track the location of medical records. The goal of the system was to allow health record employees to charge outpatient records to hospital clinical areas, be able to identify record location for subsequent requests, and monitor the length of time records were absent from the permanent files. The system was primarily a departmental system to satisfactorily meet the needs of this 300-bed facility.

Growth and Maturity

In the intervening years, the hospital has formed several alliances that have broadened the scope of the services provided. Among them is the expansion of outpatient services through acquisition of several clinics in the community, the addition of an outpatient surgery facility, and alliances with substance abuse, rehabilitation, and skilled nursing facilities. At first, the record-tracking system was able to expand to keep pace with the institution's growing needs. However, as the hospital evolved into a health care enterprise, the needs for record tracking and monitoring have changed.

Decline

The current record-tracking system, which was designed primarily for internal departmental use, does not meet today's need for a more comprehensive, enterprisewide distributed system.

Information System Life Cycle

As the record-tracking example above illustrates, information systems have a life cycle that is analogous to the general system life cycle. To be more definitive in describing what occurs at each phase in the **information system life cycle,** more descriptive labels are attached to each phase:[1]

- Design
- Implementation
- Operation and maintenance
- Obsolescence

For example, in the information system life cycle, the development phase of the general system life cycle is usually referred to as the *design* phase. This is the phase in which analysis of the requirements and design of the information system occurs. The general system life cycle growth phase is normally called the *implementation* phase. In this phase, development, testing, and implementation take place. The *operation/maintenance* activity of the information system life cycle is similar to the maturity phase of the general system life cycle. This is the functioning phase of the system in which activities to maintain, update, and operate the system occur. The fourth phase of deterioration or decline is identified in the information system life cycle as system *obsolescence*. Figure 18–1 shows a comparison between the phases of the general system and the information system life cycles.

The time over which each phase occurs varies from system to system. Large, complex systems may take months to years to design, whereas simpler, smaller systems may take a few weeks to design. The length of time over which a system can meet user needs depends on many variables. Sometimes these variables include a change in work volume, a change in strategic organizational objectives, or a change in the type of work performed. As the example above illustrates, the system became obsolete because it could not accommodate a larger volume and broader range of users in a distributed environment.

Information System Life Cycles in the Organization

An organization is composed of hundreds and perhaps thousands of interacting and interfacing information systems. For example, in a health care facility, there are information systems that support clinical functions, such as those that provide nursing care, dietary requirements, rehabilitation needs, and diagnostic testing. There are also information systems that support administrative functions, such as patient registration, collection of payments, marketing, and human resources. All of these systems use some type of information technology to assist them in carrying out their functions. Given the number of information systems in any organization, it is easy to recognize that at any one time, multiple information systems are in different phases of an information system life cycle. For example, the clinical laboratory system may be in the maintenance phase of the information system life cycle while the radiology information system is in the design phase of the information system life cycle. On the other hand, the HIM department tracking system may be in the implementation phase while the marketing information system is in the obsolescence phase. Thus, information systems throughout an enterprise are in a constant state of fluctuation. It is unlikely that at any given time, all organization information systems would be in a state of maturity. It is more likely that there will consistently be a significant level of variability in information system life cycles. Figure 18–2 shows the concept of information system fluctuation.

It is important for the health information manager to recognize this variability because this phenomenon of discontinuity causes stress within the organization. This stress can be manifested in multiple ways. One aspect of stress is the competition for resources. For example, the HIM department may be implementing a new master patient index system. At the same time, the clinical laboratory is in the process of selecting a new information system and the human resources department is requesting enhancements to its existing system. All three areas are in different phases of the information system life cycle. The HIM department system is in the implementation phase (second phase); the clinical laboratory system is in the design phase (first phase); and the human resources system is in the operations phase (third phase). Figure 18–2 shows this phenomenon of discontinuity among information system life cycle stages.

Each of these systems will be competing for some of the same sets of resources. In the scenario above, there is competition for similar resources, including technical assistance (*people*) during approximately the same pe-

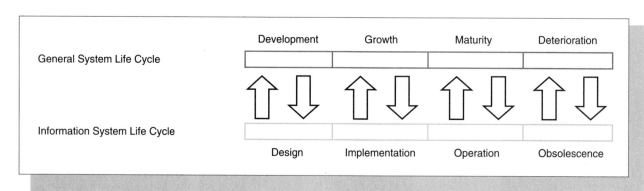

FIGURE 18–1. Comparison of general system and information system life cycle stages.

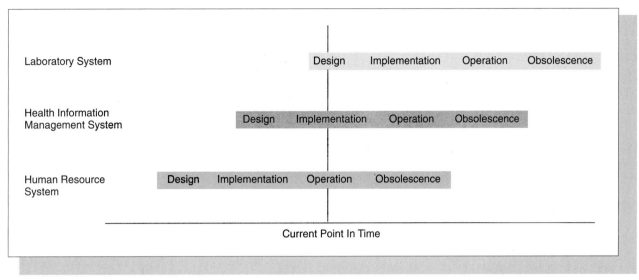

FIGURE 18–2. Comparison of departmental information systems at different life cycle stages.

riod (*time*) and use of the same hardware (*equipment*) resources. There is also competition for financial allocation (*budget*). The HIM department needs technical assistance, training, and site preparation assistance during its implementation stage. The clinical laboratory needs technical assistance in identifying system design. The human resources system requires technical expertise to perform the upgrade and may require a greater portion of the equipment resource. All systems bear some cost in regard to financial expenditure. Figure 18–3 shows the stress on resources by competing information system needs.

The juxtaposition of system life cycles constitutes the usual environment in any organization and results in competition for limited resources. Appreciating the nature of this situation allows the health information manager to understand that implementation and operation of information technology contribute to organizational stress. Prioritization of needs and suitable allocation of resources are exceedingly important to meet organiza-

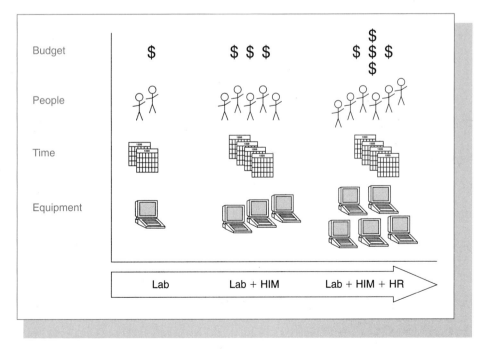

FIGURE 18–3. Stress on resources by competing systems.

tional needs. It is, however, a significant challenge for the organization to appropriately balance the allocation of resources so that maximum benefit is realized.

Aggregate Information Life Cycle of the Organization

A logical question that might arise after the discussion of information system life cycles is whether or not the organization as a whole has a life cycle of its own. In other words, can a composite picture of an organizationwide information system life cycle be visualized if all information system life cycles were aggregated into a whole? This is an appropriate question because an organization's level of experience and sophistication with information technology has an impact on how it manages the technology. For example, an organization that is just starting to automate its information functions would have a different emphasis in management of its technology than an organization in which most of the information functions were already automated.

Nolan first described the concept of organizations that have information system life cycles.[2] The view postulated by Nolan is that an organization at any given point in time is at a certain maturity or level of sophistication in deployment of information technology. Nolan postulates the following stages in his organizationwide information system life cycle:

- *Initiation,* where the organization begins to automate information functions

- *Expansion* or growth of information automation, which is usually unplanned

- *Control,* where the organization tries to manage information technology growth and control resources, primarily budget growth

- *Integration,* where the organization attempts to integrate distributed systems through organizationwide standards, policies, and procedures

- *Data administration,* where integrated databases are developed and information is considered a critical organizational resource

- *Maturity,* where growth of applications is focused on their strategic importance to the organization

At each of these stages, the organization usually takes a different approach to management of information technology. For example, in the early stages of initiation and expansion, the organization is likely to assume a laissez-faire attitude, allowing expansion of the technology with little or no organizationwide control. As the growth of technology expands, the organization becomes most concerned with budget, allocation of funds for technology expansion, and centralizing resources. In other

words, the organization tries to gain control over the resources. As time goes on, the organization becomes more sophisticated in its management of the technology. The organization grows to realize the need for integration of technology and information management. In the stages of integration and data administration the organization emphasis is to treat information and its associated technologies and management as critical to the survival of the organization. The main focus in these stages is to distribute functions but also to centralize standards for both technology and information management. In the final stage, maturity, the organization views information as a strategic resource and emphasizes development of applications that further the strategic advantage of the enterprise.

Although it is important to understand that individual information systems have their own life cycles, it is equally important to recognize that an enterprise will also be at a certain stage of information technology management maturity. Being able to identify an enterprise's point in its life cycle helps explain to the health information manager *why* certain policies exist or specific strategies are deployed. For instance, if a health information manager works in an organization that is in the integration stage of the life cycle, the manager should not be surprised to find that there are centralized standards that must be followed. This might be in areas that relate to the type of network architecture, communication protocols, or productivity tools that are allowed. On the other hand, if the health information manager is employed in an organization in which technology is newly implemented, it would not be unlikely to discover that there are few policies and procedures that help to direct information growth. Understanding at what stage of the information life cycle maturity an organization is helps the health information manager understand why or why not certain information management practices are followed.

System Obsolescence

Information systems become obsolete for several reasons. A system may be obsolete because it uses older technology that cannot meet current information-processing demands. The use of older technology in itself does not necessarily mean that the information system is obsolete. Rather, it is whether or not technology meets required needs that determines obsolescence. For example, it would be appropriate for clerical workers to use an older technology if they used their computer solely for light processing activities. In comparison, it would probably be inappropriate for them to use an older technology if their work responsibilities included heavy word processing, desktop publishing, and decision-support activities. On the other hand, a department with a local area network using a proprietary operating system might be considered obsolete if the organization was moving toward an enterprisewide network environment using an open-systems protocol and a nonproprietary operating system.

Systems can also become obsolete because they cannot handle an increase in the volume of data or cannot handle more sophisticated data management tasks. From a software perspective, for example, a system constructed using a flat file database architecture would probably be obsolete if the organization were attempting to develop an integrated architecture for data management. In this case, the use of relational database technology would probably be more appropriate. From a hardware perspective, a system could become obsolete if it could not handle an increase in the volume of data to be processed. Perhaps a newer, faster processor would need to be purchased and/or a faster and larger capacity data storage medium used.

Systems frequently become obsolete because they do not support the strategic objectives of the organization. The record-tracking system described in the first part of this chapter is a good example. The strategic objective of the organization in that example was to provide a broader range of services at multiple, diverse sites. Because of the change in strategic objective from providing only acute care services to providing acute, ambulatory, and long-term care services, the record-tracking system could not meet the needs of the organization. In other words, it became obsolete because it could not support a strategic organization change. A common example of systems that quickly become obsolete are those in the area of decision support. Decision-support systems provide a variety of tools that help management in making decisions about semistructured and unstructured problems. Because the health care environment marketplace is changing at such a rapid pace, there is a need for accurate, reliable, and user-friendly decision-support systems. Many decision-support systems and their associated tools are not flexible enough to meet current demands for information access and analysis and quickly become outdated.

Sometimes information systems become obsolete because of a change in user expectations. For example, a hospitalwide information system may provide the necessary functionality for nursing care, but users expect the functionality to be enhanced in some way. The users might have seen another system that used a graphic user interface instead of a menu interface as in the current system. Or another system might use color on the display screen to alert clinical providers of out-of-range laboratory values rather than using a two-color display with asterisks to mark such values. As users become more sophisticated about how information systems can help them to more optimally perform their daily tasks, it is likely that they will expect increased system enhancements.

In addition to changes in technology, operational functions, strategic objectives, and user expectations, information systems may become obsolete because they simply wear out, in other words, break down. Mechanical failures with storage devices, input devices, output devices, or processing components are more likely to occur as the system grows older.

INFORMATION SYSTEM DEVELOPMENT LIFE CYCLE

As systems decline or become obsolete, new systems need to be developed. In this section, a structured approach that describes various methods for handling system decline and developing an information system is presented. This approach is usually referred to as the **information system development life cycle.** This approach provides tools and techniques that essentially encompass the first two stages of the information system life cycle (the design and implementation phases).

The system development life cycle consists of the customary steps that are taken in developing an information system. Although there may be variation among authors about the names of these steps, the process usually encompasses the areas of analysis, design, implementation, and evaluation. Although the steps in the development life cycle are primarily concerned with new development efforts, they are equally appropriate with some modification for selection of already developed products from the vendor market. Modification of steps as applied to vendor system selection is noted within each section describing the various steps.

Because this chapter is concerned with the HIM professional's role in systems development, there is an emphasis on tasks associated with analysis, implementation, and evaluation support activities and a de-emphasis on purely technical activities associated with each process. The focus in the design area is more conceptual than technical and concentrates on issues that relate to general system design principles and user interface concerns associated with input and output media.

ANALYSIS

The development or selection of an information system can be an arduous and complex process. When faced with the challenge of information system development, a logical question that arises is "Where should we begin?" The beginning of any development project effort usually starts with a perceived need. For example, a supervisor in the HIM department may recognize that a new information system for case mix analysis may provide improved decision-support capabilities. Or, a perceived need may arise when a current information system, like the record-tracking system mentioned previously, enters the obsolescence phase of the information system life cycle. The launching of the development process may also be initiated by users who believe that new technology is required to support their daily tasks. Whatever the reason for initiation, the goal of the analysis step is to determine the feasibility for a new system and the scope of the developmental or selection effort. In this context, assessing system feasibility means determining the following:

- Whether there is a need for a new system
- Whether the organization can afford a new system
- Whether sufficient technical expertise exists to develop and/or operate the new system
- What general functionality is expected
- What benefits are expected from system implementation

Tools and Aids for System Analysis

Health information professionals have many tools at their disposal to assist in determining the feasibility and scope of any new information system development effort. These tools are appropriate to use whether the system is being developed internally by the organization or whether the system will be purchased from a vendor. Martin and Yourdon suggest several tools for the use in systems analysis, including the following:[3,4]

- Action diagrams
- Data analysis diagrams
- Data dictionary
- Data flow diagram
- Data navigation diagrams
- Data structure diagrams
- Decision trees and tables
- Decomposition diagrams
- Dialogue design diagrams
- Entity-relationship diagrams
- Process specifications
- State transition diagrams

The use of each of these tools depends on the desired output from the analysis and analyst preference. In this chapter, only those tools that are most likely to be needed in the set of analysis aids of the HIM professional are discussed. Table 18–1 lists each of these and a brief description of their purpose.

TABLE 18–1 STRUCTURED ANALYSIS TOOLS AND PURPOSE	
DEVELOPMENT TOOL	**PURPOSE**
Data dictionary	Data modeling technique that is a repository for all primitive-level data structures and data elements within a system.
Data flow diagram	Graphic representation of the flow of data through a system. Can be a logical or physical data flow.
Decomposition diagram	Used to break down problems into smaller levels of detail. Usually depicted in a hierarchy chart similar to an organization chart.
Entity-relationship diagram	Data modeling technique that depicts the logical design of a database schema.

Decomposition Diagrams—Hierarchy Chart

The **hierarchy chart** is a type of decomposition diagram. Its purpose is to break down problems into smaller and smaller detail. The hierarchy chart does this by identifying all the tasks in a process and grouping them into various hierarchial levels. The hierarchy chart is organized in a tree-like manner. Each task in the chart is called a *node*. Each node, except for the uppermost node, has a single *parent node*. Each parent node may have none, one, or multiple *children nodes*. *Sibling nodes* are nodes that are all on the same level of the chart. The lowest nodes on each level of the chart (i.e., nodes that have no children) are called *functional primitives*. The functional primitive nodes are eventually translated into program modules that perform the work of the system.

The following is an example of the process used by one HIM department for reviewing patient record completeness at the time of discharge. This example is used throughout the chapter to show how various analysis tools can be applied.

PATIENT RECORD COMPLETENESS REVIEW PROCESS. The Community Hospital Health Information Department uses the following manual system for reviewing the completeness of records of discharged patients.

1. When an inpatient is discharged, the patient record is received in the HIM department from various patient care areas throughout the hospital. The patient name and number from the record are matched against the daily patient discharge list. After matching the record with the discharge list, the patient name and record number are added to the daily record receipt list.

The record is then reviewed by a clerk for any deficiencies.

2. After the record is reviewed, a record deficiency data card is completed for each physician whose reports are incomplete. One copy of the deficiency card is attached to the record and one copy is filed alphabetically by the physician's last name in the deficiency file. The record is then sent to the coding analysis area for diagnostic and procedure coding. For all records sent to coding, the record number, patient name, and current date are compiled on the daily list of records sent to coders. The daily list is filed by date in the coder file.

3. An outguide data form is completed and placed in an outguide for each record that has been sent to the coding analysis area. The outguide is filed by record number in terminal digit order in the deficiency record area.

4. Once the record is coded, it is received back in the analysis area. The record outguide is removed and replaced with the record. The record number, patient name, and date sent to coders are deleted from the daily list of coder records.

To construct a hierarchy chart for this example, the first step is to list all the tasks in the order they occur. The following list enumerates the tasks that are performed once the record is received by the HIM department.

1. Reconcile the record number and patient name with the daily patient discharge list.

2. Complete the daily record receipt list.

3. Review the record for completeness.

4. Complete a deficiency card for each physician.

5. Attach one copy of the deficiency card to the record.

6. File a copy of each deficiency card alphabetically by physician's last name in the deficiency file.

7. Send the record to coders.

8. Compile a daily list of records sent to coders.

9. File the daily list of records sent to the coders in the coder file.

10. Complete the outguide data form.

11. Place the outguide data form in the outguide.

12. Place the outguide in terminal digit order in the deficiency record area.

13. Receive the record back from the coding area.

14. Remove the outguide in the deficiency file and replace it with the record.

15. Delete the record number from the daily list of records sent to the coding area.

Most of these processes are at the primitive functional level. To develop a tree structure, it is necessary to assemble the processes together in functionally similar groups. For example, the first two tasks relate to record receipt and catalog. Tasks 3 through 6 relate to deficiency review activities. Tasks 7 through 12 are associated with charging out the record to the coding area. The last tasks are related to reprocessing the receipt of the record from the coding area.

Figure 18–4 shows a completed hierarchy chart. Level 0 contains the name of the overall process. The next hierarchy level contains the categories of record catalog, deficiency review, coding charge-out, and re-

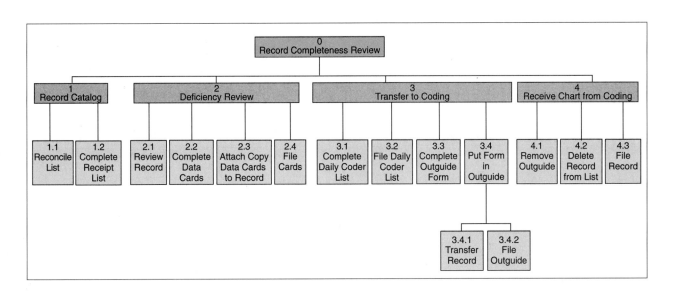

FIGURE 18–4. Hierarchy chart for record completion review.

processing record receipt. The next level contains some of the functional primitive tasks. Because review of the record (2.1) and transfer chart to coding (3.1) require additional processing, a third level is required to reach the functional primitives. The shaded areas of the hierarchy chart indicate those tasks for which program modules must be written. These areas also provide the basis for developing a data flow diagram, discussed later in this chapter.

Why would an HIM professional want to develop a hierarchy chart? Whether the information system under consideration is to be developed in-house or purchased from a vendor, a hierarchy chart of the system should be developed for the following reasons:

- The process of developing the chart forces a review of the current process. Redundancies in work patterns can be identified and inefficiencies can be corrected.
- The hierarchy chart can provide the foundation for building data flow diagrams.
- The chart provides a means of communication with developers and can also be used to assess whether or not a vendor product will meet user needs.

Data Flow Diagrams

Once tasks within a system are identified it is necessary to expand this information into a data flow diagram. **Data flow diagrams (DFD)** are used to track the flow of data through an entire system. They identify the data flow within a system, in essence providing a data map of what data go from an area, what data are received by an area, and what data are either temporarily or permanently stored in an area. In addition to tracking data flow, a DFD also identifies transformations on data (processes) and data repositories (data stores).

There are four essential concepts related to DFDs. They include *external entities, processes, data stores,* and *data flows.* An *external entity* includes people or groups of people who interact with the system but are not internal to it. For example, a patient would be considered an external entity to a system of health care delivery. *Processes* are actions performed on data. In the chart completeness review example above, processes include completing the deficiency data card and compiling the daily record receipt list. *Data stores* are repositories for data. They may be either temporary or permanent storage areas. An example of a temporary data store from the chart completeness example is the deficiency file. *Data flows* represent the movement of data through a system. Data move out of entities, to entities, between processes, and into and out of data stores.

Specific symbols are used to identify each DFD component. The external entity is represented by a square. Table 18–2 displays DFD symbols with examples of each.

Like the hierarchy chart, DFDs are constructed by going from the complex to the simple. In other words, the system as a whole is first represented and successive levels represent more and more system detail. The method and construction rules for developing DFDs vary, depending on whose recommended process is followed.[1,5,6] The description and construction of DFDs in this chapter follow general development rules. For

TABLE 18-2 DATA FLOW DIAGRAM SYMBOLS

DATA FLOW NAME	DATA FLOW SYMBOL	EXAMPLE
External entity: Person or group receiving or sending data		Admitting department
Process: Changes inputs to outputs		Complete outguide
Data store: Location of data storage		Deficiency record file
Data flow	⟶	Patient record

readers with an additional interest in developing a greater depth of tool usage, appropriate references are provided.[1,4–6]

Figures 18–5 through 18–10 represent the data flow of the record completeness review process. Figure 18–5 represents Level 0, or the context level, of the record completion review process. At this level, the process is represented in its most macro or global form. Figure 18–5 shows that data are received by the HIM department from two external entities. The admitting department sends discharge data to the HIM department and the patient care areas send the patient record. Notice that both the admitting department and the patient care areas are represented by the external entity symbol, the rectangle. The data flows (discharge data and patient record) are represented by the data flow symbol, the arrow. The record completion review system is represented by the process symbol, a rounded-corner rectangle. The permanent record file is represented by the data store symbol, the open rectangle.

The context level of the DFD provides a relatively simple picture of the system under study. In this example, the context level identifies the major external entities, data transformation, data flows, and data stores of the system. To fully understand the system, it is necessary to successively break down the process into more detailed parts. This is accomplished through explosion diagrams. Figures 18–6 through 18–10 represent first- and second-level explosions of the record completion review system.

Information contained in the hierarchy chart (can be used to help construct the successive DFD explosions. For example, in the hierarchy chart for the record completion review process (see Figure 18–4), four processes are identified. They include record catalog, deficiency review, coding charge-out, and record receipt. Figure

18–6 is the first-level explosion of the record completion review system. Notice that the four processes identified in the hierarchy chart are all represented in this diagram as transformations of data.

In Figure 18–6, the admitting, patient care, and coding areas are represented as external entities. Discharge data and the patient record are represented as data flows. The four processes and their relations to one another are also represented. Review of Figure 18–6 shows that there is a linear relation between the four processes—record catalog, deficiency review, coding transfer, and record receipt from coding. The completion of one process depends on the completion of its predecessor process. Notice that each process box is given an identifying number. For example, the record catalog process is labeled 1 and the deficiency review process is labeled 2. These numbers are used throughout successive explosion diagrams to identify each process.

Figure 18–7 is the second-level explosion for process 1—record catalog. This diagram shows the process in greater detail. Notice that the primitive functional levels represented in the hierarchy chart (see Figure 18–4) are also represented in Figure 18–7. Because they are the most detailed functions of this process, a third-level explosion diagram is not required for process 1. If the primitive functional level had not been reached in the second-level explosion, successive explosion diagrams would need to be developed until all functional primitives were represented. Figures 18–8 through 18–10 represent the second-level explosions for process 2, process 3, and process 4.

Why should an HIM professional possess the skills to construct DFDs? Like the hierarchy chart, DFDs should be developed whether the system is to be developed in-house or purchased from a vendor. An important

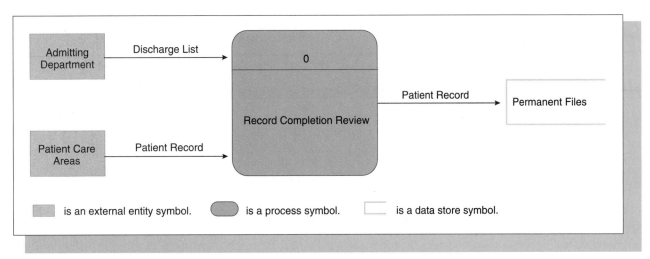

FIGURE 18–5. Context-level data flow diagram record completion review.

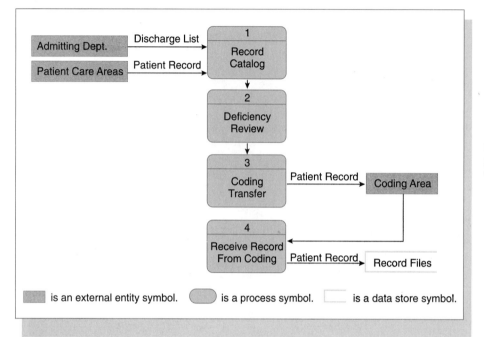

FIGURE 18–6. First-level explosion of record completion review.

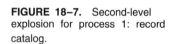

FIGURE 18–7. Second-level explosion for process 1: record catalog.

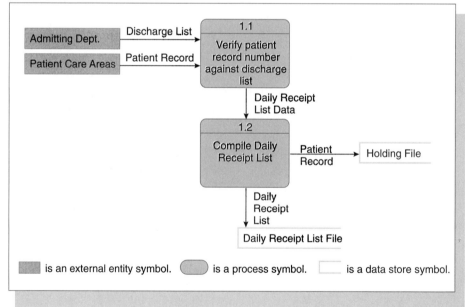

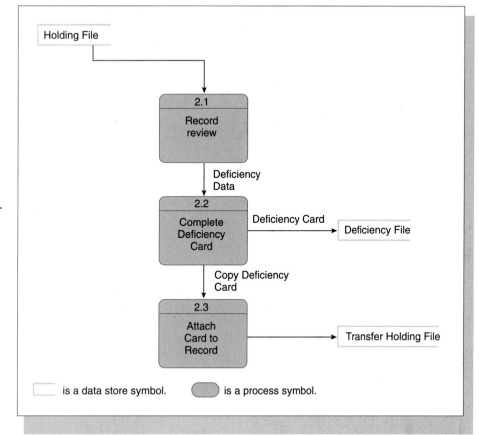

FIGURE 18–8. Second-level explosion for process 2: deficiency review.

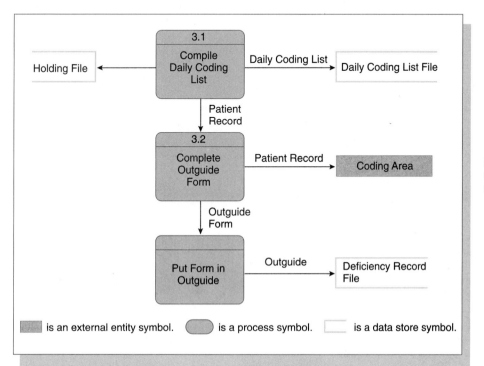

FIGURE 18–9. Second-level explosion for process 3: transfer to coding.

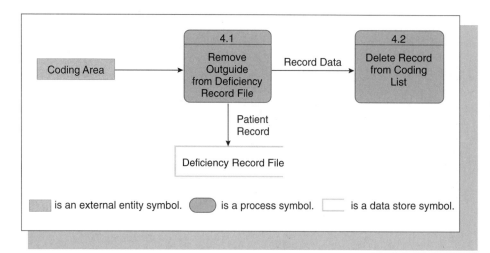

FIGURE 18–10. Second-level explosion of process 4: receive record from coding.

aspect of health information management is the design of information systems to support organizational functions and strategic objectives. To design systems, processes must be systematically described at the level of detail provided by tools such as the DFD. The construction of DFDs provides an avenue to describe the following:

- Where data originate
- How data are transformed
- How data flow
- Where data are deposited

Without this level of detail, an information system cannot be adequately designed.

HIM professionals must be able to interact with users and assist them in systematically breaking down complex systems into smaller and smaller components. They frequently serve as intermediaries between users and system developers. The processes represented in DFDs are much easier for users and developers to understand than if the processes were described in narrative or prose form. DFDs often help to resolve discrepancies in perceptions of how something is done or should be performed. Using DFDs helps to avoid confusion, which is a critical element in any system design process.

Data Dictionary

The **data dictionary** describes all the primitive-level data structures and data elements within a system. It is the central repository for all information about the database and functions as a catalog for identifying the nature of all the data in a system. It provides the central resource for ensuring that standard definitions for data elements and data structures are used throughout the system. The typical data dictionary includes information about processes, data flows, data stores, and data ele-

ments in a system. For example, in a data dictionary, the data element "sex" used in a master patient index would contain information about the data element's data type, its length, its range, allowed values, and meanings. In this case, the data element "sex" would have a data type of alphanumeric, its length would be one character, and allowed values would be "F" or "M." The meaning would be included as a notation indicating that "sex" referred to the patient's gender and that "M" meant male and "F", female.

How is the data dictionary compiled? There are several ways that a data dictionary can be notated.[1,5-7] The style used depends largely on the procedures established and the preference of individual information system departments. There usually is a unique notation for data structures, data processes, data flows, data stores, and data elements. The Visible Analyst Workbench,[8] CASE tool, provides a specific format for notation for data elements, data processes, data flows, data stores, and external entities. This notation includes identifying the following:

- Project—Name of the project to which the element, process, flow, store, or entity is related
- Label—Unique data name
- Entry type—Type of data entity, such as data element, process, data store, external entity, data flow
- Description—Used for more complete description of the data entity if the label is not self-explanatory
- Alias—Other names by which the data entity is identified
- Values and meanings—Notation depends on the data entity type. For a data element, the length, type, and values that the element can

FIGURE 18–11. Data dictionary data element notation.

Project:	Master Patient Index
Label:	Sex
Entry Type:	Data Element
Description:	Patient gender
Alias:	None
Values/Meaning:	Length: 1 character Type: alphanumeric Value: M = male; F = female

take on would be notated. For a data structure, such as patient account, all the data elements that compose the patient account data structure would be noted.

An example of how a data dictionary notation would look for the data element "sex" appears in Figure 18–11.

Figure 18–12 shows an example of a data dictionary notation for data flow. This example is taken from the record completion review system project. The label is daily discharge list, which appears in the second-level explosion for process 1 in Figure 18–7. The entry type is data flow. The description gives a more complete explanation about the data flow. There is no alias. Note that in this data dictionary entry, there is no "values/meaning" section. In its place is an area for noting the composition of the flow. In this case, the daily discharge list is composed of current date, medical record number, patient last and first name and middle initial, patient's date of birth, admission date, and discharge date. The location of the data flow is indicated in the last entry of this notation.

An example of a data dictionary notation for a data store appears in Figure 18–13. The data store used in this example is from the record completion review system, process 2 (deficiency review). The data label is physician deficiency file. The entry type is a data store. The description area adds more detail to the label name. The composition of the data store is indicated along with notations where the store appears in the DFDs.

Figure 18–14 shows an example of a data dictionary

FIGURE 18–12. Data dictionary notation for data flow.

Project:	Record Completion Review System
Label:	Daily Discharge List
Entry Type:	Data Flow
Description:	Daily list of patients discharged from the hospital
Alias:	None
Composition:	Daily Discharge List = currentdate + medrecno + ptlname + ptfname + ptmidinital + ptdob + admitdate + dischgdate
Locations:	Context- and first-level explosions; second-level explosion of Process 1, Record Catalog Data Flow → Daily Discharge List

Project:	Record Completeness Review System
Label:	Physician Deficiency File
Entry Type:	Data Store
Description:	A file containing physician deficiency data cards. Used to identify specific deficiencies by physician for a particular patient record.
Alias:	None
Composition:	Physician Deficiency File = mdno + mdfname + medrecno + currentdate + dischgdate + deficiencytype

FIGURE 18–13. Data dictionary notation for data store.

notation for a process. The process in this example is process 2.1, record review, from the record completion review system. In this notation, the label is record review and the entry type is process. The process number is notated along with the process description. Like the data flow and data store notations, the location in the DFD where the process occurs is also indicated.

Why is the development of a data dictionary important? One reason is that the data dictionary provides a central repository of standard terminology and the description of data used in all the information systems in the organization. The data dictionary helps to reduce data redundancy and increase the integrity of enterprise-wide data. Without this standardization, it is unlikely that efficient and effective information systems can be created. When used with hierarchy charts and DFDs, the data dictionary helps to fully document an information system. This type of documentation can speed up

the process of developing system programs. It also provides information that makes modification of programs and data easier. Without this type of documentation, system maintenance would be extremely difficult if not impossible. Like the development of DFDs, the development of a data dictionary helps to decrease confusion among users and analysts about the purpose and functions of a system.

Entity-Relationship Diagrams

System hierarchy charts, DFDs, and data dictionaries are all important tools in the analysis and design process. Another tool frequently used to help describe the relations among data in an information system is the **entity-relationship diagram** (ERD). The ERD is principally used to illustrate the logical design of information system databases. This is accomplished by describing

Project:	Record Completeness Review System
Label:	Record Review
Entry Type:	Process
Description:	
Process Description:	Each record of a discharged patient is reviewed by a health information department employee against standard facility criteria for patient record completeness.
Locations:	Record Review Process (2.1)

FIGURE 18–14. Data dictionary notation for data process.

diagrammatically the relation between entities and by identifying entity attributes. ERDs are composed of three categories of items:

- Entities
- Relations
- Attributes

Entities are objects such as people, places, things, or events that make up the data of a database. In the record completeness review system, entities include physicians (people), patient records (things), deficiency card (things) and patient care areas (places). In an ERD, an entity is represented by a rectangle.

Relations are links or ties that exist between or among entities. In an ERD, a relation is represented by a diamond. An example of a relation in the record completeness review system is the relation between a patient record (an entity) and a deficiency card (an entity). In this relation, a patient record can have many deficiency cards (i.e., there are many physicians, each having a card, who can have a deficiency). Another example is the relation between a physician (entity) and a deficiency card (entity). In this relation, a physician can have many deficiency cards (i.e., have deficiencies for more than one record).

Attributes describe both entities and relations. Attributes may be thought of as the data elements that need to be captured to fully describe an entity. As an example, the attributes of the deficiency card in the record completeness review system include patient number, physician name, physician number, and list of deficiencies. The attributes of the entity "physician" would include physician number and physician name.

In an ERD, entity and relation symbols are connected by straight lines. In addition to indicating a relation among entities, it is also important to indicate how frequently the occurrence can exist at any given point in time. In the example above, the relation between a patient record and deficiency cards can occur many times (i.e., a patient record can have many deficiency cards at any given point in time). This relation is referred to as a one-to-many relation. Other examples of relations include many-to-many (m to m) and one-to-one (1 to 1).

Figure 18–15 shows the use of a simple ERD. In this case, the relation between a patient record and a deficiency card is described. Note that both the entities (patient record and deficiency card) are represented by a rectangle. The relation "has" is represented by a diamond. The type of relationship (1 to many) is represented by the characters "1" and "m" on either side of the relationship symbol. This ERD is read in the following way: Each patient record can have many deficiency cards. The reverse of this is that each deficiency card can only relate to one patient record.

Another example of an ERD is shown in Figure 18–

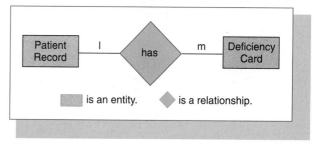

FIGURE 18–15.   Entity-relationship diagram for deficiency cards.

16. This figure shows the deficiency review process. In this case, the entities include the patient record, the review process, deficiency cards, and physicians. Starting at the left side, the diagram says that a patient record undergoes one review process at any given time. The review process generates many deficiency cards, and each deficiency card records only the deficiencies of one physician. Finally, the diagram says that each physician is associated with many patient records at one time and that each patient record is associated with many physicians at any given time. This last relation is the only many-to-many relation represented in the diagram. In this figure, attributes for the entities of patient record, deficiency card, and physician are included. Attributes, for example, for deficiency card include the key attribute of patient record number (MEDRECNO), physician identifier (MDNO), current date (CURRENT-DATE), discharge date (DISCHGDATE), and deficiency type (DEFICIENCYTYPE). The key attribute for each entity is underlined.

Why is the ERD important? Development of ERDs should be done whether the system is to be developed in-house or purchased from a vendor. In most system development projects, there are hundreds of complex ERDs that describe the entire system under development. The ERD is an important tool for the development of a logical data model of the system. The logical data model reflects a high-level, global view of information within the organization and forms the basis for the physical design of the database. As such, it prescribes physical database requirements such as a number of files, primary keys, and attributes. If the logical structure is badly designed, the databases are likely to be inefficient and ineffective. Therefore, a great deal of attention must be paid to the accuracy and completeness of the logical data model.

CASE Tools

A logical question that should arise after studying the various structured analysis tools is "How are the prod-

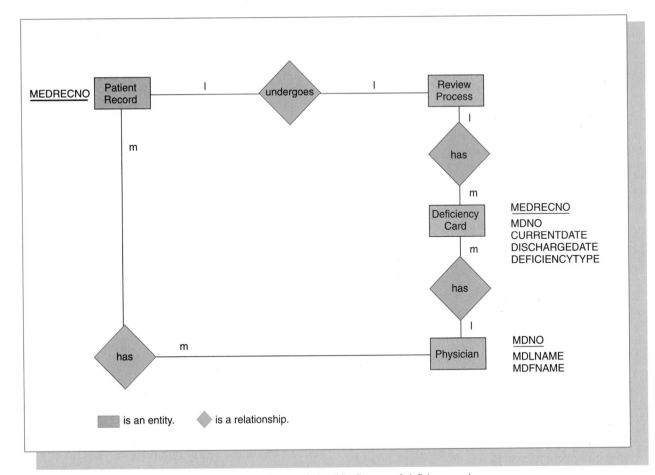

FIGURE 18–16. Entity-relationship diagram of deficiency review.

ucts that are derived from each of these tools integrated?" In other words, how are the charts, diagrams, dictionaries, and tables tied together to derive a coherent picture of system design? Until recently, most of the work to develop hierarchy charts, data dictionaries, and DFDs was done by hand. This was a time-consuming process and tended to produce fragmentation in system development. These development tools have now been computerized to improve the efficiency, accuracy, and completeness of the system development process. These computerized systems are called computer-aided software engineering (also referred to as computer-aided systems engineering) tools, or CASE.

CASE tools provide a mechanism for the electronic development of systems analysis aids such as structure charts, DFDs, ERDs, and data dictionaries. Instead of developing charts and diagrams manually, the analyst can use a computer program with a graphic interface to assist in development. CASE tools do not automatically develop the various charts and diagrams. Rather, the designer interacts with the CASE program to select the appropriate symbols, connectors, and labels and electronically draw the proper diagram. All diagrams, graphs, tables, and dictionaries that are developed are stored electronically.

CASE tools help designers relate their work electronically by organizing information about a system in a central repository. The central repository may contain data models, logic definitions, functional models, and screen and report definitions. Once it is developed, designers can query the repository for information about the system. The physical design of databases and program code can also be generated from the repository by system developers. If new processes are added or current ones extended, previously developed models, graphs, tables, and dictionaries can be reused or easily updated.

ADVANTAGES TO USING CASE PRODUCTS. There are many benefits of using a CASE product. An obvious benefit is convenience for system designers. CASE products provide an effective mechanism for development,

Advantages and Disadvantages to Using CASE Products	
Advantages	Disadvantages
Convenient for system designers to use	Expensive
Easy to alter existing charts and diagrams	Must purchase products from several vendors
Fast development of analysis tools	Problems integrating products from different vendors
Increases productivity	
Reduces design errors	

storage, retrieval, and update of charts, tables, diagrams, and dictionaries. Updates, enhancements, corrections, or extensions to already developed charts and diagrams can be easily accomplished using CASE products. CASE allows for faster development of analysis tools. Data models can be efficiently developed and results shared with other design team members and users in a more timely manner than by using manual methods. Productivity increase as a result of using CASE tools is estimated at about 15 per cent.[9] Reduction of errors is another benefit of using CASE products in the design process. Because CASE products enforce organization of system details and contain automatic consistency checks, errors in design are reduced. CASE products also increase coordination within and among projects, resulting in better standardization. Through standardization, better system documentation occurs, which can be easily maintained and updated.

DISADVANTAGES TO USING CASE PRODUCTS. Although many advantages can be realized by using CASE products, some disadvantages also exist (see Advantages and Disadvantages to Using CASE Products). CASE products can be expensive. Training costs for updating the skills of designers and analysts must also be considered. The cost of retraining designers and analysts in the use of CASE products averages between $30,000 and $50,000 per person.[9] Because one vendor does not usually provide an entire set of tools that are required to develop an information system, products from several vendors may have to be purchased. The use of several vendor products can increase costs and training time and create problems with integration.

Investigative Strategies for Analysis of Requirements

In this chapter, information life cycles and the analysis of system requirements have been discussed. The importance of developing structured tools such as hierarchy charts, DFDs, and data dictionaries when describing a system has been addressed. However, these tools require the gathering of information before they can be constructed. A legitimate question to ask is "How is the information needed for input to these tools gathered?" Various investigative strategies can be used to gather information during the analysis phase of system development. Among them are interviews with users, questionnaires, observation of tasks, and review of documents, forms, and procedures. Because HIM professionals often serve as liaisons between system developers and the end-user community, it is important that they understand and become skilled in the techniques for gathering information.

Ways of Gathering Information

INTERVIEWS. Interviews are a common method for gathering information about system requirements. The use of the interview strategy has several advantages. First, it provides an opportunity for end-users to feel as though they are co-owners in the design and development process. All too frequently, information systems are designed and selected without appropriate user input. The one-on-one interview process helps to break down barriers of user resistance by allowing the user to assume a vested interest in the process. If users are involved in the development and design of an information system, they are less likely to resist system implementation.

The type of questions asked during an interview process, the length of time that an interview takes, and the number of people to be interviewed depend on the system under development and the desired outcomes from the interview process. In general, the following factors can contribute to a successful interview process:

- Defining the target audience
- Identifying the objectives of the interview
- Developing appropriate interview questions and format
- Adequately analyzing and documenting responses

Target Audience. To be successful, the interview process must adequately identify the target audience—that is, which people are most familiar with system requirements on operational and strategic levels. For example, in the record-tracking system presented earlier, several groups of people should be interviewed. Naturally, the HIM department clerks responsible for record tracking should be interviewed because they are the direct users of the system. The interview process also should be expanded beyond direct system users and include those who are or might be remote users or secondary beneficiaries of the system. Secondary beneficiaries of the system often provide a different perspective and significant insights into system needs. In this case, employees and managers in inpatient and outpatient clinical areas as well as those in the rehabilitation, substance abuse, and skilled nursing facilities would be likely candidates for the interview process.

It is also important to identify those people in the organization who are political power brokers and whose support is essential for the system under development. For example, the director of the HIM department, although not a frequent user of a chart-tracking system, would definitely be an important power broker in successful chart-tracking system development and would be included in the roster of interviewees.

Often overlooked in the interview process are those people who have knowledge of the strategic uses of information in the organization. Too often information systems are developed from only a day-to-day operational perspective. For example, a point-of-care nursing system might be selected by nurse users because of the system's interface and support of daily tasks. This same system, however, may not support the organization's strategic objective of providing accessible data for continuous quality improvement. In this case, the system would support day-to-day operational tasks well but would be inadequate in supporting strategic information needs. Therefore, managers concerned with strategic information needs should also be included in the roster of interviewees when appropriate.

The potential number of people to be interviewed can grow to be quite large. Because the interview process can be time-consuming (between 30 and 60 minutes), the interview audience should be selected carefully. All power brokers significant to the project should be interviewed. Those managers who are knowledgeable about the strategic use of information in the organization should also be interviewed. Many times, it is not feasible to interview all end users. For example, in a 1000-bed hospital, it would not be cost-effective or efficient to interview all nursing staff for identifying requirements of a nursing care information system. If it is not possible to interview all direct users, an appropriate sample from this group should be selected.

Interview Protocol. An interview protocol should be developed and field-tested before implementing the interview process. Because interview time is limited, the analyst often has only one chance to gather information from a person. Therefore, interview questions must be appropriate, complete, and unbiased. Interview questions can be structured or unstructured. Structured questions can elicit yes or no responses to a question, or they can present the interviewee with a list of options from which to choose. Examples of structured questions are "Which of the following data are important to you in your daily work?" and "Is the current system response time adequate in meeting your needs?" Because structured questions are asked the same way from inter-

view to interview, they require limited interviewing skill by the analyst. Because there is a limited range of responses to structured questions, interviewers do not have to make judgments about what was meant in a response. Therefore, results from structured questions are usually easy to compile.

Unstructured questions allow for more probing of end users than do structured questions. Unstructured questions may be tailored to each end user and allow for a broad spectrum of response or opinion. Examples of unstructured questions might be "What are the three or four most important types of data required for you to get your job done?" and "What are the three to five most critical functions for a system to have to help you perform your daily tasks?" The responses to unstructured questions are more difficult to document, collate, and analyze. Therefore, the use of unstructured questions requires the analyst to be a highly skilled interviewer.

Scenarios and cases can also be used in the interview process. With this technique, the end user is presented with a scenario that represents an actual situation. The end user responds to questions posed by the scenario. For example, the following scenario might be presented to a end user in a clinic.

> The clinic is losing reimbursement. Claims data are not being appropriately gathered. Physicians do not consistently complete encounter forms. When forms are completed, vague ICD-9-CM and CPT codes are often assigned. Frequently, encounter forms are lost or misplaced and bills are never generated.

After the scenario is presented, several questions are posed to the end user. The following questions might be used in this example: "What functions must a new information system support to eliminate these problems? What characteristics of the current system make it difficult for physicians to complete encounter forms?"

The scenario-based interview is becoming more and more popular. One reason for this is that the end user can respond to questions in the context of a real environment. Relating responses to a current situation is thought to provide a more realistic perspective of the functionality required of a system. No matter which method of questioning is used, gathering responses from unstructured questions usually takes more time than gathering responses from structured questions. Therefore, to avoid lengthy interviews, there should be an appropriate balance between structured and unstructured questions.

Before administration, the interview protocol should be field-tested. A field test is a trial run of the questions in the protocol. Normally, the field test consists of posing the protocol questions to a sample group. Field testing is advantageous for a number of reasons. First, it allows the interview questions to be tried out on a sample group. The clarity, appropriateness, and completeness of the interview questions can be assessed during the field test process. It is much easier to make necessary modifications during field test than after the interview process has begun. Second, the field test allows the analysts to determine how much time must be scheduled for interviews during the actual interview process. Because end users selected for the interview process are probably busy people, it is important to accurately estimate the time needed for each interview. Third, the field test gives the interviewers an opportunity to develop their interview skills and hone the interview process. The importance of training the interviewers should not be underestimated. The more skilled the interviewer, the better the results from the interview.

Format. Before any interview, the end user to be interviewed should be appraised of the interview's purpose. Advance notice of the interview goals give prospective interviewees an opportunity to collect their thoughts and organize their opinions. Typically, advance notice is given by personal contact by the director of the interview team or through written communication. Adequate time for the interview should be allocated. Thirty to 60 minutes should be sufficient. If the interview drags on beyond 1 hour, results usually are nonproductive.

Although the interview format may vary from situation to situation, it usually has the following basic components:

* The number of interviewers usually consists of two or three persons. If two interviewers are present during the interview, one assumes responsibility for asking questions and the other serves as note taker.

* It is important that at least one interviewer be free from the distraction of note taking so that full concentration is devoted to the responses of the end user.

Documentation. After the interview is completed, the analysts should immediately review the interview notes. Immediate debriefing between the interviewers allows the analysts the opportunity to come to consensus on what the end user said and to add additional information to the interview notes. The interview notes should be transcribed as soon as possible—preferably the same day—after the interview. The format for the interview documentation usually includes the following:

* Interview date
* Name and position of interviewee
* Names of interviewers
* List of questions posed

* Responses to questions
* Synopsis of the interview

In some cases, copies of the interview notes may be given to the interviewee to review. In this way, the end user provides formal confirmation of responses to the interview questions and has an opportunity to correct any errors.

After all interviews are completed, an overall analysis and synthesis are developed from all interview responses. This should include the following:

* Description of the methodology
* List of all interview questions
* List of all end users who were interviewed
* Synopsis of all facts and opinions
* General synthesis of interview material with recommendations

QUESTIONNAIRES. Questionnaires are a popular method for gathering data. Questionnaire development and administration are less time-consuming and less costly than the direct interview techniques. As opposed to the interview process, questionnaires can be distributed to a larger target audience. However, the benefits of using questionnaires can be severely diminished for several reasons. Questionnaires frequently are ambiguous, poorly constructed, and too long and have low response rates. To be effective, questionnaires should primarily be used to gather facts, not opinions. Questions should be of a structured nature allowing for yes or no responses or responses to lists of multiple-choice options. If opinions are being gathered, then a structured mechanism such as a Lickert scale should be used.

Question Construction. Before preparing any questions, the purpose and goals of the questionnaire must be defined. Only questions pertinent to the purpose of the survey should be included in the questionnaire. Questions are only as good as the degree to which they measure what they are intended to measure. Therefore, the purpose of any questionnaire must be clearly identified along with a list of measures that are anticipated. For example, a customer satisfaction survey would want to assess the satisfaction with the full range of customer services offered. Measures might include data about repair response times, system downtime, system response time, degree of helpfulness of trouble-shooting personnel, and degree of availability of trouble-shooting personnel. After the measures are identified, questions specific to each can be developed. In the customer satisfaction example above, the following questions might be asked to measure repair response time:

"In the past month, how often have you had to contact customer service for computer repair—one to two times, three to four times, more than four times?"

"From the time you called the customer service unit, how long did it take a troubleshooter to respond—less than 15 minutes, 15 to 30 minutes, more than 30 minutes?"

Tabulation and compilation of survey results can be time-consuming. Before constructing any question, it is important to consider how responses to questions will be tabulated by the analyst. Responses can be nominal, ordinal, interval, or ratio data. The level of data used determines the type of tabulation and statistical techniques that can be applied to the data. As an example, nominal data refers to unordered categories. Types of nominal data include patient gender, patient third party payer type, and patient employer. Nominal data can be tabulated by category, but sophisticated statistical tests cannot be used on nominal data. Ordinal data include people or events that are ordered or placed in ordered categories along a single dimension. Examples of ordinal data include responses to the following:

"How would you rate your satisfaction with repair response time—very good, good, poor?"
"How would you rate the degree of helpfulness of system troubleshooters—high, average, low?"

Ordinal data can be tabulated by category and provide more opportunity for performing statistical tests. Interval and ratio level data are best if advanced statistical techniques on the data are desired. The level of data collected depends on what kinds of tabulation and measurement are desired outcomes of the survey.

It is important that the meaning of questions be clear to the survey respondent. A question should ask only one thing. Double-barreled questions that contain two or more concepts should be avoided. An example of a double-barreled question is "Is the daily discharge data you receive complete and accurate?" This question includes two concepts: completeness and accuracy. The data may be complete (includes all data elements), but it may not be accurate (the information associated with the data elements may be incorrect). It is also important that survey questions be nonbiased. Questions that lead the end user to a conclusion have no place on a questionnaire. An example of a leading question is "Don't you agree that the health information management department has poor customer service?" A better way of handling this question would be to ask, "How would you rate the degree of customer service of the health information management department? Excellent, good, average, poor, very poor."

The meaning of questions should be clear to the end user. Many times surveys include questions that are difficult to understand. The following is an example of an ambiguous question: "Do you favor or oppose health care legislation?" In this example, health care legislation can mean just about anything. Is it referring to a plan for national health insurance, legislation relating to security of patient data, Medicare legislation, or some other type of legislation? The answer to this question cannot be interpreted without the analyst making assumptions about what the end user is thinking.

Questionnaire Construction. Having a set of good questions is the foundation for building a questionnaire. However, certain basic principles should be followed in the construction of the questionnaire if the survey is to be successful. A poorly constructed questionnaire, even if it contains good questions, can yield a poor response rate for a variety of reasons. A questionnaire should have a pleasing appearance to the end user, directions should be easy to understand, and the document should be easy to complete. If the survey is unattractive or too difficult or time-consuming to complete, a low response rate is likely.

The following steps are guidelines for beginning questionnaire construction:

1. Choose a concise, suitable title for the survey document.
2. Clearly state the purpose of the survey in a brief paragraph at the beginning of the survey instrument followed by simple, easy-to-follow directions.
3. Order the questions.

Survey instruments usually begin with relatively easy-to-answer questions that help get the end user into the questionnaire. The questionnaire should flow easily. It is best to put questions referring to similar concepts together. This provides for easier survey completion and data tabulation. For example, in the customer satisfaction questionnaire, all questions relating to troubleshooting might be placed together. Thought-provoking or sensitive questions are usually left to the end of the survey.

A consistent, clear, and attractive format should be decided on for the survey instrument. A practical step is to divide the survey into logical sections and assign titles and numerics or characters to each. For example, the section of a survey that collects data about the end user may be titled "A. Demographics," and all questions in that section are preceded by the character A—for example, A1., A2., A3., and so on.

The length of the survey varies, depending on its purpose and objectives. No questionnaire should take more than 30 minutes to complete. Therefore, it is important to select questions carefully, including only those that are directly related to purpose and desired measurements. Like the personal interview protocol, a survey document should be pretested. The pretest should be conducted on a small sample of people. Time estimates of survey completion should be gathered and problems with question clarity, survey directions, format, and spelling errors should be identified in the pretest and corrected before general survey distribution.

Questionnaire Administration. Once the survey instrument has been developed and pretested, it is ready for general administration. A cover letter to the end user should accompany the questionnaire. The cover letter should be a vehicle for getting the end user excited about the survey. It should state the purpose of the questionnaire and what value the results will have to the end user and describe how results will be used. End users should be assured that their responses will be kept confidential. To facilitate follow-up, each questionnaire can be assigned a number. A master log of numbers with associated end user names should be maintained. As surveys are returned, their number can be compared with the master list and the end users name crossed out. If initial response is low, the master log can be consulted and users who have not returned their surveys can be sent a reminder notice or another questionnaire. To obtain a good survey response, follow-up cards or reminders usually have to be sent once or twice. The initial response rate to a survey is usually about 30 per cent. Reminders significantly increase the response rate. Analysts should strive for a response rate of 60 per cent or more to justify conclusions made from questionnaire results.

OBSERVATION. Observation is an appropriate technique for collection of information about system requirements or identifying tasks performed by end users. Observation usually is used as an adjunct to interview and questionnaire techniques. The results of observation can be used to confirm or expand on information collected from interviews and quesionnaires. Observation should not be distracting to the end users.

Conducting an observation takes a high degree of skill. It usually requires a structured technique for recording observations, the details of a system, or how users perform their tasks. When conducting an observation, the subject of the review should be narrowed down. For example, in determining order processing needs for a hospital information system, the tasks of unit secretaries might be studied. Rather than observing all the tasks performed by a unit secretary, only one or a few tasks may be observed at a time. Because observation is tedious work, the analyst should not attempt to perform observations over extended periods. Because observations can also be distracting to the end user and disruptive to regular work flow, analysts should be unobtrusive. The maximum period for a single observation should be no more than 60 minutes.

Observation can also be used to confirm whether work tasks and work flow conform to written procedures. Procedure manuals frequently are a point of reference for information gathering about system needs.

However, many times they are inaccurate or out of date. Therefore, observation of how a procedure is performed may be essential if incorrect assumptions about the process are to be avoided.

As with other information-gathering techniques, the purpose of the observation should be well defined. A structured observation protocol should be developed to facilitate easy note taking. For example, an analyst may observe how unit secretaries enter laboratory orders in the hospital information system. The purpose of the review may be to reduce duplication of work effort, ascertain if procedure is being followed, or determine if data entry flow is optimal. In this case, a list of tasks that make up the function could be compiled. As each task is observed, the analyst can note how many times the task was performed, who performed it, and how long it took to complete. Figure 18–17 is an example of an observation protocol for laboratory order entry by unit secretaries.

DOCUMENT AND FORMS REVIEW. One useful method for gathering data about information needs is to conduct a document or forms review. Review of forms can identify what data elements are routinely collected by a facility. The forms review can also help to determine information flow by identifying form origination, distribution, and archival. Health care facilities are notorious for the number of forms they use to collect data. Forms review frequently helps to uncover duplication in work effort, variation in data meanings and use, and problems with data integrity.

GROUP ANALYSIS AND DESIGN. Group analysis and design is often used in place of other traditional structured approaches to data gathering. This method is often referred to as **joint application design** (JAD). In JAD, a group of people spend a concentrated time together in determining system requirements. The group is usually composed of end users, managers, analysts, and others who may have an impact on or be affected by the system under study. The time spent together may range from several hours to several days, depending on the results desired. The group analysis process is led by a facilitator who uses various techniques to elicit facts and opinions. Brainstorming and nominal group methods are frequently used.

Group decision support software (GDSS) has been used to facilitate the JAD process. GDSS is usually a network of workstations or portable personal computers that are all located in a conference or meeting room. GDSS products typically include word processing and text and database manipulation. Other functions such as electronic worksheets, graphics, and communication capabilities are customarily included. With a trained facilitator, GDSS can be used to administer a survey or

Laboratory Order-Entry Protocol			
Unit Secretary Name: _____	_____	Date: _____	Shift _____
Task Performed	Case #/Time	Case #/Time	Case #/Time
Review MD handwritten orders			
Check date and time of orders			
Log on to HIS system			
Select patient name			
Select MD name			
Select Lab Function			
Review current lab orders against new orders to determine duplicate orders			
Select lab order entry			
Select test			
Select schedule			
Select frequency of test			

FIGURE 18–17. Observation protocol for laboratory order entry.

questionnaire to a group of people at the same time and to facilitate brainstorming or a nominal group technique. Group members can respond electronically and anonymously to survey questions or list ideas, participate in brainstorming, or answer questions posed by a facilitator through various GDSS features. The use of this kind of computer support allows for anonymity of response, minimizes bias, and speeds up the deliberative process.

There are several benefits of using the JAD process. First, the use of JAD stimulates interaction between end users and analysts in a positive, nonthreatening environment. It facilitates the development of unbiased results through the use of structured processes such as brainstorming, delphi, nominal group process, and group consensus techniques. The use of JAD usually produces results in a shorter time frame than other investigative techniques.

Analysis Document

When brought together, results from the various investigative strategies and details outlined in analysis tools depict what is required for the new information system. All of this information is synthesized and documented in a *systems analysis document*. The systems analysis report presents a logical description of what was done during the analysis phase, how it was done, and what results were obtained. In addition to describing the analysis process, strengths and weaknesses of the existing system are documented. Any resource constraints that might preclude the acquisition or development of the new system should be identified and noted in the report. These constraints may include such things as time, budget, insufficient in-house technological expertise, lack of state-of-the-art technology, and external factors. Seldom does an organization possess all the resources needed to build or acquire the ideal system. Comparing constraints to the proposed ideal system helps the facility judge what is an affordable or appropriate system, given the current situation.

The content of the systems report varies, depending on the analysis team style and scope of analysis. Martin suggests that the analysis report contain four major sections.[1]

Analysis methodology
- List of end users contacted
- Description of analysis methods used
- Procedures or processes observed or reviewed
- Records, forms, reports analyzed
- Strengths and weaknesses of methodology

Statement of user requirements
- System objectives
- Output and report requirements
- User training needs
- Impact of system on end users

Statement of system constraints
- Description of resource constraints
- Impact of constraints
- Description of realistic system, given constraints

Documentation
- Data collection instruments
- Analysis data (synopsis of interviews, tabulation of surveys)
- Hierarchy charts, DFDs, data dictionaries, ERDs

System Design

As mentioned in the introduction to this chapter, system design encompasses activities related to specifying the details of a new system. In the analysis phase, the needs and requirements of a system are specified. During the system design phase, these requirements are translated into specifications needed to build the system. During this stage, decisions about the logical and physical designs of the system are made. In today's health care environment, major systems (i.e., laboratory, radiology, order entry) are usually purchased from a vendor rather than developed by in-house systems personnel. Therefore, the following processes are usually performed within the vendor domain, particularly the physical design phase. It is still important for the HIM professional

to know about these processes and what the desired output alternatives are. Knowing both processes and preferred outputs helps the HIM professional better assess a vendor product.

Logical and Physical Designs

A specific sequence of events is used in the system design phase. This sequence usually consists of the **logical system design** and the **physical system design.** The logical design describes the functionality of the system and sometimes is called the functional specifications of a system. This is where the vision of system performance and its features are presented. In this section, the system conceptualization is stated in general rather than technical terminology.

The format of the logical design section varies, depending upon individual preferences of the design team and the scope of the project. Stair provides a traditional list of logical design outputs.[7]

Output design—Specifications, including format, content, and frequency, for all output such as forms, screens, and reports. An example of output is the display on the computer monitor of all current laboratory values with outlier values highlighted.

Input design—Specifications, including format, content, and frequency, for all input data. An example of input design for an order entry system is an automatic capability that flags drug contraindications whenever a pharmaceutical is ordered.

Processing design—Types of data manipulations required, such as calculations, comparisons, and text manipulations. An example of a processing design feature is the automatic calculation of the net fluid input and output for a patient with an intravenous line in place.

File and database design—Specifications of file and database capabilities. An example of a database capability is the real-time update of a patient file.

Controls and security design—Specifications for data access and backup. An example of security is that all users must use a log-on identification and password of six characters for entry to the system.

Another method of describing system functionality is to use a scenario-based format. This format was presented earlier in the discussion about investigative techniques. In that context, a scenario was presented to an end user and questions were posed about how an information system could alleviate the problems presented. The same format is also a good mechanism for describing system functional requirements. The following is an example of the scenario format used for a nursing point-of-care system.

> The patient pushes the call button. The nurse goes to the patient's room. The patient requests pain medication and a beverage. The nurse logs on to the patient information system from a terminal at the patient's bedside. The nurse accesses the patient record and checks to see what medication can be administered and what beverages the patient is allowed to have.

A list of general goals and features usually accompanies the scenario-based format. In the case above, for example, the general goals might include the following:

- Present data at the bedside.
- Provide for data to be entered in one place and distributed appropriately.
- Provide different formats or views of the same data to accommodate a multidisciplinary team approach.

The physical system design section specifies all the characteristics that are necessary so that the logical design can be implemented. The physical design includes details about the design of hardware, software, databases, communications, and procedures and controls.

Design Principles

Both technical and functional characteristics must be considered during system design. In the technical arena, programmers and designers are interested in the degree of modularity a program has, its cohesion within a single module, and how independent is each program module. Included among other physical design characteristics are program accuracy, augmentability, completeness, consistency, efficiency, maintainability, reliability, and reusability. The HIM professional commonly is not involved in assessing these technical design characteristics. On the other hand, the professional is frequently called on to assess the functional qualities of a system and how they comply with good design principles.

What are basic design principles for system functionality? From an end user's perspective, system functionality usually involves three things: input, output, and system performance. The basic criterion that should be used to measure all three functionalities is "How well is each integrated into the daily work task of the end user?"

Input and Output

The goals of the input process are as follows:

- To make entry of data into an information system easy so that transactions can be quickly and accurately completed.

- To integrate the process to such a degree in the employee work flow that it is transparent to the end user; in other words, the input mechanism is unobtrusive. If nursing personnel must wait in line to access a computer terminal, then the input process is not satisfactory.
- To reduce duplication in work effort while ensuring a better-quality product. If a unit clerk has to complete a source document and then re-enter that same data into the computer system, then the input mechanism is duplicative and not satisfactory. On the other hand, if a unit clerk has timely access to a computer terminal, can input data directly, and the system performs an automatic input consistency check, then the input mechanism is more likely to be satisfactory.

The goals of the output process include the following:

- To assist the end user in retrieving appropriate data at the appropriate time in the appropriate format. As with the input mechanism, the end user should be able to retrieve data unobtrusively in the regular work flow pattern. Often physicians or other care providers avoid accessing data from a computer terminal because it doesn't conveniently fit into the regular work flow process.
- To provide information that is accurate, timely, complete, and specific to the query. If a care provider queries a patient care system for all abnormal electrolyte results during the past 48 hours but the system returns results of all laboratory tests, then the output function is not satisfactory.

SCREEN DESIGN. An important part of input and output is the design of the data display screen and its ease of use. Various interface elements can be used for data display. Among them are menus, windows, dialog boxes, icons, color, and fonts. Menus present a list of options that the user can browse and then from which he or she can select a specific menu item. Menus can take several forms, including pull-down menus, hierarchial menus, and pop-up menus.

Windows can either be used as views to a document or provide utilities such as tools or commands for the user. For example, document windows contain user data and provide mechanisms for the user to interact with the data. Utility windows are usually smaller, accessory windows that provide additional tools to the user.

Dialog boxes are a special application of a window. The purpose of a dialog box is to elicit a response from the user. A common example of a dialog box is a print options box that asks the user to specify which printer is to be used, how many pages to print, and how many copies of each page to print.

Icons are graphic representations of real-world objects that help convey to the user the purpose of a command executed through the icon. In other words, the icon presents a type of picture that graphically portrays the kind of function that will be executed if the icon is selected. For example, a graphic display of a file cabinet may indicate that selection of that icon will open up a directory of files; a graphic display of an open book may indicate that the selection of that icon will initiate a thesaurus look-up function. Icons are useful devices in interface design because many end users recognize and understand pictures of things more easily than verbal commands of the same thing.

Color is an option that is often used in interface and screen display design. Although the use of color can make screen displays attractive to the user and often improve performance, there is also a danger of misuse. Color should be used conservatively and principally to enhance the identification of important data or draw the user's attention to important functions.

The HIM professional should remember that the development of data display screens is a complex process that involves knowledge of high-level theories and models from various cognitive sciences, including such disciplines as computer science, psychology, artificial intelligence, linguistics, anthropology, and sociology. It is important, therefore, that a computer interface engineer be involved in the development of data screen displays.

GENERAL DESIGN CHARACTERISTICS. Several general guidelines should be followed regardless of the type of screen or interface developed. A primary virtue of an interface is its degree of simplicity. Simple interfaces are easy to learn, easy to remember, and easy to use by a large target audience. A satisfying interface makes end users think that they are in control of the system. The system should be able to perform the following functions:

- Respond quickly to user commands.
- Provide useful and simple messages.
- Offer good navigation tools.
- Provide adequate power to perform necessary tasks.

Turoff, Whitescarver, and Hiltz,[10] Kennedy,[11] Schneiderman[12] described several human-machine interface characteristics. Input and output interfaces should provide direction and learning. An end user should be able to interact with a system without extensive training. If the interface is designed to fit the normal work pattern of the end user, extensive directions are superfluous. Screens should be layered or windowed and good navigational tools provided. Users should be able to move

within the system without getting lost in a maze of screens or commands.

Interfaces should provide the end user with a choice of style. As an example, a physician may want to review the 5-day trend in a patient's white blood cell count and compare it with the count after the administration of a chemotherapeutic agent over the same period. In this case, the system should be flexible enough to present the user with choices of a graphic, tabular, or other format for display.

Interfaces should be forgiving. This means that users should be able to recover easily from input or query errors. Error messages should be polite, meaningful, and informative. A flashing message "Error," for example, doesn't explain to the user what caused the error or how to recover from it. All interfaces should contain an escape feature. This allows the end user to interrupt a session at will or to recover from an error.

Another important part of an interface is the input device. Among input mechanisms are keyboards, light pens, touch-sensitive screens, voice recognition, pen-based systems, bar code readers, and laser scanning. The measure of utility of these mechanisms is the degree to which each comfortably augments the normal work flow of the end user. No matter how attractive a technology is, its benefit is diminished if it disrupts rather than assists employees in their normal work. For example, the choice of voice recognition may seem like an attractive alternative to using a keyboard for input. However, if such a system's ability to recognize vocabulary is limited, its use would defeat the purpose of a robust interface.

System Performance

Besides input and output considerations, the system designer must also think about system performance issues. From an end user perspective, functional system performance indicators may include such criteria as degree of data accuracy, system response rates, system efficiency, system security, and ease of system use. The HIM professional should be involved in identifying functional performance criteria and thresholds as well as developing plans for systematically auditing whether or not they are consistently met.

Criteria and thresholds for system performance vary, depending on the application. For example, response time in a clinical application may be more critical than in a billing application, or security issues may be more critical in situations that involve patient-identifiable information than in applications that deal with aggregate data. Because of this variability, system performance criteria should be developed with the application in mind. An example of functional system performance criteria for an HIM order entry system is presented in Table 18–3.

TABLE 18-3 ORDER ENTRY SYSTEM PERFORMANCE CRITERIA

PERFORMANCE ISSUE	CRITERIA	EVALUATION METHOD
Accuracy		
Input accuracy	Entry error rate	Compare physician orders to orders entered
Transaction accuracy	Errors per time period	Compare orders entered to orders received by department
Database accuracy	Error rate/record	Compare orders entered to patient database
Response Rate		
Input reponse	No. of transactions per time period	Measure transactions per time period
Output response	Amount of time for one transaction	Transaction response rate
Downtime	Downtime hours per time period	Downtime rate
Efficiency		
Input efficiency	Errorless transactions per time period	Transaction error rate
System efficiency	Errors corrected per time period	Error correction rate

In this example, three performance issues are identified. They include accuracy, response rate, and efficiency. For each issue, subissues are identified. For example, under accuracy, issues related to input, transaction, and database accuracy have been noted. For each subissue, the criteria and methods for evaluation have been enumerated. In this order entry example, accuracy has been identified as a major performance issue and is divided into three components: input accuracy, transaction accuracy, and database accuracy. The evaluation of all three of these components is essential to determine performance accuracy of the system. For example, orders may be correctly entered by unit personnel, but there may be a transaction error (system error) in processing the order. In other words, the order could be correctly entered, but the order is not received by the recipient department, such as pharmacy or laboratory. Although this type of error could occur for any number of reasons, it is nonetheless important to document the rate of such errors.

In the order entry example in Table 18–3, the criterion for measuring input accuracy is "Entry Error Rate," and the method for evaluating this error rate is to compare the physician written orders with the orders entered into the system by the unit secretaries. For transaction accuracy, the criterion for measurement is errors per time period and the method of evaluation is comparison of orders entered with orders received by the appropriate clinical department. In regard to database accuracy, the criterion for measurement is error rate per record and the method for evaluation is comparison of orders entered with the patient database.

As this example illustrates, the development of system performance criteria is a nontrivial activity. It is important that every criterion important for system performance and specific to the application is identified and that appropriate methods for evaluation are established.

ROLE OF PROTOTYPING IN SYSTEM DEVELOPMENT

Within the information systems community there has been significant debate as to whether or not the benefits of the system development life cycle outweigh the time and effort it takes to complete the process. One alternative to the system development life cycle is system prototyping. Prototyping a system usually has the following primary goals:

- To build a prototype of an information system quickly
- To heavily involve the user in the model development

Initially, the system prototype can be a preliminary model of the final system, but after several iterations of development, the prototype can evolve into the final system.

Although the prototype alternative involves investigating user requirements, it is not usually done at the depth required in the system development life cycle. The user is heavily involved in the requirements definition stage as well as all other stages of prototype development. After an initial requirements definition is compiled and analysis completed, a prototype design is developed. The first part of a prototype system usually is the development of online input and output screens and the generation of output document formats. At this stage of development, the prototype usually has little functionality. The purpose of this first step is to quickly translate system requirements into a format users can critique. The input and output mechanisms are evaluated and changed or enhanced as required.

After input and output prototyping is completed, system features are gradually added. The most important functions of a system typically are incorporated first. In a prototype of a master patient index, for example, the collection of patient data, data storage, and retrieval functions are incorporated at this stage. The end user continues to be involved in evaluation of the prototype. At this stage, there are opportunities to further define information requirements, refine system functionality, and correct defects.

The final stage of prototyping is generation of the completed prototype system. The prototype is tested and evaluated, and if changes to the prototype need to be made, the system is updated and evaluated again. If the test of the prototype is successful, then it will remain as the model for the final system. Prototype systems usually are developed in fourth-generation languages to speed up the development process. When this occurs, the final version of the prototype usually is recoded in a third-generation language for final system development.

Prototyping is gaining popularity for a number of reasons. First, prototyping provides immediate feedback to users in a format that has meaning to them. In the system development life cycle, a system may take weeks, months, or years to develop and the final product may still be unsatisfactory to end users. When the prototyping method is used, early on in prototype development users assume responsibility for approval of design and function capabilities. Second, prototypes can simulate the dynamics of the real world. It is difficult in a DFD to assess the stress incurred by an emergency department physician and the urgency as she or he attempts to locate information about a drug regimen in a patient's file. Because the prototype can simulate real-world activity, issues that relate to input and output and data manipulation can be more easily identified. A final benefit provided by prototyping is faster delivery of products than that provided by the traditional method of systems analysis.

In addition to its apparent benefits, several other factors have contributed to the increased use of the prototype methodology. First, there has been an advance in technology that has made prototyping possible. In the past, mainframe computers and third-generation programming languages were incompatible with the concept of prototyping. Today, however, microcomputers have the power that mainframes had 10 years ago. This instant power and flexibility at the desktop have contributed to prototype increase. Second, there has been a growth in prototyping tools. Fourth-generation languages, screen generators, report generators, and interactive testing systems are but a few of the tools that today's analyst has that assist in prototype development.

The prototyping process is not without its critics. In the haste to develop a product quickly, some believe that insufficient effort may be devoted to the analysis process. A quick-fix product may be developed that initially looks good but doesn't have the total function-

ality that is required. Additionally, some studies suggest that managing the prototyping process is more difficult than managing the traditional approach.[12] One reason for this is that prototyping is more ad hoc than systematic. Another potential problem is that the use of prototyping-generation tools may not produce products that are ergonomically designed. Many of these tools have rigid constraints in regard to interface design.

Prototyping, however, can be integrated into the system development life cycle. In fact, the meshing of the traditional life cycle approach with prototyping can produce positive results. Through this process, the benefits of each strategy can be achieved, including a thorough analysis derived from the traditional approach with the rapid development of a model system from the prototype approach.

SYSTEM IMPLEMENTATION

System implementation usually refers to all the tasks associated with getting the information system installed and operating. Planning for implementation should occur as soon as feasible after the initial decision is made to go forward on the design or selection of a system. System implementation can be an enormous undertaking. The key to a smooth implementation process is planning and well-executed management. Many systems fail or encounter significant problems during installation because of inadequate planning or poor execution of plans. The steps in implementing a system may vary, given the project and the scope of installation, but the following activities usually are present to one degree or another:

- User preparation and training
- Site preparation
- System testing
- System conversion
- System startup

It is important to remember that the steps in system implementation are not necessarily linear. Rather, activities associated with two or more of the categories above may be occurring concurrently. For example, system testing and user preparation activities may take place in parallel. In fact, some of the implementation processes may also be occurring during the system design phase. For example, preparations for the site may be taking place at the same time as final system design.

User Preparation and Training

User preparation and training are probably among the most underestimated tasks in the implementation process. Not only do users need to be trained how to use the system, but they also need to be educated about the system's purpose and benefits and how it supports the overall well-being of the organization. The implementation of a system should come as no surprise to end users if they have been appropriately included in the analysis and design phases. Early on in the implementation process, the system purpose, its general functionality, and its anticipated benefits should be re-emphasized to end users, managers, and appropriate others. This can be accomplished through formal or informal presentations given by an implementation team member or through brochures, newsletters, seminars, and workshops. Users should be presented with a realistic view of the system. Although the system may have many benefits, they should not be exploited so that unrealistic user expectations are developed.

The format, curriculum, and presentation materials for end user training need to be carefully developed. The format varies, given the type of end user and the complexity of the system. For example, the format for end user training for physicians is likely to be different from that for unit clerks. Format, such as time and place of training sessions, also varies. Format may consist of frequent, single sessions in small blocks of time (say, 60 minutes) or less frequent, larger concentrated sessions. System training can take place in a structured training area or room, or it can be scheduled in the end user's area of work. For instance, it may be appropriate to conduct the initial training of nursing personnel in a classroom configured with a simulated system. Once nursing personnel have gone through the initial sessions, it may be more convenient to hold one-on-one sessions with personnel on a training computer located in the work area.

The curriculum needs to be configured differently for each type of end user. One size does not fit all. The content of the curriculum should correspond to the tasks that are normally performed by each end user group. For instance, physicians do not need to know how to navigate through nursing pathways, and registration clerks do not need to know how to do order entry.

Curriculum content should begin with easy concepts and operations. As end users become proficient with each area, more difficult operations can be introduced. Competency testing is used to assess end user proficiency at each level of the training. For example, in order entry training, users may be introduced systematically to different pathways (i.e., laboratory, dietary). Before an end user can proceed to the next module, a competency test is administered to assess mastery of the current section.

The presentation method for the curriculum must match the knowledge, skills, and availability of the end users. Among presentation options are demonstration, simulation, exercises, workbooks, and lecture and discussion sessions. Each of these methods has its benefits and drawbacks. The usage of each depends on the degree of skill to be developed, the scope of the system, and the skill of the end users. For example, a demonstration might be used when the system is simple to operate and when the end user does not have to possess a great deal of skill. On the other hand, a more complex system might require demonstration as well as simulation integrated with exercises and lecture and discussion sessions.

The development of self-paced training modules is an alternative to holding large classroom-style classes. Self-paced modules can be developed so that end users can use them with minimal assistance. These modules can incorporate methods of lecture, exercise, simulation, and competency testing. They can be especially attractive in the health care environment where employees work round-the-clock shifts and may not be available to attend training sessions scheduled during the usual daytime work period.

Scheduling of training sessions can be an enormous undertaking. Take, for example, the implementation of a hospitalwide information system in a 1000-bed facility. In this case, it is likely that as many as 2000 end users will need to be trained. If each training session averages 6 hours per person and competency testing consumes another 2 hours per end user, then the total training hours would be 16,000 hours. The actual user training time needed would be calculated by determining how many end users would be in a class at one time, how many classes would be held per 8-hour shift, and how many days per week classes would be held. Hospital facilities operate round the clock and on weekends, and training scheduling must be flexible to accommodate all end users.

Another component of end user preparation is the selection and training of the trainers. Few organizations have sufficient staff available who can man the training efforts for a large-scale information system implementation. Therefore, consideration needs to be given to the selection of new staff, the number of staff required, and how these people are to be trained. Sometimes vendors or consultants are hired to develop and staff the training effort. The trade-offs of using in-house personnel versus outside contractual arrangements need to be assessed. Remember, though, that training is an ongoing process and a training staff always needs to be available.

Site Preparation

The location of the system and its associated components needs to be planned well in advance of installation. If the system is small (i.e., microcomputer-based), then management of site preparation is minimal. In larger systems, however, installation site preparation is a major activity. For example, installation of a laboratory or total hospital information system may require special wiring, special room accommodations, special cables, and sufficient room for all components. If the system involves a local area network, then site preparation is likely to require facilitywide planning. For example, plans need to be developed for network backbone wiring, locations for wiring closets and hubs, and conduit for wiring.

Analysis of end user space requirements should not be forgotten in the site preparation process. Too often when system installation occurs, it is discovered that the allotted space for end user terminals or computers is not adequate. Space may be too small, ill-configured, or inconvenient to wiring or it is not in an appropriate place to allow adequate access. This oversight can turn any installation process into a nightmare.

System Testing and Conversion

All systems must be tested to ensure that they perform in the way they were intended. It would be a disaster to install a system on an organizationwide basis and then have it fail in one or more transactions. Good system testing is a precursor to successful installation. The development of test scripts can be a tedious process. Therefore, development of tests will probably begin long before system installation. The adequacy of both the hardware and the software of a system must be assessed. Many manufacturers provide diagnostic routines to test major system components. These routines should be supplemented by organization-developed tests.

Test Phases

Several phases are used to systematically test the performance of software. First, each program is tested (*unit testing*) by providing test data or audit scripts that force the execution of all program statements. Total *system testing* is done to determine how well programs interact and execute in an integrated environment. Many times a system may work well during a test situation in which a limited amount of data are used. Most production systems, however, operate in a data-intensive environment. Therefore, it is important to determine how well the system works during actual production. This is accomplished through *volume testing,* in which large amounts of data are put through the system. Processing and response times can be more adequately assessed when volume testing occurs. Systems usually do not stand alone but are expected to interact with other systems. For example, the laboratory information system would be expected to interact with the admission and order

entry systems. To determine how well interaction occurs, the new system is tested with other information system components. This is usually referred to as *integration testing.*

System Conversion

Before a new system is implemented, files from the old system often need to be converted from one medium to another. Sometimes this means the transfer of paper records to a computer format. For example, if the master patient index has been maintained manually, information in the index needs to be placed on a computer medium before the new system can be totally implemented. Conversion can take many forms. For example, it may involve converting from one computer medium to another, from one file structure to another, or from one operating system to another. The technical issues to be addressed during any conversion can be complex. When the transfer occurs, it is extremely important to have quality control procedures in place that ensure the integrity of data and transactions. The HIM professional should be part of the team that determines the criteria and methods for quality control during the conversion process.

Startup

System startup occurs when all activities leading up to installation have been completed. This includes activities that relate to user training, site preparation, hardware installation, testing, and conversion. The following approaches to the startup phase can be used:

- Abrupt changeover
- Gradual phase in of applications in selected organizational units
- Gradual phase in of applications organization-wide

Abrupt Changeover

Abrupt changeover refers to the total rollout of a system across all organizational units at the same time. This approach is exceedingly risky unless the system is simple and does not affect a great number of organizational units. For example, an abrupt changeover may be appropriate for a utilization management system that affects a small number of people in one department. With larger, complex systems, however, abrupt changeover could prove disastrous. In an abrupt changeover, if problems occur, they are likely to impact the entire organization and potentially threaten mission-critical operations. Debugging of system problems usually is difficult in an abrupt changeover. This is because problem origin is difficult to isolate in a complex system.

Gradual Phase In of Applications

Gradual phase in of applications usually refers to bringing up one application at a time in selected units over a period of time. For example, three units in a hospital might initially bring up the order entry application. After a few weeks, the laboratory interface would be rolled out in those same units. Once the entire system was successfully operating in the selected units, organizationwide implementation would occur. This approach is risk-adverse. If problems occur during the installation, the impact on end users and the organization is minimized. Debugging any problems that occur is also easier. This is because each application is tested and debugged as it is implemented. Thus, at any one time, there are fewer modules to search for problem origin.

Systems can also be phased in application by application over the total organization. For example, the order entry application could be brought up at the same time in all patient care units throughout the facility. When the application is proved to be stable, the next module is brought on line. This approach is not quite as risk-adverse as the previous method. It does, however, provide more insurance than abrupt changeover. Allowing all organizational units to be at the same point in system installation also has its benefits from both operational and training aspects, provided all system applications are problem-free.

System Evaluation and Benefits Realization

Although system evaluation in this chapter is discussed at the end of the system development life cycle, this should not be construed to mean that the evaluation process only begins after system installation. In fact, planning for system evaluation and realization of benefits should start in parallel with the system design effort. What is system evaluation, and why is it important to begin the process early in the system development life cycle?

The purpose of system evaluation is to determine whether or not the system functions the way it was intended. All too often, systems are installed but the degree of benefit derived from them is never measured. Organizations that fail to measure system benefits cannot systematically determine whether or not expenditures on system development or purchase were justified. As a result, such organizations have no methodology to determine what impact the time, effort, and expense of a system development or selection process has had on the

organization. In today's environment of competition, continuous quality improvement, and cost justification, no organization can afford *not* to justify information system expenditures.

The following methods are used to evaluate systems:

- Benefits realization
- Cost-benefit analysis
- Cost-effectiveness analysis

Benefits Realization

In **benefits realization,** the criteria used for system evaluation evolve from the analysis and design sections of the development life cycle. Take, for example, a computerized chart-tracking system. Suppose that in the systems analysis document the goals of this system were as follows:

- Reduce errors in assignment of patient records to various hospital locations.
- Reduce employee time in locating patient records.
- Decrease response time to ad hoc record requests from patient care areas.
- Increase the percentage of delivery of requested records to patient care areas.
- Calculate daily, weekly, and monthly work volumes.

In the evaluation of the chart-tracking system, the goals above would be used as the basic criteria for determining the benefits of system installation. Using this method for evaluation of a system usually is referred to as benefits realization. In other words, has the system delivered the benefits that were anticipated? To determine the exact benefits derived from the system, good measurements must be established for each criterion. For example, the number of errors in assignment of patient records to various hospital locations before system implementation must be known. If these data are not known, then post-implementation benefits cannot be calculated.

Cost-Benefit Analysis

The benefits realization methodology is not usually economics-based. In other words, system benefits are not necessarily compared with an economic outcome. **Cost-benefit analysis** (CBA), on the other hand, attempts to measure benefits compared with system costs. Basically, the goal of CBA is to determine whether the information system decreases or increases benefits and whether or not it decreases or increases cost for the organization. Cost-benefit methodologies frequently are used before system development or selection of system alternatives. These methods are applied in an attempt to justify the selection of one alternative over another. For example, CBA would be used to justify selection of one vendor's product over another or to justify the purchase of a proposed information system.

The term cost-benefit is used somewhat loosely in the information systems field as opposed to its use by economists. Basically, CBA uses microeconomic models to assist in making good decisions. In CBA, dollar values are assigned to the cost and benefits of a proposed information system. These dollar values are then compared to help make a decision between alternative systems. Several techniques are used to evaluate alternative solutions. Among them are break-even analysis, payback period, discounted payback period, return on investment, and internal rate of return.

Break-Even Analysis

Break-even analysis is probably the simplest CBA technique. In break-even analysis, costs to operate the current system are compared with those to operate the proposed system. The point at which old system costs equal new systems cost is called the break-even point. After the break-even point, the proposed system should begin to generate a positive monetary return compared with the old system. With this analysis, a set period usually is targeted ahead of time for monetary return (e.g., 2 to 5 years).

EXAMPLE

The current software for the encoding system in the HIM department costs $10,000 per year for licensing. Maintenance of hardware for the system costs $6,000 per year. A new encoding system is being considered that initially costs $10,000 for new hardware, a licensing fee of $8,000 per year, and a maintenance fee for hardware of $8,000 per year. With the new encoder, the department expects that it will increase reimbursement by $5,000 per year.

In this case, the current system is costing $16,000 per year. In the first year, the new system will cost $26,000, but reimbursement will increase by $5,000. The net cost of the new system after the first year is $21,000, and the difference between the net cost of the new system and the old system in the first year is $5,000. In the second year, the old system would continue to cost $16,000 to operate. The new system cost will also be $16,000 ($8,000 license + $8,000 maintenance). However, the new system will continue to increase reimbursement at $5,000 per year. Thus, at the end of the

TABLE 18-4 CALCULATION OF BREAK-EVEN POINT

YEAR	NEW SYSTEM	OLD SYSTEM
Year 1		
Operation cost	$26,000	$16,000
Increase in revenue	+5,000	0
Net cost	21,000	16,000
Difference in operation and net cost	5,000	0
Year 2		
Operation cost	16,000	16,000
Difference in operation and net cost yr 1	5,000	0
Increase in revenue	5,000	0
Net cost	16,000	16,000
Difference in operation and net cost	0	0

second year, the break-even point has been achieved with the net cost of both systems being $16,000 each. Table 18–4 shows how the break-even point is determined.

Payback Period

Calculation of the **payback period** is often done to determine whether or not a new system will fully recover its investment (development) costs before the end of its life cycle. In the encoding example above, the investment cost was $10,000 (new hardware) and operating cost was $16,000. To determine the payback period, a comparison between total old system costs and total new system costs (including investment) is made. The difference between new system and old system costs is calculated on a year-by-year (cumulative) basis. When the difference between old system costs and new system costs reaches zero, the payback period has been reached. Table 18–5 shows the payback period calculation for the encoding example above.

In year one of Table 18–5, the current system cost is $16,000. The new system cost is $26,000 ($10,000+

TABLE 18-5 CALCULATION OF PAYBACK PERIOD FOR ENCODER SYSTEM

	YEAR 1	YEAR 2	YEAR 3
Current system cost	$16,000	$16,000	$16,000
New system cost	26,000	11,000	11,000
Yearly difference in costs	−10,000	+5,000	+5,000
Cumulative difference in costs	−10,000	−5,000	0

$16,000). The yearly difference in cost during the first year is a negative $10,000 ($16,000 minus $26,000). Because this is the first year of calculation, the cumulative difference remains minus $10,000. During the second year, the current system will still cost $16,000. The new system will cost $11,000 ($16,000 operating cost minus $5,000 increase in reimbursement). The yearly difference between the current and the new system costs is $5,000 ($16,000 minus $11,000). The cumulative cost difference is negative $5,000 (− $10,000 minus + $5,000). In the third year, the costs of the current system remain $16,000 and the costs of the new system remain $11,000. The yearly difference in costs is again $5,000; however, the cumulative difference in costs has reached zero (− $5,000 minus + $5,000). Thus, the payback period has been reached after 3 years.

The encoding system problem above illustrates the difference between the break-even point and the payback point. It is important to recognize how these different CBA techniques can be used to support different arguments to purchase or not purchase a system.

Discounted Payback Period

Another CBA technique is **discounted payback period.** In this method, an organization determines how much a system costs in future dollars. The basic concept underlying this approach is that today's dollars are worth more than future dollars. This is because an organization can usually invest today's dollars at a certain interest rate and receive a **return on investment** (ROI). Therefore, future dollars that are anticipated to be made by installing an information system are discounted in calculations used to determine the discounted payback period. For example, say a health care facility can invest $1 today at 8 per cent. The value of that dollar next year will be $1.08. If it is projected that an information system will earn $5,000 next year, that $5,000 in future dollars would actually have less value than today's dollars (i.e., if the facility invested $5,000 at 8 per cent interest, the amount would be $5,400 by next year). To illustrate how the discounted payback period is calculated, the encoding example discussed previously is used.

To determine the present value of today's dollar at any time in the future, the following formula is used:

$$1/(1 + ROI)^n,$$

where ROI is the facility's expected return on investment and n is the number of years into the future. Let's assume that in the encoding example above, the facility expects an 8 per cent ROI. Using the formula for present value, the discounted rate for years 1 through 5 after system startup has been calculated and is shown in Table 18–6.

What Table 18–6 indicates is that 1 year after project

TABLE 18–6 PRESENT DOLLAR VALUE, YEARS 1–5

YEARS	FUTURE DOLLAR VALUE
1	.93
2	.86
3	.79
4	.74
5	.68

start, the value of today's dollar is $.93. The value of today's dollar after year two of the project is $.86 and so on. Calculations to determine the discounted payback period for the encoding system appear in Table 18–7. Note that Table 18–7 is an extension of Table 18–5.

Table 18–7 indicates that the discounted payback period occurs sometime between years 3 and 4. To interpret the table, the discounted difference is arrived at by multiplying the discount by the yearly difference in costs. For example, during year 1, the discount is .93 and the yearly difference in cost is minus $10,000. Multiplying these figures yields the discounted difference in costs, which is minus $9,300 in year 1. All subsequent rows are calculated in the same way. To determine the cumulative difference in cost, the current year's discounted difference is subtracted from the cumulative difference. For example, in year 2, the discounted difference ($4,300) is subtracted from the cumulative difference in year 1 (− $9,300). This equals minus $5,000, which is the cumulative difference in costs between the current and new systems by year 2.

TABLE 18–7 DISCOUNTED PAYBACK PERIOD FOR ENCODER SYSTEM

	YEAR 1	YEAR 2	YEAR 3	YEAR 4
Current system cost	$16,000	$16,000	$16,000	$16,000
New system cost	26,000	11,000	11,000	11,000
Yearly difference in costs	− 10,000	+ 5,000	+ 5,000	+ 5,000
Discount (ROI = .08)	.93	.86	.79	.74
Discounted difference	− 9,300	+ 4,300	+ 3,950	+ 3,700
Cumulative difference in costs	− 9,300	− 5,000	− 1,050	+ 2,650

ROI, return on investment.

Cost-Effective Analysis

As opposed to CBA, **cost-effectiveness analysis** attempts to evaluate certain beneficial consequences in nonmonetary terms. Therefore, in cost-effective analysis, desirable benefits are not valued in monetary terms but are measured in some other unit. For example, what price could be placed on saving one life or delivering a patient's record to a patient care unit more quickly? Or, can the investment in a new information system decrease medication errors or increase more timely drug administration? The determination of how much it is worth to decrease one medication error is a social question, not a technical or economic one. Specific determination as to how much a nonmonetary item is worth is left for the specific facility to determine given current situations and constraints.

It should be obvious from review of the previous methodologies why it is important for the health information manager to have an understanding of these various techniques. As the encoding system example demonstrates, statistics can mean whatever you want them to mean. To objectively evaluate the costs and benefits of a system, a variety of analytic techniques should be used, including CBA and benefits realization.

PURCHASING PROCESS: REQUEST FOR PROPOSAL

Information system development for most health care applications is an enormous undertaking. Few health care facilities have the budget, expertise, or other resources needed to be able to develop most health care applications. Although every health care facility is unique, there are enough similarities across many functions to make the development of "vanilla" systems by vendors practical. These systems usually have general functionalities that can be modified to meet the needs of many health care facilities. For example, a health care facility would not usually develop a laboratory information system because this type of system is complex and the facility would probably not be able to justify the cost of development for benefit received. This type of system, on the other hand, is an ideal candidate for vendor development. Because most laboratories have similar functions, a general information system can be developed to meet the needs of many clinical laboratories. The cost of development, which is initially assumed by the vendor, can then be spread across many purchasers, thus making the individual cost to any one client less than if the client developed the system in-house. When a decision is made to purchase a system from a vendor rather than develop the product in-house, a **request for proposal (RFP)** process is usually undertaken. An RFP is a document that details all re-

quired system functionality, including functional, technical, training, and implementation requirements. The document is distributed to a selected number of vendors, who are invited to respond to the proposal. The vendor response to the proposal indicates to what degree the vendor's product meets the proposed system requirements.

Before any RFP is generated, functional specifications for the new system must be generated. To produce the specifications, the same techniques used in the system development life cycle should be used. This includes development of hierarchy charts, DFDs, preliminary data dictionaries, and ERDs. Many health care facilities fail to do a thorough systems analysis when developing an RFP. This results in poorly drafted system specifications. When this occurs, the facility places itself in a vulnerable position. No RFP should be generated without a thorough analysis of user needs and projected system capabilities.

Planning Steps Before RFP Preparation

When the purchase of an information system is being considered, a steering committee usually is appointed to oversee the process. Membership of the committee commonly is multidisciplinary, including users, managers, and representatives from administration and information systems. The primary responsibility of the committee is to provide overall management of the system selection and implementation process. It is the committee's responsibility to develop a work plan and time table and ensure that the process is completed. Specific tasks of the committee vary from institution to institution but broadly encompass the following:

- Development of project work plan and time table
- Oversight of systems analysis
- Development of system specifications
- Determination of costs and benefits
- Compilation and distribution of the RFP
- Evaluation of responses to the RFP
- Selection of the system
- Conducting vendor negotiations
- Oversight of system implementation

Analyzing System Requirements

Even though the decision has been made to purchase a system rather than develop a system, this does not obviate the need for an analysis effort. This process of identifying user requirements and determining system capabilities is essentially the same as in the system development life cycle. The steering committee may assign members of the committee analysis responsibilities, delegate these to in-house information system professionals, or contract with consultants to perform the function. No matter who is chosen to perform the function, the steering committee still has the final responsibility for the analysis process.

A detailed analysis document should be prepared. A benefits realization process should be identified and developed at this point as well as the feasibility of the proposed system together with estimates of cost and benefits.

The results of analysis provide the foundation from which system functionality is determined. They also provide the basis for developing the function specifications of the RFP and the criteria by which vendor products will be evaluated. Because of its importance, the analysis document should be complete and accurately reflect user requirements.

Development of System Specifications

System specifications include both the functional and the technical specifications of the system—the logical and physical descriptions of the system. Among logical system specifications are those that relate to output, input, processing, database, and security design. Physical specifications include details about hardware, database, communication, and control needs. Training needs and implementation requirements are initially identified at this time. The details of system specification will later be translated into the functional requirements section of the RFP document. Therefore, it is important that specifications be appropriate, complete, and accurate.

During the system specification process, the committee may issue a **request for information** (RFI) to vendors. Enough is generally known at this point about system capabilities so that an intelligent decision can be made about which vendor products are most likely to be competitive in a response to an RFP. The RFI basically solicits general information from vendors about their products. The RFI may state in general terms what the facility is looking for in system functionality. Vendors respond with information about their product lines and their experience in the marketplace and provide copies of their annual reports. The RFI is a good way for health care facilities to narrow down the field of vendors to whom an RFP will be sent.

Development and Distribution of the RFP

After the analysis has been performed and system specifications identified, the RFP is prepared. The RFP is

usually a lengthy document. Depending on the complexity of the system, an RFP can be several hundred pages long. Although format varies, an RFP usually includes the following sections:

- Proposal information and format
- Enterprise profile
- Conditions of response
- Functional requirements
- Technical requirements
- Training requirements
- Implementation requirements
- Vendor profile
- System costs

An RFP is a professionally prepared document. It is important that it be correct in all areas because sometimes it also functions as a legal document. Many times the RFP and the response of the vendor who wins the bid are included in the final contract. Therefore, the importance of the accuracy of the RFP cannot be overemphasized.

Disclaimer and Table of Contents

An RFP usually begins with a disclaimer that the information contained in the document is considered proprietary and is to be considered in strict confidence and that no information contained in it can be disclosed without written permission from the organization issuing the RFP. A table of contents that functions as an index to the RFP is usually included. Figure 18–18 shows the table of contents of a typical RFP.

Proposal Overview

After the table of contents, an overview of the proposal is usually presented. Here the proposal format, time table, and requirements for proposal submission are detailed. One of the most important parts of this section is the proposal time table. Here milestones of the process are listed with associated time frames. A typical time table is represented in Figure 18–19. The time frames in each proposal vary, depending on the complexity of the system being considered and organizational constraints.

Enterprise Profile

The next section of the RFP usually contains a profile of the enterprise. This consists of a brief description of the organization and its demographic data. Statistics such as bed size, occupancy rate, and number of admissions and discharges frequently are provided. These data

Table of Contents

I. General Information
   A. Proposal information
   B. Proposal format

II. Enterprise Information
   A. Description of the enterprise
   B. Hardware and software environment
   C. Departmental operations

III. Vendor Responses
   A. Specific instructions
   B. Functional requirements
   C. Technical requirements
   1. Interface requirements
   2. Processing environment requirements
   3. Support and maintenance requirements
   4. Installation requirements and approach
   5. Training requirements
   D. Vendor background
   E. System costs and financing arrangements
   F. Contractual arrangements

FIGURE 18–18. Typical request for proposal table of contents.

provide the vendor with a perspective of the facility's volume of data and transactions. General information about the facility services and organization department operations is included. The current hardware and software environments are detailed in this section as well. This includes specifics about what type of hardware is in place, what applications are running, and who the developers of each application are. This provides vendors with important information to determine whether or not their products can easily interface with current applications or operate under the current hardware environment.

This section also includes a description of activities of all departments that are planning to use the proposed information system. These descriptions provide an over-

view of current departmental operations and usually include appropriate statistics relating to work volumes that may impact system performance requirements.

Conditions of Response

In this section, guidelines to the vendors for response to the proposal are provided. This typically contains information about what format should be used, the date and time the response is to be submitted, detailed instructions for completing each section of the proposal, and the name and phone number of the person to contact if questions arise.

Functional Specifications

The functional specifications together with the technical requirements section are the heart of the RFP. In this section, all system functionality is listed. Various formats are used to allow vendors to indicate whether or not their product has the desired functionality. The format of the response usually allows the vendor to indicate whether the feature is currently developed and operational, can be custom developed, is planned to be developed, or is not available. The length and areas covered in the functional specification section depend on the system under consideration. For example, if a total hospital information system is being considered, there will be a subsection for almost every hospital department—for example, subsections for clinical laboratory, radiology, admission, HIM, and nursing. Functional specifications for a decision-support system intended to support managerial personnel specifications would be limited to such areas as cost accounting, case mix, and budgeting. Figure 18–20 shows part of a functional specification section for a pharmacy information system, and Figure 18–21 shows one for an executive decision-support system.

A recent trend for describing functional specifications is to state requirements in a scenario-based format. This format was discussed earlier in this chapter. One format

FIGURE 18–19. Time table for request for proposal process.

Proposed Time Table

The following time table is presented to facilitate a timely and orderly selection process.

Milestones	Date
1. Distribute RFP	September 1, 199x
2. Vendor Response Submission	September 28, 199x, 4:30 pm EST
3. Evaluation of Responses	September 30–October 15, 199x
4. Site Visits/Vendor Demonstrations	October 16–November 1, 199x
5. Recommendation of Vendor to Senior Administration	November 30, 199x

Application	Function Currently Available	Custom Available	Planned	Not Available
Order may be entered on any terminal by MD, nurse, unit clerk, or pharmacist				
System automatically notifies individual entering order if drug is not available in hospital formulary				
All new drug orders are automatically screened against patient's drug profile for possible interactions				

FIGURE 18–20. Sample functional specifications: pharmacy system.

of the scenario-based description is to present the goal of the ideal system followed by a scenario of current problems. Vendors are asked to explain how their systems will support the general goal and how each will address the problems presented. The following is an example of such a format of a point-of-care RFP:

> Listed below are the goals and problems for our system. Please respond to each by indicating how your system would meet each goal and how it would address each problem.
> *Goal:* Deliver information to nurse caregivers at the patient bedside.
> *Problem:* Vital signs are taken at the bedside and then written down on a scratch pad by the nurse. The nurse then takes the data to the nursing station and rewrites the data onto the vital signs sheet. The data are then retranscribed and placed in the patient health record.

Technical Requirements

Another section of the RFP is the technical requirements section. This section contains information about specifications for hardware, software, interfaces, processing environment, and communications. The following is an example of the technical interface requirements needed for a managerial decision-support system:

> 1. Explain how your system accommodates the following interfaces:
>   - Accept payroll information from a personnel/payroll system
>   - Accept cost information from a general ledger system
>   - Update general ledger system with budget information

Application	Function Currently Available	Custom Available	Planned	Not Available
System allows for user-defined product lines.				
System stores a standard treatment profile for a product.				
System allows for online review and modification of standard treatment profiles.				

FIGURE 18–21. Sample functional specifications: executive decision support system.

- Accept detail charge, payment, and patient information from patient billing, receivables, and registration systems
2. For those interfaces provided by you describe:
  - Who writes the interface
  - Who maintains the interface
  - Language used for the interface

In this section, vendors are expected to provide information about the performance of their systems. They may also be asked to submit samples of their system documentation, such as technical system, user, installation, and operations manuals. Support and maintenance details are also requested. For example, the RFP may ask the vendor to supply the following information:

- Indicate the location of personnel who would be assigned to the maintenance function.
- Describe the type of support the company is capable of providing on a continuing basis.
- Describe the means of support, such as hot lines, dial up services.
- Describe the procedure for requesting application software changes.

Installation and Training Requirements

In this section, vendors are requested to submit their installation work plans. Vendor responsibility, length of installation, customer responsibility, and skill level of installation personnel are described. Training requirements are also outlined in this section. Vendors are asked to describe the training they provide in areas of application usage, system operations, and ongoing training. A description of training techniques and samples of training materials may also be requested. Vendors may be asked to describe what resources are needed for training (e.g., type of site), the number of people they will train, and the training time. All costs associated with training should be requested.

Vendor Profile

In any selection process, it is extremely important to ascertain the stability of the vendor. Too often facilities purchase systems only to have the vendor go bankrupt or be dislodged from the marketplace for some other reason. To minimize risk to the client, a thorough background analysis of the vendor should be done.

Information requested in the vendor profile includes demographic data, such as number of employees, number of support personnel, number of employees with installation experience, years the system has been available, and the number of systems installed. Vendor an-

nual reports should be requested, including total revenues for several years, research and development expenditures, and systems contracted within the past few years. The facility may also want to ask about whether or not a user group exists, and if so, how frequently it meets and how many members it has.

System Costs and Financing Arrangements

A system cost schedule should be prepared for both lease and purchase options. For each item in the schedule, the vendor should be requested to indicate the one-time cost, annual maintenance, and total cost over a certain period (e.g., 5 years). Among the categories in the cost schedule are hardware, software, software installation, software maintenance, custom development and interfaces, training, and consulting fees.

Contractual Information, References, and Other Materials

A sample copy of all contracts and addenda that are required for the facility to contract for the proposed system should be requested. It should be noted in the RFP that the facility reserves the right to negotiate the final terms and conditions of any resulting agreements. References of facilities who are using the vendor's product should be requested. The vendor should be asked to supply a list of all installations of their product, the contact person at each of these sites, and whether or not the site can be available for a visit. Any other manuals or references that the vendor may want to provide can be added in this section.

Distribution of the RFP

Once the RFP has been developed, it is ready for distribution to the vendors. Before distribution, a short list of vendors who probably have systems that will meet functionality specifications is identified. The short list is usually compiled from information received during the RFI process. Remember that for every RFP that is sent, a potential response is possible. Because responses tend to be longer than the RFP itself, review of these can be costly and time-consuming. The facility will want to send out an RFP only to vendor candidates who are truly viable. The number of RFPs distributed depends on the vendor market, but no more than 15 usually are distributed. Once distributed, the RFP time table is invoked and the process follows the time line prescribed in the RFP document.

Evaluation Criteria

Before distribution of the RFP, the steering committee develops evaluation criteria for analyzing and comparing

Hardware/Software Configuration
• Processing options
• Ease of use
• Potential to handle projected volume increases
• Proven system
• Quality of sample documentation

Functions and Features
• Number or percentage of required functions/features currently accommodated
• Number or percentage of required functions/features that can be custom developed
• Quality of sample documentation

Economic considerations
• One-time installation costs
• Recurring costs
• Consulting charges
• Conversion costs
• Other costs

Technical considerations
• Reliability and performance
• Security
• Architecture
• Interface capabilities

Vendor considerations
• Support and training
• Contract flexibility
• Financial stability
• Management strength

FIGURE 18–22. Evaluation criteria.

vendor responses. There are many methods used for evaluation, and the type used depends on system scope and individual preference of the facility. The following general categories of evaluation are usually considered:

• Hardware and software configuration

• Application functions and features

• Economic considerations

• Technical considerations

• Vendor considerations (Figure 18–22)

Some type of weighting scheme or priority measurement is assigned to each item within a category. One method of evaluation is to develop a weighting scale. The scale may range in value from 1 to 5. Each characteristic is then assigned a weight in relation to its importance. For instance, a hospital may consider security an extremely important item for its system. In this case, on a scale of 1 to 5, security may be assigned the weight of 5, which is the highest weight on the scale. On the other hand, management strength under vendor considerations may not be a highly valued characteristic. So in this case, this item may be assigned a lower weight of 2.

In addition to weighting each characteristic, each vendor's response can also be evaluated using a Lickert scale. This is usually referred to as scoring. For example, a scale of 1 to 3 might be used. If the vendor responded that the system currently had a required feature, then 3 points would be assigned for that option. If the vendor could custom configure the feature, then 2 points would be assigned. If the vendor has plans for the feature to be developed in the future, then 1 point would be assigned. If the system does not include the feature, then 0 points would be assigned. The weighted value of each characteristic usually is multiplied by the vendor's score for that feature, resulting in a weighted score for each characteristic. The weighted score is then added across all features to arrive at a final weighted score for each vendor. Table 18–8 shows how a weighted score would be calculated for the set of sample functional characteristics for a pharmacy system.

Table 18–8 compares the products of Vendor A with those of Vendor B. The calculations indicate that overall, Vendor B's product appears to offer more functionality than Vendor A's product, given the pre-established weights.

There is not total agreement that the use of a weighting scheme such as that described above provides the best comparison method. For example, one vendor may

TABLE 18-8 WEIGHTED SCORES FOR PHARMACY INFORMATION SYSTEM VENDORS

FUNCTION	WEIGHT*	SCORE†		WEIGHTED SCORE	
		Vendor A	Vendor B	Vendor A	Vendor B
Order may be entered on any terminal by physician, nurse, unit clerk, or pharmacist	5	3	3	15	15
System automatically notifies person entering order if drug is not available in hospital formulary	3	2	3	6	9
All new drug orders are automatically screened against patient's drug profile for possible interactions	4	2	3	8	12
Total weighted scores				29	36

* Weight: 5, essential; 4, very important; 3, important; 2, somewhat important; 1, nice to have.
† Score: 3, currently has; 2, can customize; 1, plans to have.

score higher than all other contenders, but the product may in fact be mediocre in most categories. It is important, therefore, to look at the scores of each criterion individually as well as the overall weighted scores. In reality, such a weighting method is only one input into the total decision process.

Demonstrations and Site Visits

Demonstrations

After responses to the RFP have been reviewed, the steering committee culls the list of vendors. Those vendors that come out highest in the evaluation process are invited to present demonstrations of their products. The demonstrations usually take place at the facility and, depending on system complexity, may last several hours to 1 to 2 days. Before the demonstration, the steering committee should have established a demonstration schedule. This schedule should include a list of all functions to be demonstrated and a schedule of end users who will witness the demonstration. A set of evaluation criteria (e.g., apparent ease of use, interface flexibility, evaluation of inputs and outputs) should be developed by the steering committee. This criteria is then applied by the end users to evaluate the demonstration. Other methods, such as focus groups, can be used to debrief end users and gather their opinions about system functionality. All opinions and evaluations should be documented and evaluated by the steering committee. This evaluation will probably result in some vendors being eliminated from consideration.

Site Visits

After demonstrations have taken place, the steering committee usually schedules site visits to observe the vendor product in production mode. Site visits take place at facilities where the vendor product is installed. Usually 1 to 2 days is arranged for each site visit. The site visit team should have a visit protocol prepared in advance. The protocol should allow for formal and informal observations of the system and discussion with end users at the selected site. This may be the only opportunity the team has to view the system in production mode. Therefore, it is extremely important that the site protocol be complete and afford the best possible opportunity for overview of the system and its management. After each site visit, the steering committee should be debriefed. Evaluations should be compiled. Discrepancies between what was reported in the vendor response to proposal and what was observed in production mode should be noted and investigated.

System Selection and Contract Negotiation

After all data have been gathered, demonstrations held, and site visits completed, the steering committee should be ready to select a vendor product. Once a product has been selected, contract negotiations begin. The contractual process is extremely important because it lays down the rules by which the client and vendor are to operate. In complex installations, the vendor and health care facility are partners for months or even years. Therefore, it is important that the contract minimizes risk to both parties. A special team commonly is formed to carry out contract negotiation. Members of the team should have negotiation experience. Representatives from administration, information systems, legal counsel, and significant others usually are included on the facility negotiation team. It is important that the leaders of both the vendor and the facility teams be authorized to make decisions for their respective businesses.

The negotiation of a good contract is one of the most important elements in ensuring a successful system installation. The following items are usually part of any software contract:

- *Identification of products and services:* This should include detailed specifications for the software and support materials to be licensed.

- *License grant:* This includes the scope of rights to be transferred, the number of sites, and intellectual property rights.

- *Delivery terms:* This includes such things as time and date of delivery, method of delivery, schedule of delivery, recourse or damages for slippage.

- *Installation:* This includes such items as site preparation, timing of installation, and training.

- *Warranties:* This includes such items as express and implied warranties, scope and term of warranties, and conditions on warranties.

- *Remedies and liability:* This includes such items as limitations on liability and types of liability.

- *Acceptance and testing:* This includes such items as how the system will be tested, timing of testing, and specifications for testing.

- *Price and payments:* This includes method of payment, such as lump sum or spaced payments, conditional payments, royalties, taxes, and prices for updates or modifications, service, or maintenance.

- *Term and termination:* This includes such items as effective date of agreement; notice of breach, insolvency, or bankruptcy; and termination for cause.

- *Support and maintenance:* This may include such items as training, documentation, ongoing maintenance, emergency and preventive maintenance, and access to source code.

It is important to remember that a contract is a binding document. Therefore, software contracts should be negotiated by a team of people who have expertise in both legal and technologic arenas. No matter how small the contract in monetary terms, the health care facility should always seek legal advice before signing any software contract.

Key Concepts

- Information systems have a life cycle that includes system design, implementation, operation and maintenance, and obsolescence. For each life cycle stage, different activities take place that have an impact on the resources of the organization.

- An organization is composed of hundreds and perhaps thousands of interacting information systems. Given this, the number of information systems in any organization are in different phases of individual life cycles. This discontinuity of life cycle phases causes stress within the organization. This stress can be manifested in multiple ways, including competition for resources such as personnel, hardware, and financial allocations.

- Each organization as a whole has its own information system life cycle. Nolan describes six stages of an organization life cycle with each stage manifesting a different approach to management of the information technology.

- A structured approach called the information system development life cycle is commonly used to develop new information systems. This life cycle has four steps that include analysis, design, implementation, and evaluation. Structured techniques provide a tool kit for analysts as they perform system analysis and design.

- Prototyping is a recent technique that sometimes is used in place of the system development life cycle. This technique has been made possible because of advances in technology. The purpose of this method is to build a prototype or model of an information system quickly by involving the end user in repeated iterations of the design.

- System implementation is an enormous undertaking, and planning is a key to its success. Plans need to be developed that include user preparation and training, site preparation, system testing and conversion, and startup activities.

- Although often overlooked, system evaluation and development of a benefits realization process are extremely important parts of the system development life cycle. The purpose of system evaluation is to determine whether or not the system functions the way it was intended. Several techniques are used in evaluation. Among them are benefits realization, CBA, and CEA.

- When a decision is made to purchase an information system rather than develop it with in-house expertise, a document called an RFP is usually prepared. The process for developing an RFP includes the analysis of user and system requirements and development of logical and physical system specifications. The process results in the compilation of the RFP, which includes information about the enterprise and functional, technical, training, implementation, and other requirements. An RFP is distributed to likely candidate vendors with subsequent responses from vendors reviewed and evaluated. Final system selection is made after careful review of RFP responses, vendor demonstrations, and site visits to observe the product in a production environment.

References

1. Martin MP: Analysis and design of business information systems. New York: Macmillan, 1991.
2. Nolan RL: Managing the crisis in data processing. Harvard Business Review (March–April 1979).
3. Martin J: Recommended diagramming standards for analysts and programmers. Englewood Cliffs, NJ: Prentice-Hall, 1987.
4. Yourdon E: Managing the structured techniques: Strategies for software development in the 1990s, 3rd ed. Englewood Cliffs, NJ: Yourdon Press, 1986.
5. Alter S: Information systems: A management perspective. Reading, MA: Benjamin-Cummings Publishing Co., 1992.
6. Teague LC, Pidgeon CW: Structured analysis methods for computer information systems: Chicago: Science Research Associates, 1985.
7. Stair RM: Principles of information systems: A managerial approach. Boston: Boyd & Fraser, 1992.
8. Wenig RP: Introduction to C.A.S.E. technology using visible analyst workbench. New York: Macmillan, 1991.
9. Perry WE: Assessing the value of CASE technology. *In* Tinnirello PC (ed): Handbook of systems management development and support 1993–94 yearbook. Boston: Auerback Publications, 1993.
10. Turoff MW, Whitescarver J, Hiltz SR: The human machine interface in a computerized conferencing environment. Proceedings of the IEEE Conference on Interactive Systems, Man, and Cybernetics, 1978. *In* Schneiderman B (ed): Software psychology: human factors in computer and information systems. Boston: Little, Brown, 1980.
11. Kennedy TCS: The design of interactive procedures for man-machine communication. International Journal of Man-Machine Studies 6 (1974):309–334.
12. Scheiderman B: Designing the user interface: Strategies for effective computer interaction. Reading, MA: Addison-Wesley Publishing Co., 1987.
13. Henson KL, Hughes CT: The two-dimensional systems development life cycle. *In* Tinnirello PC (ed): Handbook of systems management development and support, 2nd ed. Boston: Auerbach Publications, 1992.

SECTION
VI

PERSPECTIVES ON HEALTH CARE AND HEALTH INFORMATION MANAGEMENT

19

The purpose of this chapter is to stimulate your thinking and provide food for discussion. Several authors present issues regarding the future of information in the larger context of working toward a healthier population with information systems that support practitioner, local, regional, and national goals. Some tell us what they need to work effectively. Others lay out new roles and educational models in health information management. We hope that you will enjoy reading this chapter and find that the seeds planted by these authors will stimulate health information management professionals to meet the challenges of the next century. Meeting these challenges requires teaming up with other professionals, committing ourselves to new roles, and being open to new ideas.

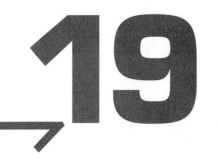

VIEWPOINTS

AN ESSENTIAL TECHNOLOGY

JON L. RUCKLE

By the time you've read this far in this book, I trust you will agree that the delivery of health care requires a great deal of information management. As a primary care internist, the flow of patients through my office generates a flow of information, and how well I manage my patients depends substantially on how well I manage their information. Some may argue that patient management *is* information management.

Looking at the health care system beyond individual patient care, many see the United States health care system as operating in a "crisis," in that the costs of health care have grown faster than other segments of our economy, and the value for these expenditures is debatable. It is widely recognized that we are faced with the challenge of how to balance the conflicting triad of maintaining "quality of care" while expanding access to care and simultaneously containing the cost of care. It is fairly easy to do any two of these things (i.e., good care for some versus expensive care for all versus poor care for all), but meeting all three demands simultaneously is very difficult.

Health care reform efforts at the legislative level apparently will not provide solutions in the near future. Ambitious proposals, including the Clinton health care plan of 1993–1994, have tried to address this problem through changing health care organization or financial structures and incentives. However, simply shifting the burden of payment from one segment of the population to another, regardless of the mechanism, does not provide an intrinsic solution. Certain experts say the Republican victories in the November 1994 national elections were partly related to the hesitancy of Americans to adopt Clinton's proposed national health care system, although alternatives which address the problems have yet to be detailed as of this writing. In early 1995, "market forces" operated to re-organize health care delivery, but political solutions were out of vogue.

Nevertheless, we cannot ignore the challenge. Our population is growing and aging. Per capita global resources are growing progressively scarce. We are unlikely to eliminate illness and suffering from this planet in the near future. It is unlikely that the public will expect and accept "less" rather than "more."

We need structural changes in the process of care delivery. Regardless of the political or organizational features, or whether change is achieved through legislation or market forces, I believe that proper health care information systems are the most crucial single component in achieving a delivery system which improves on the status quo. Information systems are *the* essential, enabling technology which allows other organizational, technical, and operational solutions to succeed.

THE GOAL

What is our ultimate goal? A "single," comprehensive, eclectic, multiprovider, longitudinal lifelong health record. The record must contain everything about a person's health and the care received regardless of provider, time, place, insurance plan, or health care delivery organization. The record must be confidential but available to and usable by individuals with a legitimate need to know. It must be a record that could be used for the multiple purposes required by our structured and complex delivery system, including anonymous statistical analysis, quality of care assessment, and clinical outcomes research as well as personal care delivery. The record must accept input from multiple sources and devices and must improve efficiency and provider productivity. The record should be linked with knowledge sources and decision support resources to assist the providers in improving care.

A "HOLY GRAIL" OR A "MAN ON THE MOON?"

As you are aware by now, the process of building a health care information system this robust is a very difficult task. Can this be done? Can we build this kind of a health care information system? Those of us who work on these tasks have doubts at times. We may feel like pilgrims walking toward a distant city, which looked so bright and almost within reach from afar. But as we travel we find we are walking against the wind, the road gets narrower, the grade steeper, the surface is more slippery, our load is heavier. Switching metaphors, some compare this effort to the search for the "Holy Grail," i.e., a noble but never-ending pursuit of an elusive goal which may or may not even exist.

But I believe this can be done. Throughout history, problems which *must* be solved eventually *are* solved. I prefer the Space Effort metaphor. Building a national health care information system is at least comparable to the American efforts to put a man on the moon in the 1960s. This too will require the best thoughts and efforts of many gifted individuals, technical breakthroughs, public and political support, organizational commitment, and substantial long-term funding. Furthermore, the ultimate goal is attained in successive stages. Neil Armstrong's "giant step for mankind" was possible only after many incremental steps, which in turn built on previous accomplishments.

It will take more than a decade—we do not have the same commitment or vision, we're concerned about privacy and confidentiality, and we ultimately see health care as an individual, personal matter and judge it on how it affects us as individuals. But I still hold the optimistic view that we will achieve the equivalent of the Apollo program in health care information. Why? I see a lot of progress, higher motivation, and growing acceptance. We now have improved software, networks, and more affordable and more powerful hardware. We are moving toward accepted standards in many areas, and many difficult problems have already been solved. We are approaching a consensus that information systems are both good and necessary.

The preceding discussion was in terms of the United States health care system, but the information needs are actually global. Fortunately, there are many people around the world who are working toward the same goals. Adequate solutions will be international solutions.

IMPLEMENTATION REQUIREMENTS

Even if we have the technology to build the system, what will it take for it to work? We can learn some important principles from information and management experience in other industries.

First, the information system must be "on the shop floor," i.e., used as an intrinsic part of the health care delivery process by providers at the point of care, at the bedside, and in the examination room. This requires not only the software tools and proper networks but also user-developer collaboration which allows "work re-engineering." We need to document the data elements that matter as efficiently as possible. This process goes beyond a simple translation of our paper systems into electronic form.

Second, the system must provide "complete" integrated data sets that contain everything relevant for the system to function, rather than jumping back and forth between paper and electronic charts or manually synthesizing data from separate subsystems on a case-by-case basis.

Third, the information must utilize standard vocabulary and database structures so we can formulate searches, queries, and reports to answer important questions, both for individuals and populations with specified clinical concerns. We must be able to do outcomes research to see what works best, and what is most cost effective.

MOTIVATION

From a motivation standpoint, how is this going to happen? We can contrast two approaches, the "carrot" and "the stick." I am a believer in the "carrot" approach. If there are natural incentives and benefits to using electronic technology, users will willingly make the transition. I believe this would be more effective than legislative or administrative requirements that force implementation, especially if it increases the cost and complexity of the care delivery process.

Similarly, "consensus" is more likely to succeed than "confrontation." We need "buy-in" from the stakeholders at all levels rather than authoritarian mandates that may provide an advantage for some at the expense of others.

STEPWISE PROCESS

As mentioned when discussing the "space program" metaphor, large-scale information systems that actually work are not going to happen in a single step, and they will not descend in final form from a central authority. We can see this from our experience so far. We can point to several examples of good information systems in certain large-scale integrated systems of care, such as the Harvard Community Health Plan, The Medical Record at Duke, the Regenstrief in Indiana, the HELP system in Salt Lake City, and the Stanford University clinics. These systems have evolved over a long period of time, and incorporate several "legacy systems" in their operations. Their continuing evolution on site is an example of the stepwise process.

Alternatively, we have a number of "niche products," which do a specific task in multiple different settings, but which do not attempt to provide global solutions. Drug interaction programs, patient education materials, bedside intensive care charting programs, clinical decision support programs, and voice transcription programs for gastroenterologic procedures represent this category. If standard programming tools, vocabulary sets, and interface standards are included in these programs, they can be incorporated into larger information systems.

Both of these approaches work because they successfully solve real world problems, but they do not have to solve all these problems to be effective in a given setting. These programs meet perhaps the most important requirement above—they are used in the process of care delivery, with proper work re-engineering, which offers a "carrot" for their users.

A national system will not come from a single source, or even a few large sources. It will emerge as many pieces from many sources that work together.

INTRINSIC CONFLICTS

Despite the potential, the effectiveness of computerized records depends on appropriate development, implementation, and utilization. Improved technology provides a foundation for better and easier solutions than we had previously, e.g., faster central processing units, better interface designs, cheaper memory and storage, better network and connectivity tools, voice technology, portable computing, handwriting recognition, imaging, and so on.

Nevertheless, there are intrinsic differences in the needs of different medical record users, and it is hard to design a system which addresses all of these concerns. Difficult problems remain—some technical, some political. Compromises are unavoidable. Will we make the right choices?

SYSTEM SECURITY: EASE OF ACCESS VERSUS CONFIDENTIALITY

Paper records are not secure, and breaches of confidentiality occur all the time; however, they are in only one place at a time and thus accessible only to a small number of users at a time. The public tends to be suspicious of computerized data because of the risk of unauthorized access, duplication, and dissemination. Security is a must, given the intrinsic confidential nature of medical data and the traditional understanding by patients that records are confidential.

In electronic systems, confidentiality and security precautions can be made extremely robust, but the tradeoff is reduced accessibility to authorized users for necessary work. How tightly do we restrict access? Answers for small offices and for nursing stations in large hospitals or clinics vary, and on-site is different from off-site or dial-in access. Security that is appropriate at the Pentagon or CIA headquarters will not work at busy hospital nursing stations where many different providers use the same terminal for many different patients in a short time.

Virtually all medical records systems have a designated set of authorized users and require at least a single-level password before the system can be used. If all records are maintained at the same level of security, the user can then exercise whatever privileges he/she is granted. Single-level password systems may deter unauthorized individuals, but they do not prevent legitimate users from viewing records that they have no need to view.

Some solutions go far beyond this, matching patients with their providers (and a provider's "call" partners), and supplying assignment of a specific security level to specific portions of the patient records, and they may selectively deny access to certain records through restriction of activity at specified terminals, multiple levels of user privileges, multiple passwords, encryption, or a combination of these and other mechanisms. This preemptive approach can be very secure, but it requires a more complex data model, usually extracts a system performance penalty, is difficult to maintain, and can be a substantial obstacle to efficient legitimate use.

An alternative is a simpler set of "confidentiality flags" for certain records. If a user wants to view such a record, the system issues a warning to the user that the record is confidential, with the choice to proceed or cancel. It would maintain an "audit trail" to track who used these records. As an additional deterrent, a record of this audit can be sent to the author of confidential records, who can question apparent unauthorized utilization. Although this type of a system relies upon the integrity of the user, it is relatively simple to maintain and still offers more security than existing paper systems.

All agree that "some" security is necessary, and almost all agree that legitimate users need reasonably easy access for routine tasks. The question is, "How many barriers to access are necessary?" Some compromise is essential, but we cannot simultaneously have tight security and easy access. The optimal compromise will vary from one setting to another, and how well the system operates in a given setting will depend substantially on how this issue is solved.

SYSTEM PURPOSE AND USE

"Translate" versus "Transform"

As alluded to above, electronic records can (and should) be more than a "translation" of paper forms onto electronic media. They should constitute a "transformation" of care delivery, with more focus on health maintenance, functional status, risk factors, and links between interventions and outcomes. Records were originally scientific documents, then increasingly became legal documents, and have become financial documents. Thus the things we include in the medical record address multiple administrative and legal concerns, and perhaps we have lost some of the original scientific value. Re-engineering the process of health care delivery with computerized records can address all these concerns in ways that paper systems cannot—*if* we do it correctly.

Management versus Practitioners

Medical systems have traditionally been accounting systems, designed to manage accounts receivable and hospital admission-discharge-transfer information. Their data and architecture focus on claims processing. Even today many systems still add only a few, if any, types of data that go beyond claims requirements. We will still need to provide accounting functions, but we also need extensive clinical data that go beyond claims. Can we do both? Discarding our existing systems and starting from scratch usually is not an option. We can either extend our current claims-based programs or integrate the current programs into systems with clinical functions.

DATA ENTRY

The limiting step in most data systems is the process of data entry itself. We need better ways to get data into electronic records, and we cannot rely on physicians for the majority of routine data entry, unlike in paper systems, in which physician entries (including transcription), communication, and reports constitute most of the chart.

Some argue that saving physician time is by far the most important factor in physician acceptance or nonacceptance of electronic record use. However, the simplest and fastest way to document encounters, given current patterns of care delivery and documentation styles, is largely based on free text and does not allow adequate query/analytic capability.

Patients and office staff can enter many key data elements, and the record will need to contain data directly imported from other systems. However, for capturing specific patient encounters, physicians still need to update prior entries, select, prioritize, and summarize the patient's history, record their physical examination findings and clinical impressions, write orders, and discuss their concerns with other practitioners.

How will they do this? Transcribed dictation is the "gold standard" for ease of use and cost in our current paper systems. In electronic systems, structured screens and menus facilitate rapid entry of coded database entries, and can be faster than dictation if designed correctly. But data modeling, concept representation in codes, and efficient context-specific screens require a lot of work by users and developers if they are to be usable

by practitioners and still meet other information system requirements. Furthermore, they work best if available immediately at the point of care, which requires portable systems or readily available workstations.

Keyboards will be with us for a long time. For rapid entry of text/character data, a skilled keyboard user will remain a valued asset. Can physicians type? Will they learn?

How about pen systems and handwriting recognition? This recognition will not happen, for lengthy text entries, unless we can convince users to print B-L-O-C-K L-E-T-T-E-R-S neatly and correctly. This takes too much time for most practitioners I know. Pen systems will work best when we use the pen as a portable pointing device to select items from structured menus. Technical advances have only so much potential—face it, if you and I cannot read each other's writing, how can a computer?

Speech recognition will get better as we have more powerful CPU's and interpretation algorithms but again will work best when applied to a specific context with limited "next word" vocabulary sets. Even today, systems are pretty good at untrained speaker independent recognition when the range of words expected is small (e.g., the menu commands in "Windows" programs). In the medical arena the speech recognition programs that work best are those that apply to specific domains, e.g., dictation of procedure reports, or when elaborate templates narrow the range of expected vocabulary in each context. And even these often require hours of voice training for specific users or require ONE . . . WORD . . . AT . . . A . . . TIME dictation rates. As trained humans, we all have some difficulty recognizing certain words of some speakers, especially if the speaker has laryngitis, has an accent, or uses terms that are unfamiliar to us. So we are a long way away from voice recognition systems that will outperform trained medical transcriptionists for general-purpose conversationally paced unrestricted vocabulary medical dictation, whichisusuallydictated— atapacethatsoundslikethislooks.

We need to keep in mind that data entry takes time and costs money, regardless of how it is obtained. Are we willing to pay the price for "complete" data sets?

COMPUTING INFRASTRUCTURE

We will depend on ongoing improvements in operating systems, high-speed and broad band width networks, connectivity tools, messaging, multimedia, and more affordable high-powered and sometimes portable hardware platforms for this to all work. Medical informatics specialists and users alike depend on the work of hardware and software engineers for these necessities.

Open versus Proprietary, Codes and Standards

In the past, many systems used codes and data structures that were unique and difficult to link with other systems. That was understandable given the lack of standards or accepted methods of solving certain problems. Of course, that made it very difficult for systems to exchange information. Our situation now is fortunately better. A huge amount of effort has gone into standards definitions, such as HL-7 and many ASTM specifications. We have coding sets such as ICD-9, CPT, and SNOMED. We have efforts to map terms from one coding system to others, such as the UMLS.

There are many advantages to building "open systems," which conform to standards and allow links with other programs. This must be done both at the programming level—with use of standard languages, operating systems, and applications program interface calls—and at the conceptual design level with use of similar concept representation.

No single vendor or system can provide the best function in all areas. We need systems that work together, because needs and preferences will vary from one care setting to another. Many providers will need to "mix and match" components or modules from different information vendors. If everyone supports common standards and builds "open systems" which can be easily linked, the pieces will fit together more easily. The problem is, how do you get everyone to agree? How do you support a standard and still allow creative/improved solutions?

Standards are a good idea but are ultimately determined not by committees but by "market share," i.e., what is actually being used. There is still much to be done in formalizing acceptable standards in many medical domains. Our existing standards, such as the HL7 and ASTM documents, represent enormous progress but will need ongoing maintenance and expansion for larger-scale implementation.

Text versus Coded Entry

As alluded to previously, medical concept representation is an even more difficult issue. As in ordinary nonmedical language, terms may include a spectrum of meanings ("pain"), vary with the context ("critical"), or be hard to specifically define consistently from one user to another ("rales"). Medical concept coding is a huge effort. The UMLS and SNOMED exemplify the scale of effort required. We have had the luxury of contextual interpretation by individual trained users reading or listening to full text records. Database queries do not allow us that luxury. We need to continue the effort to codify medical concepts and incorporate these codes into our records.

This again is harder than it sounds, and that's because we always have "lumpers" and "splitters," i.e., in some contexts a few large, coarse categories are preferable, and in other contexts we need small, finely granular categories. Different users intrinsically have different needs, and there is no way to change this. Perhaps the best we can do is map across categories so we can reliably combine finely granular sets into larger categories.

CONSENSUS REGARDING CLINICAL MEASURES AND CONCEPT MODELING

There are lots of examples here, to name just three:

Functional status is still difficult to measure objectively. We have a fair number of domain-specific questionnaires (e.g., the AUA prostatic symptom survey), and a few general-purpose survey instruments that have large normative data sets (e.g., the SF-36 and the SF-12). But we have much less experience in relating general measures to specific patient subsets and clinical interventions, and in relating domain-specific instruments to clinical interventions and global function.

"Time" is a crucial concept in medical reasoning, yet is difficult to include in most data models the way we use time clinically. Excellent research has been done in this field but is not widely implemented. Decision support tools and use of database format records for medical-legal purposes will require good functional solutions.

Physical findings significant for one specialist in a given clinical domain are very different from those of other specialists in other domains. For example, compare the respective description of heart examinations by a cardiologist and an orthopedic surgeon, and then the description of joint examinations by cardiologists and orthopedic surgeons. An individual patient might concurrently have advanced arthritis and valvular heart disease, but you have to look at the records of both examiners to see the extent of the disease. It is hard to have a unified coding system and data model that spans a wide degree of granularity and is used differently by separate providers.

SUMMARY

We have briefly described the functions desired for a robust health care information system and surveyed the problems to be solved before this can be a day-to-day reality. You probably recall that an ancient Chinese curse was "May you live in interesting times," and that the Chinese pictogram for "crisis" also means "opportunity." Our health care environment requires new delivery patterns. This is an opportunity to re-engineer the process of health care for more efficient and cost-effective delivery to a larger and more elderly population. We have made great progress yet still face difficult unsolved problems. But I believe we can and will achieve success. Like the "space race" in the 1960s, the task will require commitment, resources, and the best efforts of many people. Success will be achieved in multiple sequential steps rather than in a single bound.

No amount of yearning will bring back the simpler "good old days" of yore. Whether by choice or not, we do live in "interesting times." We may as well make the most of it.

THOUGHTS ON THE FUTURE

SUSAN HELBIG

The health information management future is unfolding as it parallels and will continue to parallel developments in the health care delivery arena. Driven by technologic innovations and the marketplace, the way in which health information is viewed and managed is rapidly changing and will continue to do so.

As important as technology advances are the purposes for which health information can or should be used. Are we moving toward a future that will become an Orwellian nightmare or toward a system designed to ensure the optimal health of individuals and communities? The choices we make about the use and abuse of health information in the present will affect the future. Health information systems can become part of a bio-regional networked system, a world networked system, or some combination of both. Health information systems can be designed to be sensitive to cultural, demographic, and environmental constructs and processes or designed to become a tool responsive to the needs of those who *have* at the expense of those who *have not.*

Designers of health information systems need to address the question of privacy and confidentiality. Will these systems protect all individuals' privacy or will they enable special-interest groups to selectively exclude people from fully participating because of certain medical conditions, genetic predispositions, or other considerations? Or will there be a complete paradigm shift in the concept and practice of privacy because technology may make privacy virtually impossible to obtain?

TECHNOLOGY DRIVES DATA—DATA DRIVES TECHNOLOGY

The technology for collecting, processing, storing, retrieving, and disseminating individual and aggregate health information is evolving from a paper-driven, labor-intensive process to one that can employ sophisticated computer and telecommunications technologies. ore than two decades ago, the introduction of computer technology to health care organizations began a journey wherein technology itself created the possibility for new and more detailed health care data. This new data pushed the invention and development of even newer technologies. For example, an x-ray film is similar to a paper record. It is a physical object that is processed in a physical space. CT scans and MRI's, however, are processed as bits of information that are formed into a visual image on a computer screen and stored as bits of information in a computer. These images are not physical objects; they are composite information bits, stored and processed in electronic form. Development of CT scans and MRI's was impossible until the computation power of computers evolved and the imagination of human beings created the demand for this kind of record.

CAPTURING PATIENT DATA

When a manual system is used to capture patient data, there is much less detailed data captured because of the time and labor it takes to both document the encounter and abstract the data at some future date. When technology evolves wherein data is generated as part of the care process itself, the amount and depth of data that can be captured increases. Generating larger and more detailed streams of data, however, is not necessarily helpful to the care provider, to researchers, or to reviewers of quality patient care unless there is some timely way of detecting changes in the patient's condition or matching patterns against a community standard. Again, it would be a labor-intensive, time-consuming task to sift through data quickly enough to make a difference in the care of that individual patient. Statistical programs can be designed to run in the background to find patterns in the data to create information that assists the provider in decision making.

Because a patient can be located in a remote rural area in which perhaps there is no physician, communications technology will make it possible to transmit almost real-time data and/or information to an expert located somewhere else on the globe. A patient can be at home hooked up to a monitoring device that communicates certain values to a home health agency. Case management for such patients becomes a combination of remote machine and human diagnostics and intervention.

Management of patient data operations at the receiving care location will mostly likely involve integrating an appointment system with the "medical record" of a specific patient. If an acutely ill patient had been "seen" before, it may mean developing systems to send the old information to the scheduled provider along with the new, almost real-time data.

In today's health care organizations, a patient who does not present physically for health care is not usually considered part of that organization's patient database even though some diagnostic services are often provided by physicians of that organization, such as radiologists. In a future scenario in which care can be diagnosed and delivered remotely, who will be considered the organization's patients?

The health information administrator in a care delivery organization will need to think through operational issues germane to setting up systems in which "expert" human providers read and interpret patient data and prescribe treatment for patients who are physically remote from the organization.

As the technology for the delivery of care develops wherein the patient does not always need to be physically with the care provider, organizational strategic planners may propose expanding their patient "community" to encompass far larger regions. This in turn generates questions about individual and aggregate patient data and information:

- What technology will be used to collect baseline data for an individual patient? Who will ensure that only accurate and authorized data are entered for that individual? What kind of language-translating capabilities are needed?

- Will patients use their own computers to answer questions or will they go to an authorized clinical data collection center for an initial evaluation? To a local physician or nurse practitioner?

- Where will this data be stored? At the collection center and the regional care center? At both? With the patient as well? Using what storage technology?

- What technology, system mechanisms, laws and policies are needed to integrate patient data derived from more than one source? Who owns this data? Where does the information reside? Who is responsible for its integrity?

HEALTH INFORMATION WITHOUT WALLS

Unlike the medical record file room, health information cyberspace has no walls. When new space is needed, it can be created by expanding the organization's data repository. Expert systems will automatically code patient diagnoses, procedures, and so on. Billing will be done automatically. Systems to measure the quality of care for an individual or group of patients will be done by computer with exceptions reviewed by a human being. To identify cases for research projects, the user will apply a combination of machine and human interventions. Access to health information stored in cyberspace is subject to only those protections placed by "owners" of that particular space and the limitations of those unauthorized persons or organizational entities who would invade or attempt to invade the space for unethical, illegal, or illicit purposes.

Data collection also knows no physical boundaries. Information can be collected from virtually any generation point on the globe and transmitted to a specific receiving facility. Future technology will make it possible to gather and store individual patient data in a cyperspace file and to add data over time to create a longitudinal record. What knowledge and skills will the health information administrator need to manage the technology and the people who use it?

MANAGING HEALTH INFORMATION CYBERSPACE

Although file rooms will disappear, the residual physical world of health information will still need to be managed, as will the people who work there and the data/information that is generated and processed. Some of the kinds of positions and functions that will need general health information management and/or influence include:

- Care providers collecting and/or entering data at the point of care

- Care providers using information for remote patient care

- Database system administrators assigning and monitoring authorization of users and managing one or more databases

- Systems analysts designing and/or improving systems

- Transcriptionists or transcription services providing text in electronic form; other data entry persons

- Researchers and reviewers of care who need access to health information
- Coders and/or coding system vendors
- Technical support specialists (either in-house or vendors or both) for software systems such as coding
- Release of information specialists
- Data validity and integrity specialists
- Privacy and confidentiality manager

Several of these functions may be carried out by one person or shared among a group.

In addition, health information administrators may share certain responsibilities with the information systems department.

SUMMARY

The future, which is unfolding as this is being written, is an exciting and challenging journey. As we begin to speed down the information highway toward health information cyberspace, we enter an increasingly complex and complicated world of technology and data streams. The core concepts and principles that began with medical record management and evolved into health information management, however, remain valid. Data are still collected, stored, processed, coded, retrieved, aggregated, and disseminated. Values relating to confidentiality are even more important. Identifying the right patient with the right record, whether electronic or paper, is still crucial to providing patient care. Managing people and machines is not going away; the kinds of machines and the types of people may change. Our terminology is expanding beyond the medical and management domains to include technology concepts and techniques. Our file rooms of the future may indeed be virtual reality in cyberspace. What an exciting time in which to practice health information administration!

FUTURE DIRECTIONS IN CLINICAL INFORMATION MANAGEMENT

MARTIN MENDELSON

Clinical medicine has lagged far behind many other fields of endeavor in the adoption of modern, automated information handling technologies. The reasons given have been many and varied, but the reality is that your bank account or your department store charge card record is far more likely to be available via computer than is your medical record. In the realm of hospital inpatient medicine there has been a long history of automation of some operations, yet hospital systems have shown remarkable resistance to the addition of hands-on clinical applications for physicians and mid-level practitioners. This has been due partly to the legacy of departmental systems and the problem of integrating these systems with one another, let alone creating a medical record that integrates them all. It has been due partly to resistance of providers to direct interaction with terminals, although this barrier is crumbling as cadres of younger, computer-savvy individuals come on the scene. And it has been due partly (perhaps largely) to unwillingness or inability of software vendors to develop a fast interactive interface that hastens rather than slows down the work of the provider. Nonetheless, the effort is well in hand, and both public (Veterans Administration and Department of Defense) and private hospital systems are involved in creating the computerized patient record. The greatest unmet need presently is in the outpatient setting, in both large multiphysician clinics and small private practices.

Outpatient medicine has slowly accepted the automation of business systems, including billing, payroll, and appointment-making functions. Yet as in the hospital, the outpatient arena also has been remarkably resistant to clinical applications for providers. I believe that the reason for this has clearly been the lack of suitable interfaces. The impact of competent automated data systems in the outpatient setting is potentially enormous, particularly with the advent of managed care and the need for primary care physicians to acquire and effectively utilize large, varied sets of patient data.

MEETING THE NEEDS OF PHYSICIANS AND OTHER PROVIDERS

For any provider engaged in an encounter with a patient, two fundamental varieties of information exist. First is information about the specific patient. Second is information about the universe of all patients who have the same set of complaints, to determine where this one particular person fits into the spectrum of problems for which help can be given. Only by making this critical match can the best possible treatment be designed and offered to the individual. The patient-specific data fall into several well-known categories. First, current problems known to have been recently active must be considered as the possible cause of any new complaints. Before being seen by the physician, a patient will have a brief, interactive conversation with a terminal to review and update symptoms already entered, as well as to add any new ones that have arisen.

Second are physical findings that may explain the new complaints. These will include results of examination at the present visit, as well as flow charts of vital signs and physician-entered findings from past encounters. The physician will be able to define the period of interest for each category of data and restrict the flow sheet to this period. Laboratory results that fit with the known condition, point to a new complaint, or point to some occult as yet unconsidered condition will be presented in a usefully structured way. Results pertinent to conditions the patient is known to have will be grouped and presented as time series to highlight trends, and all out-of-range results will be flagged. Disease-specific protocols will identify significant findings and remind the provider of tests that should be performed. Consultation reports that help explain the known problems, or that may point to some previously inapparent condition will be available. To avoid the tendency to skim long narratives, and thereby miss critical items, text analysis routines will automatically identify pertinent items that will be abstracted to create useful, brief summaries. Emergency room visits often result in laboratory tests and radiologic imaging, and the results of these investigations, including digitized images, will be sent by the hospital computer to the physician office system as soon as they are authenticated. No longer will patients seek follow-up with their primary providers only to find that their emergency room visit records are not available.

An individual's medical history stretches back over a lifetime, and with the graying of our society, more and more of those lifetimes span many decades. Much of what has happened in the past—both proximate and remote—is relevant to the present encounter. To retrieve these items may take much time. Failure to elicit these data can lead to failure to appropriately meet the patient's needs. People may selectively forget, especially if they do not fully realize the significance of an event or if the memory arouses unpleasant emotions. They may fail to disclose conditions they have had diagnosed, hospitalizations, or even surgical procedures. (In my own clinical practice I have been astonished at the number of apparently competent men who do not note on a standard questionnaire the fact that they have had a vasectomy.) Thus, advanced computer systems will scan a patient's portable historic database (see below) to extract and summarize significant items, with weighting applied for known chronic conditions, aging changes, and environmental risks. Family trees will be incorporated into the data of all patients, with pointers to the computerized records of other family members. Periodically these data sets will be linked and patterns of inherited conditions will be detected and alerts generated for persons found to be at risk.

In an earlier time primary care physicians might have known the social settings in which their patients lived, but this is infrequently the case today. Social factors such as schooling, work setting and history, family support, drinking, and smoking all are relevant to a person's proper medical care but are difficult to keep track of in today's impersonal, mobile society. With these items initially entered into a patient's record, system routines will identify and present reminders of significant risks, for example, heavy metal exposure in a former metal worker or cigarette smoking in a high-school student. Belief systems are often crucial in a patient's comprehension of a condition, as well as that patient's willingness to follow any particular course of treatment, pharmacologic or nonpharmacologic. Therefore, culture-specific beliefs, keyed to patient's ethnicity, will be flagged as they relate to exposures or risks in a specific individual.

Crucial to proper medical treatment is knowledge of medications and therapies currently being utilized, many of which will be present in the data from prior visits. But a list of prescribed drugs alone is insufficient. Over-the-counter medications and dietary supplements could be automatically entered into the database from store charge records. Exercise, physical therapy, and other similar interventions will be included. Drug-drug, drug-food (ethnic-specific), and drug-disease interactions will all be tracked, flagged, and incorporated into automatic reminders to the physician. Software will estimate the costs of therapies, and lower-cost equivalents will be presented to the provider for consideration. All product recalls and out-of-date therapies will be flagged and warnings generated. Allergies and adverse reactions must not only be tabulated but also explored in some depth so that superficial, but incorrect, conclusions do not corrupt the data. All too frequently persons will relate that, "My mom told me I was allergic to . . ." yet further questioning reveals that true allergy is very unlikely. These instances can prevent or delay the application of highly beneficial, even lifesaving treatments, so that whenever possible the reported adverse reaction must be verified, and the data system will warn if the described occurrence does not have the attributes of a true allergy.

Thus far I have been describing the kind of information that a provider would be able to retrieve from a clinical data system, assuming that these data would have been entered earlier. It is critical that at every level of this information retrieval process, the user must be able to add or correct information without having to navigate across multiple menus and screens. At any point in the process of viewing data, it will be possible —with one or two keystrokes or a mouse click—to open a window and enter new data at the relevant point in the data set. The user will not need to back out of one menu level and re-enter down another menu path to reach a data entry routine. Any such convoluted process will inevitably cause new items to be ignored or lost. Although I am sure the software developers will be quick to offer software with graphical users interfaces (GUI's), I believe that successful systems will combine GUI capabilities with keyboard input, and that any process will have to be capable of being accomplished by either method. In this way users will be able to work at their maximum effective speeds, and acceptance of automated systems will greatly increase.

Making a correct diagnosis of a person's problem involves deciding which specific subset of patients this one fits into. Clearly this will determine how to properly treat this specific person. Historical data, risk factors, current findings, and associated disorders point to a group of possible diagnoses: This list is commonly known as the differential diagnosis. From this list the physician winnows out a most-probable diagnosis, using all the facts at hand about the patient's condition to rank the likelihood of the various possibilities and ultimately arrive at the correct specific diagnosis. All physicians can generate such lists from their heads, but they are almost always incomplete and are subject to all the vagaries of remembering (and forgetting).

Several computer programs currently exist that generate ranked diagnosis lists from input of symptoms and findings, but they are of marginal utility in their present incarnations. These programs will undoubtedly be improved or superseded by vastly better routines, so that the provider will be able to utilize the output of such a program with a high degree of confidence. Of course the performance of any such routine will be greatly improved the more information it has to work with. Such information as the infectious diseases currently prevalent in the community is obviously relevant on many occasions. On a state- or region-wide scale such data are available in *Morbidity and Mortality Weekly Report,* but local conditions are often better known to the local health department. In the future, health departments will provide updated, on-line data. Individual physician's office information systems will automatically connect to the central health department database at intervals (weekly?) and update their files, so that only the most current incidence and prevalence rates will be used by the diagnostic programs. In the event of a local outbreak of some infection, the health department computer will reset the practice system to update itself more frequently and then revert when the outbreak is over. Overall, the likelihood of missing a critical diagnosis will be greatly reduced, and so will physician anxiety.

Making a correct diagnosis is generally considered to be the hardest part of any physician's job, yet having done so, the physician is not finished with the work at hand: The next job is to determine the proper course of treatment for the specific patient at hand. Just as people's individual histories, genetics, and lifestyles influence the likelihood of various diagnoses, so too do these factors influence their response to various treatment methods. Moreover, treatment guidelines and options are also constantly changing as research reveals better new treatments or newly recognized problems with old ones, so that constant updating is necessary. Useful recommendations such as those from the Agency for Health Care Policy and Research (AHCPR) or specialty society guidelines (also known as practice parameters) are reasonably current, and many are available on-line—but at present they are spread around in various locations, and the provider needs to transit through several interfaces to obtain a comprehensive set. Moreover, it is now possible to retrieve guidelines, from different organizations, that make different recommendations for the same disorder, primarily because of the fact that sufficient comparable data about the outcomes of each recommendation do not exist. However, within a few years these outcome data will become available, thanks to the linking of many clinical data systems. Large numbers of sentinel practices will automatically generate reports of treatment-outcome linkages. These will be transmitted automatically to a central repository where analytic routines will determine significant correlations. Thereafter, AHCPR will apply the newly available outcomes information to the plethora of guidelines presently in existence and will create a set of rational recommendations free of specialty or commercial bias. The use of these new guidelines will then generate additional sets of treatment-outcome data that will be used to further refine the guidelines. Unproved and experimental treatments or procedures, too often far more costly than those currently in use, will be much less likely to rapidly diffuse into common use prior to full evaluation of their effectiveness and safety. Unforeseen adverse effects as well as increasing costs will be restrained. Better analysis of outcomes will also generate clearer understanding of the kinds and rates of untoward outcomes. Recommended treatments and their likely complications will be on-line, and the provider's computer will check these regularly for updates. Every entry of a treatment choice into the record will generate a set of precautions and the follow-up needed to avoid problems. Every patient's record will carry links to the precaution and follow-up sets for each treatment in that record, and reminders will be automatically generated for all visits, as well as for the situation in which the patient does not make recommended follow-up visits.

Utilization of automated systems that competently assist in the formulation of correct diagnoses and support decision making about appropriate treatments will greatly diminish physicians' risks from litigation. A large proportion of malpractice suits revolve around failure to make a correct diagnosis or to recommend the proper therapy. Others allege that a provider failed to follow up correctly—even to the extent of claiming that the patient should have been pursued until forced to take necessary action. Although no data system will solve the problem of people who simply will not care for themselves properly, it will certainly make it possible for providers to demonstrate that they took all reasonable steps to get the right care to the patient. Adherence to recognized guidelines will become an affirmative defense to claims of negligence. Malpractice litigation will decrease in frequency, outrageous awards will be fewer when better data are available to link outcomes to treatments, and the total cost to the health care system will drop.

MEETING THE NEEDS OF PATIENTS

Although it may seem apparent that the most immediate and pressing needs and desires of patients are for effective treatment to relieve their ills, the recipients of care clearly want other things from the health care system. What they must do merely to receive the care they desire can be very important to them. To begin with, they often require information to make the decision whether to seek professional care at all. Much of what they are exposed to, in the form of entertainment or advertising, is incorrect or frankly misleading. More public medical bulletin boards, like that set up by the Department of Family Medicine at Case Western Medical School in Cleveland, will become available. Callers to the board can post a question regarding some symptom they have and within a day receive a well-researched response, from which they can decide whether to see their physician.

Having decided that an appointment is necessary, a patient has to get into the provider's office, sometimes a daunting prospect. Automated triage and appointment systems will ease this process. The computer will prompt for the reason a visit is desired, will determine the urgency of the situation, and will schedule an appointment accordingly. Systems capable of such decision making will also prevent the occasions when a patient should access emergency care, but calls the primary care office instead. Because increasing numbers of families possess personal computers with communication capability, they will be able to dial into the office appointment system, identify themselves with a password, describe their problem, and obtain an appointment. To serve those without computers, a solution just like that for those without telephones will appear: public terminals. Here 25¢ or 50¢ gets a person on-line to the doctor's computer. (If banking can be done with ATM's, this can be done too!) Because of the potential for serious injury if persons are not able to access medical care in a timely manner, such appointment systems will be able to accept collect calls from patients known to the system, presumably adding the cost to the routine bill for care. Once connected to the office's computer, a patient will be able to make an appointment without ever talking to a receptionist. (Not only will this relieve the angst of being on hold, it will also save considerable cost in receptionist time, helping to lower the overall cost of care.) Systems will incorporate methods for patients to indicate the reason for which they seek an appointment, and patients known to the system will have appointment durations adjusted for their already-known problems and their individual characteristics. Moreover, whenever a patient connects to the system to make an appointment, patient-specific reminders about screening protocols, medication refills that are due, immunizations scheduled, follow-up of previous problems, and the like will be automatically retrieved and presented. The patient will need to acknowledge these before being able to make the appointment, thus recording the fact that appropriate follow-up was offered.

People also want to be able to understand and control their own health, and part of that process is being able to keep track of their personal medical records. The creation of portable records is clearly practicable with current technology. Every individual could possess not only a complete record but also an easily carried abstract that would serve for ongoing care as well as in an emergency. CD-ROM disks, optically scanned CD-ROM cards, embedded memory chip cards, such as those conforming to the PCMCIA standard (industry standard for plug-in card for portable computers), all could be components of this personal system. The high mobility of our population will be matched by the capability for remote access to distant providers via secure on-line protocols. The person transferred cross-continent will bring his/her Boston medical record, complete with digitized images, to San Francisco either on an optical disk, or for the cost of a long distance phone call—in minutes.

The means for people to understand their own health status and needs will also be readily available. Automated, interactive patient-education systems are already here. A sophisticated computer and video disk system teaches patients about prostate surgery and helps them make informed choices among various options. The system first accepts some information about the person using it and then is able to present data about probable outcomes and risks that are statistically adjusted to the specific user. It also presents recorded interviews with patients—with the same age and risk factors—who have chosen the various options. Additional conditions are being added to the list of those available, and soon almost any procedure or surgical option will be covered. Moreover, with patient-specific data available from automated clinical record systems, the teaching systems will use those data to adjust outcome estimates, and users will not need to enter any other data than those defining their personal preferences regarding such things as risk-taking, cosmesis, and pain. These programs will provide person-specific information, at a level of technical complexity tailored to the ability of each patient to incorporate the information. They will take account of such items as education level and personal belief systems and will not inundate persons with incomprehensible terms. Patients' satisfaction with the quality of their choices will greatly increase.

In addition to the usual medications and procedures made available by medical providers, patients frequently need aid in finding other resources for use in the home and community. Often, especially when patients may come from considerable distances, knowledge of these resources is not available in the provider's office. Publicly maintained, publicly accessible computer systems will offer information about such items as where to find assistance and the agencies, both public and private, that provide it. Where to get medications and appliances, their cost and availability and eligibility for insurance coverage, will all be readily available on-line. Guidelines and suggestions for the home will also be provided. Well-documented advice regarding child safety will be ready for new parents. Information for the elderly and their caretakers about age-related changes in abilities and how to compensate for them and maintain safety will include such things as lighting needs, fall prevention, and alarm systems. In short, the use of automated informations systems will reach well beyond the traditional bounds of the hospital or doctor's office in their support of patients' health-related needs.

MEETING THE NEEDS OF SOCIETY

Beyond the individual desires and needs of patients and providers, our society as a whole needs certain kinds of information for its health care system to function at its best. Epidemiologic information is one of the first needs. How do the agencies of society best determine the prevalence and incidence of various disorders in the community, region, or nation? Traditionally, reporting has always been on a voluntary basis and has always been well short of complete, as many reports have indicated that most conditions are under-reported, almost never the converse. Difficulty of obtaining and

assembling data have necessitated limiting the conditions reported upon to the most dangerous, or the most politically expedient. But the presence of comprehensive data in automated practice systems will permit on-line, automatic collection and organization of incidence and prevalence information for all conditions of interest. Health department computers will routinely dial up and query practice site computers and extract relevant composite data, stripped of individual identifiers. Patterns and trends will be quickly identified and tracked, and the resulting composite information fed back to the practitioners' systems as noted earlier. Thus the loop of ascertainment, analysis, and corrective action will be closed in an efficient, cost-effective manner unheard of today.

As a society we also need to know about the cost and usefulness of various interventions, as well as the best ways of having them provided to patients. Having comprehensive visit/problem histories on-line will allow linking records of many patients following a given intervention and determining the rates of various outcomes. Different interventions used for the same condition would be compared for efficacy: Different patient populations may fare better with one or another treatment. Obviously if a large proportion of the recipients of a new surgical procedure were admitted to hospitals for the same (hitherto uncommon) condition within a few years, suspicion would be aroused and the procedure either modified or perhaps discarded. Once outcomes of different interventions can be better measured and compared, their costs can also be better compared. Outcomes and costs of treatments provided by various types of providers will be compiled and assessed, and rational, not political, determinations will be made of the optimal mix of provider types needed for a cost-effective and efficient health care system.

As a society we have an interest in ensuring the quality of the care we receive and in assisting providers in the maintenance of high quality. As has been shown over and again, the basis of high-quality care is high-quality information. Automated analysis of on-line outcomes data, coupled with automatic compensation for patient risk factors, will give early warning to providers when results are outside expected limits. Although the vast majority of such problems result from systemic shortcomings, it will also be possible to detect providers who consistently fall outside acceptable limits. For these individuals, targeted continuing medical education (CME) can be prescribed, or supervision and proctoring invoked. In the future, specialty certification or recertification will be based on actual day-to-day performance in addition to written and oral examinations. CME attendance records will be communicated directly to licensing bodies and specialty organizations for purposes of relicensing/reelection, so that providers will not need to maintain extensive records, and the temptation to pad reports will be eliminated. In addition to the limited sanction information now available in the National Practitioner Data Bank, credentialing and privileging bodies will be able to obtain realistic performance data on which to base their decisions. Interstate and national qualification queries will be greatly facilitated, virtually eliminating the problem of providers who move a lot to escape their mistakes or misdeeds.

Improved access to care is another benefit that automated health care systems will bring to society. Automated provider directories will be on-line with the relevant characteristics of the providers listed, as well as information about their practice patterns. Would-be patients will know about culture-specific aspects of a practice before they enlist in it. For the providers, there will be direct access to insurance or other coverage information when a patient logs in to make an appointment the first time. With much of the initial red tape eliminated, or at least greatly reduced, patients will be able to obtain care more quickly and efficiently. Because utilization data will be generated directly by the visit record and automatically sent to payers, overutilization will be discouraged and insufficient follow-up flagged to gen-

erate reminders. Thus several of the procedural problems that afflict our current nonsystem, lessening provider time available for direct patient care, will be greatly reduced, effectively increasing available access to care.

Society as a whole has critical interest in the confidentiality of medical records, a confidentiality that must be protected at all times. As more and more information goes on-line, more stringent methods of protection will have to be employed. System access will be protected not only by passwords but also by such methods as fingerprints, voiceprints, and telephone callback. Data will be encrypted using highly secure methods. Public key systems will be employed to encrypt data and protect them while in storage and while in transit. Patients will be able to access and decode their own personal records, but not those of others. Because most citizens do not want to allow access to their health records by payers or government, they will be able to grant limited decryption capability and revoke it as they desire. Compared with the degree of confidentiality now enjoyed by paper records, the future automated record will be far more secure.

PERSPECTIVES ON THE HEALTH INFORMATION MANAGEMENT PROFESSION

PAMELA K. WEAR

HISTORICAL PERSPECTIVE

The health care delivery system and health information system are inextricably intertwined. Throughout history, health information management (HIM) has met the provider needs and at other times has been at odds with the providers to meet very divergent needs. The medical cavemen demonstrated the value of documentation by drawing hieroglyphic treatments on cave walls. Documentation for patient care and research has been a natural communication tool for health care providers, ever since.

Health care was delivered and paid for by the providers and customers until 1965, when the government assumed the payment role. Since then, reimbursement, specialization, regulations, standards, and consumer awareness have exponentially increased the demand for quality health information. These health information demands put new responsibilities on providers, some positive and some negative.

Historically, HIM professionals have facilitated access to health information by designing retention and re-

trieval systems for medical records. They met the confidentiality needs of providers and patients through the development and implementation of a variety of state laws, standards, policies, and procedures. Health information management professionals took on the responsibility of assisting health care providers in fulfilling documentation requirements through the design of dictation and transcription systems and retrospective analysis and monitoring systems. They translated narrative text into data elements, abstracting them for research purposes and in the 1980s for reimbursement purposes. The source document for such activities was the paper-based patient record. Manipulating it required business, clinical, and management skills. These skills were initially obtained on the job and through colleague networking. After time, they were incorporated into academic programs, and eventually these competencies were validated through credentialing. However, the paper-based patient record and HIM delivery skills were unable to meet the increasing demands for accurate health information.

A 1991 General Accounting Office (GAO) report on automated medical records identified that medical records were not available 30 per cent of the time for patient care.[1] In 1991, reabstracting studies of medical records showed lack of documentation in the medical record for complete coding and furthermore showed that codes did not always reflect the content of the medical record.[2] The study further identified that International Classification of Disease, Ninth Revision, Clinical Modification (ICD-9-CM), designed as a system for classifying morbidity and mortality, was being used for reimbursement; there was lack of a single set of official coding guidelines, as well as human error. Although coding, like medicine, is not an exact science, it became clear that current processes for delivering health information were unable to keep up with all of the demands.

At the end of the 1980s, the leadership of the American Medical Record Association recognized the likely impact on the profession of technology, the rapidly changing delivery system, and changing management styles. The HIM initiative or Vision 2000 was launched. The focus became alliance, education, and infrastructure. HIM professionals could not afford to work in a vacuum.

1990s Perspective

The successful HIM professional today has invested in a personal professional development program to become technically competent. The goal is to acquire 1990s knowledge and leadership skills. While skills may have been acquired through continuing education programs and professional networking, more likely they were obtained through advanced education, on-the-job training and employer-sponsored programs. The vast majority of HIM managers have spent several weeks in quality improvement training.

Technically competent HIM professionals participate in, if not lead, health information systems planning and implementation committees in their facilities. They are knowledgeable about hardware, networks, standards, and the attributes of each. They have identified the health information system processing needs and the technologic solutions. They have developed strategic alliances with the information system experts and all of the users. They recognize that each user has legitimate and differing needs. They are the experts on the creation, authorship, authentication, retention, rights, and responsibilities of health information. They are the first to recognize they cannot meet the divergent needs with the paper-based patient record. The customer patient and physicians begin to perceive that information collection is more important to the hospital provider than patient care. In addition to excellent HIM competencies,

they build successful teams of knowledge workers, they are focused on the organization priorities, they are efficient and contribute to the financial viability of the organization, and they are positive. The successful professional has gained information age skills and "howls at the moon."[3]

Governmental health care reform initiatives have focused on access and reimbursement methodologies, while the providers have been dramatically changing the health care delivery system. These changes have resulted in organizational downsizing, re-engineering, mergers, and outsourcing. Many HIM professionals have assumed additional responsibilities, moved into nontraditional settings, or lost their jobs. In many instances the pace has been so frantic that competencies have not been the criteria for success. In response, the American Health Information Management Association (AHIMA) membership identified the need for national standards, the stakeholders, and the importance of volunteer and staff participation. It provided the impetus for the formation of Computer-Based Patient Record Institute (CPRI) and contributed HIM expertise to numerous standards and governmental and professional association alliance activities. The leadership educated and, more importantly, questioned the value of regulations and standards and offered alternatives. As a result, HIM expertise is increasingly sought and respected.

Perspectives Beyond the 1990s

As the information age evolves, the profession will change dramatically and there will continue to be multiple opportunities and choices for the HIM professionals.

Health Care

There will be a national health care system that rewards health rather than illness. Life expectancy and quality of life will be enhanced by human genetic programs.[4] The leadership of health care institutions will make a transition to clinical executives.[5] A standardized clinical data set will be identified and its accuracy, timeliness, and integration will continue to be crucial to health care delivery. Privacy rights and responsibilities will be integrated into the public education system. The external review system will be outcome based and incorporate patient perspectives. The legal system will continue to be a time-consuming, expensive, non–value-added check and balance. In 1985, I predicted that by 2030 all health care documentation will be pictures that represent standardized text, similar to highway signage.

AMERICAN HEALTH INFORMATION MANAGEMENT ASSOCIATION

Data Elements

Quantum leaps have been made to make these predictions a reality. AHIMA, in concert with multiple alliances, must lead the government and United States legal system to the realization that health records need to include a limited number of basic data elements, collected as a by-product of birth to death health care delivery. We need to demonstrate that narrative and dictated text adds value or does not add value to the patient care delivery process.

Creation, Authentication, Retention, Rights, Responsibilities

There needs to be a continued focus to assure that the privacy and confidentiality bills are passed; that the regulations, standards, policies, and procedures are developed; that education programs commence, and that standards are implemented nationally. In addition, the draft legislation for creation, authentication, and retention needs to be introduced and followed to implementation and postevaluation. A close alliance needs to continue with the American Bar Association's Electronic Medical Record Workgroups, for education and implementation purposes. We need them to help us change the laws.

Quality Outcomes

Many believe that quality will be improved by measurement. The major questions are:

- (1) Do the billions of dollars spent annually gathering extensive data elements, developing profiles, trends, and monitors improve patient care?
- (2) Is there additional value, when these data elements are a by-product of care, validated by the caregiver and integrated with patient perceptions?

AHIMA needs to question the value and expense and must integrate patient perceptions into the process. For example, a Harris Pollster process could be utilized to determine if a patient's physical quality of life was enhanced by laminectomy, hip replacement, or oncology therapy. Did certain prostheses or treatments have more positive results? Statistically valid samples are used in research, yet in health care the whole population is used as the sample. There could be measurable cost benefits by using statistically valid customer samples.

Computer-Based Patient Record

The vision of the computer-based patient record has been developed with all of the health care stakeholders. HIM participants can ensure that national standards address the integrity and integration of data elements, security, access, retention, and medicolegal requirements. Re-engineering and standardizing health information management at the national level is key to the ability to deliver at the community level. The AHIMA Vision 2000 action steps are vital in the future of health information management.

HEALTH INFORMATION MANAGEMENT PROFESSIONAL

Health Information Officer

What type of professionals will implement these initiatives and what will be their roles and their skills?

The Health Information Officer (HIO) is a position title that I coined when AMRA changed its name to AHIMA in 1991. These individuals will contribute to any organization that manages health information. HIOs will be masters of technical data rather than overseers of hourly workers. The HIO possesses HIM skills with the ability to apply these skills in an electronic, integrated community environment:

- Database management—clinical and financial
- Data quality—timely, accurate, organized, alerts, reminders, performance outcomes, education, training, quality improvement
- Information accessibility—stakeholder needs, standard and ad hoc
- Privacy, confidentiality, security
- Planning and implementation of a comprehensive information system

Health Information Specialist

These individuals will continue to input information into systems, until all providers have the skill to interact with the system themselves, that is, every physician might need a health information specialist (HIS). HISs will rapidly make the transition to providers of information and will have the knowledge to query comprehensive health information management databases for information for patient care, reimbursement, and so on. Their value will diminish as all care providers have the time, interest, and ability to interact with health information systems. Coding, transcription, and abstracting functions will become a by-product of the health care process.

According to a 1993 Bureau of Labor Statistics report, medical record technicians earned an annual median pay of $29,599 in 1992. There were 76,000 jobs in 1992, and the projected job growth from 1992 to 2005 is 61 per cent.[6] These figures are key to an analysis, because in 1994 there were 18,000 ART credentialed members of AHIMA, and they were not all serving in medical record technician positions. This translates to a multitude of technicians who have been potentially trained on the job and have not pursued an HIM credential. The Bureau of Labor Statistics could be counting coders, abstractors, and some transcriptionists. The Bureau of Labor Statistics forecasts demonstrate the growth and importance of the technically competent workforce. Global technical jobs have increased 300 per cent since 1950. The Bureau predicts that technical workers will represent one fifth of the total employment in the United States in the next decade.

. HIM departments are increasingly using technology to perform routine, time-consuming tasks, to eliminate errors, to speed up production, and to improve operations. As a result, HIM personnel are either laid off or retrained to tackle functions that require skill and judgment. Their value has increased in hospitals, and their competence allows departments to be lean and flat. They oversee the collection and integrity of the data and assist the users with access.

Health Information Technicians

The technicians administer the computer and telecommunications networks that keep HIM departments operating. They integrate systems. They validate the integrity of the data. They run reports. They work in concert with the health information specialists serving as a major resource to health information officers.

Technicians have varying levels of formal education and credentials. Many enter technical fields with a high school diploma and acquire training on the job. Some are coming to these careers from a trade school or a community college. And some of them have a 4-year university education or advanced degrees.

I recently visited 10 HIM departments: two of the departments had information system department liaisons, two had information system department dedicated employees, five had on-the-job trained employees reporting to the HIM department, and one director was overseeing the HIM information system. None of these individuals had an AHIMA credential. Most were in school taking information system classes and participating in hospital- or enterprise-wide information system activities. These technicians enter the labor force as hourly employees, and they quickly begin to view their jobs as the foundation of a new career. The technicians I interviewed are continually looking for the next exciting project.

Despite re-engineering health information processes and applying computer technology, health care providers have not been able to keep pace with the needs for timely, accurate, and protected health information. The vast majority of AHIMA members are busy struggling to provide these services in their institutions. Simultaneously they are fostering the development of "hands-on" information specialists. These information specialists are integrating the information system skills with traditional HIM skills that make them invaluable to their providers.

SUMMARY

The near future is bright. HIM skills are vital to health care and will continue to have value. HIM professionals have been slow to move into the information age, and as a result there will be a major fallout of current professionals. The HIM professionals who embrace technology will manage health information, perhaps as Health Information Officers. Health information specialists and health information technicians will have a 10- to 15-year period of value. The systems will then become smarter and friendlier, and these skills will rapidly become standard for all caregivers.

References

1. General Accounting Office: Medical ADP Systems: Automated Medical Records Hold Promise to Improve Patient Care. Washington, D.C., GAO, 1991.
2. Hsia DC, Ahern CA, Ritchie CO, et al: Medicare reimbursement accuracy under the prospective payment system, 1985 to 1988. JAMA 1992:268(7):896.
3. Pritchett P, Pound R: High-velocity Culture Change, a Handbook for Managers. Dallas, Pritchett Publishing Company, 1993, p. 39.
4. World in 2025. Parade Magazine, August 22, 1994, p. 21.
5. Coile C Jr: Transformation of American Healthcare. Healthcare Executive 1994; July/Aug., p. 11.
6. Bureau of Labor Statistics 1993 Report. November 1993.

HEALTH CARE AND THE NATIONAL INFORMATION INFRASTRUCTURE*

J. MICHAEL FITZMAURICE

WHAT IS THE APPLICATION ARENA?

Description of a Health Care Information Infrastructure

Implementation of wide-area, comprehensive, integrated, networked information systems is a logical response to the challenges faced by the nation's health care delivery system. These challenges arise from several sources: dissatisfaction over rising health expenditures, in both private and public health care programs; concern over the personal health security issues of access and continuity of insurance coverage; and serious questions about the uneven quality and appropriateness of health care[1,2]. These challenges are driving the health system to a cost-conscious, competitive, market-based, managed care environment. In such an environment, information systems linked to the National Information Infrastructure (NII) are destined to play a central role.

The applications of the NII have significant potential for cutting unnecessary medical costs and improving health care access and quality. With the NII in place, consumers, physicians, other practitioners, hospitals, payers, and managers could readily obtain the information needed to make informed choices about treatments, providers, institutions, and health plans. With standards for defining, collecting, communicating, and storing administrative and clinical patient care data, scientific studies could point the way to medically effective and cost-effective care. National networks would enable all persons and health care providers to access the most recent information about particular medical technologies, clinical treatments, and provider performance. Patient outcome information could be linked to medical treatment data in a variety of settings so that all interested parties could obtain a better understanding of what works in the practice of medicine in the community and where it works best.

In addition to improving clinical processes, the NII can simplify and speed up administrative processes within the health system, eliminating much duplication of paperwork and making uniform the data definitions required to make health care claims. As a result, electronic claims and payment transfers could occur rapidly over national networks and administrative costs would be significantly lowered. However, there is much infrastructure to build.

*Adapted from Agency for Health Care Policy and Research, U.S. Department of Health and Human Services, Public Health Service, AHCPR Pub. No. 94-092, June 1994

A Vision of the Future

SCENARIO 1:

In a rural area, a child awakens with severe coughing, fever, and a rash on her chest. Her mother dials the interactive telecommunication connection to access medical care support and describes her child's condition. The nurse at the other end asks for the mother to connect special probes that monitor the child's temperature, blood pressure, pulse. She then listens through an electronic stethoscope to the child's breathing. She examines the rash through the high-resolution telecommunications viewer. After consulting information through the NII about recent health events reported in the community, such as the incidence of measles, bacterial and viral infections, she recommends action to the mother. Such action could be (1) stay on the connection and the physician will be right with her, (2) remain at home and continue to monitor the child and report in, (3) come in for an appointment with the doctor, or (4) head immediately to a designated emergency department. A valid medical encounter record is documented by this system and sent to the family's longitudinal medical service file, to the community's information repository, to the family for verification, and then to the family's health plan for payment.

SCENARIO 2:

A state public health official examines the state's health profile based on encounter records (with the identifiers removed) from health plans serving the state's communities. The records are retrieved from a state-wide information network which is part of the NII. She is alerted by the information system to a statistically significant high incidence of children treated for respiratory disorders in a community. This leads her to call up the laboratory information from a sample of these children (the identifiers are removed, but the information has been linked). In one of the cases, the laboratory results confirmed a diagnosis of whooping cough (pertussis). Immediately, she queries the immunization records and finds that some children do not appear to have been vaccinated. She then calls the community's health department to verify the data in the system. Finding the data accurate, she queries the information system about the vaccine inventory in that community and, discovering it to be short of pertussis vaccine, calls four other communities with ample supplies to request that half of their vaccine be shipped to the first community. After notifying the first community of her actions and receiving their plan to resolve the problem, she returns to her examination of the state's health profile.

SCENARIO 3:

In the hospital of a major medical university in the state, Dr. Jones visits a virtual reality learning center to review procedures for a surgical removal of a portion of the prostate (prostatectomy). As she sits in the virtual reality clinical education room, she takes the electronic scalpel and feels the sensation of cutting into the patient, the texture of the skin, the hardness of the prostate as she is guided to making the proper incisions. The simulation program that guides her uses an electronic model human object obtained via the NII from a national library of reference models in conjunction with clinical measurement readings from the actual patient who will undergo the prostatectomy. Two floors up, Dr. Smith is performing a cataract surgery operation using robotics assistance. Although Dr. Smith is past middle age and has slight tremors in his hands, the robotics device with microsurgical vision enhancements eliminates the effects of his tremors. This supporting device allows his surgical productivity to continue for many years, increasing the lifelong value of his medical training and years of experience.

A Picture of Today

Other sectors of the United States economy, some even less data- and information-intensive than the health sector, have for many years centered their operations on computerized systems. Banks, airlines, stock markets, and even salvage yards use computers to communicate, maintain inventory control, allocate costs, bill, and manage their major activities in an integrated, seamless manner. All these industries have experienced operating efficiencies, improved products and services, and, most important, greater customer satisfaction.

These same benefits can be acquired for health care. The health sector, however, has lagged far behind the other sectors of our economy in applying information and communication technologies. Most hospitals and clinics have computers but relegate them to perform isolated, relatively small segments of the organizations' clinical operations. In these settings, the computer's widest use is for billing purposes and for patient admission, discharge, and transfer functions, not for clinical purposes. Few hospitals and clinics link all caregivers together over local- or wide-area networks.

As a result, patient care information is re-entered numerous times, information of value is not widely shared, and the paper outputs of these systems are manually collated in what is called a patient record. In this paper form, the patient record does not provide the basis for efficient clinical management, quality control, cost allocation, accurate billing, or clinical or health services research. Often the paper record and the information it contains is simply not available to the clinician when

needed. The course of the patient through the health system is obscured by lack of documentation of the decisions, consultations, and sequence of interventions that are experienced. Thus, it is difficult to trace longitudinally the course of an individual patient, impossible to aggregate the data across a large number of similar patients, and improbable that all useful medical knowledge can be gleaned from the ongoing treatment of patients. Without reliable, comparative, performance feedback to the provider of health care, it is not likely that improvements in the quality of care or the efficiency of operation can be effected. Reliable feedback requires uniform vocabulary and coding standards for health care conditions, diagnoses, and procedures. Further, without an active communications interface among providers of care, it is difficult to make available—especially in underserved urban and rural areas—the benefit of the rapidly developing and evolving body of knowledge arising from biomedical and health services research.

What is the Public Interest in Promoting the Application?

Health care spending is high and growing.

In 1994, the American public will spend $1 trillion on health care, nearly 15 per cent of its Gross Domestic Product (GDP). National health care expenditures have risen by 10.5 percent per year for the past 8 years—more than double the rate of increase in the consumer price index.[3]

Insufficient knowledge exists for informed decision making.

Health and medical decision-making processes are flawed by a lack of knowledge and by financial considerations. The man (or woman) on the street has less knowledge about medical treatment alternatives for a specific condition than he (or she) has about any other bought service. Therefore, people are more heavily dependent on experts in the health care industry who often have no financial incentive to refrain from ordering every service, regardless of cost, if there is the hope of a benefit, however small.

People do not pay the full price of the health care they consume.

There would be no problem with the rapid rate of growth of national health expenditures and its portion of the GDP if it adequately represented consumer preferences expressed in the marketplace. After all, how much would the GDP have grown if not for the large increases in national health expenditures? Growth by itself is not bad. There is more than a suspicion, however, that when people pay 25 per cent or less out of pocket for medical care at the time of choice, with insurance or public coffers paying the rest of the cost, there is a tendency to consume additional medical services. The value to the consumer of many of these additional services is less than the cost of the resources to produce them.

How Can the NII Help?

While the NII cannot change the United States health care system's financial incentives directly, it can support research into cost containment efforts and payment initiatives targeted at incentives to lower costs. For example, it could supply information to help appraise which payment systems in use are the most cost-effective. Further, the NII can provide information that increases knowledge about the medical effectiveness of alternative treatments and make it available to the providers and consumers of health care. The NII also can make available information consumers need to become more cost-conscious purchasers of health care services. The NII can provide an infrastructure that supports personal health improvement and medical technology assessment.

Finally, the United States is one of the world's leading manufacturers of medical technology. With increased emphasis on cost-effective technology, there is a greater need for information about how well alternative technologies work when applied (1) in an ideal setting such as an academic medical center and (2) in the average community.

The goal is to generate knowledge about which treatments and technologies work best for specific clinical conditions and under what circumstances, to have this knowledge available at the point of service (care), and to have medical decisions made jointly by caregivers and their patients. The NII can help attain this goal by supporting the analysis of large quantities of patient care and administrative data, by protecting its confidentiality, by assisting in the dissemination of information based on these data, and by adding value through the evaluation of the information gained from these data and converting it into useful knowledge.

It is well recognized that there is substantial unexplained geographical variation in medical practices. The findings of unexplained differences in decisions about the best treatment for similar patients with the same condition elevates concern about the quality of care being delivered. Analyzing of patient care data from communities and providing feedback about these findings to the caregivers and consumers can both reduce inappropriate care and increase beneficial care. It can also improve continuous, life-long learning for health care providers who have difficulty keeping up with the flood of biomedical literature and clinical practice guidelines.

By providing information access at home, schools, and the workplace, the NII can play an important role in improving public knowledge and decision making about health, thereby reducing the significant information gap between consumers and clinicians and improving clinical outcomes. National and community networks that allow consumers to obtain information about their own health care conditions and to obtain professional medical advice in their homes can empower patients to take better care of themselves.

WHERE ARE WE NOW?

In many health care settings, patient information is handwritten in paper records and stored manually. Some of this is due to "state quill pen laws" that require handwritten pen and ink signatures on paper medical records. The current health information system does not adequately support patient care, medical effectiveness and cost effectiveness, and the public health of the community. This lack of support is often a result of incompletely recording the patient's signs, symptoms, and conditions; coding the patient's medical diagnoses to maximize billed charges instead of accurately describing the patient's ailment and the treatment given; and storing this information in ways that hinder both retrieval and making comparisons among patients with similar complaints.

Consumers have insufficient information to make informed choices among the health insurance plans, health institutions, and providers available to them. Providers of care have insufficient means to keep abreast of all the information generated in their fields of specialty. Moreover, they often are unable to marshal all relevant information on a patient when making medical decisions. Health organization administrators are hampered in their ability to merge administrative and clinical information to make rational choices concerning resource allocations, quality of care, and product and service pricing. Payors of care have insufficient information to determine what package of benefits by which providers of care yield the best value for their clients.

Further, public health officials should have the ability to more rapidly detect sharp increases in the incidence of influenza, specific bacterial infections, and other public health problems and to act quickly in health crises to inform the community. Public health policymakers often have insufficient information for offering solutions to health care problems. As a result, public health decisions are made without the advantage of timely, relevant information using technology that could reduce the costs of health care and improve patient outcomes and the health status of populations.

The value of data on patient treatment and outcomes —especially automated, uniformly defined, linked, and anonymously aggregated data—is increasingly recognized and demanded throughout the health care sector.

These data are needed for clinical, quality assurance, utilization review, business planning, administrative, and public health purposes. For example, computerized ambulatory patient care data are scarce and not uniform in definition, coding, or content. Computerized hospital clinical care data are collected on hospitalized patients in a small number of settings, but often are not stored for long in retrievable form after the patient is discharged.

As valid methods for assessing the quality of care increase, so will the value of community patient care data. When the benefits from this information are shown to exceed the costs of producing it, society must find a way to pay for the resources necessary to produce it.

Confidentiality and privacy are important concerns. Society must deal with perhaps its most vital information issue: assuring the privacy, confidentiality, and security of health care data about identifiable individuals. Even though patient care data can lead to important information for health care providers and their patients, it also has potential for personal harm if disclosed inappropriately. For example, these data may be required for emergency medical treatment for telemedicine applications in rural areas. As the data are transferred across wide areas, the system that transfers the data must provide security against unauthorized access and disclosure, maintain the integrity of the data, and confirm the originators and requesters of the data. Quite possibly, most of the uses of patient care data may not require that the individuals be identified. When patient identification is necessary, the legal system must provide severe penalties for inappropriate uses of confidential patient care data. Although many states have their own privacy laws, many others do not. Moreover, uses of patient care data are not controlled uniformly from state to state. This problem must be addressed by national legislation.

WHERE DO WE WANT TO BE?

To obtain the benefits called for by the vision of the health care information system of the future, an advanced NII should support the development and evaluation of information technology applications that can improve patient care, both directly and indirectly. These achievements would improve the health status of communities and reduce their costs of health care. Applications that bring both higher benefits and lower costs should be carefully evaluated.

Patient care data describing patient's signs, symptoms, and conditions, treatment, and outcomes should be generated at the point of care delivery by the providers of health care. These data should be defined uniformly across all points of care, automated, and made available through the NII for direct patient care, public health

policy development at community, state, and national levels, and research purposes. This sharing should occur only under conditions of confidentiality, privacy, and responsibility that are acceptable to society.

Patient care data and other information necessary in the direct care of the patient should be promptly available to providers of care at the site of care.

Clinical decision support systems should incorporate research findings based on studies of these data and on other studies. The purpose is to give providers of care information about drug interaction alerts, allergy alerts, preventive screening reminders, and other prompts that improve the delivery of health care.

Personal health information should be widely available on the NII and be accessed through personal computers and telephone links, cable television, or other links to community and nationwide networks. This linkage will permit people to obtain health care information, computer assistance for analyzing health problems, and advice from medical professionals and from people with similar health conditions. The result of improving personal self-care and wellness should be more power in the hands of the people to influence their health and a more appropriate use of health care resources.

Public health surveillance and epidemiologic studies based on patient care data and social indicators should be available to inform public policy and to guide the provision of public health services. Information about the patient outcomes of care produced by health care providers and health care plans should be available to guide consumers in making health plan choices and to feed back information to providers of care about the patient outcomes their peers are achieving.

This information will benefit consumers in their homes, schools, and workplaces. Providers of care in physicians' offices, other ambulatory sites of care, and hospitals will have access to data about specific patients and the information, if necessary, to guide decisions about treatment alternatives and their expected outcomes. Health care managers and policymakers in health plans, public health departments, national health policy positions and other settings will be able to develop an overall picture of health care utilization to assess the allocation of health resources and whether private and public health needs are being met.

Achieving these benefits requires the development of several components of a health information infrastructure. These components are:

- Medical information standards for the nomenclature, coding, and structure, content of specific data sets, and electronic data interchange of patient care data. They are necessary to achieve the uniformity of definition and meaning of the patient care data used in patient care and in generating information about the outcomes of care. The standards will improve the sharing of patient care data across different computer information systems. Slowness of the development of these standards hinders the cost-effectiveness of clinical decision support systems in institutional and provider settings.

- Unique personal identification for accurate links across databases used for patient care. Although the social impact and confidentiality issues are the most important for society, technical issues still remain. Patient information must be uniquely identified and linked across databases used for patient care. Some options are thumbprints, retinal eye scan images, DNA blood typing, or personal identification numbers in digitized form. If personal identification numbers are used, they could be social security numbers (SSN) or identifiers unique to health care.

The costs and security of different techniques to ensure unique personal identity, plus confidentiality and privacy of patient care information and any information to which it may legitimately be linked, need to be investigated.

- Model development for health care information, reference requirements, and a reference architecture to define and relate patient care data and medical information and the clinical and administrative functions they serve. A concept model should be developed that serves as the guiding framework that shows the purpose, dimensions, and minimum characteristics of health information networks, computer-based patient record systems, and other concepts. The concept models may pertain to specific domains, such as hospitals, clinics, and local networks. These models, requirements, and architecture will provide a common framework that will allow software vendors and system designers to build software tools that can work together. If they work together, these tools can fill out, or build, the health care application architecture (the common framework). By supporting the design, building, and implementation of systems that can interact with each other, this framework, and tool development, will support improved patient care and build a path for the movement of existing systems to patient-centered systems.

- Federal confidentiality and privacy laws that supersede a patchwork quilt of state privacy laws. They will allow society to gain the benefits of rapid automated information transfers across States through information technology, while protecting patient care data from disclosure. They should provide penalties for inappropriate linking, use, or disclosure of patient care data and define inappropriate use.

- Health data repositories to maintain and assure the uniformity and confidentiality of patient care data and to provide access to the appropriate users of these data. These repositories might be distributed among local communities or located regionally across the United States. At the extreme, there could be one central or national data repository. Safeguarding the confidentiality of patient-identifiable data wherever it is stored is essential and must be a prime responsibility of the depository management.

- Computer-based patient record system development to capture patient data at the point of care and make it available electronically upon request of the provider for patient care. This development should extend computer-based patient record systems so they support both clinical and administrative decisionmaking.

- Health care computer laboratory (test bed) development to determine the technical usefulness of data standards and data exchanges that support specific functions. Findings from these pilot test sites should guide modifications to data standards, models, and architectures to make them suitable for commercial applications.

- Pilot tests and evaluation of health information technology in patient care settings such as the home, physician's office, hospital, and community. These pilot tests and evaluations should include rural as well as urban settings and consumer as well as provider settings. They should reveal where the most beneficial applications are likely to be.

- Community trials for applications that have been proven successful in single site settings. These trials would be linked in broad-area studies to assess their scalability (i.e., their costs and performances at different volume levels and configurations) and their success in achieving quantifiable savings that can be duplicated.

- Specific studies should evaluate the economic and medical feasibility of patient care data transfers between primary care physicians and specialists across geographic distances, of the use of personal home information systems to promote wellness and efficient use of medical services, and of administrative electronic data systems to improve the efficiency of medical claims handling and payment. These transfers include telemedicine transmissions such as medical and patient images, consumer health information and decision analyses, and consultations with experts and patients with similar conditions. Additional studies should evaluate the potential for libraries of information on standard representations of medical conditions to be accessed by providers to improve their understanding of patient conditions, disease entities, and healthy body functioning which, in turn, should improve patient outcomes of care. Studies of alternative means for professional education and training using the NII should also be undertaken.

References

1. Wennberg J, Gittelsohn A: Variations in medical care among small areas. *Scientif Am* 1982;246, 120–134.
2. Chassin M, Kosecoff J, Park RE, et al: Does inappropriate use explain geographic variations in the use of health care services? A study of three procedures. *JAMA* 1987;258, 2533–2537.
3. Health Care Financing Administration, Office of the Actuary. Personal communication, 1993.

PUBLIC HEALTH: MEETING FUTURE INFORMATION NEEDS

MARY ALICE HANKEN

PUBLIC HEALTH AND MEDICAL CARE

As we take a more overall view of health we recognize the value of lifestyles, safe and clean communities, and the myriad things we can do to prevent injuries at home, at work, and in our communities. As organizations prepare to "manage" an individual's health care, they realize that the power and payoff are not in treating individuals for expensive diseases and conditions but in preventing disease and in educating consumers to take care of themselves. This shift is the impetus needed to bring the public health sector and the medical care sectors together. The long-range goals of both groups are similar, but to many observers it appears that the two sectors are not strongly connected.

Public health provides both direct clinical services and community services. It addresses both the individual and the population being served in a community or wider region. Public health goals for the year 2000 are expressed in terms of the entire population in the United States. For example,

- Reduce outbreaks of waterborne disease from infectious agents and chemical poisoning to no more than 11 per year, (baseline: Average of 31 outbreaks per year during 1981—1988)[1] and

- Reduce nonfatal poisoning to no more than 88 emergency department treatments per 100,000 people, (baseline: 103 per 100,00 in 1986); special population target: Children aged 4 and younger (Baseline: 650 per 100,000 in 1986; target: 520 per 100,000 in 2000).[1]

POPULATION-BASED DATA

Managed care organizations who take on a group of enrollees are now asked to express their data in terms of the population they serve. The Health Plan Employer Data and Information Set (HEDIS) report card system looks at data much the same as the Healthy People 2000 goals and is using some of the Healthy People 2000 goals in its quality of care measures. These are approximate measures of meeting a quality of care goal for a given population. Employers who purchase health care need some type of feedback regarding the quality of care purchased for the dollar spent. HEDIS includes many measures in a variety of categories. At this time most of the care measures are based on data available on billing claims: for example, "Asthma inpatient admission rate. The percentage of members with inpatient admission for the care of asthma in the health plan during a calendar year. Rationale: Many, if not most, inpatient admissions for the care of asthma are thought to be preventable if enrollees receive optimal outpatient care." HEDIS details the methods for selecting the appropriate data for the numerator and denominator to calculate the rate of admission.[2]

As communities discuss and implement regional data systems, they expand the base of population data available. While most providers of care hope that these systems will also support individual direct care through coordination and reduction of duplication, most policymakers and researchers see the benefit in gaining access to more population-based data. As HEDIS and regional and national systems demonstrate, data are valuable only if they are accurate and reliable. This requires appropriate definitions for data, standards for the content, collection, and quality of the data—all skills of the health information manager.

INFORMATION NEEDS AND CORE PUBLIC HEALTH FUNCTIONS

The public health and managed care/medical care systems have similar information needs. The following discussion focuses primarily on public health because sufficient attention is focused on the medical care systems by other authors.

The goal of public health is prevention of disease, injury, disability, and premature death. . . . public health is not simply medical care funded or provided through public means.[3] Sometimes the services of public health are less visible and may be more difficult to understand than medical services. We may not think of clean water as contributing to our health, but contamination of drinking water results in sickness. Even today when areas of the United States are hit by floods or earthquakes, water supplies may be disrupted or contaminated. Leaching of chemicals from farmland fertilizer or industrial plants is another source of contamination. Public health prevention measures are designed to protect entire communities or populations from such threats as communicable diseases, epidemics, and environmental contaminants.

Public Health functions are organized around several core activities, which include:

- Assessment—collection, analysis, and dissemination of information on health status, personal health problems, population groups at greatest risk, availability and quality of services, resource availability, and concerns of individuals.

- Policy development—which uses the assessment data to consider alternatives and determine which actions and policies to pursue.

- Assurance—which monitors the actions and policy decisions of public health and other community partners to attain the goals of public health.[3]

PUBLIC HEALTH PROGRAMS

Proven cost-effective public health measures include water fluoridation to prevent tooth decay, smoking cessation among pregnant women to prevent low birth weight, immunizations to prevent measles and mumps, and health education of consumers to reduce their need for medical services.[3] We likely take public health pro-

grams for granted. However, much like the health care system, there is a cadre of trained professionals with a system in place to prevent public health problems and to respond when an epidemic breaks out or a toxic chemical is spilled. When young children were being admitted to the hospital for treatment of *Escherichia coli* infection, it was the public health department that tracked down the source of the problem as contaminated hamburger meat and undercooking of the hamburger. All states have health departments with county and city coverage. Most public health departments work together with the medical community on some aspects of care. For example, the *E. coli* outbreak was both a clinical treatment problem and a public health problem. Pediatricians and family practitioners usually work closely with the public health department in immunizing children against many childhood diseases. Both the medical care system and the public health system take an interest in prevention of injury, illness, and disease. The more intense development of those interests may be the catalyst that brings the community together.

For much of the last 40 years, public health has been defined by a series of categorical programs and problems such as AIDS, tuberculosis, sewage treatment, immunizations, foodborne illnesses, and primary care for the underserved. When a problem was identified and brought into public view, legislators enacted laws and appropriated funds to address that specific problem. Public health agencies responded by organizing themselves to carry out disease-specific or problem-specific programs.[3]

The result of these disease- and program-specific efforts and their reporting requirements is often a disconnected, dysfunctional information system—the components each built to meet a specific program need or reporting requirement without attention to the whole picture. In many states this results in program-specific data systems. In analyzing its data collection forms for all programs, one state found that it was asking for the individual's address more than 300 times. A coordinated system that allows "registration" once would be a tremendous step forward in reducing the administrative paperwork burden. The next step in the transition would be to build a coordinated database and eliminate program-specific, free-standing systems.

HEALTH PROBLEMS AND COSTS

Public health takes a long look at the real causes of health problems in the United States. It is estimated that about half of all deaths are caused by tobacco use, improper diet, lack of physical activity, alcohol misuse, microbial and toxic agents, firearm use, unsafe sexual behavior, motor vehicle crashes, and illicit use of drugs.

The element of personal and community responsibility in these causes of health problems is inescapable. With the possible exception of some microbes and toxic agents, all of the causes listed are primarily a result of human behavior.[3]

Some examples from Washington State that illustrate these principles are:

- In 1990 nearly 8000 Washingtonians died from tobacco related illness—one fifth of all deaths in the state. Direct medical costs associated with tobacco use that year were estimated at $437 million. The loss of economic productivity from people dying young or getting sick added an estimated $845 million to the costs.

- Motor vehicle crashes are the leading cause of unintentional injury and death for children aged 1–14 in Washington. Child safety seats lower a child's chance of death and injury by about 70 per cent. In 1991, child safety-seat use prevented more than 180 deaths and 70,000 injuries nationwide, for a total estimated savings of $3.5 billion.

- A 50 per cent bicycle helmet use rate would result in an estimated 840 fewer head injuries among children ages 5–9 over a 5-year period, saving approximately $9.5 million.

- Cardiovascular disease, including heart disease and stroke, is the leading cause of death in Washington, accounting for about 42 per cent of all deaths. Cardiovascular disease mortality can be reduced by controlling four major modifiable risk factors: physical inactivity, tobacco use, high blood pressure, and high cholesterol . . .

The burning cigarette, the moving car, the raw hamburger, and the failed on-site sewage system are all carriers of health threats which are best dealt with early.[3]

IMPROVING HEALTH

Public health can be a powerful tool. Its population-based focus helps to accomplish changes and evaluate the magnitude of the problem. Public health professionals also actively participate in public education efforts.

The connection between public health and better health is well established. Since 1900, the average life expectancy of United Sates citizens has gone up from 45 to 75 years. Public health improvements in sanitation, the control of diseases through immunizations, and other activities are responsible for 25 of the 30 additional years that Americans can now expect to live. In addition, population-based public health of the 1970s contributed greatly to recent improvements in reduced tobacco use, blood pressure control, diet, use of seat belts, and injury control, which in turn have contributed to declines of more than 50 per cent in deaths due to stroke, 40 per cent in deaths due to heart disease, and 25 per cent in overall death rates for children.[4]

INTEGRATING THE INFORMATION SYSTEM

To achieve the goals and to demonstrate that goals are met, public health needs an integrated information system. While some systems are in place, generally, improvements are still needed. Public health systems still need:

- Redesign of program-specific free-standing data systems into integrated systems

- An integrated, centrally managed electronic network that provides access to federal, state, and local information systems

- Data systems that facilitate the provision of services to consumers

- Data management systems that meet the local needs to systematically collect, analyze, and monitor standardized baseline data

- Linkage between local and statewide databases in both the private and public sectors

- Data use and dissemination standards

- Technical assistance to ensure a high standard of data analysis, dissemination, and risk communication

- A fully integrated, secure computer network

- Evaluation and dissemination of new health information technologies

- Tracking of clinical and environmental laboratory information.[3]

Public health professionals need good data systems to be able to provide accurate, understandable information for policymakers, community leaders, health plans, and health care providers. Outcome measures need to be tracked. Policy outcomes need data for evaluation. Through all of this data collection, analysis, and dissemination run concerns for balancing the privacy and confidentiality of the individual with the protection of the public good. Most health care providers are aware of regulations that require reporting of communicable diseases. This reporting to the public health department allows the department to take further action if necessary to prevent spread of the illness. In most instances the reporting does not endanger the privacy of the individual. Certainly the reports are not published as public

Areas of Target Goals for Public Health*

Infectious diseases
HIV/AIDS
Sexually transmitted diseases
Tuberculosis
Vaccine-preventable diseases
Cardiovascular disease
Stroke
Female breast cancer
Uterine cervix cancer
Diabetes
Tobacco use
Chemical dependency
Violence and injury
Child abuse and neglect
Homicide and aggravated assault
Youth violence
Suicide
Domestic violence
Sexual assault
Traffic crash injury and death
Falls among older adults
Bicycle crashes
Drowning
Fires and burns among children
Pedestrian injuries
Poisoning
Infant mortality
Nutrition
Adolescent health
Oral health
Emotional well-being of children
Reproductive health care
Prevention of chemical misuse
Environmental health
Drinking waters
Hazardous substances
Occupational hazard exposure
Worker compensation
Food protection
Recreational water protection

* From Public Health Improvement Plan. Department of Health, State of Washington, Nov. 1994, Appendix A, p. 86.

information. Some diseases do require follow-up with others who may have had contact with the infected individual.

Efforts to ensure access and quality of care require partnerships among many affected parties. Also needed are the sharing of data and the tracking of measurements, programs, and changes over time. Ongoing efforts are also needed to obtain community and client perspectives on quality of care and services.[3]

All states have plans and target goals for public health. The list is lengthy and may seem overwhelming (see Areas of Target Goals for Public Health). Tracking each of these goals and the assessment of progress require data.

Health information management professionals have the knowledge and skills to support the data and information systems of the public health system and can contribute to the overall health and well-being of the entire population.

References

1. Healthy People 2000, US Department of Health and Human Services. Public Health Service, Washington, D.C., 1991.
2. Health Plan Employer Data and Information Set (HEDIS), User's Manual Version 2.0. National Committee on Quality Assurance, Washington, DC 1994.
3. Public Health Improvement Plan. Department of Health, State of Washington, November 1994.
4. Health Care Reform and Public Health: A Paper on Population-Based Core Functions. Core Functions Project, US Public Health Services, 1993.

RE-ENGINEERING MEDICINE: MEDICAL DECISION MAKING AND INFORMATION TOOLS FOR MEDICAL PRACTICE*

LAWRENCE WEED AND LINCOLN WEED

RE-ENGINEERING MEDICINE

The health care reform debate and proposals do little to reform the basis of medical decision making. Policymakers may change financial incentives, but physicians will continue to make decisions based on their own knowledge. Medical decision making includes retrieving and organizing relevant information. Clinical judgment may be highly sophisticated but can yield poor results if the relevant medical knowledge and patient data are not retrieved and integrated for use with an individual patient. The burden of accessing and processing medical information in libraries and patient records has overwhelmed the physician's unaided mind. Medical decision making requires more knowledge than any physician can learn from education and experience, or remember, or extract from the medical literature and concurrently apply to each individual patient. A basic design failure in the health care system is its reliance on the mind of the physician, operating largely without external aids, to assume the burden of managing medical information. Properly designed information tools can aid both the physician and the patient by making information available for informed decision making.

In managed competition theory, the actual content of reform in medical decision making is largely undefined. The theory simply postulates that "reform of finance" will create incentives to (somehow) deliver care more efficiently without compromising quality. But this theory rests on the mistaken premise that physicians can act effectively on financial incentives. The disturbing reality is that physicians frequently are unable to do so because the complexity of managing medical information has overtaken them.

Increasing the supply of primary physicians—a major item of the current reform agenda—is no solution to the problems of complexity and narrow specialization. Primary care physicians are not equipped with the information tools necessary to grapple with the information overload that arises in primary care. In a properly functioning health care system, patients themselves will assume much of the decision-making function that the medical profession would reserve for primary care physicians. Standards of acceptable quality, economy, and individual autonomy in medical practice demand that patients be active participants in medical decision making. Active involvement of patients in their own care is

vital because patient knowledge, self-observation, and feedback to the providers is routinely needed for sound medical decision making.

Properly designed information tools enable patients to engage in an informed "conversation" with providers and assume a greater role in their own care than in the past. Such tools can couple the entire medical knowledge base with information about the unique patient. With such tools, the full range of diagnostic and treatment choices relevant to the individual patient, and the pros and cons of each choice arising from that patient's characteristics, can rapidly be made visible to the patient and provider alike. Patients can then intelligently bring to bear their own knowledge and values and evaluate the acceptability to them of each choice recommended by providers.

The intellectual process common to both diagnosis and management is one of recalling known options and potential findings relevant to choosing among those options and coupling that general information with patient-specific findings to arrive at the best options for the patient as quickly and as cheaply as possible. Medical decision making involves the following steps:

1. Gathering an initial database of patient-specific information
2. Formulating a list of problems based on the results of coupling general medical knowledge with information in the database
3. Formulating initial plans for diagnosis and/or management of each problem, again using the knowledge-coupling process
4. Follow-up action, which involves monitoring the patient's progress, reassessing the correctness of the problem list and initial plans, and taking further diagnostic and therapeutic action

This list is not controversial; however, discrepancies can be found between the professional paradigm of medical care and the reality of what good medicine requires.

INFORMATION TOOLS FOR MEDICAL PRACTICE

Knowledge Coupling Tools

What, then, are the information tools needed to address information overload in medicine? Consider that patient experiencing a problem with dizziness. The following, based on practitioners' actual use of knowledge coupling software over a number of years, describes how the process of information gathering and analysis starts.

---

* Adapted from the Federation Bulletin: The Journal of Medical Licensure and Discipline. Euless, Texas, Federation of State Medical Boards of the U.S., Vol. 81, No. 3, 1994.

STEP 1

The patient sits before a computer screen (alone or with an office assistant assigned to help those who need it) and chooses "dizziness/vertigo" from a list of symptoms. This leads to series of questions about the dizziness symptom in laymen's language that the patient easily answers by touching a key on the keyboard or pointing to it on the screen. The answer can be "yes," "no," or "I am not sure."

STEP 2

Next on the computer screen appear possible findings on physical examination that are relevant to identifying one of the 70-plus conditions associated with dizziness. A person trained to elicit such findings reliably, and whose competence in doing so should be periodically audited and certified, does the examination and enters positive findings on the computer—just as a trained technician draws blood and does a blood count. The outcome of steps 1 and 2 is a set of simple findings that are known to be useful in identifying, and discriminating among, disease conditions that cause or are associated with the dizziness symptom. This information becomes part of the patient's electronic medical record.

Comparing what typically happens in a physician's office or clinic or emergency room to these two steps is revealing.

STEP 3

The patient or provider, by simply typing "C" on the keyboard, couples the positive findings obtained in steps 1 and 2 to the list of causes in the computer. An organized index of possible causes appears, showing findings the patient had that were positive for each cause and findings that were checked and not present. This list of causes is organized into logical groups, such as causes that may require immediate action, designed to help the provider set priorities without compromising thoroughness. The software also displays comments under each cause; the comments give the patient and provider immediate access to important information from the medical literature at precisely the time and place of need. The list of possible causes and comments for each that seem to best fit the patient are available to all providers and the patient in the medical record and as a separate printout.

Again, compare this to what typically happens in a physician's office or clinic or emergency room.

The Old System	The New System
No two physicians ask the same set of questions or check the same items on physical examination. The patient, the payer, and the policymaker have no way of knowing or controlling the breadth, accuracy, and currency of the reservoir of knowledge on which the physician bases his questioning and examination.	The items examined were derived from comprehensive study of the medical literature in all specialties to determine the best means for delineating the symptom, avoiding dependence on the physician's limited knowledge.
To the extent physicians are used to gather the initial database, expense increases and quality tends to decrease, relative to using paramedical personnel. Time pressures and physicians' exercise of their clinical judgment during the process may lead them to skip over potentially important findings. In addition, due to poor training, irregular experience, and lack of evaluation of their performance, physicians may have less expertise in performing physical examinations than non-physician personnel who specialize in that function.	Knowledge coupling software to guide inexpensive, non-physician personnel in gathering the initial database promotes consistency and completeness of inputs in several ways. Non-physicians can specialize in data-gathering functions, developing the expertise that results from specialization. Moreover, such personnel are less likely to engage in unwarranted variations. In addition, such personnel can readily be made subject to audit and certification requirements to maintain the quality of their performance.
The initial database is often not readily accessible to a patient's multiple providers over time, or to the patient, due to lack of a system for maintaining a single medical record for a patient. The frequent result is expensive duplication of effort, because providers are unaware that the information they seek has already been obtained.	Using electronic information tools to record the initial database in a standardized, electronic medical record gives the patient and providers ready access to the database, permitting them to avoid duplication.
We do not have consistent input by many providers over large populations; medical science is consequently deprived of corrective feedback loops on the body of knowledge it uses to solve problems.	A structured approach facilitates a consistent, high-quality initial database of findings about the patient's problems. This is crucial to both reliable outcome studies and scrutiny of medical decision making in individual cases.

The Old System	The New System
Physicians vary greatly in their knowledge of the disease conditions associated with a positive finding or combination of findings. Yet, the patient has no way of knowing what thoughts each positive finding triggers in the physician's mind unless he or she asks the physician, and then there is no way of assessing the completeness of the physician's knowledge of causes based on the findings obtained.	Knowledge coupling software matches positive findings on the patient with a comprehensive electronic database of findings associated with every disease condition. This coupling process generates an electronic tally of exactly which causes of the dizziness symptom are "voted for" by each positive response, and, for each possible cause, which potentially associated findings are present, which are absent, and which are not yet investigated. In short, all participants in the process, including the patient, can efficiently determine possible causes for which there may be evidence and exactly what that evidence is.
Because physicians cannot remember all potentially relevant causes and findings, the physician can easily miss a diagnosis that is determinable from already available data, or can easily overlook or ignore some of the additional findings to check. As a result, physicians often order tests that cause unnecessary risk, discomfort, or expense, relative to available alternatives.	Knowledge coupling software assures that the provider can consider all potentially relevant causes and findings. This helps the provider extract the maximum amount of useful knowledge from the multiplicity of simple observations that manifest the uniqueness of the patient's situation before embarking on a course of dangerous or expensive tests.
For certain problems, the simplest and most important findings to pursue are subjective observations of his or her symptoms by the patient. The reliability and precision of these observations may be crucial to the provider's assessment of their significance. Yet, this entire process of feedback from the patient's subjective symptoms tends to become haphazard, incomplete and unreliable in medical practice because the busy physician neglects to fully educate the patient about the potential significance of the patient's own observations.	Knowledge coupling software enhances the active and honest participation of the patient because the software highlights to the patient the implications of each finding. This in turn prompts the patient to tell the provider about gradations of severity, evolution over time, and other details that may be important. Moreover, the patient's participation can lead to a continual process of checking observations against each other.
Dependence on the unaided mind of the physician necessitates a lengthy, expensive educational process that reinvents the wheel with every medical student.	The process of retrieving and organizing medical knowledge can be centralized in those who build and maintain the knowledge coupling software. Then, a single, developed system of knowledge coupling software can be used by thousands of providers. It becomes possible to bypass much of the educational process, to channel knowledge directly to the patient and providers, and to guide and facilitate their use of that knowledge, relating it directly to the patient's unique needs. The training for providers who use knowledge coupling software can be inexpensive, focused on skills and analytical ability rather than accumulating information.
Graduate medical education is unable to produce physicians whom we can trust to cope with managing medical information. The human mind is simply not well suited to retrieval and processing of large bodies of data. As a result, the mind, unlike computers, uses simplifying assumptions and other mental devices to reduce information to a manageable form. But these mental devices introduce potential for omission and error that is unacceptable in medical practice.	Knowledge coupling software takes advantage of the computer's ability to reliably retrieve and correlate massive volumes of information, freeing the mind to specialize in analytic and interpersonal functions that no computer can duplicate.
The educated physician becomes obsolete; no one can keep up with the constant flow of new medical knowledge.	A central system for maintaining knowledge coupling software can keep all providers up to date at all times because the very tools they use to do their work can have built into them the parameters of guidance and currency of information for doing that work correctly.

The Old System	The New System
Dependence on the unaided mind of the physician makes the inputs to the health care system variable and uncertain. In step 3, for example, different physicians may come up with different diagnostic possibilities from the same set of findings.	With use of knowledge coupling software, the "inputs" to the medical care system will be consistent across providers, providing a basis for corrective feedback loops on the medical knowledge that formed the basis for the questions asked and the findings examined for on physical examination.
The cost of the physician's time is exceedingly high in spite of the deficiencies described above.	Knowledge coupling software permits minimizing the use of expensively educated physicians.

The preceding describes the use of knowledge coupling software for diagnostic purposes. Couplers are equally useful to guide management of diseases. Approximately 40 diagnostic and management couplers have so far been developed, and have been in use by a few practitioners for over 10 years. One of the striking elements in that experience has been the relation between the patient and physician. Consider the following description by a psychiatrist, Dr. Willie Yee, of his experience with using a coupler on management of depression:

> The most profound alteration becomes apparent the first time the psychiatrist sits down with the patient to review the results of a Coupler. This side-by-side posture can be seen as a metaphor for the alteration in the relationship that is taking place. The psychiatrist and patient are now involved in a *collaborative* relationship, with both parties having access to the information from which a decision could be made. Since Couplers are structured to present multiple options, e.g., less frequent diagnoses or less commonly used treatments, there is no longer a "treatment of choice" for a given condition. The ambiguity which physicians, including psychiatrists, face all the time is now confronted by both patient and provider. The hierarchical structure of medicine, in which a single diagnosis or treatment is authoritatively prescribed, is replaced by a relationship which acknowledges uncertainty and the tradeoffs which must be confronted when any decision is made.
>   . . . The process of reviewing a Coupler with a patient ensures that the information on which a decision is based is accurate, and that both patient and psychiatrist are aware of the risks and benefits of a given course of action.
>   . . . This altered relationship with the patient is part of another trend in psychiatry and medicine. Consumer participation in medical decision making is now advocated as an essential process in the improved delivery of medical care. . . . In the psychoeducational treatment of schizophrenia, for example, the provision of adequate information to the patient or family members is the key to an altered relationship with the clients, one which employs them as allies, rather than passive recipients of treatment. In the field of schizophrenia, at least, the effect has been a dramatic improvement in relapse rates. . . .

Medical Records and Quality Control

The process of knowledge coupling is used at many points of decision making in the care of a patient. As explained above, the total decision making process has the following four-part structure: (1) gathering an initial database, (2) formulating a list of problems, (3) formulating initial plans for each problem, and (4) follow up action—monitoring progress, reassessing problems and plans based on that feedback and taking further diagnostic or therapeutic action based on that reassessment. The quality of care depends upon the rigor and explicitness with which that process is executed. A detailed discussion of that total process is beyond the scope of this paper. A few points, however, should be made here.

Quality of care should not be defined solely in terms of the health status outcome, for that depends partially on inputs—the nature of patient problems and the patient's actions and responses—outside the control of the health care system. Rather, quality is the excellence of each input by the health care system. Those inputs include the information tools relied upon to guide and support decision making, the decisions or recommendations by patients and providers, and the actions taken by patients and providers to execute those decisions and recommendations. At each point in the process, the participants must both "do the right thing" and "do the thing right"; that is, they must select an appropriate diagnostic or management option from the range of options available, and then execute their chosen option properly. Thus, quality can be conceived as a calculus of simple steps, of discrete inputs to the system, each of which is subject to scrutiny and improvement. In turn, quality control can be conceived of as tracing connections between unsuccessful outcomes and specific inputs, and then improving those inputs.

For example, clinical studies may reveal that a particular operation leads to few successful outcomes even when properly performed, indicating that the procedure should be removed as a management option (or at least that its failure rate should be highlighted) in knowledge coupling software. Or, peer review of an individual surgeon may show that he or she lacks skill in performing the operation. Or, review of an individual patient's case may show that the operation was properly performed, but that at an earlier stage of the disease the patient's internist ignored a symptom that, if investigated with knowledge coupling software, would have led to a diagnosis and successful, inexpensive treatment. Or, when a surgeon in a fee-for-service practice recommends an expensive operation (or an HMO physician recommends *against* the operation), the patient (and any third party payer) can use knowledge coupling software to determine what, if any, other management options are available and the pros and cons of each alternative in that patient's circumstances. Or, if a third party payer declines to pay for a procedure, the patient and provider can use knowledge coupling software to gain immediate access to information relevant to disputing the payer's decision or selecting an acceptable alternative.

These examples illustrate a few of the myriad ways in which it may become possible to gain far more control over quality and cost of health care than we have had in the past. When knowledge coupling software is used, the range of available diagnostic and management options becomes visible to all participants in the system. One result is to create checks and balances; each partic-

ipant has the information needed to intelligently scrutinize the functioning of the others.

For the health care system to operate in the manner envisioned here, a crucial element is rigorous standards for maintaining medical records. Outcome studies depend upon properly maintained records. Equally important is the fact that patient care itself depends on adequate medical records. They are the medium of communication among the various providers and the patient over time. In addition, a properly structured medical record operates as an external aid to the mind of the physician in retrieving and processing patient data, just as knowledge coupling software aids the physician in retrieving and processing general medical knowledge and coupling it with patient data. Indeed, the coupling function is hindered if medical records are incomplete and disorganized. One of the most serious deficiencies in the health care system is the lack of rigor and standards in maintaining medical records. Use of computerized medical records will naturally address this problem, for the required standards can be designed into the medical record software, reducing careless variations by physicians.

THE HEALTH INFORMATION MANAGEMENT PROFESSION IN THE 21ST CENTURY: PRACTICE AND EDUCATIONAL IMPLICATIONS

SHIRLEY EICHENWALD

HEALTH INFORMATION MANAGER'S ROLE IN THE 1990S

The 1990s must be recognized as a watershed decade in the evolution of the HIM profession. It is the decade when multiple forces converged on the health care industry providing powerful incentives for the industry to focus on its information resources. The value of information is in the contribution it makes to enhancing the quality of the decisions made by the information user. Therefore, in this new competitive environment in which successful health care organizations are required to publically demonstrate their ability to manage cost and to manage outcomes, administrators, policymakers, and care providers demand and truly need quality information to support their heightened decision-making responsibilities.

The wise application of computer technology to the information management function began to receive particular attention in the 1990s because of the potential it had for minimizing the costs associated with producing

the significantly greater volume of information now required by the health care organization on a routine basis for both internal decision making and for required transmission to numerous external policy, licensing, and/or payment agencies.

Similarly, HIM professionals began to receive increasing attention as they demonstrated to the health care organization their value in assuring the accuracy, completeness, integrity, and security of the growing electronic health care database, just as they have historically managed paper-based health care records and the information manually abstracted from them to support organizational decision makers.

The 1990s brought fundamental change to the HIM profession in the form of a simple challenge: transition of the principles and practices of the profession from a paper-based environment to a computer-based environment. In doing so the focus of the profession is clearly on obtaining quality health care data within the organization as the foundation for providing user-oriented health care information services. Specifically, health information management's primary concern is the accuracy, comprehensiveness, integrity, security, and availability of health care data on individuals and on populations. Therefore, HIM professionals are in positions with responsibility for setting standards and policies governing how health care data are collected, maintained, and disseminated within health care facilities and health-related agencies. HIMs are also in positions with responsibility for assuring that these standards and policies are operationalized on a day-to-day basis within health care organizations and agencies. HIMs act as expert advisors and internal consultants within organizations and agencies on the appropriate uses of and interpretation of health care data. HIMs are active partners with computer systems professionals and health information users (decision makers) as computer-based information systems are being planned, designed, and implemented. The HIM acts as a data quality expert in this environment and as a user advocate and trainer. HIM professionals serve in many positions of responsibility within the health care industry, but in each position the HIM's core concern is with health care data and their conversion to meaningful information that supports the needs of the decision makers internal and external to the organization they represent.

MOVING TOWARD THE 21ST CENTURY

HIM professionals must be prepared to bring a strengthened set of competencies to the health care industry in the 21st century. HIMs will be functioning in many areas of a health care organization or agency—decentralized rather than centralized in a single department location. Wherever the HIMs are located they will be functioning in at least one of the following types of roles:

- Data specialist: directly involved in data capture or data collection, in data abstracting or data retrieval, and/or in data analysis or data reporting.

- Information system analyst/designer: directly involved with the creation or modification of the software applications required to facilitate data collection, maintenance, data analysis, and reporting of information, including project management and training of application users

- Information broker: directly involved with receiving information requests from internal and external sources and coordinating the process of responding to the request in a meaningful and efficient way

- Clinical database administrator: directly involved with the day-to-day issues related to

maintaining the security of the database, including issuing of passcards/passwords, approving any modifications to the access parameters and auditing the effectiveness of the system's security protocols; receiving requests for modification in the database content and coordinating the process for responding to such requests in a timely way.

- Chief information officer: oversight responsibility for the ongoing development of an organization's information infrastructure.

For the practicing HIM professional and for the professional educator preparing the professional for practice in the future, transitions bring special opportunities for professional development and for curriculum change. The core competencies of the 21st century HIM professional will be in the areas of:

- Health care data management, specifically as it is applied to collection of standardized quality data to support the accurate reporting of services provided, the evaluation of practice patterns, the assessment of clinical outcomes, and the analysis of cost-effectiveness of services provided

- Health care statistics and research methods, including descriptive and inferential statistics, program evaluation, and survey design, as well as vital statistics, public health statistics, and library database research techniques

- Clinical practice foundations to provide a sound basis for communicating with health care providers and for understanding the clinical decision-making process, specifically so it can be applied to improve database design, enhance the quality of data collection/capture, and/or enhance the quality of data analysis

- Computer-based technologies and systems, specifically as applied to database design, systems integration, support for data analysis, data networking, and data security issues

- The health care delivery system: its mission, its structure, its players, with special emphasis on the continuum of health care and the impact of health care policy as well as societal expectations as evidenced through legislation, regulation, and community-based consumer needs

- Organizational management with special emphasis on effective communications, managerial finance, organizational behavior, and process improvement to prepare individuals to successfully lead and participate in teams to achieve ongoing systems, methods, and service modifications

While continuing acquisition of knowledge and skills in these core competency areas is crucial to the success of every HIM professional, it is equally as important that the HIM professional bring to the health care industry a dedication to the organizational mission, quality service to all internal and external customers, teaming across disciplines and departments, and quality improvement as a personal philosophy.

Prior to the 1990s, whereas change in the HIM profession was regular, it was incremental and came at a fairly comfortable pace. The 1990s heralded in a new era of professional change for the health information manager, one that requires a major shift in the basic work of the profession. During the transition period, it is important for the profession to accept that there are role conflicts as older roles coexist with newer roles. It is equally, if not more, important for the profession to embrace the transition with great fervor and to actively demonstrate its fervor within the work setting and within its continuing and formal educational activities.

References

1. Borges E: Transforming Yourselves: Pathways from Medical Records to Health Information Management. J Am Health Information Management Assoc 1994; 65(3), p. 36.
2. Brandt M: Joint Commission Standards: Management of Information Roles of Health Information Management Professionals. J Am Health Information Management Assoc 1993; 64(11), p. 41.
3. Brodnik M: Summary Report of the Education Strategy Committee of the AMRA Health Information Management Initiative, Chicago, August 19–20, 1990.
4. Eichenwald S: Our Professional Definition Sets the Boundaries of Our Practice—What Are They Today? J Am Med Record Assoc 1990; 61(8), p. 50.
5. Eichenwald S: Professional Development: The HIM Challenge of the '90s and the Key to 21st Century Career Opportunities. J Am Health Information Management Assoc 1994; 65(11), p. 48.
6. Essentials for Accredited Educational Programs for Health Information Technicians and Health Information Administrators, Definition of the Profession. Chicago, American Health Information Management Association, 1994.

HEALTH INFORMATION MANAGEMENT PROFESSIONAL EDUCATION

MELANIE S. BRODNIK

The roles and functions of health information management (HIM) professionals vary, depending on the educational background, place of employment, and job title of the individual. Typically, however, the HIM professional is concerned with health-related information and the systems used to collect, store, process, retrieve, disseminate, and communicate information for the support of operations, management, and decision making within an enterprise.

To achieve this practice level, academic programs in HIM are offered at the associate and baccalaureate degree levels and more recently at the master's degree level. For the last five years the profession has been dealing with the issues of education reform and curriculum design in order to ensure that graduates can meet the needs of a rapidly changing, information-independent and market-driven health care environment.[1] In investigating educational reform, work groups have paid attention to the content, uniqueness of the curriculum, expected knowledge and skills, tasks performed, and personal attributes needed of HIM professionals in this changing health care environment.

CURRICULUM DESIGN

A curriculum in HIM represents a blend of course work drawn from the managerial and behavioral sciences and information systems and technologies, coupled with understanding of the health care environment, health care services, and clinical knowledge. Its uniqueness as a distinct curriculum stems from the environment in which the curriculum is taught (allied health colleges or schools), the employment setting of its graduates (health care related), and how the curriculum is applied and used in a functional manner. Collectively, the HIM curriculum should provide students with the knowledge and skills necessary to capture and retrieve data, plan for and manage information, and for some, enable advancement to leadership positions in information management.

The HIM curriculum should include coursework in biomedical sciences, health care delivery systems, health data content and structure, clinical quality assessment and improvement, organization and management, health care statistics and research, information system concepts, and information technology. Each domain is composed of knowledge units that further define the content of the domain (see Knowledge Domains and Units).[2] The depth of instruction, structure, and detail of the curriculum will vary depending on the degree level of the program. For example, baccalaureate and graduate-level program curricula would require students to have more detailed understanding and skill than would be expected of students at an associate degree program level. Courses related to the liberal arts education must also be factored into the overall HIM curriculum, especially at the associate and baccalaureate program levels.

In identifying the knowledge upon which an HIM curriculum is built, work groups identified a list of task statements related to the current and future performance of HIM practitioners[3] (see Health Information Management Task Statements). Although the list appears long, it is not exhaustive, nor is it meant to suggest that all HIM practitioners must be capable of performing all tasks. An awareness of the tasks performed by practitioners, however, enables educators to design curriculum to meet the needs of the marketplace.

Health Information Management Task Statements

Health Care Delivery Systems
- Assess internal and external environments.
- Determine external information/data to be included in internal databases.
- Interpret and apply laws, accreditation, licensure, and certification standards.
- Monitor changes in federal, state, and local laws, and regulations, licensing, and/or JCAHO standards.
- Monitor accreditation, certification, and licensing survey results.
- Explain survey results or reports from outside consultants.
- Release patient-specific data to authorized users.
- Safeguard patients' right to privacy of health care information.
- Safeguard providers' interests in health information.
- Compare claims submitted to payers and explain reasons for rejections and reimbursement received.

Clinical Quality Assessment and Improvement
- Analyze data for patient-related information system needs.
- Analyze data for institutional information system needs (clinical, financial, performance-related).
- Analyze patient care data in relation to institutional performance standards.
- Analyze patient care/institutional data in relation to regulatory and accreditation standards.
- Analyze physician performance data/profiles in relation to medical staff, institutional, or regulatory/accreditation standards.
- Maintain quality assurance program.
- Compare process and outcome measurement against clinically valid standards.
- Conduct quality assessment studies utilizing appropriate research techniques.
- Analyze clinical data to identify trends.
- Analyze results of quality improvement, utilization management, risk management, and other patient care–related research studies.

Health Data Content and Structure
- Conduct quantitative analysis.
- Collect data to assure that documentation in the health record supports the diagnosis and reflects the progress, clinical findings, and discharge status of the patient.
- Maintain a database reflecting quantitative and qualitative outcomes of documentation.
- Monitor/collect data on quality/timeliness of information.
- Develop guidelines for documentation and monitor compliance.
- Collect data on status of incomplete records.
- Formulate policies regarding the collection of patient information.
- Design forms, computer screen displays, and other data collection tools.
- Assign valid diagnostic/procedure codes using ICD-9-CM, CPT, HCPCS, DSM, or other coding systems.
- Validate coding of clinical information, DRG assignment, and case mix data.
- Verify timeliness, completeness, accuracy, and appropriateness of data and data sources (patient care, management, billing reports and/or databases).
- Select appropriate classification systems.

Continued on following page

Health Data Content and Structure (*Continued*)
- Assign severity of illness categories.
- Analyze departmental/institutional case-mix and case-mix payment rates (i.e., DRG and others) to determine reimbursement optimization.
- Retrieve data from HIM indexes

Health Care Statistics and Research
- Collect data for analysis.
- Design data collection tools.
- Conduct surveys and interviews of health information customers to identify information needs.
- Analyze institutional data patterns to identify trends.
- Apply descriptive statistical techniques (i.e., mean, median, mode) to analyze patient-related data.
- Apply statistical techniques for determining data validity and reliability (i.e., correlation, Cronbach's alpha).
- Evaluate data quality, validity, reliability, methods, and adequacy of resources.
- Interpret information from other sources to determine consistency.
- Explain statistical reports.
- Interpret institutional statistics (e.g., occupancy rates, census, length of stay).
- Determine appropriate sample size and confidence levels.
- Determine clinical data needs for research studies, reimbursement, quality assurance activities, and hospital statistics.
- Present data in oral and written forms.
- Maintain professional competency by conducting literature searches, analysis.

Organization and Management
- Select personnel.
- Supervise staff.
- Counsel/discipline employees.
- Terminate employees.
- Develop and support work teams.
- Perform job analysis.
- Determine employee staffing levels.
- Monitor employee staffing levels.
- Monitor workflow/productivity under span of control.
- Benchmark employee performance data in relation to departmental/institutional performance standards.
- Utilize appropriate resources to meet workload needs.
- Inform organization staff of department/facility plans.
- Determine variation/s from established objectives and/or standards of performance.
- Collect data on employee performance.
- Develop a system for productivity control.
- Develop departmental policies.
- Develop departmental procedures.
- Develop departmental plans, goals, and objectives for area under your span of control.
- Participate in departmental and/or institutional teams/committees.
- Design ergonomically sound work environment.
- Select equipment appropriate for systems applications.
- Maintain equipment.
- Prepare budgets with appropriate justification.
- Monitor adherence to budget.
- Develop organization charts and procedural flow charts.
- Develop quality control/improvement systems.
- Apply quality improvement techniques.
- Ensure cost-effectiveness of health information systems.
- Develop cost-benefit analyses for information resources alternatives.

Organization and Management (*Continued*)
- Lead development of discipline-specific health information resources.
- Market HIM services.
- Monitor systems outcomes.
- Plan, develop, conduct, and evaluate inservice education programs for departmental or nondepartmental staff.
- Direct students assigned to facility.
- Train personnel.
- Develop job descriptions.

Information Technology
- Model data
- Maintain/administer data dictionaries.
- Develop interfaces between databases.
- Develop policies and procedures for data management.
- Input and edit patient information on database.
- Participate in database administration.
- Protect data integrity and validity.
- Assist in development of data definitions.
- Identify problems related to data and data management.
- Utilize database queries and other methods to retrieve required information from database.
- Design data quality controls/edits.
- Develop and maintain written procedure for data management.
- Track information, locate patient-specific records on-line, off-line, and in archival formats.
- Design and enforce security measures to protect information.
- Plan security systems deployed to protect databases and maintain information.
- Structure database searches and data retrieval.
- Utilize tools appropriate to data management.
- Evaluate functional objectives of electronic/nonelectronic information resources.
- Lead evaluation and selection of electronically supported information systems.
- Maintain audit trails to validate authenticity of originators of documentation.

Information Systems Concepts and Processes
- Participate in information engineering, planning, analysis, design, and implementation.
- Participate in development and maintenance of networks to share information between systems.
- Use systems analysis techniques and tools to design databases.
- Design and evaluate systems for collection, storage and retrieval of data.
- Develop systems documentation.
- Advise/train/collaborate regarding systems design/enhancement for data collection.
- Recommend systems improvement.
- Test health care data against statistical models.
- Establish priorities for design/redesign of operational and/or department level information systems.
- Develop transition plans for implementation of new or revised systems.
- Prepare requests for proposals and/or bids for vendor services.
- Evaluate vendor bids.
- Determine feasibility and constraints applicable to design/redesign of departmental operational systems.
- Manage a department local area network.
- Design operational systems for collection and processing of patient-related data.
- Recommend changes or improvements in systems.
- Determine information needs and resource requirements (i.e., staff, equipment, costs).
- Write functional specifications for information systems.
- Negotiate vendor contracts.

HEALTH INFORMATION MANAGEMENT GRADUATE LEVEL PREPARATION

The increased use of information technology in the marketplace and the demand for individuals who can manage information at both systems and knowledge levels supports the need for advanced professional preparation of HIM practitioners. Historically, the American Health Information Management Association (AHIMA) has focused its attention on supporting associate and baccalaureate degree level programs through its formal accreditation process. The recognition of a master's degree program and suggested curriculum at this time emphasizes the importance of the profession's evolutionary growth in discipline-specific content areas and the marketplace demand for individuals capable of managing health information at an executive level.

Several master's degree programs in HIM have evolved over the last 5 years in an effort to prepare individuals to assume administrative and/or technical roles in health information systems.[4–8] These programs do not require that individuals possess prior entry-level knowledge of HIM at either the associate or baccalaureate degree program levels as a prerequisite to the program. Recognizing the existence of these programs, AHIMA work groups on master's education chose to consider the establishment of advanced professional preparation leading to a Master of Science degree with prior entry-level knowledge at the baccalaureate HIM program level.[9] The Work Group recommended, however, that a prerequisite core be defined to allow other health professionals to develop the competencies needed to enter the graduate program.

The master's degree program should prepare individuals to be leaders and executives of the future. The curriculum would be designed to produce administrators who possess the knowledge, skills, and attitudes commonly found in chief administrative officers. The graduate-level HIM professional would view the environment from a broader perspective and with a wider professional scope and domain of practice than is expected of graduates at the associate or baccalaureate degree program levels. The Work Groups recognized that the graduate degree HIM professional could assume a variety of roles such as:

- Director, Information Systems and Services
- Director, Performance Assessment
- Information Engineer
- Data Administrator
- Quality Improvement Engineer or Specialist

Whatever the role title, the emphasis should be on the graduate level HIM professional's ability to use health

Knowledge Domains and Units*

Biomedical Sciences
- Anatomy
- Physiology
- Medical terminology
- Pathophysiology

Health Care Delivery Systems
- Organization of health care systems
- Health care organizations
- Standards for accreditation and licensure
- Government regulations in health care
- Methods of reimbursement
- Legal aspects and issues
- Professional ethics

Health Data Content and Structure
- Content of health record
- Health care data sets (government, private, research, etc.)
- Vocabulary standards (ASTM, etc.)
- Classification systems and nomenclatures
- Case mix/severity of illness systems
- Registries and indexes
- Medical linguistics (text processing)
- Forms and screen design

Clinical Quality Assessment and Improvement
- Quality resource management
- Utilization resource management
- Risk management
- Clinical outcomes management/research
- Critical/clinical pathway concepts

Organization and Management
- Principles of management (PODC)
- Strategic planning and forecasting
- Marketing
- Human resource management (appraisals, labor, compensation, selection)
- Education and training
- Organizational behavior
  Entrepreneurialism
  Leadership
  Motivation
  Team/consensus building
  Change management
  Negotiation techniques
- Quality improvement methods (SPC, productivity)
- Financial management
- Cost benefit analysis
- Project management
- Organizational assessment (benching marking, risk analysis)
- Cost accounting

Health Care Statistics and Research
- Vital statistics
- Descriptive statistics
- Inferential statistics (ANOVA, MANOVA, Regression, etc.)
- Epidemiology
- Data presentation techniques
- Research methods (sampling techniques)
- Data verification techniques
- Reliability and validity of data
- Computerized statistical packages
- Library research techniques
- Data search/access techniques

Information Technology
- Computer concepts (hardware, software)
- Data, information and file structures
- Telecommunications (standards and integration)
- Networks
- Microcomputer applications
  - Word processing
    - Spreadsheets
    - Graphics
    - Databases
- Databases
  - Features, functions, architecture
    - Data modeling
    - Data integrity
    - Data definitions
    - Database query languages (SQL, etc)
    - Distributed databases
    - Data administration
    - Data dictionary
- Information retrieval
  - Imaging processing
  - Hypermedia
- Automatic identification
- Expert/knowledge-based systems
- Data security

Information Systems Concepts and Processes
- Systems theory and development
- Systems planning (strategic planning)
- Systems analysis (enterprise/applications)
- Systems design (interfaces, interactions, privacy/security controls, cost, quality)
- Systems implementation and testing strategies
- Systems selection process (RFPs, contracts, etc.)
- Systems types
  - Health/hospital information systems
  - Executive support systems
  - Decision support systems
  - Office automation systems
- Systems management

* American Health Information Management Assoc.; Assembly on Education Health Information Management Curriculum Program Group, April 1994.

data and information systems for the advancement of the enterprise.

OTHER EDUCATIONAL ISSUES

Other issues that must be considered in educating the HIM professional relate to designing a curriculum that fosters the professional's ability to function as a critical thinker, problem solver, and change agent. Allied health professionals in general must prepare themselves for an environment in which managerial layers have diminished, teams have emerged, and the ability to add skills and perform multiple tasks is paramount to one's survival on the job.[10] Allied health professionals must have good communication skills, be personable and flexible, and adapt to change quickly.[11] They must also be life-long learners who are readily able to change jobs. For the HIM professional, these attributes will serve to enhance the professional's ability to maintain career resiliency in the face of constant change and increased reliance of information technology. Real-world problem solving and experiential learning must be incorporated into the HIM curriculum to foster these attributes.

References

1. Brodnik M, McCain M: The road to educational reform in health information management. J Am Health Information Management Assoc. 1995;66(1), p. 22.
2. Knowledge Clusters and Knowledge Units. Health Information Management Model Curriculum Work Group Report. Assembly on Education, American Health Information Management Association. Chicago, April 1994.
3. Task Statements. Health Information Management Model Curriculum Work Group Report. Assembly on Education, American Health Information Management Association. Chicago, April 1994.
4. Health Information Management and Systems Division, School of Allied Medical Professions. Columbus, Ohio State University.
5. Master of Science Program in Health Information Management. Birmingham, University of Alabama at Birmingham.
6. Department of Health Information Management, School of Health and Rehabilitation Sciences. Pittsburgh, University of Pittsburgh.
7. Department of Health Information Sciences, John G. Rangos, Sr., School of Health Sciences. Pittsburgh, Duquesne University.
8. Department of Health Information Management, College of Associated Health Professions. Chicago, University of Illinois at Chicago.
9. Model Graduate Curriculum. Health Information Management Model Curriculum Project. Assembly on Education, American Health Information Management Association. Chicago, April 1994.
10. Healthy America: Practitioners for 2005. A Report of The Pew Health Professions Commission. Durham, NC.
11. Stuart A: The Adaptable Workforce. CIO 1995;8(10)57.

GLOSSARY

Abstracting—Preparation of a brief summary characterizing the patient and disease. Diagnostic workup, extent of disease, treatment, and end results may also be documented on an abstract form.

Acceptance theory of authority—Theory that argues that managers have the ability to influence the behavior of employees only because employees accept the legitimacy of the influence. This view considers that authority flows up in organizations. Also known as the acceptance theory of power.

Accessibility of data—Availability of data to authorized people when and where needed.

Accession register—Listing of numbers assigned by the facility and the corresponding patient name, in numerical order.

Accession year—Year case is accessioned (entered) into the database.

Access mandates—When regulation or rules apply to the insured, or patient, in selecting which physician or facility he may choose to seek services.

Access time—Amount of time it takes for an image to be displayed on the screen after it is located on the optical disk.

Accommodation—Conflict resolution technique in which one party (the accommodator) is highly cooperative and responsive to the needs of the other party to the point of sacrificing her or his own personal needs.

Accountability—Liability for the stewardship of authority delegated to a person in an organization.

Accounting rate of return—Method used to compare the value of a capital expenditure to another. This method uses the income for a period divided by average investment during the period.

Accounts receivable—Income earned but not yet received for services provided or products sold. It is an asset of the business.

Accounts receivable turnover ratio—Patient revenues by patient accounts receivable.

Accreditation—Process by which an organization or agency performs an external review and grants recognition to the program of study or institution that meets certain predetermined standards. Certification provided a person who successfully meets criteria established by the American Health Information Management Association, including a written examination, to be an accredited record technician.

Accrual basis accounting—Accrual method of accounting that records revenues when they are expected or billed rather than when the cash has been received. The revenues are matched as closely as possible with the expenses or services rendered.

Achilles' heel—Weakness in one party's position or argument that the other party may attempt to attack to her or his advantage. The aggressive use of this tactic makes conflict resolution difficult.

Action model of problem solving—Approach to problem solving that consists of the following steps: (1) actively listening, (2) defining the issue, (3) examining the evidence, (4) identifying and analyzing biases, (5) separating cognitive and emotive understanding, (6) considering alternative solutions, (7) not oversimplifying, and (8) acting (to implement the problem resolution).

Action steps—Statements that define the date a certain activity will be completed, how much labor or funding will be required, how resources will be used, and the expected outcomes or results.

Active record—Record being used regularly with the date of last discharge or encounter within a preset period, usually 3 to 5 years.

Activity ratio—Also known as **turnover ratio.**

Acute care—Short-term care; for inpatients, acute care indicates an average hospital stay of 30 days or less; for outpatients, acute care indicates care of short duration.

Administrative organization management—School of management thought that popularized the process or functional approach to management.

Advance directive—Legal, written document that specifies patient preferences regarding future health care or the person who is authorized to make medical decisions in the event the patient is not capable of communicating his preferences; the patient must be competent at the time the document is prepared and signed. Living wills and durable power of attorney are both considered advance directives.

Adverse patient occurrences (APO)—Events that occur during an episode of patient care with the potential for adverse outcomes.

Affinity diagram—Technique for organizing information by clustering or grouping items, i.e., activities, events, resources, etc., in categories based on some empirical or logical relationship. One useful format is an outline of main headings with "bullets" for subheadings.

Affirmative action programs—Written, systematic human resource planning tools that outline goals in hiring, training, promoting, and compensation of minority groups that are protected by equal employment laws.

Aggregate—To combine or collect.

Aggregate data—Sum total of data elements; gathering individual elements into groupings; data elements assembled into a logical format to facilitate comparisons or to elicit evidence of patterns.

Aggressive problem employee—One who openly confronts management or coworkers in an aggressive, hostile, and nonproductive manner to satisfy personal needs.

Alphabetic identification—Using the patient name to identify the patient record.

Alphanumeric data—Field that uses numbers, letters, and/or symbolic characters.

Ambient lighting—Light directed toward the ceiling to provide overall lighting for a large area. It is usually insufficient to do concentrated work.

Ambulatory care—Comprehensive term for all types of health care provided in an outpatient setting; the patient travels to and from the facility on the same day.

Ambulatory patient groups—Case mix system which forms the basis for federal ambulatory care reimbursement.

American plan of office design—Inclusion of private offices in an open office design plan.

Ancillary services—(Professional service departments) Hospital diagnostic and/or therapeutic services provided to both outpatients and inpatients, excluding room and board.

Antitrust—Federal and state statutes to protect trade and commerce from unlawful restraints, price discriminations, price fixing, and monopolies.

Application—Use of computer-based routine for specific purposes such as accounts receivable, maintenance, inventory control, and new product selection; software or computer programs that process data to provide output for such a purpose.

Application software—Programs that are written to process an application such as patient registration.

Appointment/reappointment—Conferring of certain rights within a designated staff membership category and assignment to an organizational unit of the medical staff.

Arbitration—Mechanism for resolving disputes outside of court. Both parties to the dispute agree to present their arguments to a neutral party—the arbitrator—who decides the dispute. The arbitrator's decision may be either binding or non-binding upon the parties.

Architecture—Composite of specific components and the way in which they interact to form a computer system.

Assault—Deliberate threat, coupled with the apparent ability, to do physical harm to another person without that person's consent.

Asset—Future benefit or services potential that is recognized in accounting only after a transaction has occurred; an item that has value and can be traded for cash. It may be tangible or intangible, short-term or long term.

Assisted living—Long-term care facility that typically offers housing with a broad range of personal and supportive care services.

Audit—Retrospective review of selected health care records or data documents to evaluate the quality of care or services provided compared with predetermined standards.

Audit trail—Program that records the access and/or action that occurs in a computer record by logging the user identification and the file identification, recording date and time of access and the action done.

Authentication—Proof of authorship of a documented entry that may be in the form of a written signature, identifiable initials, or computer key; identification of the author of a record entry in a paper or computer-based patient record.

Authority—Rights of a manager to prohibit or require actions by employees.

Authorization—As used in this book, authorization refers to the granting of permission to release health information.

Autopsy rate—Proportion of deaths in which an autopsy was performed. It can include the gross, net, and adjusted autopsy rates.

Avoidance—Conflict resolution technique in which neither party is assertive or cooperative; instead, both parties ignore or conceal the problem.

Bailiff—Courtroom employee present to assist in keeping order, administering oaths, and performing other duties at the direction of the judge.

Balance sheet—Document that displays the organization's assets, liabilities, and fund balance or equity.

Bar graph—Method used to display nominal, ordinal, and continuous data with variables shown on the horizontal or x-axis and the frequency of the variables shown on the vertical or y-axis.

Battery—Unconsented-to touching in a socially impermissible manner. For example, operating on a patient without proper consent constitutes battery.

Bedside workstation—PC workstations that are stationed at patient bedsides and collect patient care documentation (assessments and progress monitoring) and can link to other information systems such as a computer-based patient record.

Bed size (bed count)—Total number of inpatient beds for which the facility is equipped and staffed for patient admissions.

Behavioral decision theory—Theory of decision making that attempts to describe how managers make decisions.

Behaviorally anchored rating scales (BARS)—Performance appraisal scales that are descriptive of specific desired behaviors. BARS rate employees on a scale that has specific behavioral examples on it to guide the rater.

Belt lines—Issues, words, or gestures that cross the boundary of what one party regards as acceptable. These taboo symbols or topics usually complicate conflict resolution.

Benchmark—Something that serves as a standard or reference point by which another thing can be measured.

Benchmarking—Comparison of the performance of one organization with that of another organization that is known to be excellent in that area.

Beneficiary—One who is eligible to receive or is receiving benefits from an insurance policy or a managed care program.

Benefit period—Time frame in which insurance benefits are covered; the benefit period varies from policy to policy.

Benefits realization—Methodology for determining whether or not proposed benefits of a new system have been realized.

Best evidence rule—This rule requires that the *original* evidence of a fact (such as an original document) be produced in court. If it cannot be produced (because it is not available), substitute evidence or copies can be allowed into evidence only if there is an acceptable explanation for the absence of the original.

Biomedical device—Patient monitoring device used to monitor and track signals directly from the body.

Board certified—Physicians designated as Board certified have met the standards of certification established by their specialty examining bodies.

Borrowed servant—Doctrine referring to situation in which an employee is temporarily under the control of another. The temporary "employer" of the borrowed servant may be held responsible for the negligent acts of the borrowed servant under the doctrine of **respondent superior** (also defined below).

Bottleneck—Slowdown that occurs because certain activities or operations in the processing of data are lagging behind. Common bottleneck areas are data preparation, input, and output.

Bounded rationality—Limits of information available to the manager under behavioral decision theory.

Brainstorming—Group process designed to facilitate the generation of ideas by the leader's encouraging uninhibited expression by group members and the avoidance of criticism. The typical cycle includes (1) identifying the problem or issue, (2) structuring the task, (3) recording all individual responses, (4) clarifying ambiguous responses, (5) expanding or linking responses, and (6) repeating the cycle to generate additional ideas or to address a related issue.

Break-even analysis—Methodology used to determine at which future point in time the costs of the current system will equal the costs of the proposed system.

Budgets—Numerical documents that translate the goals, objectives, and action steps into forecasts of volume and monetary resources needed; comprehensive plan of operation that formally expresses management's broad and specific objectives and sets standards for the evaluation of performance.

Burden of proof—Refers to the obligation of parties to a lawsuit to prove their contentions. Normally, a plaintiff bears the burden of proof. Unless he can show that his version of events is more likely than the defendant's version, he will lose. However, in many medical malpractice cases, the burden of proof shifts to the defendant. See the chapter's discussion of *res ipsa loquitur* for the circumstances under which the burden of proof shifts.

Bureaucracy—School of management thought that focuses on the structure of organizations and emphasizes the importance of hierarchy and impersonality of procedures and rules.

Business plan—Formal, written document evolving from input of others that lists objectives that support the organizational goals.

Cache memory—Process of reserving a section of the main memory (RAM) or a special bank of high-speed memory that is used to improve computer performance.

Cafeteria benefit plan—Employees may choose benefits according to their specific needs (e.g., child care, health insurance, dental insurance, tax-deferred annuity accounts).

Capital budget—Plan of proposed outlays for acquiring long-term or expensive assets and the sources of capital to finance these acquisitions.

Capital expenditure—Typically, an expenditure for equipment, furniture, or another asset that has a life of more than 1 year or a cost that exceeds an amount defined by the organization.

Capital expenditure committee—Committee of administrative or management members who evaluate requests for items or services.

Capitation—Fee that providers receive for each person enrolled in a managed care setting; fixed amount paid by a health maintenance organization per member to a provider as compensation for providing health care services for the period; reimbursement method that is a prepaid, fixed amount paid to the provider for each person (per capita) served, regardless of how much or how often resources are used.

Capitalization ratio—The amount of long-term debt to the amount of assets that the organization can convert to cash.

Captain of the ship—Doctrine that imposes liability on surgeons in charge of operations for the negligence of his or her assistants during the period when those assistants are under the surgeon's control—even if those assistants are not employed by the surgeon. This is a surgery-specific adaptation of the **borrowed servant** doctrine defined above.

Capture of data—Entry of data into an information system.

Care—Management of, responsibility for, or attention to the safety and well-being of someone else.

Career counseling—Assisting employees in finding appropriate career goals and paths according to ability and desires.

Career planning—Process by which one selects career goals and the paths to those goals.

Carpal tunnel syndrome—Swelling of the tendons through the carpal tunnel (located in the front part of the wrist), which puts pressure on the median nerve, causing pain and weakness.

Case-control retrospective study—Study in which characteristics or risk factors are collected from cases or from patients with the disease under study as well as from controls or people without the disease under study by looking back in time.

Case eligibility—Case that meets criteria for inclusion into the data base. Criteria vary with registry type.

Casefinding, case identification—Method for locating and identifying every reportable case eligible for inclusion in the data base.

Case mix—Method by which patients are grouped together based on a set of characteristics, e.g., resource consumption, diagnosis, or procedure.

Cash—Results from the collection of payments for services rendered.

Cash basis accounting—Accounting method in which each transaction is recorded when cash is exchanged, similar to one's personal finances. Revenues are recognized when money is received for services provided, and expenses are recognized when money is paid out for the resources used to provide those services.

Cash budget—Management tool that predicts for management when cash will be received and when cash will be disbursed.

Catchment area—Defined geographic area that is served by a health care program, project, or facility.

Categorical/text data—Information that is classified or labeled by text, number, or other coding system.

Census—Listing of all patients occupying beds in an inpatient facility.

Census statistics—Statistics that examine the number of patients being treated at specific times, length of their stay, and number of times a bed changes occupants.

Centralization and decentralization—Cornerstone concept of classical management theory relating to where decisions are made in an organization. If they are made at the top, the organization is said to be centralized. The more decisions are forced to lower levels in the organization, the more decentralized it is said to be.

Certificate of Need—State-directed program that requires facilities to submit to a state review committee detailed plans and justifications for the purchase of new equipment, new building, or new service offerings that cost in excess of a certain amount. The committee determines whether the proposed service or structure is needed. If so, a certificate to proceed is extended.

Certification—Process by which an agency or organization evaluates educational programs, health care facilities, and individuals as having met predetermined standards; indicates that standards established by a profession to measure the competence of a person seeking entrance to the profession have been met.

Character assassination—Situation in which one party turns a legitimate issue at dispute into a personal attack against the other, thereby avoiding the real issue.

Charge master (charge description master)—Report that reflects the charge for each item that may be used in the treatment of a patient and the charge for most services (e.g., respiratory therapy treatments, physical therapy services, laboratory tests).

Charismatic leadership—Aspect of leadership that involves the attraction of personality (charisma) exerted by the leader over followers.

Charitable immunity—This legal doctrine, which developed out of the English court system (and no longer applies to health care organizations in the United States), protected nonprofit hospitals from liability as a result of harm to patients.

Chart of accounts—Systematically arranged listing of revenue, expense, asset, and liability accounts giving account numbers and titles.

Claim—Bill for health care services submitted to a third party payer for payment of benefits under a health care insurance plan.

Classification—A system of assigning diseases and operations to code numbers covering groups of related diseases.

Clerk of the court—Administrative manager of the court, handling the paperwork associated with lawsuits. Complaints are filed with the clerk, as are other pleadings and documents.

Clinical data—Data related to a patient's or resident's medical or surgical care.

Clinical data management—Clinical data as it is maintained for use by physicians or health care providers in peer or quality review.

Clinical data repository—Collects clinical data from diverse sources to support individual practitioner inquiry in ad hoc formats, stores data longitudinally, and is designed to support monitoring and analysis of patient care outcomes. It may be a component of an institutional information warehouse and/or community and state health information systems.

Clinical information system—Systems that contain clinical information; may be limited to a single area or a more comprehensive treatment of clinical information appropriate for a computer-based patient record.

Clinical pertinence documentation—Refers to the evaluation of the completeness, adequacy, appropriateness, accuracy, and quality of documentation rather than to quality of care.

Clinical privileges—Permission granted after meeting certain standards by the governing board to licensed practitioners to provide services in the granting institution, based on licensure, education, training, experience, competence, health status, and judgment [JCAHO, 1994].

Clinical trial—Experimental study in which an intervention or treatment is given to one group in a clinical setting and the outcomes compared with a control or comparison group who did not have the intervention or treatment or who had a different intervention or treatment.

Closed system—Organizational system that does not actively interact with its environment.

Code of ethics—Ethical statement formulated and adopted to guide the conduct of the members of the AHIMA profession.

Coding—Process of assigning a number to a data element.

Coding specialist—Professional title of coding practitioners certified as certified coding specialist by AHIMA.

Coefficient of variation—Comparison of two groups' standard deviations expressed as a percentage of the mean.

Coinsurance—Health insurance term indicating that the insured is responsible for a portion or percentage of the health care cost.

Collaboration—Method of conflict resolution considered most likely to be successful for all parties. Both parties are highly assertive and cooperative in working toward an equitable solution in which the needs of each party are fully met.

Color coding—Use of color schemes to promote ease in visual recognition.

Common law—Body of principles that evolves over time from court decisions. American common law has its roots in English common law. Although these principles are not written into law as are statutes, they are used to guide court decisions.

Communication—Transference of understanding between two or more persons through verbal, nonverbal, or written messages.

Community health information network—Collects health data from participating organizations such as hospitals and clinics and feeds into a central repository capable of supporting financial, analytical, research, and health planning needs.

Community trial—Experimental study similar to the clinical trial in which an intervention or a treatment is tested on a group or population as a whole in the community rather than in a clinical setting.

Comorbidity—Condition present at admission, in addition to the principal diagnosis, which increases the patient's length of stay by one day in 75 per cent of the cases.

Competition—Conflict resolution technique in which one party (the competitor) is highly assertive and aggressive in meeting her or his own personal needs while ignoring the needs of the other party.

Complaint—Initial written pleading, or statement, or a plaintiff in a civil action. It sets forth the plaintiff's claim(s) for relief and commences the action against the defendant(s).

Completeness of data—All required data are present in the information system.

Complication—A condition, arising during hospitalization, which increases the patient's length of stay by one day in 75 per cent of the cases.

Compounding effect—Additional income that results when one leaves interest received on deposits with the initial deposit, thus increasing the base value of the deposit.

Compromise—Conflict resolution technique in which both parties are moderately assertive but also cooperative and each party has partial satisfaction of personal needs.

Computed fields—Fields/columns that receive their value from the computation of data in other fields.

Computer-aided software engineering (CASE)—Computer programs used to assist in the analysis, design, development, and maintenance of information systems.

Computer-based patient record (CPR)—Electronic patient record that resides in a system specifically designed to support users by providing accessibility to complete and accurate data, alerts, reminders, clinical decision support systems, links to medical knowledge, and other aids; also called electronic health record; all financial, administrative, and clinical information that pertains to patient care entered into the computer at the time service is provided.

Computer output microfiche (COM)—Process of transferring computerized data to microfilm for use or storage.

Computer output to laser disk (COLD)—Automatic transfer of computerized data to a laser disk for use or storage.

Concurrent review—Evaluation of the appropriateness and necessity of services provided to a patient during the episode of care.

Conditions of participation—Regulations that health care institutions must follow to receive Medicare reimbursement.

Confidential communications—Communications made with the expectation that they will be held in confidence.

Confidentiality—The ethical and legal concept endorsed by health professionals to meet the expectation of patients that their information, when provided to an authorized user, will not be redisclosed.

Confidentiality of data—Data that are protected from unauthorized access.

Conflict resolution—Method of dealing with or solving disagreement between individuals or organizations through avoidance, accommodation, competition, compromise, or collaboration.

Confounding variables—Variables, such as age and sex, that have an effect on the independent variable (characteristic or risk factor) and the dependent variable (disease under study) and that may, therefore, influence or bias the results of the study.

Consent—Voluntary agreement to allow someone to do something. For this book's purposes, it refers to granting permission to health care providers to perform surgery or render other treatment.

Contemporaneous documentation—Documentation made while care is being provided, while the information is fresh in the provider's mind.

Contingency plans—Plans that allow for conditions different from those assumed to provide the foundation for the primary plan of an organization. Organizations may have a number of contingency plans to allow for various conditions.

Contingency theory—School of management thought that emphasizes the importance of the organization's interaction with its environment; theory of leadership that focuses on the influence of situational or environmental factors in determining leadership effectiveness—for example, nature of the task and power of the leader.

Continuous data—Data that can assume an infinite number of possible values and the number has real meaning (e.g., height, weight, cost/charges).

Continuous quality improvement—Aspect of total quality management that emphasizes the need to implement long-range planning and continuous monitoring of performance.

Continuum of care—Full range of health care services provided, moving from the least acute and least intensive to the most acute and most intensive or vice versa.

Contract—Legally enforceable agreement. It need not be written but often is.

Control chart—Statistical method of monitoring performance over time based on charting deviation from an expected or target range of performance.

Controlling—Management function that is designed to detect and correct variances from desired behavior; monitoring effect made by management to ensure that what was predicted or planned is occurring or adjusted to meet the organization's needs.

Cooperating parties—Group of four organizations which cooperate in the development and maintenance of the ICD-9-CM coding system, training in its use and provision of coding advice. These parties are the National Center for Health Statistics, the Healthcare Financing Administration, the American Hospital Association, and the American Health Information Management Association.

Copayment—Type of cost-sharing in which the insured (subscriber) pays out of pocket a fixed amount for health care services.

Cornerstone concept of classical management—Specialization of labor, unity of command, span of control, departmentalization, and centralization versus decentralization.

Corporate negligence—Refers to the ability to hold organizations responsible for monitoring the activities of the people who function within their facilities, whether those people are employees or independent contractors, such as physicians. This concept is increasingly used to hold health care organizations responsible for ensuring that their professional staff members provide an acceptable quality of care.

Corrective discipline—Action that follows a rule infraction and tries to discourage repeat offenses so that future employee behavior meets the standards.

Correlation analysis—Statistical method of measuring the strength of association between two variables, commonly using the Pearson product-moment correlation (rho). Correlation (rho) values range from -1.0 to $+1.0$ with these boundary values representing a perfect inverse relationship and a perfect direct relationship, respectively.

Cost-benefit analysis—Benefits compared with system costs.

Cost-effective analysis—Evaluate systems benefit in nonmonetary terms.

Counseling—Discussion of employee problems or deficiencies with the objective of correcting the problem or helping the employee adapt or cope.

Court order—Order given by the judge for, something to occur outside of the court room.

Court reporter—Is responsible for creating a verbatim transcript of court proceedings.

Courtroom—Strategy in which a third party is brought in by one party to validate that party's position and to refute the position of the other party.

Credentialing—For this book's purposes, refers to the act of granting professional or medical staff membership; includes gathering of historical information and verifying the applicant's degrees, training, and other background data; any process by which a professional is evaluated with the intent to effect control over professional practice.

Criteria—Objective statements that describe the desired standard against which actual practice is measured.

Critical incident method—Performance evaluation method that requires the evaluator to report statements that describe positive or negative behaviors by the employee during a given period. The statements are used as examples of good or bad performance to substantiate the evaluation.

Critical path or pathway—Sequence of activities on a PERT network that takes the greatest amount of time to complete.

Critical success factors—Relatively few essential things that organizations and individuals must accomplish to be successful as compared with the trivial thousands of things that often consume the time and energy of managers.

Cross-reference—Method of indicating the previous location of a record when it has been permanently moved, as with a name change.

Cross-sectional prevalence study—Study that describes characteristics and health outcomes or disease concurrently or at one point or period in time.

Current—Data that are recorded at or near the time of the event or observation.

Current ratio—Current assets divided by current liabilities. What this ratio tells a manager is whether there are sufficient cash and cash-like assets to cover the immediate liabilities (bills) that will come due in the short term (1 year).

Data (singular datum)—Characters or symbols that can be stored and processed by computers; things known, given, or assumed as the basis for decision making; collection of elements on a given subject; the raw material of information systems expressed in text, numbers, symbols, and images; facts, ideas, or concepts that can be collected and represented electronically in digital form; may be in the form of characters (A through Z), numbers (0 through 9) on which arithmetic operations can be performed, an alphanumeric combination, as well as special symbols (e.g., $+$, $-$, \$, #, *). Data can be captured, communicated, and processed electronically. Contrast with **information.**

Database—All the data (bits, bytes, fields, rows, and files) of all the patients or subjects for all related applications that are stored independently of the software programs that use the data; collection of data that are related to a particular purpose; collection of stored data, typically organized into fields, records, and files, and an associated description; generalized, integrated collection of data structured to model the natural relations in the data; set of data processable by several computer programs.

Database management system—Computer software program that processes information, either storing or retrieving data from a database; system that stores and retrieves information in a database; integrated set of programs that manages access to the database.

Data dictionary—"Super catalog" that provides for each data field or element a list that describes such information as the field, where the data originates, edits or rules that apply to that field, type and width of the field, security levels applicable to the field, codes used (if any), and what applications or reports use that data element; catalog and central repository for identifying the nature of all data in a system; dictionary that contains definitions for all the entities, attributes, and relations the user view of the data and denotes the physical system in which the data item resides.

Data flow diagram (DFD)—Structured analysis tool used to track the flow of data through an entire system, identify transformations on data, and identify data repositories.

Data integrity—Accuracy and completeness of data.

Data item—Smallest unit of data stored in a computer system. The stored representation of a fact or value.

Data redundancy—Data entered more than once, either in the same file management or database management program or in different programs within the same facility.

Data security—Technical and procedural methods by which access to confidential information is controlled and managed.

Data set—A group of data elements relevant for a particular use. The data elements are defined to promote uniform collection of data, e.g., Uniform Hospital Discharge Data Set.

Data steward—Person to whom the facility has given the responsibility and authority to protect and control access to specific data items or databases as well as to promote data sharing throughout the organization.

Days of revenue in patient accounts receivable ratio—Measure of the average time that receivables are outstanding or the period that a health care organization extends credit to its debtors.

Decision grid (or matrix)—Chart used to compare various alternatives in a decision with criteria that are the basis for making the decision.

Decision making—Management function that involves selecting among alternative methods of goal accomplishment.

Decision support system—System in which data are combined with analysis tools to understand current activities and perform "what if" questions that enable future optional scenarios to be posed.

Decision table—Analytical tool that provides a means of communication of the logical sequence of an operation.

Decision tree—Used to chart alternative courses of action for solving a problem and subsequent consequences from each course of action.

Deductible—Amount of cost that the beneficiary must incur before the insurance will assume liability for remaining costs.

Deemed status—According to the Medicare act, those health care facilities accredited by the Joint Commission on Accreditation of Healthcare Organizations or the American Osteopathic Association are considered to be in compliance with the Medicare *Conditions of Participation* for hospitals and, therefore, receive deemed status.

Defamation—Act of harming another person's reputation or character by communicating false statements to a third person. If done verbally, it is called *slander,* if in writing, *defamation.*

Defendant—In criminal cases, refers to the person accused of the crime. In civil litigation, refers to the party against whom the lawsuit is brought.

Delegation—Act of passing one's rights or authority to prohibit or require actions on the part of another to others.

Delineation of privileges—Act of granting specific permission to perform certain activities upon patients within the health care facility. For example, surgeons may be granted privileges to perform specific types of surgeries.

Delinquent record—Incomplete record that has not been finished within the time as specified in the medical staff or facility bylaws, rules, or regulations.

Delphi process—Method to tap the expertise of a group of experts while controlling for the distorting effects of group process. A panel of experts that never meet face to face is asked to make individual predictions (estimates) about some future event (e.g., rate of inflation in the year 2001). The leader compiles the results, provides the panel with statistical summaries of the responses, and asks each member to either confirm or revise the original estimate and to justify that prediction. The process continues while the variability in responses decreases until a consensus judgment has been achieved.

Demographics—Population statistics; data related to a study of the human population.

Demotion—Moving an employee from one job to another that is lower in pay, responsibility, and organizational level.

Departmentalization—Cornerstone concept of classical management theory relating to the various ways organizations can be structured or divided into departments.

Deposition—Sworn out-of-court oral testimony. A transcript is made of the testimony. Depositions are used by lawyers to discover facts about the case prior to trial. Depositions may also be admitted into evidence if the witness cannot attend the trial in person.

Depreciation—Systematic allocation of the cost of a capital asset over a predetermined time frame in a rational manner.

Destruction letter—Letter of proof that records have been destroyed and are no longer available, signed by two witnesses. It usually includes a detailed manifest of the records that were destroyed.

Diagnosis related group (DRG)—Method of case mix adopted by the federal government and some other payers as a prospective payment mechanism for hospital inpatients. A classification system which places diseases into related groups. Related diseases and treatments tend to consume similar amounts of health care resources and incur similar amounts of cost. DRGS are used to determine reimbursement for hospitalized patients with health care coverage under Medicare.

Differentiation—Describes how much or how little a tumor resembles the normal tissue from which it arose.

Direct method of age adjustment—Uses a standard population and applies age-specific rates available for each population to determine the expected number of deaths in the standard population.

Direct pay, self-pay, out-of-pocket—Interchangeable terms meaning the patient himself or herself is paying for health care services.

Discharge analysis—Statistical reports based on discharged patient data, which describe the professional activities of the medical staff and the services provided by the health care organization.

Discharge planning—Coordination and communication among care providers to assure that a patient has a planned program of continuing or follow-up care post discharge.

Discipline—Management action to encourage compliance with organizational, departmental, or professional standards.

Discounted payback period—Methodology to determine at what future point in time a system will fully recover in present dollars its investment costs.

Discounting—Amount needed to be deposited today to have a designated amount at the end of a term.

Discovery—For this book's purposes, discovery refers to the pretrial methods that can be used by each party in a lawsuit to investigate the facts of the case. Depositions and interrogatories are forms of discovery.

Discrete data—Data that can assume numerical values; usually whole numbers and the number has real meaning (e.g., number of records that are coded, number of children in a family).

Disparate impact—Occurs when the results of an employer's actions have a different effect on one or more protected classes.

Disparate treatment—Occurs when members of a protected class receive unequal treatment.

Document imaging—Practice of scanning documents into a system. Medical record pages can be scanned and later retrieved for further processing.

Domiciliary (residential)—Facility that provides supervision, room, and board for people who are unable to live independently. The resident is usually in need of assistance with activities of daily living (bathing, eating, dressing).

Double-distribution method—Method of cost allocation that allows costs to be allocated to a unit from other units for services/products and by that unit to other units within an organization.

Double-entry method—Method of transaction recording used in accrual-based accounting systems.

Downloading of data—Electronic transfer of data from one database to another, often from the main database to a personal computer or a local area network.

Due process—Refers to the safeguards built into procedures so that individual rights are protected. For example, before stripping a physician of his or her medical staff membership, "due process" must be given—that may mean that certain hearings must take place, and steps prescribed in the medical staff bylaws must be followed so that the physician is not treated unfairly.

Duplicated patient count—Patient is counted more than once in a report during the same reporting period. If the same patient is discharged twice during the month, the report reflects two patients discharged.

Durable medical equipment—Equipment such as wheelchairs, oxygen equipment, walkers, and other devices prescribed by the physician for use in the home.

Durable power of attorney for health care—Person named, in writing, by a competent adult to make medical decisions on his or her behalf in the event he or she becomes incapacitated.

Dysmorphologist—Specialist in dysmorphology, a branch of clinical genetics concerned with structural defects.

Edit, rule—Condition that must be satisfied in order for the data to be added to the database, along with a message that will be displayed in case the data does not satisfy the condition.

Effective listening—Ten-step process to facilitate understanding of the message received from the sender.

Effectiveness—Extent to which an organization does the right things to ensure its survival in the larger system; sometimes contrasted with efficiency or doing things right.

Electronic data interchange (EDI)—Electronic exchange of data between computers and the standardization of electronic language used; exchanging business transaction data between organizations using electronic communications. Data are in specified formats understood by both organizations.

Electronic mail—Communication system in which computers are connected through networks. It may be local to an institution or extend to national and international users.

Emancipated minor—Persons (generally under 18 years of age, or the state's age of majority) who are considered by the court to be independent, self-supporting, or otherwise responsible to make their own decisions.

Emergency department—Hospital unit or department equipped to provide patient care that is urgent for a life-threatening or potentially disabling disease or condition.

Employee assistance program—Company-sponsored program to help employees through personal problems by direct company assistance, outside referral, or personal counseling.

Employee handbooks—Explains key benefits, policies, and general information about the employer.

Employment "at will"—Legal concept in which an employment arrangement that is not for a specified period can be terminated by either party without cause.

Empowerment—Process of facilitating the individual's optimal development and effective application of her/his skills, knowledge, and abilities as mediated through the work group or team process.

Encoder—A computer program which assists the coder in assigning diagnosis and procedure codes.

Encounter—Contact between a patient and a provider who is responsible for the assessment and evaluation of the patient at a specific contact, exercising independent judgment; contact may be face to face or per phone, video transmissions, or other communication medium; professional contact between a patient and a provider during which services are delivered.

Entity-relationship diagram (ERD)—Data modeling tools used to illustrate the logical design of an information system database by describing diagrammatically the relation between entities and identifying entity attributes.

Environmental assessment—Process of determining which issues in the environment of an organization are significant enough to warrant continuous evaluation. This is an important aspect of strategic planning.

Environmental forecasting—Process of predicting the expected direction of key factors in the environment of organizations. This is an important aspect of strategic planning.

Environmental monitoring—Process of observing and continuously monitoring the direction of key elements in the environment of organizations. This is an important aspect of strategic planning.

Environmental scanning—Process of surveying the environment of organizations in an effort to determine the important issues that should be systematically forecasted and monitored. This is an important aspect of strategic planning.

Episode of care—Health care services received by a patient during a period of relative continuous care by health care providers regarding a particular clinical problem or condition.

Equal opportunity employment—Giving all people a fair chance to succeed without discrimination based on factors unrelated to job performance, such as age, sex, disability, religion, race, or national origin.

Equity—A category on a financial balance sheet used to show the fund balance (or equity). It is the difference between the assets and the liabilities.

Ergonomics—Study of relationship of people to their work environment, including the construction and adjustability of equipment and furniture, arrangement of workstation, and design of work processes.

Essentials—Document which describes standards for approval of educational programs for health information administrators and health information technicians established by AHIMA in collaboration with the Commission on the Accreditation of Allied Health Educational Programs (CAAHEP).

Etiology—Study of cause(s) or origins of a disease or disorder.

Evidence—Refers to information legally presented at trial, which is offered to prove or disprove an issue under contention. If that information is allowed to be used at trial, it can be "admitted into evidence." Both the Federal government and individual states have rules of evidence, which are interpreted and applied by the judge in deciding what information may fairly be admitted into evidence.

Exchange time—Amount of time it takes the jukebox to locate the optical disk containing the requested image and place it in the disk drive.

Executive information system—System that typically draws a limited amount of data from contributing systems and offers analysis for strategic questions for high level executives.

Expert system—System that incorporates concepts derived from experts in a field and uses their knowledge to provide problem analysis through programs available to clinical practitioners.

Face validity—Evaluation of data to determine if it is logical, if the results appear accurate on the surface.

Factor comparison—Job evaluation system that allocates part of each job wage to key job factors. The result is a relative evaluation of the organization's jobs.

False imprisonment—Unlawful restraint of an individual's personal liberty. These claims sometimes occur in health care facilities using restraints to prevent patients from falling or injuring themselves, or when detaining an intoxicated patient because the staff feel that he or she is in no condition to leave safely.

Feedback controls—Controls that allow a discrepancy to develop between planned and desired and actual performance before identifying the variance. These controls may be self-correcting or non–self-correcting.

Feedback loop—Process of clarifying information (message transmitted) by questioning the sender of the message to facilitate further communication and/or to take appropriate action.

Fee-for-service—Payment method in which the cost is based on the provider's estimate of the cost for services rendered; method of payment to health care providers whereby a payment is made for each service provided.

Field—Smallest meaningful storage unit for data. Usually aligned vertically on a list.

File—All the records on all the patients or subjects for a single application. Equivalent to one table.

File guide—Card in a filing system used to mark major divisions and subdivisions and help the user locate the correct record.

File management system/flat file system—Program to manage the files of one application.

File server—Computer in a local area network that stores programs and data files shared by the users connected to the network.

Financial accountant—Fiscal services professional responsible for recording events that have incurred or will incur expense or revenue.

Financial accounting—Accounting method in which the financial transactions of the organization are recorded and reported.

Financial analysis—Management process of formulating judgments and decisions from the relation between the numbers represented on two reports—the statement of revenues and expenses and the balance sheet; also known as **ratio analysis.**

Fishbone diagram—A method of cause and effect analysis using a schematic technique for analyzing factors which cause or contribute to a problem situation. The spine and bones of a fish-like diagram reflect the organizing principle of this technique.

Fiscal intermediary—Organization that serves as the claims processor for Medicare hospital services.

Fists and tears—Situation in which one party uses raw emotions so that the other party's position is weakened through either intimidation or sympathy.

Flexible budget—Budget predicated on volume. All supplies, labor, and other variable expenses are budgeted in proportion to the anticipated volume.

Flextime—Method of scheduling staff that allows the employee to be flexible in start and stop times as long as a specific number of core hours are worked and/or the accountabilities of the position covered.

Flowchart—"Road map" that shows the logical steps and sequence involved in a procedure.

Flow process chart—Chart used to list each step in a work process; identifies the distance traveled and the time consumed by each delay. It is useful to collect information about a manual process, analyze it, and improve it.

Focused review—Investigation of an identified problem through analysis of a few critical variables.

Follow-up—Continued medical surveillance through patient contact either directly or indirectly (e.g., patient's physician, relatives).

Force field analysis—Similar to a fishbone analysis, a graphic technique for quantifying and displaying the relative influence of various factors which contribute to or impede the development of a problem, trend, or other outcome of interest.

Form—Structured document, typically paper, designed to collect and store data.

Formal theory of authority—Theory of authority based on rights that suggests authority always flows down in an organization.

Fraud—Intentional distortion of the truth that could cause harm or loss to a person or his or her property.

Frequency distribution—Method used to group nominal, ordinal, and continuous data into specific categories and in which the total number of observations in each category is recorded.

Frequency polygon—Method of presenting a frequency distribution with continuous-interval data by joining the midpoints of the top of each bar with a straight line; effective when comparing two or more data sets because multiple lines can be displayed on the graph.

Full-time equivalent—Equivalent of one employee working full time (i.e., 2080 hours per year). For example, two employees working half-time are one full-time equivalent.

Functional managers—Managers who are responsible for administering a single function like management information systems as contrasted to general managers.

Fund balance—A category on a financial balance sheet used to indicate the equity. It is the residual category that shows the difference between the assets and the liabilities or the difference between the revenues and expenses.

Gantt chart—Scheduling and progress chart that emphasizes work time relations necessary to meet a defined goal.

Gatekeeper—Refers to the primary care physician who participates in a comprehensive managed care plan and is responsible for the care provided to the managed care enrollee (patient).

General managers—Managers who are responsible for administering two or more distinct functions, like management information systems and marketing, as contrasted to managers of a single function.

General system life cycle—Usual stages of the life cycle of any system, including development, growth, maturity, and deterioration.

Genetics—Study of genes and their heredity.

Goal—Statement of what the organization wants to do.

Goal setting—Process of establishing the targets that organizations will pursue and the standards that will be used to gauge their success.

Good loser—Strategy in which one party shifts responsibility to the other through projected guilt; indicated by such statements as "No, it's all my fault," "I take full responsibility for this even though . . . ."

Grade—A grade from 1 to 4 assigned to a malignant tumor by a pathologist. Grades are used to designate degrees of differentiation.

Grievance procedure—Multistep, predefined process that the employer and union jointly use to resolve disputes that arise under the terms of a labor agreement. In nonunion organizations, this may be called a complaint procedure.

Gross patient revenue—All patient services at charges not reduced by discounts, allowances, or other adjustments.

Group decision support software (GDSS)—Computer program used to facilitate the group decision-making process.

Grouper—Computer program that assigns based on several factors including principal diagnosis and principal procedure.

Group maintenance—Process of maintaining the group's viability and effectiveness through recruiting and placing new members, providing orientation and training, establishing goals, communicating performance expectations, monitoring and evaluating performance, providing rewards and incentives, managing conflict, and supporting personal empowerment.

Group process—Intragroup activity or behavior of relevance to organizational effectiveness (e.g., socialization of new members, conflict resolution).

Gunny sacking—Unproductive conflict strategy in which one party stores up grievances and hold them in readiness to dump on the other party.

Halo effect—Bias that occurs when a performance evaluator or hiring manager allows some information to disproportionately prejudice the final evaluation.

Hardware—Physical equipment that makes up computers and computer systems.

Hawthorne studies—Famous management studies that took place at the Western Electric Company's Hawthorne Works outside Chicago and that ushered in the era of human relations thought in management.

Health—The World Health Organization defines health as a state of complete physical, mental and social well-being and not merely the absence of disease or infirmity. (WHO, 1946).

Health care data network—Electronic network that provides access to an individual's healthcare information to care providers, payors, employers, vendors, and other support organizations through centralized and distributed data bases.

Health care services—Processes that contribute to the health and well-being of the person; can be provided in the hospital or in an ambulatory or a home setting and includes nursing, medical, surgical, or other health-related services.

Health information administrator—Professional title of one of the three specialized practitioners with the credential of registered record administrator (RRA) granted by the American Health Information Management Association.

Health information technician—Professional title of one of three specialized practitioners certified by AHIMA associated with the credential ART (accredited record technician).

Healthy People 2000—Report published by the U.S. Department of Health and Human Services that established goals and objectives promoting health and prevention of disease.

Hearsay rule—Rule of evidence restricts the admissibility of evidence or statements that are not the personal knowledge of the witness. There are some limited exceptions to the rule. For example, an HIM professional would be barred from testifying about the contents of the medical records under the hearsay rule, because the statements in the records are not the personal knowledge of the HIM professional. However, in many jurisdictions (but not all), patient records are admissible as an exception to the hearsay rule.

Hierarchy chart—Type of decomposition diagram whose purpose is to break down problems into smaller and smaller detail.

Histogram—Method of presenting a frequency distribution with continuous-interval data; similar to the bar graph except the horizontal or x-axis includes continuous-interval categories rather than discrete categories used in the bar graph.

Histology—Structure, composition, and function of tissues.

Hit 'n run—Situation in which one party attacks the other personally and then "leaves the scene" before the other can respond.

Home health care—Provision of medical and nonmedical care in the home or place of residence to promote, maintain, or restore health or to minimize the effect of disease or disability.

Hospice—Multidisciplinary health care program responsible for the palliative and supportive care of terminally ill patients and their families, with consideration for their physical, spiritual, social, and economic needs.

Hospital—The definition of a hospital that is most commonly used was established by the American Hospital Association. It defines a hospital as a health care institution with an organized medical and professional staff and with inpatient beds available round-the-clock, whose primary function is to provide inpatient medical, nursing, and other health-related services to patients for both surgical and nonsurgical conditions, and that usually provides some outpatient services, particularly emergency care.

Hospital ambulatory care—Hospital-directed health care provided to patients who are not admitted as inpatients and for which the hospital is responsible, regardless of the location of health care.

Hospital inpatient—Person receiving health care services provided by the hospital who is admitted for an overnight stay and is provided room, board, and nursing service in a unit or area of the hospital.

Hospital patient—One who is receiving and/or using health care services for which the hospital is liable or held accountable; includes inpatient, observation patient, outpatient, and any other patient of the hospital.

Human diversity (in the workplace)—Management philosophy of personal empowerment in which individual differences are seen as a source of organizational strength in improving workplace performance.

Human relations—School of management thought that focuses on the importance of the individual and interpersonal relationships in organizations.

Human resource audit—Evaluates the personnel activities used in an organization.

Human resource planning—Plan that systematically forecasts the organization's future supply of and demand for employees.

ICD-9-CM Coordination and Maintenance Committee—Consists of the federal government users of ICD-9-CM, which recommends changes in the ICD-9-CM system.

Inactive record—Record that no longer meets the active record criteria established by the organization. Inactive records do not need to be as readily available as active records but do need to be available when needed.

Incidence—Number of new cases of a specific disease occurring during a certain period.

Incidence rate—Number of new cases of a disease at a specific time period divided by the population at a specified time period; the quotient is then multiplied by a constant.

Incident report—Written account of an unusual event; written description of any event not consistent with routine operational procedures or patient care activities that has an adverse effect on a patient, employee, or facility visitor.

Income statement—Statement of revenues, expenses, gains, and losses for the period ending with net income or loss for the period. The earnings per share amount is usually shown on the income statement for for-profit entities. The reconciliation of beginning and ending balances of retained earnings or fund balance may also be shown in a combined statement of income and retained earnings or fund balance.

Incomplete file area—Location in the health care facility where physician incomplete records are stored until missing reports and signatures are obtained.

Incomplete record—Patient record that is missing content reports or authentications, as defined by facility policy.

Inconsistency of data—Contradictions in data in the same content field for the same patient or subject in two or more databases, e.g., date of birth is 12/24/90 in one database and 12/25/90 in another.

Independent living facilities—Facilities, including apartments and condominiums, that allow people to live independently but do offer dietary, health care, social service, and other services as needed by the resident.

Index—Numerical listing by diagnosis or procedure code number of the cases treated in a facility.

Indicator—An important factor in service provision; competent performance of key factors is indicative of quality.

Indicator focus—Topic, subject, or item measured in an indicator monitoring program.

Indicator monitoring program—An indicator-based performance monitoring system for accredited organizations that, when integrated into the accreditation process, will provide the Joint Commission with a continuous picture of organizational performance, allowing for monitoring between triennial on-site surveys.

Indigent—One who is without the means for subsistence; the poor or impoverished.

Informal organization (unwritten organization)—Composed of two or more persons who develop mutually satisfying interactions pertaining to personal and/or job-related matters. These relationships are not depicted on an organization chart.

Information—Human interpretation of data; data that has been processed for use; collection of data that contain meaning; data that have been processed into a meaningful form. Information adds to a representation and tells the recipient something that was not known before. What is information for one person may not be information for another. Information should be timely, accurate, and complete. Information reduces uncertainty. Contrast with **data**.

Information highway—Exchange of electronic information through a computer system.

Information system life cycle—Usual stages of the life cycle of an information system, including design, implementation, operations, and obsolescence.

Information warehouse—System organized to receive clinical data from transaction systems such as a pharmacy system or a radiology system and combines it with other organizational data; and made available for a variety of access and analysis tools. It can also present data in a series of clinical views and can be designed to deliver the CPR content to users.

Informed consent—Patient or legal representative granting permission for treatment or testing after receiving appropriate information about the benefits, risks, and alternatives.

Inpatient—Hospital patient receiving health care services and who is provided room, board, and continuous nursing service in a unit or area of the hospital.

Input/input device—To submit data or instructions to the computer system for processing, in a general systems context, input is anything that enters the system from the environment. Devices include: keyboards, mice, scanners, voice input units, etc.

Input validation—Performance of tests and checks on input to ensure that the input operation is legal and the input itself is correct. A wide variety of tests can be applied to ensure the correctness of data being input to a computer system.

Institutional review board (IRB)—Generally is a multidisciplinary board established to review proposed research projects for their compliance with sound and ethical research practices.

Insurance—Purchased contract (policy) in which the purchaser (insured) is protected from loss by the insurer's agreeing to reimburse for such loss.

Intelligence factor—Process of employing external research, quality monitoring, diagnostic aids in combination with patient record data to provide medical care.

Intensity of service/severity of illness criteria—Standard criteria used by a medical review entity to justify admission to an inpatient facility.

Intentional torts—Act that is contrary to civil—not criminal—law, which the perpetrator does knowingly. For example, false imprisonment, defamation of character, invasion of privacy are torts that are done with the intention to harm.

Interface—The point at which one system's functioning ends and another system takes over; a shared boundary between two systems. Graphical user interfaces (GUIs), such as windows, use a pointing device to select icons.

Internet—A telecommunications international computer network that serves as gateway to thousands of users.

Interrogatories—A form of discovery that includes answering, under oath and in writing, a written list of questions submitted by the opposing party.

Invasion of privacy—For the purposes of this book, this refers to the publicizing of another's private affairs, with which the public has no legitimate concern, or wrongful intrusion into another's private affairs in such a manner to cause a person shame, embarrassment, or mental suffering.

Job analysis—Systematic collection, evaluation, and organization of information about jobs.

Job description—Formal statement of the nature of the responsibilities in a particular task; written document that explains duties, working conditions, and requirements of a specified job.

Job enrichment—Adding more responsibility, autonomy, and control to a job.

Job evaluation—Systematic procedure to determine the worth of a job to the organization compared with other jobs.

Job grading—Form of job evaluation that assigns jobs to predetermined classifications according to the job's relative worth to the organization. This technique is also called the job classification method.

Job performance standards—Work requirements that are expected from an employee on a particular job.

Job ranking—Form of job evaluation that subjectively ranks jobs according to their overall worth to the organization.

Job sharing—Arrangement in which two or more persons share one full-time position.

Joint application design (JAD)—Group process used in the analysis and design of an information system.

Jukebox—Device that holds and retrieves the individual disks in an optical disk system.

Jurisdiction—Refers to the right of a court to hear and decide given controversies; for example, Federal courts have "jurisdiction" over certain cases, e.g., cases concerning questions of Federal law or concerning citizens of differing states, and state courts have jurisdiction over certain cases.

Key field—Field containing redundant data which links two or more tables in a relational database; a sort field.

Kitchen sinking—Interpersonal approach in which one part to the conflict dwells on past grievances to strengthen her or his current position.

Knowledge—Collected information about an area of concern.

Knowledge base—Collection of stored facts, heuristics, and models that can be used for problem solving.

Lag time—Time period between discharge of a patient or a patient's encounter and billing of the services to the payor.

Layoffs—Separation of employees from the organization for economic or business reasons.

Layout—Specifies the location of each item of information on an output document or visual display, and specifies any headings, titles, or page numbers that appear.

Leadership—Reciprocal relationship in which one person (the leader) influences others (followers) to accept and act on the vision, values, and goals communicated by the leader.

Leading—Management function that motivates and inspires employees to pursue organizational goals.

Legality of data—Data that are created, authenticated, stored, and corrected according to law or regulation.

Legibility of data—Data that are decipherable or readable.

Liability—Obligation to pay a certain amount at a specified time for a current benefit; amount owed to another.

Libel—False writing, intended to injure the reputation of another, that is published to a third person (or more).

Licensed—Right to practice an occupation or provide a service granted by a public state-level agency; for individuals, generally based on examination and proof of specified educational requirements; for facilities, based on demonstrated compliance with specified regulations.

Licensure—Legal approval for a facility to operate or for a person to practice within his or her profession.

Life care centers—Retirement communities that provide living accommodations and meals for a monthly fee; facilities that offer a variety of services, including housekeeping, recreation, health care, laundry, and exercise programs.

Life table analysis—Examines survival times of individual subjects that tend to enter a study sample at different times.

Line graph—Also known as a run chart, a simple but visually powerful method of displaying the relationship between two variables or the trend in one variable over time. The latter is typically referred to as a time series or trend line.

Liquidity ratios—Measure the ability of the health care organization to meet its short- and long-term obligations.

Living will—Written document that allows competent adults to indicate their wishes regarding life-prolonging medical treatment in case they should be incapacitated and unable to voice their wishes themselves.

Local area network (LAN)—Connects multiple devices together via continuous cable and is located within a small geographic area.

Logical record/view—Collection of data items that are used or looked at together, independent of their mode of physical storage.

Logical system design—First stage of the system design process in which the functionality of the system is described in general terms.

Logic field—Field for Yes/No entries.

Longitudinal—Documentation of the healthcare status for patient(s) over a period of time.

Longitudinal records—Records which include all health and illness data collected on an individual from birth until death.

Long-term care—Health care provided in a non–acute care setting in which the patient resides; includes personal care, social, dietary, and housing services provided to the residents who do not have the ability to live independently.

Long-term debt/total assets ratio—Compares the amount of long-term debt the organization has (bills that will come due in a period more than 1 year from now [e.g., mortgages]) with the amount of assets (things the organization can convert to cash [e.g., furniture, land, inventories, marketable securities]) it has to pay those debts.

Magnification ratio—Number of times a microfilmed image must be increased to return it to the original size; inverse of reduction ratio.

Mainframe computers—Machines used for major applications, to maintain large databases and for high volume work.

Malpractice—Professional negligence or misconduct, such as failure to meet the prevailing standard of care for that profession, that results in harm to another. For malpractice to be proven, four elements must be shown: duty, breach, cause, and harm. See the book's discussion on negligence and malpractice for an explanation of these elements.

Managed care—Group that contracts with providers to give a range of medical services to an enrolled population; generic term for a payment system that manages cost, quality, and access to health care; system of controlling cost in health care by presetting reimbursement amounts and regulating patient access to participating physicians and health care institutions.

Management—Process of coordinating individual and group activity toward the accomplishment of organizational goals in a manner that is acceptable to the larger society.

Management by objectives—Approach to management that involves participative goal setting and evaluations based on results.

Management functions—Planning, organizing, and controlling activities that managers perform in accomplishing their jobs.

Managerial accountant—Fiscal services professional who compares what is happening presently or previously (variance analyses) with what was anticipated and what is still anticipated to happen (the budget).

Managerial finance officer—Health care administrative officer charged with planning for the future.

Managerial grid—Descriptive model of leadership behavior developed by Blake and Mouton that characterizes leadership styles on the dimensions of "concern for production" and "concern for people."

Master budget—The overall operating budget for an organization, combining budgets from all units (revenues and expenses) into one.

Master charge list—List that reflects the charge for each item that may be used in the treatment of a patient and the charge for most services (e.g., respiratory therapy treatments, physical therapy services, laboratory tests); also known as the charge master or charge description master.

Master patient index (MPI)—Alphabetical file of all patients who have received services from the facility. Whether manual or computerized, it contains basic patient demographic information and the patient identification number, if one is assigned.

Matching principle—States that revenues should be matched with the expenses incurred to produce the revenue.

Matrix—See **Decision grid.** Multidimensional tool used to organize, categorize, and reduce both qualitative and quantitative data into a more usable form. As an organization and reduction tool, the matrix may be used in the decision-making process by weighing information or in the evaluation of performance over an extended period.

Mean—Average number of observations calculated by adding up the values of all observations and dividing the total by the number of observations.

Meaning of data—Data conveys understandable information; is consistent when naming or describing the same findings or treatment; is relevant and useful to the provider, patient, health care institution, and public.

Median—Midpoint or the middlemost value when values are arranged in numerical order.

Medicaid—Jointly funded program between the state and federal governments to provide health care to welfare recipients in the different states; originally titled the medical assistance program; established by Title XIX of the Social Security Act;

entitlement program (Title XIX) that provides health care for low-income people.

Medical decision support systems—Systems that provide diagnostic investigation tools, clinical guideline advice, and expert system resources to clinicians.

Medical informatics—Field that concerns itself with the cognitive, information processing, and communication tools of medical practice, education, and research, including the information science and the technology to support these tasks.

Medical information system—Set of formal arrangements by which the facts concerning the health or health care of individual patients are stored and processed in computers.

Medically indigent—Those whose incomes are above what would normally qualify for Medicaid, but their medical expenses are high enough to bring their adjusted income to the poverty level.

Medical record administrator—See **Health information administrator.**

Medical record librarian—Professional title of early members of the American Association of Medical Record Librarians (AAMRL).

Medical record technician—See **Health information technician.**

Medical staff organization (MSO)—Self-governing entity that operates as a responsible extension of the governing body and exists for the purpose of providing patient care.

Medicare—Government program funded through taxation that provides payment for health care services for the elderly and certain categories of illnesses; federally funded program that provides health insurance for the elderly and certain other groups; established in 1965 by Title XVIII *Health Insurance for the Aged* of the Social Security Act of 1935, now referred to as Medicare; entitlement program (Title XVIII) enacted by the U.S. Congress and effective July 1, 1966, as an amendment to the Social Security program. It provided health care payment for all participants 65 years of age or over.

Memo or note fields—Field using narrative information that is difficult to code.

Methods improvement—See **Work simplification.**

Microcomputer (PC)—Computer used in individual applications such as a single user donor registry and as a workstation for large systems.

Microfiche—One of three forms: a copy of a microfilm jacket, an original film produced by a step-and-repeat camera, or a computer output microfiche produced by a COM recorder.

Microfilm jacket—4″ × 6″ Mylar holders having channels, or narrow sleeves, formed by fusing two panels of transparent material together. The channels hold pieces of microfilm cut from the roll.

Microfilm reader—Projection box that magnifies the microfilmed image, passes light through it, and displays it on a screen; also called a viewer.

Microform—Generic term for any format of microfilm.

Minicomputer—Machine often used in departmental systems such as laboratory or radiology.

Mission—Statement of the organization's purpose in broad terms—what it is and what it does.

Mode—Value that occurs most frequently in a given set of values.

Model/data model—Plan or pattern for an information system including database structure and content, methods to input, store, retrieve, analyze, and display data.

Monitoring and evaluation—Ongoing review of routinely collected data regarding critical indicators of quality care or service.

Moping—Situation in which one party adopts an "ain't it awful" approach to win the conflict by smothering the other party with guilt or pity.

Morbidity—Extent of illness, injury, or disability in a given population.

Morbidity rates—Complication rates, such as community-acquired, hospital-acquired, and postoperative infection rates; includes comorbidity rates and the prevalence and incidence rates of disease.

Morphology—Form and structure of a particular organism, organ, or part.

Mortality—Death rate in a given population.

Mortality rates—Death rates, including gross death rate, net death rate, cause-specific death rates, and neonatal and infant death rates.

Motion to quash—Motion, made to the court, to invalidate or set aside a subpoena or subpoena duces tecum.

Movement diagram (layout flowchart)—Graphically represents the movement of paper or people in the physical environment where the processes are performed.

Multihospital system—Health care system composed of two or more hospitals that are owned, managed, or leased by a single organization.

Multimedia—Term used to specify capability of computer systems to process data, voice, and image and video to communicate through a PC workstation.

National Labor Relations Act—Basic foundation in federal law governing labor relations, employee rights of representation and collective bargaining, and restrictions against unfair labor practices. This legislation established the National Relations Board as the federal "watchdog" to enforce national labor relations policy by conducting representation elections, certifying appropriate bargaining units, and adjudicating unfair labor practice complaints.

National practitioner data bank (NPDB)—A data bank containing information about actions taken against physicians and other health care professionals, and any settlements or claim payouts. Health care organizations query the NPDB at the time of initial appointment and reappointment of members to the medical/professional staff.

Negligence—Omission or commission of an act that a reasonably prudent person would or would not do under similar circumstances. Negligence is a form of carelessness that represents a departure from the standard of care imposed on members of society.

Negotiation—Interpersonal or intergroup process in which each party involved in a conflict attempts to advance its own interests while recognizing the other's claims. Within the framework of labor relations negotiation, it refers to the fundamental process of collective bargaining that results in the written agreement (contract) between management and the employees' representative (the union or employee association).

Net—Reduced by all relevant deductions.

Not-for-profit—Organizational category that implies that the organization will use its excess funds after expenses to enhance services to the community the organization serves rather than distribute the excess to owners of the organization.

Net income—Excess of all revenues for the reporting period over all expenses of the period.

Net loss—Negative net income. The excess of all expenses for the reporting period over all revenues of the period.

Net operating revenue—Amount of revenues *expected* to be received or total charges less those deductions expected by third party payers.

Net present value—Discounted or present value of all cash inflows and outflows of a project at a given discount rate.

Net working capital—Current assets less current liabilities.

Niche vendors—Vendors that supply a single component or group of components of information systems to meet limited objective.

Nomenclature—List of proper names for diseases and operations which may include a code number for each listing.

Nominal data—Includes numerical values assigned to categories such as sex or race; also referred to as categorical or qualitative data.

Nominal group process—Extension of brainstorming to incorporate the development of a group consensus judgment through ranking priorities or preferences among alternatives.

Normative decision theory—Approach to decision making that provides managers with prescriptions for how decisions ought to be made when the goals are clear.

Numeric identification—Using a number to identify the patient record.

Nursing facility—Comprehensive term for long-term care facility that provides nursing care and related services for residents who require medical, nursing, or rehabilitative care; a sufficient number of nursing personnel must be employed on a 24-hour basis to provide care to residents according to the care plan.

Objectives—More specific statements that define the expectations or outcomes given by the goal statements.

Observation patient—Patient who needs assessment, evaluation, and/or monitoring because of a significant degree of unsteadiness or disability but does not require admission to hospital as an inpatient; observation period not to exceed 48 hours.

Occasion of service—Specific identifiable act of service involved in the care of the patient that is not an encounter (e.g., test such as urinalysis ordered during the encounter).

Occurrence report—See **Incident report**.

Occurrence screening—Procedure for reviewing health records and other data to identify documentation of adverse events for which the hospital could be held liable.

Odds ratio—Estimate of the relative risk a person has of acquiring a disease or condition if exposed to a certain characteristic or risk factor.

Office landscaping—Another term for **open office design plan**.

On-line—Equipment or devices connected to or directly communicating with the central processing unit.

Open office design plan—Design for an office arrangement that features open space free of permanent walls. Workstations that are created with the use of partitions and furniture. The open plan focuses on work groups, traffic patterns, and work flow.

Open system—Organizational system that actively interacts with its environment by taking inputs in, performing transformations on them, and providing desirable goods and services back to the environment; technology system that incorporates all types of devices, regardless of the manufacturer or model, with standard communication facilities and protocols; refers to the use of computers based on industry-standard hardware and software components; also called a public domain system.

Operating budget—Predicts the labor, supply, and other expenses required to support the work volume predicted.

Operating margin ratio—Shows the relation between the net revenues received and the expenses required to supply the revenues.

Operating room procedure—Procedure in the DRG system which, by its presence, causes a case to be grouped into a surgical DRG.

Operating system—Programs that include the set of instructions that direct actual computer operating functions.

Operation flowchart—A graphic representation of the logical sequence of activities in a procedure. It shows the decision points encountered in carrying out that function.

Opportunity costs—Benefits that would be received from the next best alternative use of the funds being used for the project or purchase.

Optical character recognition (OCR)—Machine recognition of printed characters.

Order communications/order entry—Hospital information system component that enables orders to be transmitted through communications directly to the departments responsible for carrying them out. Data noting date, time, conditions, and required functions are included; automatic linkage to charges occurs.

Ordinal data—Ranked data according to some specific criterion.

Organizational culture—Term coined by Schein that refers to a prevailing set of norms of behavior, values, ethical standards, symbols, customs, and beliefs shared by members of an organization. This approach to understanding organizational behavior emphasizes the difficulty of introducing organizational change without addressing the underlying cultural assumptions and commitments.

Organizational structure—Structure of an organization established to plan work, to fix responsibility, to supervise work, and to measure results.

Organization chart—Illustrates the hierarchical relationships between various individuals, lines of authority, accountability, and responsibility; identifies the organization's primary functions and the subfunctions within each primary function.

Organizing—Management function that converts organizational goals into actions; consists of defining the activities necessary to achieve goals, logically grouping the goals, and assigning responsibility to someone for accomplishment.

Osteopath—Physician licensed to practice in osteopathy. The philosophy of osteopathy focuses on the whole body with emphasis on prevention and health and the interrelationship of structure and function.

Outcard—Card placed in the active files that lists the new location or media of an inactive record removed from the files.

Outcome—End result of treatment or intervention; compared to preestablished criteria defining desired outcomes.

Outguide—Plastic folder used in a paper filing system that holds the place of the record when it is removed from the file. It includes information about where the record is currently located and allows for accurate placement of the record on its return to the file.

Outlier—Data point that falls far outside the expected value; might include a length of stay greater than the 95th percentile of a regional norm or costs for an inpatient stay more than twice the diagnosis-related group reimbursement rate.

Out-of-pocket—Moneys that the patient pays directly to a health care provider.

Outpatient—Patient receiving health care services at a hospital without being hospitalized, institutionalized, and/or admitted as an inpatient.

Output/output device—Data or information that results from processing and are made available to users. In a general systems sense, output is anything that is produced by a system and movement across the boundary into the environment. Devices include printers, display screens, voice output devices, and the like.

Palliative care—Health care services that relieve or alleviate patient symptoms or discomforts, such as pain or nausea; is not curative.

Paradox of planning—Confusing situation that explains why the very areas in which plans are most likely to be inaccurate are the areas in which they are most needed and the areas in which plans are most accurate are those in which they are less essential.

Parallel processing—Duplicate processing of the same data at the same time in two separate information systems.

Pareto chart (analysis)—Graphic technique for analyzing and displaying the causal factors contributing to a problem, event, or trend of interest. The chart is presented as a series of histograms arrayed in (usually) descending order of apparent influence and overlaid with a cumulative frequency line graph. This method facilitates clear identification of the most significant factors to be addressed in resolving the problem. Similar in form to bar charts and histograms.

Passive problem employee—One who seeks to satisfy personal needs through use of passive resistance—for example, the silent treatment, gunny sacking, moping, the good loser, or avoidance.

Password—Word or series of characters that must be entered by a person into the computer to have access to all or specified portions of the database.

Path-goal theory—Model of leadership that focuses on the leader's instrumental role in motivating and facilitating the worker's efforts to attain individual and organizational goals. Key components of leadership effectiveness are worker's perceptions of effort needed to perform the task, probability of attaining desired outcomes, and value placed on those outcomes.

Patient—Person, including one who is deceased, who is receiving and/or using or has received health care services.

Patient assessment—Systematic collection and review of patient-specific data.

Patient care evaluation—Formal process used to evaluate the adequacy of care given to a specific patient population.

Payback method—Method used to compare the value of a capital expenditure with another; calculates the time frame that must pass before inflow of cash from a project equals or exceeds outflow of cash.

Payback period—Methodology used to determine at what future point in time a system will fully recover its investment (development) costs; the time in which a project or equipment saves enough money to pay for itself; time frame that must pass before inflow of cash from a project equals outflow of cash.

Peer review—Evaluation of professional performance by other people of equal standing within the same profession.

Peer review organization (PRO)—Medical review entity under contract to the Health Care Financing Administration to monitor the medical necessity, quality, and appropriateness of services provided to Medicare beneficiaries.

Pen-based device—Hand-held device that builds in communications and organizer software. These are used in some health care settings for data capture purposes.

Per case—When services are charged based on the total service being rendered rather than by each component of the service—for example, charging for transplantation services when all of the following have been performed: the organ has been procured, the transplant has been made, and aftercare has been rendered.

Per diem—Established payment for a day's worth of services.

Performance appraisal—Used interchangeably with performance evaluation to describe the process by which managers determine if the requirements of a particular job have been successfully accomplished by the person being evaluated; process of evaluating how a person is doing on the job.

Performance ratio—Used to evaluate the effectiveness of resource use to deliver services and products.

PERT network—Acronym for *p*rogram *e*valuation *r*eview *t*echnique; diagram that illustrates the dependency relation of several projects leading to a larger nonroutine goal (e.g., building project); tool used to plan and coordinate the smaller projects and accomplish the larger goal; used to give likely completion times.

Physical system design—Details the design of hardware, software, databases, communication procedures, and controls.

Picture archiving and communication system—Integrated computer system that acquires, stores, retrieves, and displays digital images.

Pie chart—Method to display qualitative, ordinal, discrete, or continuous data in which a circle is drawn and divided into sections that correspond to the frequency in each category.

Placement—Assignment of an employee to a new or different job.

Plaintiff—Party who initiates the civil suit seeking monetary damages or some other form of relief.

Planning—Management function that is futuristic in nature and involves thinking about and preparing for possible alternative "futures." The result of management planning is a set of clear and concise goals.

Planning flexibility—Characteristic of an effective plan that makes it adaptable to changing organizational conditions.

Platter—Optical disk made of special material that is written and read by a laser beam.

Players—Individuals or organizations with key roles; stakeholders.

Pleadings—Document filed in court by either a plaintiff or defendant, either to commence the action, or in response to the initial pleading. Pleadings set forth the nature of a plaintiff's claim or the defendant's answer to the plaintiff's claim(s). Pleadings that commence actions are called complaints, petitioners, or bills. A responsive pleading is generally called an answer or affidavit of defense.

Point-of-care documentation—Data entry at the time and location of service.

Point-of-care system—System of data capture at the place where the service of care is provided.

Point of service—Component of managed care plans in which the patient is required to use a primary care physician (gatekeeper) who is responsible for the care provided.

Point system—Form of job evaluation that assesses the relative worth of the job's key factors to arrive at the relative worth of jobs.

Political subsystem—System of bargaining and negotiating that determines to a great extent how work is actually done in organizations.

Population-based central registries—Registries operated to assess trends, conduct cancer control or research in a defined population, usually a geopolitical entity such as a county or state.

Potentially compensable event (PCE)—Occurrence that could result in financial liability at some future time.

Power—Ability of one person in an organization to influence the behavior of another.

Practice guidelines—Parameters that help physicians make clinical decisions.

Practitioner—Identifying data elements on individuals licensed or certified to deliver care to patients, who had face-to-face contact with the patient and who had provided care based on independent judgment.

Precedent—Earlier court decision or course of conduct which is considered to furnish an example of how similar cases or situations should be decided or handled in the future. Courts attempt to decide cases on the basis of principles established in prior cases.

Pre-existing condition—Any disease, injury, or condition identified as having occurred before a specific date.

Preferred provider organization (PPO)—Network of physicians who enter into an agreement to provide health care services on a discounted fee schedule.

Prevalence rate—Number of existing cases of a disease at a specific time period divided by a specific population at that time; quotient multiplied by a constant.

Preventive controls—Controls that attempt to keep a discrepancy from developing between desired and actual performance.

Preventive discipline—Management action taken to encourage employees to follow standards and rules so that infractions are prevented.

Primary care—Care provided at first contact with the health care provider in an ambulatory care setting; care is continuous and comprehensive.

Primary data—Original data; direct result of patient care (e.g., medical record).

Primary health data—Original source data; the patient's original record.

Principal diagnosis—Reason after study which caused the patient to enter the hospital.

Principles of management—Guidelines for management behavior. These "principles" have been developed as the result of theory and experience.

Privacy—Right of an individual to control disclosure of their personal information.

Privileged communications—Statements made to attorneys, priests, physicians, spouses, or others in a legally recognized position of trust. The confidentiality of these statements are generally protected by law from being revealed, even in court.

Privilege delineation—Definition of a professional's scope of practice within an individual institution.

Proactive human resource management—Exists when decision makers anticipate problems and take steps to minimize the impact rather than waiting for problems to occur and then taking action.

Problem solving—Characteristic and arguably most important activity of the manager. Most decision making in organizations both by individuals and by groups can be characterized as relevant to the analysis and resolution of some organizational problem to be addressed.

Process—Specific actions taken, events occurring, and human interactions in the delivery of health services.

Processual change—Refers to evolutionary and incremental change resulting in the gradual development or expansion of the organization.

Process view of management—Conceptualization of management as a process or series of functions.

Productive time—Time a person is present and working.

Productive unit of work—An item produced that meets established levels of quality.

Productivity—Process for converting the resources of an organization (labor, capital, materials, and technology) into products and/or services that meet the organization's goals.

Productivity standards (work standards)—Tools used to specify the expected performance and to measure actual performance.

Profession—An occupation needing training and advanced study in a specialized field.

Profit—Represents the amount of money (cash) actually received from the payer (patient or insurance company) less the actual cost to do the service, assuming the cost is less than the cash received.

Progressive discipline—Protocol for supervision using a system of stronger penalties for repeated offenses. Its purpose is to allow the employee to correct the behavior before the stronger penalties must be assessed.

Progressive responsibility—Customary career path of managers in which progression takes place from first-line supervisor to middle manager to top-level executive.

Project management—Group of people with expertise in a variety of functions lead by a project manager who work to accomplish a single goal.

Promotion—Moving an employee from one job to another that is higher in pay, responsibility, and/or organizational level.

Proprietary system—Technology system that is owned or copyrighted by an individual or a business and that is available for use only through purchase or by permission of the owner.

Prospective/cohort/incidence study—Study in which people with the characteristic or risk factor but free from the disease at the beginning of the study and people without the characteristic or risk factor and free from the disease at the beginning of the study are followed forward in time to determine if they develop the disease under study.

Prospective payment system—Government reimbursement system in which the amount of payment to the hospital is fixed in advance of services rendered; established annually; based on the discharge diagnosis. The payment for each diagnosis is determined prospectively based on the types of cases treated at the hospital.

Protected groups or classes—Groups of people who fall into categories protected by civil rights legislation, e.g., African Americans, women, Hispanic Americans, Catholics, and persons over 40 years of age.

Prototype—Initially the system prototype is a preliminary model of the final system, but after several development phases, it can evolve into the final system.

Providers—Individuals or organizations that provide health care services to individual patients or the community; all-inclusive, generic term for individuals or institutions that provide health care.

Proximate cause—That which, in a sequence unbroken by intervening causes, produces injury, and *without which* the injury would not have occurred; in other words, the primary or substantial cause of an injury. Whether or not an action or omission is the proximate cause of an injury is sometimes a difficult question involved in negligence/malpractice litigation.

Proximity chart—Matrix that provides information useful in work space design; shows the desirability of having work areas close to or far apart from one another.

Purge—Process of removing inactive records from the active files.

Qualitative analysis—Review of records for accuracy and completeness of the record content, rather than for the presence of forms and signatures.

Quality—Degree of excellence of a thing; a required character or property that belongs to a thing's essential nature.

Quality assessment—Process of measuring quality to define existing levels.

Quality assessment and improvement—Continuous monitoring, evaluation, and improvement of the processes of providing health care services to meet the needs of the public.

Quality assurance (QA)—Activities designed to measure the quality of a service, product, or process with remedial action as needed to maintain a desired standard.

Quality improvement (QI)—Activities designed to increase the quality of a product or service through process or system changes that increase efficiency or effectiveness.

Quality indicator—Important factor in service provision; competent performance of key factors indicates quality intensity of service criteria.

Quality management—Cultural commitment to high-quality performance, service, and outcomes through the empowerment of all workers in a process of continuous quality improvement through the application of scientific methods of data collection, analysis, and interpretation.

Quality data/data quality—Data that are correct, valid, reliable, legible, current, timely, have meaning, are accessible, confidential, secure, and legal.

Quantitative analysis—Review of a patient record to determine if specified reports and authentications are present.

Quantitative data—Measurement information; numerical information that can be computed in some way.

Query—Question, asked by the user, the answer to which is in the database.

Range—Difference between the highest and lowest values.

Rating scale—In performance appraisal, requires the rater to provide a subjective evaluation of a person's performance along a scale from low to high.

Ratio analysis—Management process of formulating judgments and decisions from the relation between the numbers represented on the various reports; also known as financial analysis.

Rationality—Extent to which a decision maker has knowledge or information relative to alternatives available and the outcomes associated with each alternative.

Reappointment—Conferring of certain rights with designated staff membership category; an assignment to the organizational unit of the medical staff; following an initial appointment.

Reasonable accommodation (in terms of the Americans with Disabilities Act)—Changes that an employer would make in the work processes, furniture, equipment, or building structure to accommodate a disabled worker.

"Reasonable man" standard—Standard that one must observe to avoid liability for simple negligence. A defendant's actions are judged as to whether a "reasonable man" would act in a similar way. This is not the standard used for professional negligence (malpractice).

Record—Group of data items that are stored together and/or used together in processing. A collection of related data items treated as a unit. See also **logical record.**

Record linkage—Ability to electronically relate records regarding a single patient which have been created and stored in discrete locations.

Record location tracking system—Means of pinpointing the flow of records.

Record, rows—All the related data, all the fields of information, about a single patient or a single subject.

Record tracking—Maintaining information about the current location of a record.

Recruitment—Process of finding and attracting capable people to fill jobs.

Reduction ratio—Number of times the image has been reduced from the original size; inverse of magnification ratio.

Redundancy—Same data are collected and stored inadvertently several times.

Re-engineering—Fundamental rethinking and radical redesign of business processes to achieve dramatic improvements in performance, such as cost, quality, service, and speed; management theory in which the way business is usually performed is re-evaluated and radically changed to achieve dramatic improvement in performance.

Reference date—Beginning date of data collection.

Reflective calculator—View of management that pictures the manager as a systematic planner, organizer, decision maker, and controller.

Registration—Certification provided an individual who successfully meets criteria including a written examination required by the American Health Information Management association to be a registered record administrator.

Registries—Statewide and nationwide collections of data used to make information available to improve quality of care and measure the effectiveness of a particular aspect of health care delivery, i.e., trauma, cardiac.

Regulation—Dictates of agencies charged with enforcing and implementing legislation in a particular area; these dictates are designed to carry out the intent of the law.

Rehabilitation—Processes of treatment and education that lead the disabled person in achievement of maximum independence and function and a personal sense of well-being.

Reimbursement formula—Factors used to determine the payment for health care services, e.g., percentage of charges and/or the cost of living in a certain community.

Relational database management system—Related information is grouped in tables within the database and is accessed by a series of key fields. Redundant data entry is minimized.

Relative humidity—Percentage of moisture in the air.

Relative risk (RR)—Measures the degree of association in epidemiological studies; obtained by dividing the incidence rate of the exposed group by the incidence rate of the unexposed group; used with prospective and/or experimental studies.

Reliability—Measures how often data are classified in the same manner; reproducibility; accuracy of the picture provided by the information. For example, the same survey conducted randomly among 1000 persons will be more reliable than one conducted among 10 persons.

Reliability of data—Data that yield the same results on repeated collection, processing, storage, and display of information in the same database; data that are consistent when entered into two or more databases.

Replacement charts—Visual presentations of who will replace whom in the organization when a job opening occurs.

Request for information—Information requested from vendors regarding their products in selection process of vendors to whom an RFP will be sent.

Request for proposal (RFP)—Document distributed to vendors that specifies functional, technical, training, implementation, and other requirements for an information system.

Requisition—Request for a record and an acknowledgment that the borrower has the record and intends to return it.

Res ipsa loquitur—"The thing speaks for itself"—doctrine applied to cases where the defendant had exclusive control of the thing that caused the harm and where the harm ordinarily couldn't have occurred without negligent conduct.

Resource-based relative value scale—Scale of reimbursement in which services are priced in relation to a reference or standard service.

Respondent superior—"Let the master answer"–this means that the master (e.g., employer) is liable in certain cases for the wrongful acts of his servants/agents (e.g., employees), as long as those actions were within the scope of the employment/agency relationship.

Restraint of trade—Contracts or agreements that tend to or are designed to eliminate or stifle competition, create a monopoly, artificially maintain prices, or otherwise hamper or obstruct the course of trade and commerce.

Results reporting—Application designed to retrieve diagnostic and treatment results from feeder systems such as laboratory, radiology, and other departmental settings and present them directly on inquiry by the care provider.

Retention period—Number of years a record will be kept before destruction.

Retrospective payment system—Payment method in which the cost to provide the health care is figured after the health care is provided and is based on the provider's statement of cost.

Retrospective record completion—Documentation in the patient record is completed after the patient care is rendered.

Return on investment (ROI)—Amount an organization can earn by investing today's dollars at a certain interest rate. Today's dollars are worth more than future dollars.

Revenue—Result from performing the services; charges for the services provided.

Risk management—Activities intended to minimize the potential for injuries to occur in a facility and to anticipate and respond to ensuing liabilities for injuries that occur.

Role ambiguity—Uncertainty about the content of a particular role or job.

Role conflict—When two or more behavioral requirements of a job are in conflict with one another.

Rolling budget method—This method allows for continuous updating of the budget by dropping the oldest month of data and adding a new month of projected data.

Roll microfilm—Continuous filmstrip that holds several hundred miniaturized document images; readable only with magnification.

Round robin—Situation in which both parties reassert their positions and arguments over and over again, usually resulting in a stalemate; can also mean taking an idea from each person in a group in turn.

Run chart—See **line graph.**

Sample size—Number of subjects chosen for a research study to represent the population under study.

Satellite clinic—Primary care facility owned and operated by a hospital or other organization that is located in an area that is convenient to the patients or in an area that is closer to a specific patient population.

Satisficing behavior—Outcome of decision making visualized by behavioral decision theory.

Scanner—Device that reads text, images, and bar codes into an electronic format.

Scanning—Using a scanner to digitize graphics or text for input to a computer system for storage, retrieval, and editing.

Scientific management—School of management thought that focuses on work as its element of analysis and uses such tools as time and motion study.

Secondary care—Generic term for health care services provided by a specialist at the request of the primary care physician.

Secondary data—Data collected for internal use, such as diagnostic and procedure indexes.

Secondary health data—Individual or aggregate patient data found in reports that are summarized from the source or primary patient record.

Security of data—Data that are guarded to prevent misuse, corruption, or loss as a result of accidental or fraudulent acts.

Security of health information—Refers to the physical safety and protection of health information, e.g., protection from the elements, from loss, and from alteration or destruction.

Selection process—Process of steps used to decide which applicants or recruits should be hired.

Self-pay—This category, when used with payer categories, indicates that the patient or patient's family, rather than a third party payer (e.g., insurance company) will pay the bill for care.

Seniority—Length of a worker's service with the organization in relation to other employees.

Sensitivity—Percentage of all true cases correctly identified; used in tests of validity.

Sentinel event—Undesirable occurrence of such magnitude that it warrants comprehensive investigation.

Sequential search—Random generation of successive alternative solutions to a problem as visualized by behavioral decision theory.

Serial numbering—System in which a new number is assigned to the patient for each encounter with the facility.

Serial-unit numbering—System in which a new number is assigned to the patient for each encounter with the facility, but all former records are brought forward to the most recently assigned number.

Severity of illness system—Database established from coded data on diseases and operations used in the hospital for planning and research purposes.

Sexual harassment—In the workplace, when sexual favors are required for work benefits, such as a promotion or even maintenance of one's position, or when the performance is affected by an intimidating, hostile, or offensive work environment.

Significant procedure—Procedure that is surgical in nature or carries a procedural risk or carries an anesthetic risk or requires specialized training.

Silent treatment—Situation in which negative emotions, such as anger, humiliation, or frustration, are communicated through nonverbal means.

Simultaneous-equations method—Method of allocating costs to a department; uses complex equations to allocate the cost of nonrevenue-generating departments to revenue-generating departments; also known as reciprocal method.

Situational theory—Belief in leadership theory that leaders emerge as a result of the situation that is presented.

Slander—False oral statement about another, made to a third person (or more), that injures the subject's character or reputation. If done in writing, it is libel. Slander and libel are the two forms of defamation.

Sliding scale fee—Cost of health care services based on the patient's ability to pay.

Small computer system interface (SCSI)—Parallel interface for high-speed access to peripheral devices such as scanners and disk drives.

Social subsystem—Informal system that "is not on the organization chart" but describes the patterns of social interaction in an organization.

Socioeconomic data—Data elements that describe patient characteristics, such as name, address, date of birth, next of kin, race, sex, marital status.

Software—Set of instructions and documentation required to operate computers and their applications.

Solo practice—Practice in which the physician is self-employed and is legally the sole owner of the practice.

Span of control—Cornerstone concept of classical organization theory that suggests that managers are capable of supervising only a limited number of employees.

Specialization of labor—Cornerstone concept of classical management theory that states that the most productive way to organize work is for everyone to train for and concentrate on doing what they do best; sometimes called the division of work.

Specificity—Percentage of all true noncases correctly identified; used in tests of validity.

Sponsors—People and organizations who authorize, endorse, and fund information systems.

Staffing table—Table of anticipated job openings for each type of job.

Standard deviation—Statistic that demonstrates how values are spread around the mean; square root of the variance.

Standardized mortality ratio (SMR)—Indirect method of age adjustment in which standard rates are applied to two populations to calculate the expected number of deaths, which is compared with the observed number of deaths.

Standardization movement—Effort sponsored by the American College of Surgeons to improve the care of patients by establishing standards for surgery performed in hospitals in the United States. The movement led to the improvement of medical records and the establishment of the hospital accreditation program.

Standard of care—Conduct expected of an individual in a given situation. Used as a measure against which a defendant's conduct is evaluated.

Standard query language—Programs designed to apply to standard questions used when accessing a database.

Stare decisis—Translates as "let the decision stand." A legal principle stating that courts should decide similar cases similarly. In other words, cases that have similar facts and questions should ordinarily be decided in the same way.

Statement of revenues and expenses—Document in which the revenues and expenses are reported.

Statistical process control—Management philosophy developed by Tagucchi that grounds managerial decision making on the application of statistical analysis and industrial control methods to ensure ongoing quality control in production.

Statistics budget—Budget based on historical data regarding the volume and type of health care services provided, data about the community, and future projections of need for health care services. All available data is used to estimate types and volumes of health care services needed for the projected budget period.

Statute—Act of the legislature—state or federal; legislatively created laws.

Statute of limitations—Law that determines the period in which a legal action can be brought against a facility for injury, improper care, or breech of contract; legal limit on the time allowed for filing suit, usually measured from the time of the wrong or from the time when a reasonable person should have discovered the wrong. Proceedings brought after this time limit are subject to dismissal by the court.

Step-down method—Forward allocation of costs of non-revenue-producing centers to other non–revenue-producing centers that use their services as well as to the revenue-producing centers to which they render services.

Strategic planning—Planning activities that are directed toward positioning the organization effectively in its environmental context; process of matching environmental opportunities and threats with the organization's strengths and weaknesses.

Style of leadership—Way a leader may lead, including free reign, participative, and autocratic styles.

Subpoena—Court- or governmental agency-sanctioned order commanding someone to appear in court to testify. In some jurisdictions, attorneys may be authorized by the court or agency to issue a subpoena. Subpoenas are not always reviewed by a judge prior to issuance.

Subpoena duces tecum—Court- or governmental agency-sanctioned order commanding someone to appear in court with certain specified documents. As is true with subpoenas, judges do not always review the subpoena duces tecum prior to issuance.

Surveillance—To monitor incidence and trends.

Symbology—Manner in which a bar code is designed.

System—Series of elements that are interrelated according to a plan for achieving a well-defined goal.

System design—Translation of system requirements identified in the analysis phase into specifications used to build the system.

System development life cycle—Customary stages of development of an information system, including analysis, design, implementation, and evaluation.

Systems analysis and design—Defined and accepted methodology for gathering and analyzing great quantity of data in a logical, documented format to improve an existing system or implement a new one.

Systems flowchart—Depicts the flow of data through all or part of the system, the various operations that take place within the system, and the files that are used to produce various reports or documents.

Tables/file—Columns (fields) and rows of related information in a database. Many tables are incorporated into one database.

Tactical planning—Operational and budgetary planning designed to accomplish intermediate and short-term plans.

Task (accent) lighting—Light fixtures that are built into the furniture or workstation to illuminate specific work areas.

Task-ambient lighting—Combination of general light with light directed to the work surface.

Task-oriented subsystem—Formal system of job descriptions, policies, procedures and rules, and related facts that prescribe how work would be done in organizations.

Tax Equity and Fiscal Responsibility Act (TEFRA)—Legislation enacted by the Congress of the United States in 1983 designed to bring about prospective pricing Medicare in inpatient health care. Prospective pricing sets the fees for hospital care in advance of the care.

Team building—Process of developing the effectiveness of the team in decision making, problem solving, and planning and implementing activities. This can be described as a cycle of (1) coming to task, (2) coming unglued, (3) coming around, (4) coming home, and (5) becoming (empowered).

Telemedicine—Employs telecommunications to link providers and patients together from diverse geographic locations and transmits text and images for medical consultation and treatment.

Temper tantrums—Situation in which one party applies emotions to blackmail the other, with the effect of interrupting or terminating conflict resolution efforts.

Terminal—Device (usually keyboard based) connected to information systems and used to enter and retrieve information.

Terminal digit filing—A method of filing in which a number is divided into two digit pairs and read in those pairs from right to left rather than left to right for filing purposes.

Tertiary care—Generic term for highly specialized care provided by specialists who use sophisticated technology and support services (e.g., neurosurgeon, fertility specialist, immunologist).

Tests of significance—Statistical tests used to determine that the difference between two groups of people relative to a characteristic are real or due to sampling variability.

Text processing—Computer processing of natural language.

Theory X—One of two contrasting sets of managerial assumptions about the nature of human behavior in the workplace articulated by McGregor; contends that employees are inherently lazy, dislike work, are self-absorbed, avoid responsibility, and resist applying their energies to further organizational goals. Consequently, management must apply either "the carrot" (bribes) or "the stick" (coercion) to elicit positive worker behavior.

Theory Y—One of two contrasting sets of managerial assumptions about the nature of human behavior in the workplace articulated by McGregor; contends that work itself and the opportunity to use intellect, skills, knowledge, and energy are basic human needs. Workers will seek out responsibility and respond positively to challenge as long as their personal needs are being addressed in the process.

Thinning—Process of removing inactive records from the active files.

Third party payer—System whereby an entity other than the patient pays for services rendered to the patient, e.g., an insurance company, is a third party.

Threshold—Tolerance limit in monitoring and evaluation; point at which a process is subjected to intensive review to determine the need for corrective action.

Timeliness of data—Length of time is minimized between an event or observation that produces data, the recording of the data, and when the data become available to those who need the data.

Time-out—Negotiated interruption of active conflict resolution in which both parties separate to cool off, consider alternatives, or reevaluate their positions.

Time value of money—Concept that states that money received today is worth more than the same amount received 1 year or some period from today.

Topography—Description of an anatomic region or of a specific part; site of origin of a neoplasm.

Tort—A civil—not criminal—wrong, in which one party alleges that another party's wrongful conduct has caused harm. The party bringing suit seeks compensation for the harm.

Total quality management—Management philosophy popularized by the work of Deming that focuses on quality, excellence, commitment, worker participation, and customer service.

Training—Activities that teach employees how to perform their jobs.

Trait theory—Belief underlying early leadership theory that leaders possessed certain biological and/or psychological traits.

Transaction—Event taking place during the course of routine business activities (for example, registering a patient or ordering laboratory tests). Transaction processing uses information technology to increase volume, accuracy, or consistency in processing data about business transactions.

Transactional leadership—Role or aspect of leadership that involves the day-to-day interactions between the leader and followers (employees) that characterize the supervisory relationship; includes structuring the task, setting goals, clarifying performance expectations, providing feedback and incentives, and performing other behavior shaping and control activities.

Transfer notice—Message sent to the file telling that a record has been given to another requester without returning to the file first.

Transformational leadership—Role of leadership in re-creating and renewing organizational culture by providing employees a vision of the transformed organization, by creating an expectation of change, and by modeling the capacity to deal with changing environment effectively.

Translational leadership—Role of leadership in communicating (translating) the vision and energy of the transformational leader into policies, systems, plans, and procedures to direct activity at the operating level of the organization.

Trauma center—Emergency care center that is specially staffed and equipped to handle trauma patients; most are equipped with an air transport system.

Triage—Process of sorting out for the purpose of early assessment to determine the urgency and priority for care and to determine appropriate source of care.

Trip frequency chart—Matrix that represents the number of times employees interact with one another in a specified period of time; used in designing a work space.

Truncate—Eliminating some information or characters in a field due to lack of sufficient character space.

Turnaround document—Computer-generated summary containing clinical information such as a problem list and medications and space to capture current encounter information. The document is then "turned around" for updating the information on the document and entering new data from the encounter.

Turnover ratio—Uses data from the balance sheet and the statement of revenues and expenses; measures the organization's ability to generate net operating revenue in relation to its various assets; also known as **activity ratio**.

Type I recommendations—A recommendation or group of recommendations that addresses insufficient or unsatisfactory standards compliance in a specific performance area. Resolution of Type I recommendations must be achieved within stipulated time frames in order for an organization to maintain its accreditation.

UB-92—Uniform Bill, 1992 version (HCFA 1450); standardized form developed by the National Uniform Billing Committee for billing and payment transactions.

Unbundling—Process in CPT coding of using several codes for each part of a procedure rather than the one comprehensive code which covers all the parts.

Undue hardship (in terms of Americans with Disabilities Act)—Action taken to accommodate a disabled worker that would require significant difficulty or expense when considered in light of the nature and cost of the accommodation in relation to the size, resources, nature, and structures of the employer's operation.

Unduplicated/unique patient count—Statistical report that counts a patient only once, even though he or she is readmitted during the same reporting period.

Uniform hospital discharge data set—List of data items and their definitions that make up the minimum fields of information which should be collected on discharged hospital patients.

Uninterruptable power supply (UPS)—Battery-operated device used to keep a system running during a power failure or to protect the system from the power surge associated with power outages.

Unit numbering—System in which one number is permanently assigned to a patient for use in tracking all services provided at that facility.

Unit record—All records of a patient are filed together in one location in the files.

Unity of command—Cornerstone concept of classical organization theory that states that no one should have more than one boss at a single time.

Uploading of data—Electronic transfer of data from a personal computer or local area network to another database.

Users—Health care team, clerical and technical personnel, analysts, and managers that rely on computer systems to perform their job.

Usual, customary, and reasonable charge—Charge for health care services based on a community norm or on a norm developed by a third party payer.

Utilization management (UM)—Systems and processes to assure that facilities and resources, both human and nonhuman, are used maximally but consistent with patient care needs.

Utilization review (UR)—Activities intended to assure that all health services provided to a patient are medically necessary and provided in the most appropriate setting.

Validity—Correctness, completeness, accuracy, and relevance; measures how well an instrument measures what it should measure; characteristic of information. Valid information is meaningful and relevant to the stated purpose. Information may be invalid if applied to a different purpose than that for which it was collected.

Validity of data—Numbers, characters, or symbols stored, processed, and displayed are exact and conform to known standards. Data represent what was intended by the original source. Data are supported by objective truth or generally accepted authority.

Variance—Discrepancy between planned and desired and actual performance in control theory; statistic that demonstrates how values are spread around the mean; computed by squaring each deviation from the mean, summing them, and then dividing the sum by one less than the sample size (n).

Variance report—Control report that shows what was budgeted (planned or predicted) and what has actually been expended.

View, logical—Logical view is the user's view of data, focusing on data needed for application rather than on details of storage or access.

Viruses, computer—Hidden, unlawful computer instructions designed to delete or corrupt data or interfere with computer operations in some way.

Vision—A statement of where an organization (or an individual) wants to be in the future. This is usually one component of an organized planning process.

Vital statistics—Data collected from births, deaths, fetal deaths, marriages, and so on; displayed as rates, proportions, ratios, and percentages.

Voice recognition—Technology in which the computer system recognizes and accepts voice input through limited or speaker-independent vocabularies.

Whole service—When facilities or individuals are paid for all services rendered at the rate the facility or individual charges with no discount applied.

Wide area network—Used for extensive, geographically larger environments—often connecting separate institutions.

Win-win—Bargaining strategy that encourages an outcome in which both parties achieve net gains and experience satisfaction with the process.

Work breakdown structures—Divides a project into major objectives, partitions each objective into activities, and further divides the activities into subactivities; creates work packages that must be done to complete the project.

Work distribution chart—Matrix that illustrates the tasks being performed in a work group, the employees who perform them, and the amount of time spent on each task by each employee and the work unit as a whole.

Work sampling—Method of measuring work that collects data about the work being performed on randomly selected times of observations.

Work simplification—Organized approach to determine how to accomplish a task with less effort, in less time, or at a lower cost while maintaining or improving the quality of the outcome.

Workstation—Collection of desks or work surfaces, equipment, storage facilities, and chairs shaped by technology, the tasks to be performed, and various human needs; personal computer that is connected to an information system; when appropriately configured, data can be received from the system and additional functions can be performed at the local level.

Write once read many (WORM)—Method of recording data on an optical disk by which it can be recorded only once and cannot be altered.

Zero-based budget—Budgeting technique that requires the justification of all activities performed by a department before allocating any funding.

Zero defects—Concept introduced by Crosby, who defines quality as the achievement of "zero defects"—that a commitment to quality management requires doing it right the first time with no tolerance for errors.

INDEX

Note: Page numbers in *italics* refer to illustrations; page numbers followed by (t) refer to tables.

A

AAMRL (American Association of Medical Record Librarians), 54
AAMRS (automated ambulatory medical record systems), 587–588
Abbreviated Injury Scale, 277
Abbreviations, in form/view design, 103
Abstracting, in AIDS registry, 266
  in birth defects registry, 267–268, *269*
  in coding, 218, *218, 219*
  in diabetes registry, 270, *273, 274*
  in hospital-based cancer registry, 244–246, *248*
  in trauma registry, 277
Acceptance theory of authority, 410
Access time, of jukebox, in optical image processing, 204
Accessibility, of data, 140, *140*
Accession register, computer-generated, 244, *245*
  of hospital-based cancer registry, 242–244, *244*
Accession year, 244
Accommodation, on conflict resolution, 438
Accountability, in management, 409–410
Accountant, financial, duties of, 517, 518(t)
  managerial, duties of, 517, 518(t)
Accounting, accrual basis, 517–518
  cash basis, 517–518
  financial, 517
Accounting rate of return, 538–539
Accounts receivable, 519
Accounts receivable turnover ratio, 521
Accreditation, advantages of, 13
  definition of, 13
  of health care facilities, 49
  of health information management educational programs, 55
  standards for, compliance with, documentation of, 77
Accreditation Manual for Hospitals (AMH), 73
  in quality assurance, 323
Accredited record technician (ART), 55
  continuing education of, 57
  credentials of, 56
Accredited Standards Committee (ASC) X3, in health care information processing, 614
Accredited Standards Committee (ASC) X12, in health care information processing, 614

Accrual basis accounting, 517–518
Accuracy, of data, factors in, 141
  of reports, in database design, 149–150
ACF (Administration for Children and Families), 11, *11*
Achilles' heel, identification of, in conflict resolution, 441
ACR-NEMA (American College of Radiology–National Electrical Manufacturers Association) Imaging Standards, 79, 615
ACS (American College of Surgeons), as external data source, 74, 75(t)
  purpose of, 6, 8
Action model, of problem solving, 445–447
  active listening in, 446
  alternative solutions in, 446
  bias/assumption analysis in, 446
  cognitive/emotive reasoning separation in, 446
  evidence examination in, 446
  issue definition in, 446
Active records, 187
Activity ratio, 521
Acute care, data collection in, 122–124
  forms/views in, 123–124
  issues in, 124
  Uniform Hospital Discharge Data Set in, 122–123
Acute Physiology and Chronic Health Evaluation (APACHE), 234
ADA (American Dental Association), in health information processing, 615
Addenda, to health information, 368–369
ADEA (Age Discrimination in Employment Act), in human resources management, 478
Administration for Children and Families (ACF), 11, *11*
Administrative agencies, rules/regulations of, 361
Administrative forms, 110–112, 111(t)
Administrative organization, 399
Admission audit review procedure, in long-term care, 169–170
Admission data review criteria, in long-term care, 171–173
Admitted, discharged, and transferred (ADT) list, 165
Advance directive, 110, 111(t), 387
  definition of, 13

Adverse patient occurrences (APOs), 345
Affinity diagrams, in quality management, 453–454, *454*
Affirmative action, in human resources management, 474(t), 477–478
Age, adjustment for, in mortality rates, direct method of, 287–288, 287(t), 288(t)
  indirect method of, 287–288, 287(t), 288(t)
Age Discrimination in Employment Act (ADEA), in human resources management, 474(t), 478
Agency for Health Care Policy and Research (AHCPR), 10, 330–331
  as external data source, 74, 75(t)
Agency for Toxic Substances and Disease Registry, 10
Agenda for Change, 323
Aggregate data, 67
  in cost containment, 581–582
AHA (American Hospital Association), as external data source, 73, 75(t)
  in *International Classification of Diseases, 9th Edition, Clinical Modification* updating, 217
  purpose of, 5, 8
AHCPR (Agency for Health Care Policy and Research), 10, 330–331
  as external data source, 74, 75(t)
AHIMA. See *American Health Information Management Association (AHIMA)*.
AIDS registries, 263–266
  automation of, 266
  data from, use of, 266–267
  database management in, 263–266
    abstracting in, 266
    case eligibility in, 263, *264, 265*
    casefinding in, 263
    coding in, 266
    staging in, 266, *266*
AJCC (American Joint Committee on Cancer) Manual for Staging of Cancer, 246
Alcohol, abuse of, record of, confidentiality of, 371–372
Allied health professionals, definition of, 34–35
  in health care team, 34–35
Allocation(s), cost of, 539–542
  importance of, *541*, 541–542
  methods of, 540–541
    double-distribution, 540–541